WATSON-JONES
Fractures and Joint Injuries

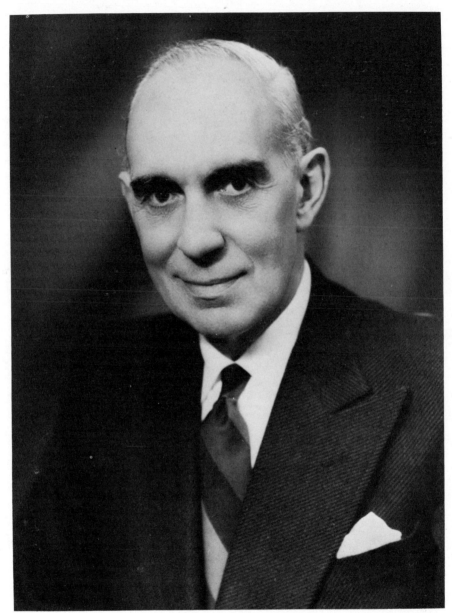

Sir Reginald Watson-Jones, 1902–1972

WATSON-JONES

6n. ed.

Vol. 2.

WATSON-JONES
Fractures and Joint Injuries

Edited by

J. N. Wilson, Ch.M., F.R.C.S.

Consultant Orthopaedic Surgeon, Royal National Orthopaedic
Hospital, London, and The National Hospitals for Nervous
Diseases, Queen Square and Maida Vale; Surgeon in Charge of
the Accident Unit, Royal National Orthopaedic Hospital,
Stanmore; Honorary Orthopaedic Surgeon, Garston Manor
Medical Rehabilitation Centre; Recognised Clinical Teacher,
Institute of Orthopaedics, University of London; Fellow of the
British Orthopaedic Association and the Royal Society of
Medicine; Hon. Member of the Egyptian Orthopaedic
Association; President of the World Orthopaedic Concern

Volume II

SIXTH EDITION

CHURCHILL LIVINGSTONE
EDINBURGH LONDON MELBOURNE AND NEW YORK 1982

CHURCHILL LIVINGSTONE
Medical Division of Longman Group Limited

Distributed in the United States of America by Churchill
Livingstone Inc., 19 West 44th Street, New York, N.Y. 10036,
and by associated companies, branches and representatives
throughout the world.

First Edition 1940
Second Edition 1941
Third Edition 1943
Fourth Edition, Volume I 1952
Fourth Edition, Volume II 1955
Fifth Edition 1976
Sixth Edition 1982

ISBN 0 443 02082 5

British Library Cataloguing in Publication Data
Watson-Jones, *Sir* Reginald
   Fractures and joint injuries.—6th ed.
  1, Fractures
  I. Title   II. Wilson, J. N.
  617′.15   RD101

Library of Congress Cataloging in Publication Data
Watson-Jones, R. (Reginald), 1902–1972.
  Watson-Jones Fractures and joint injuries.

  Half title: Fractures and joint injuries.
  Fifth ed. published as: Fractures and joint injuries.
  Includes bibliographical references and indexes.
    1. Fractures. 2. Joints—Wounds and injuries. I. Wilson, J. N.
(James Noel) II. Title. III. Title: Fractures and joint injuries.
[DNLM: 1. Fractures. 2. Joints—Injuries. WE 175 W343f]
RD101.W28   1982   617′.15   82-1260
                    AACR2

Printed and bound in Great Britain by William Clowes (Beccles) Limited, Beccles and London

Contributors

N. J. Barton FRCS
Consultant Surgeon, Nottingham University Hospital Group and Harlow Wood Orthopaedic Hospital.

Sir George Bedbrook Kt, OBE, OStJ Hon, MD(WA), MS(Melb), DPRM(Syd), FRCS, FRACS
Senior Orthopaedic Surgeon and Senior Spinal Surgeon, Royal Perth Hospital and Royal Perth Rehabilitation Hospital. Previous Director of Spinal Injuries Unit Royal Perth Hospital and Royal Perth Rehabilitation Hospital.

A. Benjamin FRCS
Consultant Orthopaedic and Traumatic Surgeon, St Albans City Hospital and West Herts. Hospital, Hemel Hempstead; Hon. Lecturer, Institute of Orthopaedics, University of London.

M. A. Birnstingl MS, FRCS
Consultant Surgeon, St Bartholomew's Hospital, London; Surgeon (Peripheral Vascular Diseases), Royal National Orthopaedic Hospital, London.

Doreen R. G. Browne MB, BS, DObsRCOG, DCH, FFARCS
Consultant Anaethetist, Royal Free Hospital, Hampstead, London.

Donal Brooks MA, MB, BCh, FRCSI, FRCS
Consulting Orthopaedic Surgeon, Royal National Orthopaedic Hospital, King Edward VII Hospital for Officers; Consulting Orthopaedic Surgeon, University College Hospital; Civilian Consultant Orthopaedic Surgeon in Hand Surgery, Royal Navy and Air Force.

C. L. Colton FRCS
Consultant Orthopaedic Surgeon, Nottingham University Hospital and City Hospital.

A. Catterall MChir, FRCS
Consultant Orthopaedic Surgeon, Royal National Orthopaedic Hospital, London and Charing Cross Hospital Group.

H. A. Crockard FRCS
Consultant Neurosurgeon, National Hospital for Nervous Diseases and University College Hospital, London.

G. R. Fisk MB, BS, FRCSEng, FRCSEdin
Consulting Orthopaedic Surgeon, Princess Alexandra Hospital, Harlow; St Margaret's Hospital, Epping; Hunterian Professor, Royal College of Surgeons.

Lipmann Kessel MBE, MC, FRCS
Consulting Orthopaedic Surgeon, Royal National Orthopaedic Hospital, London. Emeritus Professor of Orthopaedics, University of London.

L. Klenerman ChM, FRCS
Consultant Orthopaedic Surgeon, Northwick Park Hospital and Clinical Research Centre, Harrow.

S. Mattingly TD, FRCP, DPhysMed
Late Consultant Physician and Deputy Director, Department of Rheumatology, Middlesex Hospital, London; Medical Director, Garston Manor Medical Rehabilitation Centre.

B. McKibbin MSc, MD, FRCS
Professor of Traumatic and Orthopaedic Surgery, Welsh National School of Medicine, Cardiff. Consultant Orthopaedic Surgeon, South Glamorgan A.H.A.(T).

B. C. O'Riordan FDS, RCS
Consultant Oral Surgeon, Faciomaxillary Unit, Mount Vernon Hospital, Northwood, Middlesex.

R. Sanders BSc, FRCS
Consultant Plastic Surgeon, Mount Vernon Hospital, Northwood, Middlesex; Royal National Orthopaedic Hospital, London.

E. L. Trickey FRCS
Consultant Orthopaedic Surgeon, Royal National Orthopaedic Hospital, London and Edgware General Hospital. Dean of the Institute of Orthopaedics, London University.

Contents *Volume II*

34. Injuries of the Foot

Soft tissue injuries; plantar fascial strain; tendonitis; fractures of calcaneum, classification, clinical features; treatment of fractures of the calcaneum—conservative and operative; late disability and summary of treatment; fractures and dislocations of the talus, peritalar dislocation; instability of subtalar joint; dislocation of calcaneum; total dislocation of talus; fracture of neck of talus; fracture of talus with dislocation; avascular necrosis of body of talus; fractures of the navicular; fracture-dislocations of the mid-tarsal joint and tarso-metatarsal joints; metatarsal and toe fractures.

35. Pathological Fractures

General principles of management; developmental disorders of bone; nutritional and vitamin deficiencies; hormonal imbalance causing pathological fracture; atrophic conditions of bone; fractures through infected bone; cystic disorders and fibrous dysplasia; Paget's disease; primary and secondary tumours; pathological fracture from marrow cell disorder; hydatid disease; neurotrophic dystrophies; iatrogenic fractures; fatigue fractures.

Contents *Volume I*

20

Injuries of the Shoulder

Lipmann Kessel

The shoulder differs from other joints at least in one important respect: its functional efficiency depends on interrelated synchronous action at five sites. The term 'shoulder joint' is often used to denote the scapulo-humeral joint alone, but from the point of view of the surgical anatomy of the shoulder region, the scapulo-humeral joint is only one component of a complex system of articulations which normally function synchronously to produce smooth, rhythmic and co-ordinated movements of the upper limb. The shoulder joint is effective at five different places (i) the glenohumeral joint (ii) the 'sub-acromial joint' (iii) the acromioclavicular joint (iv) the sternoclavicular joint (v) the movement of the scapula across the thoracic cage. The smooth function of the shoulder, in particular rhythmic elevation of the arm, require that all five parts of the mechanism work normally. Although it is possible for some 90 degrees of abduction to take place at the glenohumeral joint alone, this is an artificial movement.[1]

The commonest sites in the shoulder region which present problems in clinical practice are the acromioclavicular joint, and the subacromial joint between the acromioclavicular arch above and the head of the humerus and tuberosities below, with the intervening large sub-deltoid bursa acting as a joint cavity.[2] the supraspinatus and other tendons of the abductor-rotator cuff are attached to the tuberosities of the humerus and impinge against the margins of the acromion with every movement of the limb—or at least would do so without the protection of the sub-deltoid bursa. With increasing age and continuous physical effort the bursal protection may become inadequate. The area of the supraspinatus tendon immediately proximal to its insertion is particularly vulnerable to ischaemic degeneration.[3] Progressive degenerative changes occur and give rise to the clinical syndrome known variously as 'subacromial bursitis', 'supraspinatus tendinitis', the 'subacromial painful arc syndrome'.[4-8]

Before considering the special problems of the shoulder, including the acromioclavicular joint, supraspinatus tendinitis, ruptures of the rotator cuff and of the tendon of the biceps, let us consider first the shoulder joint which is stiff after injury, exactly as any other joint may become stiff after injury.

POST-TRAUMATIC STIFFNESS OF THE SHOULDER

In considering the management of post-traumatic stiffness of the shoulder it is important to distinguish it clearly from the condition of periarthritis or 'frozen shoulder'.[9] The distinction is made on the history and subsequent progress of events. 'Frozen shoulder' occurs without previous significant injury and is characterised by severe pain at rest. The pain of a post-traumatic stiff shoulder is felt only on attempted movement.

The more vigorous and energetic the treatment of an injured shoulder by early passive movement, stretching and repeated manipulation with the object of preventing stiffness, the more certain it is that the joint will become stiff.

It is unwise to urge movement within the first few days when torn tissues are still bleeding and pouring out sero-fibrinous exudate—the glue of which adhesions are made. It is still more unwise after that to use forced passive movement which stretches young repairing tissue and causes recurrent bleeding and exudation. Even elderly patients who sustain dislocation of the shoulder with torn ligaments, regain full movement if the joint is left completely at rest for two or three weeks, with the encouragement thereafter in the ordinary activities of dressing, eating or washing. That is the way to make the most complete recovery.

The best exercises are those which the patient does himself, without the aid of relatives, friends or physiotherapists, and with no passive stretching or forceful endeavour. There are four simple movements, which are best done standing up (Figs 20.1 to 20.4). First the arms are turned into the laterally rotated position, trying to reach backwards as far as possible; then the hands are crossed behind the neck, and the elbows are slowly and gently stretched back; the hands are then placed in the small of the back and reach upwards, the bad arm competing with the good. Finally the patient faces a wall and reaches upwards, 'walking' with his fingertips up the wall to reach a marked point, each day above the day before.

These exercises should be done for a few minutes at a time, but must be done several times each day.

When a shoulder is stiff from injury, the limb has usually been held with the forearm across the chest in a sling at rest in the position of full medial rotation.

Lateral rotation must be regained as well as abduction, and these are interrelated. Abduction of the upper limb is accompanied by lateral rotation of the humerus; if an arm is held in full medial rotation it cannot be abducted beyond the right angle. Thus all shoulder exercises must restore lateral rotation and abduction as one combined movement. This is best taught to the patient by simple personal exercises.

Manipulation under anaesthesia. Post-traumatic stiff shoulders should rarely be manipulated under anaesthesia, and then only when the patient has reached maximum improvement by his own efforts. It should be explained to the patient that the manipulation will do no more than make it easier to do his own exercises. Manipulation of a stiff shoulder

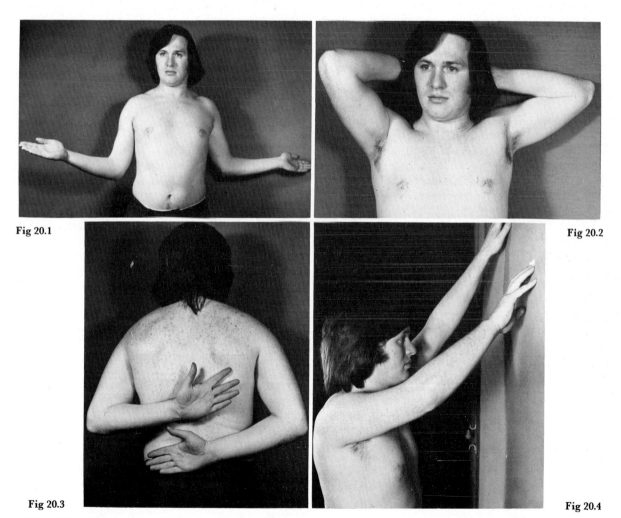

Fig 20.1

Fig 20.2

Fig 20.3

Fig 20.4

Figs 20.1 to 20.4 The patient does his own shoulder exercises.

in an elderly patient must be carried out with extreme caution. *It is only too easy to turn a nuisance into a total disaster by damaging the axillary vein or artery.* Manipulation under anaesthesia should rarely be used more than once. A few patients require a single manipulation under anaesthesia to help their own endeavour.

The gloom expressed in many surgical conferences regarding the problem of stiffness of the shoulder arises from the fact that no distinction is made between the stiffness of a spontaneous 'frozen shoulder', and a post-traumatic stiff shoulder. The two behave quite differently and respond quite differently to manipulation. Whereas occasionally a highly satisfactory result can be achieved by the manipulation of a 'frozen shoulder', during the correct phase of the disease, it is only rarely that manipulation under anaesthesia will significantly improve the range of movement following trauma.

THE SUBACROMIAL PAINFUL ARC SYNDROME (SUPRASPINATUS TENDINITIS)

The subacromial region comprises a functional joint between the acromioclavicular arch above, the tendinous cuff and tuberosities of the humerus below, and the intervening subacromial bursa acting as a joint cavity. Affections of this region are the most common and the most characteristic disorders of the shoulder girdle. Pain is referred to the lateral aspect of the upper arm in the region of the insertion of the deltoid muscle or just above it. The pain can be experienced at rest, but is typically felt only within a certain arc of movement.

The painful arc of movement is between about 80 degrees and 120 degrees of abduction and varies with the position of rotation of the arm (Fig 20.5). This sign can be caused by several different lesions all of which have one thing in common: there is loss of normal gliding between the acromion and coraco-acromial ligament above, and the tuberosities below. Damage or disease of the supraspinatus or one of its related tendons characteristically causes this symptom complex. The greater the associated effusion into the subdeltoid bursa, the more severe is the pain. It is most severe in supraspinatus tendinitis with calcification.

Movement which is limited as a result of glenohumeral trauma or a 'frozen shoulder', is limited and painful *throughout* the range of abduction and is increasingly painful as further movement is attempted.

Diagnosis may be assisted by the injection of 1 ml of 1 per cent local anaesthetic solution into the damaged area. The immediate relief of pain is often dramatic and the painful arc of abduction is abolished.[10] A diagnosis having been established, the local anaesthetic may be supplemented with 40 mg of Depo-Medrone or other hydrocortisone preparation in order to provide longer lasting relief.

The clinical differentiation between supraspinatus tendinitis and spontaneous rupture of the tendon may be established by local anaesthetic test and confirmed by arthrography.[11–12] The persistence of symptoms despite conservative treatment will be discussed in later pages.

Supraspinatus tendinitis with calcification. This condition is responsible for about one-tenth of patients exhibiting a subacromial painful arc syndrome.[13–14] Calcareous or calcific tendinitis has been described in relation to almost every extra-articular site in the body, but its most frequent occurrence is in the subacromial region of the shoulder where it involves particularly the supraspinatus tendon (Figs 20.6 and 20.7). The deposit consists of a collection of a variety of amorphous calcium salts, principally

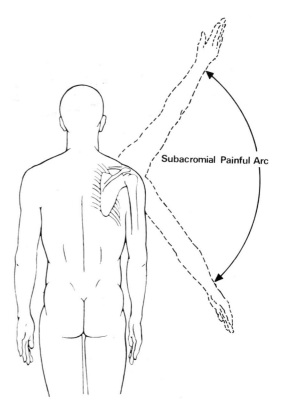

Subacromial Painful Arc

Fig 20.5 The subacromial painful arc

calcium apatite in the same proportion as in bone. The cause of the deposition has not yet been established but it seems likely that trauma does play some part in the precipitation of the material within the substance of a damaged and relatively avascular tendon. A surrounding inflammatory reaction occurs in the tendon and the intimately associated subacromial bursa into which an effusion develops. The onset may be dramatic and intense, often at night. The pain may be of such severity that continued expectant treatment is not justified.

In acute cases evacuation of the deposit through a wide-bored aspirating needle under local anaesthesia should be attempted. It is a procedure which must be carried out with kindness and precision. It is better to use two needles so that the material may be observed flowing out of one needle as local anaesthetic is injected into the other. If the deposit has been successfully needled, one needle is withdrawn and 40 mg of hydrocortisone is injected by way of the other needle. If the needling procedure is unsuccessful it is advisable to explore the lesion through a short deltoid-splitting incision and remove the grey-yellow toothpaste-like substance with a curette.

Surgical treatment of chronic supraspinatus tendinitis. The persistence of pain, in particular the painful subacromial arc syndrome, may occasionally require surgical treatment. For several years the most widely practised operation for this condition was excision of the acromion.[15–17] This is a destructive procedure with uncertain and sometimes harmful consequences. It is possible to relieve the obstruction by excision of the anterior edge of the acromion, or— better still—by deliberate division of the coraco-acromial ligament under direct vision.[18]

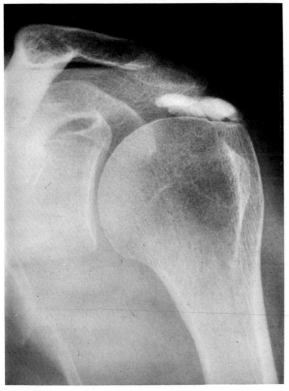

Fig 20.6 The deposit of calcium apatite appears as a radio-opaque mass in the subacromial region.

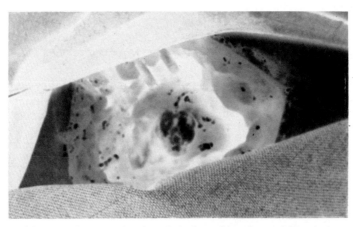

Fig 20.7 Calcific deposit exposed at operation presenting through the floor of the subacromial bursa. (Same patient as in Fig 20.6).

RUPTURE OF THE ROTATOR CUFF OF THE SHOULDER (SUPRASPINATUS TENDON RUPTURE)

The clinical signs of a rupture of the rotator cuff of the shoulder are so little understood that almost every patient with this injury experiences considerable delay in receiving adequate treatment. This is perhaps not surprising because the physical signs may develop after a comparatively trivial injury. The curious movement caused by reversal of the scapulo-humeral rhythm which leads to hunching of the shoulder, and the trick movements to achieve abduction combined with the presence of a full range of passive movements, may cause the surgeon to suspect a functional, hysterical disorder. Following the pioneering work of Codman of Boston, several surgeons have continued the analysis of this injury, so that at the present time diagnosis may be made early and with precision. Nevertheless, many patients with even total rupture of the whole rotator cuff are still being treated conservatively, although there is no hope of improvement.

Diagnosis of rupture of the rotator cuff. The symptoms and signs of rupture of the supraspinatus and associated tendons of the rotator cuff may be difficult to distinguish from other afflictions of the subacromial region. There is the same unwillingness to raise the arm beyond the right angle by reason of pain in the middle third of the arc of abduction, whereas having passed the range of painful movement the limb is again comfortable in full elevation. The movement of raising the limb and once more lowering it to the side may be accompanied by postural circumduction trick movements to avoid pain and to bring into action undamaged parts of the conjoint tendon. *The management of these patients by a policy of 'wait and see' is no longer justifiable.* The diagnosis can now be made early and with certainty.

It is very rare for normal tendons to rupture by injury alone, and age degeneration of the tendon is therefore a constant predisposing factor. It is considerably more common in men than in women by a ratio of approximately 10:1. The distinction between incomplete and complete ruptures is not as important as it was thought to be. The real issue is whether or not sufficient continuity of the conjoint tendon remains to effect active muscle action (Figs 20.8 and 20.9). Even a complete rupture extending throughout the substance and allowing direct continuity between the subacromial bursa and the shoulder joint, whilst causing pain, might cause only very little functional disability. An estimate of the size of the rupture is

more important. Small ruptures, although completely through the substance of the tendon, can heal around the margins and so provide adequate continuity for normal or near normal activity of the shoulder. The less common complete rupture with discontinuity of the whole of the tendinous cuff leads to permanent serious incapacity unless it is surgically repaired.

On examination after a recent injury, palpation of the subacromial region will be tender, and in some patients it may be possible to palpate a gap in the tendon. When the patient attempts to abduct his arm, characteristic hunching occurs by reversal of normal scapulo-humeral rhythm (Figs 20.10 and 20.11). He may be able to abduct his arm to about 20°, but closer examination shows that this is due to rotation of the scapula, little or no movement occurring at the gleno-humeral joint. Full range of passive movement is possible. If the arm is passively abducted above the right angle the patient may be able to sustain it in the erect position, but on asking him to lower his arm it characteristically will suddenly give way. If a rupture of the rotator cuff is suspected on clinical grounds, the damaged area is injected with local anaesthesia. By abolishing pain and muscle spasm the power of voluntary active abduction may be restored and a major lesion of the tendinous cuff is unlikely; treatment may be carried out conservatively with good expectation of recovery. If the injection of traumatised tissues with local anaesthetic does not permit the patient to abduct his shoulder, arthrography of the shoulder joint is carried out (Figs 20.12 to 20.14). If the contrast medium enters the joint and immediately flows out to fill the subacromial bursa, there must be a communicating tear. In these cases operative repair may be considered. There is no place whatever for conservative treatment of a major rupture of the rotator cuff. The disability should be consciously accepted as permanent, or surgical treatment should be undertaken. Delay means retraction of the tendon, adhesion formation, and a much more serious problem.

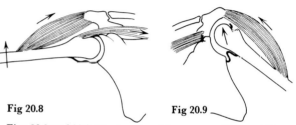

Fig 20.8   Fig 20.9

Figs 20.8 and 20.9 The function of the rotator cuff is to stabilise the head of the humerus while the deltoid elevates the arm. If the tendon is ruptured or avulsed, abnormal and weak elevation by scapular movement only occurs.

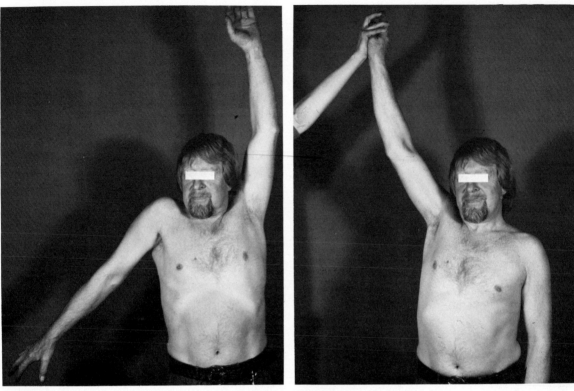

Fig 20.10   **Fig 20.11**

Figs 20.10 and 20.11 Rupture of the rotator cuff leads to hunching of the shoulder and reversal of the normal scapulo-humeral rhythm of elevation (Fig 20.10). Passive movements remain full (Fig 20.11).

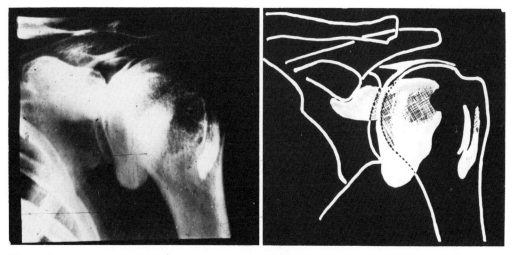

Fig 20.12   Fig 20.13

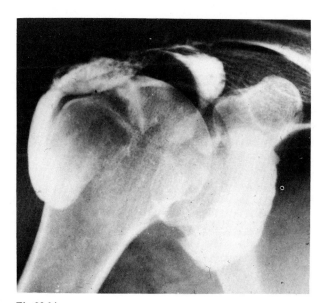

Fig 20.14

Figs 20.12 to 20.14 Arthrograph of the shoulder joint. Fig 20.12: Normal arthrograph. Fig 20.13: Line drawing of normal arthrograph. Fig 20.14: Arthrograph in a case of rupture of the rotator cuff showing a leak of the contrast medium from the shoulder joint into the subacromial bursa.

Surgical treatment: the transacromial approach[19–20] (Figs 20.15 to 20.20)

The skin incision runs in the coronal plane across the middle of the acromion just behind the acromioclavicular joint. The line of the incision is conveniently located by pressing the index finger into the supraspinous fossa, when one side of the finger palpates the back of the clavicle and the other is in contact with the spine of the scapula. The incision extends 5 centimetres both proximally and distally from the acromion process. Trapezius and deltoid muscles are split in the line of their fibres up to the acromion. The line of the incision across the acromion is coagulated and *short flaps of conjoint aponeurosis, periosteum and bone are raised with an osteotome in continuity with the trapezius and deltoid muscles.* The acromion is split with an oscillating saw. Retraction of the two halves of the acromion with a self-retaining retractor exposes the sub-deltoid bursa through a gap of some 3 centimetres. The roof of the bursa is then formally opened. By medial and lateral rotation of the arm the whole of the rotator cuff may be paraded into direct vision. The edges of the ruptured tendon must now be carefully sought for and defined. They are picked up in tissue forceps or sutures, and gradually brought into view. The tendon is freqently adherent to the overlying bursa and it must be fully mobilised by freeing of all adhesions. It is essential to mobilise the tendon so that the repair can be effected without tension, a process which requires careful and painstaking dissection. The tendon is repaired either by direct suture or by insertion into a freshly cut trough into the anatomical neck of the humerus. After repair, the self-retaining retractor is released and the wound edges fall together for simple interrupted suture of deltoid, trapezius and the intervening osteo-periosteal flap of acromion. Post-operatively the arm is held in abduction in a simple roller towel sling and passive mobilisation may start on the day following operation.

Advancement of supraspinatus. An operation has been proposed[21] by which the muscle belly of supraspinatus is separated from the supraspinous fossa, care being taken to protect its nerve and blood supply, in order to advance the retracted muscle to the site of its avulsion of the tendon. The author has no experience of this operation but has never found that the retracted muscle could not be advanced after mobilising the tendon fully, and the more extensive operation does not, therefore, appear to be necessary.

RUPTURE OF THE BICEPS TENDON

Degenerative changes occur in various anatomical sites of the shoulder more or less simultaneously as a result of a variety of manual occupations. Comparatively trivial injury may then lead to damaged tendons. Not only does the acromioclavicular joint exhibit degenerative arthritis, but the underlying coracoacromial ligament becomes thickened and obstructs the anterior part of the rotator cuff during rotation and abduction. The cuff in the region of the bicipital groove, as well as the margins of the groove, undergo fibrotic changes, and the biceps tendon is at hazard. In association with degenerative changes in the margins of the bicipital groove, the tendon undergoes attrition and may rupture spontaneously or from trivial muscular effort. These predisposing factors explain why the long tendon of biceps is ruptured much more commonly than the short muscle origin from the coracoid or the distal tendon at its insertion to the bicipital tuberosity of the radius. The distal tendon is exposed to similar strains but is not subject to pathological degenerative changes, and only about 40 cases of avulsion of the biceps tendon from the radius have been recorded.[22–24]

Clinical features of rupture of the long head of biceps. The warning symptoms of pain and stiffness of the shoulder have often been present for some months or even years. At the moment of injury there is a sharp snap and thereafter pain and sometimes ecchymosis. In many cases, however, the patient may have come for an orthopaedic opinion on an entirely different matter, and is noted to have a total rupture of the proximal tendon of the biceps.

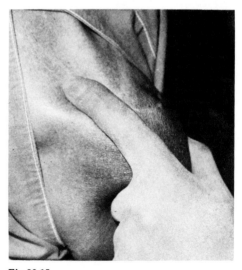

Fig 20.15

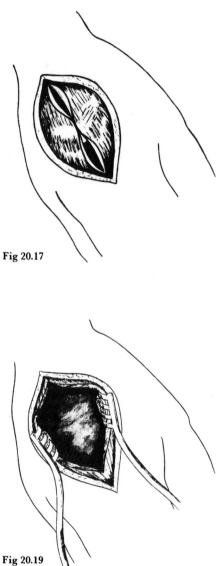

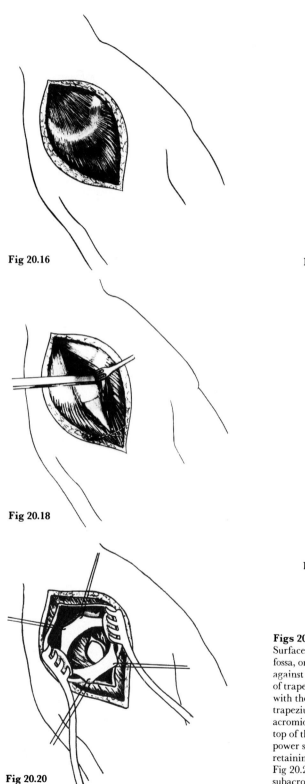

Fig 20.16

Fig 20.17

Fig 20.18

Fig 20.19

Fig 20.20

Figs 20.15 to 20.20 The transacromial approach. Fig 20.15: Surface marking. The index finger presses into the supraspinous fossa, one side abuts against the back of the clavicle, the other against the front of the spine of the scapula. Fig 20.16: Insertion of trapezius and origin of deltoid form a single sheet in continuity with the periosteum of the acromion. Fig 20.17: The fibres of the trapezius are split above and the fibres of deltoid below the acromion. Fig 20.18: A thick osteo-periosteal flap is lifted off the top of the acromion. Fig 20.19: The acromion is divided with a power saw in the coronal direction and then spread with a self-retaining retractor to reveal the underlying subacromial bursa. Fig 20.20: the rotator cuff lesion is not revealed until the subacromial bursa has been formally opened.

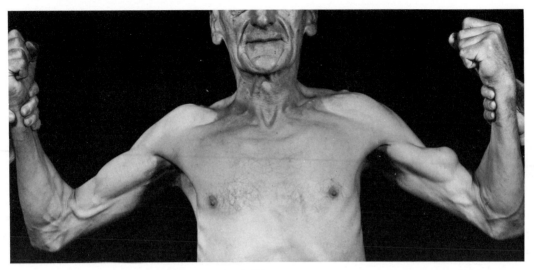

Fig 20.21 Spontaneous rupture of the tendon of the long head of biceps.

He has never had any shoulder trouble and is entirely unaware of it. Typical hollowing in the upper arm is seen, and when the patient supinates the forearm or flexes the elbow against resistance, the belly of the muscle retracts down to the middle third of the arm (Fig 20.21). There is little loss of power because the short head of biceps, brachialis anterior and flexor muscles of the forearm combine to produce near normal power of elbow flexion.

Treatment. The disability caused by rupture of the proximal long tendon of biceps is rarely sufficient to require treatment. Nevertheless, since there is slight loss of power and cosmetic disfigurement, and occasionally a degree of persistent pain, it may be wise in selected cases of recent rupture of the tendon to bring it back to its normal level, suturing it either to bone at the level of the bicipital groove, or simply to the short head of the tendon. In late cases, when several months have elapsed, it is usually better to reassure the patient and not to undertake any operation.

Treatment of rupture of the distal tendon of biceps (Fig 20.22). When the distal tendon is ruptured there is no underlying problem of degenerative change and the injury occurs in younger and more athletic patients, and causes complete loss of function of the biceps brachii, so that a much stronger case can be made for operative repair. Through an anterior approach the avulsed and retracted tendon is pulled down and held by suture passed through the radius in the region of the bicipital tuberosity.

FRACTURES OF THE CLAVICLE

This is a very common injury. Fractures of the clavicle usually occur in the middle third of the bone from falls on the outstretched hand. The lateral fragment is displaced forwards and downwards by the weight of the limb, while the medial fragment is held at a higher level by the sternomastoid muscle. The essential treatment is to support the weight of the limb by a sling tied over the opposite shoulder. Nearly always the fracture is clinically united within three weeks and functional recovery is complete within about two months.

About one in a hundred fractures of the clavicle need primary operative treatment. Sometimes there is comminution with severe upward tilting of the medial fragment and a sharp spur of bone that threatens to perforate the skin. Still more rarely a fragment may be displaced backwards and endanger the subclavian vessels. Sir Robert Peel, who established the police force of Great Britain, died of a fractured clavicle which ruptured the subclavian

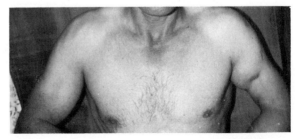

Fig 20.22 Rupture of the tendon of insertion of biceps.

vein. He was attended by Sir Benjamin Brodie who wrote 'the haemorrhage itself was the consequence of the subclavian vein having been lacerated by splinters of the fractured bone'.[25]

Treatment by figure-of-eight bandage. The patient sits on a stool, the operator standing behind with his knee between the patient's shoulder blades. Over large pads of felt or wool in each axilla, several domette bandages 15 cm wide are bound in front of the shoulders and cross between the shoulder blades in such a way that both shoulders are braced back (Fig 20.23). The limb is supported by a triangular sling under the elbow and forearm, tied over the opposite shoulder. Movements of the fingers, wrist and elbow joints are practised frequently throughout the day. The bandage is removed after about three weeks and the support of the sling is discarded in four weeks. There will then be clinical evidence of union, though of course radiographic evidence of consolidation is more delayed.

Although figure-of-eight bandaging is a universal and time-honoured treatment for fractures of the clavicle, it should not be used as a routine in every case. In the simplest fractures, for example an undisplaced subperiosteal crack, only a sling is necessary. In elderly patients the figure-of-eight bandaging can be hazardous by causing pressure upon the axillary vessels and nerves. *The treatment may cause more damage than the condition for which it is being employed.* Figure-of-eight bandaging, therefore, whilst generally useful should be employed with circumspection and not routinely in every case.

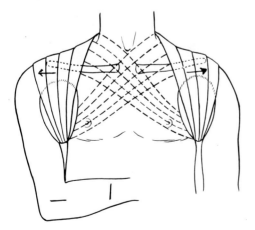

Fig 20.23 A figure-of-eight bandage pulls the outer fragment of the clavicle backwards and upwards, and the weight of the arm over the axillary pad maintains distraction.

Treatment by early operation. In the very few cases where sharp spurs of bone endanger the vessels or threaten to perforate the skin, a slender pin should be driven in a retrograde direction through the medulla of the bone of the outer fragment, then from without inwards across the fracture site into the medial fragment (Figs 20.24 and 20.25). The bone should be exposed with minimal stripping of soft tissues so that its blood supply will be preserved. The intramedullary pin will be needed only for the first 8 or 10 weeks and will always be removed. It is a dangerous situation in which to leave a sharp pointed wire which has been known to get loose and migrate even into the lung. It is for this reason that threaded wire should be used. The Crawford Adams pin has threads on the outer half which are wider than the core-diameter, designed to prevent migration of the intramedullary pin.

The patient whose radiographs are shown in Figures 20.26 and 20.27 was a famous jockey who several years before had sustained a fracture of the clavicle united with considerable thickening of the bone; he was again thrown and sustained a grossly comminuted fracture with wide displacement of the fragments. It was dealt with by open operative reduction and intramedullary fixation, the pin being removed after three months.

The intramedullary pin itself must not be relied upon. The limb should still be supported by a triangular sling so that the fracture site is protected. Indeed, in so far as operative exposure with its stripping of soft tissues must inevitably delay repair, such support should be continued for rather longer than the usual period, and seldom less than for about six weeks.

Un-united fracture of the clavicle. Non-union of this fracture is very unusual.[26-27] It may occur by reason of early operative procedures for internal fixation which strips its blood supply. In these exceptional cases late operative treatment is needed. The incision is made in the line of the skin crease below the clavicle, so that the scar will heal without disfigurement. The sclerosed bone ends are freshened and brought into apposition. A threaded intramedullary pin is driven through the medulla of the lateral fragment, emerging in the region of the acromion process, and then back into the medulla of the medial fragment. The protruding pin is cut to the level of the skin, bent over and left buried under the skin. Cancellous bone taken from the crest of the ilium is implanted between and around the freshened bone ends, care being taken to place the grafts principally

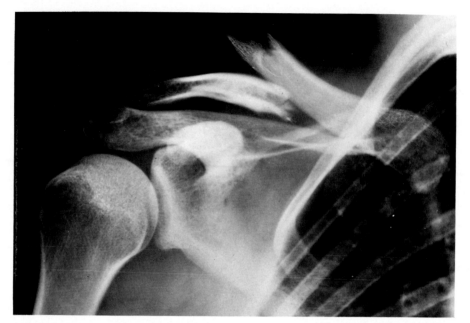

Fig 20.24

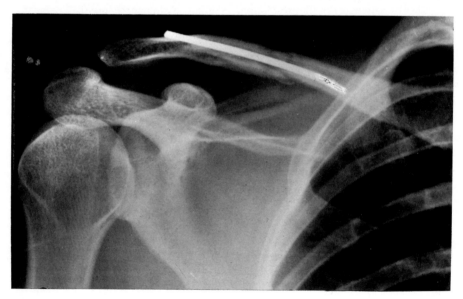

Fig 20.25

Figs 20.24 and 20.25 Fracture of the clavicle with severe displacement treatment by intramedullary pinning.

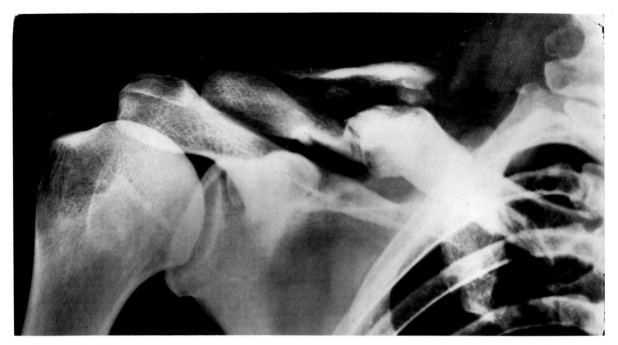

Fig 20.26

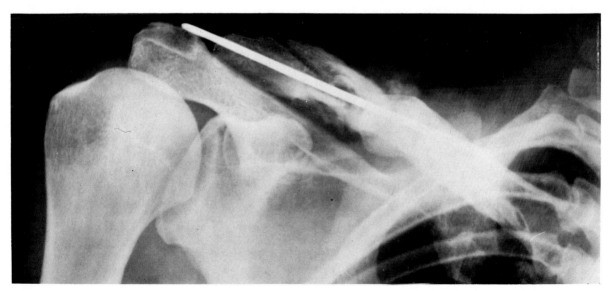

Fig 20.27

Figs 20.26 and 20.27 Comminuted repeated fracture of the clavicle of a steeplechase jockey treated by intramedullary pinning, removed after 3 months.

on the inferior aspect of the bone rather than on the subcutaneous surface, so that there will be no cosmetic disfigurement from bone thickening. The intramedullary wire is removed when union of the fracture is judged to have taken place, at about 12 to 16 weeks following operation. Alternatively bone fixation can be achieved by small-fragment plate and screws.

Cleido-cranial dysotosis. In giving a prognosis for un-united fracture of the clavicle the surgeon must be sure that it is a straightforward un-united traumatic fracture and not the congenital lesion of cleidocranial dysostosis in which, from birth, there is inherent failure of bone fusion between the two centres of ossification of the clavicle.

DISLOCATIONS OF THE STERNO-CLAVICULAR JOINT

The medial end of the clavicle may be dislocated forwards and downwards. Sometimes it is displaced upwards and in rare cases there is backward and retrosternal displacement with dyspnoea from pressure on the trachea.[28-29]

Swelling of the sterno-clavicular joint due to synovitis may exactly mimic a forward dislocation of the joint. Radiographs of this joint are notoriously difficult to obtain or interpret; but if an accurate history is taken and the possibility of sternoclavicular arthritis is kept in mind, the diagnosis should not be in doubt.

It is seldom difficult to replace the forwardly displaced sternal end of the clavicle by pulling the shoulder girdle upwards and bracing it backwards, exactly as for fractures of the clavicle; but it is difficult to prevent redisplacement. Reasonably good position may be maintained by a figure-of-eight bandage with large axillary pads over which the weight of the limb maintains distraction; but if reduction is unstable, operative fixation should be considered. In acute injuries, the torn tissues are repaired as found at operation, but in later cases such repair must be reinforced with adjacent muscle and fascia, or by stitching the meniscus of the joint across the front of the bone. Strips of fascia lata have been used to anchor the clavicle to the first or second rib or to the sternum,[30-33] and Jackson Burrows has suggested tenodesis of the subclavius.[34] It should be understood, however, that unreduced sternoclavicular dislocation may not cause any disability (Fig 20.28). The bone often becomes stable in its displaced position without causing serious pain or limitation of movement.

Retrosternal dislocations are rare but they deserve

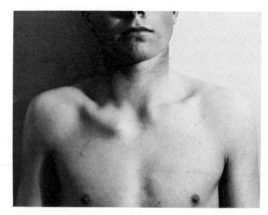

Fig 20.28 Dislocation of the right sterno-clavicular joint. Failure of reduction of the dislocation does not limit the shoulder movement and in this case accounts for no disability.

special consideration because of the serious complications that may accompany them. There may be severe pain at the base of the neck, pressure on the trachea, the oesophagus and the great vessels behind the sternum. A retrosternal dislocation of the clavicle may be a real emergency, the patient exhibiting marked respiratory embarrassment, and traumatic shock. Manipulative reduction should be attempted under conditions in which an open operation can be performed if manipulation is not successful. A sandbag is placed between the scapulae of the anaesthetised patient with the arm of the affected side hanging over the table. An assistant applies steady downward and outward traction to the arm while the surgeon will attempt manipulative reduction by direct manual manoeuvring of the medial end of the clavicle. If it is not successful immediate open reduction should be undertaken.

SUBLUXATION AND DISLOCATION OF THE ACROMIOCLAVICULAR JOINT

The acromioclavicular joint may seem to be a very unstable joint between two small articular surfaces although it is, with its associated ligaments, the main support of the upper limb from the trunk. The stability of this joint depends on muscle attachments and joint ligaments for a few millimetres on each side of it, and principally on the strong ligaments attached between scapula and clavicle—the conoid and trapezoid or coraco-clavicular ligaments—which pass from the whole length of the coracoid process to the inferior surface of the outer shaft of the clavicle (Fig 20.29). When these ligaments are ruptured or avulsed,

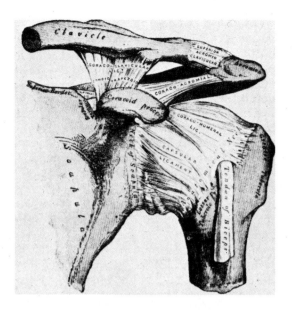

Fig 20.29 The ligaments of the shoulder girdle.

the weight of the limb depresses the scapula and its acromial process below the outer end of the clavicle. The displacement is further increased by the action of the trapezius which elevates the clavicle. The traumatic anatomy of injury of the acromioclavicular joint is one of degree ranging from the simplest disruption of deltoid and trapezius muscle attachments which merge with the capsule of the joint, to

the severest form in which the periosteum is stripped from the inferior surface of the clavicle and the continuing force disrupts the acromioclavicular ligaments (Figs 20.30 to 20.32).

Subluxation of the acromioclavicular joint. The injury usually arises from a rolling fall with impact on the outer side of the injured shoulder, as for example when the patient is thrown from a horse or is tackled in football. There is tenderness and some swelling of the joint but little or no difference in level as the examiner's finger passes from the outer end of the clavicle to the acromion. The joint is stable as tested by passively moving the clavicle to and fro on the acromion. These clinical signs may reveal minor stretching of the joint capsule and the immediate joint ligaments.

Radiographs should be taken in a manner which will allow strict comparison between the two damaged acromioclavicular joints. This is best performed with a single film centred on the manubrium sterni and encompassing both shoulders. Comparison is then reliable. Not only should the acromioclavicular joints be carefully compared, but the distance between the coracoid and clavicle on each side should be measured. The use of films taken in a standing position while the patient holds a weight in each hand is a time-honoured procedure, but of doubtful value.

Clinical tests are more reliable. It is usually suggested that the stability of the joint is tested by thrusting the arm up and down against the examiner's

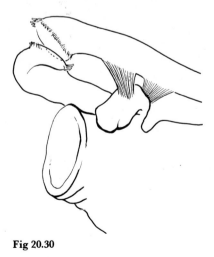

Fig 20.30

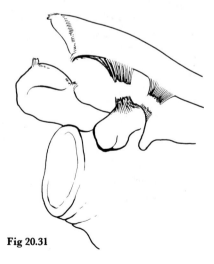

Fig 20.31

Figs 20.30 and 20.31 Stages in dislocation of the acromioclavicular joint. Fig 20.30: The capsule of the acromioclavicular joint is ruptured. Fig 20.31: The periosteum is stripped from the undersurface of the clavicle, and complete dislocation occurs when the ongoing forces are sufficient to rupture the conoid and trapezoid ligaments.

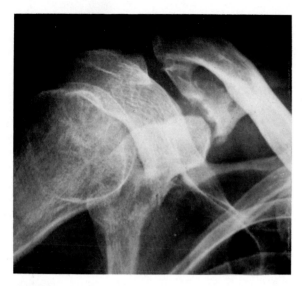

Fig 20.32 In late cases ossification of the haematoma occurs due to avulsion of the periosteum and rupture of the coracoclavicular ligaments.

resistance over the clavicle. The reverse test is, however, more reliable. If the damaged arm is steadied and the clavicle itself is depressed or moved to and fro by the other hand, the mobility of the outer end of the clavicle can in this way be more certainly seen and felt. The to-and-fro movement of the outer end of the clavicle in relation to the acromion in the antero-posterior plane is particularly useful as a test for stability. In doubtful cases instability of the acromioclavicular joint becomes most obvious in the position of forced adduction of the arm held behind the patient's body.

Dislocation of the acromioclavicular joint (Fig. 20.33). If clinical examination is confirmed by radiography so as to make it clear that the important coracoclavicular ligaments have been disrupted, a diagnosis of dislocation of the acromioclavicular joint must be made.

Treatment of injuries to the acromioclavicular joint. Minor injuries of the joint require minimal protection for a few weeks to prevent distraction of the joint by the weight of the arm. It is by no means certain, however, that the current *laissez faire* attitude with regard to more severe injuries can be justified. Fortunately, this

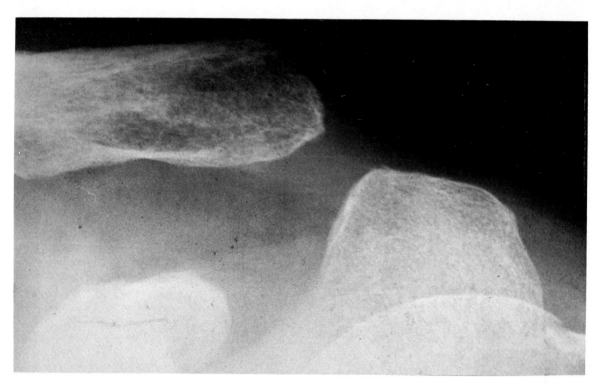

Fig 20.33 Acute dislocation of the acromioclavicular joint.

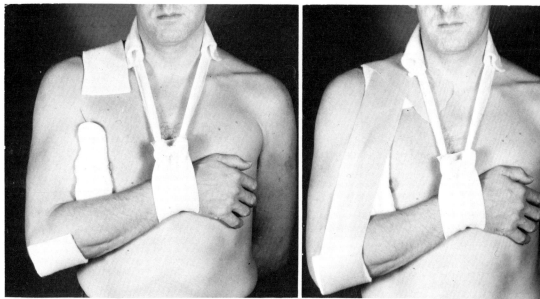

Fig 20.34   Fig 20.35

Figs 20.34 and 20.35 Method of strapping an acromioclavicular joint injury. The humerus and scapula are elevated and the clavicle is depressed while strapping is tightly applied over pads of adhesive felt.

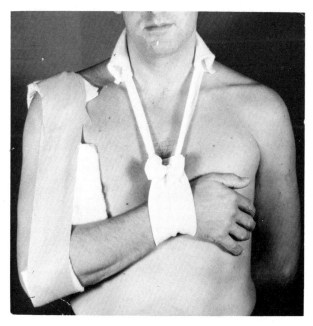

Fig 20.36 Wrong method of strapping for acromioclavicular injury.

long cherished view is being increasingly challenged and surely it must be true that an injury to the acromioclavicular joint should be clinically evaluated in all its aspects, like an injury to any other joint: if the injury is a minor one in an elderly person, entirely conservative treatment is appropriate; if the injury is a major disruption in an active young person, the best result will certainly be obtained by early operative treatment. It is a matter of total clinical judgement: the age of the patient, whether he is right or left-handed, his occupation, etc. must all be considered.

Protection by bandage and strapping. The joint can be

supported by strapping which encircles it from the middle third of the clavicle around the elbow joint[35] (Figs 20.34 to 20.36). Too often the strapping is applied to the length of the shaft of the humerus from elbow to shoulder; this is not only entirely useless but can be dangerous. Very careful padding is required, particularly around the elbow joint, in order to avoid pressure on the skin and even pressure paralysis of the ulnar nerve.

Acute acromioclavicular dislocation. A lack of understanding of the traumatic anatomy of this injury and the consequent poor surgical repair is largely responsible for the pessimistic attitude which is current regarding operative treatment[36]. The treatment is to repair the lesion displayed at operation, and to do this properly the traumatic anatomy must be understood

(Figs 20.37 and 20.38). The most striking feature present in every case is the damage sustained by the deltoid and trapezius muscles. The deltoid is avulsed from the anterior end of the outer clavicle leaving it stripped bare; the trapezius is split in the direction of its fibres so as to leave a gap between the superior segment gaining insertion into the clavicle and the inferior segment inserted into the spine of the scapula and acromion. In some cases the deep fascia overlying the muscle is intact and conceals the lesion until it has been incised. The short capsular fibres of the acromioclavicular joint are disrupted and from the inferior surface the periosteum is stripped off the clavicle for a variable distance, the force of disruption running on into the conoid and trapezoid ligaments which are damaged to a varying degree.

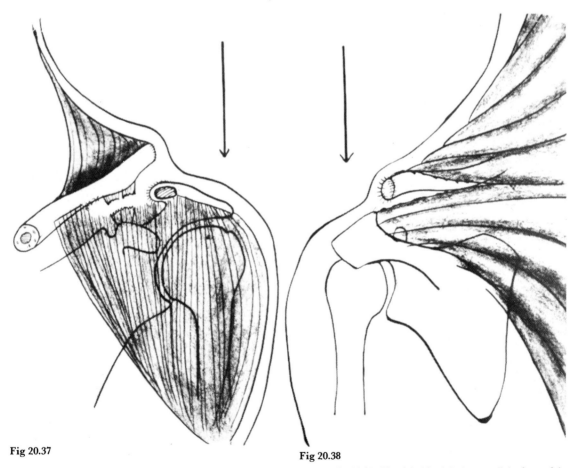

Fig 20.37

Fig 20.38

Figs 20.37 and 20.38 Traumatic anatomy of acromioclavicular dislocation. Fig 20.37: The deltoid origin is torn off the front of the clavicle. Fig 20.38: The trapezius fibres are split, the joint capsule is disrupted, the coraco-clavicular ligaments are torn. (From Horn J. S. (1954). The traumatic anatomy and treatment of acute acromioclavicular dislocations. *Journal of Bone and Joint Surgery*, 36-B: 194. Reproduced by kind permission of the editor and the author).

Operative treatment for acute acromioclavicular dislocation. The object of the operation is to repair the damage systematically at each layer. Simply driving an intramedullary pin across the joint, or fixing clavicle to coracoid by a screw, without careful attention to the disruption of muscle attachments, ligaments and joint capsule will not give a good result.

The incision follows the outer third of the acromion, across the acromioclavicular joint and runs medialwards along the horizontal fibres of the trapezius. The full extent of the injury is displayed once the deep fascia has been opened in the line of the skin incision. The essential dissection of the operation has been done by the violence of the injury: the deltoid is avulsed from the outer end of the clavicle, leaving it stripped and bare for a varying distance; the trapezius is split in the direction of its fibres so as to leave a gap between the superior segment of the muscle gaining insertion to the clavicle, and the segment immediately below it gaining insertion to the spine of the scapula and the acromion. When the full extent of the injury has been displayed by dissection, the integrity of the coracoclavicular ligaments is established, if necessary by extending medially the gap between clavicle and avulsed deltoid muscle, leaving a fringe of muscle attached to the clavicle to facilitate suturing. Any obstacle to reduction that may be in the acromioclavicular joint is removed. Fringes of capsule and intra-articular disc are excised. A suture is passed to and fro through the torn ends of the coracoclavicular ligaments and the ends of the suture are left long. Two holes are drilled vertically through the clavicle to accept the suture which is not tied at this stage. Whilst the dislocation is held reduced by the assistant, a threaded wire is passed across the joint (Fig 20.39), or a Bosworth lag screw is passed from clavicle to coracoid, and tightened (Fig 20.40). The suture is then tightened, and secured. The layers of soft tissue are then serially repaired; joint capsule, deltoid and trapezius, each in layers. Suction drainage is advisable. The screw is removed at ten weeks, during which time all movements except the extremes of abduction are encouraged.

Late acromioclavicular joint injuries. Although persistent subluxation and even persistent dislocation does not always require treatment, no form of conservative treatment helps patients who

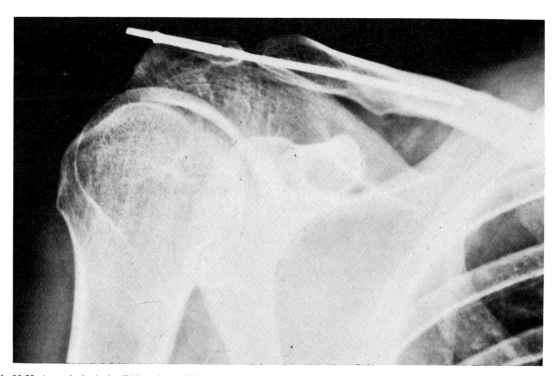

Fig 20.39 Acromioclavicular Dislocation stabilised by a threaded intramedullary pin. (Case treated by Mr J Crawford-Adams).

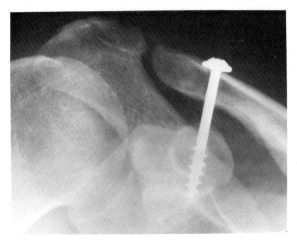

Fig 20.40 The Bosworth lag screw is probably the most effective method of temporary fixation of an acromioclavicular joint. It must be removed when the soft tissues have fully healed.

complain of pain or limitation of movement. In cases of persistent subluxation where the coracoclavicular ligaments are intact, the most effective method is an excision of the lateral 1 cm of the clavicle.[37-38] This simple operation gives excellent results.

In cases of persistent dislocation it is often justifiable to reconstruct the coracoclavicular ligaments. The ligaments may be refashioned either by strips of fascia lata or by using a length of conjoint tendon of the coraco-brachialis and short head of biceps muscles, or by transferring the coracoid with its attached muscles to the clavicle.[39-43]

After operation for both acute and late acromio-clavicular joint injuries it is essential that the joint is temporarily stabilised by some form of internal fixation, but permanent fixation of the acromioclavicular joint by any technique should never be done because of the subsequent restriction of elevation of the arm which requires rotation of the clavicle. Horn used wire sutures passed through the clavicle and acromion which held for several months—long enough for healing to occur—before the wire became fragmented by movements of the joint. This is an acceptable technical procedure but rather difficult and late radiographs are unaesthetic! One satisfactory method of temporary fixation is by a threaded metal pin across the joint, the end of which remains buried deep to skin. Crawford Adams has devised a suitable pin whose threads are of a larger diameter than the pin, which prevents migration (Fig 20.39). It is removed through a small stab wound.

Reconstruction of late acromioclavicular dislocation. Of the many operations which have been devised for this condition, transfer of the coraco-acromial ligament to replace the ruptured acromioclavicular ligaments is the most physiologically appropriate procedure[44] (Figs 20.41 and 20.42). An oblique incision is made

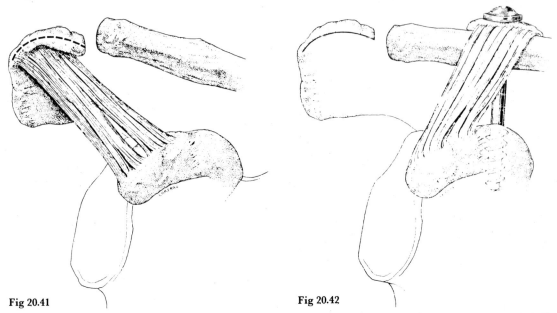

Fig 20.41

Fig 20.42

Figs 20.41 and 20.42 Transfer of the coracoacromial ligament with a small sliver of bone at its insertion is the most physiologically appropriate procedure for the reconstruction of late acromioclavicular dislocation.

in the line of the fibres of the deltoid muscle centred over the coraco-acromial ligament and exposes the ligament in its entire length. The ligament is detached with a large sliver of bone from the full width of the undersurface of the acromion. The acromioclavicular joint is exposed and the intra-articular meniscus and other obstructing soft tissue tags are removed. The clavicle is now brought forwards and downwards to its normal anatomical position where it is held firmly with a Bosworth screw passed from clavicle to coracoid under direct vision. The clavicle immediately adjacent to the screw is scarified to receive the bony attachment of the transposed coraco-acromial ligament. With the ligament held taut, the Bosworth screw traps the flake of bone with its attached ligament. The acromioclavicular joint is now mechanically stabilised by the screw until biological stabilisation can take place by the transposed ligament. The screw is removed at about 10 weeks.

FRACTURES OF THE SCAPULA

Fractures of the body of the scapula are caused by direct crushing injury and may be associated with fractures of the ribs. The bone is comminuted but the fragments are so completely surrounded by muscles and fascia that displacement is unimportant. Firm bandaging relieves the discomfort.

Fractures of the neck of the scapula. A fall on the outside of the shoulder, or on the outstretched hand, may cause fracture of the neck of the scapula. It extends from below the glenoid fossa to the base of the coracoid process, or through the whole width of the neck of the scapula. The glenoid fragment is often impacted downwards and inwards but the displacement is seldom sufficient to cause disability and there is no need to attempt to reduce it. The limb should be supported in a sling, active exercises of the shoulder being encouraged within 10 to 14 days. There is no need for operative treatment.

Fracture of the coracoid process. When there is dislocation of the acromioclavicular joint the coracoclavicular ligaments sometimes tear a fragment of bone from the coracoid which is displaced upwards with the clavicle. Late radiographs show ossification of the haematoma within the avulsed coraco-clavicular ligaments, which is indeed a stabilising safeguard.

The coracoid process may also be fractured near its base. In one unusual injury this was the result of direct upward violence from a heavy fall on the point of the elbow while the limb was near the trunk which drove up the whole humerus together with the coracoid, clavicle and acromion process. It may complicate anterior dislocation of the shoulder.

The coracoid may be avulsed and displaced downwards by muscular traction of the three muscles attached to it. There is no need to correct this displacement; in fact Oudard[45] and Bristow[46] produced it deliberately by osteotomy, transferring the displaced coracoid to the front of the neck of the scapula to reinforce the capsule of the shoulder as a protection against recurrent anterior dislocation.

PROXIMAL HUMERAL FRACTURES

In all previous editions of this book fractures involving the upper end of the humerus have been considered in relation to their anatomical site and the presumed direction of violence causing presumed direction of displacement as seen on an antero-posterior radiograph. We thus classified various types of fracture of the tuberosities, abduction and adduction fractures of the surgical neck of the humerus, and a variety of fracture-dislocations. These descriptions were a useful guide to the general management of these injuries. However, time does not stand still, and even the most hallowed concepts must give way to better ideas.

There are two principal reasons why it has become important to use a completely new and improved classification for these fractures, leading to a new approach to facilitate their management.

Firstly, we now realise that radiographs can, and do, give a spurious appearance of angular deformity (Figs 20.43 and 20.44). The fallacy of the terms 'abduction' fracture and 'adduction' fracture has now become apparent: although there is some angulation, the principal deformity is almost always in a rotational direction. Moreover, in fractures of the surgical neck of the humerus, the angular deformity is not mainly in abduction nor in adduction, but rather directed forwards or backwards in the sagittal, and not in the coronal plane.

Secondly, The work of Charles Neer of New York demands a fundamental reappraisal of the classification of proximal humeral fractures, in particular displaced fractures. As a result of his observations on 300 cases, Neer has provided us with a completely new classification.[47–48] This classification is based both on the anatomical site of the fracture and the number of principal fragments with their muscle attachments: two-part, three-part, and four-part fractures, as well as fracture-dislocations. Most importantly, the classification is related to the muscles

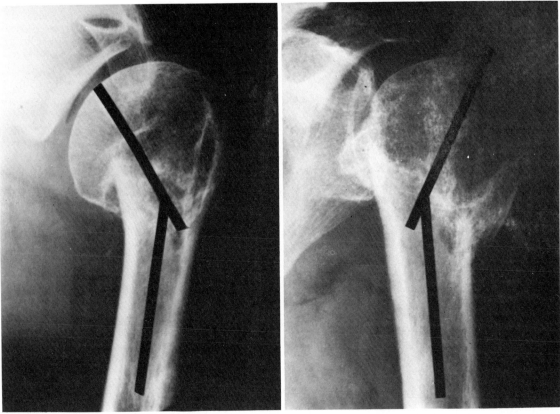

Fig 20.43

Fig 20.44

Figs 20.43 and 20.44 Two radiographs of the same fracture showing spurious angular deformity: with the arm in internal rotation (Fig 20.43) the fracture looks like an impacted adduction fracture; with the arm in external rotation (Fig 20.44) the same fracture looks like an impacted abduction fracture.

which are attached to each fragment. The muscle attachments are a principal guide to displacement, and consequently the appropriate treatment to be followed. Neer's concept provides an excellent basis for the management of these fractures. What follows here is based on Neer's work but does not exactly correspond to it.

STABLE PROXIMAL HUMERAL FRACTURES WITH MINIMAL DISPLACEMENT

Fractures involving the articular surface of the head of the humerus. These occur either by direct impaction violence or more commonly in association with anterior or posterior dislocation (see p 549 and 554).

Greater tuberosity of the humerus. This may occur by direct contusion from a fall on the side of the shoulder. The comminuted fragments are held in good position by periosteal attachments and the only treatment needed is to support the limb in a sling for a week or two encouraging active movements of fingers, wrist, and elbow from the beginning, with guarded assisted movements of the shoulder within a few days. If strenuous activity by the patient and physiotherapist is avoided, full movements and normal restoration of power will be regained within a few weeks (Figs 20.45 to 20.47).

Surgical neck of the humerus. This group of fractures previously described as impacted abduction, and impacted adduction fractures of the surgical neck of the humerus are more accurately designated as stable two-part fractures of the neck of the humerus with minimal displacement. This classification does not prejudge the direction of the displacement. A single antero-posterior radiograph does not define the displacement. A lateral radiograph, preferably a

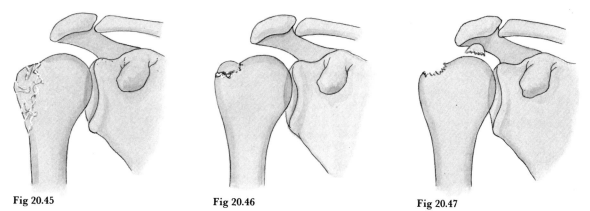

Fig 20.45   **Fig 20.46**   **Fig 20.47**

Figs 20.45 to 20.47 Types of fractures of the greater tuberosity. Fig 20.45: Stable contusion of the great tuberosity. Fig 20.46: Avulsion without significant displacement but stable due to the attachment of soft tissues. Fig 20.47: Avulsion with displacement and retraction by the rotator cuff muscles.

trans-axillary projection taken at right-angles, will enable one to judge with more accuracy the direction and degree of angulation, which is a consequence of rotational force. After a few days when the acute episode has passed it is possible with gentleness to make a reasonable assessment of the degree and direction of rotation which has occurred. In children a similar fracture may be sustained through the metaphysis (Figs 20.48 and 20.49); the angular component of the deformity will correct itself by remodelling, the rotational deformity will not correct by remodelling but is functionally of little importance.

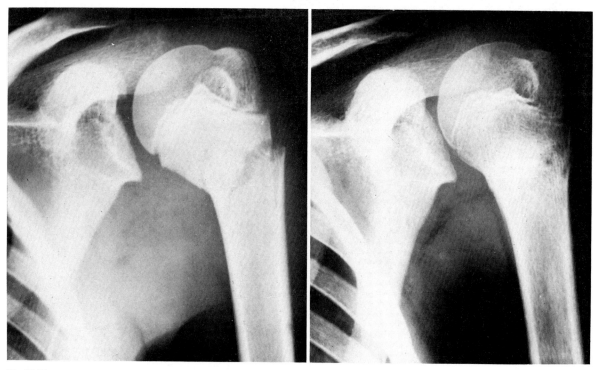

Fig 20.48   **Fig 20.49**

Figs 20.48 and 20.49 Fracture of the surgical neck of the humerus in a child treated by manipulative reduction.

Stable fractures of the neck of the humerus are treated by a simple sling and early active movements to hand, wrist and elbow. Nothing must be done to prejudice the stability of the fracture. After about two weeks the patient is instructed in gentle active exercises of the shoulder. Full functional recovery is usual.

It is exceptional for greater degrees of displacement to arise, perhaps with the interposition of periosteal fibres, or trapping of the biceps tendon, needing operative reduction.

In the very rare case in which the deformity has caused a final limitation of movement sufficient to impair the patient's ability to carry out his normal work or take part in his particular sport, corrective osteotomy may be considered as a secondary procedure later (Figs 20.50 and 20.51). It is in every way unwise and prejudicial to attempt a correction of the deformity of these stable fractures at an early stage.

UNSTABLE PROXIMAL HUMERAL FRACTURES WITH DISPLACEMENT

The classification of these fractures based on the work of Neer provides a far more precise basis than hitherto on which to understand this often complicated injury, and consequently to plan treatment suitable for each case (Fig 20.52). Most fractures of the proximal

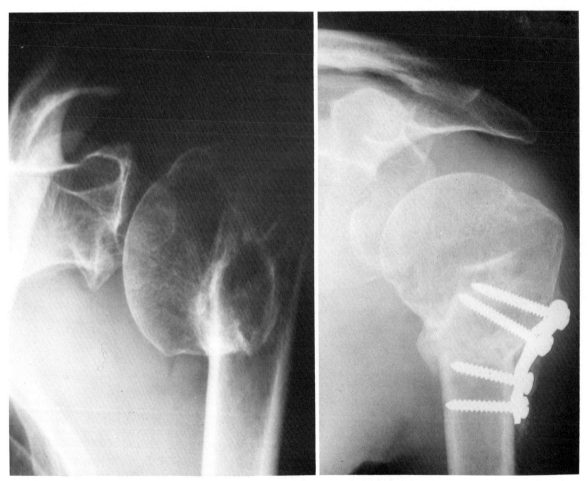

Fig 20.50   **Fig 20.51**

Figs 20.50 and 20.51 Fracture of the surgical neck of the humerus impacted but with very considerable displacement (Fig 20.50). Although the displacement appears to be principally into adduction, the internal rotation and extension displacements of the fragments are the most important. The acute fracture was treated by simple rest and early mobilisation. Later when the patient found that his loss of movement—in particular outward rotation and flexion—was a serious handicap to him, a formal corrective osteotomy was performed (Fig 20.51).

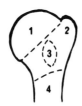

	Two-part	Three-part	Four-part
Anatomical Neck			
Surgical Neck			
Greater Tuberosity			
Lesser Tuberosity			
Fracture Dislocation			

Fig 20.52 Classification of unstable proximal humeral fractures (after Neer).

humerus consist of either two, three, or four fragments. These fragments each carry important muscle insertions. The four major segments consist of the articular surface of the humeral head, greater tuberosity, lesser tuberosity, and surgical neck of the humerus. It is essential to have at least two-plane radiographs in order to assess the injury accurately.

Treatment of unstable two-part fractures
1. Greater tuberosity. The unstable variety of fracture of the greater tuberosity should really be thought of as an avulsion of the attached rotator cuff insertion (Figs 20.53 and 20.54). Usually periosteal and capsular fibres remain intact so that there is minimal displacement and there is then no need for treatment other than simple protection of the limb in a sling. If, however, the fragment is completely avulsed and displaced either at the time of the accident or by subsequent injudicious exercising, so that it lies above the head of the humerus and is medially retracted, the injury is much more serious. Operative replacement of the avulsed fragment by the transacromial approach (p 520) is imperative.

Fracture of the greater tuberosity with anterior dislocation of the shoulder. Anterior dislocation of the shoulder may be complicated by a fracture of the greater tuberosity with its attached rotator cuff muscle insertion. After reducing the dislocation (Figs 20.94 to 20.96), the treatment for this fracture is as for the avulsion fracture of the greater tuberosity as already described, either conservatively if judged to be stable, or by open operation and internal fixation if judged to be unstable.

2. Lesser tuberosity. This is a rare injury but important because complete avulsion of the lesser tuberosity carries with it the insertion of the subscapularis and may lead to significant disability (Figs 20.55 to 20.58). A displaced fragment should be replaced into its bed and fixed by a nail or screw. A direct deltoid-splitting approach is usually satisfactory for this purpose.

3. Surgical neck of the humerus. On the basis of the age and occupation of the patient as well as the degree of displacement of the fragments, a clinical judgement must be made as to whether the fracture is treated by simple immobilisation until it has become stable, after which graduated exercises are resumed, or by immediate open reduction and internal fixation (Figs 20.59 to 20.60). This judgement should be made within the first week because delay considerably increases the difficulties and hazards of operation. This fracture is most conveniently held in place by a screw or a Rush Nail (Figs 20.61 to 20.64). Subsequent treatment depends on the degree of stability which has been achieved by operation. Postoperatively the arm is held in a roller towel abduction sling for a few days; active exercise is commenced at a time appropriate to each individual case.

4. Two-part fractures of the surgical neck of the humerus with anterior dislocation (Figs 20.65 and 20.66). One single attempt should be made at manipulative reduction of the dislocation. If this is successful the associated fracture can be treated conservatively or by open internal fixation according to the degree of displacement. The manipulative reduction should be attempted with great caution in conditions which would allow the surgeon to proceed to open operation if it proves necessary.

Treatment of unstable three and four-part fractures and fracture-dislocations of the shoulder
These are complex injuries which usually require operative reduction and internal fixation except in

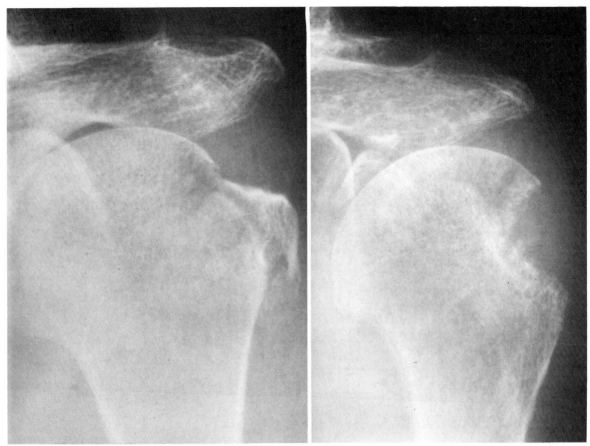

Fig 20.53   **Fig 20.54**

Figs 20.53 and 20.54 If there is insufficient soft tissue attachment to retain the greater tuberosity, it will be pulled off by the rotator cuff muscles and may come to lie several centimetres medial to its normal insertion.

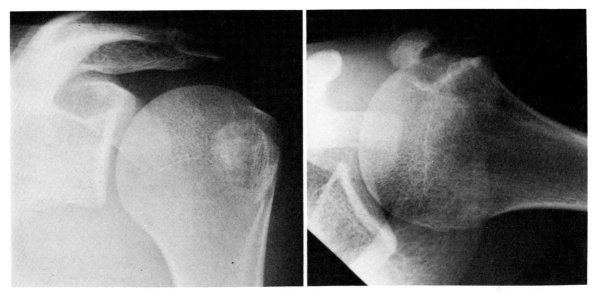

Fig 20.55

Fig 20.56

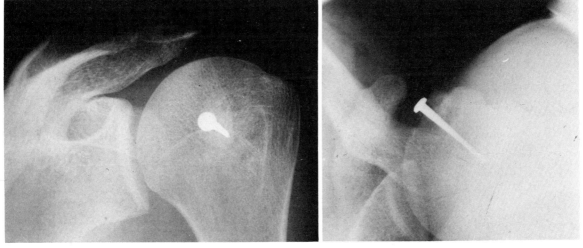

Fig 20.57

Fig 20.58

Figs 20.55 to 20.58 Avulsion fracture of the lesser tuberosity displaced by the pull of subscapularis (Figs 20.55 and 20.56). It has been replaced into its bed and held there by a Stuck nail (Figs 20.57 and 20.58).

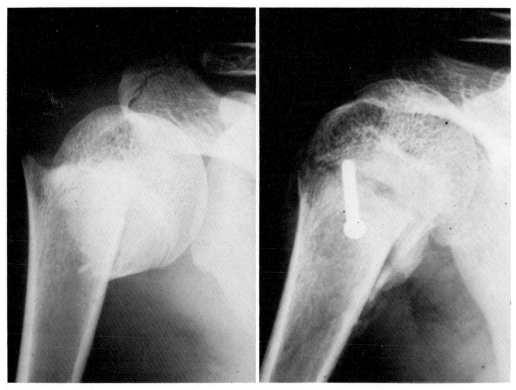

Fig 20.59   **Fig 20.60**

Figs 20.59 and 20.60 Unstable fracture of the surgical neck of the humerus with displacement. An attempt at closed reduction failed because the biceps tendon was interposed. At open operation the fragments were fixed by a screw. (Acknowledgement to Mr W N Laurence).

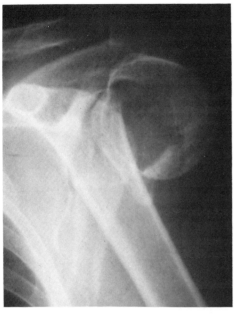

Fig 20.61

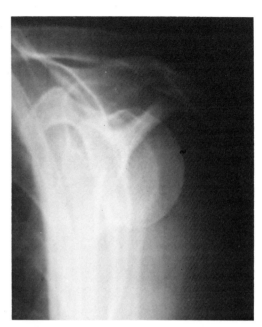

Fig 20.62

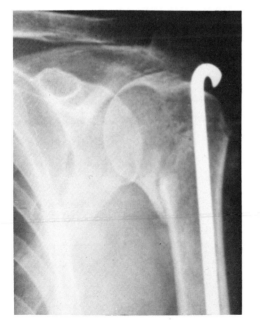

Fig 20.63

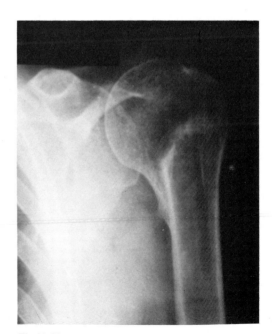

Fig 20.64

Figs 20.61 to 20.64 Instability and displacement of this fracture of the surgical neck of the humerus is due to unopposed muscle action on the two fragments: the upper fragment is rotated outwards by the rotator cuff muscles; the lower fragment is adducted and rotated inwards by pectoralis major. Open reduction and fixation by Rush pin is an appropriate treatment. (Courtesy of Mr E L Trickey).

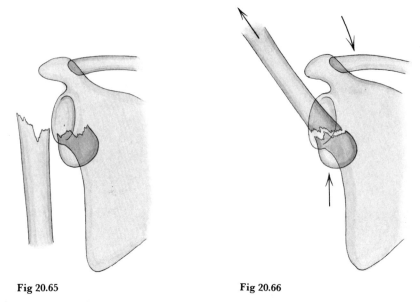

Fig 20.65   **Fig 20.66**

Figs 20.65 and 20.66 It is occasionally possible to carry out a closed manipulative reduction of this difficult fracture-dislocation. The attempt should be made *once* only and with great caution under conditions which would allow immediate open operation to be carried out if necessary.

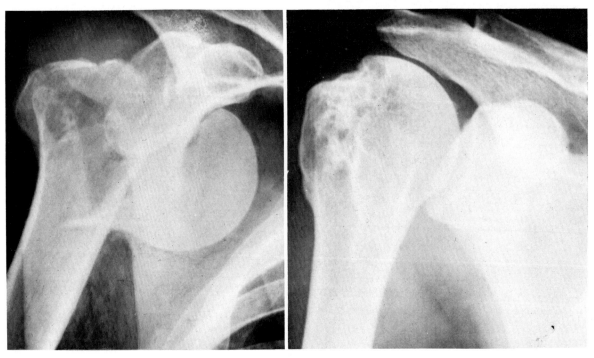

Fig 20.67   **Fig 20.68**

Fig 20.67 and 20.68 Fracture-dislocation of the shoulder reduced by traction applied to the limb by the side of the trunk together with direct manual pressure beneath the head of the humerus. One attempt only is justifiable at closed manipulative reduction.

patients who are too old and infirm, or in those cases in which such great comminution has occurred that it is beyond the surgeon's skill to reconstitute the fragments and muscle attachments. It is justifiable to make one single attempt at manipulative reduction, relying on the presence of residual periosteal attachments to carry the fragments into an improved position (Figs 20.67 and 20.68).

If this does not succeed, open reduction and internal fixation using screws, wire suture or Rush pinning is carried out according to circumstance (Figs 20.69 to 20.71). It is essential that the decision to operate is not delayed beyond the first two weeks, after which the operation becomes exceedingly difficult, and the result correspondingly poor. The surgical approach used for fractures of the greater tuberosity or lesser tuberosity are suitable, but occasionally a full anterolateral deltopectoral exposure is required. It is important to preserve any blood supply to the head of the humerus, in particular muscle, capsular and periosteal attachments to the fragments. The ascending branch of the anterior circumflex artery carries the main residual blood supply to the head of the humerus and should be protected from injury. Kirschner wires are unsuitable for internal fixation because they impair early post-operative mobilisa-

tion. The object of the operation is to secure re-attachment of the more important muscles around the shoulder (Figs 20.72 and 20.73), serially to reduce each displacement (usually rotation) of each fragment, and hold it in place with screws or sutures. Thus the greater tuberosity fragment which has usually been displaced proximally and rotated upwards by the rotator cuff muscles inserted into it is replaced and fixed to the major humeral head fragment; the lesser tuberosity fragment similarly displaced by subscapularis is replaced and fixed (Figs 20.74 and 20.75). When necessary the reconstituted proximal fragments are then held to the shaft of the humerus by a Rush nail or wire sutures.

In a three- or four-part fracture-dislocation, when the head of the humerus is entirely devoid of any blood supply, it can be replaced by a humeral prosthesis. This procedure must be reserved for the humeral head fragment totally devoid of any soft tissue attachment. If there is any doubt, it is better to replace the humeral head and await developments.

Most of the poor results following open operation and internal fixation of three-part fractures are due to imperfect technique; most of the poor results following four-part fractures are due to avascular necrosis of the head of the humerus.

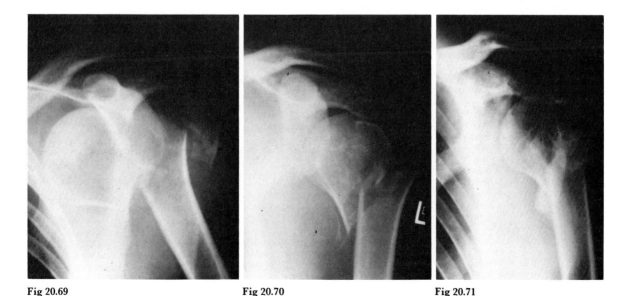

Fig 20.69   **Fig 20.70**   **Fig 20.71**

Fig 20.69 to 20.71 Unstable three-part fracture-dislocation treated by closed reduction of the dislocation and open reduction and fixation of the greater tuberosity with its attached rotator cuff muscles (Figs 20.69 and 20.70). The fracture of the neck of the humerus was thereafter treated conservatively in a simple collar-and-cuff. Union in good position was obtained (Fig 20.71). (Courtesy of Mr E L Trickey).

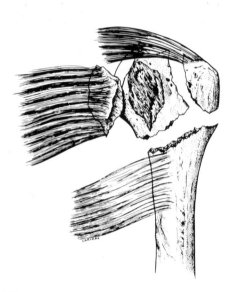

Fig 20.72 The key to an understanding of these complicated fractures is the principal muscle attachment to each major fragment.

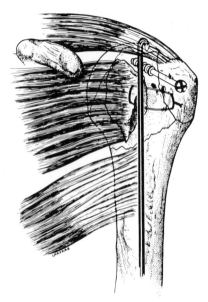

Fig 20.73 Each major fragment is reduced and held in position by a screw, wire suture, or intramedullary pin as appropriate. The precise details vary from case to case, but the principle is the same in all cases. (After Neer).

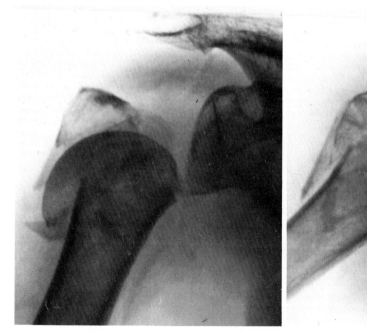

Fig 20.74   **Fig 20.75**

Fig 20.74 and 20.75 Unstable four-part fracture of the proximal humerus before and after operative reduction. The re-attachment of each principal fragment with its muscle insertion is the key to operative reduction. In this case silk sutures were used and cannot therefore be seen on the radiographs.

DOWNWARD SUBLUXATION OF THE HEAD OF THE HUMERUS FOLLOWING INJURY

When fractures of the shoulder girdle and other injuries of the arm have been treated by suspension in a collar-and-cuff sling it will often be found after several weeks that there is downward subluxation of the head of the humerus from the glenoid. One should be immediately suspicious of a circumflex nerve injury leading to paralysis of the deltoid when downward subluxation may be severe. However, even with an unparalysed deltoid, the degree of displacement may be considerable and give rise to alarm. The fact is that displacement arises from the weight of the heavy limb suspended from the shoulder at a time when muscles are hypotonic and may be augmented by a traumatic effusion into the shoulder joint.

The problem was clarified by the studies of T. J. Fairbank[49] who demonstrated the degree of subluxation which is possible from traction on the normal shoulder joint of an anaesthetised individual whose muscles are fully relaxed. If, after fractures or dislocations, the limb is left unsupported, such traction arises simply from limb-weight which is of course increased if there is a plaster cast and still more so if the discarded notion of adding weights to the cast makes it even more heavy. There need be no alarm, because once the limb is supported and particularly when muscle tone is regained by exercise, the displacement will correct itself.

The patient shown in Figures 20.76 to 20.78 was threatened with real danger. He had sustained a fracture of the neck of the humerus which had been slow in uniting and radiographs showed a severe degree of downward subluxation. The surgeon responsible for treatment thought that there was both an ununited fracture of the neck of the humerus and an unreduced dislocation, and had to be dissuaded from operating on what was thought to be a severe and difficult fracture-dislocation. Not only did the fracture consolidate soundly but the subluxation corrected itself and the patient had a normal limb. Do not be disturbed by temporary downward subluxation of the head of the humerus arising solely from muscle hypotonicity and corrected by active exercise.

DISLOCATIONS OF THE SHOULDER

Although dislocations of the gleno-humeral joint do not differ in basic pathological anatomy from dislocations of other joints, there are certain features of the traumatic anatomy which predisposes the shoulder joint to recurring dislocation. The traumatic anatomy of acute dislocation and recurrent dislocation of the shoulder is precisely the same: it is really a matter of the degree of the injury rather than its nature. If the initial injury is protected fully from undue early mobilisation, in particular outward rotation, and if the limb is held long enough for capsular injury to repair, recovery will usually be complete without recurrence. Primary dislocations which have been treated with full protection of the anterior joint capsule for at least three weeks rarely recur; whereas patients with recurrent dislocation almost always did not have appropriate treatment at the time of their first injury.

Mechanism of injury. The most common injury is a fall on the outstretched hand with the limb in lateral rotation, so that the head of the humerus is forced against the anterior capsule which is therefore torn or avulsed from bone. It is not just an abduction injury; it is more particularly a lateral rotation injury. Usually the patient falls to the ground and tries to save himself. If the outstretched hand is level with or behind the plane of the trunk the forward drive of the head of the humerus against the anterior capsule is obvious; but even when falling with the limb in front of the trunk there is such obliquity of the plane of the gleno-humeral joint, 30 degrees forwards, that the force is still translated into a forward thrust of the head of the humerus against the anterior capsule. This force, combined with outward rotation, causes the anterior dislocation.

Anterior dislocation: pre-glenoid, sub-coracoid and sub-clavicular.

When the anterior capsule is torn or avulsed from bone and the joint is dislocated, the head of the humerus may come to lie in front of the glenoid fossa of the scapula, or if the force is stronger it is driven further forwards to lie in the sub-coracoid or sub-clavicular position (Figs 20.79 and 20.80). In one patient reported by Bankart[50] the head of the humerus was driven between the clavicle and the first rib.

In a still more remarkable displacement recorded by West[51] the humeral head was driven into the chest between the third and fourth ribs (Fig 20.81). It was pulled out like a cork from a bottle and the patient made a complete recovery.

In the usual displacements, the head of the humerus comes to lie in front of the glenoid, in the sub-coracoid or sub-clavicular position. The head of the humerus may lie within the capsule of the shoulder joint which

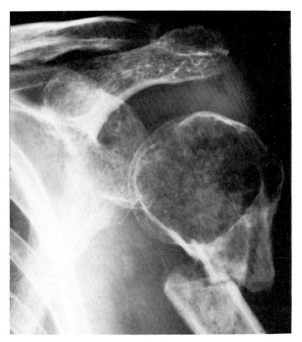

Figs 20.76 to 20.78 Downward subluxation of the shoulder after fracture of the neck of the humerus or other injuries. The film taken 4 months after injury was incorrectly thought to show a fracture-dislocation with non-union of the fracture and non-reduction of the dislocation (Fig 20.76). The fracture was, however, clinically united and the 'dislocation' was a simple consequence of muscle atrophy and gravitational dependence of the limb. After active exercises the end result was a functional normal shoulder (Figs 20.77 and 20.78).

Fig 20.76

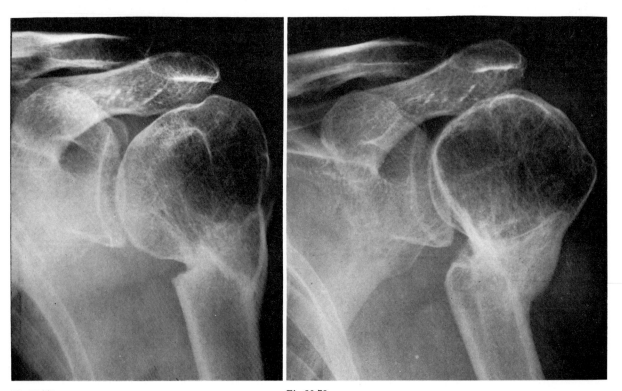

Fig 20.77

Fig 20.78

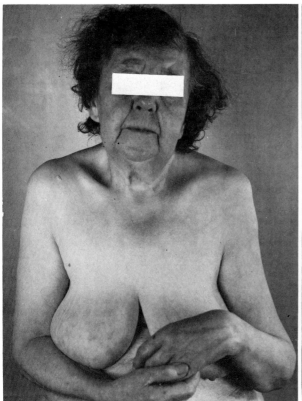

Fig 20.79

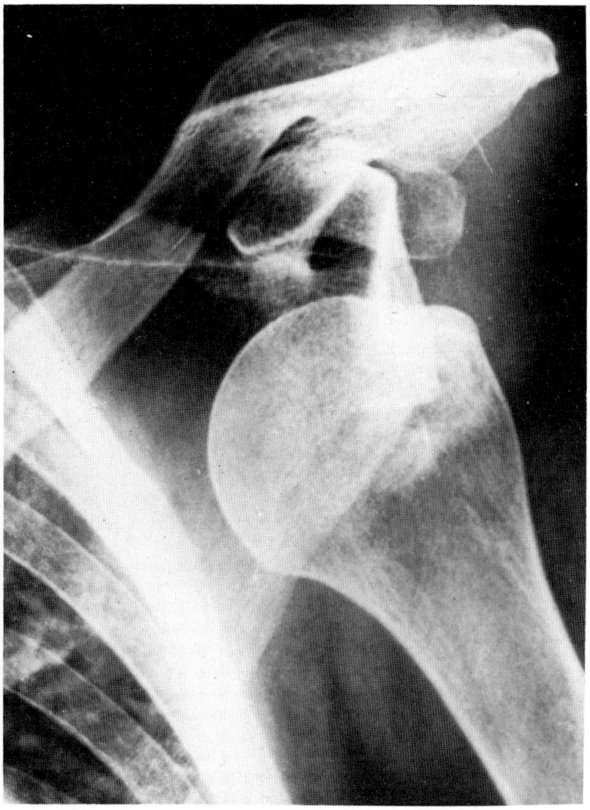

Fig 20.80

Figs 20.79 and 20.80 Sub-coracoid dislocation of the shoulder. Note the loss of contour of the shoulder and the projection of the elbow from the side.

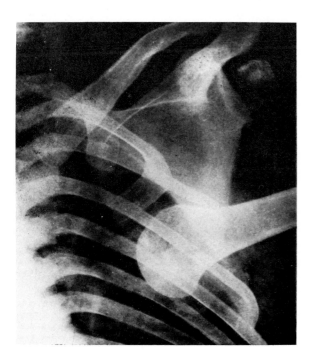

Fig 20.81 Intra-thoracic dislocation of the shoulder.

has been stripped off the front of the glenoid and neck of the scapula, or it may lie outside the capsule which has been torn.[52–53] Although this variation of traumatic anatomy may have some bearing on future recurrent dislocation, the same considerations of treatment apply initially whether the capsule has been stripped from the neck of the glenoid, or torn, or carries a fragment of bone (Figs 20.82 and 20.83).

Downward dislocation: sub-glenoid or luxatio erecta. In rare cases, at the moment of falling the limb is strongly abducted so that the head of the humerus is driven down to a sub-glenoid position. Then, instead of the limb being held rigidly in slight abduction, it is held rigidly in full abduction because the head of the humerus is displaced downwards. The patient comes with his arm fixed almost by the side of his head. This is *luxatio erecta.*

Posterior dislocation. Falls on the outstretched hand with lateral rotation drive the head of the humerus forwards. The opposite injury of forceful medial rotation seldom arises from falls, but occurs from the bizarre positions produced by muscle spasm during epileptic attacks, from a severe electrical shock, or during electroconvulsive therapy when muscle relaxants have not been used. Such stresses may tear the posterior capsule, or avulse the capsular attachment from the posterior margin of the glenoid with stripping of the periosteum from the sub-spinous fossa, so that the head of the humerus is forced back into posterior dislocation by powerful medial rotation of the arm.

Posterior dislocation of the shoulder can also rarely occur as a result of a direct blow over the front of the joint. Zadik[54] recorded the case of a young enthusiast who sparred with a lightweight champion of Great Britain and 'in this unequal contest retreated until his back was against the wall-bars whereupon the champion delivered a heavy blow to the front of his right shoulder, knocking the head of the humerus directly back from the glenoid fossa of the fixed scapula'.

Such posterior dislocations are much less usual than

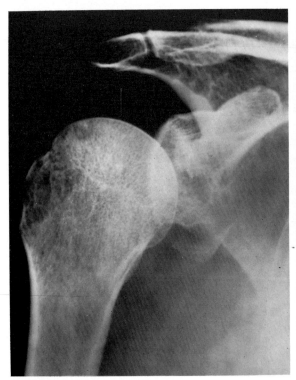

Fig 20.82

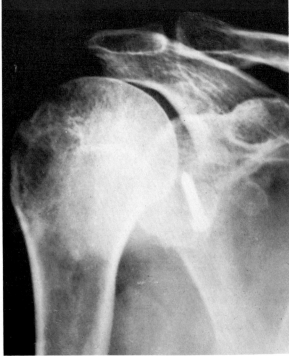

Fig 20.83

Figs 20.82 and 20.83 Anterior dislocation of the shoulder with avulsion of the glenoid labrum carrying a fragment of attached bone. Repair by a single screw.

anterior dislocations; but we shall see later that the apparent infrequency often arises from failure to recognise the displacement because the clinical and radiographic signs are seldom obvious. In fact, posterior dislocation of the shoulder was well known in the middle of the last century, the first being recorded as long ago as 1814.[55] Posterior dislocation caused by an epileptic seizure was recorded by Sir Astley Cooper in 1824.[56]

ANTERIOR DISLOCATION OF THE SHOULDER

Some people display generalised laxity of capsule and ligaments so that all their joints move through an abnormally large range. These are the people who claim to be 'double-jointed'. In the shoulder, the head of the humerus is easily displaced forwards or backwards without injury or tear of capsule. In adolescent children the growth plate of the head of the humerus is more vulnerable to injury than the capsule, so that the joint is seldom dislocated and the more usual injury is displacement of the upper humeral epiphysis.

We are now concerned with traumatic dislocations in young adults, middle-aged and elderly patients.

Traumatic anatomy. Apart from those cases with rare congenital laxity of ligaments or underdevelopment of the glenoid, there is always an injury to the anterior capsule and often an accompanying injury to the head of the humerus. In young adult patients aged from 15 to 30 years the lesion of the anterior capsule is most commonly an avulsion from its glenoid attachment; the capsule may be torn from the glenoid labrum which remains firmly attached to bone, or it may strip off and carry the labrum with it, or it may be avulsed with the labrum and underlying fragment of bone (Figs 20.84 to 20.87). In older patients there is a rupture through the substance of the capsule. All these lesions are capable of sound healing if shearing and twisting strains are prevented from the time of injury and for a period of not less than three weeks. As age increases, the capsular fibres undergo degenerative change with areas of fibrosis or even calcification and with consequent increasing fragility. Thus in patients from middle-age onwards who sustain dislocation of the shoulder, rupture of the capsule is more common than avulsion from bone.

Sometimes the capsule together with subscapularis is avulsed from the lesser tuberosity of the humerus. In this distal capsular avulsion it is either torn trimly from the bone or carries fragments of bone with it.

The capsular and muscle avulsion may involve not only subscapularis but also the adjacent supraspinatus and the rotator cuff of the shoulder as a whole. Moreover, bone fragments torn from the humerus may include the whole of the greater tuberosity. Separation of bone fragments is easily seen in radiographs; but corresponding avulsion of musculotendinous insertion is recognised only by clinical examination. This is one reason why *after reduction of dislocation of the shoulder it is important to test clinically not only for nerve injuries but for avulsion of muscles and in particular the rotator cuff.*

The forward dislocation is the same whether the capsule is avulsed proximally from the glenoid, torn within its length, or avulsed distally from the tuberosities. The only difference is that tears within the substance of the capsule in the elderly heal more rapidly than avulsions from the glenoid in the young. When the shoulder capsule has been avulsed from its proximal attachment it may be separated from the glenoid fibro-cartilage which remains in normal position, or it may avulse the labrum from bone, in each case stripping up an area of periosteum from the front of the neck of the scapula so that the capsule and periosteum remain as a continuous sheet. Occasionally the capsule not only avulses the fibro-cartilage but also an underlying fragment of bone from the anterior margin of the glenoid. Quite often there is an associated injury to the postero-lateral section of the head of the humerus with a compression fracture sustained by impact during displacement against the

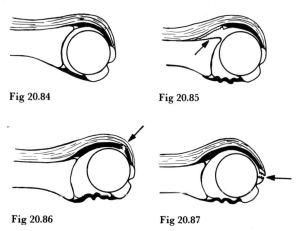

Fig 20.84   Fig 20.85

Fig 20.86   Fig 20.87

Figs 20.84 to 20.87 Traumatic anatomy of anterior dislocation of the shoulder. Fig 20.84: Normal. Fig 20.85: The glenoid labrum and adjoining periosteum are stripped from the front of the neck of the scapula. Fig 20.86: the anterior capsule is ruptured. Fig 20.87: The anterior capsule is torn with a fragment of bone from the lesser tuberosity.

anterior margin of the glenoid. This is more fully discussed below in the section dealing with recurrent dislocation of the shoulder joint.

Clinical signs of forward dislocation. The shoulder loses its rotund outline because the head of the humerus does not occupy its normal position and is displaced not only forwards but also medially. There is a depression over the joint which even if it cannot be seen because of general swelling can certainly be felt as the examiner's fingers explore below the acromion. The arm is held in a slightly abducted position with the elbow away from the side because the upper end of the humerus is locked in its medially displaced position. Movements are almost completely restricted and are painful. The head of the humerus may be felt in front of the glenoid, below the coracoid process, or below the clavicle.

Nerve Injuries. It is wise to examine the limb for possible nerve injuries before reducing the dislocation, and again after reduction. The management of nerve injuries is described in Chapter 12. Lesions of the inner cord of the plexus are recognised by paralysis of the small muscles of the hand with loss of sensation on the medial side of the hand and forearm; lesions of the posterior cord including the radial nerve are recognised by paralysis of the extensors of the forearm with wrist drop. It is more difficult to recognise injuries of the outer trunk of the plexus, or of the circumflex nerve itself, which is the most common nerve injury. The frequency of circumflex nerve injury is accounted for by the short fixed course of the nerve from the back of the plexus, round the medial side of the neck of the humerus to the back—a course which makes it difficult to escape traction when the humerus is displaced forwards. It is, however, possible to recognise deltoid paralysis even before the dislocation has been reduced and without moving the limb, by gently and carefully palpating the muscle whilst the patient tries to contract it against the examiner's resistance. Such isometric contraction is palpable and causes no pain. Muscle paralysis due to nerve injury has to be carefully distinguished from loss of action due to avulsion of the rotator cuff which may accompany dislocation of the shoulder.[57]

Vascular Injuries. The limb must be examined for injuries to the axillary vessels which may be compressed or even ruptured.[58] The hand may be cold and blue with the loss of the radial pulse. Dislocation of the joint should of course be reduced promptly and this may relieve the circulatory embarrassment; but we must be alerted. The possible complications and the treatment are discussed in Chapter 11.

TREATMENT OF ANTERIOR DISLOCATION

It is not only of historic interest to recall that two centuries ago endeavours were made to force the dislocated head of the humerus back into its socket by a variety of mechanical apparatus of an inquisitorial type (Figs 20.88 and 20.89). We should remember this because some surgeons are unnecessarily forceful, although a reduction can be better achieved with gentleness and with such freedom from pain that very often there is no need for a general anaesthetic. Although, of course, anaesthesia produces such good muscle relaxation that it should always be used unless there is some definite contraindication.

Kocher's Manipulation. The patient lies on a couch with the surgeon standing at his side. For a dislocation of the right shoulder the surgeon takes the elbow in his right hand and the wrist in his left. Gentle firm traction is applied to the humerus in the line in which it is lying, by pulling with the right hand. While traction is maintained the humerus is gently and smoothly rotated laterally by moving the forearm out to the extreme of rotation (Figs 20.90 to 20.93). By this manoeuvre the subscapularis muscle is gently but firmly stretched.[59–60] While the limb is held in lateral rotation, the elbow is brought forward to the front of the chest, into the position of adduction. Finally the arm is put into full medial rotation. The manipulation is performed so gently and smoothly that the head of the humerus should glide into position, and often the surgeon does not know the moment at which the dislocation is reduced. There is no need to elicit any click or jerk.

Hippocrates' manipulation. If Kocher's manoeuvre fails to reduce the dislocation, the Hippocratic method of traction against counter-pressure of the surgeon's stockinged foot in the axilla should be employed. This is essentially the same as Kocher's manipulation except that it is reinforced by increased counter-pressure using the leverage of the head of the humerus over the surgeon's foot. The foot is used not to thrust into the axilla but as a fulcrum to lever the head into the glenoid. It is important to examine for nerve lesions prior to this manoeuvre so that the method is not subsequently blamed for producing nerve damage.

Reduction of luxatio erecta. By applying traction to the limb, in the position of deformity in which it lies, and using counter-traction over the chest by an assistant, the luxatio erecta is easily reduced when the arm is brought down gently to the side.

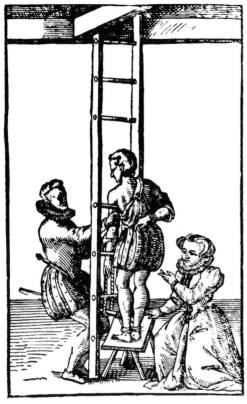

Fig 20.88

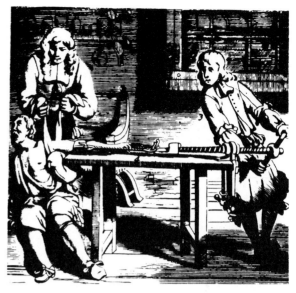

Fig 20.89

Figs 20.88 and 20.89 Ancient techniques of reducing dislocation of the shoulder.

After-treatment of acute dislocation of the shoulder. A small pad of wool dusted with talcum powder is placed in the axilla and a collar-and-cuff sling is applied. Some form of bandaging is used so that the arm cannot be moved more than a few degrees in the direction of lateral rotation or abduction and this must be continued for three weeks without interruption. This is achieved either by bandaging or by strapping, or more simply by incorporating the entire damaged arm under a vest; the patient's own vest or one made from elasticated gauze is convenient and comfortable. The patient can wash around the arm but must dress over it. Of course the fingers, hand and wrist, must be left entirely free and exercised actively from the beginning. Static, isometric deltoid muscle contraction should also be practised at this time.

By protection of the shoulder joint in a position of medial rotation by the side of the body for three weeks the probability of recurrence of the dislocation is diminished. An exception to this rule may be made for the elderly and infirm who are given a simple sling to wear underneath the outer garments, and allowed normal use of the arm in their everyday activities.

Dislocation with Fracture of the Great Tuberosity. In many dislocations of the shoulder there is also a fracture of the great tuberosity from avulsion or possibly shearing impact against the margin of the glenoid. This fracture usually does not add to the difficulties of treatment because the large fragment retains periosteal attachment at its base so that it is incompletely separated from the humerus, and after manipulative reduction of the dislocation the fragment resumes its anatomical position (Figs 20.94 to 20.96). Sometimes, however, the fragment remains in an unsatisfactory position after manipulative reduction of the dislocation and is unstable.

It cannot be emphasised too strongly that the fracture of the great tuberosity seen on a radiograph is evidence of the functional disinsertion of the attached rotator cuff (Figs 20.97 and 20.98). Treatment must therefore be directed to maintaining

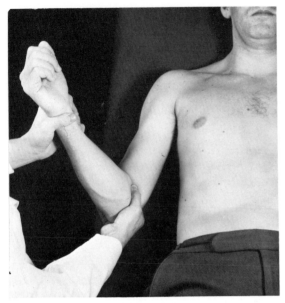

Fig 20.90

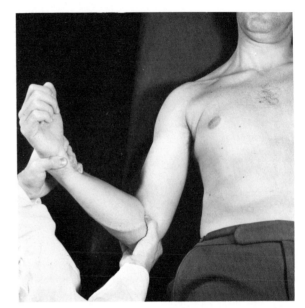

Fig 20.91

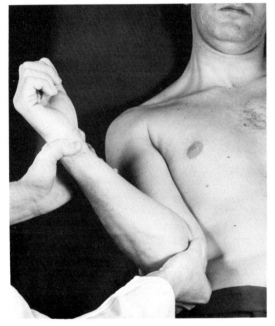

Fig 20.92

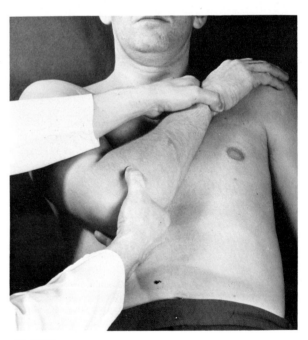

Fig 20.93

Figs 20.90 to 20.93 The four stages in the Kocher method of reducing anterior dislocation of the shoulder. Each stage should be done gently and with deliberation. First traction is applied (Fig 20.90); the limb is then gently and slowly rotated outwards (Fig 20.91), the elbow is brought forward in front of the trunk (Fig 20.92), and finally the shoulder is internally rotated (Fig 20.93).

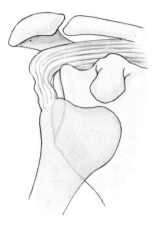

Fig 20.94 Simple anterior dislocation of the shoulder.

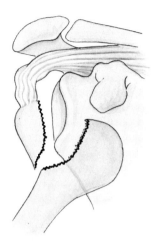

Fig 20.95 Dislocation with fracture of the greater tuberosity.

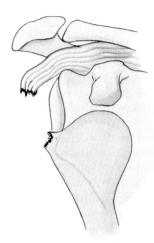

Fig 20.96 Dislocation with avulsed supraspinatus.

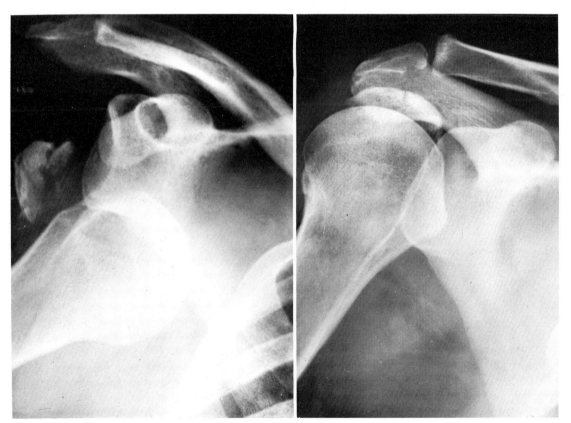

Fig 20.97   **Fig 20.98**

Figs 20.97 to 20.98 Anterior dislocation of the shoulder with fracture of the great tuberosity (Fig 20.97). After reduction of the dislocation, the fragment usually returns by residual soft tissue attachment to its normal position. In this case, however, it has not done so and lies above the head of the humerus, pulled medially by the rotator muscles (Fig 20.98). The displaced fragment must be reduced and fixed by open operation.

integrity of the tendon insertion. The same treatment in principle is indicated whether there has been a visible fracture of the tuberosity or whether the rotator cuff tendons have ruptured proximal to their insertion without avulsion fracture. If the great tuberosity has been avulsed and has been accurately repositioned by closed manipulation there is a very good chance that it will heal without surgical intervention. If there has been rupture of the rotator cuff without fracture, the diagnosis is less evident but can be confirmed by arthrography.[11–12, 61–62]. In case of doubt operative reposition and fixation of the displaced tuberosity, or repair of the ruptured rotator cuff is indicated. The earlier that this is done within reason the easier will be the procedure and the better the final result. The transacromial approach is ideal for the surgical management of this injury (p. 520).

Late unreduced anterior dislocation of the shoulder. With progress in the development of organised accident services it is now unusual to see a patient several weeks or even months after dislocation of the shoulder which is still unreduced. If the problem does arise it is formidable. Not only is the head of the humerus displaced with the formation of adhesions, capsular contraction and shortening of subscapularis, but these adhesions involve the axillary artery and vein and the nerves of the axillary plexus.[63–65] Attempted manipulative reduction carries a grave risk of fracture of the porotic humerus; or worse still a rupture of axillary vein or artery or one of its branches; or a traction injury of one of the cords of the plexus. It is better not to attempt manipulative reduction of uncorrected dislocation after the first three weeks.

In elderly patients with dislocations still unreduced after three or more weeks, provided that there is no disability from compression of axillary vessels or nerves, it is usually best to leave well alone. Despite the displaced position and gross restriction of movements, reasonably good function may be regained.

Operative reduction. In younger patients operative reduction should be undertaken; but again we must beware. The results may be disastrous. If operation is undertaken, the incision should be so planned that control of the vessels proximal to the clavicle may be secured if it proves necessary. The operation is designed as an exposure of the axillary vessels and nerves rather than an exposure of the head of the humerus. Once the vessels and nerves have been defined and retracted, the head of the humerus is exposed by dividing the tightened subscapularis and anterior capsule. The head of the humerus is then guided outwards and backwards to the glenoid fossa. After protection in a sling with the arm bound to the body for three weeks, movement is regained by the patient's own activity.

POSTERIOR DISLOCATION OF THE SHOULDER

The head of the humerus may be displaced backwards by powerful internal rotation of the arm when strong general muscle spasm occurs, as for example, in epilepsy (Figs 20.99 and 20.100). Less commonly it is forced backwards by a direct blow over the front of the joint[66] (Fig 20.101). We have mentioned an example of posterior dislocation from direct injury while boxing (p. 548).

In posterior dislocation the head of the humerus lies behind the scapula in a subspinous position. It is almost the exact counterpart of anterior dislocation. The capsule is torn or avulsed from the posterior margin of the glenoid, usually with the posterior part of the labrum or with the labrum and a fragment of attached bone. As in anterior dislocation, there may be an associated compression fracture of the head of the humerus sustained as it is impacted against the posterior margin of the glenoid. The defect is in the antero-medial sector of the head and not, as in forward dislocation, the postero-lateral sector.

Posterior dislocation is often overlooked because the clinical signs are not usually obvious. There may not be significant flattening of the contour of the shoulder as there is when the humeral head is displaced forwards, and swelling may obscure hollowing over the front of the joint and the prominence of the coracoid process. The characteristic physical sign is loss of lateral rotation of the shoulder which is locked in medial rotation.[67]

Unless radiographs are of good quality the displacement is often concealed. In antero-posterior projections there may not appear to be loss of congruity between the head of the humerus and the glenoid; though in fact if films of good quality are examined with care the displacement can be seen even in this unsatisfactory projection. It is of course confirmed quite certainly by axial projection taken from the axilla with a cassette over the top of the shoulder.

Treatment of posterior dislocation. The dislocation is reduced by traction to the limb and rotating it outwards. After reduction the stability is tested by medial and lateral rotation. If the joint is stable on reduction, a simple sling worn for two or three weeks will suffice as aftercare. If, however, after reduction

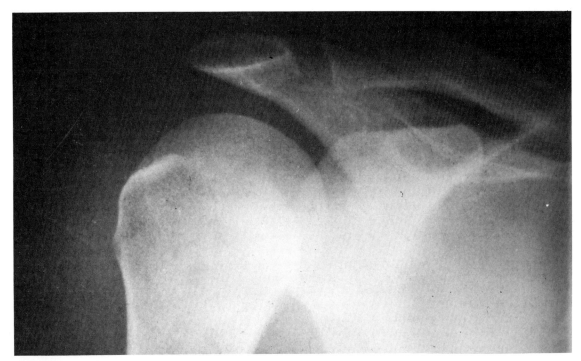

Fig 20.99

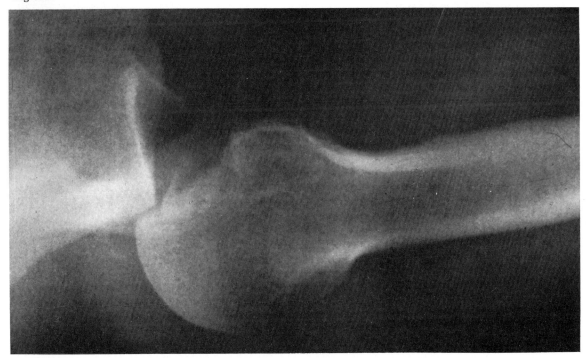

Fig 20.100

Figs 20.99 and 20.100 Posterior dislocation of the shoulder sustained during convulsive therapy three months earlier. Careful scrutiny of the antero-posterior radiograph shows an overlap of shadows of humerus and glenoid. This is easily missed. The lateral axillary view makes the diagnosis obvious.

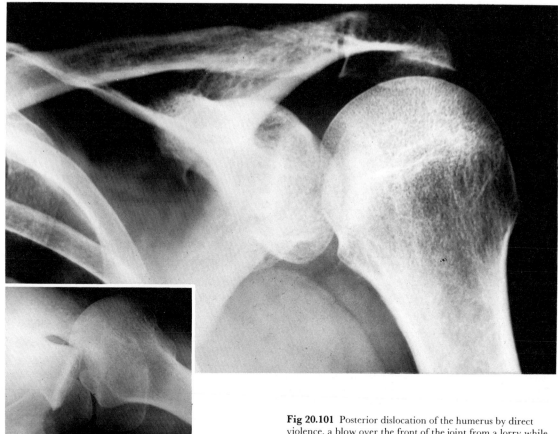

Fig 20.101 Posterior dislocation of the humerus by direct violence, a blow over the front of the joint from a lorry while cycling. The displacement is disguised in the antero-posterior radiographs but clear in the axial view (inset). (Reproduced by kind permission of C K Warrick and the Editors of the *Journal of Bone and Joint Surgery* (1948), 30-B, 651).

there is clearly instability of the joint, it is necessary to apply a plaster spica with the limb in a position of about 40 degrees of abduction, with the elbow behind rather than in front of the plane of the trunk, but essentially in 30 degrees of lateral rotation. After three weeks movements are commenced.

Late unreduced posterior dislocation. Being so commonly overlooked, late operative reduction of unreduced posterior dislocation is required in an unduly high proportion of cases. Fortunately this presents less difficulty and danger than operative reduction of late unreduced anterior dislocation. The operation should be done from *the front*. Through a standard delto-pectoral approach the shoulder joint is entered and the impacted humerus is levered forwards into place with the aid of a Bankart skid. In this type of case, the largest cleavage fractures of the humeral head are to be found and this may cause particular technical difficulties not only in carrying out the reduction, but in maintaining it. Once reduction has been accomplished the technique described by McLaughlin,[68] whereby the insertion of subscapularis is transferred into the depths of the cleavage defect, considerably enhances the stability. Post-operative immobilisation of the limb depends on the stability as determined at operation; if there is any doubt the limb should be immobilised in a plaster spica in a position of 30 degrees of lateral rotation for six weeks.

RECURRENT ANTERIOR DISLOCATION OF THE SHOULDER

Although it has been emphasised that dislocation and recurrent dislocation of the shoulder do not differ in basic pathological anatomy from dislocation and recurrent dislocation of any other joint,[69] the fact that the shoulder joint depends to such a large extent on surrounding capsular strength and that it has such a great range of circumduction, makes it more liable than any other joint to suffer recurrent dislocation. In all dislocated joints the capsular injury may be tearing of ligament fibres in the middle of their course, or avulsion of ligaments from proximal of distal bone attachments.[70] In the shoulder, the commonest injury in young adults is avulsion of capsule with or without the labrum from the anterior glenoid margin.[71–73] In more elderly patients the capsule is more often ruptured about 2.5 cm proximal to the humeral attachment. Occasionally the capsule with tendon of subscapularis is avulsed from the lesser tuberosity of the humerus. Each of these injuries sustained at the time of initial dislocation may cause recurrent dislocation if healing and repair is unsound. Since capsular repair is more difficult when it has been avulsed from bone, recurrence of shoulder dislocation occurs most commonly in healthy and vigorous young men with good muscle development. Incidentally it is exactly this type of patient who is least tolerant of immobilisation of the limb for three weeks after first dislocation, which has been shown to diminish considerably the probability of recurrence.

In anterior dislocation the head of the humerus which is driven forcefully over the anterior margin of the glenoid often sustains compression injury in its postero-lateral sector. There may be a deeply depressed segment of bone involving as much as one-quarter of the head of the humerus. Recognition of the humeral head defect, its size and position, may influence the planning of operation.

Thus three factors are concerned in the traumatic anatomy of recurrent anterior dislocation of the shoulder[74] (Figs. 20.102 and 20.103) ; (i) a detachment of the anterior capsule of the joint with or without the labrum ; (ii) a defect of bone in the back of the head of the humerus from compression fracture of the postero-lateral sector ; and (iii) a range of lateral mobility which in some individuals may be such as to allow the compression fracture to engage on to the bared anterior glenoid rim and lever the head of the humerus out of the joint.

Clinical diagnosis. The diagnosis should easily be made from the history. After the first dislocation there may be recurrence from any sudden lateral rotation of the abducted arm and subsequent dislocations occur with increasing freqency and ease, as for

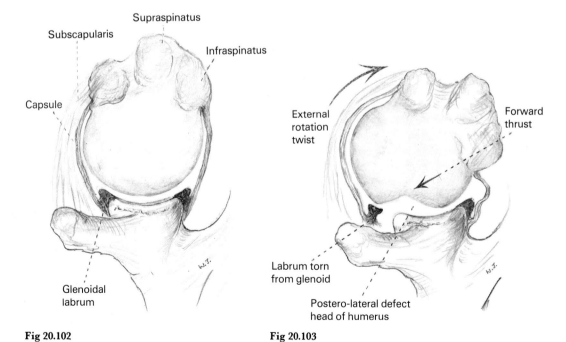

Fig 20.102   **Fig 20.103**

Figs 20.102 and 20.103 Diagram showing the position of the glenoid labrum in the normal shoulder (Fig 20.102), and the displaced position in recurrent dislocation, where there is usually also a compression of a sector of bone in the postero-lateral aspect of the humeral head (Fig 20.103). In these circumstances the head of the humerus slides forwards and levers outwards whenever the limb is externally rotated.

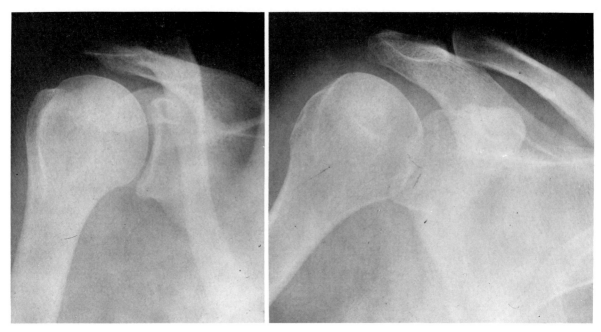

Fig 20.104   Fig 20.105

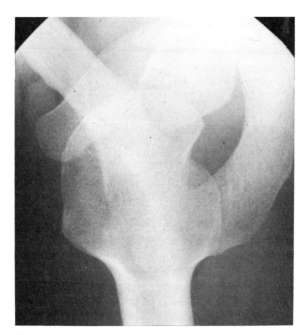

Fig 20.106

Figs 20.104 to 106 The compression defect in the postero-lateral aspect of the humeral head in recurrent dislocation of the shoulder arises from impaction against the anterior margin of the glenoid. It can only be visualised in profile. Standard projection shows no abnormality (Fig 20.104); radiograph in medial rotation shows an abnormal contour (Fig 20.105); lateral axillary view clearly reveals the defect (Fig 20.106).

example: reaching with the hand to the back of the neck; putting the arm through the sleeve of a coat; swimming with an overarm stroke, or even turning over in bed. A history of 20 or 30 dislocations is not unusual. There may be frequent subluxation without actual dislocation.

Occasionally there is some doubt as to whether or not the dislocation is anterior or posterior. Such doubt arises when—as so often happens—the dislocation is self-reducing or has been reduced by a lay bystander and no radiograph is available in the dislocated position. If there is doubt as to the diagnosis it can be confirmed at clinical examination by rotating the limb outwards with the elbow to the side. It is not necessary to dislocate the joint; the patient's anxiety when it is about to displace is obvious. This 'apprehension sign' is diagnostic.

Radiological diagnosis. A good deal of additional information can often be obtained by appropriate radiographs, particularly when there is some doubt as to the precise diagnosis. Standard anteroposterior and axillary lateral views are obligatory. In most cases of recurrent anterior dislocation there will be no lesion seen in the anteroposterior view, but a compression defect on the postero-lateral aspect of the head of the humerus is usually seen in the axillary lateral projection. If the lesion is not shown in these two projections, an anteroposterior view taken with the arm in 60 degrees of internal rotation is likely to reveal the defect in profile[75] (Figs 20.104 to 20.106), and as a final resort the Stryker view[76] will reveal a minor defect which may not be evident in all the other views.

OPERATIVE TREATMENT OF RECURRENT ANTERIOR DISLOCATION

The recurrence of dislocation of the shoulder which in some patients can be numbered in scores is matched only by the number and variety of operations which have been devised for its cure. More than 100 different operations are recorded in literature!

Historical survey. Although pathologists had already described how often there was a defect of bone in the back of the head of the humerus, the nature of the lesion was not understood. Some believed it to be the cause and not the consequence of the first displacement, a congenital abnormality. Even as late as 1929 Tavernier[77] wrote that 'this singular lesion is the most enigmatic of all lesions in recurrent dislocation'. He recorded abnormalities of

shape of the humeral head 'la tête en hachette' and 'la tête en maillet' revived again recently as the 'hatchet head' (Figs 20.107 and 20.108). These are all simple variations of the same lesion, depending on its precise size and shape, and seen on radiographs taken with different centering of the ray in different positions of rotation of the joint. Although it varies in size and shape, the compression fracture is always in

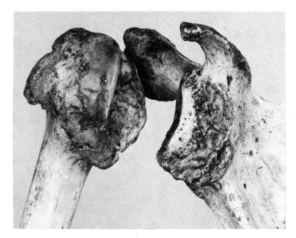

Fig 20.107 Museum specimen to show the basic lesions in recurrent dislocation of the shoulder. (Reproduced by kind permission of Dr A G Stansfeld of St Bartholomew's Hospital).

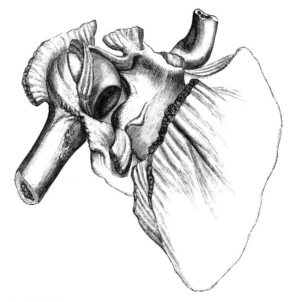

Fig 20.108 Traumatic anatomy of recurrent dislocation of the shoulder. (Reproduced by kind permission from a paper by S F Eve 1880) *Proceedings of the Royal Society of Medicine* 5: 51).

the postero-lateral segment of the head. In recent years the compression fracture of the head of the humerus has become known, particularly in the American literature, as the Hill-Sachs lesion.[75] However, if the lesion requires an eponym it should surely be called the Broca lesion, since he had described it in detail 50 years earlier[87] (Fig 20.109). Eve[88] had described the lesion in a single case ten years before Broca.

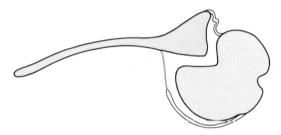

Fig 20.109 Diagrammatic representation of the 'hatchet' deformity (after Broca and Hartman 1890 In *Bulletins de la Société Anatomique de Paris*, 5me serie 4 : 312).

Excision of the head of the humerus. In the last century almost the only operation practised was excision of the head of the humerus. This avoided the embarrassment of recurrent locking but left the limb so weak that it was abandoned.

Capsular division, resection and capsulorrhaphy. In the first 20 years of this century the emphasis on operative procedures was on division, tightening, and strengthening the anterior capsule. It was done by subcutaneous tenotomy or by exposing the capsule at operation and cutting it vertically throughout its length. Overlapping flaps of divided capsule was advocated and attempts were made to reinforce it with strips of fascia from various sources. The tendon of biceps and other available tendons or fascia in the region was threaded in and out. These operations were done in the most readily available part of the capsule, and no surgeon was so adventurous as to reach into the deep recess of the anterior capsular attachment of the glenoid. Recurrence of dislocation frequently followed. Occasional successes were due to restricting abduction and lateral rotation of the arm. Ironically the most successful operations were due to the high incidence of post-operative infection with consequent scar tissue which restricted movements. Basically these operations were essentially following the technique of Hippocrates who centuries earlier had seared the front of the joint with a hot cautery and said 'then above all should the arm be continually

bound to the side both night and day, for so would the cavity into which the humerus is mostly displaced be best cicatrised up and cut off'.

Correction of muscle imbalance. Because of the failure of operative repair a theory was born that recurrent dislocation arose from imbalance of power of the shoulder muscles. Subscapularis was divided—then the insertion of pectoralis major or of latissimus dorsi or of all three. These operations were all performed through an anterior exposure and in so far as scarring restricted lateral rotation movement, they sometimes succeeded.

Muscle transplantations. Impressed with the theory of muscle imbalance and the belief that dislocation was produced by abduction, Ehrlich in Europe and Clairmont[78] in America decided to transplant the posterior part of the deltoid from back to front under the neck of the humerus, so that at the moment when the remaining part of the deltoid abducted the arm, the transplanted part also contracted to prevent displacement. This ingenious procedure appealed to surgical dexterity so that it was warmly approved by many leading surgeons. Finsterer[79] used coracobrachialis cut from its origin and passed through the axilla from front to back under the neck of the humerus.

But since recurrent dislocation does not arise from unbalanced active abduction, these operations failed.

Tendon Suspension. Free fascial grafts or transplanted tendons were then used to sling the head of the humerus to the scapula. Kirschner[80] used fascia 'as a sort of cravat', encircling the neck of the humerus and fixed to the acromion. Carrel[81] used the long tendon of biceps as an acromial sling, and as recently as 1947 Gallie[82] in his Moynihan lecture to the Royal College of Surgeons of England advised free fascial grafts, passed through the scapula and neck of the humerus. The most popular of these procedures was devised by Heymanowitsch[83] of Germany and popularised by Nicola[84-85] in the United States. They used the biceps tendon to form an intra-articular ligament, like the ligamentum teres of the hip. It was a neat operation and experienced a short-lived vogue.

Anterior bone blocks. Attention being turned from the inadequacy of excision of the humeral head, tendon division, capsular reinforcement or muscle transplantation, endeavours were made to create bone blocks in front of the joint. The same principle is used to this day by Moseley[86] of Montreal, who has spent most of his surgical life on this problem, and advises that the glenoid cavity be deepened in front by implanting a prosthesis. The first attempt at an anterior bone block, and the most successful, which gained approval in France for many years was that of Oudard,[45] who used the lengthened coracoid process to block exit from the antero-medial aspect of the joint. Subsequently Helfet[46] described the bone-block procedure taught to him by Bristow at which the coracoid process with its attached muscle origins is transferred through subscapularis to the bared neck of the scapula. Such anterior bone block procedures still have a limited place in the treatment of recurrent anterior dislocation when one is faced with recurrence after a failed previous operation.

The essential lesions. With this long story of astonishing surgical endeavour we must get back to the fact that any reconstructive operation should be designed to deal with the traumatic anatomy of the two basic lesions of recurrent anterior dislocation of the shoulder: the anterior capsular-labrum injury, and the compression defect on the postero-lateral aspect of the head of the humerus. The anterior capsular-labrum injury allows the head of the humerus to move forwards, and the postero-lateral compression defect encourages its leverage out of the joint when the arm is placed in outward rotation.

Recurrence of forward dislocation of the shoulder arises from failure of healing of disrupted or avulsed capsule, usually from its anterior glenoid attachment with or without the fibro-cartilaginous labrum, most often in vigorous young men with good muscle development. It was recognised in England by Bankart[71–73] and in Germany by Perthes.[89] Both these surgeons made an anterior surgical approach exposing the margin of the glenoid fossa and drilled holes through its bone for sutures to secure the capsule. Even at the extreme of outward rotation of the arm the posterior defect in the head of the humerus could no longer engage onto the front of the glenoid and lever the humeral head out of joint.

Bankart's operation

Although Perthes devised his operation independently, it was not published until three years after Bankart's first contribution in 1923, and it is to Bankart of London that every credit is due for the true solution of the problem of operative correction of recurrent anterior dislocation of the shoulder. He insisted on the essential lesion and said 'It is a constant, straightforward, uncomplicated anatomical condition which can be observed at any time by any competent surgeon who cares to expose the anterior margin of the glenoid cavity.' The variation of anterior detachment was recognised by Bankart: in his first publication of 1923 the emphasis was on

capsular avulsion; in 1938 he laid stress on the glenoid fibro-cartilage detachment; in 1948 he said 'the fibro-cartilage or glenoid labrum may be torn from the bone, or the capsule may be torn from it;'

Technique of Bankart's Operation (Figs 20.110 to 20.115). The patient is towelled so that the limb is free to be manipulated in any direction. Two assistants are helpful, one being entirely concerned with holding and manipulating the arm. Classically the incision, 12 cm long, is made from below the clavicle over the coracoid process in the line of the delto-pectoral groove as far as the axillary fold. However, if the skin incision is curved and placed medial to the line of the delto-pectoral groove, it gives a more aesthetic scar and prevents keloid development. In young women the incision can be placed just below the anterior axillary fold with considerable cosmetic advantage; this incision increases the technical difficulties, but with adequate retraction of the skin and subcutaneous fat, access is obtained to the delto-pectoral groove, after which the operation proceeds in the usual fashion. The cephalic vein indicates the line of separation of deltoid laterally and pectoralis major medially. A variety of measures have been suggested to avoid the cephalic vein, but there is no doubt that it is better to ligate and excise it formally throughout the length of the exposure.

Pectoralis major is retracted medially and deltoid laterally. In muscular subjects it may be necessary as an aid to exposure to divide 2 to 3 cm of the anterior fibres of origin of the deltoid just below the clavicle, leaving a fringe for subsequent closure. In this area one or more small branches of the acromio-thoracic artery and accompanying veins may be encountered. By retracting the delto-pectoral interval the coracoid process is exposed with its musculo-tendinous attachment of short head of biceps, coraco-brachialis and pectoralis minor in one sheet. The bone is divided with an osteotome about 1 cm from its tip, and the distal fragment with attached tendons is retracted downwards by a stay suture.

At this stage the limb is rotated outwards and the well delineated transverse fibres of subscapularis come into full view. Its lower margin is identified by three humero-circumflex veins crossing the field transversely. They should be formally divided. Two or three overlapping mattress sutures are inserted into subscapularis approximately 4 cm from its insertion in order to prevent its medial retraction. The entire subscapularis is then divided by vertical section at a level 3 cm short of its insertion. The capsule may or may not be attached to subscapularis

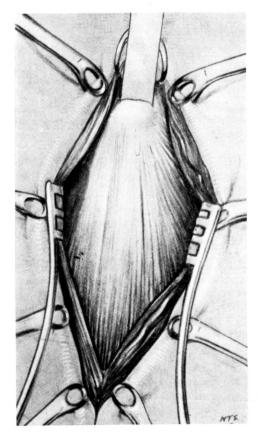

Fig 20.110

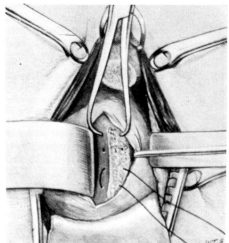

Fig 20.111

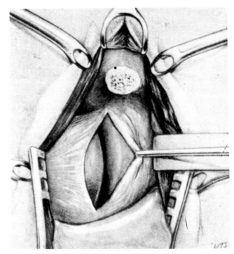

Fig 20.112

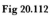

Fig 20.113

Figs 20.110 to 20.115 Bankart's operation (from the original publication by Bankart A S B (1938) *An operation for recurrent dislocation.* British Journal of Surgery 26: 320).

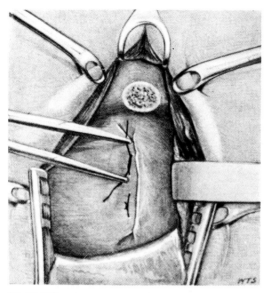

Fig 20.114

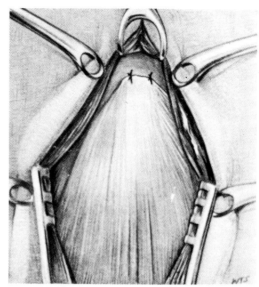

Fig 20.115

at this point and need independent division in the same line.

Then comes the most important duty of the first assistant. With one hand gripping the elbow to control rotation, the other hand on the inner aspect of the upper arm, he pulls the head of the humerus laterally to show clearly the depth of the wound and the anterior margin of the glenoid. A broad skid-retractor is inserted over the front of the humeral head with prongs behind the glenoid fossa. This aid is indispensable and is the secret of success.

The lesion is now exposed. Essentially there are three varieties: (i) the anterior capsule is stripped with a large gap leading to the sub-scapular fossa, the labrum itself is intact and still firmly attached to bone. (ii) The labrum may be lifted from bone and quite loose, sometimes displaced like the bucket-handle tear of a meniscus in the knee joint, and sometimes torn so that it is in several fragments. (iii) There may appear to be no labrum at all, either because it has retained firm contact with the capsule and has been displaced forwards with it, or because it has been worn away by repeated dislocation. The anterior margin of the glenoid is rounded on to the front of the neck of the scapula, exposing a smooth surface of eburnated bone.

Operative repair consists of (i) any tags of torn labrum are excised and the underlying bone is rawed and freshened. (ii) Two or preferably three sutures are passed from holes drilled through the bone of the anterior margin of the glenoid to the cut edge of the lateral flap of capsule, the sutures being tightened while the limb is held in full medial rotation. Pins or staples, which often in time become loose, may wander dangerously. The medial flap of capsule is then stitched over with double-breasting. This double-breasting of capsule was always an essential part of Bankart's operation.

The muscle belly of subscapularis which meanwhile has been held by its three mattress sutures, is then stitched to its distal tendon, the limb being held in the position of neutral rotation—not in full medial rotation as was essential during the capsular repair. The coracoid fragment with its muscles is sutured back into position using a drill hole passed through the stump of the coracoid. The wound is then closed in layers. Vacuum drainage is desirable. In closing the wound each layer should be carefully sutured including the subcutaneous fascia and fat, because operation scars in this area have a marked tendency to keloid change. After operation, as Bankart said: 'Keep the arm bandaged to the side for one month. Then begin active movement. Full movement should be regained in about a month. The dislocation does not recur.'

Putti-Platt operation (Figs 20.116 to 20.125). Some years after Bankart published his operation in 1923, Valtancoli[90] and then in 1938 Boicev,[91] recorded a similar operation done by Putti of Bologna.

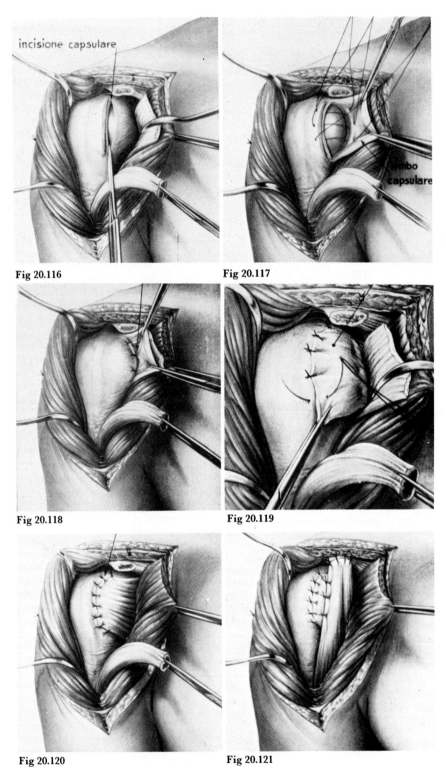

Fig 20.116

Fig 20.117

Fig 20.118

Fig 20.119

Fig 20.120

Fig 20.121

Figs 20.116 to 121 The Putti operation described by his pupil Boicev in 1938. (Taken from the original publication by Boicev B (1938) in *Chirurgia degli Organi di Movimento*, 23 : 354. Compare these figures to Figs 20.122 to 20.125).

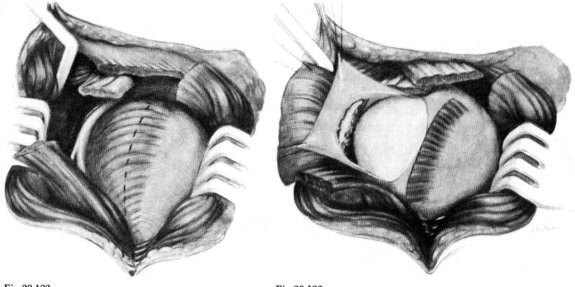

Fig 20.122

Fig 20.123

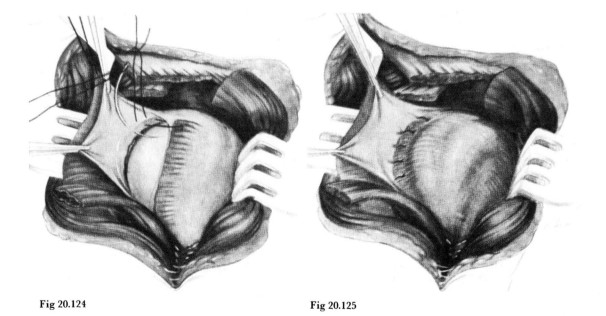

Fig 20.124

Fig 20.125

Figs 20.122 to 20.125 The Putti-Platt operation. Fig 20.122: Coraco-brachialis has been divided close to the coracoid process and retracted downwards, but it is easier to osteotomise the coracoid as in Fig 20.116. Note the line of division of subscapularis and the underlying capsule which is about $\frac{3}{4}''$ (2 cm) medial to the insertion of the tendon. Fig 10.123: The medial part of the subscapularis and the capsule being retracted inwards, the detachment of the glenoid labrum (Bankart's lesion) is exposed. Fig 20.124: The tissues in front of the neck of the scapula, including labrum, periosteum and deep capsule, are sutured to the lateral stump of subscapularis. Fig 20.125: The four or five sutures are tied while the limb is in internal rotation. The medial part of the capsule and subscapularis are then overlapped and sutured to the region of the tuberosity. After repair of coraco-brachialis and closure of the wound, the limb is held in internal rotation for four weeks.

The operative exposure was the same but no attempt was made formally to repair the lesion at the anterior margin of the glenoid. The lateral flap and joint capsule were sutured to such soft tissues as remained in front of the neck of the scapula, and greater emphasis was laid on repair by double-breasting not only the capsule but also of subscapularis. The sutures were all placed in position before being tied with the arm held in medial rotation. Capsule, and double-breasted subscapularis were sutured in consecutive layers, the limb thereafter being bandaged to the side in medial rotation for three weeks.

In Great Britain the operation has been popularised by Osmond-Clarke and labelled the Putti-Platt operation, not because either Putti or Platt ever recorded it (though Putti's pupils did), but because he had seen his chief, Harry Platt, do it; and also for the sake of euphony rather than to indicate precedence.[92]

It is claimed that the Putti-Platt operation is undesirable in so far as it imposes a severe degree of restriction of lateral rotation movement of the shoulder. The patient should, however, regain a range of movement so normal that he is unaware of the slight restriction. It is true that lateral rotation, as tested with the elbow to the side with the forearm pointing forwards and then turned outwards, will be less on the operated than on the unoperated side, usually about 40 degrees, but that is exactly its purpose. Lateral rotation movement beyond that range is not needed and may cause recurrence because if there is a serious bone defect in the back of the head of the humerus it is excess lateral rotation that will re-dislocate the joint. In many patients it is possible and desirable to combine the two operations so that the basic principles of the Bankart repair are carried out, followed by the Putti-Platt reconstruction when the wound is being closed.

Treatment of the failed operation. In almost every reported series of operations for recurrent anterior dislocation of the shoulder there are a number of failures. The highest number of failures undoubtedly follow any of the operations relying on fascial or tendon slings. The lowest recurrence after operation follows the Bankart procedure, the Putti-Platt operation, or a combination of the two. Excellent results are also reported from the Magnuson-Stack operation,[93] in which the lesser tuberosity carrying the insertion of subscapularis is transferred laterally and downwards across the bicipital groove. It is a less extensive procedure and possibly suitable for the older patient. If any operation for recurrent disloca-

tion has failed, a careful study must be carried out and this should include arthrography of the shoulder. Often a large anterior subscapularis pouch is found into which the head still dislocates. It is in this type of case that one of the anterior bone block procedures such as recommended by Eden,[94] Hybbinette,[95] or the Bristow procedure described by Helfet,[46] may usefully be considered.

RECURRENT POSTERIOR DISLOCATION OF THE SHOULDER

Nearly all injuries to the shoulder joint tend to thrust the head of the humerus forwards, but occasionally the force is in the opposite direction and a backward drive with internal rotation displaces the head of the humerus behind the glenoid. The traumatic anatomy of this injury is the exact converse of forward dislocation. The capsule is detached with or without the labrum from the back of the joint; there may be a fracture of the posterior margin of the glenoid; and there is often a severe cleavage fracture of the front of the head of the humerus in the antero-medial sector (Fig 20.126).

There are four clinical types of posterior dislocation of the shoulder (i) acute traumatic (ii) late unreduced (iii) recurrent (iv) habitual recurrent.[96–97] The first two types have been described on pages 554 to 555.

Operation for recurrent posterior dislocation of the shoulder.[98] An incision is placed running along the spine of the scapula and outwards following the outer border of the acromion. The origin of trapezius is raised to expose the belly of infraspinatus. This muscle is retracted downwards using a lever under the neck of the glenoid. An osteotomy is carried out through the neck of the scapula levering the glenoid forwards and into this defect a wedge of bone which has been removed from the back of the acromion is inserted, thereby increasing the ante-version of the glenoid. The soft tissues are repaired by overlapping infraspinatus in a manner reminiscent of the anterior Putti-Platt procedure. In muscular subjects, glenoplasty and infraspinatus overlap may be deemed inadequate and a full thickness bone-block from the iliac crest should be used to act as a barrier to further posterior dislocation.[99] The limb is immo-bilised in a plaster cast in at least 40 degrees of outward rotation for four weeks.

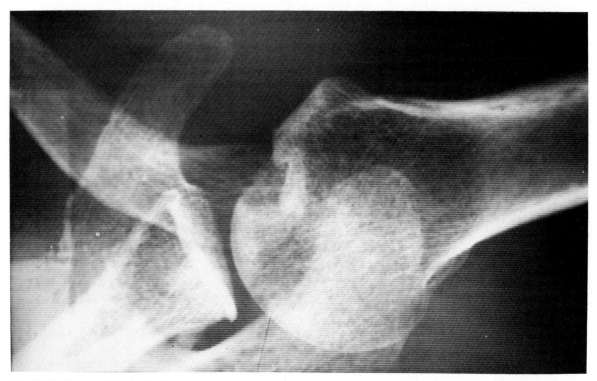

Fig 20.126 Fracture of the head of the humerus accompanying posterior dislocation occurs in the anterior rather than in the posterior segment of the head (compare with Figs 20.104 to 20.106).

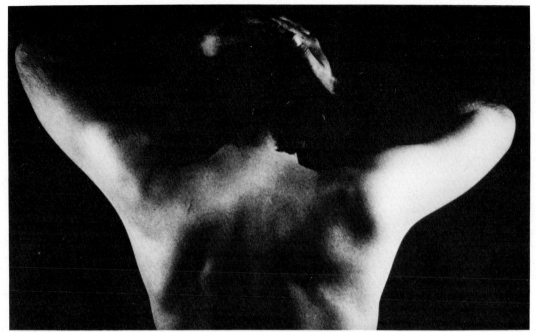

Fig 20.127

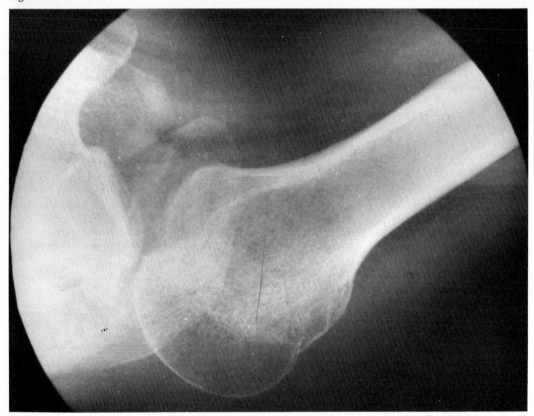

Fig 20.128

Figs 20.127 and 20.128 The patient could dislocate his right shoulder backwards by abnormal muscle contraction. He could do so at will in the position of abduction and internal rotation, and replace it by outward rotation with a painful thud. The differentiation between an involuntary and a habitual recurrent posterior dislocation is difficult. It can only be made on general clinical evaluation.

Habitual posterior dislocation (Figs 20.127 and 20.128). The importance of making a precise diagnosis of habitual posterior dislocation of the shoulder,[100-101], lies in the fact that surgeons must be warned that the disorder is often an expression of general psychiatric disturbance and the results of operation can consequently be extremely disappoint-ing. Whereas the operative treatment for recurrent posterior dislocation of the shoulder uncomplicated by psychiatric disturbance is very rewarding, the same operation carried out on a patient with habitual recurrent posterior dislocation will almost inevitably lead to failure.

REFERENCES

1. Kessel L 1967 The shoulder. In: Rob C, Smith R (ed) Clinical surgery. Butterworth, London, vol. 13, p 389
2. Diamond B 1964 The obstructing acromion. Thomas, Springfield, Illinois
3. Rathbun J, Macnab I 1970 The microvascular pattern of the rotator cuff. Journal of Bone and Joint Surgery 52-B: 540
4. Codman E A 1931 Rupture of the supraspinatus tendon. Surgery, Gynecology and Obstetrics 52: 579
5. Codman E A 1934 The shoulder. Todd Boston
6. Harrison S H 1949 The painful shoulder. Journal of Bone and Joint Surgery 31-B: 418
7. Keyes E L 1935 Anatomical observations on senile changes in the shoulder. Journal of Bone and Joint Surgery 17: 953
8. Meyer A W 1937 Chronic functional lesions of the shoulder. Archives of Surgery 35: 646
9. Lundberg B J 1969 The frozen shoulder. Acta Orthopaedica Scandinavica, Suppl 119
10. Brown J T 1949 Early assessment of supraspinatus tears. Journal of Bone and Joint Surgery 31-B: 423
11. Ellis V H 1953 The diagnosis of shoulder lesions due to injuries of the rotator cuff. Journal of Bone and Joint Surgery 35-B: 72
12. Kessel L 1950 Arthrography of the shoulder joint. Proceedings of the Royal Society of Medicine, 43: 418
13. Hamilton A R 1951 Calcinosis. Journal of Bone and Joint Surgery 33-B: 573
14. Codman E A, Akerson I B 1931 Pathology associated with rupture of supraspinatus tendon. Annals of Surgery 93: 348
15. Watson-Jones R 1955 Fractures and Joint Injuries, 4th edn. Livingstone, Edinburgh, footnote p 449
16. Armstrong J R 1949 Excision of the acromion in treatment of the supraspinatus syndrome. Journal of Bone and Joint Surgery 31-B: 436
17. Moseley H F 1951 Ruptures of the rotator cuff. British Journal of Surgery 38: 359
18. Watson M 1978 The Refractory Painful Arc Syndrome. Journal of Bone and Joint Surgery 60-B: 544
19. Kessel L, Watson M 1977 The Painful Arc Syndrome, Clinical Classification and Guide to Management. Journal of Bone and Joint Surgery 59-B: 166
20. Kessel L, Watson M 1977 The transacromial approach to the shoulder for rupture of the rotator cuff. International Orthopaedics 2: 153
21. Debeyre J, Patte D, Elmelite E 1965 Repair of ruptures of the rotator cuff of the shoulder. Journal of Bone and Joint Surgery 47-B: 36
22. Platt H 1931 Observations on some tendon ruptures. British Medical Journal i: 611
23. Sonnenschein H D 1932 Rupture of the biceps tendon. Journal of Bone and Joint Surgery 14: 416
24. Rogers S P 1939 Avulsion of tendon of attachment of biceps brachii. Journal of Bone and Joint Surgery 21: 197
25. Holmes T 1898 Sir Benjamin Collins Brodie. Fisher Unwin, London
26. Berheiser E J 1937 Old ununited clavicular fractures in the adult. Surgery, Gynecology and Obstetrics 64: 1064
27. Ghormley R K, Black J R, Cherry J H 1941 Ununited fractures of the clavicle. American Journal of Surgery 51: 343
28. Niessen H 1931 Zur Behandlung der retrosternalen Luxation der Clavicula. Deutsche Zeitschrift für Chirurgie 231: 405
29. Kennedy J C 1949 Retrosternal dislocation of the clavicle. Journal of Bone and Joint Surgery 31-B: 74
30. Richard M 1930 Zur Behandlung der Luxationsterno-clavicularis. Zentralblatt für Chirurgie 57: 1660
31. Allen A W 1928 Living suture grafts in the repair of

fractures and dislocations. Archives of Surgery 16: 1007

32. Lowman C L 1928 Operative correction of old sternoclavicular dislocation. Journal of Bone and Joint Surgery 10: 740

33. Bankart A S B 1938 An operation for recurrent dislocation (subluxation) of the sternoclavicular joint. British Journal of Surgery 26: 320

34. Burrows H J 1951 Tenodesis of subclavius in the treatment of recurrent dislocation of the sternoclavicular joint. Journal of Bone and Joint Surgery 33-B: 240

35. Jones R 1924 Injuries to joints. Oxford University Press, London p 57

36. Horn J S 1954 The traumatic anatomy and treatment of acute acromioclavicular dislocation. Journal of Bone and Joint Surgery 36-B: 194

37. Gurd F B 1941 The treatment of complete dislocation of the outer end of the clavicle. (An hitherto undescribed operation). Annals of Surgery 113: 1094

38. Mumford E B 1941 Acromioclavicular dislocation. Journal of Bone and Joint Surgery 23: 799

39. Watkins J R 1925 An operation for the relief of acromioclavicular luxations. Journal of Bone and Joint Surgery 7: 790

40. Bunnell S 1928 Fascial graft for dislocation of acromioclavicular dislocation. Surgery, Gynecology and Obstetrics 46: 563

41. Schneider C C 1933 Acromioclavicular dislocation: autoplastic reconstruction. Journal of Bone and Joint Surgery 15: 957

42. Meyerding H W 1937 Treatment of acromioclavicular dislocation. Surgical Clinics of North America 17: 1199

43. Dewar F P, Barrington T W 1965 The treatment of chronic acromioclavicular dislocation. Journal of Bone and Joint Surgery 47-B: 32

44. Copeland S, Kessel L 1980 Disruption of the acromio-clavicular joint—Surgical Anatomy and Biological Reconstruction. Injury 11, 208–214.

45. Oudard O 1924 La luxation récidivante de l'épaule (variété antérointerne): procédé operatoire. Journal de Chirurgie 23: 13

46. Helfet A J 1958 Coracoid Transplantation for recurrent dislocation of shoulder. Journal of Bone and Joint Surgery 40-B: 198

47. Neer C S 1970 Displaced proximal humeral fractures, Part I: classification and evaluation. Journal of Bone and Joint Surgery 52-A: 1077

48. Neer C S 1970 Displaced proximal humeral fractures. Part II: Treatment of three-part and four-part displacement. Journal of Bone and Joint Surgery 52-A: 1090

49. Fairbank T J 1948 Fracture-subluxations of the shoulder. Journal of Bone and Joint Surgery 30-B: 454

50. Bankart A B S 1928 Robert Jones birthday volume. Oxford University Press, p 309

51. West E F 1949 Intrathoracic dislocation of the humerus. Journal of Bone and Joint Surgery 31-B: 61

52. Reeves B 1966 Arthrography of the shoulder. Journal of Bone and Joint Surgery 48-B: 424

53. Reeves B 1968 Experiments on the tensile strength of the anterior capsular structures of the shoulder in man. Journal of Bone and Joint Surgery 50-B: 858

54. Zadik F R 1948 Recurrent posterior dislocation of the shoulder joint. Journal of Bone and Joint Surgery 30-B: 531

55. Demersay J J 1814 Dissertation sur la luxation primitive de la tête de l'humerus en dehors ou en arrière. Thèse de Paris, No. 55

56. Cooper Sir Astley 1824 A treastise on dislocations and on fractures of joints, 3rd edn. Longman, London

57. Watson-Jones R 1938 Injuries in the region of the shoulder joint. (ii) Bone and joint injuries. British Medical Journal ii: 80

58. Kirker J R 1952 Dislocation of the shoulder complicated by rupture of the axillary vessels. Journal of Bone and Joint Surgery 34-B: 72

59. Kocher T 1870 Eine neue Reductionsmethode für Schulterverrenkung. Berliner Klinische Wochenschrift 7: 101

60. Nash J 1934 The status of Kocher's method of reducing recent anterior dislocations of the shoulder. Journal of Bone and Joint Surgery 16: 535

61. Lindblom K 1939 Arthrography and roentgenography in ruptures of tendons of the shoulder joint. Acta Radiologica (Stockholm) 20: 548

62. Nelson D H 1952 Arthrography of the shoulder. British Journal of Radiology 25: 134

63. Bennett G 1936 Old dislocations of the shoulder. Journal of Bone and Joint Surgery 18: 594

64. Dollinger J 1911 Die veralteten traumatischen Verrenkungen der Schulter, de Ellenbogens und der Hufte. Ergebnisse der Chirurgie und Orthopédie 3: 83

65. Cubbins W, Callahan J, Scuderi C 1934 Reduction of old or irreducible dislocations of the shoulder joint. Surgery, Gynecology and Obstetrics 58: 128

66. Warrick C K 1948 Posterior dislocations of the shoulder joint. Journal of Bone and Joint Surgery 30-B: 651

67. Michaelis L S 1950 Internal rotation dislocation of the shoulder. Journal of Bone and Joint Surgery 32-B: 223

68. McLaughlin H L 1952 Posterior dislocation of shoulder. Journal of Bone and Joint Surgery 34-A: 584

69. Watson-Jones R 1948 Recurrent dislocation of the shoulder (editorial). Journal of Bone and Joint Surgery 30-B: 6

70. Eyre-Brook 1948 Recurrent dislocation of the shoulder joint. Journal of Bone and Joint Surgery 30-B: 39

71. Bankart A S B 1923 Recurrent or habitual dislocation of the shoulder joint. British Medical Journal ii: 1132

72. Bankart A S B 1928 Robert Jones birthday volume. Oxford University Press, p 307

73. Bankart A S B 1948 Discussion on recurrent dislocation of the shoulder. Journal of Bone and Joint Surgery 30-B: 46

74. Adams J C 1948 Recurrent dislocation of the shoulder. Journal of Bone and Joint Surgery 30-B: 26

75. Hill H A, Sachs M D 1940 The grooved defect of the humeral head. Radiology 35: 690

76. Stryker W S cited by Hall R A, Isaac F, Booth C R 1959 Dislocations of the shoulder with special reference to accompanying fractures. Journal of Bone and Joint Surgery 41A: 491

77. Tavernier L 1929 Les luxations récidivantes de l'épaule. Revue d'Orthopédie 16: 575

78. Clairmont P, Ehrlich H 1909 Ein neues Operationsverfahren zur Behandlung der habituellen Schulterluxation mittels Muskelplastik. Archiv für Klinische Chirurgie 89: 798

79. Finsterer H 1917 Die operative Behandlung der habituellen Schulterluxation. Deutsche Zeitschrift fur Chirurgie 141: 354

80. Kirschner E 1914 Die freie autoplastische Faszientransplantation. Mentioned in Kleinschmidt O 1914 Ergebnisse der Chirurgie und Orthopedie 8: 207, 273

81. Carrel W B 1928 Habituell Schulterluxation. Zentralblatt für Chirurgie 55: 2034

82. Gallie W E 1948 Recurrent dislocation of the shoulder. Journal of Bone and Joint Surgery 30-B: 6

83. Heymanowitsch Z 1927 Ein Beitrag zur operativen Behandlung der habituellen Schulterluxationen. Zentralblatt für Chirurgie, 54: 648

84. Nicola T 1929 Recurrent anterior dislocation of the shoulder. Journal of Bone and Joint Surgery 11: 128

85. Nicola T 1934 Recurrent dislocation of the shoulder. Journal of Bone and Joint Surgery 16: 663

86. Moseley H F 1961 Recurrent dislocation of the shoulder. Livingstone, Edinburgh

87. Broca A, Hartmann H 1890 Contribution a l'étude des luxations de l'épaule. Bulletins de la Societé Anatomique de Paris, 5me Série 4: 312

88. Eve F S 1880 A case of sub-coracoid dislocation of the humerus, with the formation of an indentation on the posterior surface of the head, the joint being unopened: Abstracted in the Proceedings of the Royal Society of Medicine 8: 511

89. Perthes G C 1925 Uber Ergebnisse der Operationen bei habitueller Schulterluxation. Deutsche Zeitschrift für Chirurgie, 194: 1

90. Valtancoli G 1924 Sulla lussazione abituale di spalla. Chirurgia degli Organi di Movimento 9: 131

91. Boicev B 1938 Sulla lussazione abituale della spalla. Chirurgia degli Organi di Movimento 23: 354

92. Osmond-Clarke H 1948 Habitual dislocation of the shoulder. Journal of Bone and Joint Surgery 30-B: 19

93. Magnuson P B, Stack J K 1943. Recurrent dislocation of the shoulder. Journal of American Medical Association 123 (14): 889

94. Eden R 1918 Operation for recurrent dislocation of shoulder (in German). Deutsche Zeitschrift der Chirurgie 144: 269

95. Hybbinette S 1932 Transfer of a bony fragment for treatment of an anterior dislocation of shoulder (in French). Acta Chirurgie Scan 71: 411

96. Bayley J I L, Kessel L 1978. Posterior dislocation of the shoulder. Abstracted in Journal of Bone and Joint Surgery 60-B 440

97. Bayley J I L, Kessel L 1978 Posterior dislocation of the Shoulder—The Clinical Spectrum. Journal of Bone and Joint Surgery 60–B: 3, 440.

98. Scott D J 1967 Treatment of recurrent posterior dislocation of the shoulder by glenoplasty. Journal of Bone and Joint Surgery 49-A: 471

99. Adams J C 1976 Glenoplasty by posterior bone block for recurrent posterior dislocation of shoulder. Standard orthopaedic operations. Churchill Livingstone, Edinburgh, p 125

100. Rowe C R, Yee L 1944 Recurrent posterior dislocation of the shoulder. Journal of Bone and Joint Surgery 29: 582

101. Rowe C R, Pierce D S, Clarke J G 1973 Voluntary dislocation of the shoulder. Journal of Bone and Joint Surgery 55-A: 445

21

Injuries of the Arm

L. Klenerman

FRACTURES OF THE SHAFT OF THE HUMERUS

Fractures of the shaft of the humerus are usually easy to treat, no matter whether spiral from rotational strain, oblique or transverse from angulation, or comminuted from direct injury. The blood supply is so vigorous that union is rapid, and the fracture is clinically firm within about six weeks. There is no tendency to over-riding; on the contrary, the only danger is that the fragments may be allowed to distract by the weight of the limb and cause delayed union. The management of the closed fracture of the shaft and its complications, delayed union, the infected fracture and radial nerve palsy will be considered. Soft tissue injuries to the arm such as rupture of the biceps tendon and myositis ossificans have been considered in other chapters (see chapters on the shoulder, elbow and joint stiffness).

Anatomical features. The shaft of the humerus is almost cylindrical and can be fractured by bending or twisting forces or combinations of the forces producing transverse, spiral or oblique fractures. These are almost equally frequent in clinical practice.[1] The middle third of the bone is the most vulnerable in relation to delayed or non-union. This is because the main nutrient artery enters the bone very constantly at the junction of the middle and lower thirds or in the lower part of the middle third,[2] and the foramina of entry are concentrated in a small area of the distal half of the middle third of the shaft on the medial side of the bone. Thus fractures through the shaft of the humerus at the junction of the middle and lower thirds may destroy the main nutrient artery at the time of injury. The radial nerve is another structure at risk from fractures or operations on the humerus. It does not travel along the spiral groove of the humerus next to the bone as is commonly described; instead along most of its course it is separated from the humerus by a variable layer of muscle, and lies close to the inferior lip of the spiral groove, but not in it. It is only for a short distance near the lateral supracondylar ridge that the nerve is in direct contact with the humerus and it is in this area that it pierces the lateral intermuscular septum before passing on to the surface of the brachialis muscle.[3] This explains why the radial nerve escapes injury in so many of these fractures, for it is clear that in most cases the nerve is protected from the sharp bone edges by a layer of triceps or brachialis muscle. It is in fractures at the junction of the middle and lower thirds where the nerve is tethered to the bone as it pierces the lateral intermuscular septum that damage is most likely to occur.[4]

General principles of treatment

In general treatment of the fractured shaft of the humerus is not usually difficult. The fractured ends whether oblique, transverse or spiral can be readily aligned with the patient sitting or standing, when the weight of the forearm on the distal fragment will usually achieve an acceptable position. Support of the wrist with a collar and cuff or narrow sling, allowing the elbow to lie free and unsupported may be all that is required. In the early stages when there is considerable pain a well padded plaster of Paris U-slab passing from the region of the acromion down to the olecranon and up the inner side of the arm to the axilla and bandaged in place is usually effective in relieving discomfort. In the words of Sir John Charnley: 'It is perhaps the easiest of major long bones to treat by conservative methods'. A 'hanging cast' which has sometimes been advocated, i.e. a heavy plaster cast suspended from the neck and passing from the knuckles to the axilla is not recommended because it may distract the fracture and produce delayed union.

Most fractures of the shaft of the humerus treated conservatively are clinically united by about six weeks, a fact which was known as far back as the time of Hippocrates. Union may occur with some angulation but one of the advantages of conservative management is that a moderate degree of deformity can be accepted without an obvious cosmetic blemish or functional impairment, and anterior bowing of 20°, or varus angulation of 30° results in little obvious angulation of the arm (Figs 21.1 to 21.4). The slight loss of elbow flexion or extension is hardly noticed and the muscle bulk of the arm hides any bony deformity.

Unfortunately not all fractures of the humerus behave in this way. Union may not be clinically firm at six weeks and if not given appropriate treatment the fracture can go on to a state of established non-union. The need for other methods of treatment may also arise when there are compound injuries, and the use of external skeletal fixation may be valuable if the soft tissue damage is extensive. Internal fixation may be required for patients with more than one fracture in the same limb, for double fractures, or where there are multiple fractures of the humerus or multiple fractures elsewhere in the body. Lastly, fractures with radial nerve injuries which follow manipulation of the fracture should be explored.

It is a pity that in some parts of the world the trend of recent years has been to operate more and more readily on recent fractures of the shaft of the humerus, sometimes relying on totally inadequate techniques of internal fixation without sufficient external protection, thus causing established non-union of the fracture (Figs 21.5 to 21.9). When this stage of indolence is reached with sclerosis of the bone ends and mature fibrous tissue laid down between the fragments, treatment becomes more difficult. It is then necessary not only to refreshen the bone surfaces but to immobilise them as rigidly as possible, which cannot be done by a simple plaster cast and not even by a shoulder spica. In a spica the patient can still shrug his shoulder up and down, rotate the fragments and move them to and fro; sound intramedullary fixation or a heavy duty compression plate is needed, and if necessary a spica may be applied for supplementary support.

The conservative treatment of recent closed fractures. A collar or cuff applied with the patient in the sitting or standing position will usually correct deformity by traction on the distal fragment from the weight of the forearm. Distraction of the fracture

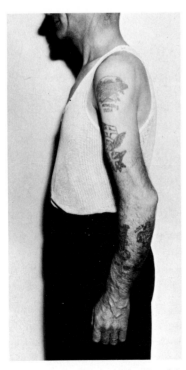

Fig 21.1 Patient with little apparent deformity of the left arm.

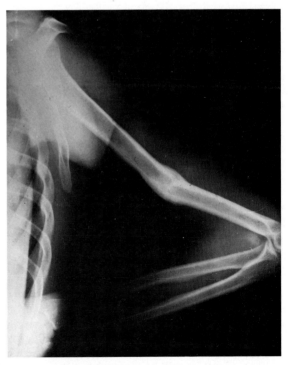

Fig 21.2 Radiograph of the humerus showing 20 degrees of anterior bowing.

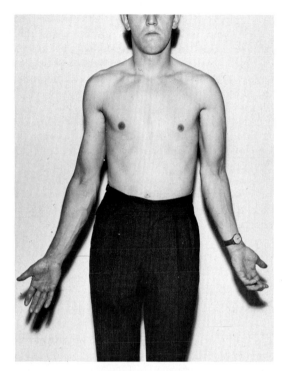

Fig 21.3 Patient showing just perceptible varus of the left arm. (Reproduced by kind permission of the Editor of the *Journal of Bone and Joint Surgery* from Klenerman L. (1966) Fractures of the shaft of the humerus. *Journal of Bone and Joint Surgery*, 48-B, 108.)

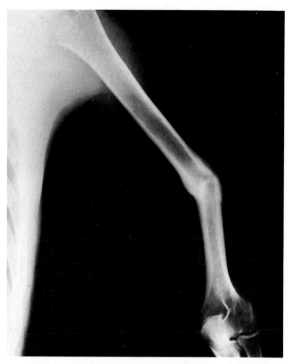

Fig 21.4 Radiograph of the humerus showing 30 degrees of varus. (Reproduced by kind permission of the Editor of the *Journal of Bone and Joint Surgery* from Klenerman L. (1966) Fractures of the shaft of the humerus. *Journal of Bone and Joint Surgery*, 48-B, 108.)

surfaces is not a problem because it is controlled by the compressive forces of the biceps, brachialis and triceps. A plaster U-slab passing down the outer side of the arm from the acromion and up the inner surface to the region of the axilla and bound on to the arm with careful padding of bony prominences such as the medial epicondyle is useful for support in the early stages (Fig 21.10). Once the initial acute discomfort has subsided the patient is encouraged to exercise the hand, wrist and even the shoulder of the injured limb. By keeping the hand within the collar and cuff the patient can bend forward towards the injured side and exercise his shoulder holding on to a support with the good arm if necessary. In this way, with the elbow held away from the trunk, the patient can swing the injured arm in circles, while elbow movements can be carried out standing after removal of the hand from the collar and cuff. By six weeks with this regime the fracture is usually clinically united, but even if there is still slight mobility it is unlikely that there will be serious delayed union and the fracture with further immobilisation should still go on to consolidation. If, however, by eight weeks the fracture is still completely mobile it can be concluded that union will not occur without operative treatment.

Primary operative treatment of recent fractures. There are some circumstances in which open reduction and internal fixation are indicated as part of the early treatment of closed fractures of the shaft of the humerus. For example, in multiple injuries the patient may be recumbent for many weeks and the simple U-slab fixation which depends upon the upright position to hold the fracture reduced loses its effectiveness. Also, as part of a multiple injury there may be severe damage to the soft tissues of the arm such as occurs in burns, or in severe skin loss which require frequent dressings, and possibly early skin grafting procedures. In these conditions stabilisation of the fracture by means of internal fixation facilitates the more urgent treatment of the soft tissues. Secondly, some fractures of the shaft of the humerus may demand internal fixation because of associated injuries

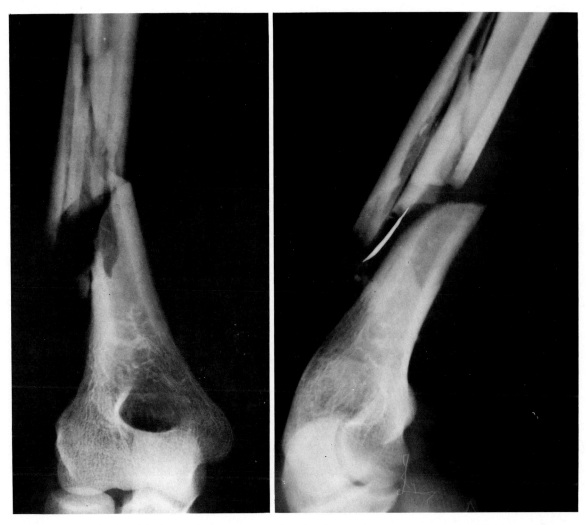

Fig 21.5 The comminution of the fracture does not matter at all; in fact the comminution encourages union. All that is needed is to maintain reasonable alignment with a simple plaster slab, and support the limb to prevent distraction. There is no need for a surgical operation.

in the forearm or elbow which without stabilisation of the humerus make the management of the combined injuries even more difficult. Thirdly, a double fracture of the humeral shaft may be difficult or impossible to control by conservative means and require early intramedullary nailing: and lastly, open fractures which are complicated by a radial nerve injury, or radial nerve injuries which occur after manipulation of the fracture should be explored.

Operative approach. If primary internal fixation is indicated the humerus should be exposed through an antero-lateral incision (see Chapter 15—Operative Approaches). An essential first step is to locate the radial nerve so that it can be retracted safely, and this is most easily done by defining the muscle interval between brachialis and brachio-radialis in which the nerve lies. This interval is not always easy to define, but it can be identified by taking the line of the lateral epicondyle and lateral intermuscular septum thus exploring the nerve distally and then tracing it proximally. Only when the nerve has been retracted safely should the operative exposure be developed and the bone fragments dissected free and prepared for internal fixation.

Methods of internal fixation. Fractures of the shaft of the humerus can be fixed either by a bone plate or an

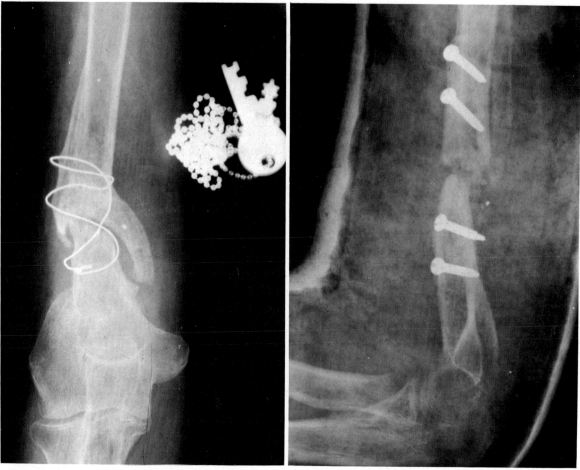

Fig 21.6   **Fig 21.7**

Figs 21.6 and 21.7 The same fracture of the humerus shown in Fig 21.5 which might have united perfectly well if left alone with no more than protection from movement and support to prevent distraction. Instead an operation was performed with the insertion of two or three loops of wire (Fig 21.6). The chain and keys are not in the limb; they are in the patients pyjama jacket. The fracture failed to unite—of course. The next effort was a tibial graft with four screws but no immobilisation in a plaster spica (Fig 21.7). Again the fracture failed to unite.

intramedullary nail. If rigid internal fixation is achieved it should not be necessary to supplement it with a shoulder spica, but to obtain this degree of fixation a heavy duty compression plate, or a closely fitting intramedullary nail must be used. On the whole because of the cylindrical nature of the humeral shaft intramedullary nailing is easier to perform than plating. However, when the fracture is very oblique, or spiral the use of an intramedullary nail may not be reliable and a plate gives more effective fixation. Kuntscher nails provide the most rigid intramedullary immobilisation and although less easy to insert are preferred to the more flexible Rush nail. They are

best introduced into the bone through the olecranon fossa as there is thus no interference with shoulder movement and this approach results in only minor restriction of the elbow range. It must be remembered that nailing through the lower end of the humerus can be difficult if the elbow cannot be fully flexed. Nails inserted at the proximal end of the humerus are easier to introduce but almost always restrict shoulder movement.

To insert the nail from the region of the elbow, an incision is made in the middle of the posterior surface of the lower third of the arm, extending proximally from the tip of the olecranon for about 7.5 cm, and

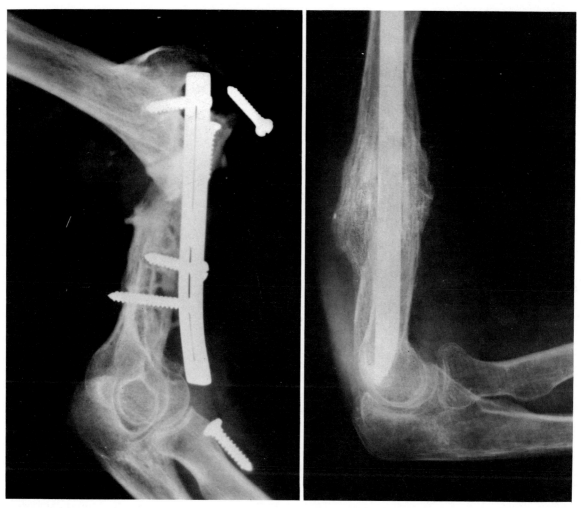

Fig 21.8   **Fig 21.9**

Figs 21.8 and 21.9 A more strenuous endeavour was made with a slotted plate and five screws, but still without the protection of a plaster spica. Fig 21.8: The fracture remained un-united. Not until the sclerosed bone surfaces were refreshed to reproduce the conditions of the original fracture, together with the sound fixation of intramedullary nailing and protection in a plaster spica for three months did the fracture finally unite (Fig 21.9).

the triceps aponeurosis is split to expose the olecranon fossa. Starting at the apex of the fossa a hole is made into the medullary canal. This is gradually enlarged and after the fracture has been exposed and reduced a guide wire is passed from the distal into the proximal fragment. With the fracture held reduced by bone holding forceps and the guide wire in place reaming is carried out until the largest possible diameter reamer does not stick (9 to 10 mm is common). The length of the humerus is carefully measured and a nail of the correct length and diameter is then inserted and a screw fixed just below the protruding portion of the nail to prevent the nail from backing out. After closure of the wound a wool and crepe body bandage is applied with a supporting collar and cuff. Within a few days of operation the bandages can be released and active exercises of the fingers, wrist, elbow and shoulder are commenced. If the fixation is rigid the patient should regain good function of the arm very rapidly. However, he should be discouraged from taking heavy strain before bony union has occurred.

Fractures associated with radial nerve injury.
Injury to the radial nerve, either axonotmesis or

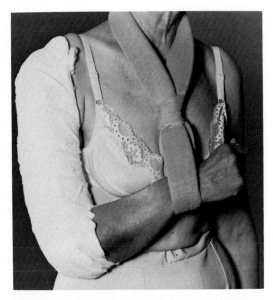

Fig 21.10 A useful method of external splintage.

neurapraxia, in association with fractures of the shaft of the humerus is the commonest peripheral nerve injury complicating a closed fracture.[5] Fractures at the junction of the middle and lowest third of the bone are the most likely to be associated with nerve palsy as the nerve has least mobility where it passes through the lateral intermuscular septum from the posterior to the anterior compartment of the arm. Fractures at this level are often spiral and the lower fragment is angulated to the radial side sometimes causing the nerve to be trapped between the fracture surfaces (Figs 21.11 and 21.12). Spontaneous recovery can be expected in the majority of radial nerve injuries and with few exceptions the initial treatment should be conservative. A lively splint supporting the wrist and metacarpo-phalangeal joints of the fingers should be provided and this will allow the patient to exercise his hand effectively and maintain some functional use. The surgeon awaiting signs of recovery in the nerve should allow for distal growth at the rate of 1 mm per day until the brachioradialis, the most proximal muscle has been reached, remembering that the point of entry of the radial motor branch is about 2 cm above the lateral epicondyle. Where electromyography is available this will simplify the problem of forecasting recovery.

One of the exceptions to the conservative management of a radial nerve injury after a closed fracture is that following a manipulation to reduce the fracture, particularly when the fracture is in the lower third of the shaft and this demands early exploration to free the nerve from between the fracture surfaces. Another rare exception is the radial nerve palsy which may occur as a delayed phenomenon due to involvement of the nerve by callus. This should be treated by neurolysis.

Operative nerve palsy. In a surgical exposure of the humeral shaft the radial nerve is particularly at risk where it passes behind the humerus in the line of the spiral groove, and if open reduction is necessary it is best to begin by a formal exposure of the nerve. The danger is not only that the nerve may be cut if the exposure of the humerus traverses tissues distorted by swelling or scarring; but it can also be stretched and injured by the overenthusiastic use of subperiosteal retractors. Always remember the radial nerve is particularly vulnerable in any surgery on the upper arm and give it the respect it demands.

UN-UNITED FRACTURES OF THE SHAFT OF THE HUMERUS

Un-united fractures have a notorious reputation for being resistant to treatment and to lead to a series of unsuccessful operative procedures often ending in persistent non-union. A basic fault of many surgical techniques of the past has been a lack of rigid internal fixation, and Hicks has shown convincingly that a number of non-unions will consolidate by bone without grafting provided they are rigidly fixed.[6]

Non-union of shaft bones may be of the 'elephant foot' type with a marked proliferative reaction of bone at the site of the pseudarthrosis, and these are the cases which do well with internal fixation alone; or of the atrophic type where the ends of the bone at the pseudarthrosis show no bone reaction and the addition of a bone graft is necessary before union is achieved. The humerus more than any other bone produces the atrophic type of pseudarthrosis. Casual and ill-conceived surgical treatment of pseudarthrosis of the humeral shaft is still associated with a relatively high complication rate which includes joint stiffness, nerve injuries, infection of the donor graft area and a noteworthy rate of non-union.

It is tempting to rely entirely on rigid internal fixation, but if in doubt use a bone graft. Even if the pseudarthrosis is of the hypertrophic type the proximal fragment is frequently osteoporotic and the addition of a graft is advisable. Thus the four essential principles of treatment for the care of established non-union of the humerus are:

1. To freshen the fractured surfaces for 2 to 3 cm above and below the fracture.

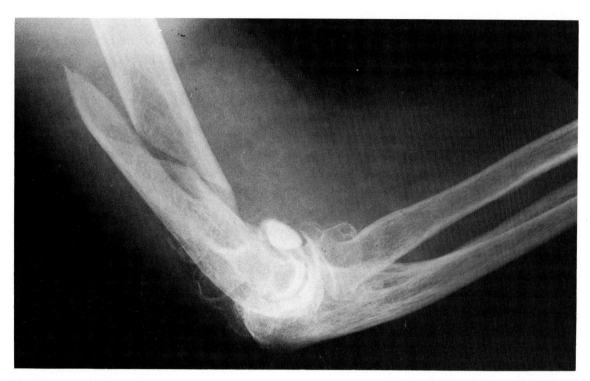

Fig 21.11

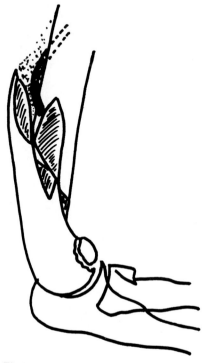

Fig 21.12

Figs 21.11 and 21.12 Fig 21.11 shows a spiral fracture of the lower third of the humerus with typical displacement. The line diagram of the radiograph, Fig 21.12, shows how the radial nerve is tethered close to the lower third of the humerus by the intermuscular septum and can be easily drawn between the fracture surfaces.

2. To use an intramedullary nail or 6 to 8 hole compression plate for internal fixation.
3. To lay cancellous strips of bone from the iliac crest over the prepared decorticated fragments.
4. If there is any doubt about the rigidity of the internal fixation to supplement this with external splintage either by means of a U-slab or shoulder spica (Fig 21.13).

External skeletal fixation of fractures of the shaft of the humerus. Undoubtedly external skeletal fixation has a place in the treatment of fractures of the shaft of the humerus, particularly with infected fractures, severely comminuted fractures, bone defects or considerable skin loss in compound fractures. There are a variety of systems of external fixation available some involving application of apparatus to both sides of a limb such as that of Hoffmann, and others which are applied to the outer side only, such as that devised by Sukhtian and Hughes[7] (Figs 21.14 to 21.17).

Antero-lateral exposure for un-united fractures of the middle third of the humerus (see Chapter 15). As previously described the radial nerve must first be exposed and retracted safely. When non-union is established with fibrosis and scarring around the fracture site, especially when there have been previous operations, the radial nerve may be anywhere other than in its normal position. Even the introduction of spike-retractors while the bone ends are being exposed, or the gripping of bone fragments with lion-jaw forceps while they are freshened, realigned and nailed, endangers the nerve. It is therefore an essential prelude to the operation on the bone to find, trace and retract the nerve. It can usually be found where it lies between brachialis and brachioradialis in front of the lateral epicondyle and lateral intermuscular septum. It is then traced proximally and all adhesions divided so that it can be held away from the site of fracture by soft saline-soaked linen or rubber tapes.

Eburnated bone at the end of the fragments is removed with bone-cutting forceps and the medullary canal of each fragment opened with small gouges. The proximal and distal fragments of the bone are reamed, and the widest reamer that the medullary canal can accept indicates the width of the intramedullary nail to be selected. Measurements are taken of the length of reamer between the fracture site and

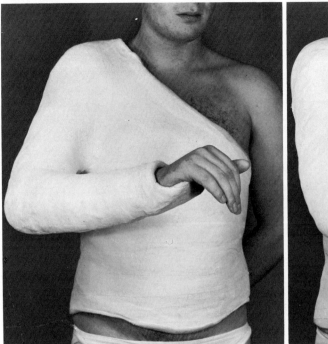
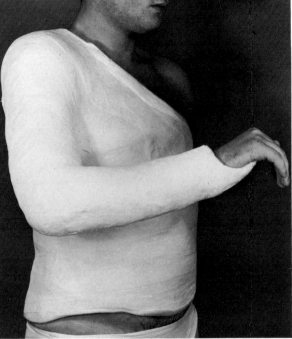

Fig 21.13 When there is slow and delayed union or need for primary operative reduction, a shoulder spica is helpful in improving the quality of immobilisation.

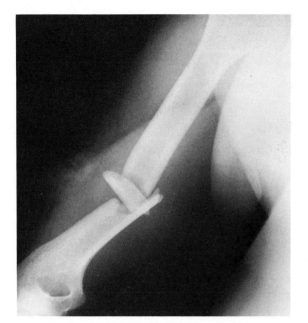

Fig 21.14

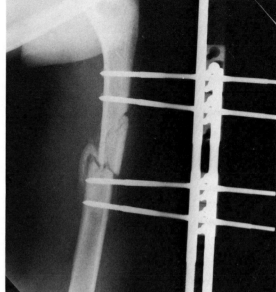

Fig 21.15

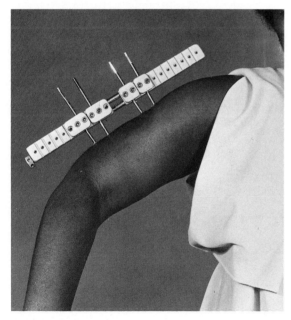

Fig 21.16

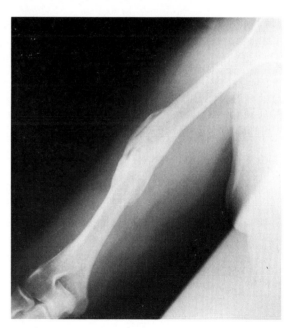

Fig 21.17

Figs 21.14 to 21.17 The use of external skeletal fixation for a compound comminuted fracture of the humerus. Fig 21.12 shows the initial displacement before reduction. A satisfactory position of the large comminuted fragment was obtained at open reduction and rigid fixation with good alignment maintained by using an external fixation device (Figs 21.15 to 21.16). There was sound bone union by three months (Fig 21.17). (Reproduced by kind permission of Professor S. P. F. Hughes, Princess Margaret Rose Orthopaedic Hospital, Edinburgh.)

the resistance of the tuberosity above, and that of the sub-articular region of the elbow below. The exact width and length of the nail needed is thus determined. As previously described the nail is best inserted through the distal end of the bone. Meanwhile an associate surgeon has exposed the crest of the ilium and has taken slivers of cancellous bone to lay around the fracture site. After the operation the limb is immobilised by a U-slab and collar and cuff. When the would has healed if there is any doubt about the rigidity of the internal fixation a shoulder spica should be applied.

Posterior exposure for un-united fractures of the lower and upper thirds of the shaft (see Chapter 15). If the fracture is in the upper or lower third of the humeral shaft it is probably best to use a posterior approach to the bone. In the lower third a mid-line posterior incision is safe without need first to expose and retract the radial nerve. For more extensive exposure it is best to remember that if one takes a line from the postero-lateral margin of the acromion to the olecranon process, the midpoint corresponds to the oblique course of the radial nerve across the posterior surface of the humerus into the region of the deltoid tuberosity. An incision starting distal to this point and continues towards the olecranon avoids the radial nerve. If more of the shaft is to be exposed the incision is extended proximally. Further longitudinal splitting of the triceps muscle is done until the radial nerve and profunda brachii artery are identified, bearing in mind that the course

of the radial nerve and the vessel is towards the lateral border of the humerus.

INFECTED FRACTURES OF THE SHAFT OF HUMERUS WITH NON-UNION

The treatment of infected un-united fractures is difficult, often requiring prolonged periods of hospitalisation.[8] The first essential is to remove dead and sequestrated fragments of bone. Open irrigation drainage is invaluable. One or more irrigation drains is placed in the focus of infection and a further tube is connected to a suction pump.[9] It is probable that irrigation is effective mainly because of mechanical cleansing, and therefore appropriate systemic antibiotics are needed, particularly if there is severe infection of soft tissues or signs of toxaemia. It may be necessary to continue the irrigation for several weeks until there is a layer of healthy granulation tissue at the base of the wound, and during this time external fixation is probably the most effective and safest method of obtaining rigid stabilisation of the fracture. Cancellous bone grafts are sometimes required to stimulate bone growth at the site of non-union and to establish bony continuity if there is a defect. But these should be delayed until healthy granulations have developed at the fracture site. If a suitable external fixation is not available it may be necessary to use an intramedullary nail, although this technique carries the grave risk of introducing infection through the medullary cavity. However, if this should occur the nail can easily be removed through a short incision remote from the fracture site.

REFERENCES

1. Klenerman L 1966 Fractures of the shaft of the humerus. Journal of Bone and Joint Surgery 48-B: 105
2. Carroll S E 1963 A study of the nutrient foramina of the humeral diaphysis. Journal of Bone and Joint Surgery 45-B: 176
3 Whitson R O 1954 Relation of the radial nerve to the shaft of the humerus. Journal of Bone and Joint Surgery 36-A: 85–88
4. Holstein A, Lewis S B 1963 Fractures of the humerus with radial nerve paralysis. Journal of Bone and Joint Surgery 45-A: 1382
5. Seddon Sir Herbert 1972 Surgical disorders of the peripheral nerves. Churchill, Livingstone, Edinburgh, Ch 5, p 84

6. Hicks J H 1963 Rigid fixation as a treatment for non-union. The Lancet 211: 272
7. Sukhtian W, Hughes S 1979 External fixation of fractures. Journal of Royal Society of Medicine 72, 831–834.
8. Meyer S, Weiland A J, Willenegger H 1975 The treatment of infected non-union of fractures of long bones. Journal of Bone and Joint Surgery 57-A: 836
9. Taylor A R, Maudsley R H 1970 Installation-suction technique in chronic osteomyelitis. Journal of Bone and Joint Surgery 52-B: 88

22

Injuries of the Elbow

The dangers of passive stretching and forcible manipulation after joint injuries have already been fully discussed in Chapter 4 but it would be negligent not to re-emphasise these dangers when considering the elbow joint in particular. This joint, with its complex mechanism of flexion, extension and rotation is dependant not only on perfect gliding action of its collateral ligaments, but also on free extension of the anterior and posterior capsule. It is no small wonder then that the elbow joint is slow in regaining movement sometimes even after the most trivial injury. One thing is certain, and that is that passive stretchings can only do harm at this early stage (Fig 22.1). Every effort must be made to prevent well meaning parents, physiotherapists, occupational therapists and young residents from embarking upon manipulative methods. They will only make matters worse and may be responsible for producing, or aggravating, myositis ossificans in the brachialis insertion.

Although it hardly seems credible that this form of maltreatment still takes place, that it does so is undoubtedly true, and it may be that it is a more common cause of disability than we would be led to believe. The explanation probably lies in the desperately slow rate of improvement in joint movement after some elbow injuries. There are few parents, and even some physiotherapists who, when faced day after day with a stiff joint, can resist the temptation to use passive treatment. There is very little a physiotherapist can do that the patient cannot do himself, and if there is any danger that passive stretchings are to be used it would be wiser to allow the patient to exercise at home. However, sometimes no attendance at the physiotherapy department may be wrongly interpreted by the relatives as neglect and may lead to the worst forms of passive stretchings by parent or patient; in these circumstances attendance in the department during the early stages of mobilisation can be valuable not only to instruct the patient in a regime of active exercices, but to warn him against the dangers of passive movement. Even attendance once a week is valuable for it allows the

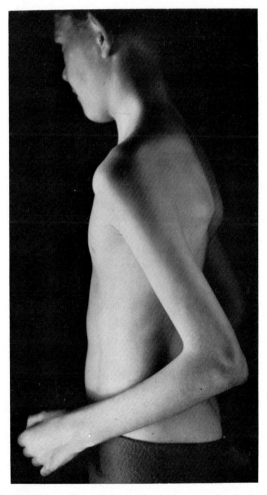

Fig 22.1 Range of extension movement two years after simple strain of the elbow. The serious stiffness arose solely from passive stretching.

physiotherapist to monitor progress. From the beginning it should be explained that although recovery may be slow it will be gained most rapidly by the unaided activity of the patient. The range should be measured month by month because movement is often restored so slowly that only by regular measurement can the gain be recognised, and the anxiety allayed. If dislocations are reduced and fractured bones replaced, a full range of movement will indeed be regained provided only that passive force, painful stretching and repeated manipulations are avoided.

CLASSIFICATION OF ELBOW INJURIES

The components of the elbow joints are the lower end of the humerus, the head of the radius, and the articular surface of the upper end of the ulna. These are bound together by a complex ligamentous structure which is almost inevitably damaged in every injury to the joint. Any classification must therefore take into account soft tissue injuries in addition to fractures and joint disorders. Elbow injuries will therefore be considered under the following headings:

1. Soft tissue injuries (sprains, tennis elbow etc.).
2. Fractures of the capitellum in the adult.
3. Supracondylar fracture of the humerus.
4. Intercondylar and single condylar fractures of the humerus.
5. Epiphyseal injuries (whole epiphysis; capitellum epiphysis; epicondylar epiphysis).
6. Dislocations.
7. Unusual injuries.

It will be noted that fractures of the head and neck of the radius and fractures of the olecranon have not been included in this list. They are fully discussed in the following chapter on forearm injuries.

SOFT TISSUE INJURIES OF THE ELBOW

Traumatic synovitis of the elbow joint. Minor strains and contusions often cause traumatic synovitis of the elbow joint in children and may sometimes be associated with ruptures of the collateral ligaments. Radiographs rarely show any bony abnormality unless there has been avulsion of bone as a result of ligament damage; but an effusion may be demonstrated in the lateral radiograph by displacement of the anterior and posterior fat pads which normally lie against the lower end of the humerus.[1,2] If there has been a ligament rupture there will be local swelling, tenderness and discolouration over the site of the rupture. Instability is sometimes present, and under these circumstances an arthrogram* will demonstrate escape of the radio-opaque fluid through the defect.[3] If a ligament rupture is diagnosed the elbow should be immobilised in a plaster cylinder from the upper arm to the wrist for two to three weeks, with the joint extended 40 to 60 degrees below the right angle. In this position the collateral ligaments are on tension[4] and are less likely to produce troublesome contractures. It is much easier for the patient to regain flexion from the half extended position than it is for him to restore extension from the time-honoured position of immobilisation at a right angle. Where there are no local signs of ligament rupture active movement should be encouraged in the joint just as soon as the acute symptoms have settled. A few days rest in a collar-and-cuff, however, is beneficial

Tennis elbow—lateral epicondylar tendinitis. The condition known as tennis elbow often arises from strain of the fibres of the common extensor tendon at its origin from the lateral epicondyle of the humerus. Sports, such as golf and tennis, which involve striking a ball with club or a racquet, tend to produce a varus strain at the elbow, and this may lead on to damage of the common extensor origin.[5] In tennis players this is often the consequence of a mistimed backhand stroke. When the forearm is semi-pronated and the muscles are tensed, a fast ball hits the racquet more quickly than was expected, and sudden flexion of the wrist stretches the extensor muscles of the forearm at their epicondylar attachment. Thus the injury is often sustained from one sudden movement; but it may arise also from a series of minor pronation-supination strains in those whose work demands hammering, screwing, ironing or wringing. The patient finds it difficult to turn a door-knob, hold a teapot, or grasp any weight in the semi-pronated position of the limb. There is tenderness on pressure over a very localised spot on the lateral side of the joint immediately below the epicondyle. Pain is often referred to the forearm, and it is increased by the clinical test of lateral strain of the elbow with adduction of the forearm, especially in the pronated position. Because of the radiation of pain lower down the forearm, and because of weakness of grip which always results from this condition, it has been

*Arthrography of the elbow; 50 per cent Conray in normal saline is injected under local anaesthetic through a postero-lateral approach with X-ray control.

suggested that some resistant cases of tennis elbow are due to an entrapment lesion of the posterior interosseus nerve as it passes beneath the heads of the supinator muscle,[6,7] although a more recent electromyographic study has not supported this view.[8] Others consider that degenerative changes in the orbicular ligament and superior radio-ulnar joint are important.[9,10]

Tennis elbow and the Fibrilosis Syndrome.[11,11a] Although it is accepted that there may be other causes for pain over the outer side of the elbow in addition to tendinitis of the common extensor origin, there is little doubt that the vast majority of the cases are due to a simple tendon abnormality. Very often the tendinitis is lighted up by relatively minor strains and is only one manifestation of similar collagen disorder at many tendinous origins from bone, and also in the fibrous sheaths of tendons. Many patients with 'tennis elbow' have also had, or will develop, de Quervain's stenosing tendo-vaginitis at the radial styloid, trigger fingers or trigger thumb from fibrous thickening of the flexor tendon sheaths, carpal tunnel compression of the median nerve from fibrosis of the anterior retinaculum, supraspinatus tendinitis, and many other examples of the 'fibrilosis syndrome'. Cervical spondylosis, which, after all that, is only another example of degenerative disease of fibrous tissue, is not uncommonly associated with tennis elbow, and on occasions may present as referred pain at this site. The painful heel resulting from a fascial strain at the site of the plantar musculo-tendinous origin and the degenerative strain of the medial collateral ligament of the knee are just other examples of the same condition.

Conservative treatment. The constitutional background to 'tennis elbow' or epicondylar tendinitis explains why relief is so often complete without local injection, manipulation or operation. Recovery is accelerated by salicylates (Butazolidin and other 'anti-rheumatic' drugs). Local infiltration of the tender area with 2 ml of a mixture of 1 per cent lignocaine, 1500 units of Hyalase and 25 mg of hydrocortisone will usually bring complete relief; but if one, or perhaps two, such injections fails to cure the pain it is unwise to continue infiltration. Sometimes the pain will be relieved for a few weeks but returns when the patient resumes full work, and it is an important part of the after treatment to warn the patient that for at *least three months* he should not persist with a movement which provokes pain. This may require an alteration in work patterns: even a period of rest in plaster may be indicated.

Manipulative treatment. Manipulation under anaesthesia has been advised. With the forearm in full pronation and the elbow extended the joint is then sharply adducted in such a way as to stretch the lateral aspect of the joint and the common extensor tendon. It is difficult to be convinced that this manipulation does any good at all. Of course many patients get better; just as they would have done without manipulation. However, it is sometimes worth a trial in resistant cases before resorting to operation.

Operative treatment. In a very few patients symptoms persist despite adequately supervised conservative treatment. The diagnosis in these cases should be critically reviewed to exclude other causes, such as referred pain from cervical spondylosis, derangement of the superior radio-ulnar joint, or even entrapment of the posterior interosseus nerve. Re-X-rays of the elbow should be taken to exclude any intra-articular or bony explanation for the persisting symptoms. If the site of local tenderness still remains strictly confined to the apex of the lateral epicondyle and the pain is brought on by resisted extension of the wrist, release of the tendinous origin of the extensor carpi radialis brevis from the epicondyle should be successful in relieving the pain. This is done through a longitudinal incision centred on the lateral epicondyle. The origin of the muscle is only exposed by retraction of extensor radialis longus; an important step which may explain the occasional failure of the Bosworth operation where the origin of extensor carpi radialis brevis is not exposed.[11a] It is important to divide the fibres of origin *strand by strand*; quite often the lesion will be demonstrated as a tiny area of granulation, or degenerative cyst formation, *within* the tendinous origin itself, suggesting that the condition could be due to degenerative change in collagen tissue. Only the origin of extensor carpi radialis brevis is divided in the operation and it is interesting to note that the same relief of pain can be obtained by lengthening the tendon of this muscle at its lower end.[12] Following operation the patient must be warned that for several months he must not engage in work which previously was known to provoke symptoms.

'Pitcher's elbow'.[13] Valgus strain of the elbow is more likely to occur in throwing sports, such as baseball or javelin throwing.[14] Under these conditions maximum strain is felt at the flexor origin on the medial side of the joint; it is increased by sudden contraction of the finger and wrist flexors at the moment when the projectile is released: sometimes a bad golf swing can produce the same effect (*Golfer's elbow*). Although pain and tenderness may be strictly localised to the medial epicondyle, it is sometimes more diffuse than in tennis elbow. Treatment by local injections of cortisone, followed by a period of rest from the aggravating strain is usually successful; operative measures are rarely needed.

Acute calcification around the elbow. This is a rare condition which can occur in association with either the lateral or medial muscle origins. It presents as a hot tender area over the site of calcification with gross limitation of movement. The clinical and radiological signs in the case illustrated in Figures 22.2 and 22.3 were so gross that they were mistaken for those of osteosarcoma. Treatment by rest in plaster

gives dramatic relief of pain and a quick resolution of the calcified plaque.

Pulled elbow. There are surgeons who deny the existence of this syndrome, but they are, of course, quite wrong. It is a very definite clinical entity, and has been demonstrated in cadaveric experiments on the still born to be due to the orbicular ligament jamming over the radial head.[15] It is usually caused by pulling up the arm of a recalcitrant young child, or swinging a child by both arms as part of a game. The condition presents as a painful elbow, a useless arm and limitation of active and passive rotation of the forearm. It responds dramatically to a quick

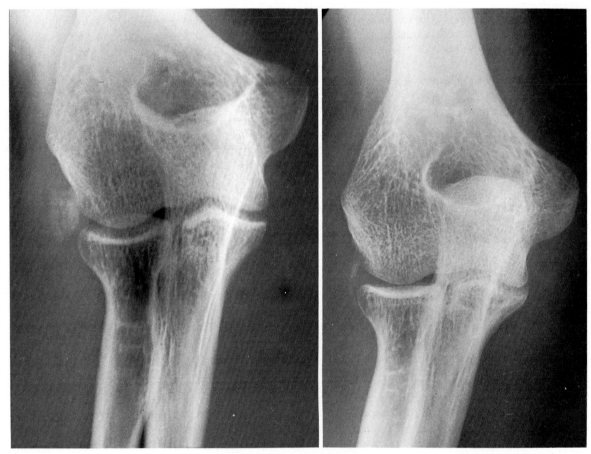

Fig 22.2

Fig 22.3

Figs 22.2 and 22.3. The patient whose elbow is shown in Figure 22.2 presented with severe pain and redness on the outer side of the elbow for the previous two to three days, with a history of intermittent aching for several weeks previously. The house surgeon who first saw her diagnosed either acute infection or osteosarcoma. Fortunately a short period of rest in plaster quickly resulted in resolution of symptoms and an X-ray taken three weeks later showed considerable reduction in size of the calcified plaque (Fig 22.3).

movement of the forearm into full pronation and supination.

Snapping elbow. Snapping elbow caused by the ulnar nerve subluxating out of its groove during flexion is a well known entity and in one survey of 2000 elbows was found to occur in over 16 per cent.[16] It has already been fully described in Chapter 12. A more rare cause due to forward dislocation of the medial head of the triceps has also been described.[17, 18] The medial head is found to dislocate over the medial epicondyle when the elbow is flexed. It is associated with pain and paraesthesia of the ulnar nerve. Separation of the muscle from its attachment and rerouting it through the lateral part of the tendon will cure the symptoms. Anterior transposition of the ulnar nerve may also be necessary.

Olecranon bursitis. A troublesome effusion into the olecranon bursa may result from a direct blow on the point of the elbow, or from chronic irritation produced by leaning on the elbow for long periods. Not uncommonly a spur of bone over the tip of the olecranon predisposes to the condition. The patient usually presents with a 'baggy' swelling the size of a pigeon's egg overlying the whole of the olecranon. Sometimes the swelling is reddened and tense suggesting infection. Treatment of the uninfected case is by aspiration and the injection of 0.5 ml of hydrocortisone (12.5 mg) with 1500 units of hyaluronidase. Infected cases should be incised and drained. Recurrent effusions can be treated by excision of the bursa, or preferably by aspirating or incising it, and then removing the underlying prominent tip of the olecranon. By careful splitting of the triceps without disturbing its distal fibres it is possible to remove a wedge of bone from the olecranon thereby reducing the prominence under the bursa.[19]

FRACTURES OF THE CAPITELLUM IN THE ADULT

There is a frequent association of fracture of the head of the radius with injury to the cartilage of the capitellum. The radius is driven upwards and forwards by a fall on the outstretched hand and it delivers a shearing blow to the front of the capitellum which may injure the bone as well as the articular cartilage.[20] Any size of fragment may be broken off but it is convenient to distinguish three degrees of injury:

1. Bruising of the articular cartilage of the capitellum.

2. Marginal chip fracture of the capitellum where small fragments of cartilage and bone are completely detached.
3. Fracture of half the capitellum and part of the trochlea.

Bruising of articular cartilage of the capitellum. This injury of articular cartilage is responsible for the limitation of extension movement that is sometimes unavoidable in fractures of the head of the radius. It may also occur as an isolated injury without associated fracture of the head of the radius, causing localised avascular necrosis and osteochondritis dissecans.

Marginal chip fracture of the capitellum. This fracture is more common in women than in men, an incidence which suggests that Bohler's view is correct, i.e. that it is due to a hyperextension injury in an unusually valgus elbow.[21] If the detached fragment consists only of cartilage it is not disclosed by radiographic examination, and the lesion may be discovered only when the joint is opened for treatment of the associated fracture of the radial head.[20] The fragment may consist largely of cartilage but also include a thin flake of bone. In other cases cartilage covers a large fragment of bone. The defect in the outline of the capitellum may be too small and too shallow to be seen in radiographs but the source of the loose fragment is proved by its typical elliptical or moon shape (Figs 22.4 and 22.5); there is no other articular surface in the elbow with a similar contour. On one occasion the fragment was found firmly imbedded within a fragmented head of radius.[20] Since the fragment is completely detached and avascular, it should be removed through a short incision on the lateral side of the joint.

Fracture of half the capitellum. The front half of the capitellum may be broken off by a vertical fracture line in a sagittal plane coinciding with the front of the shaft of the humerus. The fragment is pushed upwards but is seldom tilted or rotated, and its fractured surface usually remains in close contact with the humerus immediately above the bed from which it has been broken. For this reason the displacement is often overlooked and serious restriction of elbow movement then remains.

The fragment is much larger than it appears to be in lateral radiographs; it includes the whole of the front half of the capitellum and a considerable part of the trochlea, so that it carries almost half the articular surface of the humerus. Involvement of the

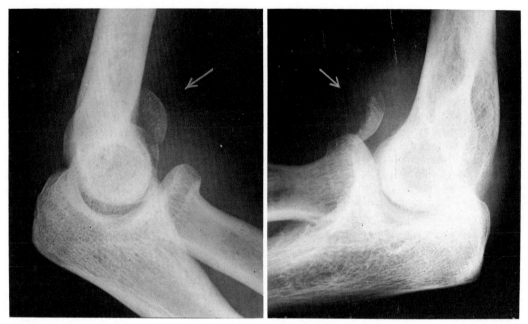

Fig 22.4   **Fig 22.5**

Figs 22.4 and 22.5 Two examples of marginal fracture of the capitellum. In the injury shown in Figure 22.4 a crack fracture of the head of the radius became obvious in later X-rays. In Figure 22.5 the capitellar fragment is rotated and is back to front. These fragments involve only a small part of the articular surface and have no blood supply; they should be excised.

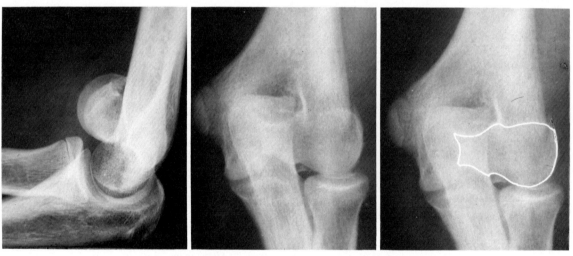

Fig. 22.6   **Fig 22.7**   **Fig 22.8**

Fig 22.6 Fractures of the anterior half of the capitellum. The injury is obvious in the lateral radiograph. In this case even more than half the capitellum has been broken off and displaced upwards. It is a very severe intra-articular injury.

Figs 22.7 and 22.8 Antero-posterior radiograph shows that the displaced fragment includes not only a large part of the capitellum but also of the trochlea (Fig 22.7). It is not always easy to interpret this antero-posterior projection because of overlap of bone shadows. The same projection is reproduced in Figure 22.8 with the fragment outlined. Radiographs of high quality are needed because accuracy of reduction is imperative.

trochlea as well as the capitellum is recognised only in the antero-posterior radiograph which is often difficult to interpret because the shadow of the displaced fragment overlies that of the humerus (Figs 22.6 to 22.9). If so large a part of the joint is removed the result will be no better than that of an excision-arthroplasty. Every effort should be made to replace rather than excise the bone, especially since its blood supply is usually preserved by capsular attachments.

Manipulative reduction. It is essential to secure absolutely accurate replacement with a perfectly smooth articular surface. This can sometimes be achieved by closed manipulation done under radiographic control in the theatre, the surgeon being prepared to proceed to open reduction if manipulation fails. With the elbow held by an assistant in the extended position both thumbs are used to press the

fragment down into its bed. If reduction is stable, as confirmed by antero-posterior and lateral radiographs, it may be safe to immobilise the joint in plaster at the right angled position, or even acutely flexed as advised by some authorities;[22] but there need be no fear in immobilising it fully extended for two weeks if the reduction is acceptable only in this position. Gentle active movements are started in the third week, and there is little difficulty in regaining full flexion over the next three or four months.

Operative reduction. More often than not manipulation will fail to secure an adequate and stable reduction and under these circumstances there should be no delay in opening the joint so that pressure can be applied directly to the bone fragment itself under visual control. There is, of course, the added hazard of dissecting the soft tissues too freely and, by

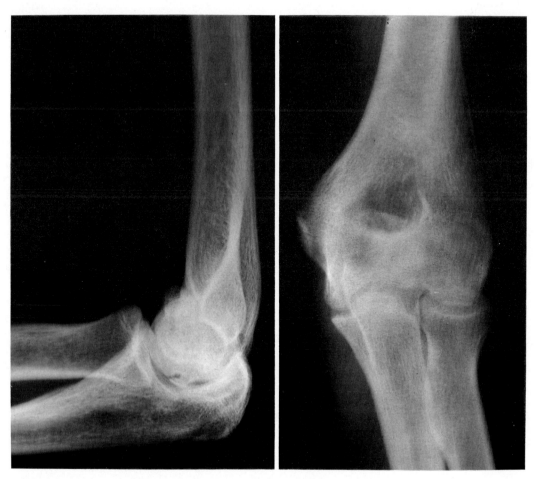

Fig 22.9 The fragment was replaced after operative exposure and secured with two catgut sutures. After six months movement was from 60 to 140 degrees with the range slowly increasing.

removing capsular attachments, imperilling the blood supply of the bone fragment with its large articular surface. However, through a lateral incision, with no more exposure than is essential, blood clot can be evacuated, bone spicules or interposed soft tissues removed and the fragment pressed into its bed. There is often no need for internal fixation and two or three catgut sutures suffice (Figs 22.10 to 22.13). If more fixation is necessary the fragment can be stabilised by one or two Kirschner wires inserted percutaneously. These should be removed after two to three weeks.

Excision of the fragment. The ideal time for operative reduction is within the first two or three days when replacement can be achieved with hair-line accuracy. But this view is by no means unanimous amongst orthopaedic surgeons, some of whom advise early excision of the fragment.[23] Probably both methods give equally good results provided that the operation is carried out early. Every week of delay increases the difficulty. If two or more months have elapsed it is probably best to leave the joint alone; but sometimes when displaced bone is blocking flexion movement it may be excised.

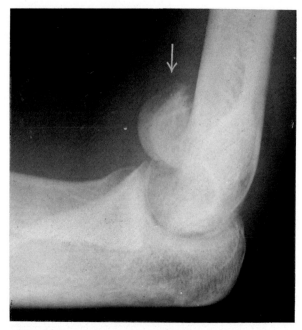

Fig 22.10

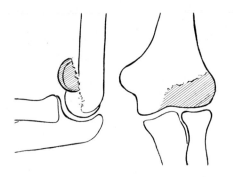

Fig 22.11

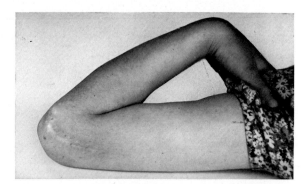

Fig 22.12

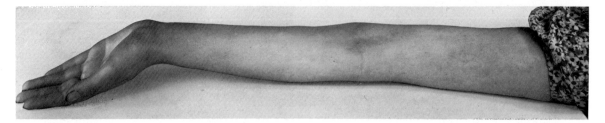

Fig 22.13

Figs 22.10 to 22.13 Fractures of the anterior half of the capitellum and trochlea; the detached fragment includes at least half the articular surface of the humerus. The fragment was replaced by open operation and normal movement was regained.

SUPRACONDYLAR FRACTURE OF THE HUMERUS

Supracondylar fracture of the humerus is one of the commonest elbow injuries in children. It becomes progressively more uncommon as the child approaches adolescence—the average age group of patients being $7\frac{1}{2}$ years. The line of fracture is usually oblique from the front of the bone upwards and backwards, the small distal fragment being displaced backwards (Fig 22.14). After traction has been applied the displacement can be corrected by flexing the elbow and, by reason of the obliquity of the fracture line, reduction is stable in this position.

Less commonly a supracondylar fracture is oblique in the opposite direction (Fig 22.15); the distal fragment is then displaced forwards and its displacement is increased by flexing the elbow. It is clearly wrong to treat every supracondylar fracture in the flexed position: this is the correct position for the usual fracture, but the opposite type of fracture may require to be extended.

Importance of accurate reduction. Extension of the elbow joint is limited by the olecranon process locking in the olecranon fossa of the humerus. If supracondylar fractures unite with the lower fragment of the humerus, carrying the olecranon fossa, tilted forwards 30 degrees, this locking occurs 30 degrees before the normal limit of extension movement is reached. Angulation of the bone from forward tilting of the lower fragment is shown in a corresponding degree of permanent limitation of extension. Similarly, uncorrected backward tilting of the lower fragment causes permanent limitation of flexion. Moreover, if the fracture unites with lateral tilting of the lower fragment, the forearm bones are carried laterally with it and there is a corresponding degree of cubitus valgus or cubitus varus. None of these angulations is corrected by later growth of bone. Lateral and antero-posterior displacements without angulation grow straight in children (see Figs 22.31 to 22.34), but limited flexion or extension movement and alteration in the carrying angle from angulation of the bone persist into adult life. Correction of any

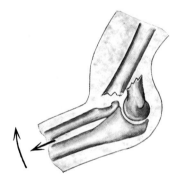
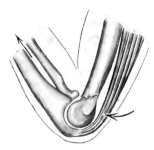

Fig 22.14 In a supracondylar fracture the small fragment is usually displaced backwards; after traction this is corrected by flexing the joint.

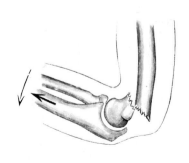
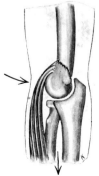

Fig 22.15 Occasionally there is forward displacement of the lower fragment; after traction the fracture is usually corrected by extension.

rotatory deformity is of equal importance to the reduction of antero-posterior and lateral tilt, and can easily be missed unless reduction X-rays are carefully assessed. If rotatory mal-alignment is not corrected it may result in an apparent cubitus varus; or it can accentuate the deformity of a valgus or varus tilt. It is important, therefore, in supracondylar fractures to secure perfect realignment of the fragments as far as angulation and rotation are concerned. Lateral or medial shift and antero-posterior displacement alone are not important.

Manipulative reduction. The elbow is usually so swollen that it is impossible to feel the bony outlines, and the perfect position that should be insisted upon cannot always be achieved by the first manipulative manoeuvre. Nevertheless, with the patient under a general anaesthetic, and a portable X-ray machine in the theatre, two or three adjustments of position can be made and usually an acceptable reduction can be achieved. There is rarely any need for traction and operative reduction should be confined to the rare compound injury, or fractures where ischaemic complications demand exploration. This management of supracondylar fractures has sometimes been misunderstood and often been misrepresented. Repeated manipulation to secure perfect position means repeated manoeuvrings under X-ray control *in the course of one manipulative procedure under one anaesthetic*. It does not mean that the patient should be brought back to the theatre day after day for repeated anaesthetics and repeated manipulations. That would be harmful and might be dangerous—there is no need for it.

An important part of the manipulation is traction in the long axis of the humerus, but this must *never* be applied as a long straight pull with the elbow fully extended, because in this position the brachial artery and median nerve will be angulated over the fracture site. For the same reason the elbow must not be forced into flexion without first disimpacting the fragments. Traction should be applied to the forearm with the elbow in a position 30 to 40 degrees short of full extension (Fig 22.16). The thumb of the other hand

Figs 22.16 to 22.18 Reduction of a supracondylar fracture of the humerus. Traction is applied with the elbow flexed 30 to 40 degrees from the fully extended position. With the other hand the antero-posterior displacement is reduced and the elbow gradually flexed to 30 degrees above the right angle. Lateral displacement can be corrected in this position and held while a posterior plaster slab is applied.

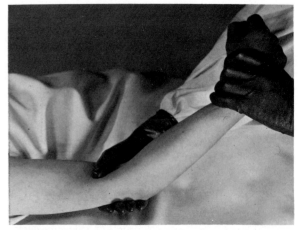

Fig 22.16

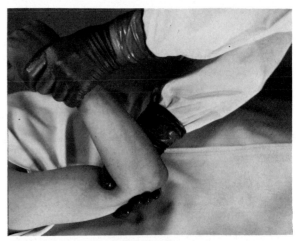

Fig 22.17

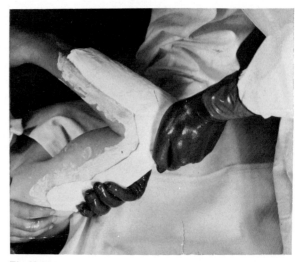

Fig 22.18

is then placed over the front of the proximal fragment with the fingers behind the distal fragment. While traction is continued the small fragment of the humerus is pulled forward and the elbow gradually flexed to about 30 degrees above the right angle (Figs 22.17 and 22.18). Lateral displacement, rotation and tilt are then corrected. An assistant takes the limb by the wrist and holds the elbow flexed. The surgeon applies direct lateral pressure with one hand over the side of the lower shaft of the humerus, and the other hand on the opposite side over the displaced fragment. If the lower fragment is displaced outwards it is pushed inwards. If it is displaced inwards it is pushed outwards; it really should be no more difficult than that. But, of course, there are times when it can be very difficult to obtain a satisfactory reduction. Sometimes gently rocking the lower fragment into position with two thumbs over the back of the lower fragment, while maintaining traction on the flexed elbow with the fingers pushing against the forearm, can correct the antero-posterior deformity, rotation and lateral displacement in one movement (Fig. 22.19).

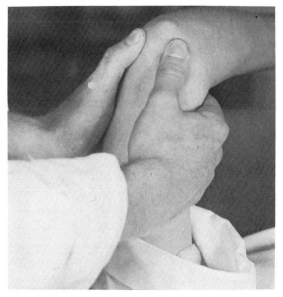

Fig 22.19 It is sometimes easier to obtain the final reduction of a supracondylar fracture by gently rocking the lower fragment into position with the thumbs, while traction is maintained by pressure of the forefingers against the flexed forearm. The elbow and shoulder should be flexed to a right angle and counter-traction may be needed at the shoulder. A remarkably fine control of the small fragment is often possible using this manoeuvre which allows correction of the three primary deformities due to antero-lateral, lateral and rotatory displacement.

Maintenance of reduction. The reduction of the posterior displacement of the common supracondylar fracture is only stable with the elbow flexed to about 30 degrees above the right angle (the hand coming to lie on the opposite shoulder (see Figs 22.20 and 22.21)) and it is said that with pronation of the forearm the lateral ligament tightens up and prevents varus tilt.[24] However, as most supracondylar fractures occur proximal to the capsular and ligamentous attachments this explanation is unlikely and displacement is probably controlled by releasing the tension of the flexor-pronator muscle group.[25] In the same way a valgus tilt is corrected by supinating the forearm. With the arm in this position a posterior plaster slab is applied from the axilla to the wrist, wide enough at the elbow to control lateral displacement. After check X-rays have been taken the arm is bound to the side with crepe bandages and Elastoplast strapping—the wrist and hand being left exposed to allow a constant check on the circulation (Fig 22.22). Close observation is necessary for the first 24 hours after reduction and it is always preferable to admit the child to hospital over this period. The arm is then left undisturbed in this position for three weeks: by that time X-rays will invariably show sufficient union to allow mobilisation within the limits of a sling.

Check X-rays. The taking of lateral check X-rays with the elbow in acute flexion presents no difficulty, but obtaining a good antero-posterior view can sometimes be a problem. It is not possible to extend the elbow without losing the reduction, so that it is necessary to take a 'shoot through' film, superimposing the radius and ulna over the front of the humerus (Fig 22.23). The lower end of the humerus is nearer to the X-ray plate and will usually be seen in sharp focus. Provided there is no rotatory deformity direct lateral or medial displacement is acceptable and will mould perfectly. It is tilt which will not correct by moulding and may sometimes cause gross alteration of the normal carrying angle. The amount of tilt can be estimated by comparing *Baumann's angle* on the two sides.[26, 27] This is the angle subtended between a transverse line drawn along the lower border of the lateral humeral metaphysis and a line drawn at right angles to the long axis of the humerus (Fig 22.24). Unfortunately these lines can sometimes be difficult to draw, especially when the antero-posterior view is taken by the 'shoot through' method. If it has not been possible because of swelling to flex the elbow into a stable position, X-rays must be repeated after a few days (see Fig 22.21). If displacement has recurred, or if the fracture is unstable because the elbow could not be acutely flexed initially, one more

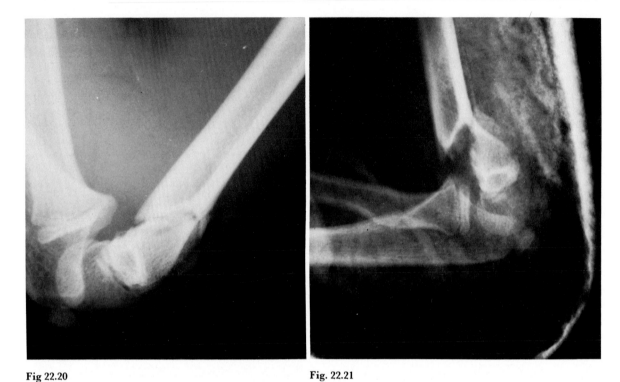

Fig 22.20   Fig. 22.21

Figs 22.20 and 22.21 Reduction of a supracondylar fracture is only stable when the forearm is flexed well above the right angle (Fig 22.20). An accurate reduction was lost when this fracture was immobilised with the elbow at a right angle (Fig 22.21).

attempt at reduction is justifiable, but repeated manipulation for further displacement only leads to permanent joint stiffness and is to be discouraged. Far better to accept deformity, and correct later by osteotomy if it proves necessary. It is important to keep one's nerve when faced with persistent deformity and constantly remember that even the most horrifying displacements are not incompatible with an excellent functional result (see Figs 22.25 and 22.26).

Prognosis. The final appearance and function of the elbow following a well reduced supracondylar fracture are usually excellent. Even when there is severe displacement and gross swelling it is usually possible to secure a good result. It is essential, however, to achieve correct alignment, to allow movement to recover at its own rate, even though this may take several months, and to avoid any passive stretchings or manipulations.

Complications. The primary complications of supracondylar fracture which cannot be avoided include Volkmann's ischaemic contracture from brachial artery contusion or rupture, and primary lesions of the ulnar, median and radial nerves. The secondary complications can be avoided. They include vascular obstruction from forcing the elbow into flexion or from the application of a tight encircling bandage; and increased stiffness, scattered traumatic ossification and secondary nerve lesions from passive stretching or forcible manipulation in the endeavour to accelerate recovery of movement.

Vascular complications. Any hint of vascular impairment in the distal part of the limb must put the surgeon immediately on guard. An absent radial pulse alone, without other signs of ischaemia, is not necessarily of serious consequence,[28] but it should always be regarded as a warning that vascular damage has occurred. It may be possible to restore the pulse by accurate reduction of the fracture, but very often swelling around the elbow makes it impossible to safely flex the joint beyond the right angle, and in these circumstances it is wiser to treat the fracture in Dunlop traction (see next section). Certainly if a secondary vascular impairment occurs after manipulative reduction all constrictive bandages should be removed immediately and the arm put

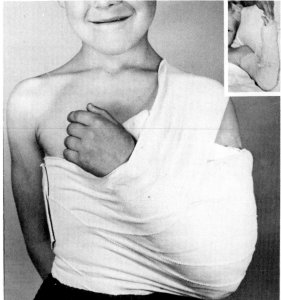

Fig 22.22 The reduction of a supracondylar fracture with posterior displacement is only stable with the elbow acutely flexed and the arm bound to the chest, with the hand on the opposite shoulder. The limb should *never* be allowed to swing free, as this will inevitably lead to recurrence of lateral tilt and rotatory deformity (see inset).

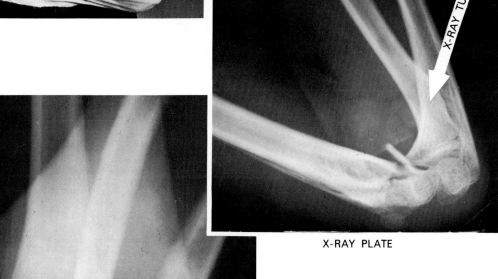

X-RAY PLATE

Fig 22.23 The antero-posterior check X-ray of the reduced supracondylar fracture cannot be taken by the orthodox method without losing position; a 'shoot through' view brings the lower end of the humerus into sharp focus with the radius and ulna superimposed over it (see inset).

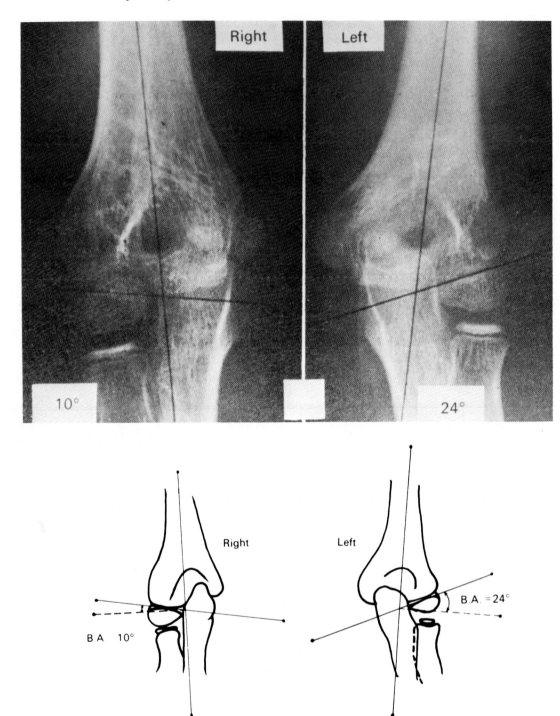

Fig 22.24 Antero-posterior views of comparison elbows with outline tracings of the X-rays showing how Baumann's angle is calculated. (From Mr David Jones' paper (1977) *Proceedings of the Royal Society of Medicine*, 70, 624. Reproduced by kind permission of the author and the Editor of the *Proceedings of the Royal Society of Medicine*.

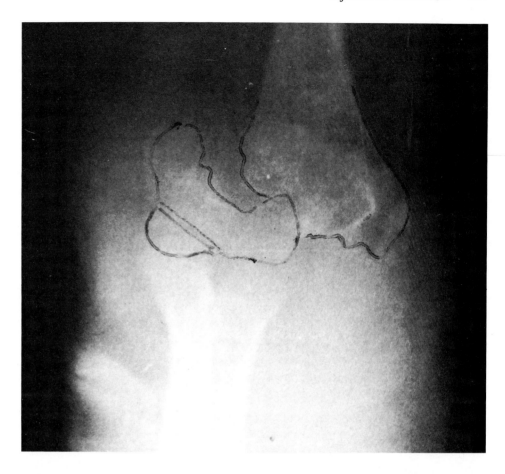

Fig 22.25

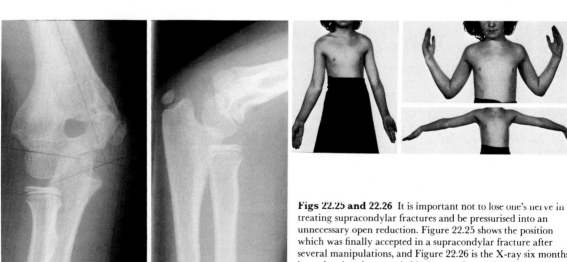

Fig 22.26

Figs 22.25 and 22.26 It is important not to lose one's nerve in treating supracondylar fractures and be pressurised into an unnecessary open reduction. Figure 22.25 shows the position which was finally accepted in a supracondylar fracture after several manipulations, and Figure 22.26 is the X-ray six months later showing the remarkable degree of moulding. This child regained a full range of movement with only a minor valgus tilt deformity (inset).

into traction. Where there are signs of a full ischaemia, with pain in the forearm, inefficient peripheral circulation and sensory and motor impairment in the distal part of the limb, the surgeon must be prepared to expose the brachial artery, openly reduce the fracture and carry out a wide fasciotomy, unless there is rapid improvement when the arm is put in traction (see Chapter 9). Fortunately decompression of this type will usually restore an adequate circulation without having to resort to arterial reconstruction.[29] The wounds must, of course, be left open, but can be closed by secondary suture in a few days. During this period the arm is conveniently immobilised in traction.[22, 27]

Nerve complications. The nerve most commonly affected is the median; radial palsies are rare; and the ulnar nerve is only involved when the fracture displacement is anterior. The nerve injuries are nearly always in continuity and recover without operative interference. Neurolysis of the median nerve is occasionally necessary if signs of recovery are delayed for more than two to three months.

Myositis ossificans. This is a rare complication, but can result from over-enthusiastic exercises during the period of early rehabilitation, and should be imme-diately suspected if movement diminishes and the joint becomes painful and swollen. The treatment is by rest in a sling and a plaster back splint for a few weeks, followed by a gradual return to active exercises. Under no circumstances should the child be submitted to passive exercises, massage or manipula-tion. Surgical removal of residual spurs of bone is rarely necessary.

The use of Dunlop traction. When there is circulatory embarrassment it is commonly worsened by flexing the elbow to reduce the fracture, and in these circumstances simple skin traction on the forearm as described by Dunlop[30] is a safe and valuable method of treatment. With the child recumbent the arm is abducted to a right angle at the shoulder, the elbow put over the side of the bed and flexed through about 60 degrees; skin traction is applied in the line of the forearm using about 3 lb (1.5 kg) suspended from a convenient overhead beam or a drip stand; the elbow is prevented from extending by a vertical sling placed over the fracture site, to which is attached a weight of 2 lb (1 kg) (Fig 22.27). To prevent a tendency to varus tilt the child should

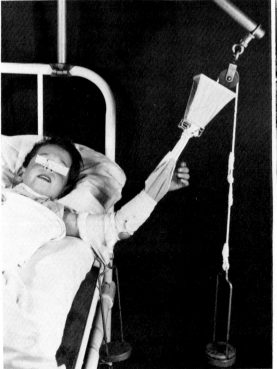

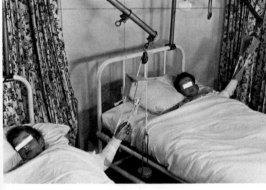

Fig 22.27 Dunlop traction for supracondylar fractures of the humerus. Skin traction of 3 lb (1.5 kg) is applied to the forearm and 2 lb (1 kg) to the supracondylar sling. *Inset:* Problem fractures never come singly! The child on the left had an exploration of the brachial artery for impending Volkmann's ischaemia.

be encouraged to keep the forearm pronated.[24] Particular care must be taken to pad the margins of the sling in order to avoid sores over the supracondylar area. Apart from this minor difficulty children tolerate this treatment very well (see Fig 22.27 inset) and can be nursed in this position until there is sufficient radiographic evidence of callus formation to allow the application of a plaster (usually in about two weeks).

There is a growing tendency to use this form of treatment for all difficult supracondylar fractures,[27, 31] but it must be emphasised that the reduction obtained is by no means perfect (Figs 22.28 to 22.30) and although varus or valgus tilt is usually corrected a significant amount of backward angulation may persist. A well reduced fracture, held by flexing the elbow to above the right angle, is still the treatment of choice for this fracture. Dunlop traction should be used only for the irreducible fracture, or where there are associated vascular complications.[32]

Mal-united supracondylar fracture. A supracondylar fracture with displacement first seen after one or two weeks can still be treated by attempted manipulative reduction rather than by embarking upon a hazardous operative replacement. It is true that it will be impossible at this stage of the fracture to achieve a replacement with accurate apposition of the fragments, but it is alignment that matters rather than apposition. A clear example is shown in Figures 22.31 to 22.34. The original injury was a supracondylar fracture with wide displacement of the fragments and considerable injury to soft tissues with vascular damage (Fig 22.31). The best position secured by manipulation is seen in Figure 22.32—the reduction was far from perfect but the fragments were in good alignment with no backward or lateral tilting. It was therefore decided, quite rightly, to accept the position and not to embark on a difficult and perhaps dangerous operative reduction. The later remoulding of bone by normal growth is seen in Figures 22.33 and 22.34. Within 18 months the elbow was clinically indistinguishable from normal, and within about another year it was radiographically indistinguishable from normal. But it must be emphasised that alignment has been corrected by manipulation and there was no *angulation* of the supracondylar fragment. Again it must be repeated that it is angulation, rotation or tilt which will not correct by moulding and will go on to produce permanent deformity. There was no residual backward *tilting* which, although of fairly minor importance, would have caused some permanent limitation of flexion movement, but far more important, there was no residual lateral tilting which would have caused the ugly permanent deformity of cubitus varus or valgus.

Compare this last case with that illustrated in Figures 22.35 to 22.37. Here the fracture has been allowed to unite with a residual varus tilt (Fig 22.35) which inevitably results in at least some loss of the normal carrying angle and more than likely an ugly cubitus varus or 'gunstock' deformity (Fig 22.37). In this case the effect of varus tilt has been increased by an internal rotation deformity of the lower fragment (Fig 22.36) shown by the tell-tale anterior spike formed by the medial supracondylar ridge of the humerus[33] (see also Figs 22.39 to 22.41). Unlike lateral or antero-posterior shift, rotation and tilt deformities are never fully corrected by subsequent moulding and must always result in some degree of permanent deformity.[34]

Operative reduction of supracondylar fractures. In the past decade there has been a resurgence of interest in open reduction of supracondylar fractures.[35, 36, 37, 38] It is considered by those advocating the method that the results are as good as closed reduction;[36] or that the incidence of loss of function compares favourably with conservative treatment.[38] The blame for bad results is put on the use of a posterior approach, or the selection for surgery of only the cases which have had multiple manipulations. It is claimed that by using an antero-lateral approach and carrying out the operation early the problem of limitation of movement is minimised. However, study of the results[38] reveals that the loss of movement in the various series of operative cases varies from 0 to 90 per cent with an average of 40 per cent loss compared with an overall 30 per cent loss in patients treated by closed reduction, and residual varus deformity is about 24 per cent in both operative and conservative series. Where then is the advantage? The answer is none. Moreover, open reduction of a supracondylar fracture is not an easy procedure, and although possibly safe in the hands of those treating every displaced fracture by this method it could be disastrous for the occasional operator dealing only with the irreducible case. It has been said many times before, and it is repeated again, that a difficult open reduction, with the extensive dissection needed, may cause capsular contraction, subsequent ossification and permanent stiffness. Most fresh displaced supracondylar fractures can be manipulated into an acceptable position and the only justification for open reduction is in compound fractures or in association

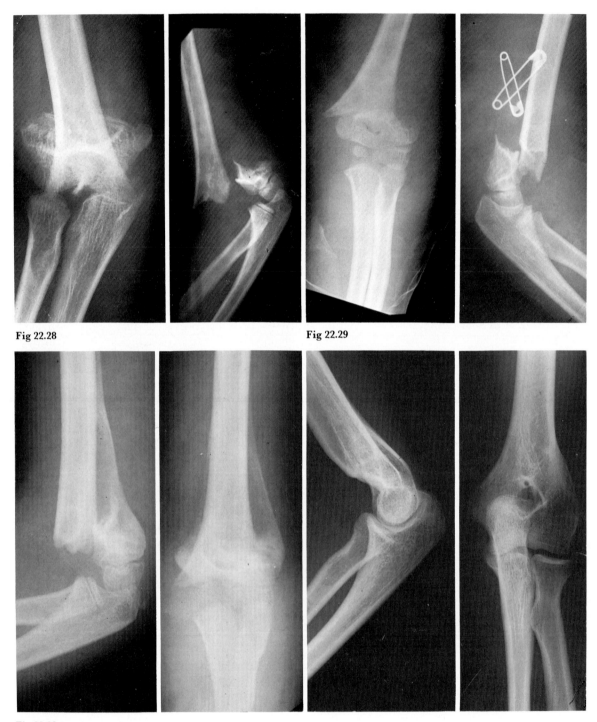

Fig 22.28

Fig 22.29

Fig 22.30

Figs 22.28 to 22.30 Figure 22.28 shows the initial X-rays of a supracondylar fracture complicated by vascular impairment which was treated by Dunlop traction. Figure 22.29 is an X-ray in traction and Figure 22.30 the position at one month and at eight years. Note that although there was marked backward and lateral shift there was no tilt deformity. This patient had no permanent disability.

Fig 22.31

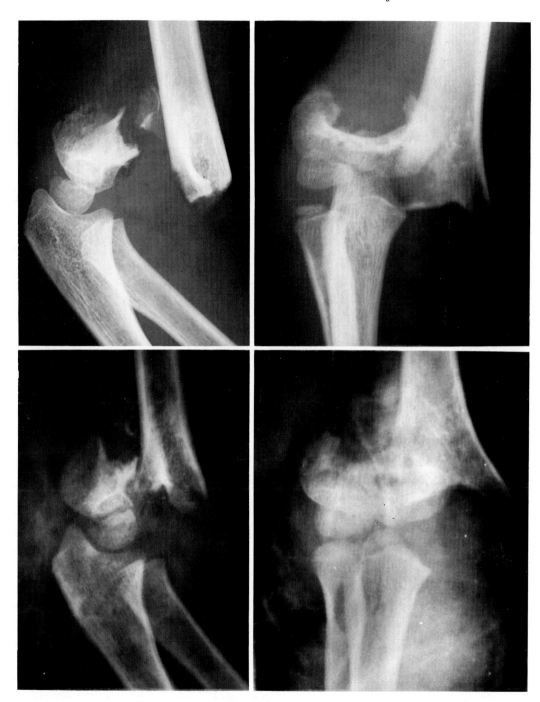

Fig 22.32

Figs 22.31 to 22.34 In recent supracondylar fractures of the humerus it is always important to correct angulatory displacement which causes persistent cubitus valgus, cubitus varus, or limitation of flexion or extension movement; but lateral displacement without angulation will grow straight. In this difficult supracondylar fracture (Fig 22.31) the reduction was not as good as it might have been, but the residual displacement was not angulatory (Fig 22.32), and since the soft tissue injury and vascular damage was great, it was decided to accept the position knowing that the bones would grow straight in time. Subsequent radiographs (Figs 22.33 and 22.34) show how perfectly the bone was remodelled because although there was imperfect apposition the displacement of the fragments was not angulatory. (Treated by the late Mr C. G. Attenborough when he was a Registrar at The London Hospital).

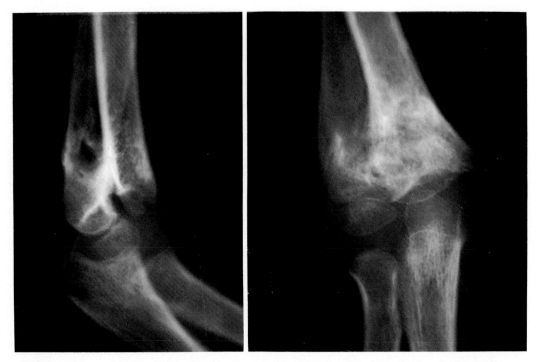

Fig 22.33

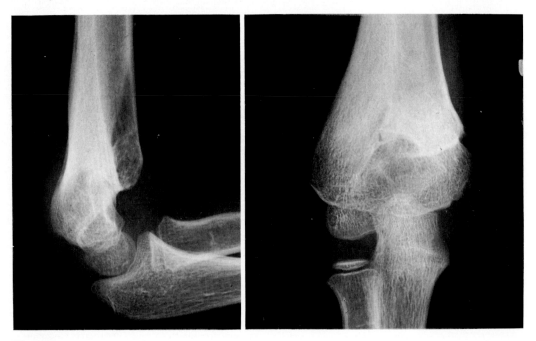

Fig 22.34

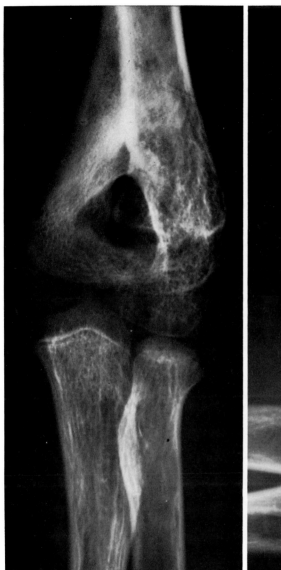

Fig 22.35

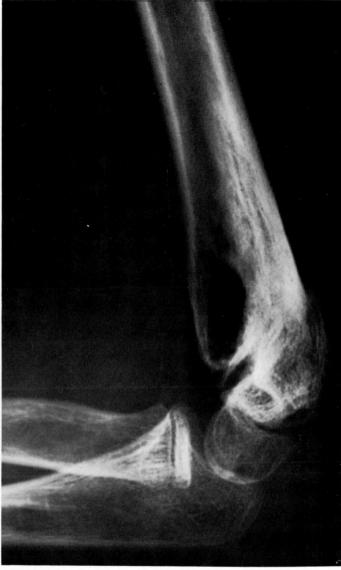

Fig 22.36

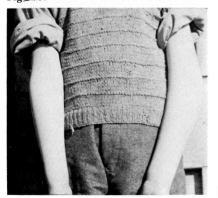

Fig 22.37

Figs 22.35 to 22.37 Residual varus tilt of the lower fragment after supracondylar fracture (Fig 22.35). In the lateral view the anterior spike of the medial supracondylar ridge indicates that there has been an internal rotation deformity of the lower fragment (Fig 22.36). The combination of these two displacements inevitably results in a cubitus varus or 'gunstock' deformity (Fig 22.37).

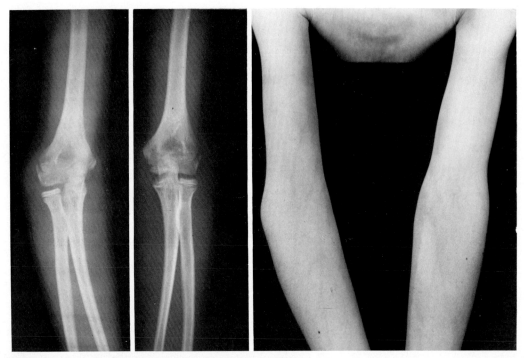

Fig 22.38

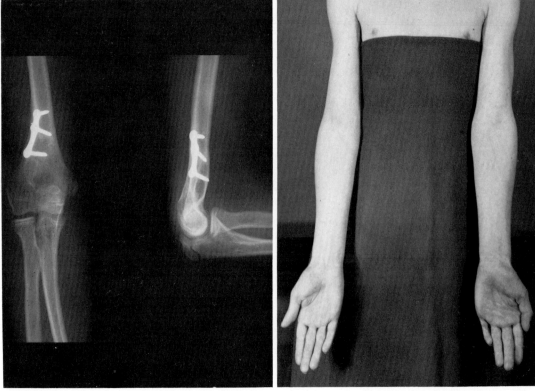

Fig 22.39

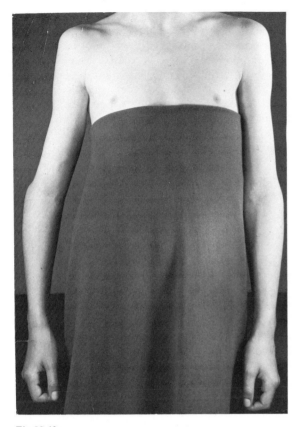

Fig 22.40

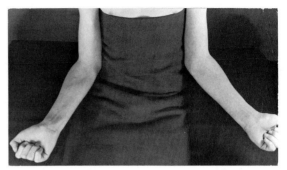

Fig 22.41

Figs 22.38 to 22.41 This patient developed an obvious varus deformity as a result of mal-union after supracondylar fracture (Fig 22.38). This was corrected by a supracondylar wedge osteotomy (Fig 22.39). Unfortunately an associated internal rotation deformity was not corrected and the patient still had an apparent varus deformity (Fig 22.40). The degree of rotatory deformity can be appreciated by measuring the relative external and internal rotation of the shoulder (Fig 22.41).

with an exploration of the brachial artery for vascular insufficiency. It is a disastrous exercise in the case of fractures which arrive late and are already well on the way to bony union. It is far better to allow the fracture to unite in its displaced position and to correct any residual deformity when growth has ceased. Apart from minor limitation of movement there is no functional disability from mal-union, and even the loss of movement may disappear, for as the child grows any residual bony prominence recedes from the vicinity of the elbow.[34] Late osteotomy to correct the cosmetic deformity brought about by rotatory mal-alignment or lateral tilt is an easy operation which does not involve extensive dissection round the joint and there is therefore no capsular contraction, or peri-articular ossification.

Kirschner wire fixation after closed reduction. Blind pinning of the fracture with crossed Kirschner wires has been suggested as a method of internal fixation for the difficult fracture in which the elbow cannot be flexed to a stable position.[39, 40, 41]

After closed reduction of the fracture Kirschner wires are inserted into the lower fragment just lateral to the olecranon. Two wires should always be used, one passing almost vertically up the medulla of the proximal fragment for 4 to 5 centimetres, the other inserted at an angle of 30 degrees just traverses the medial cortex of the humeral shaft. The distal ends of the pins must be bent over to prevent migration and may be left outside the skin.[40] Another, but more difficult technique is to insert the wires from either side at angles of 45 degrees.[39] In either case the pins must be removed in four to five weeks. This method has the advantage that the fracture is made stable with the elbow flexed at a right angle or below and this method of fixation could be useful in the management of fractures with vascular complications. It requires, however, an accurate closed reduction and a fairly high degree of technical skill to insert the Kirschner wires correctly. It is not a method to be used by those unfamiliar with the technique of blind pinning. Also, the technique is not without its complications. In one series of 110 patients there were five which developed nerve lesions after reduction and pinning, three had infections of the elbow, and there were five pin track infections.[40]

The use of skeletal traction. It is claimed that overhead olecranon traction, with either a threaded pin,[24] or a special traction screw,[42] allows the forearm to be pronated, preventing the tendency to varus deformity.[24] It is suggested that the incidence of varus deformity is higher when Dunlop traction is used because the forearm usually lies in supination.* Although the surgeons advocating this method of traction report a very small incidence of pin track infection, pins through the olecranon are known to have caused disastrous stiffness as a result of infection and it is doubtful if the small gain is worth the risk of complications from pin track infection. Dunlop traction produces the same results with less hazard.

Osteotomy for cubitus varus or valgus. If, when normal movement has been regained, there is a significant lateral tilt of the lower fragment this can be corrected by wedge osteotomy of the lower end of the humerus. It is unusual for a valgus tilt to increase the carrying angle to such a degree that it produces a cosmetic deformity, or endangers the ulnar nerve, but even a small amount of cubitus varus can result in an ugly 'gunstock' deformity which is not corrected by growth (Fig 22.37). As there is no functional disability during childhood and correction is easier to carry out when the bones are fully grown, operation is preferably deferred until adolescence. With careful technique the osteotomy can be done a few months after the fracture provided a full range of movement has been restored,[43] but the fragments are very small and it may be difficult to assure an adequate correction. It must also be remembered that the effect of lateral tilt of the lower fragment can be increased by rotatory mal-alignment and that any corrective osteotomy which does not take this into account may fail (Figs 22.38 to 22.41). In one series of 15 cases where in most instances no attempt had been made to correct the rotation there was a 30 per cent failure to eradicate the varus deformity.[44] Clinical measurement of this deformity is easily carried out by simply comparing the arc of rotation of the two shoulders[45]— if internal rotation is increased and external rotation is decreased then there is an internal rotation deformity which must be corrected. Through a lateral

or posterior triceps splitting approach the lower end of the humerus is exposed, an appropriate wedge of bone removed from just above the olecranon fossa and the lower fragment rotated to correct any rotation deformity. The elbow must be extended at this stage to insure that the deformity is corrected, and it is sometimes useful to to temporarily fix the fragments with a Kirschner wire while this is being done.[43] If possible, the osteotomy should then be stabilised by internal fixation, using either crossed Kirschner wires, or a small plate (Fig 22.39) and the arm immobilised in an above elbow plaster with the elbow flexed to just below the right angle for six weeks. Immobilisation of the elbow in full extension should only be used if it has not been possible to obtain stable internal fixation.

Supracondylar fracture with forward displacement. The flexion type of supracondylar fracture where the distal fragment is displaced forward is an uncommon injury and has an incidence of 4 per cent of all supracondylar fractures.[46] Reduction usually presents no difficulty. It is necessary only to apply traction to the limb and extend it fully. In the extended position it is easy to judge the carrying angle and under X-ray control to apply lateral pressure to correct tilting of the lower fragment. A posterior plaster slab is applied and lightly bandaged in position. While the patient is up and about the limb hangs by the side, but swelling of the fingers and hand should be avoided by elevating the limb on cushions when the patient sits or lies. The plaster is removed after three weeks. If reduction is perfect, full movements are regained easily (Figs 22.42 to 22.45). There are however some fractures, particularly in adults (who lack the child's thick periosteum to maintain reduction in extension), which are not stable in the extended position. Also, immobilisation in full extension, although safe in the young child, may result in permanent loss of flexion when used in the adult. To overcome this difficulty and to allow the elbow to be immobilised in flexion, Soltanpur in Tehran has devised an ingenious technique of manipulation and applying a plaster cast in two stages (Figs 22.46 to 22.49).[47] The fracture is first disengaged by traction and then the forearm held in supination with the elbow at a right angle while an assistant applies a plaster cylinder to the upper arm terminating at the fracture site (Fig 22.46). When this is thoroughly hard the forearm may be pushed backwards against the resistance of the upper arm cast (Figs 22.47 to 22.49) and the immobilisation completed by applying plaster to the

---

*This, however, is not true. It is just as easy to have the arm pronated in Dunlop traction as it is for it to be supinated. Similarly, in overhead traction the forearm can equally lie in supination or pronation. Try it yourself if you still do not believe it!

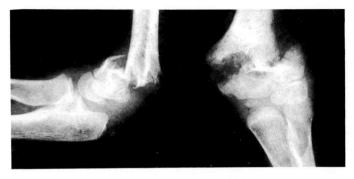

Fig 22.42 Flexion type of supracondylar fracture of the humerus with forward displacement.

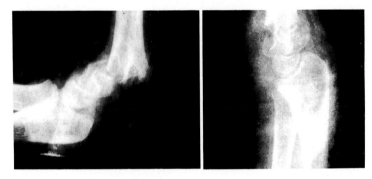

Fig 22.43   **Fig 22.44**

Figs 22.43 and 22.44 The displacement remained uncontrolled in flexion (Fig 22.43). It was satisfactorily reduced in the position of full extension (Fig 22.44).

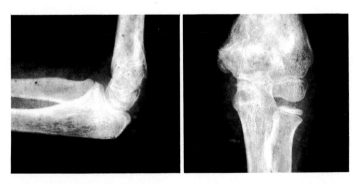

Fig 22.45 If the fracture unites without displacement full movement of the joint is regained without difficulty despite immobilisation in extension.

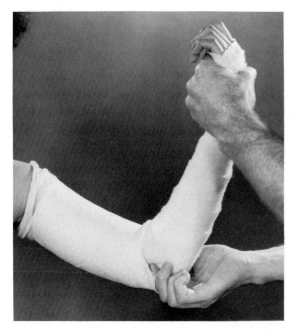

Fig 22.46

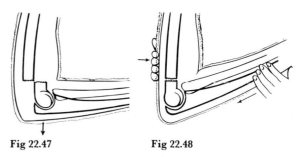

Fig 22.47   **Fig 22.48**

Figs 22.46 to 22.49 Soltanpur's two-stage technique for manipulation of an anterior supracondylar fracture.

Stage 1. (Fig 22.46)—The surgeon with one hand grasps the condylar mass and with the other keeps the forearm in supination and the elbow flexed while an above elbow cylinder is applied to the upper arm by his assistant. As the plaster sets the surgeon's fingers prevent the front edge cutting into the skin and keep the condylar mass free of immobilisation. Figures 22.47 and 22.48 show diagramatically the movements necessary to obtain reduction.

Stage 2. (Fig 22.49)—The fracture is reduced by placing one hand under the hard plaster cylinder and the other pushes the forearm firmly backwards. The forearm part of the plaster is then completed to immobilise the elbow at a right angle.

(Reproduced by kind permission of the Editor of the *Journal of Bone and Joint Surgery* and Professor A. Soltanpur from his paper in the *Journal of Bone and Joint Surgery* (1978) 60–B, 383).

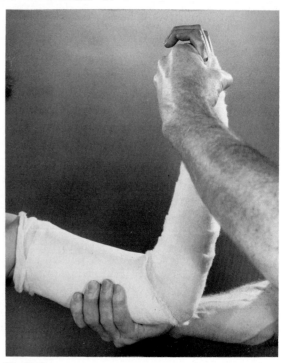

Fig 22.49

forearm. Although this method was primarily designed to treat the adult fracture, it has also been used successfully in children.[47]

INTERCONDYLAR FRACTURES AND SINGLE CONDYLE FRACTURES OF THE HUMERUS

Intercondylar fractures of the humerus are sustained more often by adults than children, often in the very elderly whose bones are porotic. They usually occur from falls direct on the back of the elbow. The wedge-shaped olecranon process is driven between the condyles which are fractured from each other and from the shaft by a T- or Y-shaped fracture. The condyles are usually tilted and rotated away from each other, and both are displaced forwards in relation to the shaft (Fig 22.50). The joint surface is distorted, and there is often comminution with separation of other smaller fragments.

Few injuries of the elbow are more difficult to treat. It may be impossible to secure any degree of accuracy in reduction by manipulation alone; and operative reduction with internal fixation presents very considerable problems of surgical technique. Indeed some-times in elderly patients when the bone is shattered it is best to accept the inevitability of restricted joint movement and attempt neither manipulative nor operative reduction.

Conservative management. Since it is a flexion injury with forward displacement of the fragments the joint must not be held in the acutely flexed position. Under anaesthesia the fragments are moulded together by the pressure of the palms of the hands, one on each side, and a posterior plaster slab is applied with the elbow at or just below the right angle. The limb is supported in a sling, finger and shoulder exercises being started from the beginning. The plaster cast is discarded in two to three weeks and the joint mobilised by the patient's own activity. Despite gross comminution the results are surprisingly good,[48, 49] at least half the normal range of movement can be expected and, being a non-weight-bearing joint, even severe damage of the articular surface causes relatively little disability. It is the treatment of choice in the elderly. An alternative conservative regime for the young adult is to encourage active exercises immediately by putting the arm up in

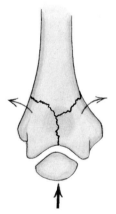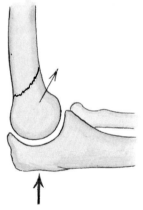

Fig 22.50 Intercondylar T fractures are due to the olecranon being wedged between the condyles, which are rotated laterally and displaced forwards.

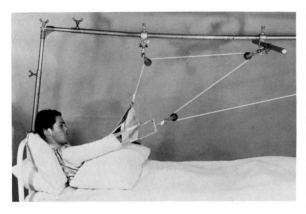

Fig 22.51 Traction for intercondylar fractures of the humerus. Skin traction with a spreader has been applied to the lower end of the humerus. The advantage of using skin extensions in this injury is that there is some compressive force applied to the displaced condylar fragments which helps to maintain the articular alignment. By using only one traction cord and a double pulley it is possible to produce a dynamic system which allows the patient to move the elbow while still maintaining his traction.

Dunlop traction or one of its modifications (Fig 22.51).

Theoretically, because the fracture is a flexion injury, manipulation and immobilisation should be carried out in full extension, and Figures 22.52 and 22.53 illustrate the excellent result which can sometimes be obtained. However, in practice immobilisation of the adult elbow fracture in full extension is not without its hazards as far as limited motion is concerned, and immobilisation in the mid-flexed position after moulding the lower end of the humerus is probably the safest conservative measure.

Operative reduction with internal fixation. This is indicated for open fractures and fractures where external splintage is not possible.[50] It should also be considered when the fracture occurs in a young adult, although there is little evidence that, except in the most expert hands, open reduction gives a better functional result than the conservative regimes outlined above. This is a difficult operation, not to be undertaken lightly. The problems are summarised in this quotation from a well known text book on fractures: '*anyone who has operated upon these badly broken and comminuted fractures of the lower end of the humerus must have been impressed by the extreme difficulty of fixing the fragments in their proper position*'.[51] The injury may be exposed through a mid-line incision either splitting the triceps, or by osteotomy of the olecranon

and refraction of the triceps insertion,[52] or through two incisions one on the lateral and the other on the medial aspect. There should be minimal dissection and separation of soft tissue attachments to the condyles. Small, completely loose interposed fragments of bone are removed to ensure accurate apposition of the main fragments. It is essential to replace the two condyles accurately in relation to each other and fix them with a screw transversely just below the epicondyles. Mervyn Evans[53] suggested that this was all that was needed, thus converting the injury to a simple supracondylar fracture relatively easy to manage. He described a simple technique of exposing the fracture through a medial or lateral incision, slipping the index finger across the joint to control the fragment on the opposite side, and inserting a transverse screw across the intercondylar fracture under X-ray control (Fig 22.54). However, having embarked on open reduction and internal fixation it seems better to complete it either by using crossed Kirschner wires, or as is shown in the case in Figures 22.55 and 22.56. Through a lateral incision the lateral condyle was replaced and fixed to the shaft of the humerus with a nail; then through a medial incision, after protecting the ulnar nerve, the medial condyle was screwed in position. After the simple support of a sling for two weeks, movements were started and good function regained.

Representatives of the Swiss A.O. group advise open reduction and internal fixation of these injuries and demonstrate very beautifully how accurate reduction can be achieved by the use of two or three cancellous screws, with sometimes a plate to control the transverse element of the fracture.[52] No long term follow-up is available but the immediate results reveal a 50 per cent full recovery which is an improvement on results from conservative treatment. However, against these results must be weighed the considerable time and technical skill necessary to achieve them and the complications of any open fracture procedure. On balance, conservative management is less likely to give trouble in the long run and is no more likely to be the cause of later degenerative arthritis.

Fractures of single condyles. These fractures are relatively uncommon and usually occur in adults. When one or other condyle is displaced sufficiently to interfere with the normal joint line open reduction and internal fixation is the treatment of choice and should be carried out as soon as possible. Figure 22.57 illustrates such a case where the medial condyle is displaced superiorly, laterally and anteriorly. If uncorrected this may lead to subluxation of the elbow,

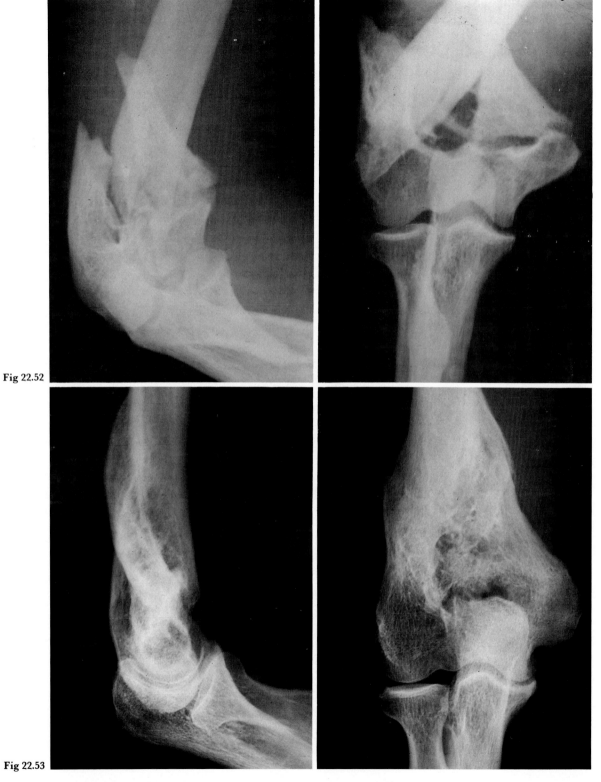

Fig 22.52

Fig 22.53

Figs 22.52 and 22.53 Intercondylar fracture before and after manipulative reduction and immobilisation in full extension of the elbow. The patient regained extension movement to 180 degrees and flexion to 45 degrees.

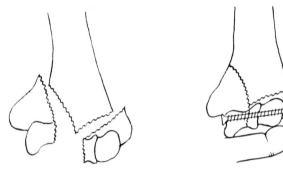

Fig 22.54 Diagram of the Mervyn Evans' method of fixation of the condylar fragments of a Y-shaped supra-condylar fracture of the humerus. The fragment on the far side of the incision is held with the index finger inserted across the joint while a screw is inserted to stabilise the separated condyles. Thereafter the management is that of a supracondylar fracture. (Reproduced by the kind permission of the Editor of the *Journal of Bone and Joint Surgery* and Mr Mervyn Evans from his paper in the *Journal of Bone and Joint Surgery* (1953) 35–B, 381).

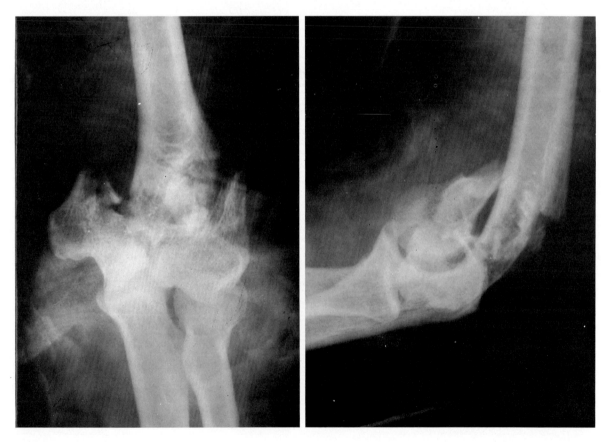

Fig 22.55 Typical T-shaped intercondylar fracture of the humerus with forward displacement of both main condylar fragments, tilting and rotation of the condyles away from each other, distortion of the joint surface and separation of several small fragments.

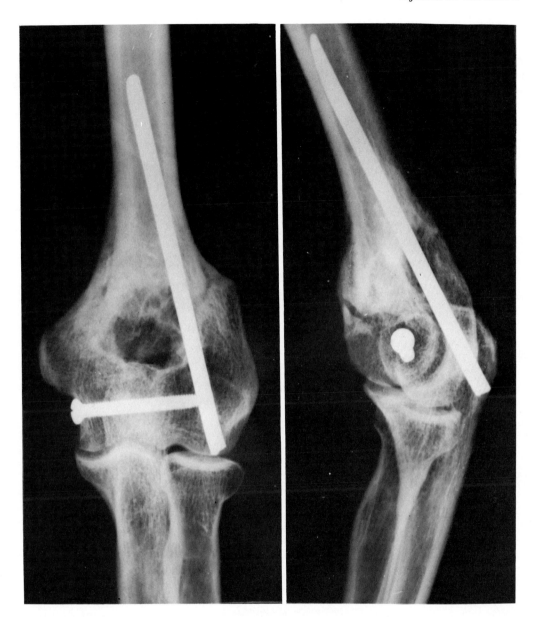

Fig 22.56 After operative reduction and internal fixation. Through a lateral incision the lateral condyle was replaced and fixed to the shaft with a short Rush nail. Through a medial incision, after protecting the ulnar nerve, the medial condyle was replaced and fixed with a transverse screw. Full movement was regained with normal function.

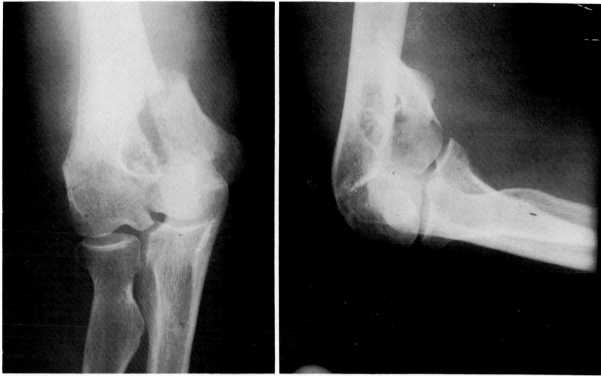

Fig 22.57

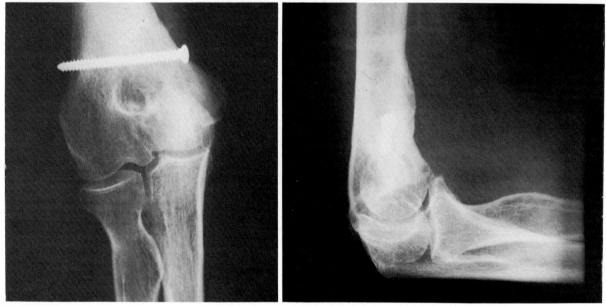

Fig 22.58

Figs 22.57 and 22.58 A 54-year-old lady fell on to the point of her elbow and sustained a fracture of the medial condyle of the humerus with disruption of the ulnar-humeral joint. Already there is anterior subluxation of the loose fragment. Through a medial approach a reasonable, although not perfect, reduction was obtained and fixed with a screw. Six months later the patient was only restricted in the last 30 degrees of extension.

and certainly degenerative arthritis will be inevitable at a later date. Figure 22.58 shows the elbow six months after internal fixation using a transverse screw. Even at that stage the patient had regained full flexion and was only limited in the last 30 degrees of extension. No conservative measures could be expected to produce as satisfactory a result.

EPIPHYSEAL INJURIES OF THE LOWER END OF THE HUMERUS

The epiphysis at the lower end of the humerus includes three main centres of ossification, one appearing during the second year for the capitellum, and two appearing several years later, a double centre for the trochlea and one for the medial epicondyle. There is occasionally a small separate centre for the lateral epicondyle (Fig 22.59). The

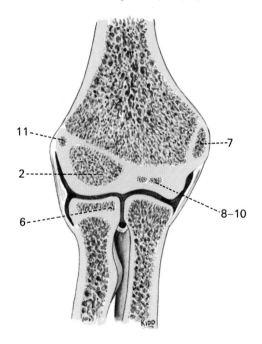

Fig 22.59 The epiphyses at the elbow joint, the figures indicating the year of appearance of each centre of ossification.

medial epicondyle soon separates from the rest of the epiphysis by an extension of the shaft between it and the trochlea. The capitellum and trochlea fuse to each other shortly after puberty, and to the shaft a year or two after puberty. The medial epicondyle fuses one or so years later and can be as late as 17 years of age.

A fall on the point of the flexed elbow may displace the whole of this epiphysis forward, the separated

fragment including the ossific centres of the capitellum, the trochlea and sometimes the medial epicondyle. More often, as a result of a fall on the outstretched hand, there is a fracture through the cartilage and one of the centres is pulled from the rest by muscle traction. When the joint is forced into valgus the epiphysis of the medial epicondyle may be avulsed by the common flexor group of muscles which are attached to it. Similarly when the joint is forced into varus the capitellum may be avulsed by the common extensor origin. The lateral epicondyle has such a small and inconstant ossific centre that it is seldom avulsed independently of the rest of the condyle, except when associated with dislocation of the elbow.

Displacements of the epiphyses at the elbow joint show the feature that characterises nearly all epiphyseal displacements. The line of fracture does not coincide exactly with the epiphyseal line but lies close to it on the diaphyseal side. The displaced fragment includes the epiphysis, the epiphyseal line and a triangular fragment from the metaphysis. The triangular fragment is always separated from the margin of the diaphysis over which the epiphysis is displaced. As in other epiphyseal injuries retardation of growth is rare unless there is a compression or segmental injury.

Summary of epiphyseal injuries of lower end of humerus. The epiphyseal injuries at the elbow include:

1. Displacement forwards of the whole of the lower humeral epiphysis.
2. Compression injury of the trochlea or capitellum.
3. Displacement of parts of the lower humerus epiphysis.

Which include:

1. Displacement of the lateral condyle of the humerus which may be rotated out of the joint and cause serious disability unless recognised and corrected.
2. Separation of the epiphysis of the lateral epicondyle which is seldom important.
3. Separation of the epiphysis of the medial epicondyle which is common and very important, often with inclusion of the fragment within the joint.

All these will now be discussed in the succeeding pages.

Forward displacement of the lower humeral epiphysis.
The detached fragment consists of the whole of the cartilage of the lower end of the humerus including the epiphyses of the capitellum and trochlea and sometimes of the medial epicondyle. A clear recognition of this injury is important because it is

easily overlooked. The epiphysis is normally tilted slightly forwards in relation to the shaft of the humerus, and displacement may amount to no more than slight exaggeration of this normal tilt. If it is not recognised, and treatment is carried out as for simple traumatic synovitis by immobilising the joint in the flexed position with a collar-and-cuff sling, the epiphysis unites with forward tilting, and extension movement of the elbow is then limited permanently by a corresponding degree.

Radiographic diagnosis. The difficulty of diagnosis is shown in Figure 22.60. These radiographs might easily be passed as showing no bone injury, and yet there is forward displacement of the epiphysis sufficient to cause permanent limitation of movement. If there is doubt, radiographs should be taken of the opposite elbow for comparison (Figs 22.61 and 22.62). The axis of the humerus is determined by dropping a line down the front of the shaft—if the axis of the epiphysis is compared with this, it is found that whereas the normal tilt is no more than about 25 degrees, on the injured side there is a tilt of nearly 60 degrees. Moreover, in the normal elbow at least two-thirds of the epiphysis lies behind the line of the front of the humeral shaft, whereas on the injured side the greater part of the epiphysis is in front.*

Treatment. The injury is a flexion fracture with forward displacement and it must not be treated in the flexed position. The elbow should be extended fully, and immobilised in the extended position by means of a plaster slab for three weeks. A normal range of movement will then be regained (Fig 22.63).

Epiphyseal separation with medial and posterior displacement.[55a]

This is a rare type of epiphyseal displacement which may be mistaken for a supracondylar fracture, a dislocation of the elbow, or a lateral condylar fracture. The whole of the lower humeral epiphysis is displaced medially, and usually posteriorly in relation to the humeral shaft. It can be distinguished from a dislocation or a lateral condyle fracture by observing that the radial head maintains

---

*Cohn's Line. In the young child a line bisecting the shaft of the humerus, projected vertically downwards lies behind the posterior limit of the capitellum.[54] Ghosh, in West Bengal has made a further extensive survey of this subject[55] and has found that in over 200 observations on Indian children more than half of the lower humeral epiphyses normally lie in front of the anterior humeral line, and that the humeral diaphyseal-epiphyseal angle varies from 30 to 80 degrees. There is therefore a wide difference between normals and it does seem clear that at least half the capitellum can lie in front of the anterior humeral border. But it is not the normal variation that matters, for this could be due to racial differences, it is the difference between normal and abnormal which is important.

its normal relationship with the capitellum. A small spike of bone is usually separated from the postero-lateral aspect of the humeral metaphysis and this may lead the unwary to suppose that the injury is part of an isolated fracture of the lateral condyle. Treatment should be conservative, as for a supracondylar fracture. There is no advantage to be gained by operative intervention.

Compression injury of the lower humeral epiphysis. Supracondylar fractures are rarely complicated by retardation of growth of the lower end of the humerus, and when this does occur it is always due either to segmental damage, or to compression. The 'fishtail' deformity which may result from an injury to the lateral condyle and epiphysis for the capitellum (see Fig 22.73) is probably due to segmental damage to the small part of the trochlea which is avulsed with the capitellum. Figure 22.64 shows the X-rays of a 7-year-old child with an incomplete supracondylar fracture which was virtually undisplaced. Figures 22.65 and 22.66 are comparison views of the elbows 18 months later, when it is already clear that there is retardation of trochlear growth and some irregularity of the capitellar epiphysis, suggestive of traumatic osteochondritis. X-rays taken 12 years later at the end of growth (Fig 22.67) showed gross deformity of the trochlear notch and some mal-formation of the capitellum. There was broadening of the elbow joint, limited full extension, and already attacks of pain brought on by athletic activity. There is little doubt that the X-ray changes of retardation of epiphyseal growth are due to a compression injury of the epiphysis for the trochlea and are similar in those seen in the ankle, the knee and sometimes the wrist (see Chapter 19). Sometimes the damage to the trochlear epiphysis is very localised producing a narrow 'hatchet' defect within which the olecranon will mould itself a new articulation (Fig 22.68). If most of the trochlear epiphysis is involved traumatic arthritis in later life is inevitable (Fig 22.69) and this may be associated with ulnar nerve weakness.

Displacement of the epiphysis of the lateral condyle. This injury occurs between the ages of 5 and 15 years. Post-mortem studies[56] have shown that the injury can be produced by forced adduction with the forearm fully extended and supinated. The separated fragment is the whole lateral condyle of the humerus including the epiphysis of the capitellum, adjacent part of the trochlea, and part of the metaphysis immediately above the capitellum to

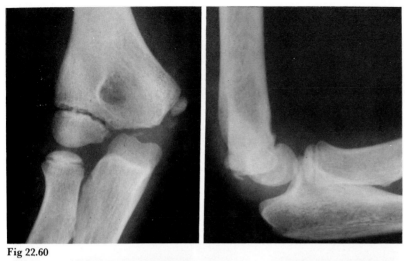

Fig 22.60 This patient fell on the point of the elbow. On first inspection of the radiographs there appears to be no bone injury or displacement.

Fig 22.60

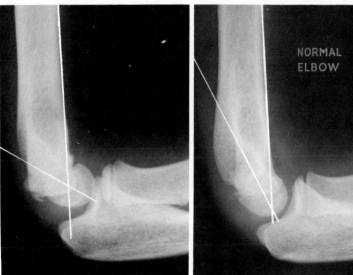

NORMAL ELBOW

Fig 22.61   Fig 22.62

Figs 22.61 and 22.62 Comparison with the normal elbow (Fig 22.62) (print reversed for easier comparison) shows that the lower humeral epiphysis is tilted and displaced forwards.

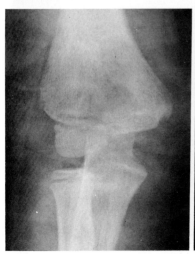

Fig 22.63 When the elbow is fully extended, the displacement is corrected. The joint must be immobilised in plaster in the position of full extension.

Fig 22.63

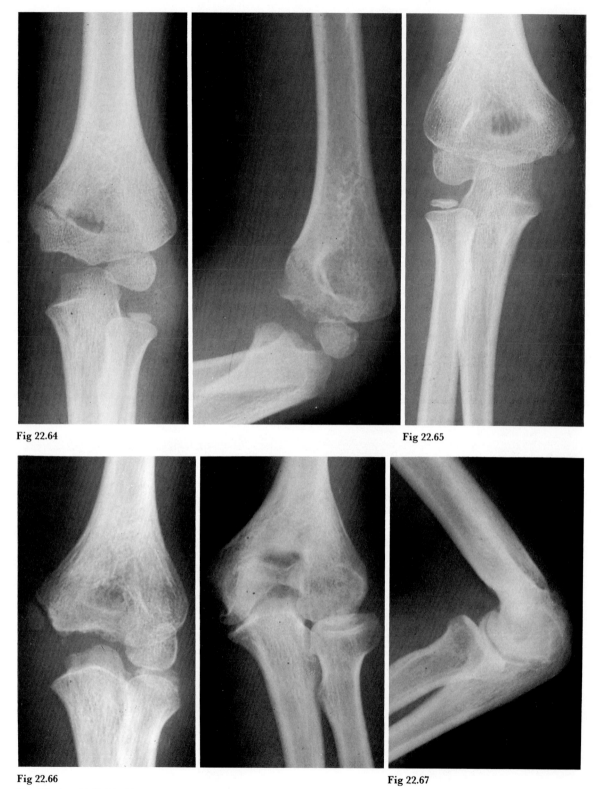

Fig 22.64

Fig 22.65

Fig 22.66

Fig 22.67

Figs 22.64 to 22.67 The X-rays shown in Figure 22.64 are those of a 7-year-old child who sustained a fracture of the supracondylar region with minimal displacement. Eighteen months later, however, the X-rays compared with the normal side suggest that there is retardation of trochlear growth (Figs 22.65 and 22.66), and this is confirmed in X-rays taken 12 years later (Fig 22.67).

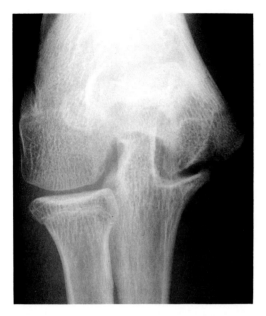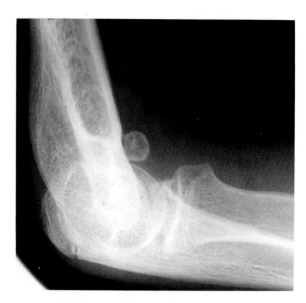

Fig 22.68 This 14-year-old boy sustained a supracondylar fracture of the humerus at the age of 5½. There was a very localised epiphyseal arrest of the lateral trochlear epiphysis which has resulted in a 'hatchet like' defect in the articular surface. Note how the olecranon has moulded itself to the narrow articular area. However, even at this age the boy has limited extension and pain from an arthritic loose body lying anteriorly.

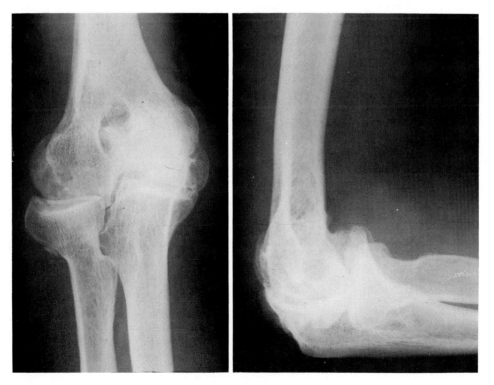

Fig 22.69 This patient had a supracondylar or external condylar fracture as a child. There was an extensive epiphyseal arrest of the trochlea which resulted in deformity of the ulnar-humeral joint. Osteoarthritic change was the inevitable late result.

which the lateral ligament of the elbow and the common extensor origin of muscles are attached (Fig 22.70). The fragment may be stabilised by an intact hinge of trochlear cartilage, not displaced, but the addition of axial strain will break the hinge and produce the typical unstable fracture. Sometimes the injury is part of a fracture dislocation of the elbow joint (see Fig 22.82). If this has been a subluxation and is reduced it can easily be missed unless the joint stability is tested.[57] The radiograph shows only the ossific nucleus of this large piece of incompletely ossified cartilage, and this may account for the frequency with which the injury is overlooked or the displacement misinterpreted. Nevertheless if the normal shape of the epiphysis of the capitellum is recalled three degrees of displacement can easily be recognised.

1. The musculo-tendinous origin of the common extensor muscles of the forearm with the periosteum overlying the fragment may be torn incompletely in which case the condyle is displaced laterally but not rotated, and its fractured surface remains in apposition with the fractured surface of its bed. These fractures usually unite by bone whether or not the slight lateral displacement is corrected.

2. The soft tissue attachments may be ruptured completely, but without tilting the condylar fragment with gross malalignment. Radiographically these cases resemble the first degree fracture, but they are very unstable when examined under anaesthetic and can go on to non-union. This type should be treated by internal fixation.[58]

3. The tendinous origin and periosteum may be completely ruptured so that the common extensor muscles avulse the fragment and rotate it from the joint with its fractured surface directed laterally and its articular surface medially (Fig 22.71). There may be more than 90 degrees of rotational displacement and the fragment lies almost upside down. Moreover, it is rotated not only round a horizontal axis, but also round a vertical axis, so that the outer part of the epiphysis and the metaphyseal fragment lie on the inner side, and the medial part of the epiphysis on the lateral side. There is no contact between the fractured surfaces and, unless the displacement is corrected, bony union cannot take place. Repair is by fibrous tissue which is not strong enough to resist the continued thrust of the radius. Displacement of the condylar fragment increases gradually. Cubitus valgus deformity develops and the carrying angle may become as much as 40 or 50 degrees. Delayed ulnar palsy often arises in adult life. The ulnar nerve is normally relaxed when the elbow is extended, and

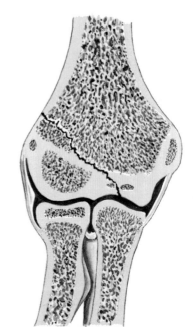

Fig 22.70

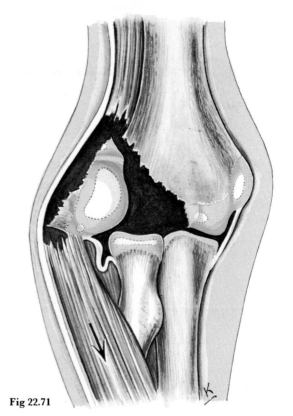

Fig 22.71

Figs 22.70 and 22.71 Line of fracture in separation of lateral condylar epiphysis (Fig 22.70). The epiphysis is rotated out of the joint by the pull of extensor muscles (Fig 22.71).

relatively taut when the joint is flexed. In the presence of marked cubitus valgus deformity the lengthened course of the nerve round the medial side of the joint makes it taut even in extension and if the joint is flexed the nerve is overstretched. Vigorous flexion movements of strenuous activity cause tension and friction neuritis, with incomplete or even complete paralysis necessitating anterior transposition of the nerve. These complications are to be avoided by accurate reduction at the time of the original bone injury.

Manipulative reduction. When there is lateral but no rotatory displacement complete reduction can easily be secured by manipulation. The difficulty is in maintaining it. The fragment should be pressed into its bed by direct lateral compression of the elbow between the surgeon's two hands. Even with a rotatory deformity it is said to be possible in some cases to carry out a closed reduction.* After reduction the elbow is flexed to just above the right angle and immobilised with a plaster back-slab for three weeks. That reduction can be achieved is proved by Figures 22.72 and 22.73; but it must be appreciated that this is potentially a very unstable fracture, and that with conservative management it may end up either as a non-union, or as in this case, mal-union due to a fishtail deformity (Fig 22.73). For this reason all unstable external condylar fractures should be treated by open reduction and internal fixation.

Operative reduction. It has already been made clear that this fracture can be unstable, and it is important,

*'An assistant holds the limb by the wrist with one hand, with his other hand on the inner aspect of the elbow, and gently opens the joint on the lateral side so that there is slight cubitus varus, the surgeon then places both thumbs under the fragment and pushes it upwards and inwards, tilting it into the joint.' (R.W.-J.)

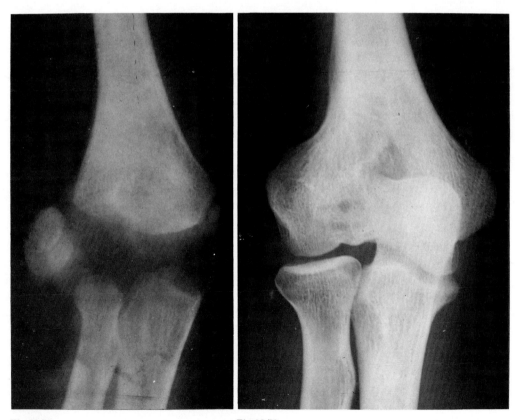

Fig 22.72   **Fig 22.73**

Figs 22.72 and 22.73 Displacement of lateral condyle epiphysis before and six years after manipulative reduction. Union has occurred but with some broadening of the lower end of the humerus—the so-called 'fish-tail' deformity (Fig 22.73).

if the initial treatment has been conservative, to have X-rays at weekly intervals to check the position of the fragments. Beware of a progressive forward tilt of the fragment associated with forward subluxation of the radial head, for this may progress on to non-union (Figs 22.74 to 22.76). If post-reduction radiographs do not show perfect reposition, or there is evidence of lateral instability or progressive forward tilt, operative reduction must be undertaken without delay.[58, 59, 60]

Through a direct lateral approach the fragment should be exposed with the minimum of dissection and care be taken not to detach the muscles and ligaments because they carry the blood supply, and division of these tissues may cause necrosis of bone and stiffness of the joint. Blood clot, bone spicules and capsular tissue which may be filling the bed of the bone are removed. The muscles arising from the condyle are gripped with forceps and the fragment is pulled upwards and rotated into position. Reduction should be maintained by internal fixation using a pin or Kirschner wire. Catgut sutures and the like have an uncanny knack of either stretching or coming undone, and several cases of non-union have been reported after using this technique[58] (Figs 22.77 and 22.78). It is preferable therefore to fix the fragment with a screw, two Kirschner wires, or a similar device such as a Smillie pin. The arm should be immobilised

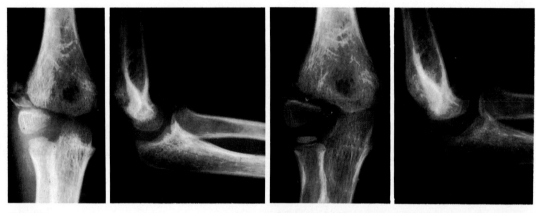

Fig 22.74   **Fig 22.75**

Figs 22.74 to 22.76 Non-union of lateral condylar fracture. Figure 22.74 shows the appearance after one month (conservative treatment). There is clearly no union. A month later (Fig 22.75) the union is even less obvious and the radial head is displacing anteriorly. Figure 22.76 shows established non-union four years later. (Reproduced by kind permission of the *British Journal of Surgery* from J. N. Wilson's article (1955) Fractures of the external condyle of humerus in children. *British Journal of Surgery*, 43, 88).

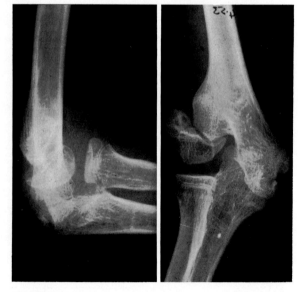

Fig 22.76

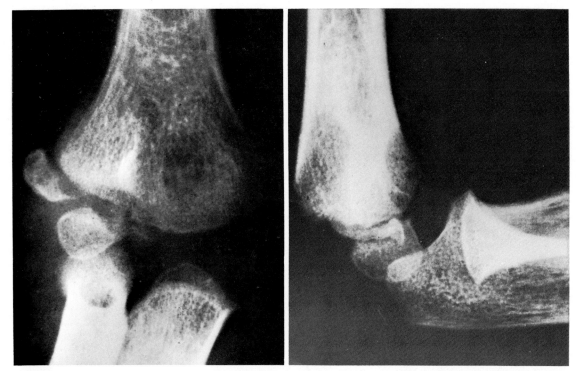

Fig 22.77

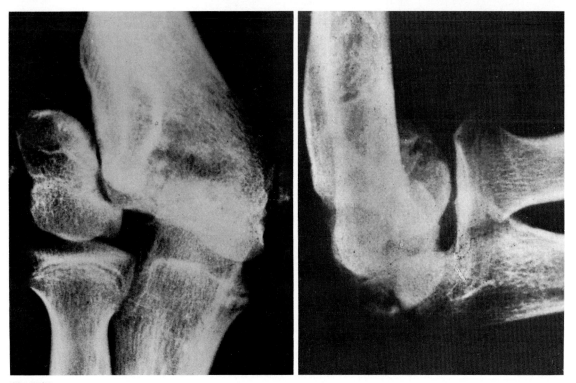

Fig 22.78

Figs 22.77 and 22.78 Figure 22.77 shows the appearance of a lateral condylar fracture one month after open reduction and soft tissue suture. Note the lateral subluxation of the condylar fragment. Figure 22.78 shows the established non-union eight years later. (From Mr C. C. Jeffrey's paper (1958) *Journal of Bone and Joint Surgery*, 40–B, 396. Reproduced by kind permission of the author and the Editor of the *Journal of Bone and Joint Surgery*).

in plaster with the elbow at a right angle for three to four weeks and the pins are removed at three months (Figs 22.79 to 22.81).

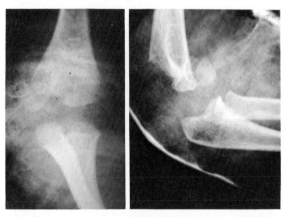

Fig 22.79   Fig 22.80

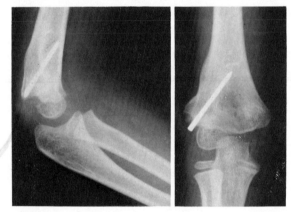

Fig 22.81

Figs 22.79 to 22.81 Figures 22.79 and 22.80 show the radiographs of a widely displaced condylar fracture prior to open reduction. Figure 22.81 shows the same case four months after fixation with a bone pin. (Reproduced by kind permission of the *British Journal of Surgery* from J. N. Wilson's article (1955) Fractures of the external condyle of humerus in children. *British Journal of Surgery*, 43, 88).

Treatment of old ununited fractures of the lateral condyle. Although the difficulties of operative reduction are very much greater after the first few weeks, it may be possible to reduce the displaced fragment even up to a year after injury. However, the longer the delay before reduction the greater is the risk of avascular necrosis of the fragment and stiffness of the elbow, both of which can be the result of the extensive soft tissue release necessary to obtain any sort of acceptable position of the fracture. This has led some surgeons to the view that no open reduction should be attempted after as short a period as three weeks, and if non-union and its inevitable cubitus valgus deformity is a certainty a prophylactic anterior transposition of the ulnar nerve should be carried out.[56] Either procedure is preferable to excision of the fragment which does little or nothing to improve the range of movement or stability of the joint. Through an extended lateral approach the fractured surfaces are cleared and freshened, packed with autogenous cancellous bone, and fixed with a screw or nail (Figs 22.82 to 22.84). In cases where the fracture has only occurred a few months ago successful union has been obtained by drilling across the fracture and packing the drill hole with cancellous bone.[58]

A useful distinction has been made between non-union in good position and non-union in poor position.[60a] Operative treatment for non-union in good position is always worthwhile, but it has been rightly pointed out that the stripping necessary to reduce the badly positioned fracture may seriously damage its blood supply with premature closure of its epiphysis. This will cause a progressive valgus deformity and little will be gained from surgery. Moreover after several years, owing to secondary contracture of soft tissues and distorted growth of the condylar fragment, operative reduction is impossible. The fragment should still not be excised because even in its displaced position it augments stability of the joint. The exaggerated carrying angle may be corrected by osteotomy, but as a rule the disability is not sufficient to warrant operation unless delayed ulnar palsy supervenes and this can be relieved by anterior transposition of the nerve.

Delayed ulnar palsy in old ununited fractures of the lateral condyle. This was discussed in the first volume. The nerve is stretched round the inner side of the deformed joint and it should be transposed to the front. Anterior displacement superficial to the flexor muscles is often successful, but it is better to bury the nerve deep in the muscles and at the same time divide the medial supracondylar septum to prevent kinking.

Displacement of the epiphysis for the medial condyle. This very rare injury is the mirror image of the fracture on the lateral side.[61] The fragment usually consists of a triangular piece of bone detached from the medial humeral metaphysis containing the

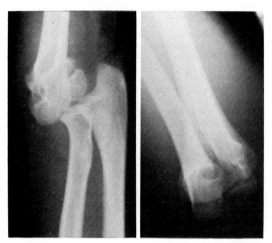

Fig 22.82

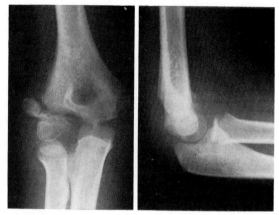

Fig 22.83

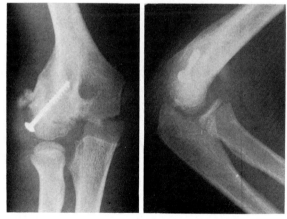

Fig 22.84

Figs 22.82 to 22.84 This boy's condylar fracture of the humerus was part of a fracture-dislocation of the elbow (Fig 22.82) and was still ununited six months after the injury (Fig 22.83). The fracture surface was freshened and packed with bone chips taken from the ilium The fragment was fixed with a cancellous screw. Three months later the fracture was soundly united (Fig 22.84).

cartilaginous trochlea and the ossified medial epicondyle (Figs 22.85 and 22.86). It is displaced and rotated in the vertical and horizontal planes so that the medial epicondyle faces distally while the articular surface faces anteriorly. Only sporadic cases have been reported in the literature.[62] It seems to be most likely to occur between the ages of 8 and 12 and is possibly caused by a fall on to the extended arm with the elbow forced into varus,[62] although associated valgus fractures of the olecranon lend support to the view that a valgus strain on an extended elbow may be the causative force.[62a] The diagnosis can be easily missed if it occurs before the ossific nucleus for the trochlea has been calcified and can be mistaken for an avulsion of the medial epicondyle.[63, 64, 65] The diagnosis should be suspected if there is a very wide displacement of the medial epicondyle at, or below the joint line, in a patient whose trochlear epiphysis is not yet ossified (Figs 22.87 and 22.88). Treatment by open reduction is essential and should be carried out without delay. In order to avoid the risk of avascular necrosis muscle attachments to the fragment should be preserved. Kirschner wire fixation should be used and the elbow immobilised in a plaster with the forearm flexed to 90 degrees for four to six weeks.

Displacement of the epiphysis of the lateral epicondyle. The lateral epicondyle is usually ossified by extension from the epiphysis of the capitellum, but occasionally there is a separate centre of ossification appearing at the age of 11 and fusing to the main epiphysis at the age of 13 or 14. During this short

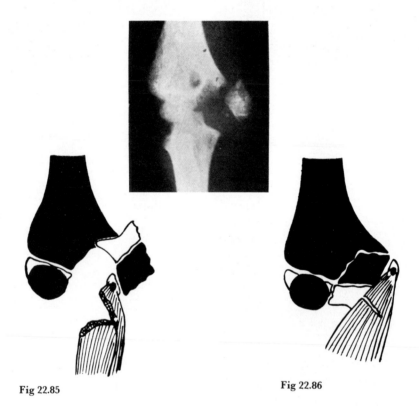

Fig 22.85   Fig 22.86

Figs 22.85 and 22.86 Figure 22.85 shows diagrammatically the displacement which occurs in fracture separation of the medial condylar epiphysis of humerus. The fragment consists of a block of bone avulsed from the metaphysis, along with the ossified epiphysis for the medial epicondyle and the cartilaginous trochlea epiphysis (in white). The radiological appearance is shown in the inset. There is usually a tear in the common flexor origin and the fragment is rotated through 90 degrees in the vertical and horizontal axis. The reduced position is seen in Figure 22.86. (Reproduced by the kind permission of the Editor of the *Journal of Bone and Joint Surgery* and Professor Chacha from his paper in the *Journal of Bone and Joint Surgery*, 52–A, 1453[62]).

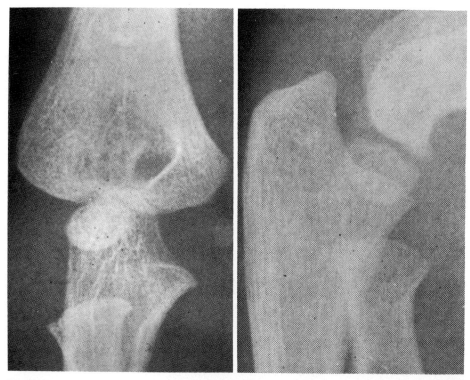

Fig 22.87

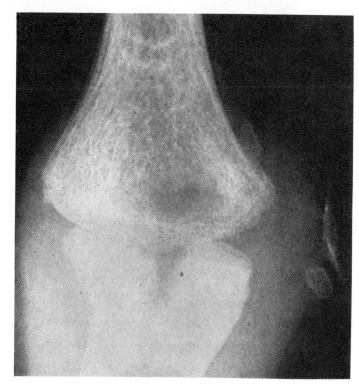

Figs 22.87 and 22.88 Fracture-dislocation of the medial condylar epiphysis should be suspected if there is wide separation of the medial epicondyle in a child whose trochlea has not yet ossified (Fig 22.87). A film taken six weeks later shows calcification at the site of separation making the diagnosis clear (Fig 22.88). (Reproduced by the kind permission of the Editor of the *Journal of Bone and Joint Surgery* and Miss Cothay from her paper in the *Journal of Bone and Joint Surgery*, 49–B, 766[63]).

Fig 22.88

interval there is a separate ossicle of bone to which the common extensor origin of muscles is attached, and traction of these muscles from varus strain of the joint may avulse the epicondyle instead of the whole condyle. Since the lateral epicondylar epiphysis is inconstant, and in any event exists as a separate ossicle only for a year or two, it is obvious that such avulsion must be unusual. Two very rare cases of avulsion of the lateral epicondyle with inclusion of the fragment in the elbow joint are illustrated in Figures 22.89 and 22.90. It must be understood that whereas avulsion of the epiphysis of the medial epicondyle, often with inclusion within the joint, is quite common, corresponding injury to the lateral condyle is very rare indeed.

Displacement of the epiphysis of the medial epicondyle. Under the age of 18, when the medial epicondyle fuses to the humerus, the epiphyseal line is a potential source of weakness. Avulsion of the epiphysis by traction of the common flexor muscles from valgus strain of the joint is one of the commonest injuries of the elbow joint in adolescents.

Four clinical types. There are four degrees of displacement of the epiphyseal fragment of bone (Fig 22.91).

1. The least serious injury is slight separation of the epiphysis with minimal displacement.
2. If the strain is more forcible the fragment is pulled down to the joint level and there is traumatic synovitis of the joint.

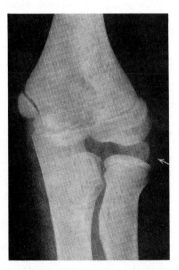

Fig 22.89 Inclusion of lateral epicondyle epiphysis in elbow joint after reduction of a dislocation in a boy aged 12.

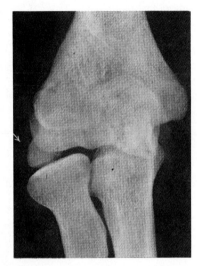

Fig 22.90 Youth aged 19, who at the age of 13 displaced the lateral epicondyle into the elbow without actually dislocating the joint.

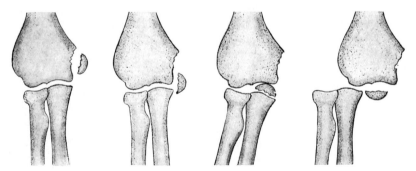

Fig 22.91 The four degrees of displacement of the epiphysis of the medial epicondyle.

3. If the valgus strain is still greater the fragment is avulsed, the joint is momentarily opened on the medial side, and as the humerus and ulna snap together again the epiphysis is included within the joint on the medial side.

4. If valgus strain continues the fourth degree of displacement arises, avulsion of the epicondyle being associated with complete lateral dislocation of the elbow; unless such a dislocation is manipulated carefully, the epiphysis may be included within the joint.[66]

The degree of displacement of the medial epicondyle is an index to the degree of stretching of all structures on the medial side of the joint, including the ulnar nerve. With increasing displacement we find an increasing incidence of traumatic ulnar neuritis. Complete lateral dislocation of the elbow and subluxation with inclusion of the epicondyle are nearly always associated with complete or incomplete ulnar paralysis. Not only is the nerve stretched and bruised but it may be kinked or distorted, and cases have been reported where it was displaced into the elbow joint with the bone fragment.[67]

Treatment of displacement of the medial epicondyle. Operative treatment is unnecessary for the first two degrees of displacement of the medial epicondyle.* The bone is pulled from its bed and the fracture haematoma may be obliterated by adjacent soft tissues so that fibrous union develops. Nevertheless the common flexor muscles gain a new attachment to the humerus through scar tissue which surrounds the bone fragment and encloses it like a sesamoid. The elbow becomes just as strong as if bony union has been secured. Indeed the most important part of the treatment of these cases is the treatment of the associated traumatic synovitis. The joint should be rested for three weeks in a plaster with the elbow extended about 60 degrees below the right angle.[68] It is always extension which is difficult to regain after this injury, whereas flexion returns quickly. Immobilisation below the right angle, therefore, speeds up the restoration of motion. It is often many months before full extension is regained, and on no account should forcible passive measures be used or permanent limitation of movement may be the result.

Diagnosis of inclusion of epicondyle in joint. The clinical diagnosis is seldom difficult despite the marked

---

* But beware of the widely displaced epicondyle at, or below the joint line. If the trochlear epiphysis has not yet ossified the epicondylar fracture may be associated with the more serious injury of separation of the medial humeral epiphysis (see Figures 22.87 and 22.88).

swelling of the joint and the oedema and ecchymosis on the inner side. When the elbow is compared with the normal joint of the opposite side it is usually obvious that the epicondyle has disappeared from its usual position. If there is also a complaint of tingling or numbness in the ulnar distribution, on the inner side of the fingers and hand, the diagnosis is almost certain. The radiographic evidence is equally obvious. Every patient between the ages of 7 and 17 should have a separate centre of ossification in the position of the medial epicondyle. If there is no ossicle in that position it should be searched for on the medial side of the joint; it will be found overlapping the shadow of the trochlea, or between the trochlea and the ulna. The fragment may be turned to one side or it may lie upside down. Even when antero-posterior radiographs are difficult to take without anaesthetising the patient, the diagnosis can be made from lateral radiographs. Patrick pointed out that if the epicondylar fragment can be seen at all in a lateral X-ray, it must be in the joint.[69]

Treatment of inclusion of medial epicondyle. It is essential to remove the fragment from the inner side of the joint or there will be serious and permanent limitation of movement, and kinking of the ulnar nerve may interfere with recovery from the paralysis. In recent injuries the fragment should be replaced as near to its normal position as possible by operative or manipulative reduction.

Manipulative reduction. In recent cases it may be possible to extract the epiphysis from the joint by manipulation[63] (Figs 22.92 and 22.93). The valgus deformity is slightly increased by abducting the forearm so that the medial side of the joint is opened. With the forearm fully supinated, and the wrist and fingers extended so that there is tension on the flexor group of muscles, the elbow is extended and the epicondyle may be felt to slip out of the joint.

Operative reduction. A short incision is made on the medial side of the joint. As soon as the deep fascia is divided it is seen that the inner aspect of the humerus below the raw bed of the epicondyle is uncovered, and that the muscles and fascia which normally cover it are turned into the joint. It is an easy matter to hook the muscles out, and with them the epicondyle. The bone is secured as close to its normal position as possible by one or two catgut sutures through adjacent soft tissues. It is unnecessary to nail or pin the fragment to the shaft. Any ulnar nerve weakness will usually recover without treatment and there is no necessity for an immediate anterior transposition. Provided the elbow joint is stable in extension it should then be immobilised for two or three weeks

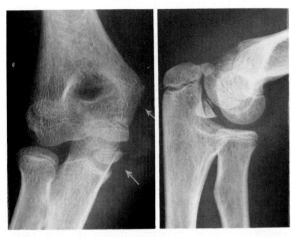

Fig 22.92

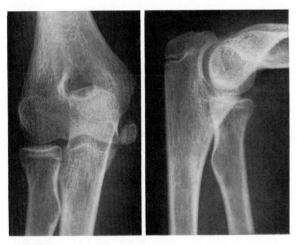

Fig 22.93

Figs 22.92 and 22.93 Inclusion of the medial epicondylar epiphysis within the elbow joint before and after reduction (by Mr Norman Roberts, Liverpool). There is only fibrous union, but movement and strength are normal.

with the forearm extended 60 degrees below the right angle.

DISLOCATION OF THE ELBOW JOINT

While supracondylar fractures of the humerus and some other injuries of the elbow occur with particular frequency in patients of certain age groups, dislocations of this joint may be sustained at any age, and in one series of 60 patients the age range was 5 to 76 years.[70] In the majority of cases the injury results from a fall on the outstretched hand, and the non-dominant arm is affected almost twice as often as the dominant side.[70, 71] Although the forearm bones are displaced backwards and laterally in about 80 per cent of the dislocations,[71] sometimes the displacement is purely backwards, or backwards and medially, and the brachialis anticus is torn from the coronoid process (Fig 22.94). Such avulsion encourages the formation of a haematoma beneath the displaced periosteum. In this subperiosteal haematoma bone is laid down and continues to be laid down until the periosteum is replaced in normal contact with bone by reduction of the displacement. Abnormal ossification is, of course, increased if the haematoma is scattered by repeated passive stretching or forcible movement. Thus, the first principle of treatment of dislocations of the elbow joint is prompt reduction of the displacement with immobilisation of the joint flexed to a right angle for about ten days and recovery of movement by active exercise alone without passive stretching or repeated forcible movement.

Clinical features. The deformity of backward dislocation of the elbow joint is to be distinguished from that of backwardly displaced supracondylar fractures by the relative immobility of the dislocated bones, and by the abnormal relationship of the olecranon to the epicondyles. The diagnosis must be confirmed by radiographic examination because otherwise it is impossible to know whether or not the dislocation is accompanied by fractures of the radial head, the epicondyles, or the condyles of the humerus.

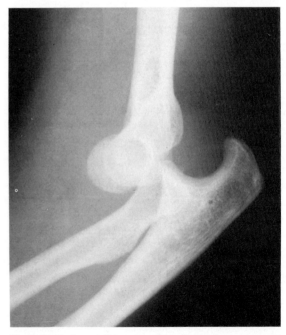

Fig 22.94 Backward dislocation of the elbow joint.

Manipulative reduction. If there is no associated fracture it is easy to reduce a dislocated elbow joint. There need be no violent traction, and certainly there should be no full extension of the joint as a preliminary to reduction by flexion. Still less is it wise to hyperextend the joint—this is a dangerous manoeuvre. Gentle traction should be applied to the forearm in the position in which it lies. While traction is maintained the joint is flexed and if there is lateral displacement appropriate pressure is applied.

After-treatment. A simple collar-and-cuff sling is applied with the elbow comfortably flexed to a right angle. Radiographs must be taken to confirm the accuracy of reduction. Reduction is usually stable but if not, a posterior slab of plaster of Paris may be applied to prevent redisplacement. It is important to check the stability of the joint *immediately* after reduction and if there is suggestion of instability X-rays should be taken within a few days and then at weekly intervals until the plaster is discarded (Figs 22.95 and 22.96). Shoulder and finger exercises are begun at once. If there is any instability movement of

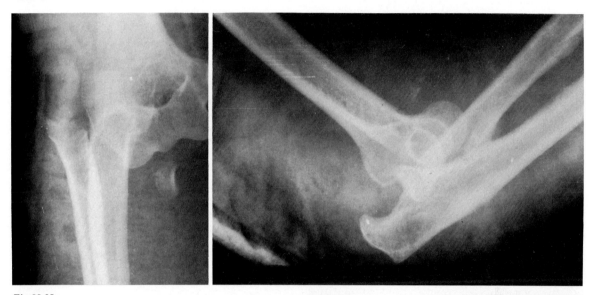

Fig 22.95

Figs 22.95 and 22.96 This elderly patient sustained a posterior dislocation of the elbow with a fracture of the neck of the radius. After reduction it was noted to be unstable but no further check X-ray was taken for two weeks. By then the dislocation had recurred—despite immobilisation (Fig 22.95). It was eventually stabilised by immobilisation for four weeks in acute flexion (Fig 22.96).

If a dislocated elbow is recorded as unstable at time of reduction X-ray again within a few days and then at weekly intervals.

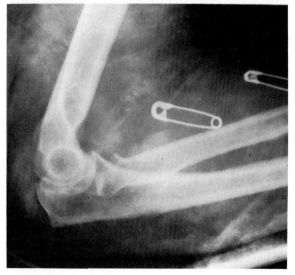

Fig 22.96

the elbow should not be instituted for three weeks, and it is then restored by the patient's unaided activity. There must be no massage and no passive or forcible movements. Such treatment causes increased stiffness and may produce myositis ossificans. In simple, stable dislocations immobilisation in a sling or collar-and-cuff should be discontinued after 10 to 14 days. There is good evidence to suggest that permanent stiffness in the uncomplicated case is directly related to the length of immobilisation.[71]

Myositis ossificans. This complication of traumatic subperiosteal ossification used to be very common in the days when vigorous physiotherapy was used in after-treatment with the object of accelerating recovery. The vigorous early movement when the joint should have been at rest, and the passive stretching in succeeding weeks, separated still more the torn anterior capsule and avulsed periosteum, thus increasing the volume of subperiosteal haematoma and the area of subperiosteal ossification in front of the joint. Now that such forceful after-treatment has been abandoned, this type of traumatic myositis ossificans is very unusual. However, beware of the over keen athlete, such as the 'intercollegiate football player who, without our knowledge, forcibly tried to gain full passive extension so that he could return to competition'.[71] As in all sporting injuries firm management is essential to protect the athlete from overdoing his efforts to restore function.

But even without such vigorous after-treatment, traumatic ossification can still occur when reduction has been delayed or when manipulative reduction on the day of injury has failed and a second manipulation is needed several days later. Especially is this so if the biceps and brachialis muscles have been avulsed with their periosteal insertions (Fig 22.97), or if there have been associated intra-articular fractures, particularly the head of the radius.[70]

The essential treatment is to protect the joint in a sling, usually with a posterior plaster slab incorporated in the dressing, for the usual period of three weeks, but no longer. If there is no massage or passive stretching, the patient's own guarded use within the limits of pain does no harm and does not aggravate the traumatic ossification. As months go by, the abnormal new bone matures to a relatively small mass and a full range of movement may be regained despite it. At its worst, the small area of consolidated bone may need to be dissected out and removed through a short incision 12 or more months after the original injury.

There is, however, a more common form of post-traumatic ossification which occurs in association with the attachments of the collateral ligaments. Fortunately, it very rarely causes any permanent loss of function.

Treatment of old unreduced dislocations. Although unreduced dislocations presenting many weeks or months after the injury are rare in Western societies, they are commonplace in the undeveloped countries. Manipulative reduction may still be possible three to four weeks after injury and is always worth a trial. Steady prolonged traction is necessary while the elbow is gradually flexed. If reduction is successful the joint should be immobilised in flexion for three or four weeks. Active movements are then permitted whether or not there is evidence of traumatic subperiosteal ossification. Abnormal bone

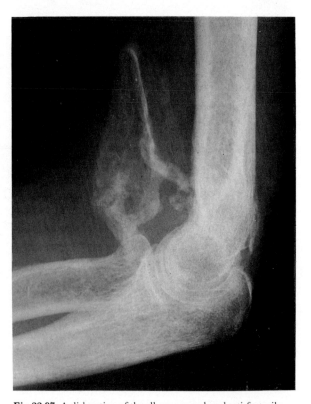

Fig 22.97 A dislocation of the elbow was reduced satisfactorily but three days later check X-rays showed that there was recurrent subluxation, probably from interposition of capsule in front of the joint on the lateral side. A second manipulation was confirmed to be successful by X-rays in the theatre. One week later there was induration in front of the lower arm. Later radiographs showed clear evidence of traumatic subperiosteal ossification ('myositis ossificans'). At no time had there been massage or passive stretching. The ossification is in the subperiosteal haematoma at the site of avulsion of biceps and brachialis. (Treated by Mr A. Ronald, Barrow-in-Furness).

formation is promoted by passive stretching but not by active exercise, and it consolidates just as rapidly when gentle exercise is permitted as when the joint is immobilised rigidly for many months. Moreover, a far better range of movement will be regained if active exercises are encouraged after three or four weeks.

Open reduction. This is a difficult procedure, but if closed manipulation fails it is the only surgical treatment available for a late dislocation in the growing child, where the presence of open epiphyses prevent an arthroplasty being performed. It has less place in the management of late dislocations in the adult where after a lapse of eight weeks excision arthroplasty, or sometimes arthrodesis, is to be preferred.

Technique of open reduction (after Speed[72]). The operation is best carried out through a postero-lateral approach (for details see below under arthroplasty). By splitting the muscles of the triceps the whole of the back of the lower end of the humerus can be exposed. There is usually extensive new bone and thick scar tissue filling in the olecranon fossa and the defect between the humerus and the displaced forearm bones (Fig 22.98). This should be completely removed by subperiosteal dissection. The capsular and muscle attachments anteriorly and laterally, as well as posteriorly must be detached from the humerus by subperiosteal dissection, until the lower end of the bone is completely exposed. If this dissection is kept deep to the periosteum the ulnar nerve should not be at risk, but if there is any doubt about its location the nerve should be formally exposed and retracted out of harm's way. With the humerus displayed and the head of radius defined it is usually possible to twist the forearm and, by pressure, reduce the radio-humeral joint. Once this is reduced the upper end of the ulna will often slide over the trochlea, completing the reduction. After repair of the triceps, muscle and skin the arm is immobilised in plaster for two weeks with the elbow at 90 degrees. A long period of physiotherapy may be required to restore a useful range of movement and a night splint is necessary for several months to prevent contractures.

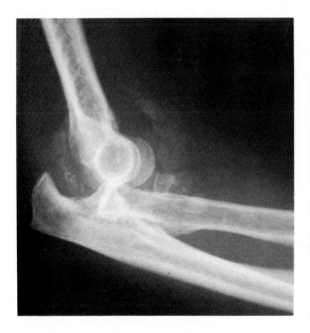

Fig 22.98 Two-month-old dislocation of the elbow. Failure to reduce the dislocation and so to replace the periosteum has caused myositis ossificans. Manipulative or operative reduction is therefore contraindicated and arthroplasty may offer the best prospect.

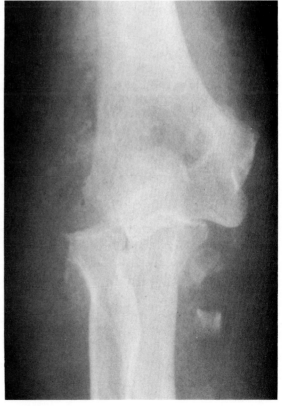

Arthroplasty of the elbow for old unreduced dislocations. When a dislocated elbow joint has been unreduced for many months and there is painful stiffness, arthroplasty is usually the best treatment. Through a long postero-lateral approach, extending from 3 inches (7.6 cm) above the olecranon to a point 2 to 3 inches (5.1 to 7.6 cm) distal to the head of the radius, the tendinous insertion of triceps is turned down as a tongue-like flap based on its olecranon attachment. The deep fibres of the triceps are then split to expose the back of the humerus. The dissection of the considerable scar tissue and callus in the olecranon fossa presents a difficulty at this stage and it is wise to isolate the ulnar nerve before embarking on this clearance. The lower end of the humerus should be removed at the level of the epicondyles; the olecranon process, coronoid and head of the radius are also excised. The forearm bones are brought forward into normal relationship with the humerus and the limb immobilised by means of a plaster cast in about 90 degrees of flexion for three weeks before active exercises are begun. It is important to realise that

brilliant as are the results of arthroplasty of the elbow in rheumatoid arthritis and old infective arthritis where fibrosis around the joint promotes stability, too free excision of bone in a recently injured elbow, and too early mobilisation after excision, may cause severe disability from the weakness of an almost flail limb.

The new surgical techniques for arthroplasty of the elbow using a hinged prosthesis with intramedullary fixation in the humerus and the ulna are a considerable advance over the simple excision arthroplasty just described. The purpose is of course to preserve stability as well as mobility (Figs 22.99 and 22.100). The results in the treatment of arthritis and traumatic stiffening of the elbow joint are encouraging; but it must be emphasised that these appliances should only be used where the operating theatre facilities are beyond reproach—conditions which are often lacking in the countries where late unreduced dislocation of the elbow is prevalent.

Arthrodesis of the elbow for old unreduced dislocations. The preference of most surgeons in the treatment of old unreduced dislocations of the elbow joint is always for

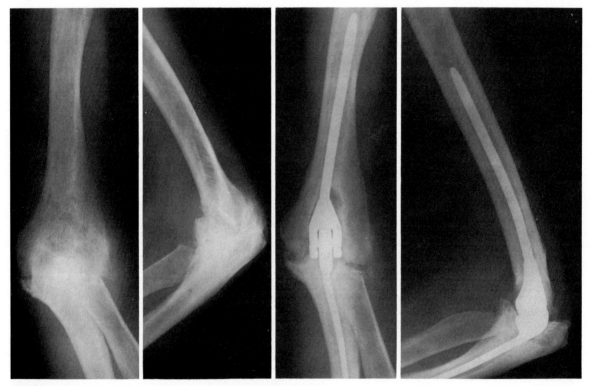

Fig 22.99   **Fig 22.100**

Figs 22.99 and 22.100 Elbow joint replacement using a hinged prosthesis may replace excision arthroplasty in the treatment of late unreduced dislocation. Figures 22.99 and 22.100 demonstrate a method used after old fracture-dislocation of the elbow.

arthroplasty, which if done carefully and with suitable after-treatment usually gives a joint with good movement and reasonable stability. But a good argument can be made for arthrodesis in the case of men who must pursue arduous labour and who have a full range of movement in the opposite joint. Certainly an elbow which is fused soundly is painless and strong, and in certain circumstances it may be better. Through the same approach used for open reduction or arthroplasty the joint surfaces of the humerus and ulna are denuded of cartilage and held in apposition by one or two bone screws. The joint should be fused with the forearm extended about 60 degrees below the right angle—an optimum working position and one which is cosmetically acceptable (Figs 22.101 and 22.102). Bony consolidation of an arthrodesis of the elbow can be slow and three months or more of immobilisation in a shoulder spica is usually essential. In order to preserve full radio-ulnar movement of the forearm it is often wise to excise the upper end of the radius, either at the time of the original arthrodesis of the humero-ulnar joint or sometimes at a secondary operation some months later.

FRACTURE-DISLOCATIONS OF THE ELBOW

Dislocation of the elbow joint with fracture of the coronoid process. In many dislocations of the elbow joint the injury to the insertion of the brachialis anticus is shown by a chip fracture of the coronoid process. Small fragments of bone may be retracted from the ulna. The injury is of no significance, and if the usual after-treatment is carried out by immobilising the joint in flexion the fracture will unite and cause no disability. When larger fragments of the coronoid are broken off the reduction may be less stable, and to guard against the possibility of redisplacement a posterior plaster slab should be used as well as a collar-and-cuff sling.

Forward dislocation of the elbow joint with fracture of the olecranon. The elbow is seldom dislocated forwards unless there is also a fracture of the olecranon. This injury is usually caused by a fall on the back of the upper forearm which fractures the ulna and drives both forearm bones forward (Fig 22.103). The ulnar nerve may be damaged by traction over the lower end of the humerus. The fracture-dislocation of the elbow is easily reduced by applying traction, extending the joint, and pressing backwards on the front of the upper forearm (Fig

22.104). Although the reduction is stable in extension and the olecranon fracture will unite given time, a better result will be obtained if the olecranon fragment is reduced and fixed by a screw or Rush nail. Sometimes a third fragment comprising the coronoid and part of the ulna immediately adjacent to it is separated anteriorly. This rarely gives trouble provided the olecranon is properly stabilised, and usually it falls back to an acceptable position. This operation should be followed by three to four weeks in an above elbow plaster (Figs 22.105 and 22.106), with the joint immobilised at a right angle. Alternatively the olecranon fracture can be fixed with Kirschner wires and a figure-of-eight tension suture (see Chapter 23).

Side-swipe fracture-dislocation of the elbow, or 'baby-car fracture'. This is a fracture-dislocation of the elbow with forward displacement of both forearm bones, fracture of the olecranon, fracture of the lower shaft of the humerus and fracture of the upper shaft of the ulna, sustained by drivers of cars who while resting an arm with the elbow projecting through the window met oncoming cars too closely (Fig 22.107). Originally it was thought that the injury was the particular penalty of small 8-horse-powered cars of pre-war days in which there was no room to move, and thus it was described as 'the baby-car fracture'. But the same fracture-dislocation occurs in the roomy and luxurious cars of the present era. These drivers also indulge in putting their elbows out too far, and the Americans have found a better title— the *side-swipe fracture*.

The combination of injuries is quite typical, and it presents a serious problem of treatment. There may be danger in trying to correct all displacements at once and succeeding in correcting none. The important displacement on which the surgeon should focus his attention is the forward dislocation of both forearm bones at the elbow joint. The fractures of the shafts of the humerus, ulna and sometimes the radius can always be dealt with successfully by later operative treatment, but unless the forward dislocation of the forearm bones at the elbow joint is reduced promptly there will be permanent disability with no better end-result than that of arthroplasty or arthrodesis of the joing. It may be possible to push back the upper ends of radius and ulna until the small curved articular surface at the front of the upper end of the ulna is in normal relation with the condyle of the humerus. But even if the dislocation is thus reduced, only immobilisation in full extension is likely to have any chance of preventing redisplacement and, as we have already said, this position in the adult may lead to unacceptable stiffness. Combine this problem with the difficulty of managing a humeral shaft fracture in the extended position and conservative treatment becomes a surgical nightmare. The fracture of the olecranon must be dealt with as soon as possible by reconstruction and internal fixation, or by excision of the fragment and repair of the triceps. The dislocation of the radius may reduce spontaneously when the ulnar fracture is stabilised, but sometimes reduction is obstructed by infolding of the orbicular ligament and requires open reduction. There is still some time after that to realign the fragments of the fractured humerus and the fractured forearm bones by open operation and internal fixation with intramedullary nails.

Dislocation of the elbow joint with fracture of the head of the radius. Dislocation of the elbow may be accompanied by a marginal or comminuted fracture of the head of the radius. One patient fell forward on both outstretched hands and sustained bilateral dislocation of the elbow joints with symmetrical marginal fractures of both heads of radius. There is no difficulty in reducing the dislocation. The fracture of the radius should then be treated as if it was an isolated injury. If there is a widely displaced marginal fragment this should be removed; but if there is comminution of the bone, the whole head must be removed. These operations should be performed two or three weeks after reduction of the dislocation.

A patient once showed his surgeon a scar on the inner side of his elbow and said that the head of the radius had been removed from it. It was pointed out that he meant the medial epicondyle but he insisted that it was the head of the radius. When the surgeon still showed disbelief the patient delved into his pockets and produced from his waistcoat—the head of the radius! One case has been reported of ulnar paralysis from the pressure of a displaced fragment of the head of the radius. This curious displacement is more readily understood when it is recognised that the primary injury was a dislocation of the elbow.

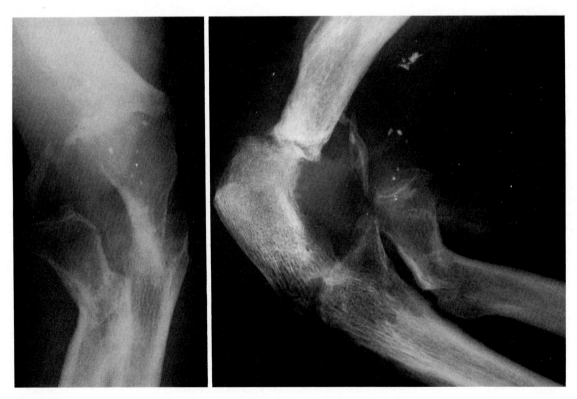

Fig 22.101

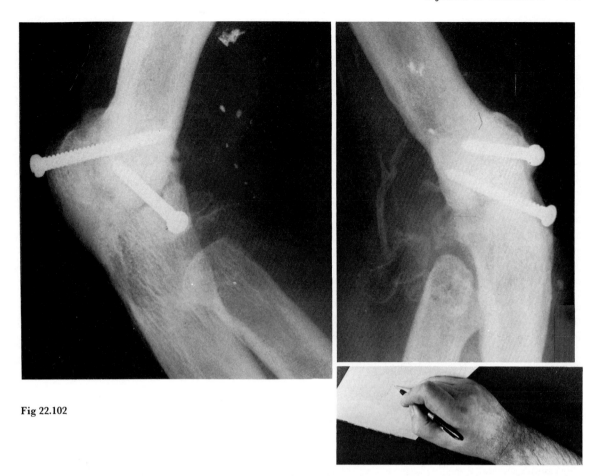

Fig 22.102

Figs 22.101 and 22.102 Figure 22.101 is the X-ray of a patient who sustained a severe compound fracture-dislocation of the right elbow a year before. The joint was flail and painless. Arthrodesis was successfully achieved with the forearm extended about 20 to 30 degrees below the right angle (Fig 22.102). The inset shows the patient writing completely naturally with the right forearm in the partly extended position.

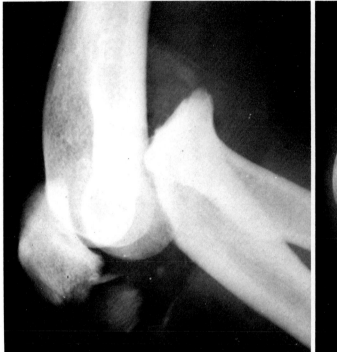

Fig 22.103 Forward dislocation of the elbow with fracture of the olecranon process—an injury that is sometimes complicated by paralysis of the ulnar nerve.

Fig 22.104 Same case as that of Figure 22.103 after manipulative reduction of the dislocation and suture of the olecranon. Repair of the fracture is usually slow.

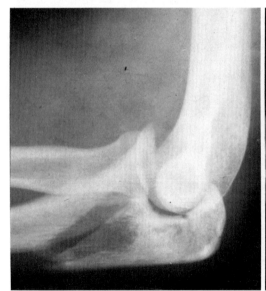
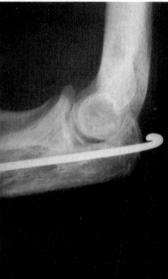
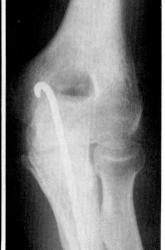

Fig 22.105 Forward subluxation of the elbow with an oblique fracture through the base of the olecranon.

Fig 22.106 Sound bony union three months after open reduction and Rush nailing of the olecranon fracture shown in Figure 22.105.

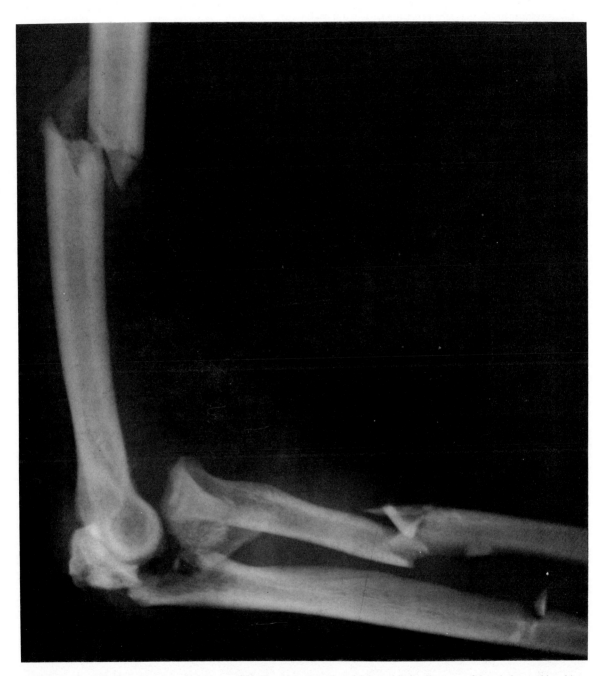

Fig 22.107 The typical combination of injuries produced by side-swipe when driving with the elbow out of the window and brushing too close to an oncoming car. There is always a comminuted fracture of the olecranon, forward dislocation of both bones, fracture of the mid-shaft of the humerus and fracture of the shaft of the ulna; in this case there was also a fracture of the shaft of the radius.

Figure 22.108 shows a backward dislocation with comminution of the radial head. After manipulative reduction some of the fragments lay near their normal position, but half the head of the radius was left stranded on the medial side of the joint. All fragments were removed through incisions on the medial and lateral side of the joint, and an almost normal range of movement was regained (Figs 22.109 to 22.111).

Dislocation of elbow joint with avulsion of the medial epicondyle. Lateral dislocation of the elbow joint may be associated with avulsion of the epiphysis of the medial epicondyle—these injuries have been discussed on page 629. There is often ulnar paralysis from traction injury of the nerve, and on rare occasions the nerve may even be trapped within the joint. Care must be taken in reducing the dislocation to avoid inclusion of the epiphysis on the side of the joint. Inclusion of the medial epicondyle within the joint after reduction of an elbow dislocation may be suspected if there is only a small amount of movement after a satisfactory manipulation. Usually after simple reduction the range of movement under anaesthetic is full.[73] Later treatment is the same as for uncomplicated dislocations; operative replacement of the epiphysis is not needed despite the frequency of fibrous and not bony union, but if included in the joint the fragment must be removed as early as possible. Operation is almost always necessary, although there are reports of extraction of the fragment by applying faradism to the flexor muscles.[69]

Dislocation of the elbow joint with posterior marginal fracture of the condyles. When the forearm bones dislocate backwards they may break off and carry with them the posterior margin of the lateral condyle of the humerus. Such a case was reported by Howard[74] in an Italian labourer; the displacement was unreduced and there was almost complete ankylosis of the joint. In the case of the patient whose radiographs are shown in Figure 22.112 reduction was made difficult not only because 11 days had elapsed since injury but because he had no hand or lower forearm—it had been amputated some years before. Despite the amputation he had worked as a general labourer and was anxious to get back to his job after this injury. By sustained traction on the stump for several minutes, and then gradual flexion of the elbow, a satisfactory reduction was gained (Fig 22.113). Eight weeks later the patient discharged himself from the clinic and went back to work at the docks; he had full flexion movement, and at that time limitation of extension by 30 degrees. Transcondylar fracture-dislocation of the elbow has also been described. In one reported case[75] the displaced articular fragment comprised both trochlea and capitellum and rested on the front of the humerus within the capsule. Open reduction and Kirschner wire fixation is the management of choice.

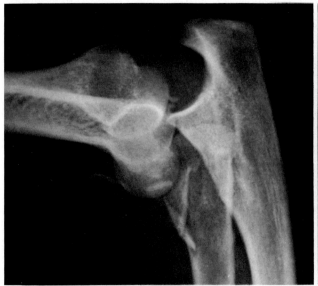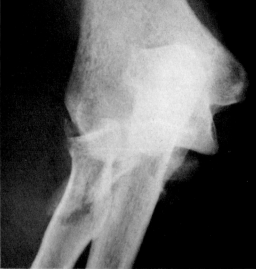

Fig 22.108 Dislocation of the elbow with comminuted fracture of the head of the radius (see Figs 22.109 to 22.111).

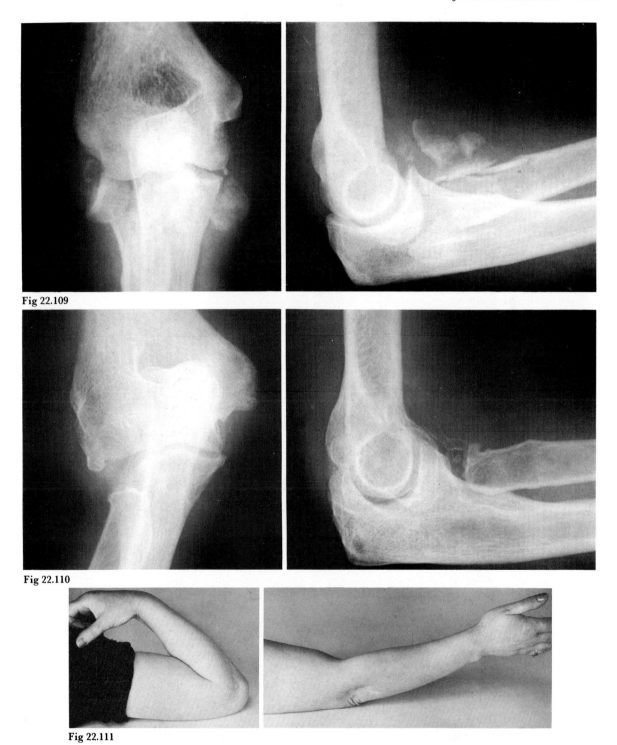

Fig 22.109

Fig 22.110

Fig 22.111

Figs 22.109 to 22.111 The original injury is seen in Figure 22.108. After reduction of the dislocation there are many fragments of the head of the radius on the antero-lateral aspect of the joint, and one on the medial aspect (Fig 22.109). All these fragments must be excised at an early stage of treatment (Fig 22.110). A good range of painless movement may then be expected (Fig 22.111).

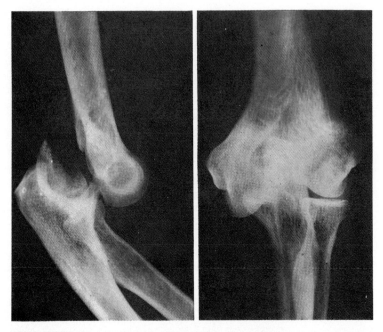

Fig 22.112 Ten-day-old fracture-dislocation of the elbow joint. The posterior margin of the lateral condyle of the humerus has been broken off and displaced posteriorly with the ulna. Incidentally, the patient had previously had an amputation through the lower forearm.

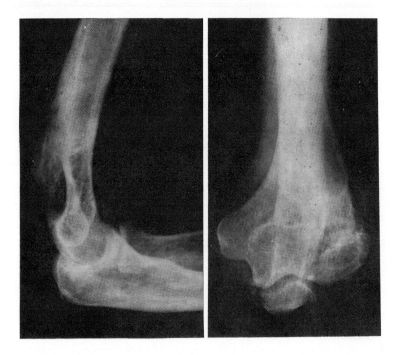

Fig 22.113 Manipulative reduction and after-treatment were the same as for a simple posterior dislocation. The condylar fragment bedded down in normal position and united without need for any operation. The patient discharged himself and was back at work in the docks in eight weeks.

RECURRENT DISLOCATION OF THE ELBOW JOINT

Recurrent or habitual dislocation of the elbow joint is very rare indeed; but of course recurrence after a first dislocation may occur in any joint if its stability is impaired by unsound healing of avulsed capsule or fractured marginal fragments of bone. It is possible that there may sometimes be predisposition to recurrent displacement by abnormal shallowness of the trochlear notch of the ulna, but probably recurrent backward dislocation of the elbow joint results from unsound healing of the capsule and ligaments, the effect of which may be worsened by an ununited fracture near the base of the coronoid impairing the integrity of the trochlear notch. Most of the operations designed to cure the condition depend upon strengthening the anterior joint structures,[76, 77] or reconstructing the collateral ligaments.[78] Osborne and Cotterill and others[79, 80] consider instability to be due to a failure of repair of the postero-lateral capsule and the lateral triangular ligament. Patients have been treated successfully by repair of the lateral capsular and ligamentous laxity. Through a lateral approach the bone of the lateral epicondyle and lateral side of the capitellum is scarified and the postero-lateral capsule sewn down tightly to the bone using catgut sutures passed through the lateral epicondyle (Figs 22.114 and 22.115). The capsule should be made to adhere to the humerus as close to the articular margin as possible. Usually only the lateral side of the joint requires attention, but if there is clinical evidence of marked laxity of the medial ligament this should be repaired in the same way. Following operation the elbow is immobilised extended below the right angle at about 40 degrees for four weeks.

UNUSUAL DISLOCATIONS AND FRACTURE-DISLOCATIONS OF THE ELBOW

Isolated dislocations of the head of the radius. Reports of traumatic dislocation of the head of the radius without other bone injury must be accepted with caution. Almost invariable there is an associated fracture of the shaft of the ulna—the Monteggia fracture-dislocation which will be discussed in Chapter 23. There may of course be congenital subluxation or dislocation of the head of the radius, but this should be easily recognised by the dome shaped appearance of the radial head and the reversed concave posterior border of the upper third of the ulna.[81, 82] There may

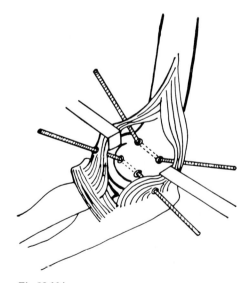

Fig 22.114

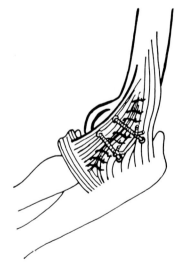

Fig 22.115

Figs 22.114 and 22.115 Drawings to illustrate repair of the postero-lateral capsule for recurrent dislocation of the elbow (Osborne-Cotterill operation). Figure 22.114 shows catgut sutures passed through transverse holes bored in the lateral epicondyle close to the articular margin. These sutures are used to draw the postero-lateral capsule on to the scarified bone thereby obliterating the postero-lateral capsular defect (Fig 22.115). Reproduced by kind permission of the *Journal of Bone and Joint Surgery* and of G. Osborne and P. Cotterill from their article (1966) Recurrent dislocation of the elbow. *Journal of Bone and Joint Surgery*, 48–B, 340).

also be paralytic subluxation or dislocation when over a period of months or years the radial head gradually displaces in consequence of the muscle imbalance of poliomyelitis. Finally, if there is failure of development of the ulna as in dyschondroplasia, or premature fusion of the ulnar epiphyses, while the radius continues to grow so that it becomes relatively longer than the ulna, the head of the radius subluxates and then completely dislocates. Theoretically, the rotational strain of forced pronation could tear the orbicular ligament and displace the radial head as an isolated injury. But beware if the radial head is normal in shape. Look for the associated fracture of the ulna.

Dislocations of the elbow with fracture of the shaft of the radius. When a patient falls on the outstretched hand and dislocates the forearm bones backwards at the elbow, there may be at the moment of weight-bearing impact a rotational strain on the forearm with forced pronation or supination. This is the underlying mechanism of the Monteggia injury, to be considered in the next chapter, in which the head of the radius is dislocated and the upper shaft of the ulna is fractured.

The converse of that injury is shown in Figure 22.116 where the ulna is dislocated backwards, the upper shaft of the radius fractured, and the proximal third of the radius displaced downwards. The spiral shape of the fracture of the radial shaft confirms that it arose from rotational strain—probably forced pronation of the distal part of the forearm. Traction was applied and the forearm supinated; this corrected the over-riding of radial fragments and restored normal relationship of the radial head to the sigmoid notch of the ulna. Flexion of the elbow then corrected the backward dislocation (Fig 22.117). The shaft fracture united with a trace of angulation causing slight impairment in the range of radio-ulnar movement; but flexion-extension movement of the elbow was normal.

A similar fracture-dislocation is shown in Figures 22.118 and 22.119 but in this case the fracture, again a spiral fracture, was at the junction of the middle and *lower* thirds of the shaft. Good reduction was again secured by manipulation without open operation.

Although in both of these injuries an acceptable result was obtained by manipulation alone, there should be no hesitation in carrying out internal fixation of the radial fracture with a plate or a Rush nail, if the position is not acceptable.

REFERENCES

1. Corbett R H 1978 Displaced fat pads in trauma to the elbow. Injury 9: 297
2. Smith D N, Lee J R 1978 The radiological diagnosis of post-traumatic effusion of the elbow joint and its clinical significance: the 'displaced fat pad' sign. Injury 10: 115
3. Johansson O 1962 Capsular and ligament injuries of the elbow joint. A clinical and arthrographic study. Acta Chirurgica Scandinavica, suppl 287
4. Tucker K 1978 Some aspects of post-traumatic elbow stiffness. Injury 9: 216
5. Bodnar L M, Zobol Z W, Troyer M L, Krizman D, Scherer J 1971 Epicondylitis as an athletic injury. Journal of Bone and Joint Surgery 53-A: 1228
6. Capener N 1966 The vulnerability of the posterior interosseus nerve of the forearm. Journal of Bone and Joint Surgery 48-B: 770
7. Rolfs N C, Maudsley R H 1972 Radial nerve tunnel syndrome. Journal of Bone and Joint Surgery 54-B: 499
8. Van Rossum J, Buruma O J S, Kamphuisen H A C, Onvlee G J 1978 Tennis elbow—a radial tunnel syndrome? Journal of Bone and Joint Surgery 60-B: 197
9. Bosworth D M 1955 The role of the orbicular ligament in tennis elbow. Journal of Bone and Joint Surgery 37-A: 527
10. Newman J H, Goodfellow J W 1975 Fibrillation of the head of the radius—one cause of tennis elbow. Journal of Bone and Joint Surgery 57-B: 115
11. Watson-Jones Sir Reginald 1961 Surgery is Destined to the Practice of Medicine. (Hunterian Oration—The Royal College of Surgeons of England). Livingstone, Edinburgh
11a. Nirschl R P, Pettrone F A 1979 Tennis elbow. The surgical treatment of lateral epicondylitis. Journal of Bone and Joint Surgery 62-A: 52
12. Garden R S 1961 Tennis elbow. Journal of Bone and Joint Surgery 43-B: 100
13. Brewer B J 1962 Athletic injuries; musculotendinous unit. Clinical orthopaedics. Lippincott, Philadelphia, vol 23, ch 4, p 31 & 35
14. Miller J S 1960 Javelin thrower's elbow. Journal of Bone and Joint Surgery 42-B: 788
15. McRae R, Freeman P A 1965 The lesion in pulled elbow. Journal of Bone and Joint Surgery 47-B: 808
16. Childress H M 1975 Recurrent ulnar nerve dislocation at the elbow. Clinical Orthopaedics and Related Research 108: 168
17. Rolfsen L 1970 Snapping triceps tendon with ulnar neuritis. Acta Orthopaedica Scandinavica 41: 74
18. Dreyfuss U, Kessler I 1978 Snapping elbow due to dislocation of the medial head of the triceps. A report of two cases. Journal of Bone and Joint Surgery 60-B: 56
19. Qayle J B, Robinson M P 1978 A useful procedure in the treatment of chronic olecranon bursitis. Injury 9: 299
20. Milch H 1931 Unusual fractures of the capitulum humeri and capitulum radii. Journal of Bone and Joint Surgery 13: 882
21. Bohler L 1930 Der Bruch des Oberarmköpfchen und der Bruch der Oberarmrolle mit dem Köpfchen, typische anatomisch—Konstitutionell bedingte Verletzungen. Arch Orthop u Unfallchir 28: 734

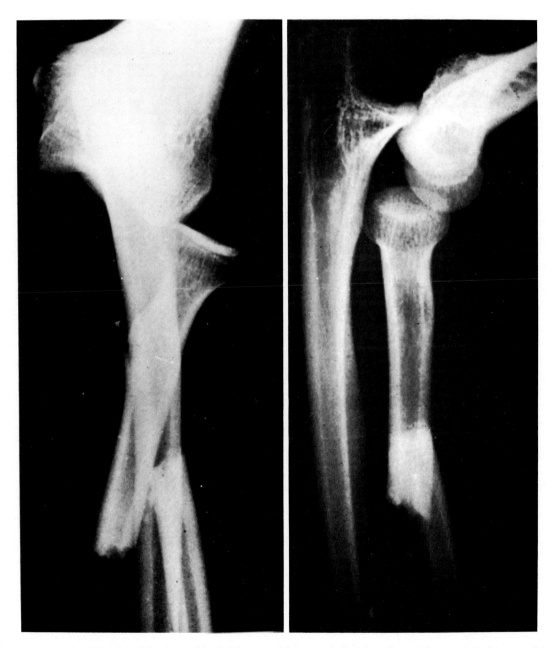

Fig 22.116 Posterior dislocation of the elbow with spiral fracture of the upper shaft of the radius and downward displacement of the upper third of the radial shaft. (This is more or less the converse of the Monteggia injury in which there is dislocation of the radial head with fracture of the upper shaft of the ulna).

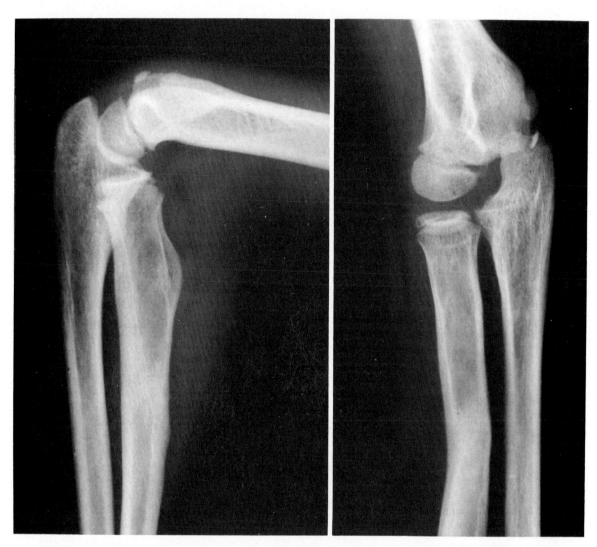

Fig 22.117 After traction and supination of the forearm the displacement and over-riding of the radial shaft fragments was corrected and the radial head restored in normal relation to the sigmoid notch of the ulna. Flexion of the ulna then corrected the dislocation.

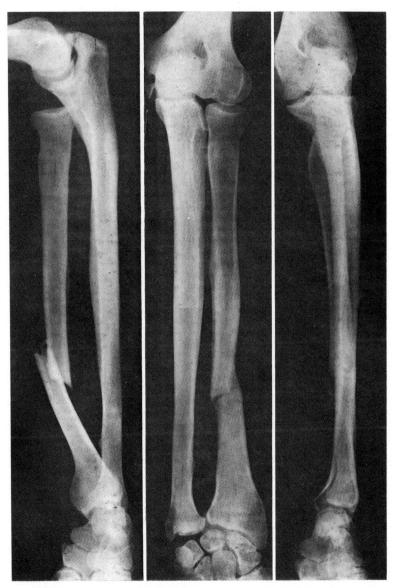

Fig 22.118   **Fig 22.119**

Figs 22.118 and 22.119 Unusual fracture-dislocation of radius. The elbow joint had been dislocated and apparently reduced, but there is independent downward dislocation of the upper two-thirds of the radius (Fig 22.118). It was necessary to redislocate the ulna before the displacement could be reduced by manipulation (Fig 22.119). Note the avulsion of the internal epicondyle which gives the clue to the mechanism of injury. Recovery was complete, all joints regaining normal movement.

22. Van Gorder G W 1958 In: Cave E F (ed) Fractures and other injuries. The Year Book Publishers Inc, Chicago, ch 19, p 321

23. Fowles J V, Kassab M T 1974 Fractures of the capitulum humeri. Treatment by excision. Journal of Bone and Joint Surgery 56-A: 794

24. D'Ambrosia R D (1972) Supracondylar fractures of the humerus—prevention of cubitus varus. Journal of Bone and Joint Surgery 54-A: 60

25. Arnold J A, Nasca R J, Nelson C L 1977 supracondylar fractures of the humerus. The role of dynamic factors in prevention of deformity. Journal of Bone and Joint Surgery 59-A: 589

26. Baumann E 1929 Beiträge zur Kenntnis der Frakturen am Ellbogengelenk. Unter besonderer Berücksichtigung der Spätfolgen. Allgemeiner und Fractura supracondylica. Beiträge zur Klinischen Chirurgie 146: 1–50

27. Jones D 1977 Transcondylar fractures of the humerus in children: Definition of an acceptable reduction. Proceedings of the Royal Society of Medicine 70: 624

28. Lawrence W 1956 supracondylar fractures of the humerus in children—a review of 100 cases. British Journal of Surgery 44: 143

29. Brown J J M 1952 Supracondylar fractures with circulatory impairment. Journal of Bone and Joint Surgery 34-B: 155

30. Dunlop J 1939 Transcondylar fractures of the humerus in childhood. Journal of Bone and Joint Surgery 21: 59

31. Dodge H S 1972 Displaced supracondylar fractures of the humerus in children—Treatment by Dunlop's traction. Journal of Bone and Joint Surgery 54-A: 1408

32. Powell H D W 1973 Dunlop traction in supracondylar fractures of the humerus. Proceedings of the Royal Society of Medicine 66: 515

33. French P R 1959 Varus deformity of the elbow following supracondylar fractures of the humerus in children. Lancet ii: 439

34. Attenborough C G 1953 Remodelling of the humerus after supracondylar fractures in childhood. Journal of Bone and Joint Surgery 35-B: 386

35. Ramsey R H, Griz J 1973 Immediate open reduction and internal fixation of severely displaced supracondylar fractures of the humerus in children. Clinical Orthopaedics and Related Research 90: 130

36. Nassar A, Chater E 1976 Open reduction and Kirschner wire fixation for supracondylar fractures of the humerus. Journal of Bone and Joint Surgery 58-B: 135

37. Hart G M, Wilson D W, Arden G P 1977 The operative management of the difficult supracondylar fracture of the humerus in the child. Injury 9: 30

38. Weiland A J, Meyer S, Tolo V T, Berg H L, Mueller J 1978 Surgical treatment of displaced supracondylar fractures of the humerus in children. Journal of Bone and Joint Surgery 60-A: 657

39. Flynn J C, Matthews J G, Benoit R L 1974 Blind pinning of displaced supracondylar fractures of the humerus in children. Journal of Bone and Joint Surgery 56-A: 263

40. Fowles J B, Kassab M T 1974 Displaced supracondylar fractures of the elbow in children. A report on the fixation of extension and flexion fractures by two lateral percutaneous pins. Journal of Bone and Joint Surgery 56-B: 490

41. Arino V L, Lluch E E, Ramirez A M, Ferrer J, Rodriquez L, Baixauli F 1977 Percutaneous fixation of supracondylar fractures of humerus in children. Journal of Bone and Joint Surgery 59-A: 914

42. Palmer E E, Neimann K M W, Vesley D, Armstrong J H 1978 Supracondylar fracture of the humerus in children. Journal of Bone and Joint Surgery 60-A, 635

43. Nassar A 1974 Correction of varus deformity following supracondylar fractures of the humerus. Journal of Bone and Joint Surgery 56-B: 572

44. Sweeney J G 1975 Osteotomy of the humerus for malunion of supracondylar fractures. Journal of Bone and Joint Surgery 57-B: 117

45. Smith L 1960 Deformity following supracondylar fractures of the humerus. Journal of Bone and Joint Surgery 42-A: 235

46. Siris I E 1939 Supracondylar fracture of the humerus. Surgery, Gynecology and Obstetrics 68: 201

47. Soltanpur A 1978 Anterior supracondylar fracture of the humerus (flexion type). Journal of Bone and Joint Surgery 60-B: 383

48. Brown R F, Morgan R G 1971 Intercondylar T-shaped fractures of the humerus. Results in ten cases treated by early mobilisation. Journal of Bone and Joint Surgery 53-B: 425

49. Riseborough E J, Radin E L 1969 Intercondylar T-fractures of the humerus in the adult. A comparison of operative and non-operative treatment in twenty-nine cases. Journal of Bone and Joint Surgery 51-A: 130

50. Merle D'Aubigne R, Meary R, Carlioz J 1964 Fractures sus et intercondyliennes recentes de l'adulte. Revue de Chirurgie Orthopedique 50: 274

51. Conwell H E, Reynolds F C 1961 Key and Conwell's management of fractures, dislocations and sprains, 7th edn. Mosby, St Louis, p 478

52. Scharplatz D, Allgower M 1975 Fracture dislocations of the elbow. Injury 7:143

53. Evans E M 1953 Supracondylar Y-shaped fractures of the humerus. Journal of Bone and Joint Surgery 35-B: 381

54. Cohn I 1921 Observations on the normally developing elbow. Archives of Surgery 2: 455

55. Ghosh D P 1970 Radiological observation on the relationship of the lower humeral epiphysis with its shaft. Indian Journal of Surgery 32: 71

55a. Holda M E, Manoli A, Lamont R L 1980 Epiphyseal separation of the distal end of the humerus with medial displacement. Journal of Bone and Joint Surgery 62-A: 52

56. Jakob R, Fowles J V, Rang M, Kassab M T 1975 Observations concerning fractures of the lateral humeral condyle in children. Journal of Bone and Joint Surgery 57-B 430

57. Martini M, Hallaz N, Daoud A, Descamps L 1978 Les luxations traumatique récentes du coude. A propos de 94 observations. Acta Orthopedica Belgica 44: 542

58. Jeffrey C C 1958 Non-union of the epiphysis of the lateral condyle of the humerus. Journal of Bone and Joint Surgery 40-B: 396

59. Wilson J N 1955 Fractures of the external condyle of humerus in children. British Journal of Surgery 43: 88

60. Conner A N, Smith M G H 1970 Displaced fractures of the lateral humeral condyle in children. Journal of Bone and Joint Surgery 52-B: 460

60a. Flynn J C, Richards J F, Saltzman R I 1975 Prevention and treatment of non-union of slightly displaced fractures of the lateral humeral condyle in children. Journal of Bone and Joint Surgery 57-A: 1087

61. Potter C M C 1954 Fracture-dislocation of the trochlea. Journal of Bone and Joint Surgery 36-B: 250

62. Chacha P B 1970 Fracture of the medial condyle of the humerus with rotational displacement. Journal of Bone and Joint Surgery 52-A: 1453

62a. Fowles J V, Kassab M T 1980 Displaced fracture of the medial humeral condyle in children. Journal of Bone and Joint Surgery 62-A: 1159

63. Cothay D M 1967 Injury to the lower medial epiphysis of the humerus before development of the ossific centre. Report of a case. Journal of Bone and Joint Surgery 49-B: 766

64. Fahey J J, O'Brien E T 1971 Fracture-separation of the medial humeral condyle in a child confused with fracture of the medial epicondyle. Journal of Bone and Joint Surgery 53-A: 1102

65. Fowles J V, Rizkallah R 1976 Intra-articular injuries of the elbow: pitfalls of diagnosis and treatment. CMA Journal 114: 125

66. Watson-Jones R 1930 Primary nerve lesions in injuries of the elbow and wrist. Journal of Bone and Joint Surgery 12: 121

67. Cotton F J 1929 Elbow dislocation and ulnar nerve injury. Journal of Bone and Joint Surgery 11: 348

68. Wilson J N 1960 The treatment of fractures of the medial epicondyle of the humerus. Journal of Bone and Joint Surgery 42-B: 778

69. Patrick J 1946 Fracture of the medial epicondyle with displacement into the elbow joint. Journal of Bone and Joint Surgery 28: 143

70. Roberts P H 1969 Dislocations of the elbow. British Journal of Surgery 56: 806

71. Protzman R R 1978 Dislocation of the elbow joint. Journal of Bone and Joint Surgery 60-A: 539

72. Speed J S 1925 An operation for unreduced posterior dislocation of elbow. Southern Medical Journal 18: 193

73. Purser D W 1954 Dislocation of the elbow and inclusion of the medial epicondyle in the adult. Journal of Bone and Joint Surgery 36-B: 247

74. Howard N J 1935 Epiphyseal fracture-dislocation of the elbow joint. Journal of Bone and Joint Surgery 17: 123

75. Grantham S A, Tietjen R 1976 Transcondylar fracture-dislocation of the elbow. Journal of Bone and Joint Surgery 58-A: 1030

76. Reichenheim P P 1947 Transplantation of the biceps tendon as a treatment for recurrent dislocation of the elbow. British Journal of Surgery 35: 201

77. Wainwright D 1947 Recurrent dislocation of the elbow joint. Proceedings of the Royal Society of Medicine 40: 885

78. Spring W E 1953 Report of a case of recurrent dislocation of the elbow. Journal of Bone and Joint Surgery 35-B: 55

79. Osborne G, Cotterill P 1966 Recurrent dislocation of the elbow. Journal of Bone and Joint Surgery 48-B: 340

80. Symeonides P P, Paschaloglou C, Stavrou Z, Pangalides Th 1975 Recurrent dislocation of the elbow. Report of three cases. Journal of Bone and Joint Surgery 57-A: 1084

81. McFarland B 1936 Congenital dislocation of the head of the radius. British Journal of Surgery 24: 41

82. Almquist E E, Gordon L H, Blue A I 1969 Congenital dislocation of the head of the radius. Journal of Bone and Joint Surgery 51-A: 1118

23

Injuries of the Forearm

A. Benjamin

The articulation between the radius and the ulna is in three parts; the proximal and distal radio-ulnar joints, and the interosseous membrane which is the intermediate radio-ulnar joint. The behaviour of forearm fractures varies with the extent to which the radio-ulnar articulation is involved. The aim of treatment is the return of normal function, and this often, but not always, coincides with re-establishment of normal anatomy. The forearm is subservient to the hand, and the mobility of the joints of the hand, shoulder and elbow must be preserved. Rehabilitation commenced on the day of injury prevents much disability.

Forearm fractures in children seldom need open operation and even less frequently need internal fixation. These injuries are generally due to a fall on the hand or forearm and in a child who is not yet walking must be considered possibly the result of non-accidental injury.

CLASSIFICATION OF FOREARM FRACTURES

Fractures of the proximal ulna without radio-ulnar dislocation
Fracture of the olecranon.
Fracture of the coronoid.

Fractures of the head and neck of the radius
Fracture of the head of the radius.
Fracture displacement of the upper radial epiphysis.
Dislocation of the head of the radius without fracture of the ulna.

Fractures of the shafts of both forearm bones

Fractures of the shaft of the ulna
Without radio-ulnar joint disruption.

With dislocation of the head of the radius which comprise flexion, extension and adduction Monteggia fractures and the Hume fracture.

Fractures of the shaft of the radius or ulna with dislocation of the elbow

Fractures of the shaft of the radius
With disruption of the interosseous membrane.
With dislocation of the distal radio-ulnar joint.
The Galeazzi fracture.

Fractures of the radial head with dislocation of the distal radio-ulnar joint
The Essex-Lopresti fracture.

Fractures of the lower end of the radius with dislocation of the distal radio-ulnar joint
Colles' fracture.
Smith fracture.
Barton fracture.
Fracture displacement of lower radial epiphysis.

FRACTURES OF THE PROXIMAL ULNA WITHOUT RADIO-ULNAR DISLOCATION

Fracture of the olecranon
Fractures of the olecranon may be transverse, with wide separation of the fragments due to avulsion by the triceps muscle; or comminuted, due to a fall on to the point of the elbow, often associated with contraction of the triceps again resulting in wide separation of the fragments. As separation of the fragments of a fractured patella causes quadriceps insufficiency, so in the elbow the separated olecranon fragment causes triceps insufficiency. An isolated fracture of the patella, however, never results in subluxation of the knee, whereas a large olecranon fragment can be associated with anterior displacement of the elbow (Figs 23.6 and 23.7). The aims of treatment are three-fold:

1. To restore the power of active extension.
2. To restore mobility.
3. To restore stability of the joint should this be lost.

If a separated olecranon is allowed to repair by fibrous tissue movement is preserved and it may appear that active extension is satisfactory, because of gravity, but the lack of power in an elbow so treated produces a real disability. There is inability to extend the elbow against gravity as in reaching up above the head (Fig 23.1), and it is almost impossible to cut a loaf of bread as the holding hand is unable to steady the loaf and the cutting hand unable to apply pressure (Fig 23.2).

Treatment. The treatment is influenced by the state of the triceps insertion. If detached, repair of the tendon is the primary concern. The separated bony fragment must be reduced by open operation and fixed internally. There is seldom place for conservative treatment, as closed reduction would need to be

followed by immobilisation in full extension of the elbow for five to six weeks, a position which, except perhaps in children, risks permanent stiffness. Comminuted fractures without separation are treated by immobilisation in plaster with the elbow at just below 90 degrees for three weeks followed by gentle mobilisation. Fractures of the olecranon, although involving the articular surfaces of the elbow, do not cause sufficient degenerative change to warrant excision of the separated fragment. Previously, a widely separated olecranon fragment too small to take a screw was an indication for operative excision followed by tendon repair (Figs 23.3 to 23.5). Now, excision of the fragment, however small, is rarely indicated owing to the introduction of internal fixation by tension band wiring (Figs 23.8 and 23.9).

Operative reduction with internal fixation. Operative reduction with internal fixation is the treatment of choice whenever there is separation of fragments. Through a posterior mid-line incision the fracture is exposed, blood clot evacuated and interposed soft

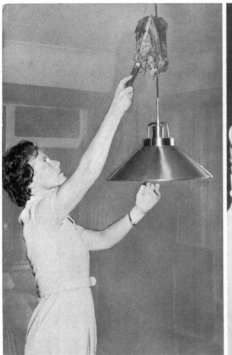
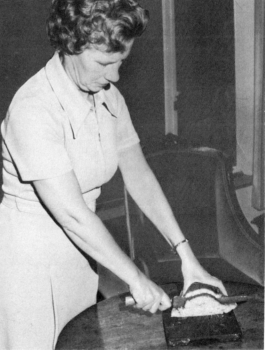

Fig 23.1   **Fig 23.2**

Figs 23.1 and 23.2 Activities requiring triceps muscle action. Fig 23.1: Extension of the elbow against gravity. Fig 23.2: Active extension of the elbow is needed in simple everyday activities. The left arm is extended to steady the loaf, while the right puts pressure on the bread knife.

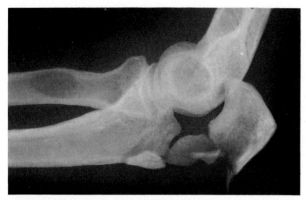

Fig 23.3

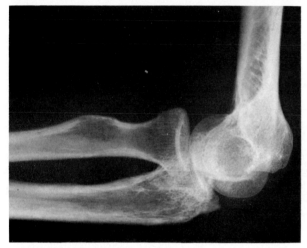

Fig 23.4

Figs 23.3 and 23.4 X-rays of a fracture of the olecranon
(Fig 23.3) treated by excision of the fragment and repair of
the triceps tendon to the shaft of the ulnar (Fig 23.4).

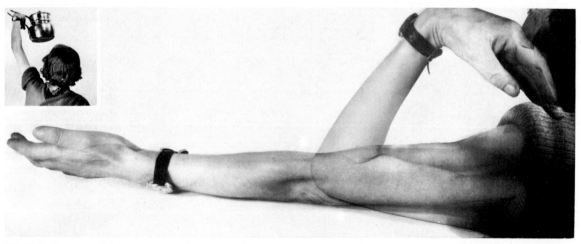

Fig 23.5 The range of elbow movement after excision of the olecranon. The inset shows the ability to extend the elbow against
gravity. Although the result in this case is extremely good, the fracture could have been treated equally well by internal fixation, with
less probability of instability.

tissue removed. In the absence of severe comminution a reduction of hairline accuracy should be achieved. The position is held temporarily by a bone or towel clip. The method of internal fixation chosen depends upon the type of fracture and the preference of the surgeon. A large olecranon fragment may be fixed by means of a screw (Figs 23.6 and 23.7), but tension band wiring is the treatment of choice. Two Kirschner wires are introduced into the fragments parallel to each other and to the long axis of the ulna. A transverse drill hole is made distal to the fracture and a 1.2 mm wire is threaded through the hole and crossed over at the fracture site in a figure-of-eight and passed around the protruding ends of the Kirschner wires. The first throw of the knot is made and whilst still loose a loop is fashioned in the wire on the side of the olecranon opposite to the knot. The knot is now tightened and completed and the wire on

the other side is tightened by turning the previously fashioned loop. Finally the Kirschner wires are bent over and hammered into the bone in order to secure the tension wire (Figs 23.8 and 23.9).

Post-operative management. The elbow is immobilised in a plaster backslab at 75 degrees. This prevents the firm pull of the triceps muscle when the elbow is in more flexion. During immobilisation the hand and shoulder are exercised and used for all normal activities such as writing and eating. The plaster is removed after three weeks and movement is gained by the patient's own gentle efforts; physiotherapy is rarely necessary. If the surgeon considers the internal fixation at the time of operation is adequate, there is a case for immediate mobilisation.

Patella cubiti. Occasionally the centre of ossification for the olecranon does not fuse to the proximal

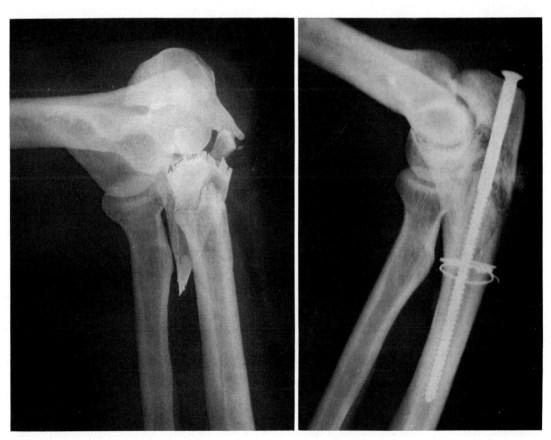

Fig 23.6   Fig 23.7

Figs 23.6 and 23.7 X-rays of a comminuted fracture of the olecranon with instability of the elbow treated by a long intramedullary screw and circumferential wiring.

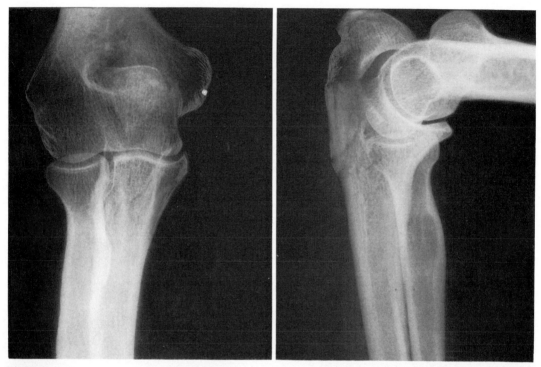

Fig 23.8

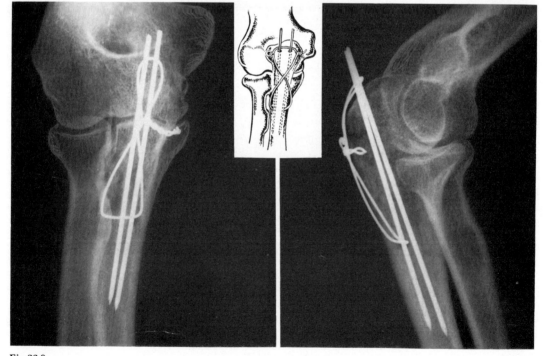

Fig 23.9

Figs 23.8 and 23.9 X-rays of an olecranon fracture treated by tension band wiring. The wires were about to be bent over and hammered home. The inset shows an extra loop to facilitate tensioning of the wire on the side away from the knot.

end of the ulna but remains separate (Fig 23.10). This condition may be mistaken for a fracture of the olecranon. However, there are a number of distinguishing points: (1) the shape of the olecranon is complete apart from the patella cubiti; (2) the separation is minimal; (3) the adjacent bone surfaces are smooth; and (4) the condition is bilateral.

Fracture of the coronoid. This fracture is usually associated with dislocation of the elbow and rarely requires treatment except when a large fragment results in elbow stability.

INJURIES OF THE HEAD AND NECK OF THE RADIUS

Fracture of the head of the radius
Fracture of the head of the radius is due to a fall on the outstretched hand, forcing the elbow into valgus and impacting the head of the radius against the capitellum (Figs 23.11 and 23.12). The valgus strain may damage the medial aspect of the elbow avulsing the medial epicondyle. The ulna may also be damaged, in which case there is dislocation or instability of the radio-ulnar joint; and every case of fractured head of radius must be examined to exclude these complications.

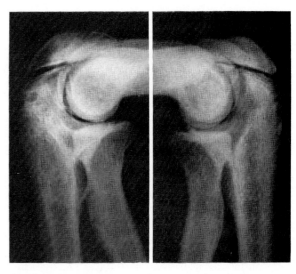

Fig 23.10 In each elbow joint of this patient there is a large fragment of bone lying above the olecranon. These are not fractures—the condition is sometimes described as patella cubiti. The ossicles are developed in the triceps tendon from secondary centres of ossification. The distinction from a fracture can be made by the completeness of the shape of the olecranon in each joint and the smoothness of the surfaces between the olecranon and the ossicle.

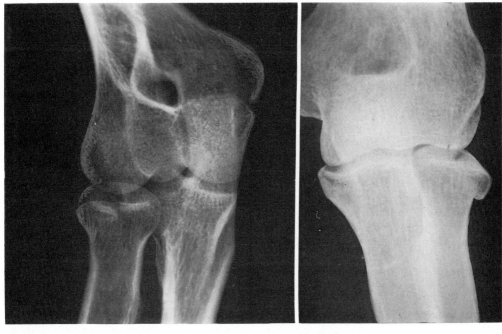

Fig 23.11   **Fig 23.12**

Figs 23.11 and 23.12 Segmental fractures of the head of the radius.

Diagnosis. The clinical signs of this fracture can be minimal. Careful examination of the elbow joint will show some swelling due to an effusion into the joint filling the posterior sulci. The grip is grossly weakened, and any attempt to use the hand is accompanied by pain over the outer side of the elbow. The diagnostic sign, however, is acute local tenderness over the head of the radius when it is rotated under the examining thumb. If this sign is present the elbow must be X-rayed to exclude fracture.

Treatment. At one time many fractures of the head of the radius were treated by excision, but the pendulum has swung towards conservative rather than operative treatment of these injuries.[1] Most fractures are best treated by immobilisation in a plaster backslab with the elbow at 90 degrees and the forearm in mid-pronation for 10 days. The forearm is mobilised by gradual return to normal use. Physiotherapy is contraindicated and so also is manipulation. During the subsequent two to three years the elbow and forearm usually regain a satisfactory range of movement and the head of the radius remoulds to a surprising extent. There is considerable evidence to suggest that conservative treatment associated with aspiration of the haemarthrosis at twenty four hours gives even better results than conservative measures alone.[2] These conservative measures generally are satisfactory even in the comminuted fracture involving the whole of the radial head.[3, 4] Early excision results in more stiffness, less stability and an unnecessary scar. Several papers have been published in recent years recommending excision of the head of the radius with or without prosthetic replacement. Many of these do not compare the results of resection with conservative treatment and consequently their conclusions are of limited value. However, if the head of the radius is comminuted and large fragments are severely displaced, excision is indicated. The optimum time for operation is two to three weeks after injury. Early excision of the head of the radius is followed by high incidence of subluxation of the inferior radio-ulnar joint due to proximal migration of the radius.[5, 6] This may be prevented by replacement of the radial head with a silastic prosthesis. Figs 23.13 to 23.15.

Technique of excision of a fractured head of radius. A short longitudinal incision is centred over the radial head, which may be located by repeatedly pronating and supinating the forearm with an examining finger over the lateral side of the joint. Care is taken not to extend the dissection so far distally as to imperil the posterior interosseous nerve. The common extensor tendon and underlying capsule are divided without dissection into planes. Strachan has pointed out that the posterior interosseous nerve is less in danger when the forearm is pronated.[7] The bone is cut with a sharp osteotome through the neck of the radius at the level of the orbicular ligament. The surgeon pronates and supinates the forearm during the operation to ensure a good view of the entire circumference of the radial neck. Every loose piece of bone is removed from within the joint, and it is a wise precaution to put all the pieces together after excision in order to make sure that the whole radial head has been removed. Sometimes the head of radius should be replaced by a prosthetic implant. This is not advised as routine, but it may be indicated in those rare cases when the head is excised in the young, when early excision is necessary or when the injury has disrupted the interosseous membrane as in the Essex-Lopresti fracture.[8] Further experience is needed to indicate the advisability of prosthetic replacement (Figs 23.13 to 23.15).

Fracture displacement of the upper radial epiphysis

A fall on the outstretched hand is the cause of the displacement of the upper radial epiphysis in children. The displaced fragment includes the epiphysis, the epiphyseal plate and a triangular fragment of bone from the metaphysis (Figs 23.16 to 23.18). The head is displaced laterally and anteriorly and it is tilted so that its humeral articular surface faces laterally. Slight displacement is unimportant, and satisfactory remoulding of the bone will occur (Figs 23.16 to 23.18). If the head of the radius is significantly tilted then reduction is advisable either by manipulation or by operation. The acceptable degree varies with the age of the child. The younger the skeletal age the greater the degree of displacement that will be corrected by remodelling. A displacement of 45 degrees should probably always be corrected. This fracture displacement may be associated with an unrecognised dislocation of the elbow. It may be unrecognised due to spontaneous reduction of the dislocation. Close observation is necessary less the dislocation recurs during the first weeks of treatment. Figs 23.19 to 23.22.

Manipulative reduction. It is often possible to correct the displacement by extending the elbow, adducting the forearm and pressing firmly over the head of the radius. The extension of the elbow and the adduction of the forearm is best maintained by an

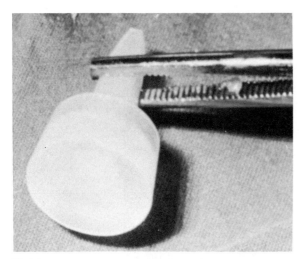

Fig 23.13

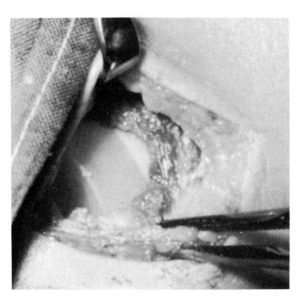

Fig 23.14

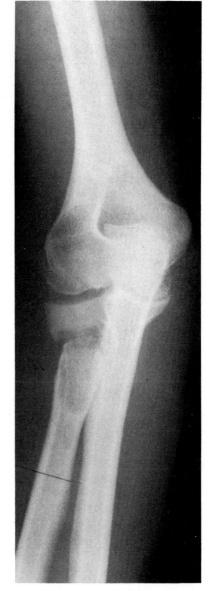

Fig 23.15

Figs 23.13 to 23.15 Some surgeons have advocated the use of a prosthetic device to replace the radial head removed for fracture. Figure 23.13 shows the type of prosthesis used and Figure 23.14 shows the prosthesis *in situ* at operation. The X-ray appearance is shown in Figure 23.15. This procedure is not advised for the straightforward case requiring excision of the head of the radius at three weeks following the fracture, but there may be a case for it when upward displacement of the radius can be expected.

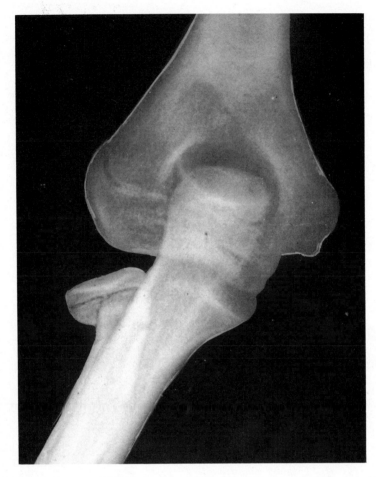

Fig 23.16 X-ray of a fracture displacement of the upper radial epiphysis with a large triangular metaphyseal fragment.

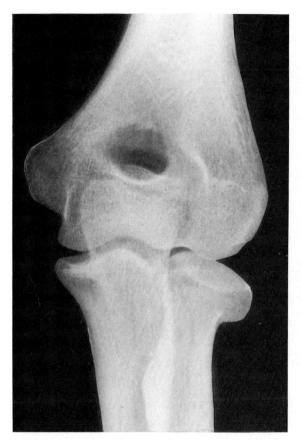

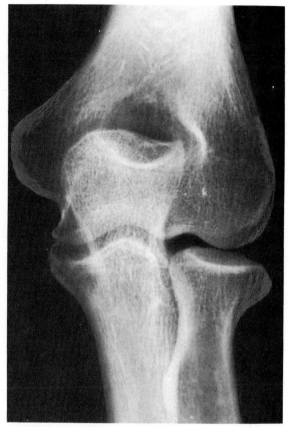

Fig 23.17 Fracture displacement of the upper radial epiphysis immediately after union in a 14-year-old girl.

Fig 23.18 The same elbow six months later after complete correction by the moulding of growth.

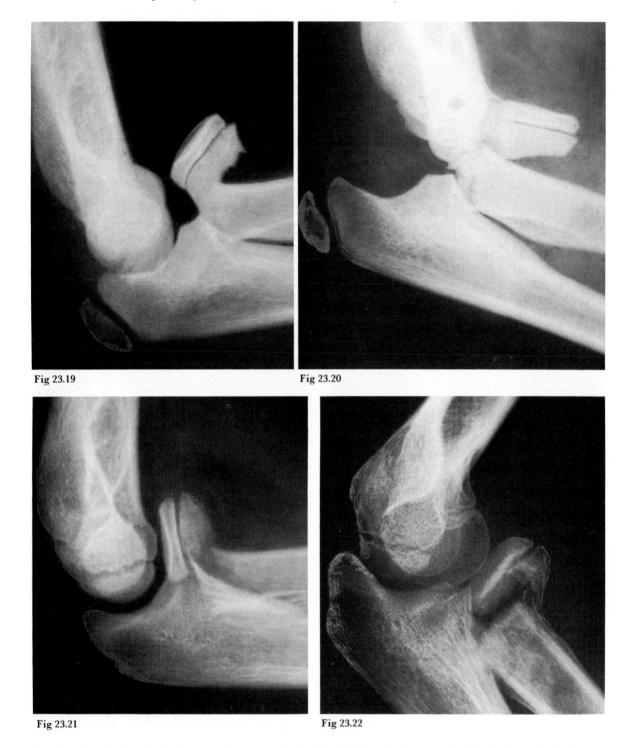

Fig 23.19

Fig 23.20

Fig 23.21

Fig 23.22

Figs 23.19 to 23.22 Fracture displacement of the upper radial epiphysis. Fig 23.19: The apparently isolated injury. Fig 23.20: During manipulation the elbow tended to dislocate giving a clear indication of the mechanism of the injury. Fig 23.21: The radial head and capitellum are congruous following reduction. Fig 23.22: Three months later there is union, moulding is taking place and clinically a full range of movement has been regained.

assistant whilst the surgeon presses over the head of the radius, the forearm being alternately pronated and supinated. The deformity can be palpated, and by palpation one can recognise when it is reduced. This is checked by X-ray. So long as the angulation is significantly improved the last few degrees will correct by remodelling.

Operative reduction. Through a short incision the head of the radius is exposed, a pad of gauze is placed over the head and with thumb pressure it is pushed back into place. Reduction is usually stable (Figs 23.23 to 23.25) and it is rarely necessary to use internal fixation to maintain the reduction (Figs 23.26 and 23.27). The treatment following both manipulation and operation is the same as that for conservative treatment, namely a plaster backslab for 10 days and then mobilisation without physiotherapy or special exercises.

Pulled elbow

Pulled elbow may be caused by a child falling when its hand is being held by an adult. The body weight being taken at the elbow results in the head of the radius being pulled down into the annular ligament which normally surrounds the neck of the radius. The elbow is painful the X-ray normal and the condition is usually relieved by a sharp supination of the forearm without an anaesthetic. The possibility of non accidental injury must be considered.

FRACTURES OF THE SHAFTS OF FOREARM BONES

A fracture of the shaft of one forearm bone is likely to be associated with either fracture of the other or dislocation of some part of the radio-ulnar joint. Whenever this type of fracture is diagnosed it is essential that the rest of the forearm is examined and

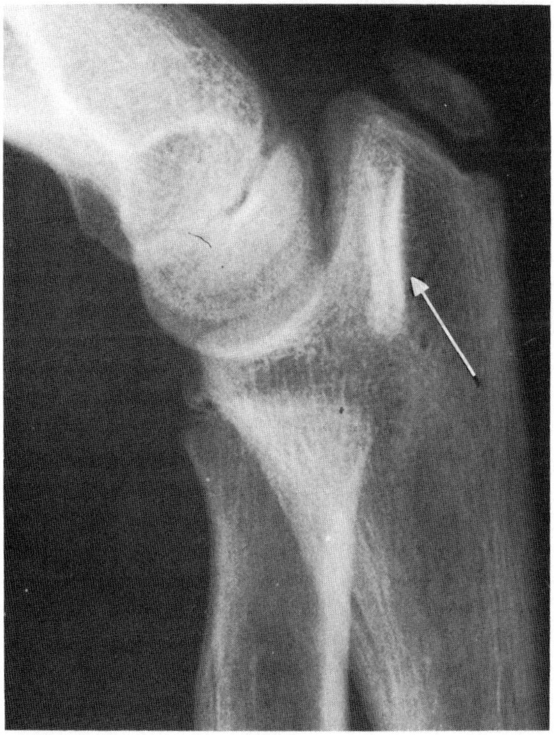

Fig 23.23

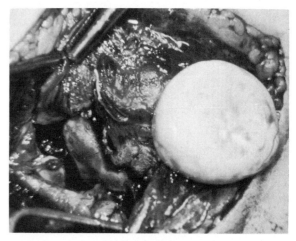

Fig 23.24

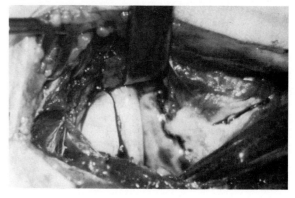

Figs 23.23 to 23.25 The X-ray shown in Figure 23.23 is of a child who sustained a complete displacement of the upper radial epiphysis (see arrow). The displacement was confirmed at operation (Fig 23.24). Reduction was stable without internal fixation (Fig 23.25).

Fig 23.25

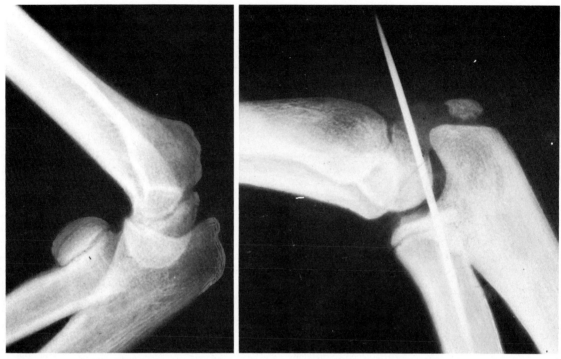

Fig 23.26   Fig 23.27

Figs 23.26 and 23.27 This totally displaced radial epiphysis (Fig 21.26) was reduced by open operation and fixed by an intramedullary wire (Fig 23.27).

usually that the full length of both forearm bones is X-rayed. If the fracture of the shaft of one forearm bone is associated with overriding or angulation, but without corresponding fracture of the other forearm bone, there must be, of necessity, a dislocation of one of the radio-ulnar joints. Failure to recognise this simple fact may result in serious disability.

FRACTURES OF SHAFTS OF BOTH RADIUS AND ULNA

When reducing fractures of the forearm it is important that both the angulation and rotation deformities are corrected. Equal shortening due to overriding of the two bones can sometimes be accepted, particularly in children, so long as there is neither angulation nor rotation. There is, therefore, a place for the conservative management of these fractures particularly if there is comminution, if the fracture is compound, and in children. The axis of rotation of the forearm bone extends from the centre of the head of the radius to the insertion of the triangular fibro-cartilage at the base of the styloid process of the ulna. If the relation

of the forearm bones to this axis is altered by angulation the mechanics of the radio-ulnar joint are deranged and permanent limitation of rotation is inevitable.

Rotational deformity will also limit radio-ulnar movement. The supinator muscles are inserted proximally and the pronators distally; consequently in a fracture of the mid-shaft of the radius the proximal fragment supinates and the distal fragment pronates. This rotational displacement is shown clearly in Figure 23.28, in which the fragments appear to be in good position in the lateral X-ray while the antero-posterior X-ray shows a striking discrepancy in the width of the interosseous space between the distal and proximal fragments. The proximal fragments are supinated and the distal fragments pronated, resulting in 90 degrees of rotational displacement. Open reduction and internal fixation are nearly always recommended in this type of fracture although skilful manipulation and plaster immobilisation offer an excellent alternative. The reduction of a fracture under direct vision is a relatively easy technical procedure whereas the closed

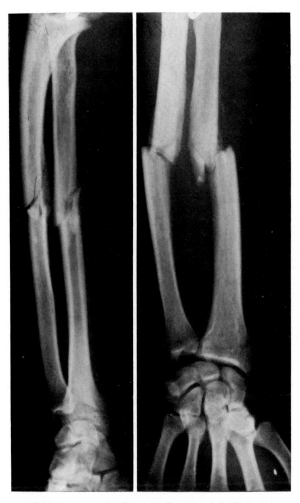

Fig 23.28 Radiographic diagnosis of rotational displacement may be difficult in fractures of the shafts of the femur and humerus, but it is easy in fractures of the forearm and leg bones where it is disclosed by the unequal width of the interosseous space in proximal and distal fragments. In Figure 23.28 the position appears satisfactory in the lateral view, but in the antero-posterior view it is obvious that the distal radial fragment is much more pronated than the proximal.

treatment of fractures generally requires considerable skill and vigilance.

Manipulative reduction. After careful study of the anatomy of the fracture the deformity is reduced by sustained traction and manipulation, sometimes angulating the bone ends in order to engage the projecting spikes at the fracture site. The fracture is normally manipulated with the elbow flexed to a right angle, with counter-traction over the front of the arm just above the elbow. The position is checked

by X-ray and when it is acceptable a plaster cast is applied while the traction is still maintained (Fig 23.29). This plaster should be well padded, particularly at the front of the elbow; it is applied first with a plaster slab extending from the heads of the metacarpals to just below the shoulder, and anchored

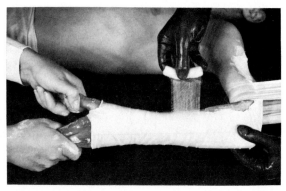

Fig 23.29 Reduction and immobilisation of fracture of the shafts of the forearm bones. Traction is maintained against the counter-pull of a sling. After reduction a plaster slab and cast are applied.

by lightly applied encircling plaster bandages (Fig 23.30). Further X-rays should be taken to ensure that the fracture has not redisplaced, and a window is made over the radial artery at the wrist to allow the pulse to be checked in the first 24 to 48 hours. An alternative plaster cast encloses the arm and the forearm leaving the elbow and cubital fossa free, the two sections of plaster being connected by plaster

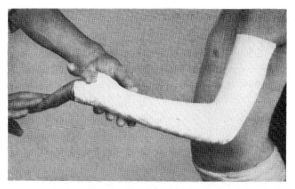

Fig 23.30 Completed plaster for fracture of the forearm bones. The operator is testing for flexion contracture of the fingers, one of the signs of ischaemic contracture of the muscles which can be due to a tight plaster.

struts, one on either side (Figs 23.31 and 23.32). Manipulation and early functional bracing with a cast which allows both wrist and elbow movement has been suggested as a form of treatment which provides sufficient stability for the fracture to heal while the upper limb joints continue to function.[9]

After treatment. X-rays are taken weekly for four weeks and then two-weekly. Union is often present at eight weeks but the fractures will not, in the adult, be consolidated by then. If at any time an X-ray shows significant displacement then the fractures are reduced and fixed by open operation.

Circulation and Volkmann's contracture. After manipulation and application of plaster the patient is admitted and for 24 hours the hand is elevated; for the first day a half-hourly pulse chart is kept, the nursing staff being instructed to take the pulse through the window in the plaster cast. Hand and shoulder exercises are begun at once and practised regularly during the period of immobilisation. The circulation and movement of the fingers must be watched with special care in this early period as ischaemic contracture of the forearm muscles can occur in fractures of the shafts of the radius and ulna. If there is any suspicion of ischaemia, the plaster must at once be cut throughout its whole length from the wrist to the shoulder. Sometimes there are obvious signs of ischaemia, with persistent cyanosis, pallor of the fingers, lack of sensation, or lack of capillary return. It is important to realise that there may be ischaemia of the muscles though none of these signs is present. A good radial pulse should be palpable at all times, and if not, this alone is an indication for splitting the plaster.

The earliest indications of incipient Volkmann's contracture are pain and limitation of passive extension of the fingers. Unfortunately forearm fractures themselves cause flexor muscle pain when the fingers are passively extended. Nevertheless, increasing limitation of passive extension must be regarded as an urgent indication of forearm muscle ischaemia, and immediate action must be taken to split the plaster. It is essential that underlying padding or dressing is also cut so that the skin can be seen through the entire length of the split. Blood-caked wool acts just as much like a tourniquet as does a plaster cast. If, after removal of all constriction, the circulation still does not return to normal the deep fascia must be incised.[10] (see Chapter 9). Loss of pulse is an indication for fasciotomy but fasciotomy may be necessary without the loss of pulse.[11]

Duration of immobilisation. In children, fractures of the radius and ulna are usually united in six weeks. If the fractures are transverse and both at the same level, then longer immobilisation is advisable. In adults immobilisation should be continued for at least 10 weeks. Shorter periods of immobilisation, which are often recommended, may result in non-union or re-fracture.

Complete plaster until the fracture is united. At no stage before the fracture is firmly united should the plaster be reduced to below the level of the elbow. A

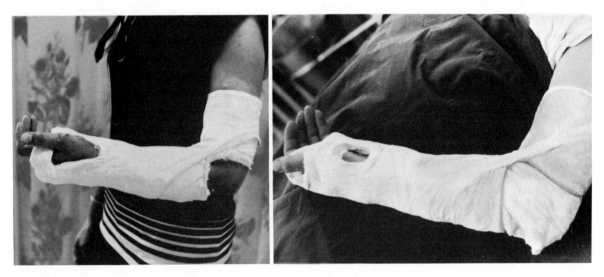

Fig 23.31 A plaster cast for immobilisation of the forearm leaving the elbow and cubital fossa exposed and with a window for palpation of the radial pulse.

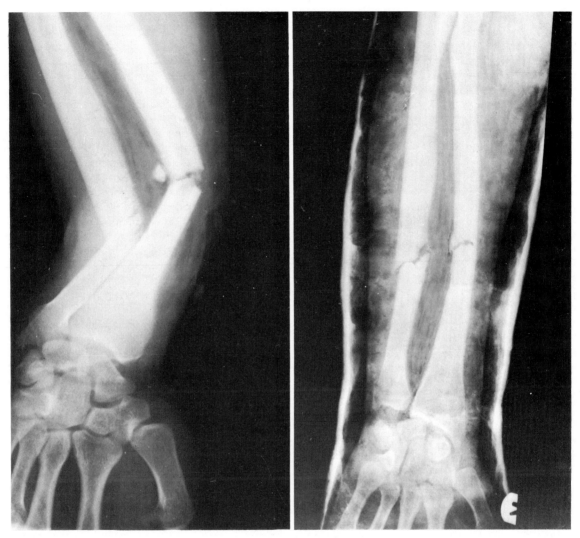

Fig 23.32 A fracture of both forearm bones treated successfully by closed manipulation and plaster immobilisation.

conventional short forearm plaster increases rotational strains on the fracture by limiting movement at the distal radio-ulnar joint and allowing it at the proximal. Both the conventional above elbow plaster and the Sarmiento functional cast brace prevent pronation and supination.

Fractures in children. Forearm fractures in children may be complete, but are often greenstick. There may be no significant displacement, or no more than a few degrees of angulation, which is often easily corrected by firm moulding under anaesthetic. Greenstick fractures should not be over-reduced and

completely broken during reduction* as they can be corrected sufficiently by gentle controlled manipulation, and residual angulation will correct by moulding in the years following the fracture. Immobilisation is needed for only three weeks in most greenstick fractures and five to six in complete fractures. A plaster cast is applied from the metacarpal heads to just below the axilla with the elbow at right angle and the forearm in mid-pronation.

* There is still much controversy about whether greenstick fractures should be completed, and many surgeons feel strongly that they should be broken in order to prevent unnecessary recurrences of angulation (see Chapter 19).

Fractures of the lower third of the shafts of the radius and ulna in children may be of the 'kink' greenstick variety and require little treatment other than a protective forearm plaster; but sometimes they can be severely displaced, and prove difficult to reduce and very difficult to keep reduced (Figs 23.33 and 23.34). The persistence with which the surgeon should repeat manipulations of such a fracture depends on the age of the patient and the degree to which one can expect growth moulding. Under eight years of age considerable moulding can be expected (Figs 23.35 and 23.36), whereas over 12 years of age moulding is much less. If in the older age group this fracture cannot be reduced, the radius can be levered into place through a small incision and without internal fixation, immobilised in an above elbow plaster, either in the supinated or pronated position, whichever is the more stable. Contrary to popular teaching, these fractures tend to be more stable in full supination.[12]

Treatment of forearm fractures with the elbow fully extended. If full extension of the elbow is the only position in which the fracture can be controlled then open reduction is indicated. Fractures of the forearm bones should never be immobilised with the elbow fully extended.

Operative treatment of fractures of the shaft of the forearm bones

There are proponents for conservative and for operative treatment, and there are arguments as to the operative technique of choice. Willenegger has summed up the aims as follows:

'1. To give the injured patient the best possible functional end result without regard to the surgeon's personal ambitions.
2. To have an open mind about the choice of method of treatment in every individual case.
3. To maintain a self-critical attitude.
4. To be acquainted with all methods of treatment so as to be free to choose the proper method in each case. One should consider not only the intrinsic dangers and difficulties of a particular method but also one's own ability and limitations.'

Open reduction and internal fixation is the treatment of choice of most surgeons in the majority of unstable fractures of the shafts of both forearm bones in the adult. Fractures during growth seldom require open operation. If conservative treatment has been selected for an adult regular X-rays must be taken, and if the position is not entirely satisfactory conservative treatment should be discontinued and open reduction and internal fixation performed. This decision should be taken and the operation carried out within a few weeks of the fracture. The presence of associated soft tissue injury may well influence the timing of operation. In a compound fracture it is better to await skin healing before open reduction and internal fixation. It is important that the internally fixed bones be covered by viable soft tissue, including skin. Should a fracture caused by a crush injury be associated with devitalisation of muscle and loss of skin the latter must be replaced before open reduction. Even fracture blisters are a contra-indication to immediate operation. A delay is not always detrimental; a 45-year-old man with a fracture of the mid-shafts of both bones of the forearm had been treated two weeks previously by manipulation and an above elbow plaster, the X-ray was unsatisfactory and the patient was admitted for open reduction and internal fixation. The plaster was removed, but the skin was found to be unsatisfactory and the arm was rested on a pillow to await healing. When, three weeks later, conditions were satisfactory to proceed with the operation, X-ray showed the bones united in good position. The end result was a forearm with good contour and full range of movement. In contrast, sepsis after open reduction and internal fixation is a disaster. If theatre conditions are such that significant numbers of deep infection are occurring then open operation in that unit is contra-indicated.

Timing of operation. There is much to be said in favour of carrying out an open reduction and internal fixation of forearm fractures between 7 and 14 days from the time of the injury. By that time the initial oedema will have subsided, much soft tissue damage will have healed, the operation can be performed on a routine list in the best available conditions; there will have been time for thought and discussion as to the best technique to be used, and the appropriate instrumentation will have been made available. There is also some evidence that a better rate of union can be expected from late operation.[13]

Aims of operation. The aims of open reduction and internal fixation are:

1. To attain a more satisfactory reduction than is possible by conservative means.
2. To improve the probability of bony union.
3. To produce internal fixation of such a standard that, if required, plaster can be discarded and mobilisation be commenced immediately post-operatively, thus assuring rapid return of joint mobility

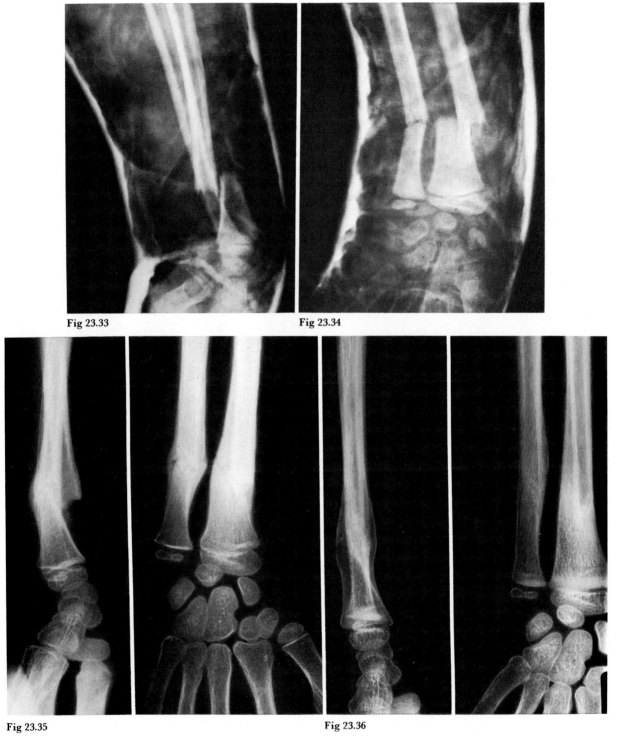

Fig 23.33

Fig 23.34

Fig 23.35

Fig 23.36

Figs 23.33 to 23.36 The fracture of the lower end of the radius and ulna in a child shown in Figure 23.33 could not be reduced and the position shown in Figure 23.34 was accepted. Two months later the fracture had united soundly (Fig 23.35), and by 12 months the forearm was indistinguishable from normal (Fig 23.36). The case illustrates the remarkable moulding ability of the child.

Intramedullary nailing. Intramedullary nailing for unstable forearm fractures has been abandoned by some surgeons following the unfavourable reports at the Salzburg meeting of the Austrian Association for Accident Surgery in 1965. It is certainly unsuitable where there is gross comminution. Nevertheless, this is a useful technique, particularly where there is a double fracture of one or both bones. It is a comparatively simple operation and inflicts minimal damage at the site of the fracture (Figs 23.37 and 23.38). The radial fracture is usually reduced first and is exposed through a small antero-lateral incision. A second incision is then made over the dorsum of the wrist joint near to Lister's tubercle and a small hole drilled from a point immediately distal to the tubercle in the direction of the medullary cavity of the radius. No harm is done if the wrist joint is opened; in fact exposing the wrist joint often facilitates the insertion

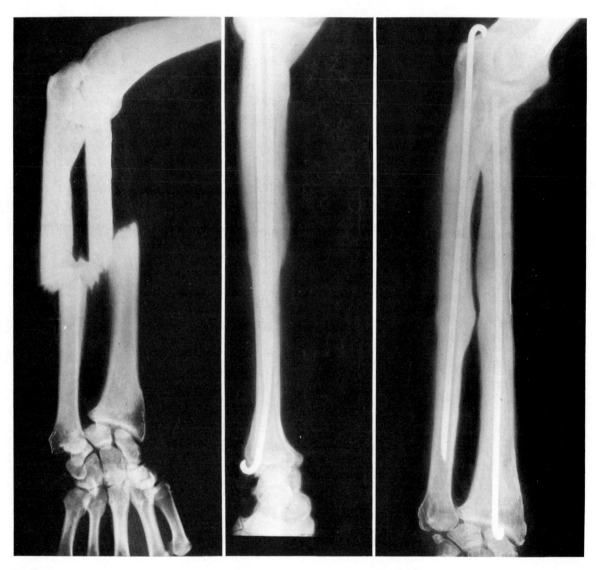

Fig 23.37   **Fig 23.38**

Figs 23.37 and 23.38 This fracture of the mid-shafts of the radius and ulna (Fig 23.37) was internally fixed by means of intramedullary Rush nails. Figure 23.38 shows the sound bony union one year later.

of the nail. The reamer for a narrow gauge Rush nail is then passed up the radius until it is seen to cross the fracture site, and the fixation checked. After removal of the reamer a Rush nail of suitable length is inserted along the intramedullary track. The ulnar fracture is then exposed through an incision along its subcutaneous border and reduced. A Rush nail is passed down the shaft of the ulna through a small incision over the olecranon. After skin closure the forearm is immobilised in an above elbow plaster cast. Plaster fixation is maintained until union is complete.

Plating of both bones of forearm. More rigid fixation can be obtained by the use of plates of which there are many varieties. One excellent plate is the type devised by Hicks (Figs 23.71 and 23.72), in which the screw holes are offset and do not impair the strength of the plate itself. There are many plates which give satisfactory fixation of the radius and ulna, but probably the most effective method of producing rigid internal fixation is by the use of compression plates, developed by the AO School in Switzerland[14, 15, 16] Whichever device is used the fractures must be adequately exposed through separate incisions. The ulnar fracture is reduced first and a plate fixed to one of the two main fragments by screws and held to the other by a temporary clamp. The radius is then reduced; and at this stage it is often desirable to allow the ulnar fracture to displace again to allow perfect reduction of the radius. The radius should then be temporarily fixed and pronation and supination tested. The plating of the two bones can now be completed, using three screws on each side of the fracture whenever possible. At every stage supination and pronation should be checked to make sure that the range is full. A separate compression device may be used with compression plates (see Chapter 16), but in the forearm this involves unnecessarily long incisions and extensive dissection. The dynamic compression plate (DCP) first described by Bagby[17,18] and Denham[19] and more recently developed by the AO School[20] has an intrinsic compression device making extensive dissection unnecessary. The plate depends upon the obliquity of cylindrical screw holes for compression which is produced as the screws are driven home (see Chapter 16).

Technique of internal fixation by DCP plate. The fracture is reduced and the DCP plate placed across the fracture site. A first hole is drilled half an inch (1.3 cm) from the fracture and a screw is inserted, but not driven home. A second hole is drilled through the hole in the plate closest to the fracture on the other

side, using a load guide. The load guide ensures eccentric positioning of the drill hole so that the head of the screw applies pressure to the edge of the cylindrical hole as it is driven home, causing the plate to shift slightly and thus producing compression at the fracture. X-rays may be taken at this stage before the other holes are drilled and the screws inserted. Occasionally these other screws may be used to increase the compression by inserting them with the load guide, but if additional screws are so used, the previous ones must be partly unscrewed before applying compression with the next screw.

Post-operative management. Provided there is excellent rigid fixation, plaster is unnecessary and active movements can be started 48 hours post-operatively. If the fixation is not rigid then a full arm plaster should be applied until union is complete.

Open operation without internal fixation. Sometimes after operative exposure of a forearm fracture the fragments can be locked together so securely that it is tempting to leave them without internal fixation. This is only justifiable in the growing child where moulding takes care of any residual deformity. In the adult, however satisfactory the fracture may appear at operation, it is highly likely that displacement will recur in plaster afterwards unless internal fixation is used, with the grave possibility of permanent disability.

COMPLICATIONS OF FRACTURES OF THE FOREARM

Open fractures of the forearm. Open fractures of the forearm are frequently from within out, and this applies especially to the ulna which is subcutaneous throughout its length. They should be treated by exploration and excision of non-viable tissue, followed by skin closure whenever possible and systemic antibiotics. Serious infection including gas gangrene may complicate a forearm fracture with a small wound from within. The mechanism of injury is frequently a fall on the outstretched hand and when the proximal fragment protrudes through the skin it may be contaminated by soil.[21] Open forearm fractures may be treated in an above elbow cast with an extensive window for observation and dressing of the damaged skin (Fig 23.39). After skin healing an open fracture may be treated in the same way as a closed injury either by continuing closed immobilisation or by open reduction and internal fixation. The preference of the surgeon, the facilities available as well as the type of injury dictate which method is employed. Severe trauma with extensive soft tissue

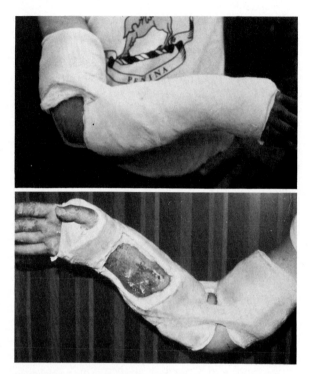

Fig 23.39 An above elbow plaster cast for an open fracture of both forearm bones. The wound has been observed and dressed through a large window, it is now healed. The elbow has been left free to reduce the harmful effects of swelling. It has been bridged by a plaster strut on either side connecting the arm and forearm cylinders.

injury as well as fractures present special difficulties. Whereas such fractures are often treated satisfactorily with plaster cast fixation only, fixation of very unstable fractures is often necessary to ensure adequate soft tissue healing. This fixation may be internal or by external skeletal apparatus.[22, 23] Sir Reginald's wartime case of severe forearm injury is still relevant. A pilot in 1941 fractured his forearm and returned to flying duties 10 months after the injury. He sustained a double fracture of the radius with splitting of the central fragment, a comminuted fracture of the head of radius and a delayed dislocation of the inferior radio-ulnar joint. His soft tissue injuries were more serious, a radial nerve paralysis and avulsion of skin from the elbow and upper half of forearm. The wound was excised after resuscitation, but there was no possibility of closing it, and the next day 48 square inches of split skin graft were transferred to the denuded area. Two months later three bone operations were undertaken. First the fragment of ulna was

fixed by onlay bone graft, then the fractured head of radius was excised and the fragments of radial shaft replaced by an onlay graft. Lastly the dislocated lower end of ulna was excised (Figs 23.40 and 23.41). This case was under the care of Murray Meekison of Vancouver when he was serving in the R.A.F. Orthopaedic Service.

Infected fractures of the forearm. If deep infection occurs after operative treatment of forearm fractures any metallic implants should be removed. It is usually undesirable to remove the metal immediately, and wiser to leave it *in situ* until some bony stability at the fracture site has been achieved. In the meantime the infection is treated with the appropriate antibiotics and surgical drainage, with effective decompression of tension and the removal of non-viable tissue, including sequestra. Large portions of bone, even an entire diaphysis, can sequestrate

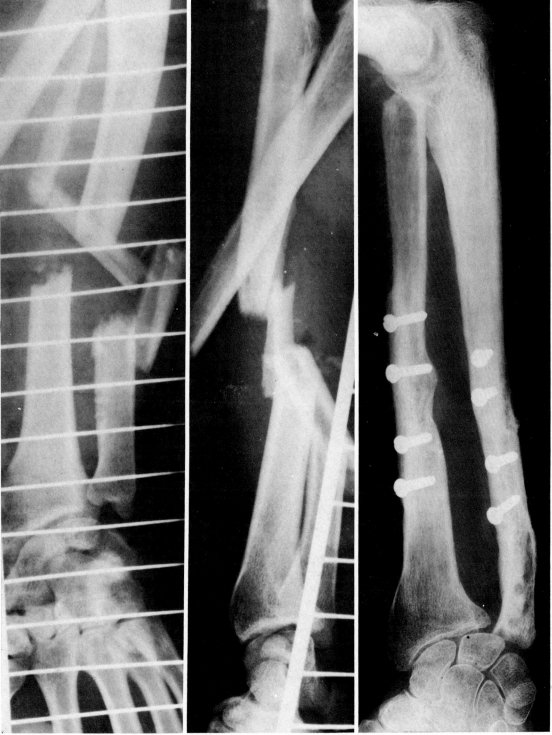

Fig 23.40

Fig 23.41

Figs 23.40 and 23.41 Grossly comminuted fracture of the shafts of both forearm bones with destruction of the skin from above the elbow to the lower third of the forearm (Fig 23.40). The first problem was the replacement of the skin; the second was the realignment of the forearm bones with onlay grafting from the tibia; the third was reconstruction by excision of the head of the radius and the lower end of the ulna (Fig 23.41; see text).

(Figs 23.42 to 23.44). Figure 23.45 shows a double fracture of the shaft of the radius in which operative reduction with wiring of the fragments had been complicated by infection, so that a large part of the shaft of the radius was exposed in the wound. The extensor muscles of the forearm were destroyed and there was a wrist drop. After the dead bone had been removed, most of the radius was missing and the remaining fragments were so porotic that it would have been difficult to secure sound fixation of bone grafts (Fig 23.46). In this type of injury the operation originally described by Hey Groves of constructing a single bone out of the radius and ulna may be applicable.[24, 25, 26] In this particular case the lower shaft of the ulna was impaled into the distal radial fragment. Following the Hey Groves procedure all forearm rotation is of course lost, so that care was taken in this case to fix the new single forearm bone slightly on the pronated side of the mid-position (Figs 23.47 to 23.49). The flexor-carpi-ulnaris was later transplanted to the distal extensor tendons of fingers and thumb, and function was so good that the boy took over most of his father's arduous duties as a farmer (Figs 23.48 and 23.49).

Un-united fractures of the forearm bones
Occasional non-union of fractures of the forearm bones is inevitable, but its incidence is reduced by correct treatment. Inadequate internal fixation, with plates which are too small, or with single screws, is a potent cause of non-union. Repeated manipulation during conservative treatment, particularly after 10 days, combined with the use of an inadequate plaster cast, may also cause this complication. It is important to recognise the difference between delayed union and non-union, for so long as established non-union has not occurred further immobilisation may still result in a united fracture. Loss of substance of the radius or ulna such as occurs in gunshot wounds with infection invariably leads to non-union. The treatment of the un-united fracture without a bony defect is by adequate internal fixation reinforced by a cancellous onlay bone graft (see Chapter 18). Internal fixation may be by plating or intramedullary nailing. An advantage of a nail is that the limited space around the pseudarthrosis may be taken up entirely by bone graft rather than in part by the plate. Although it is usual to take cancellous slivers from the iliac crest, the upper end of the ulna is a useful source of cancellous bone, and if the fracture is not too near this site, it may be preferable to take the graft from there. Large defects in the radius or the ulna, however,

must be filled by appropriately shaped blocks of cancellous bone taken from the ilium (Fig 23.44).

Radio-ulnar synostosis from cross union.
Cross union of the radius and ulna results from a continuous haematoma between the two fractures. Such a haematoma may arise from the injury, or it may be due to operative intervention (Fig 23.50). It is of paramount importance in open reduction that the surgeon keeps the two haematomata separated. This can be done by making separate incisions for the exposure of the two fractures and by gentle technique during the operation to avoid joining the two haematomata internally. If cross union occurs, the bridge of bone joining the radius and ulna will prevent pronation and supination, but surprisingly this often produces little functional disability and the patient should always return to work to see if he can manage. Only those cases in which there is severe disability justify operation and then not before 12 months after union, when recurrence of synostosis is less likely. The bridge of bone should be excised, the forearm immobilised in mid-pronation for 10 days and gentle mobilisation commenced. The interposition of a silastic membrane between the two bones may prevent cross union recurring. However, it should be made clear to the patient before operation that the bridge of bone may re-form.

FRACTURES OF THE SHAFT OF THE ULNA

Fractures of the shaft of the ulna without radio-ulnar joint disruption
This fracture usually results from a direct injury to the bone, occurring when the forearm is raised to protect the face. With the increased incidence of 'mugging' attacks the fracture is becoming more common. It frequently occurs at the junction of the lower and middle thirds of the ulnar shaft and is occasionally not visible on the initial X-ray. If diagnosed clinically a further X-ray should be taken a week later when the fracture is usually clearly visible (Fig 23.51). The treatment is immobilisation in an above-elbow plaster or by functional bracing[27] until the fracture is united. Check X-rays should be taken as angulation sometimes occurs, associated with subluxation of the lower radio-ulnar joint. If this happens internal fixation may become necessary. Surprisingly, non-union is not uncommon and is treated by internal fixation and an onlay cancellous graft. If the fracture is within two inches (5.1 cm) of the lower end of the ulna, the lower fragment may

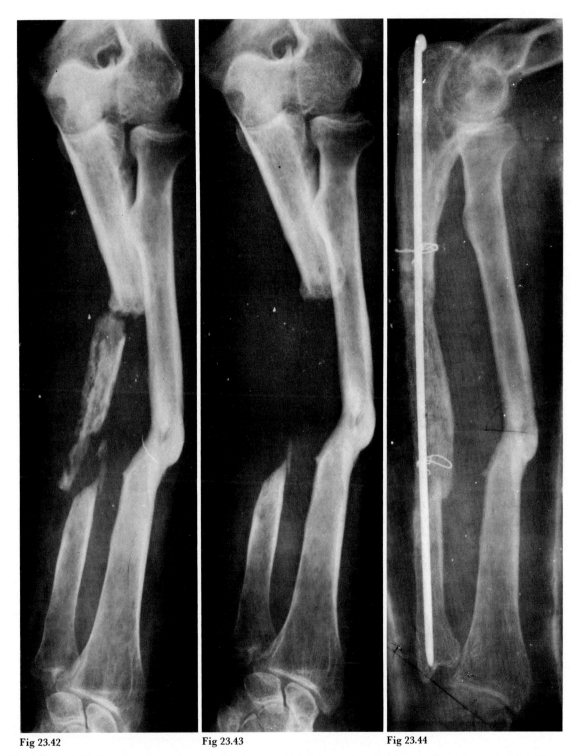

Fig 23.42   **Fig 23.43**   **Fig 23.44**

Figs 23.42 to 23.44 Comminuted open fracture of the forearm with infection and massive sequestration of the middle third of the shaft of the ulna (Fig 21.42). Sequestrectomy was followed by iliac cancellous bone graft fixed with a Rush nail and circumferential wiring (Fig 23.43 and 23.44).

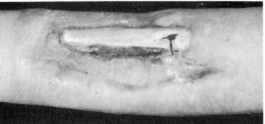

Fig 23.45 Fracture of the shaft of the radius at two levels with infection and sequestration of the central fragment.

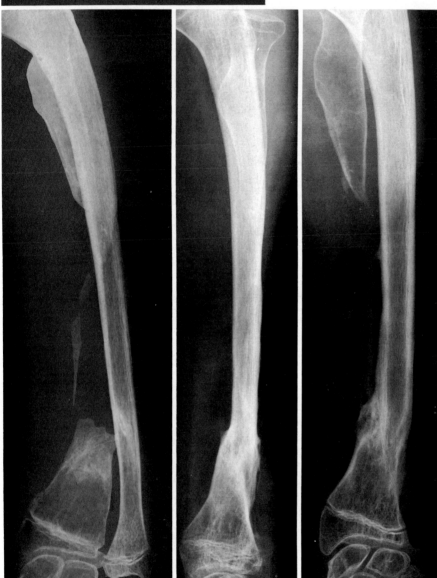

Fig 23.46

Fig 23.47

Figs 23.46 to 23.49 The problem of destroyed bone was met by radio-ulnar transference (grafting the distal fragment of the radius into the shaft of the ulna— Hey Groves). There was still the problem of complete destruction of all extensor muscles which was met by a transfer of a flexor muscle (Figs 23.48 and 23.49).

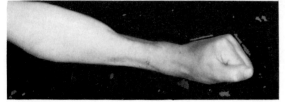

Fig 23.48

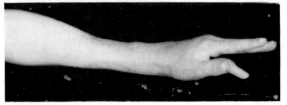

Fig 23.49

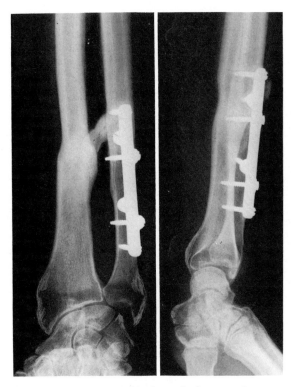

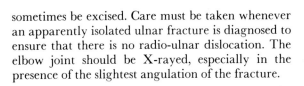

Fig 23.50 Cross union possibly the result of too extensive a dissection at open reduction causing a single fracture haematoma.

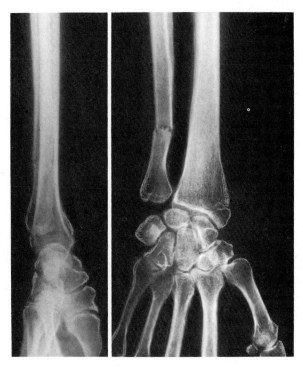

Fig 23.51 Fracture of the distal ulnar shaft which had been invisible immediately following the fracture two weeks previously.

sometimes be excised. Care must be taken whenever an apparently isolated ulnar fracture is diagnosed to ensure that there is no radio-ulnar dislocation. The elbow joint should be X-rayed, especially in the presence of the slightest angulation of the fracture.

Fracture of the shaft of the ulna with dislocation of the head of the radius (Monteggia fracture)

This fracture of the upper third of the ulna with dislocation of the head of the radius was first described by Monteggia in 1814.[28] The head of the radius is dislocated both from the radio-ulnar articulation and from the elbow joint. It may be displaced anteriorly, posteriorly or laterally according to the angulation of the ulnar fracture. More than a century elapsed before a solution was found to the problems of treatment of this injury. Until 1940, the overall results of treatment were abysmal. In a series of 34 Monteggia fracture-dislocations treated by many surgeons* there were only two good results, and 32

* Reviewed by R.W.-J.

out of 34 patients had serious permanent disabilities. From this study arose the principles of treatment which have resulted in a solution to most of the problems of this fracture. Internal fixation has become the treatment of choice.

Diagnosis. Every fracture of the upper shaft of the ulna without a fracture of the radial shaft should be considered to be a Monteggia fracture until proved otherwise. The first X-ray may show the head of the radius in its correct position, but this can be fortuitous, for if dislocation has occurred and there is instability, the head of the radius may redisplace later. *Repeated X-rays over the first few weeks are mandatory to avoid missing this important fracture-dislocation.* It must be emphasised that in a fracture of the upper shaft of the ulna with angulation or over-riding of the fragments and without corresponding injury to the radius, there must be a dislocation of the proximal or distal radio-ulnar joint, usually the proximal.

Three types of displacement. Monteggia fracture-dislocations may occur from either flexion, extension or adduction forces and there are three corresponding types of injury.

The flexion injuries account for only 10 to 15 per cent of cases. The fractured ulna is angulated with the convexity posteriorly and the head of the radius is dislocated backwards (Figs 23.52 and 23.53). *The extension injury* is the common type of Monteggia fracture accounting for 85 to 90 per cent of cases. The fractured ulna is angulated with its convexity anteriorly and laterally, and the head of the radius is dislocated forwards and to the lateral side (Figs 23.54 and 23.55).

The adduction injury is rare and caused by an adduction strain at the elbow. The ulna is angulated laterally and the radial head displaced laterally. (Figs 23.56 and 23.57).

The Hume fracture. In 1957 Hume described three cases of fracture of the proximal ulna associated with forward dislocation of the head of the radius occurring in children.[29] This fracture is a high Monteggia injury, but it is frequently misinterpreted in the initial X-ray when the dislocated head of the radius is mistakenly thought to be an isolated injury.

Mechanism of injury. It has been suggested by Mervyn Evans that these fracture-dislocations are sustained from a fall on the outstretched hand with twisting of the trunk, forcibly pronating the forearm.[30] If this is correct then supination is essential for reduction and a safeguard against recurrence of displacement. This injury does not always arise from forced pronation, and immobilisation in supination is not always successful in preventing displacement. A Monteggia fracture can result from a direct injury. It is a common fracture in Africa, where the usual cause is a direct blow on the back of the forearm with a stick while the arm is raised warding off an attacker. The ulna fractures, angulates forwards, and the head of the radius is driven anteriorly. It may be that a Monteggia fracture-dislocation is sometimes caused by the mechanism described by Mervyn Evans and sometimes by direct violence. In this fracture, what matters is that the need for reduction of both the ulnar fracture and the displaced head of radius is recognised.

Treatment of the Monteggia fracture-dislocation.

Conservative treatment. Manipulation and plaster immobilisation is advocated by some surgeons.[30, 31] These conservative measures are justifiable in a child, but a close watch must be kept for a recurrence of the deformity and, if this occurs, open reduction and internal fixation of the ulna is advisable within two weeks of the initial injury. The extension fracture dislocation is reduced by longitudinal traction on the forearm with the elbow flexed. It may be necessary to apply pressure over the radial head and the ulna in order to reduce the deformity. The upper limb is immobilised in a well padded plaster cast, with the elbow flexed as much as possible without impeding the circulation. Generally the forearm is stable in supination. The plaster is windowed to observe the radial pulse. The flexion injury is reduced by traction on the forearm with the elbow extended, and as the reduction is only stable with the elbow extended it is never desirable to use this method in the adult. The adduction injury is reduced by traction on the forearm with the elbow extended and pressure over the head of the radius, and after reduction this fracture dislocation is stable with the elbow flexed, and as a rule with the forearm supinated. (Figs 23.52 to 23.57).

Operative treatment. The degree of skill and vigilance necessary to achieve good results in the Monteggia fracture, using conservative means, is such that it is generally advisable in the adult to treat this lesion by open reduction of the fracture of the ulna and rigid internal fixation, preferably with a plate, although an intramedullary nail may be satisfactory. Less rigid fixation using wires and screws alone is useless.

Dislocation of the head of the radius generally reduces spontaneously when the deformity of the ulna has been reduced. If the radial head is not in perfect position it should be exposed and reduced under direct vision.

Operative technique. The fracture of the ulna is exposed, reduced and fixed by a compression plate, an intramedullary nail or other appropriate device. During the operation it is advisable to take elbow X-rays in two planes. If the head of the radius is perfectly reduced the position is accepted and a well-padded plaster cast is applied from the metacarpal heads to the axilla, with the elbow at right angles and the forearm supinated. If the X-ray shows that the head of the radius is not reduced it must be exposed and reduced under direct vision. Very often the annular ligament is the cause of the obstruction and may need to be incised before the radial head can be reduced. Reconstruction of this ligament may be of value, but it is usually unnecessary, as full reduction of the radial head is maintained by the rigid fixation of the ulnar fracture.

Danger of early excision of the head of the radius. It has been suggested that in order to avoid limitation of radio-ulnar movement the head of the radius should

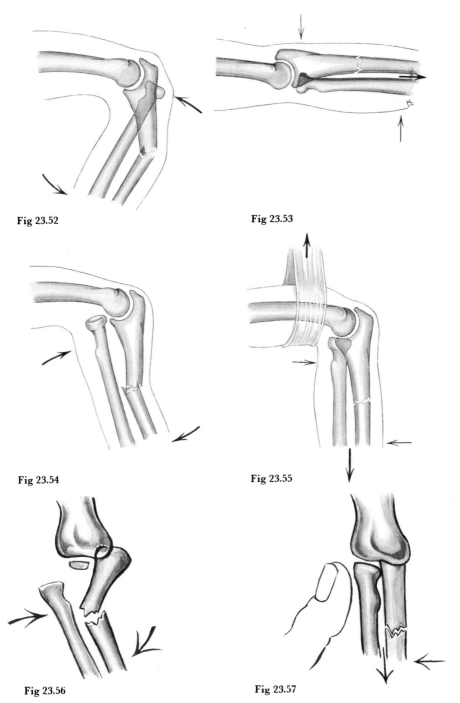

Fig 23.52

Fig 23.53

Fig 23.54

Fig 23.55

Fig 23.56

Fig 23.57

Figs 23.52 to 23.57 Types of Monteggia Fracture.

Figs 23.52 and 23.53 The flexion injury. Fracture shaft of the ulna with backward dislocation of the head of the radius. The displacement is reduced by traction in extension.

Figs 23.54 and 23.55 The extension injury. Fracture shaft of the ulna with forward dislocation of the head of the radius. The displacement is reduced by traction in flexion.

Figs 23.56 and 23.57 The adduction injury. Fracture of the shaft of the ulna with lateral displacement of the head of the radius. The displacement is reduced by traction in extension and with pressure over the head of the radius and at the same time correcting the ulnar deformity.

be excised at the time that the ulna is reduced and plated. This is bad advice. The head of the radius should be left *in situ*, partly because of the danger of traumatic ossification, but also early excision, before the torn annular ligament and interosseous membrane have healed, may allow the shaft of the radius to move proximally, with consequent dislocation of the distal radio-ulnar joint. The stump of the upper end of the radius impacts against the capitellum once more and excision of more bone may be required (Figs 23.58 to 23.61). When the head of the radius is fractured as a complication of a Monteggia fracture, the indications for excision of the fragments are the same as those for simple fracture of the head of the radius. If the fracture is severely comminuted with displacement of the fragments excision should be delayed until the fractured ulna is united or the excised radial head immediately replaced by a prosthesis.

Treatment of the complications of Monteggia fracture-dislocations. *Un-reduced dislocation of the head of the radius.* Late unreduced dislocation is best treated in adults by excision of the displaced head of the radius. This may result in increased elbow flexion by removing the obstructing block of bone and usually restores a good range of pronation and supination. Excision of the head of the radius is not justified in children because it involves removal of the upper radial epiphysis with increasing inequality in the length of the forearm bones and further dislocation of the radio-ulnar joints, both superior and inferior. Attempts to reposition the head of the radius and reconstruct the annular ligament have been reported. Figures 23.62 to 23.64 show one of two cases in which tendon grafts were used in the repair, the palmaris longus in one and the peroneus tertius in another. The tendon was passed around the neck of the radius and through a drill hole in the ulna. The effects of pressure on the newly constructed ligaments can be seen in the ridging of bone in the final radiograph taken three years after operation. The position of the radial head is not perfect, but good stability and a normal range of movement were maintained. This can be a difficult operation and the radial head seldom remains in its correct position.

Traumatic ossification around the radial head. When traumatic ossification around the head of the radius has followed early operative reduction of the dislocation, excision of the head of the radius and the block of bone attached to it may be indicated (Figs 23.65 to 23.67). Unfortunately, there is a tendency for such ossification to recur. The probability of

recurrence may be reduced provided that the operation is delayed for 6 to 12 months following the injury and the elbow is immobilised after operation for at least two weeks. Physiotherapy, manipulation and passive exercise must be avoided during the rehabilitation period.

Posterior interosseous nerve palsy. This nerve lesion more frequently accompanies the adduction fracture dislocation than other types. The prognosis in early cases is excellent, so long as the head of the radius is fully reduced. Occasionally, late posterior interosseous nerve lesions may be due to inadequate reduction of the radial head.[32]

Cross union between the radius and the ulna. The problem of cross union complicating Monteggia fracture-dislocations is more difficult to treat than that following fractures of the mid-shaft and the radius and ulna. The bony fusion is between the neck of the radius and the fracture site in the upper third of the ulna (Fig 23.68). This is a difficult area to deal with surgically, owing to the proximity of the elbow joint and the posterior interosseous nerve and the probability of recurrence is high. The alternative and probably more advisable course of action is to accept the permanent limitation of radio-ulnar movement, the disability of which is minimised if the forearm is slightly on the pronated side of the mid-position.

Dislocation of the lower end of the ulna. This usually reduces spontaneously with reduction of the ulnar shaft fracture but may occur if the head of the radius is excised. If there are wrist symptoms the distal inch of the ulna should be excised.

Un-united fracture of the ulna. Fractures of the ulna are notoriously slow in uniting but union usually follows adequate fixation. Should non-union occur the treatment is by rigid internal fixation and cancellous onlay grafting.

Dislocation of the head of the radius. Dislocation of the head of the radius is rarely an isolated lesion. It is usually associated with fracture of the ulna. Whenever dislocation of the head of the radius is diagnosed the entire length of the ulna must be X-rayed. It should be remembered that the head of the radius normally articulates with the capitellum. Anterior dislocation seen on the lateral X-ray can easily be missed by the junior Casualty Officer. (Figs 23.71 and 23.72)

FRACTURE OF THE SHAFT OF THE RADIUS OR ULNA WITH DISLOCATION OF THE ELBOW. (Figs 23.69 and 23.70). This rare and serious injury must be treated by reduction of the

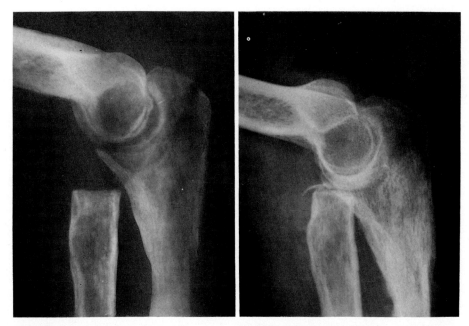

Fig 23.58 Immediately after operation.   **Fig 23.59** Three months after operation.

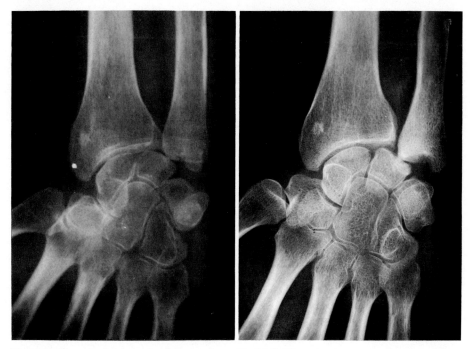

Fig 23.60 The wrist three months after operation.   **Fig 23.61** The wrist nine months after operation.

Figs 23.58 to 23.61 Case illustrating the danger in Monteggia fracture-dislocations of too early excision of the radial head—thus causing subluxation of the inferior radio-ulnar joint. Early excision of the radial head may not only cause myositis ossificans, but if it is performed before the orbicular ligament and the interosseous membrane have healed it allows sliding of the radius and dislocation of the lower end of the ulna (Figs 23.60 and 23.61). Moreover the stump of the radius impacts once more against the capitellum (Fig 23.59) and a second excision may be needed.

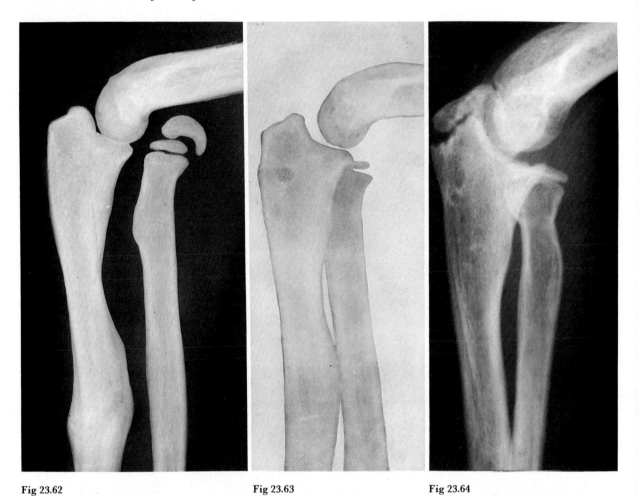

Fig 23.62   **Fig 23.63**   **Fig 23.64**

Figs 23.62 to 23.64 Monteggia fracture-dislocation and unreduced dislocation of the radial head in a child (Fig 23.62). A free graft of palmaris longus was used to maintain reduction of the dislocation (Fig 23.63). Three years after the operation slight redisplacement has occurred but the elbow remains clinically satisfactory. Ridging of the bone from pressure of the newly constructed ligament can be seen (Fig 23.64).

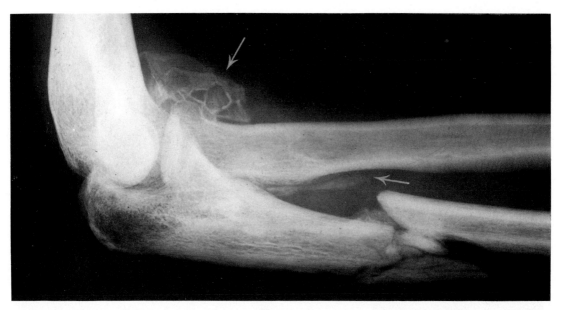

Fig 23.65 Monteggia fracture-dislocation treated by open reduction of the ulna without internal fixation (which was a mistake) and by open reduction of the dislocated radial head (which was also a mistake because it caused traumatic ossification).

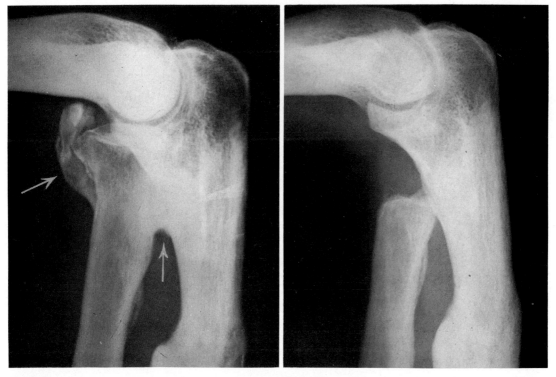

Fig 23.66   **Fig 23.67**

Figs 23.65 to 23.67 Case illustrating the danger in Monteggia fracture dislocation of failing to secure sound internal fixation of the ulna—and the dangers of traumatic ossification. End result in the case shown in Figure 23.65. Traumatic ossification around the head of the radius caused serious limitation of movement (Fig 23.66). Note how extensively the upper end of the radius must be excised to restore the radio-ulnar movement when this complication has arisen (Fig 23.67).

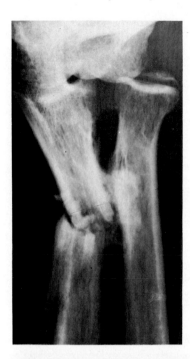

Fig 23.68 Result of operative reduction of a Monteggia fracture-dislocation without internal fixation. There is redisplacement and cross union.

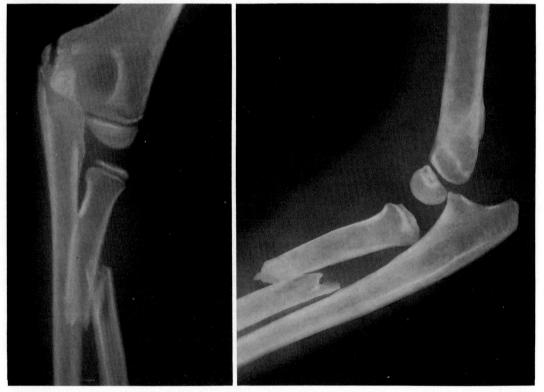

Fig 23.69   Fig 23.70

Figs 23.69 and 23.70 Fracture of the shaft of the radius associated with dislocation of the elbow.

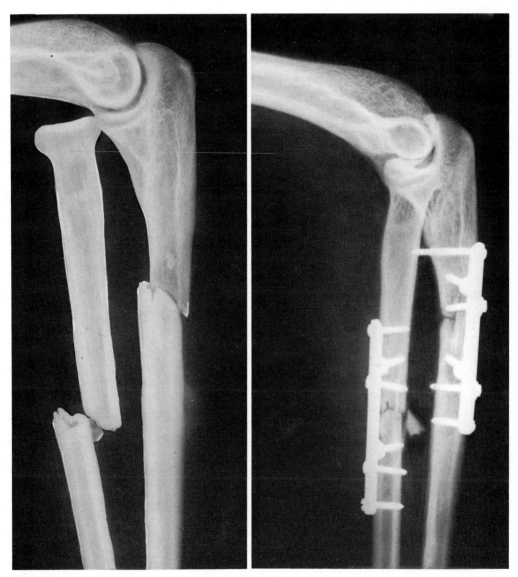

Fig 23.71   **Fig 23.72**

Figs 23.71 and 23.72 An unusual fracture of both radius and ulna with dislocation of the head of the radius treated by fixation with Hicks plates.

dislocation and internal fixation of the fractured bones. A dislocated elbow may sometimes be associated with fracture of the shaft of the ulna and such a fracture is usually compound.

FRACTURES OF THE SHAFT OF THE RADIUS

Fracture of the shaft of the radius with disruption of the interosseous membrane (intermediate radio-ulnar joint)

In this fracture muscular action results in rotational displacement. The biceps and the supinator muscles, both of which are supinators, are inserted into the upper third of the shaft of the radius; the pronator teres is inserted into the middle third of the bone, and the pronator quadratus into the lower third. A fracture of the shaft of the radius at the junction of the upper and middle thirds is therefore situated between the two groups of muscles. The proximal fragment has only supinator muscles inserted into it and the distal fragment only pronators (Figs 23.73). The proximal fragment is therefore supinated and the distal fragment pronated. There may be from 90 to 180 degrees of rotational displacement and Figure 23.75 shows a typical clinical deformity. Fractures of the upper third of the radius, therefore, should usually be immobilised with the hand and forearm supinated, so that the distal fragment is rotated into the same axis as the proximal fragment. If the fracture is at, or below, the middle third of the bone the proximal fragment has both supinator and pronator muscles attached to it (Fig 23.74). It therefore takes up the mid-position halfway between full supination and

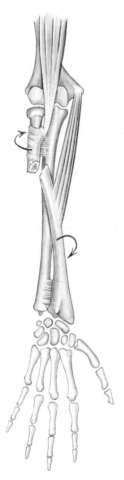

Fig 23.73 In a fracture of the upper shaft of the radius the proximal fragment is supinated and the lower fragment pronated.

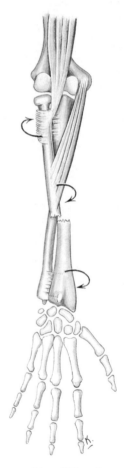

Fig 23.74 In a fracture of the middle or lower third of the shaft the proximal fragment is in the mid-position and the lower fragment pronated.

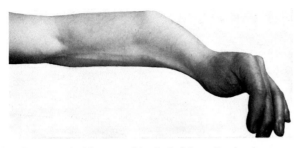

23.75 Mal-united fracture of the shaft of the radius showing typical displacement with pronation of the lower fragment and backward angulation.

full pronation, and this forearm fracture should usually be immobilised with the hand and lower forearm in the mid-position. A method of assessing the rotatory deformity of these fractures has been described by Mervyn Evans.[33] The normal forearm is X-rayed in various degrees of pronation and supination. In one of these X-rays the tuberosity of the radius will show the same contour as that on the fractured side. This is an indication of the degree of supination or pronation of the upper radial fragment, and the forearm on the fractured side can be placed in the appropriate position of rotation before plaster immobilisation. Unstable fractures of the shaft of the radius alone are best treated by operative reduction and internal fixation.

Fracture of the shaft of the radius with dislocation of the lower radio-ulnar joint—Galeazzi fracture.[34]

As fractures of the upper shaft of the ulna are associated with dislocation of the upper end of the radius, so fractures of the lower shaft of the radius are associated with dislocations of the lower end of the ulna (Fig 23.76). This fracture-dislocation, with angulation of the radius and dislocation of the inferior radio-ulnar joint, shows the same tendency to redisplacement after reduction as does the corresponding fracture-dislocation of the upper forearm. The fibrocartilage of the inferior radio-ulnar joint may remain intact, it may be ruptured, or it may avulse the styloid process of the ulna.

Treatment. Rarely this fracture may be treated by manipulation and plaster immobilisation only. It is reduced in supination. A well-padded, full arm plaster of Paris cast with the elbow at right angles is applied and maintained until union is complete, usually eight weeks. If the fracture is selected for conservative treatment weekly X-rays are mandatory, and should the position become unsatisfactory open reduction must be undertaken without delay.

The treatment of choice for the Galeazzi fracture is open reduction and internal fixation (Figs 23.76 and 23.77). The fracture is exposed through an anterior incision, and after hairline reduction, rigid fixation is achieved by means of a plate or by an intramedullary nail. As soon as the radius has been dealt with, X-rays are taken to ensure that the lower radio-ulnar joint is satisfactorily reduced. If the ulnar styloid has been avulsed the AO School have advocated fixation with a small screw[14] but this is probably unnecessary. Fig 23.77. If the rigidity of the internal fixation is adequate, early mobilisation without plaster may be allowed; otherwise a full arm plaster cast is maintained until bony union of the fracture.

Mal-union and non-union of the Galeazzi fracture with unreduced dislocation of the inferior radio-ulnar joint. When the dislocated lower end of the ulna has remained unreduced for many months and there is angulation of the radius with or without union, the first step is to excise 1 inch (2.5 cm) of the lower end of the ulna. If the radial fracture is united this may be all that is required to restore the movements of pronation and supination and to regain good function in the wrist. However, if the degree of angulation is unacceptable, osteotomy may be performed, either immediately following excision of the lower end of the ulna, or several months later after the patient has assessed the function of his forearm. If there is non-union of the radial fracture preliminary excision of the lower end of the ulna facilitates reduction of the fracture, which can be reduced and fixed, either by a compression plate or an intramedullary nail. In addition, onlay cancellous bone grafts cut from the upper end of the ulna or the iliac crest should be used.

Persistent instability of the lower radio-ulnar joint. Occasionally, in spite of reduction of the fracture of the radius with rigid internal fixation and the apparent complete reduction of the lower radio-ulnar joint, there may be persistent instability of the lower radio-ulnar joint. This can be diagnosed more easily clinically than radiographically, and it is sometimes the cause of symptoms. A radiograph will occasionally demonstrate the instability (Figs 23.78 and 23.79).

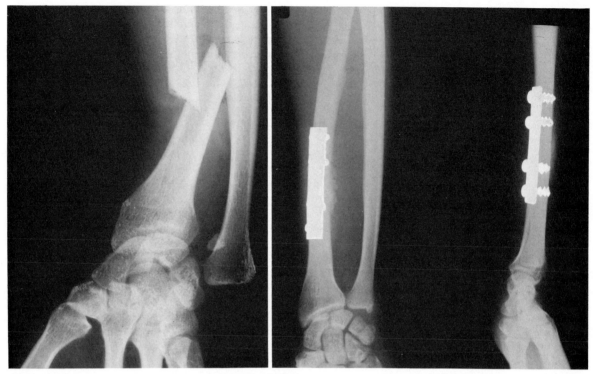

Fig 23.76   **Fig 23.77**

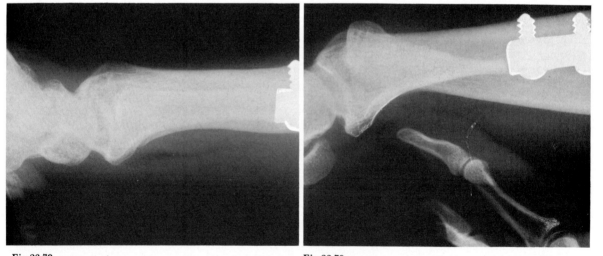

Fig 23.78   **Fig 23.79**

Figs 23.76 to 23.79 Fig 23.76: Galleazzi fracture with avulsion of the styloid process of the ulna. Fig 23.77: Eight weeks later the fractures of both the radius and the ulnar styloid are united in good position, the radius having been plated. Figs 23.78 and 23.79: One year later showing that in spite of good positioning of the lower radio-ulnar joint digital pressure on the palmar aspect of the head of the ulna will displace it dorsally indicating instability.

Fractures of the radial head with dislocation of the distal radio-ulnar joint—the Essex-Lopresti fracture.[8]

Sometimes the upper end of the radius is fractured by longitudinal (axial) compression of the forearm as is shown in Figure 23.80. This is an X-ray of the elbow of a man who was pushing a loaded truck with his wrist dorsiflexed and his elbow extended when the truck suddenly stopped. The radius was driven forcibly against the capitellum and the head of the radius fractured; at the same time the ulna was dislocated at its lower end (Fig 23.81). The true nature may sometimes be disclosed in radiographs of the elbow alone which show impaction of the neck of the radius into the middle of the comminuted fragments of the head with shortening. Radiographs of the inferior radio-ulnar joint will confirm the displacement and must be taken in every comminuted fracture of the head of the radius. If the interpretation of these radiographs by an inexperienced casualty officer is in doubt, X-rays of the other wrist should be taken for comparison. If the head of the radius is excised early there can be further displacement of the radial shaft proximally and the deformity at the lower radio-ulnar joint will increase (Fig 23.82).

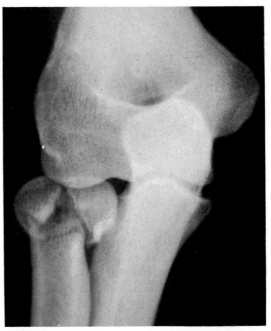

Fig 23.80 Comminuted fracture of the head of the radius sustained not by a valgus strain of the joint but by longitudinal compression of the forearm.

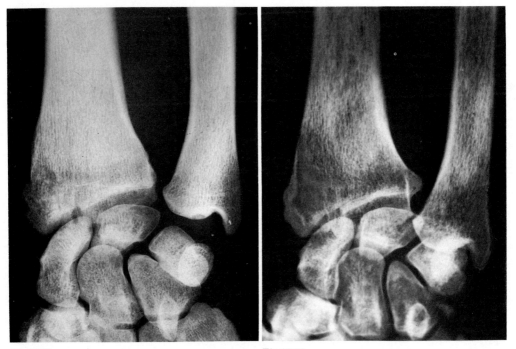

Fig 23.81   **Fig 23.82**

Figs 23.81 and 23.82 Radiographs of the inferior radio-ulnar joint at the time of the initial injury (in the same case as shown in Fig 21.80) prove that there had been longitudinal compression with subluxation of the inferior radio-ulnar joint—the Essex-Lopresti type of fracture-dislocation (Fig 23.81). The significance was not recognised so that, of course, early excision of the radial head increased the displacement at the inferior radio-ulnar joint (Fig 23.82). The lower end of the ulna then had to be excised.

Excision should be delayed long enough for the damage to the interosseous membrane and inferior radio-ulnar ligaments to heal. Replacement of the excised radial head by a silicone rubber prosthesis may prevent this complication (Figs 23.13 to 23.15).

FRACTURES OF THE LOWER END OF THE RADIUS WITH DISLOCATION OF THE DISTAL RADIO-ULNAR JOINT

Colles' fracture

This common injury is a fracture dislocation of the lower radio-ulnar joint, not of the wrist joint as is sometimes taught. The injury was first described in 1814 by Abraham Colles of Dublin who pursued his studies in Edinburgh and at the astonishingly early age of 29 was elected President of the Royal College of Surgeons in Ireland. His article on fracture of the lower end of the radius was published in the *Edinburgh Medical and Surgical Journal*[35] (Figs 23.83 and 23.84).

Incidence. A Colles' fracture is a fracture of the elderly, occurring more commonly in women than in men. There is some seasonal variation in that the fracture is more common in icy weather.

Diagnosis. The injured wrist is swollen and painful and may show the typical 'dinner fork' deformity (Fig 23.85). Clinical examination must include palpation of the styloid processes of the radius and ulna. If they are at the same level, or if the ulnar

styloid is more distal, then a Colles' fracture is the likely diagnosis. The possibility of an old Colles' fracture which has united in the displaced position must also be considered.

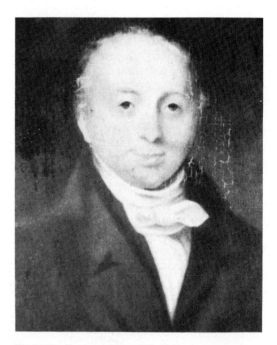

Fig 23.83 Abraham Colles 1773–1843.

V.

On the Fracture of the Carpal extremity of the Radius. By A. Colles, M. D. one of the Professors of Anatomy and Surgery in the Royal College of Surgeons in Ireland.

THE injury to which I wish to direct the attention of surgeons, has not, as far as I know, been described by any author ; indeed the form of the carpal extremity of the radius would rather incline us to question its being liable to fracture. The absence of crepitus, and of the other common symptoms of fracture, together with the swelling which instantly arises in this, as in other injuries of the wrist, render the difficulty of ascertaining the real nature of the case very considerable.

Fig 23.84 *Edinburgh Medical Journal.* April 1814.

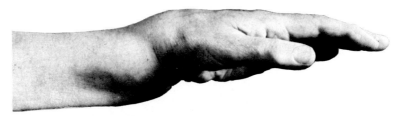

Fig 23.85 A Colles' fracture of the radius showing the typical 'dinner fork' deformity due to backward displacement and tilting of the lower fragment.

Mechanism of injury and displacement. The Colles' fracture is caused by a fall on the outstretched hand. So many upper limb fractures are caused in this way it would be of benefit if we could develop a reflex to fall on the outer aspect of the arm and shoulder with the elbow tucked into the side as do gymnasts and parachutists. An irate general surgeon once accosted his orthopaedic colleague saying 'I did what you have been advising for years and look what has happened'. He had a fracture dislocation of his elbow! Having avoided a fall on the outstretched hand he had fallen instead on the point of his elbow.

On falling onto the outstretched hand the prominent thenar eminence takes the brunt of the force. The fracture of the lower end of the radius occurs while the triangular fibro-cartilage is still intact; thus there is a rotary element, with the centre of rotation at the ulnar styloid, the lower end of the radius rotating into supination. If the force continues, the ulnar styloid is avulsed. Six deformities occur. These are: impaction; lateral displacement; lateral rotation; dorsal displacement; dorsal rotation; and supination (see Figs 23.86 to 23.91).

Treatment. The aim is to restore a fully functional hand and forearm, with a full range of movement and no deformity. It must be remembered that a Colles' fracture if left untreated will usually result in a fully functioning hand and forearm, but with displacement and some limitation in movement. It is important, therefore, to ensure that the end result following treatment is better than leaving well alone.

Timing of reduction. It is wise to allow six hours to elapse after food before giving a general anaesthetic. X-ray facilities should be available for immediate checking of the reduction. It may be justifiable, although undesirable, to apply a temporary splint and reduce the fracture on the following morning.

Anaesthesia. Either a general anaesthetic or a Bier's regional anaesthetic block gives satisfactory analgesia and relaxation. Local anaesthesia injected into the fracture haematoma often does not relieve pain and is not recommended.

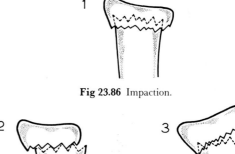

Fig 23.86 Impaction.

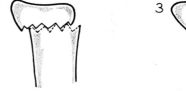

Fig 23.87 Lateral displacement.   **Fig 23.88** Lateral rotation.

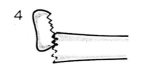   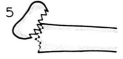

Fig 23.89 Dorsal displacement.   **Fig 23.90** Dorsal rotation.

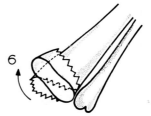

Fig 23.91 Supination.

Figs 23.86 to 23.91 Diagrams to show the six displacements of the typical Colles' fracture.

Manipulative reduction. It has been said in the past that after suitable treatment it should be impossible to know which wrist has been fractured.[36] This is desirable, but is not always possible. A house surgeon (A.B.) working for a well-known orthopaedic surgeon (R.W.J.) was asked to review a series of cases to show at a clinical meeting. He chose the Colles' fracture. When the end results were assessed residual deformity was present in almost every case. Function was excellent, but the houseman was advised not to present this series!

When manipulating the fracture the surgeon must keep in mind the six deformities. With the patient supine, the shoulder abducted and the elbow flexed, traction is applied to the thumb with counter-traction above the elbow, by an assistant or by using a roller towel attached to a hook in the wall. The fracture is disimpacted by a direct and firm pull, it is seldom necessary to increase the deformity to disimpact. Traction alone reduces the lateral displacement and rotation and should be maintained by an assistant while the surgeon manipulates to correct any residual deformity. When manipulating a right Colles' fracture the right-handed surgeon places his right thenar eminence over the dorsal and lateral aspect of the patient's radial styloid and his left thenar eminence on the ulnar and palmar aspect of the limb, just proximal to the fracture line (Fig 23.92). It is important that the right hand applies pressure to the lower end of the radius and not to the carpal bones. With the hands in this position and by pushing the lower radial fragment into pronation, it is also possible to correct the supination deformity. If the dorsal displacement and rotation are not corrected

by this manoeuvre forcible hyperflexion of the wrist may be necessary. Over-correction is said to be impossible, but it does happen sometimes (Figs 23.93 to 23.95). X-ray control is desirable. The use of an image intensifier is not advisable unless there is accurate monitoring of irradiation during the procedure.

Immobilisation. After reduction the assistant maintains traction on the thumb while a plaster backslab 6 inches (15.2 cm) wide is applied over a thin layer of orthopaedic wool (Fig 23.96), special care being taken to pad the styloid process of the ulna. The slab extends from the metacarpal heads to just below the elbow and surrounds two-thirds of the circumference of the forearm. It is held in position with a wet cotton bandage. The slab must maintain the ulnar deviation of the hand, by a tongue of plaster shaped to the radial side of the index metacarpal. The plaster cast should not extend over the radial side of the thumb metacarpal for fear of an adduction deformity of the thumb. While the plaster is setting the surgeon moulds the wrist in the same way as when reducing the fracture, holding the wrist in a few degrees of flexion and full ulnar deviation. Sometimes the reduction is not maintained in this position and some surgeons immobilise the wrist well flexed (the Cotton-Loder position). If this position is used care must be taken that the wrist does not stiffen in flexion and it is important that after 10 days the wrist is brought into a less flexed position.[37] Others have used above elbow casts with the forearm fully pronated in an attempt to prevent recurrence of the supination deformity, but it is doubtful if either of these methods is justifiable. Immobilisation of the arm in an above

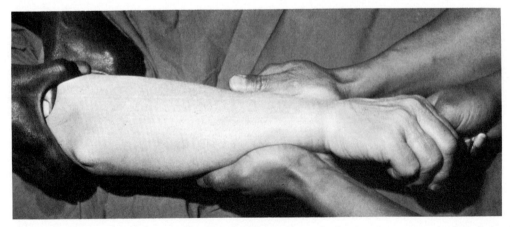

Fig 23.92 Manipulation of a Colles' fracture while an assistant applies traction to the thumb and counter traction is applied to the elbow.

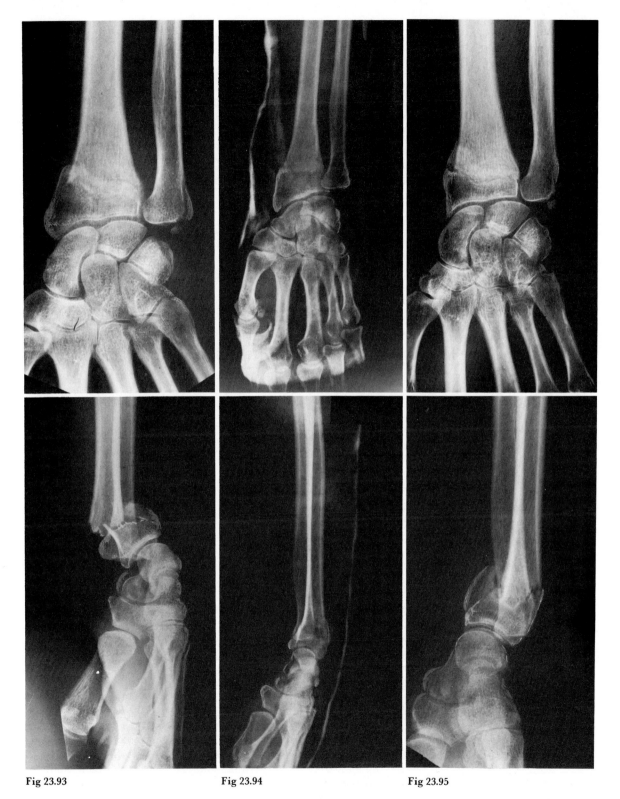

Fig 23.93   **Fig 23.94**   **Fig 23.95**

Figs 23.93 to 23.95 A curious example of Colles' fracture which has over-corrected. Fig 23.93: The original displacement. Fig 23.94: In plaster after satisfactory reduction. Fig 23.95: After removal of the plaster spontaneous overcorrection has occurred.

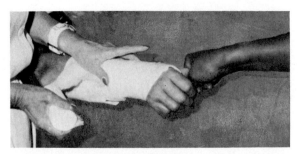

Fig 23.96 Traction is maintained while padding and plaster are applied and until after the plaster is set.

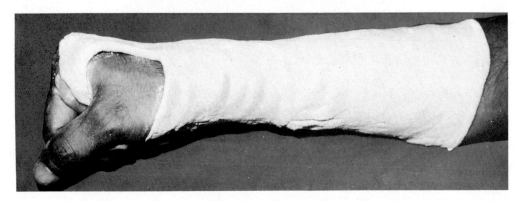

Fig 23.97 A Colles' plaster showing the metacarpo-phalangeal joints fully flexed. This wrist, however, has been immobilised with the joint too straight. After reduction of a Colles' fracture the wrist should be immobilised in about 10 degrees of palmar flexion and in ulnar deviation.

elbow cast with the elbow in flexion, the forearm in supination and the wrist in moderate ulnar and volar flexion may give more satisfactory results.[38]

After treatment. Rehabilitation commences as the patient recovers from the anaesthetic. Clear instructions both verbal and printed, to return to hospital immediately in the event of any complications must be given. In the post-anaesthetic period the patient may not remember these instructions and they must be given also to any accompanying relative.

An old lady arrived at her first fracture clinic appointment following a Colles' fracture with her fingers swollen, blue and numb. She assured the surgeon that no instructions had been given her. On being asked whether she had been given anything, she delved into her handbag and produced a slip of paper neatly folded. On it was printed the standard hospital instructions! 'But no one told me that I should read them, they just told me I should put them in my bag.' This story of a rather foolish old lady emphasises

the doctor's responsibility to make instructions clear to his patient.

Continuation of normal household activities or 'light work' while in plaster is the best form of rehabilitation.

Plaster check. On the morning following the manipulation the condition of the fingers and plaster is checked at hospital and an appointment is made for the next fracture clinic.

Fracture clinic visits. The plaster cast can be completed by replacing the cotton bandage with plaster of Paris. The completed cast must allow free movement of the elbow joint and the metacarpo-phalangeal joints (Fig 23.97). The next fracture clinic appointment should be about 12 days from the time of the injury, when the fracture must be re-X-rayed through plaster. If there is significant displacement, manipulation under anaesthetic should be carried out. Remanipulation before this time is not advised because the same conditions are present which allowed the original redisplacement. By waiting 12 days the fracture is 'sticky' and should not redisplace.

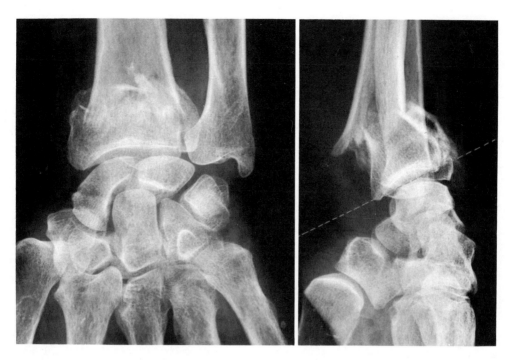

Fig 23.98 A Colles' fracture with dorsal displacement and rotation, lateral displacement, and impaction of the distal fragment.

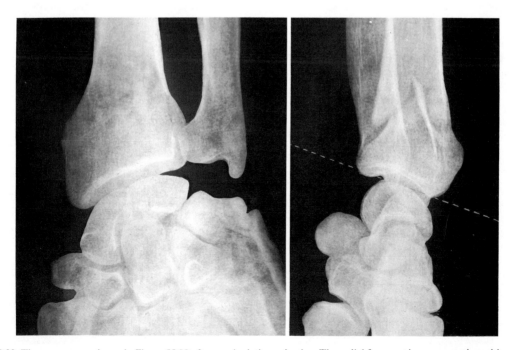

Fig 23.99 The same case as shown in Figure 23.98 after manipulative reduction. The radial fragment is now correctly positioned with its articular surface directed slightly forward.

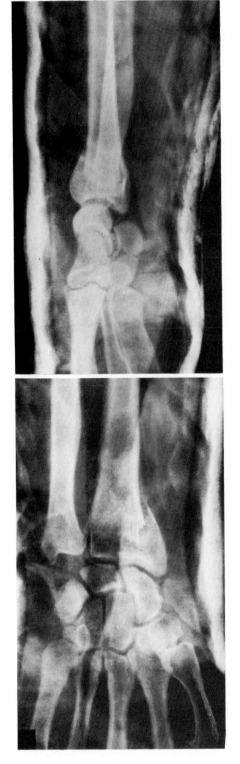

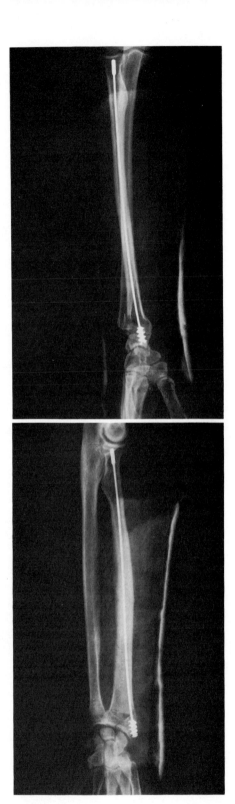

Fig 23.100

Fig 23.101

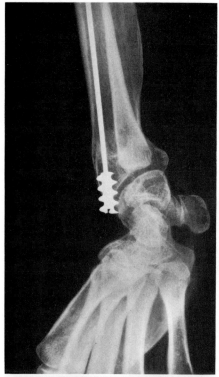

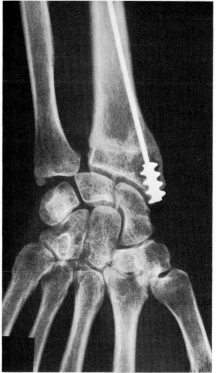

Fig 23.102

The plaster cast is removed at between five and six weeks. There is a common misunderstanding that the period of immobilisation should be measured from the date of the last manipulation. Remanipulation of a Colles' fracture within three weeks of the injury has little effect on the time taken for it to unite. On removal of the plaster cast the range of wrist and forearm movement should increase with normal activity, and physiotherapy is rarely necessary.

Acceptable position. In the young adult a perfect position is aimed for so that the final result will be a wrist indistinguishable from normal. The lower radio-ulnar joint must be fully reduced, and the palmar angulation of the articular surface must be correct on lateral X-ray (Figs 23.98 and 23.99). In the elderly patient, unless very infirm, an attempt should be made to reduce deformity. If the displacement recurs the question of remanipulation can be discussed with the patient. In the unlikely event of forearm rotation being significantly limited 12 months after the fracture, excision of the lower end of the ulna will restore movement.

Operative treatment. Incomplete correction of deformity is often accompanied by adequate function, nevertheless there is a correlation between the residual deformity and a poor functional result.[39] Many comminuted Colles' fractures present severe difficulty in maintaining reduction by cast support. External skeletal fixation with a double pin Roger Anderson apparatus has been used to maintain stable reduction. An ingenius intramedullary rod has been devised which maintains the length of the radius by one end being screwed into the radial styloid and the other applying counterpressure on the subchondral bone of the radial head. Figures 23.100 to 23.102.[40, 41]

Complications of the Colles' fracture
Carpal tunnel compression. In the rare event of early signs of median nerve damage, carpal tunnel decompression should be carried out forthwith, as early decompression allows rapid recovery to take place. The carpal tunnel syndrome occurring late is treated as though unassociated with a fracture.[42, 43]

Figs 23.100 to 23.102 Internal fixation of Colles' fracture with the Myles intramedullary flexible rod. Fig 23.100: One week after a satisfactory initial reduction showing redisplacement of the fracture. Figs 23.101 and 23.102: The expanded proximal end of the flexible rod rests on the subchondral bone of the radial head, the distal end is attached to radial styloid by a thread. Note that the flexible rod tends to straighten within the bone thus holding the fracture reduced.

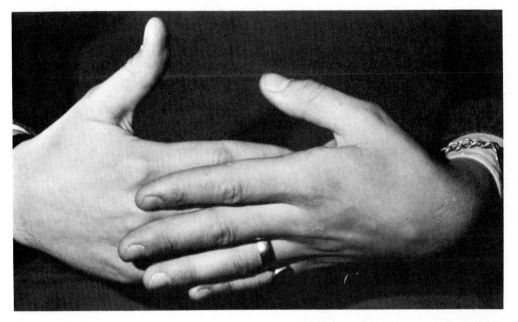

Fig 23.103 Rupture of the left extensor pollicis longus tendon eight weeks after a Colles' fracture. Always examine the two hands together.

Rupture of the tendon of the extensor pollicis longus. Rupture of this tendon complicating a Colles' fracture commonly occurs about the fourth week although it sometimes presents much later (Fig 23.103). There are two theories as to the cause:

1. That the initial injury impairs the blood supply to the tendon resulting in necrosis and rupture.

2. That rupture is due to attrition in the damaged groove by Lister's tubercle.

The first theory seems untenable as it would suggest that free tendon grafts having no blood supply would rupture. The second theory is more likely and is comparable to the lesion described by Vaughan-Jackson.[44] Operative treatment may be by direct repair, bridging the gap with nylon sutures as proposed by Trevor,[45] or by the transplant of extensor indicis proprius. The results of these operations are functionally identical, although in a personal review of 45 cases careful examination revealed that when the extensor indicis proprius had been transplanted there was some permanent loss of extension of the index metacarpo-phalangeal joint. What is more surprising was the finding that several patients left untreated for various reasons, when seen a year or more after the injury, had no functional disability from the tendon rupture, and a few had spontaneously regained active extension of the interphalangeal joint of the thumb. None of these patients were pianists and the question of spanning an octave did not arise. A ruptured extensor pollicis longus may cause very little permanent disability, there is no urgency to repair it.

Mal-union. This is more common than some surgeons would like to suggest. Usually there is no significant functional disability and the appearance of the wrist is, as a rule, accepted by the patient. Functional disability, when it does occur results from dislocation of the inferior radio-ulnar joint, which may cause painful limitation of pronation and supination. This can be relieved by excision of the distal $\frac{1}{2}$ inch (1.3 cm) of the ulna. A silastic cap has been designed to replace the excised ulnar head[46] (Fig 23.106), but it is unnecessary and only complicates an otherwise simple operation. If the radial deformity also has to be corrected, the lower end of the ulna is excised followed by osteotomy of the radius. Even at eight weeks, if the lower end of the ulna is excised first, the radius can sometimes be corrected by manipulation (Figs 23.104 and 23.105).

Non-union. This is so rare that at six weeks the plaster cast should be removed whether there is X-ray evidence of union or not. The harm from

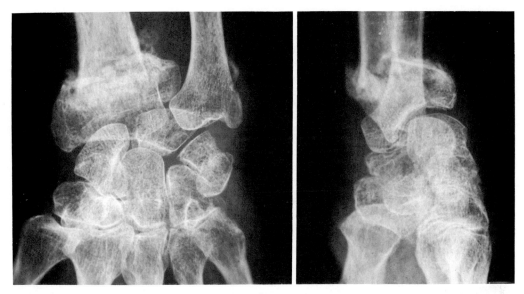

Fig 23.104

Fig 23.106

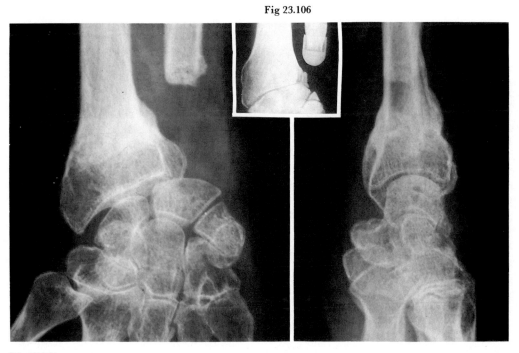

Fig 23.105

Figs 23.104 to 23.106 A Colles' fracture mal-united after eight weeks in an elderly doctor's widow who resented the deformity and disfigurement just as much as the loss of function. After eight weeks it is easy to correct displacement if the head of the ulna is first excised (Fig 22.105). A silastic cap has been advised by some surgeons after excision of the lower end of the ulna (Fig 23.106 inset). It is an unnecessary complication of an otherwise simple operation so long as no more than ½ in (1.3 cms) of ulna has been excised.

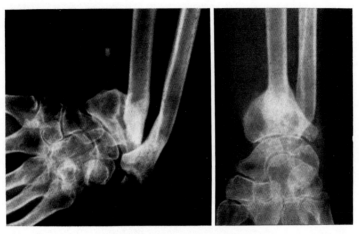

Fig 23.107   **Fig 23.108**

Figs 23.107 and 23.108 Un-united Colles' fracture. An extremely rare complication. Figure 23.108 shows union after excision of the lower end of the ulna, impaling the shaft of the radius into the distal fragment and cancellous grafting.

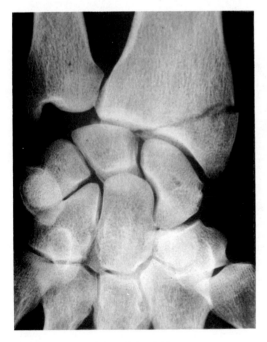

Fig 23.109 Fracture of the radial styloid process.

prolonged immobilisation is greater than the risk of this complication. Reconstruction after non-union is illustrated in Figures 23.107 and 23.108.

Sudeck's atrophy. Osteo neuro dystrophy.[47] Sudeck's atrophy is characterised by pain, stiffness in the wrist and fingers, red shiny skin and osteoporosis of the bones of the wrist and hand. Sometimes it is unavoidable but often it is due to inactivity following the fracture. The main problem is the finger joint stiffness which once established is soon irreversible, and treatment must be directed to maintaining finger mobility by active exercise. Paradoxically, reapplication of a forearm plaster sometimes relieves pain sufficiently to allow active finger exercises. If the metacarpo-phalangeal joints are stiff in extension a manipulation of these joints to 90 degrees under anaesthetic and immobilisation in this position for three weeks, with the interphalangeal joints extended, may retrieve this difficult situation. Recovery from Sudeck's atrophy is prolonged and painful both for the patient and the surgeon. Three years usually elapse before the bones are remineralised and it is rare that a full range of finger movement returns. Sympathectomy is of doubtful value but a Bier's type regional block, with the addition of hydrocortisone to the local anaesthetic injected intravenously sometimes hastens recovery.*

* Encouraging results have also been obtained by using Guanethidine as an intravenous regional sympathetic block (see Chapter 4).

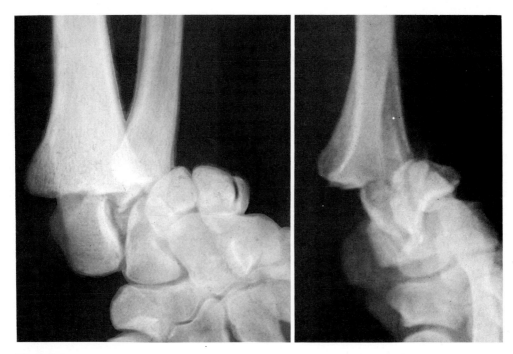

Fig 23.110

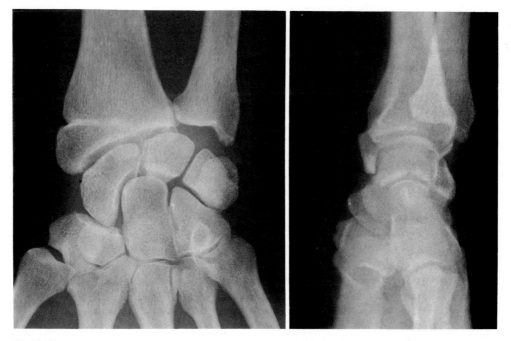

Fig 23.111

Figs 23.110 and 23.111 Even when there is a wide displacement of a fracture of the radial styloid process it can be reduced by manipulation.

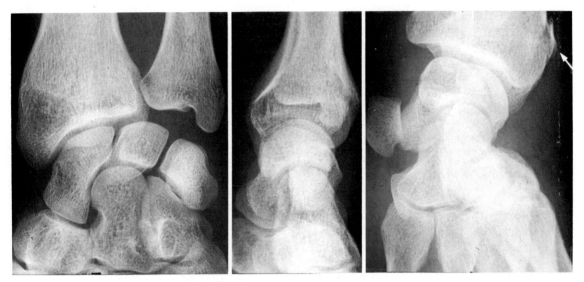

Fig 23.112   **Fig 23.113**

Figs 23.112 and 23.113 Posterior marginal fracture of the lower end of the radius. Antero-posterior and lateral radiography show no evidence of the injury (Fig 23.112), but it is disclosed by an oblique view (Fig 23.113). In this case the extensor pollicis longus tendon ruptured spontaneously six weeks later.

The shoulder-hand syndrome. This condition may be related to Sudeck's atrophy. It is characterised by a swollen, painful, stiff hand and a 'frozen' shoulder. The patient refuses to use the upper limb and there is probably always a psychological basis, a mental amputation having been performed by the patient. The shoulder-hand syndrome is difficult to treat and usually requires prolonged and gentle attention from an understanding physiotherapist. In extreme cases the patient may even exert pressure upon the surgeon to amputate one or more digits. Amputation should be resisted, as the patient may not be satisfied until the entire upper limb is removed.

Fracture of the radial styloid process

Fracture of the radial styloid process is caused by a fall on the outstretched hand. In the days when cars had starting handles this fracture sometimes resulted from a backfire. The fracture enters the wrist joint between the scaphoid and lunate bones (Fig 23.109). Very often there is minimal displacement, and immobilisation of the wrist in a plaster cast for four weeks is all that is needed. If there is displacement reduction is by traction on the hand and direct pressure on the fragment (Figs 23.110 and 23.111). Internal fixation is advocated by some surgeons but is usually unnecessary.

Posterior marginal fracture of the lower end of the radius

In this injury a small fragment is chipped from the back of the articular margin of the radius by forcible dorsiflexion of the wrist. It may occur as an isolated injury, often overlooked and only disclosed in oblique radiographs (Figs 23.112 and 23.113); but not uncommonly careful examination of the lateral X-ray shows that the normal palmar angulation of the articular surface has been lost and that the injury is in fact a Colles' fracture (Fig 23.114). Treatment is simple—the wrist is immobilised in a Colles' plaster for four weeks. The important point to remember about this fracture is that it is sometimes complicated by a late rupture of the tendon of extensor pollicis longus.

Smith fracture

This fracture was first described in 1847 by Smith[48] who wrote: 'I cannot speak with accuracy as to the anatomical characters of the injury, having never had an opportunity of examining after death the skeleton of the forearm in those who had during life met with this accident'. Nevertheless he was satisfied that the injury was a fracture of the lower end of the radius with palmar displacement of the distal radial

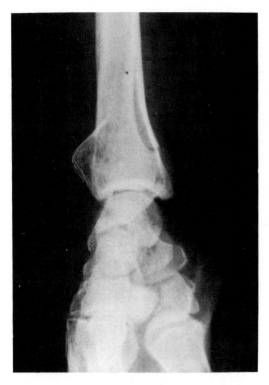

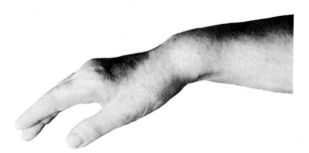

Fig 23.115 Smith fracture (or reversed Colles' fracture) through the whole thickness of the radius not extending into the joint.

Fig 23.114 This lateral X-ray shows what is apparently a posterior marginal fracture of the radius. But it is a Colles' fracture, as indicated by the dorsal rotation of the articular surface.

fragment, and with a dislocation of the inferior radio-ulnar joint. The injury described by Smith may have been what we now know as a Barton fracture[49], but the fracture associated with Smith's name is as he described it and is a reversed Colles' fracture, caused by a fall onto the dorsum of the flexed wrist (Figs 23.115 to 23.117). Treatment is by manipulation and immobilisation in an above elbow plaster cast with the elbow at right angles, the wrist dorsiflexed and the forearm supinated. Union is complete in six weeks. If closed manipulation is unsuccessful then open reduction from the palmar aspect is followed by fixation with the buttress plate described by Ellis[50] (Fig 23.118).

Barton fracture

In 1838 Barton described 'a subluxation of the wrist consequent upon a fracture through the articular surface of the carpal extremity of the radius.[49] He described two types—one with a dorsally displaced fragment and a rare type with a palmar fragment. Like Smith nine years later, Barton was without the benefit of X-rays and his dorsal type was probably a Colles' fracture.[50] The fracture now associated with his name is an anterior marginal fracture of the radius with subluxation both of the wrist and inferior radio-ulnar joints (Fig 23.119). The carpus and the hand displace forwards with the large anterior marginal fragment, the fracture extending into the wrist joint. The treatment is similar to that for the Smith fracture, but closed reduction is often difficult to maintain and fixation with a buttress plate is necessary more frequently (Fig 23.118).

Fracture displacement of the lower radial epiphysis

This injury occurs in the older child whose lower radial epiphysis is not yet fused and results from a fall on the outstretched hand. The displacement is similar to that of a Colles' fracture. Epiphyseal separations are essentially fractures adjacent to the epiphyseal disc and not through the disc, the line of cleavage being on the metaphyseal side of the epiphyseal plate so that cartilage cells are undamaged. The displaced epiphysis always carries with it a small triangular fragment of bone from the margin of the metaphysis.

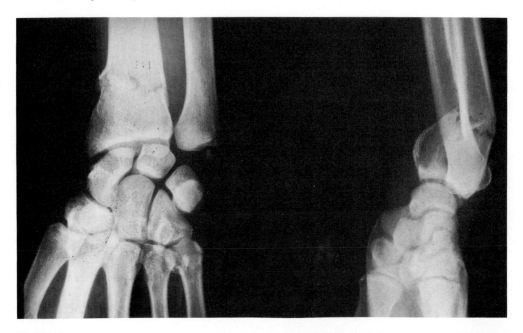

Fig 23.116

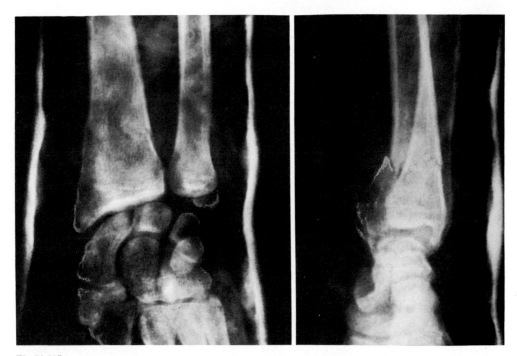

Fig 23.117

Figs 23.116 and 23.117 Smith fracture. The entire distal radial articular surface displaces palmarwards. Figure 23.117 shows the position after reduction.

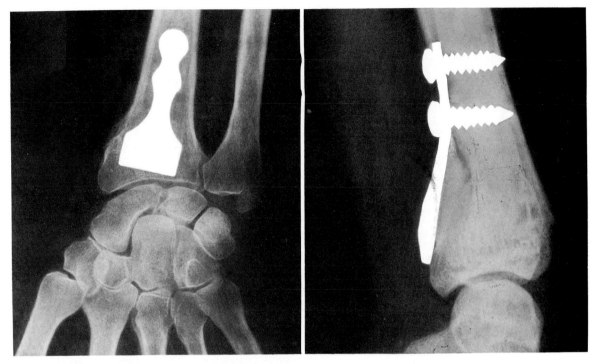

Fig 23.118 The Ellis buttress plate used in the fixation of a Smith fracture.

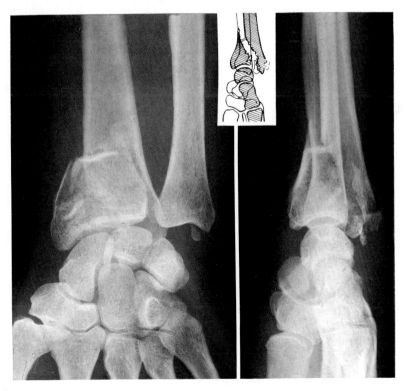

Fig 23.119 Barton fracture.

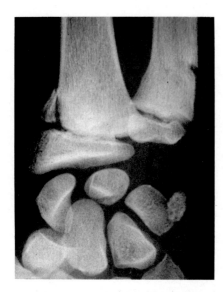

Fig 23.120 Displacement of the lower radial epiphysis showing the triangular metaphyseal fragment with a greenstick fracture of the ulna.

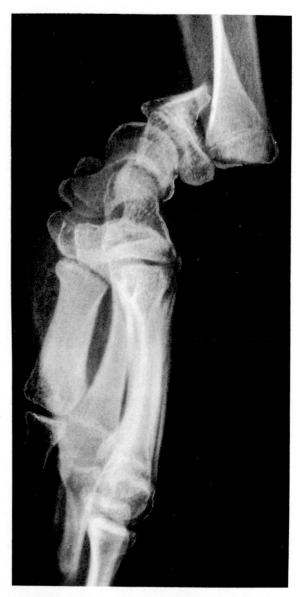

Fig 23.121 Rare palmar fracture displacement of the lower radial epiphysis, comparable to the Smith fracture. The triangular metaphyseal fragment is clearly seen.

If it is a simple dorsal displacement the bone fragment is detached from the back of the metaphysis. If there is both dorsal and lateral displacement it is detached from the dorso-lateral aspect (Fig 23.120). Rarely the displacement is palmar with a palmar triangular metaphyseal fragment (Fig 23.121). No matter how slight the degree of epiphyseal displacement there is always an injury to the metaphysis; in fact, minor epiphyseal separations are often disclosed more clearly by the greenstick buckling of the back of the metaphysis than by any obvious displacement of the epiphysis. As in the Colles' fracture the inferior radio-ulnar joint is subluxed, with avulsion of the styloid process of the ulna, or tearing of the ulnar collateral ligament. Occasionally the radio-ulnar joint is not dislocated, in which case there is displacement of the lower ulnar epiphysis, or a greenstick fracture of the lower shaft of the ulna (Fig 23.120). Any displacement should be reduced by the same manipulation as is used for a Colles' fracture. Immobilisation in a forearm cast for three weeks is usually all that is required. Any residual displacement usually corrects by the moulding of growth (Figs 23.122 to 23.125).

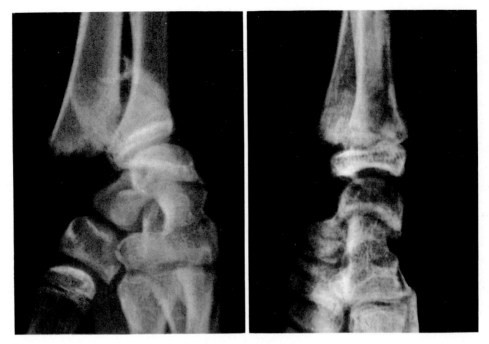

Fig 23.122   **Fig 23.123**

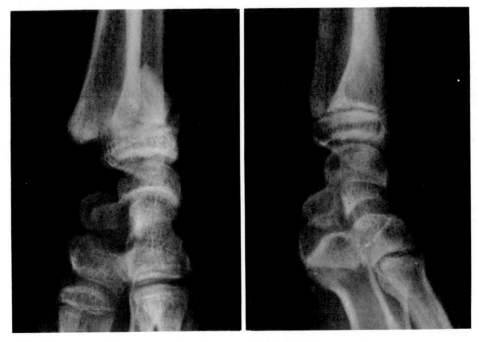

Fig 23.124   **Fig 23.125**

Figs 23.122 to 23.125 Backward displacement of the lower radial epiphysis (Fig 23.122). It was almost completely corrected (Fig 23.123) but displacement recurred (Fig 23.124), nevertheless alignment was restored in this growing child by later remodelling with resorption of the projecting anterior margin of the radial metaphysis (Fig 21.125).

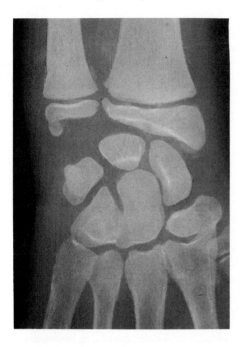

Fig 23.126 Radiographs of the wrist the day after a fall on the outstretched hand. There is a fracture of the ulnar styloid process but only a suspicion of injury to the central part of the lower radial epiphysis.

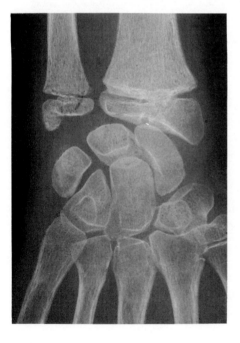

Fig 23.127 The same wrist two months later. There is more definite evidence of abnormality of the central part of the lower radial epiphysis, with early obliteration of a part of the epiphyseal line.

Crushing of the lower radial epiphysis with premature fusion and arrested growth. When a child falls on the outstretched hand the wrist is usually in a position of slight dorsiflexion so that the carpus and the lower end of the radius are driven backwards. The shearing stress which is produced by this injury displaces the lower radial epiphysis, without damage to the epiphyseal plate and there is no interference with growth. If the impact occurs when the wrist is fully dorsiflexed the shearing stress is minimal and the crushing force damages the epiphyseal plate itself. This injury can cause prema-ture fusion of the epiphysis with arrested growth. At the time, there may be little or no evidence of bone damage; the epiphysis is in its usual position and the possibility of damage can be surmised only from the radiographic appearances. A few months later the signs become more obvious, and after several years there is arrested growth of the radius with continued growth of the ulna, which dislocates at its lower end (Figs 23.126 to 23.128). If this condition is recognised it is advisable to wait until the age of 18 or 19 years and then excise the lower inch of the ulna.

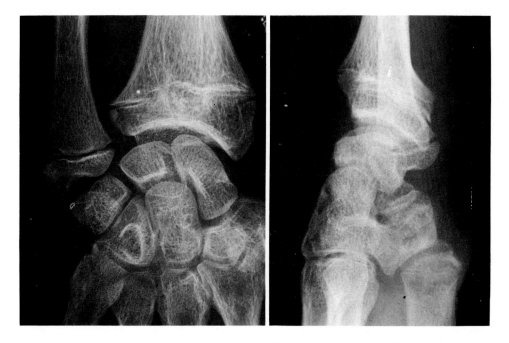

Fig 23.128 The same wrist six years later showing premature fusion of the lower radial epiphysis. The ulna continued to grow and has dislocated at the inferior radio-ulnar joint. This is not a complication of ordinary epiphyseal displacement but of crushing of the epiphyseal line. Excision of the lower end of the ulna is indicated.

REFERENCES

1. Bakalim G 1970 Fractures of the radial head and their treatment. Acta Orthopaedica Scandinavica 41: 320
2. Fleetcroft J 1980 Personal communication
3. Mason J A, Shutkin N M 1943 Immediate active motion treatment of fractures of the head and neck of the radius. Surgery, Gynecology and Obstetrics 76: 731–737
4. Johnston G W 1962 A follow-up of 100 cases of fracture of the head of the radius with a review of the literature. Ulster Medical Journal 31: 51–56
5. McDougall A, White J 1957 Subluxation of the inferior radio-ulnar joint complicating fracture of the radial head. Journal of Bone and Joint Surgery 39-B: 278–287
6. Taylor T K F, O'Connor B T 1964 The effect upon the inferior radio-ulnar joint of excision of the head of the radius in adults. Journal of Bone and Joint Surgery 46-B: 83–88
7. Strachan J C H, Ellis B W 1971 Vulnerability of the posterior interosseous nerve during radial head resection. Journal of Bone and Joint Surgery 53-B: 320
8. Essex-Lopresti B 1951 Fractures of the head of the radius with distal radio-ulnar dislocation. Journal of Bone and Joint Surgery 33-B: 244–247
9. Sarmiento A, Cooper J S, Sinclair W F 1975 Forearm fractures early functional bracing, a preliminary report. Journal of Bone and Joint Surgery, 57-A: 297–304
10. Benjamin A 1957 The relief of traumatic arterial spasm in threatened Volkmann's ischaemic contracture. Journal of Bone and Joint Surgery 39-B: 711
11. Mubarak S J, Carroll M C 1979 Volkmann's contracture in children, aetiology and prevention. Journal of Bone and Joint Surgery 61-B: 285–293
12. Pollen A G 1973 Fracture and dislocations in children. Churchill Livingstone, Edinburgh
13. Smith J E M 1959 Internal fixation in the treatment of fractures of the shafts of the radius and ulna in adults. The value of delayed operation in the prevention of non-union. Journal of Bone and Joint Surgery 41-B: 122
14. Muller M E, Allgower M, Willenegger H 1970 Manual of internal fixation. Springer-Verlag, Berlin, Heidelberg and New York
15. Burwell H N, Charnley A D 1964 Treatment of forearm fracture in adults with particular reference to plate fixation. Journal of Bone and Joint Surgery 46-B: 405–425.
16. Dodge H S, Cady G W 1972 Treatment of fracture of the radius and ulna with compression plates. A retrospective study of one hundred and nineteen fractures in seventy-eight patients. Journal of Bone and Joint Surgery 54-A: 1167–1179
17. Bagby G W, Janes J M 1957 An impacting bone plate. Proceedings of Staff Meetings of the Mayo Clinic 32: 55
18. Bagby G W 1968 Clinical experience of a simplified compression bone plate. American Journal of Orthopaedic Surgery 10: 302
19. Denham R A 1969 Compression and coaptation. Journal of Bone and Joint Surgery 51-B: 177
20. Allgower M, Perren S, Matter P 1970 A new plate for internal fixation—the dynamic compression plate. (DCP). Injury 2: 40
21. Fee N F, Dobranski A, Bisla R S 1977 Gas gangrene complicating open forearm fractures. Journal of Bone and Joint Surgery 59-A: 135–138
22. Elstrom J A, Pankovich A M, Egwele R 1978 Extra articular low velocity gun shot fractures of the radius and ulna. Journal of Bone and Joint Surgery 60-A: 335–341

23. Jackson R P, Jacobs R R, Neff J R 1978 External skeletal fixation in severe limb trauma. Journal of Trauma 18: 201–205
24. Groves E W Hey 1921 Modern methods of treating fractures, 2nd edn. John Wright, Bristol, p 320
25. Greenwood H H 1932 Reconstruction of the forearm after loss of the radius. British Journal of Surgery 20: 58
26. Watson-Jones R 1934 Reconstruction of the forearm after loss of the radius. British Journal of Surgery 22: 23
27. Sarmiento A, Kinman P B, Murphy R B, Phillips J G 1976 Treatment of ulna fractures by functional bracing. Journal of Bone and Joint Surgery 58-A: 1105–1107
28. Monteggia G B 1814 Instituzioni Chirurgiche. Maspero, Milan, vol 5, p 130
29. Hume A C 1957 Anterior dislocation of the head of the radius associated with undisplaced fractures of the olecranon in children. Journal of Bone and Joint Surgery 39-B: 508
30. Evans E M 1949 Pronation injuries of the forearm with special reference to the anterior Monteggia fracture. Journal of Bone and Joint Surgery 31-B: 579
31. Bado J L 1967 The Monteggia lesion. Clinical Orthopaedics and Related Research 50: 71
32. Yamamoto K, Yanase Y, Tomihara M 1977 Posterior interosseous nerve palsy as a complication of Monteggia fractures. Archiv für Japanische Chirurgie (Kyoto) 46: 46–56
33. Evans E M 1951 Fractures of the radius and ulna. Journal of Bone and Joint Surgery 33-B: 548
34. Galeazzi R 1935 Uber ein besonderes Syndrom bei Verletzungen im Bereich der Unterarmknochen. Archiv für Orthopädische und Unfallchirurgie 35: 557
35. Colles Abraham 1814 On the fracture of the carpal extremity of the radius. Edinburgh Medical & Surgical Journal 10: 182
36. Platt H 1932 Colles' fracture. British Medical Journal ii: 288
37. Taylor G W, Parson C L 1938 Fracture of the lower end of the radius. Surgery, Gynecology and Obstetrics 67: 249
38. Sarmiento A, Pratt G W, Berry N C, Sinclair W F 1975 Colles' fractures, functional bracing in supination. Journal of Bone and Joint Surgery 57-A: 311–317
39. Hollingsworth R, Morris J 1976 The importance of the ulnar side of the wrist in fracture of the distal end of the radius. Injury 7: 263–266
40. Cooney W P, Linscheid R L, Dobyns J H 1979 External pin fixation for unstable Colles' fractures. Journal of Bone and Joint Surgery 61-A: 840–845
41. Myles J W 1978 A new device for the internal fixation of wrist fractures. Preliminary communication. Journal of the Royal Society of Medicine 71: 186–188
42. Lynch A C, Lipscombe P R 1963 The carpal tunnel syndrome and Colles' fractures. Journal of the American Medical Association 185: 363–366
43. Lewis M H 1978 Median nerve decompression after Colles' fracture. Journal of Bone and Joint Surgery 60-B: 1095–1096
44. Vaughan-Jackson O J 1948 Rupture of the extensor tendons by attrition at the inferior radio-ulnar joint. Report of two cases. Journal of Bone and Joint Surgery 30-B: 528
45. Trevor D 1949 Rupture of the extensor pollicis longus after Colles' fracture. Journal of Bone and Joint Surgery 31-B: 477
46. Swanson A B 1972 The ulnar head syndrome and its treatment by implant resection arthroplasty. Journal of Bone and Joint Surgery 54-A: 906

47. Sudeck P 1900 Ueber die akute entzundliche Knochenstrophie. Archiv. für Klinische Chirurgie 62: 147

48. Smith R W 1847 A treatise on fractures in the vicinity of joints and on certain accidental and congenital dislocation. Hodges and Smith, Dublin, p 162

49. Barton J R 1838 Views and treatment of an important injury of the wrist. Medical Examiner 1: 365

50. Ellis J 1957 Smith's and Barton's fractures. A method of treatment. Journal of Bone and Joint Surgery 47-B: 724

24

Injuries of the Wrist

G. R. Fisk

Fractures near the wrist joint from falls on the outstretched hand make up one of the largest of all groups of bone injuries. Displacements of the lower radial epiphysis are sustained by children and adolescents; fractures of the carpal scaphoid bone occur in young men with greater frequency than is generally recognised; fractures of the bases and shafts of the metacarpals are amongst the commonest injuries of working men; and fractures of the lower end of the radius are often sustained by middle-aged and elderly women. Much of the time of a surgeon who treats fractures will be spent on injuries of the wrist, but although fractures near this joint are quite usual, sprains are often disregarded.

SPRAINS OF THE WRIST

In the past soft tissue injury of the wrist joint has been dismissed as rare and unimportant, and carpal fractures and dislocations so common and so easily overlooked that, quite rightly, diagnosis of 'sprained wrist' has been accepted only with reserve. However ligamentous and capsular injury of the wrist is now better appreciated as the cause of continued disability of aching, tenderness, weakness of grip and alarming bony displacement.

Ligamentous rupture may form part of an articular or bony injury and its effects visible on X-ray. Colles' fracture, for instance, is often associated with avulsion of the tip of the ulnar styloid where the ulnar collateral ligament of the carpus is inserted. It is rare for this tiny avulsed fragment to unite, and although in most cases this gives rise to no disability persisting tenderness is not uncommon. Similarly with forced ulnar flexion the tip of the radial styloid may be avulsed by traction upon the radial collateral ligament and internal fixation may be necessary to obtain bone union. Rupture of the volar carpal ligaments is invariable in fracture-dislocations of the carpus, and the disability following some of these complicated injuries results not so much from bone damage as to the distortion of the carpal articulations. Even in Colles' fracture pain and swelling of the wrist may arise not only from the fracture but also from the hyperextension injury to the volar ligaments. Instability of the carpus associated with fracture of the carpal scaphoid alters the prognosis in this injury, and will be dealt with in a later section. Flexion and rotation injuries to the wrist may result in avulsion of ligamentous and capsular attachments to the dorsum of the carpal bones and metacarpals. These result in bony prominences and tenderness while the ligament itself is subject to horizontal splits, such injuries being sometimes confused with the common dorsal ganglion of the wrist joint. Most sprains of the wrist will recover after simple immobilisation in a plaster cast or strapping, but surgical repair is occasionally necessary especially if diastasis or carpal malalignment is observed by X-ray examination.

Carpal instability.[1,2] The carpus consists of a jointed strut comprising three elements: the radius, the proximal carpal row and the distal carpal row. The scaphoid bridges the two carpal rows and its long axis lies directed some forty degrees volarwards. The long axes of the radius, lunate and capitate normally lie in line or parallel and these relationships are not significantly affected in flexion or extension of the wrist except at the extremes of movement. The wrist is inherently an unstable structure in which the proximal row is an 'intercalated' segment. Concertina or zigzag deformity[3] will occur if the position of these bones is not maintained by the resilience of the soft tissues (Fig 24.1). In about 75 per cent of cases the lunate extends and the capitate hyperflexes, whereas in the remainder the reverse deformity is seen.[2]

Side-to-side movement occurs in two different ways: ulnar flexion takes place at the radio-carpal level, the axis of rotation being located in the neck of the capitate; indeed all carpal movements have this

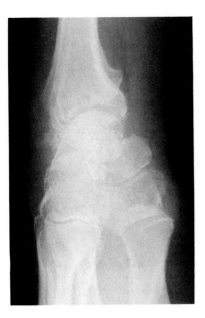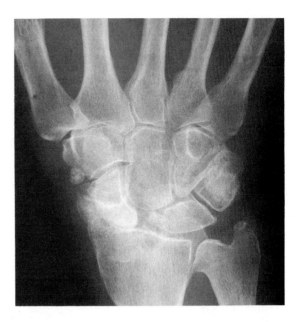

Fig 24.1 Scapho-lunate diastasis with the formation of an exostosis on the radial styloid and 'concertina' deformity of the carpus.

common axis. Radial flexion of the carpus takes place at the midcarpal joint and the scaphoid rotates so that its long axis comes to lie at some eighty degrees to that of the radius. Where ligament damage has induced carpal instability the scaphoid assumes this more horizontal position (Fig 24.2). Carpal stability depends upon long tendons, particularly flexor carpi radialis, the extrinsic ligaments of the carpus, the joint capsules and the interosseous ligaments. The shape of the bones and their articulations are designed

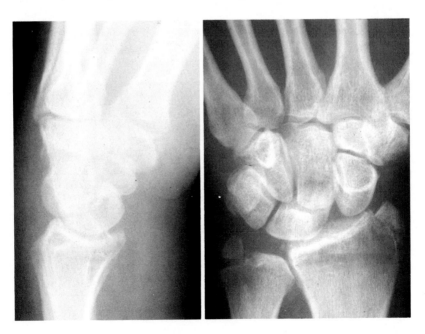

Fig 24.2 Collapse of the carpus, scapho-lunate diastasis and 'horizontal' scaphoid after open reduction of the dislocated lunate.

for mobility and they contribute little or nothing to stability. The most important structure in maintaining carpal stability is the volar radio-carpal ligamentous complex. These ligaments arise from a ridge on the radius just proximal to its articular surface and stout bands attach distally to the scaphoid, the lunate, the capitate and the triquetral bones.[4] Other ligamentous bands radiate from the neck of the capitate to the trapezium, triquetral and hamate bones. Most soft tissue injuries of the wrist are caused by falls on the outstretched hand and it is in dorsiflexion that the carpus is at its most vulnerable, since this places the volar structures on the stretch. In some subjects who have generalised joint laxity there is an increased antero-posterior excursion of the carpus which may be detected on the image intensifier screen or by ciné-

radiography. If the normal hand is placed in a neutral position and antero-posterior forces are exerted upon the wrist the capitate is seen to rock backwards and forwards at its articulation with the lunate, clearly displaying the mechanism of intra-carpal dislocation. If after injury an abnormal excursion is observed then there will have occurred stretching or rupture of the luno-capitate articulation. If the scapho-lunate interosseous ligament is also ruptured, diastasis takes place between these two bones and a gap can be seen on an antero-posterior X-ray film. This gap is further enhanced by the transverse posture adopted by the scaphoid within the carpus since the silhouette of the scaphoid is narrower than in its usual oblique position. If in addition the capito-hamate ligaments are damaged the capitate intrudes its proximal pole

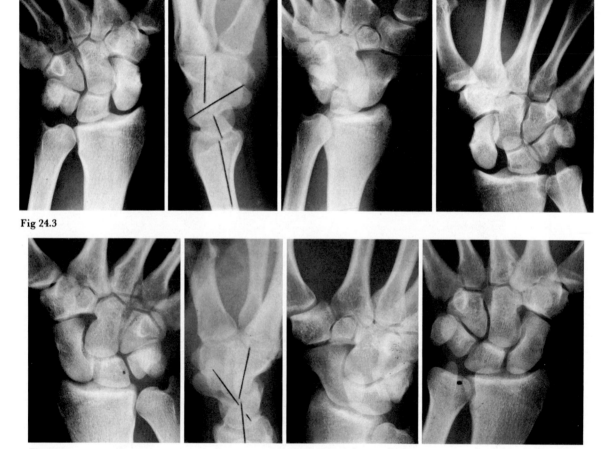

Fig 24.3

Fig 24.4

Figs 24.3 and 24.4 Figure 24.3 are of the X-rays of a patient who sustained a hyperextension injury of the wrist while playing football. Note the increased gap between the scaphoid bone and the lunate, indicating a break in the stabilising link system of the carpal bones. These X-ray findings are easily missed unless the X-ray of the damaged wrist is compared with the normal side (Fig 24.4).

between the scaphoid and the lunate. If the distal attachment of radial collateral ligament and the capsule between the scaphoid and trapezium are ruptured the scaphoid now becomes free to move within the carpus and this produces recurrent intracarpal dislocation of the scaphoid (rotary subluxation) when a compression force, such as a firm grip, is exerted upon it (see Figs 24.56 and 24.57).[5] This gives rise to a painful and alarming snap in the wrist and seriously prejudices the function of the hand. Lastly, rupture of the dorsal ligaments of the carpus allows the proximal pole of the scaphoid to sublux over the dorsal lip of the radius (see page 731).

Ligamentous disruption of the carpus can be treated successfully if it is recognised within the first four weeks (Figs 24.3 to 24.6). The concertina deformity should be corrected with the aid of the image intensifier, a padded plaster is applied and the cast is carefully moulded in the corrected position until it is set. Reduction is maintained in plaster for some eight weeks. Care must be taken not to produce vascular or neural compression or pressure sores by indenting the plaster. In persistent instability and in cases seen late, ligamentous reconstruction is to be preferred to arthrodesis or carpectomy (Figs 24.7 to 24.9). Degenerative changes is a contra-indication to

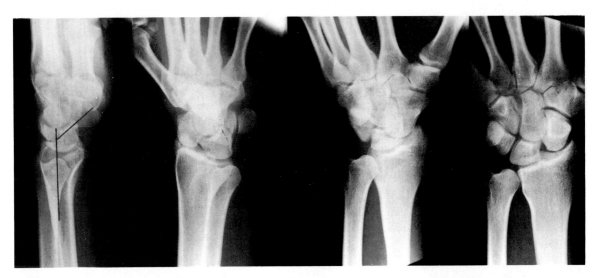

Fig 24.5

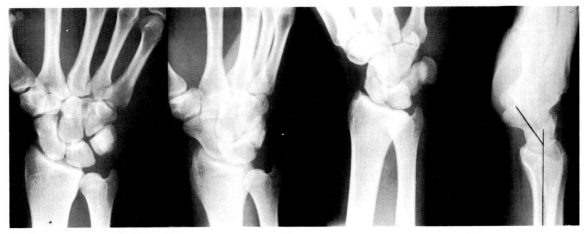

Fig 24.6

Figs 24.5 and 24.6 Films taken six years after injury of the wrists shown in Figures 24.3 and 24.4. Although the patient had no disability apart from occasional pain on exercise, the abnormal gap between the scaphoid and lunate is still present and there is increased forward tilt of the scaphoid compared with the normal side (Fig 24.6).

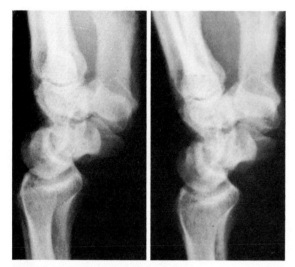

Fig 24.7

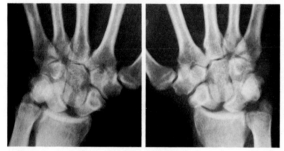

Fig 24.8

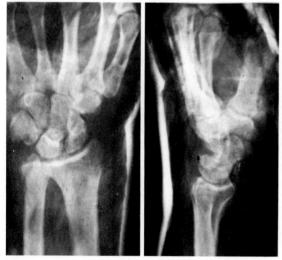

Fig 24.9

Figs 24.7 to 24.9 Gross instability of the carpus (Figs 24.7 and 24.8). Stabilisation by open reduction, ligamentous repair and plaster immobilisation (Fig 24.9).

ligamentous reconstruction. Surgical stabilisation is often difficult to achieve and may involve reefing the dorsal capsule and repairing the volar radio-carpal ligament through separate incisions. Scapho-lunate fusion has been advocated but this has the disadvantage of seriously limiting carpal movement, since this joint is essential in midcarpal movement and radial flexion.

Operative treatment. Under a pneumatic tourniquet an incision is made along the thenar crease, curving across the chaplet creases of the wrist and along the centre of the forearm. The transverse carpal ligament is incised throughout its length, the flexor tendons and the median nerve are gently retracted ulnarwards and the flexor carpi radialis and flexor pollicis longus to the radial side. Diastasis can be usually identified and it is sometimes possible to carry out direct suture with a non-absorbable material. Unhappily this sometimes results in persistent pain and tenderness. Palmaris longus or other tendon may be taken as a free graft and threaded through the capsule overlying the lunate, the capitate and the scaphoid as a purse-string repair. Alternatively holes may be drilled through the lunate and the proximal pole of the scaphoid and a strip of tendon passed through them using a small dorsal incision to tighten and fix the tendon ends.[6]

Traumatic tendinitis around the wrist, especially the extensor-abductor tendons of the thumb (de Quervain's disease) sometimes develops from repeated and stereotype movements as in painting, farming, working on the assembly line or from other actions involving repeated grasping between the fingers and thumb with a rapid pronation-supination movement of the forearm.[7,8,9] Newcomers to such jobs and workers recently returned from holiday or sick leave are especially vulnerable. Over-anxiety, tension and an inability rhythmically to relax the hand while it is being used is probably the underlying cause. In de Quervain's disease there is aching pain with slight swelling over the lower quarter of the radius situated where the short extensor and abductor of the thumb cross the radial extensor of the wrist and movements of the thumb are sometimes accompanied by 'wash leather creaking' at this site. The essential treatment is temporary rest from repetitive movement. Relief is usually obtained by applying a dorsal plaster slab for about ten days followed by an elastic bandage. This clinical picture may herald the onset of rheumatoid arthritis.

It has recently been suggested that traumatic tenosynovitis of the radial extensor of the wrist is due to hypertrophy of the long abductor and short extensor muscles of the thumb where they cross the radial extensor tendons. It is claimed that decompression of the sheath of these two muscles eliminates the patient's symptoms within a few days of operation.[10]

Tendovaginitis of extensor digiti minimi. This has been described in adults following a Colles' fracture[11] and presents as pain and tenderness of the tendon just distal to the radio-ulnar joint. It is usually relieved by a local injection of cortisone.

Tenosynovitis of extensor carpi ulnaris.[12] There is commonly a history of a twisting injury to the wrist prior to the onset of this condition. Pain is felt over the distal end of the ulna, and the tendon sheath of extensor carpi ulnaris may be enlarged. If local cortisone injections fail to give lasting relief, the tendon should be decompressed where it passes through a tunnel on the dorsum of the ulna.

Tenosynovitis of flexor carpi radialis. This condition is found almost exclusively in middle-aged women and is often associated with degenerative changes in the joint between the scaphoid and the trapezium.[13] Pain is felt on the radial side of the wrist near the base of the thenar eminence, especially with actions requiring wrist flexion against resistance, such as supporting a weight, with the forearm supinated. Decompression may be necessary if local cortisone injection is ineffective.

Tendo-vaginitis stenosans.[14,15] Traumatic tendinitis of the abductor-extensor tendons of the thumb (de Quervain's disease) may proceed to thickening and constriction of their sheaths. The pain is localised to a point half an inch proximal to the tip of the radial styloid process which is exquisitely tender. Radiographs may show osteoporosis of the bone subjacent to the radial styloid, movements of the wrist are usually full but when the thumb is flexed and adducted to the ulnar side the patient experiences excruciating pain. Careful palpation of the lower end of the radius discloses a small hard nodule about the size of a pea (Fig 24.10). There is considerable anatomical variation in the way in which the tendons of extensor pollicis brevis and abductor pollicis longus are enclosed as they pass through the fibrous tunnel over the radial styloid.[16] In 50 per cent of patients the tendon of abductor pollicis longus may be reduplicated and the tendons may even lie in separate tunnels. They may be inserted into the trapezium, the origin of abductor pollicis brevis or the transverse carpal ligament. It has been suggested that the alteration in excursion occasioned by these aberrant tendons is the cause of pain but as such anomalies are so common and a well recognised anatomical variant

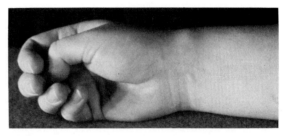

Fig 24.10 Stenosing tendovaginitis at the radial styloid process. A fibrous nodule involving the sheath of the extensor tendons of the thumb can be felt, and in this case seen, on the radial side of the wrist.

it is difficult to accept this explanation.[17] In the early stages the condition can be relieved by injection of hydrocortisone into these synovial sheaths but if this is unsuccessful or the condition is seen late, surgical decompression should be undertaken, care being taken to decompress all the tendons. It is of the greatest importance to preserve the dorsal cutaneous branches of the radial nerve which lie subcutaneously in the line of the tendon. Damage or division of this nerve will give rise to unpleasant paraesthesia and the formation of tender neuromata, the after-effects often being worse than the original disease. A transverse incision may allow the tendon sheaths to be divided leaving an invisible scar, but to avoid nerve damage it is safer to expose the tendon sheaths along their length through a longitudinal incision.

The extensor indicis proprius syndrome.[18] Cases have been recorded of pain over the extensor retinaculum due to a synovial reaction around the musculotendinous junction of the extensor indicis. When the wrist and fingers are flexed this part of the muscle usually lies in the extensor tunnel and swelling of it can provoke general pain over the back of the wrist. Although the condition has been described mainly in athletes, it is possible that it is also the explanation of the extensor tendinitis experienced by typists. If the pain is not relieved by hydrocortisone, decompression of the extensor retinaculum is indicated.

Peritendinous fibrosis of the dorsum of the hand. (Secrétan's disease).[19] This is an intractable disability not yet fully understood which may develop from a blow on the back of the hand with thickening of the soft tissues which does not pit on pressure. The patient complains of severe pain and tenderness and he is reluctant to use the hand to make a fist or to grip. X-ray examination does not reveal any alteration in bone appearance or texture. If the swelling is explored it is found to consist only of thickened hyperaemic fringes around the extensor tendons but excision of the inflamed tissues does not relieve the aching pain; the thickening usually recurs and the patient now has the benefit of a surgical scar. Vander Elst in 1961[20] and other authors concluded that this was invariably a case of self-mutilation, there was always a compensation case of some kind, the initial accident was often trivial, there was no clear pathology and all investigations were negative. Improvement was obtained only by protecting the dorsum of the hand by a plaster cast or dressing from further damage. Vander Elst felt that the patient had a poor level of education and intelligence and that psychiatric examination was often illuminating.

Acute calcification around the wrist. The commonest site is the insertion of flexor carpi ulnaris tendon into the pisiform bone.[21] Tenderness is so severe that the condition is sometimes misdiagnosed as an infection. X-rays will show a hazy patch of calcification at the site of the tenderness which rapidly disappears on resolution of symptoms. Acute calcification can occur at other sites.

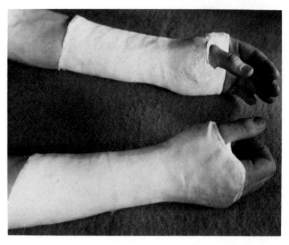

Fig 24.11 Bilateral fracture of the scaphoids showing the type of plaster cast used. It extends to the metacarpal heads and includes the whole of the first metacarpal. The hand is tightly gripped so that there cannot be any trace of wrist movement, but the plaster in the palm does not extend beyond the transverse skin creases.

FRACTURE OF THE CARPAL SCAPHOID BONE

This is perhaps the fracture which is most commonly overlooked in the accident department or doctor's surgery. Indeed the patient may think that he has simply suffered a sprain of the wrist and may never seek treatment. The fracture usually occurs from a fall on the outstretched hand or less commonly a backfire injury when hand-starting an engine. The level of the fracture depends upon the degree of ulnar flexion at the moment of impact, and like Colles' fracture it is a supination-dorsiflexion injury.[22] There is swelling and tenderness in the region of the anatomical snuffbox; passive dorsiflexion to the radial side is painful, grip is weak and the release of the grip gives transitory pain, resisted pinch between the thumb and index finger is uncomfortable. Where some or all of these tests are positive a fractured scaphoid should be presumed until proved otherwise. The wrist should be immobilised in a plaster cast extending from the proximal phalanx of the thumb to the upper third of the forearm with the wrist in a little dorsiflexion and radial flexion (Fig 24.11). X-ray examination in four planes (antero-posterior, lateral, pronation-oblique and supination-oblique) should be carried out in all suspected cases.[23] However, it is common for the fracture not to be visible at first but resorption of the fracture line demonstrates the injury when the X-rays are repeated two or three weeks later (Figs 24.12 to 24.15).

Diagnosis of recent from old fractures. Recent and old fractures of the carpal scaphoid bone must be distinguished because the age of the fracture has an important bearing on treatment. The history given by the patient is often unreliable. Very often the original injury has been overlooked or forgotten and symptoms arise only after several months or years when a second injury is sustained. A patient with an old fracture often believes that he sustained it only two or three days before. Recent fractures of the scaphoid are nearly always fine cracks; resorption at the fracture site may be visible on an X-ray but the articular cartilage may have united and the fracture may be impossible to detect at operation. This is the so-called 'peanut' fracture where the shell represents the intact articular cartilage and the two kernels the unhealed bone fragments. Where the scaphoid remains totally ununited the fractured surfaces sclerose—sometimes with cyst formation—since they are bathed in synovial fluid which inhibits endosteal replacement and the callus undergoes a metaplasia into fibrous tissue or fibro-cartilage. However cyst formation may be an illusion since the X-rays may simply show an oblique view of the fractured surfaces. If further resorption occurs a pseudarthrosis may be established so that the two fragments move independently, each with a carpal row. If the carpus is unstable (see below) the anterior margins of the fracture will resorb so that the scaphoid becomes progressively flexed within the carpus or 'hump-

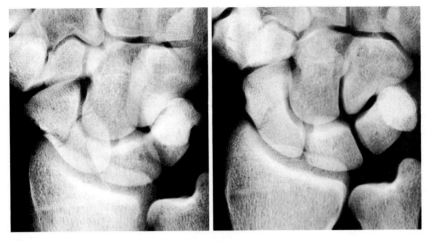

Fig 24.12   **Fig 24.13**

Fig 24.12 and 24.13 Few days old fracture of the scaphoid. The crack is much more obvious in the oblique view (Fig 24.12) than in the anteroposterior view (Fig 24.13). The fracture united after six weeks' immobilisation.

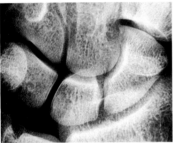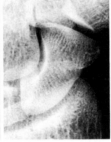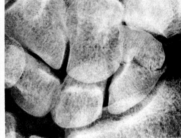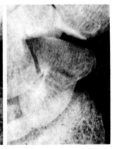

Fig 24.14 The clinical signs suggested a probable fracture of the scaphoid, but careful examination of the X-ray films, even with a magnifying lens, failed to show evidence of bone injury.

Fig 24.15 Radiographs taken three weeks later show the fracture very clearly. This occurs far too often for there to be any doubt that the fracture was actually present at the time of injury three weeks earlier.

backed' so that in the anterior-posterior view the scaphoid appears foreshortened and the distal extremity of the scaphoid is seen end-on (Fig 24.16).

Differentiation of old fractures from congenital bipart scaphoid. Old ununited fractures of the scaphoid with smooth and rounded fragments must be distinguished from congenitally bipart scaphoids, a distinction that is often difficult (Figs 24.17 and 24.18). There are three types of this developmental anomaly: separation of an os centrale (which is represented in the normal carpus by the interosseous ligament running between the scaphoid and capitate bones) which is the most frequent (Figs 24.19 and 24.20); separation from an os radiale externum corresponding to the os tibiale externum of the tarsus; and an equal division into a bipartite bone divided across the waist. It is the last type which is the most difficult to distinguish from

ununited fracture (see Figs 24.17 and 24.18) and may have important medico-legal significance. The literature is confusing because many cases reported as bipart scaphoids are almost certainly ununited fractures.[24,25,26] It has often been assumed that separation of a fragment from the scaphoid must be of congenital origin if the patient remembers no injury and if the other wrist joint shows similar changes, but both these assumptions are wrong. Many patients cannot recall the injury which first caused the fracture and bilateral scaphoid fractures from one injury or two successive injuries are not at all uncommon. It is usually possible to establish the distinction by noting the texture of the bone. If separation arises from developmental anomaly each fragment has a normal blood supply, there is no evidence of avascular necrosis and the subchondral

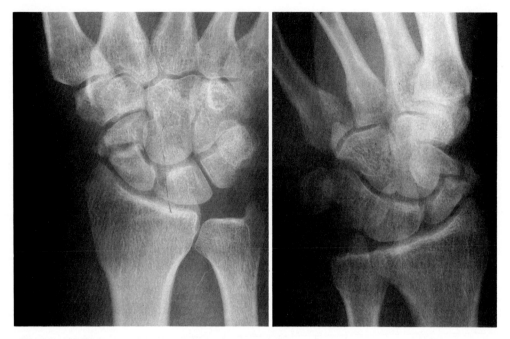

Fig 24.16 Ununited fractured scaphoid with 'hump-backed' appearance.

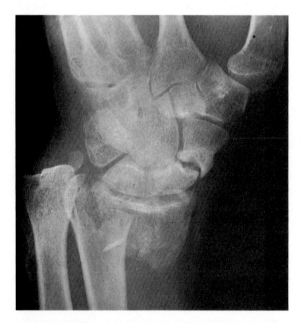

Fig 24.17 This young man sustained a Colles' fracture. The oblique radiograph revealed a scaphoid in two parts. Is this an old ununited fracture or a congenital bifid scaphoid?

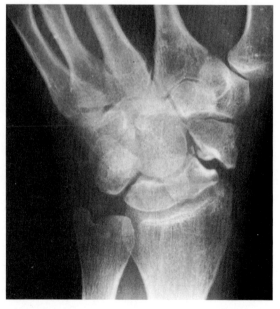

Fig 24.18 An X-ray of the opposite wrist showed a similar appearance. Both wrists hitherto had been symptom-free suggesting a congenital anomaly.

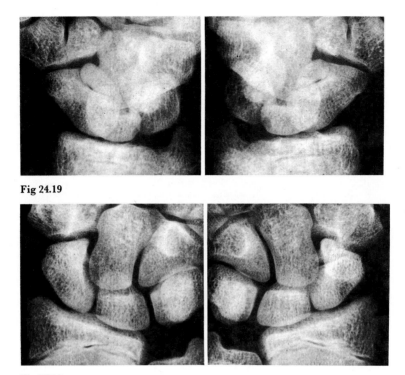

Fig 24.19

Fig 24.20

Figs 24.19 and 24.20 Oblique and antero-posterior radiographs of both wrist joints in a patient with bilateral os centrale. Other member of the family had normal scaphoids.

cortex runs smoothly round the whole bone. If the line of demarcation is irregular and the texture is abnormal with adjacent surfaces sclerosed the separation has almost certainly arisen from fracture—whether or not the patient remembers an injury or whether the lesion is unilateral or bilateral.

Three anatomical types of fracture of the scaphoid.

The bone may be fractured at any of three levels; the distal pole (10 per cent) the waist (70 per cent) or the proximal pole (20 per cent). The level of the fracture depends on the degree of ulnar flexion present at the moment of injury. A fourth type—fracture of the tubercle—is a distinct variety since this is a traction avulsion of the bony attachment of the transverse carpal ligament. The difference in behaviour of these three types of fracture is explained by variations in the blood supply of the bone. Examination of a large series of scaphoid bones shows that the vascular foramina, which are situated in the ligamentous ridge between the two main articular surfaces, conform to two types of distribution[27] (Figs 24.21 to 24.31). In two-thirds of the bones the vessels are distributed equally throughout the length of the ligamentous ridge (Fig 24.21). In the other third, there are no vessels directly entering the proximal half. They pierce the cortex of the distal half and travel backwards in the bone. The foramina may be

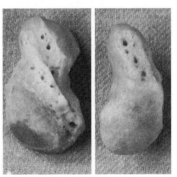
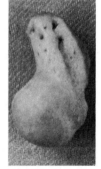

Fig 24.21   **Fig 24.22**

Figs 24.21 and 24.22 The blood vessels of the scaphoid are usually distributed throughout the length of the bone (Fig 24.21); but in one-third of scaphoids all the blood vessels enter the distal half (Fig 24.22).

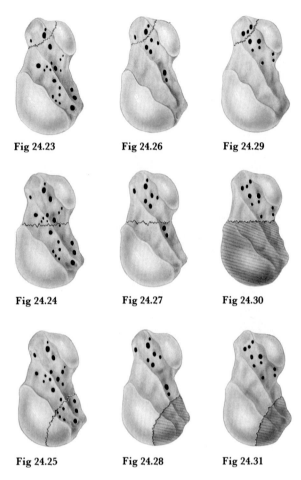

Fig 24.23

Fig 24.26

Fig 24.29

Fig 24.24

Fig 24.27

Fig 24.30

Fig 24.25

Fig 24.28

Fig 24.31

Figs 24.23 to 24.31 With the first type of blood supply, in which vessels enter the bone throughout its length (Figs 24.23 to 24.25), there is no danger of avascular necrosis from any fracture; it occurs only after dislocation. With the second type of blood supply, necrosis of the fragment sometimes occurs in waist fractures (Figs 24.26 to 24.28) and always in proximal pole fractures (Figs 24.29 to 24.31).

confined to the tubercle or there may be a few small, or one or two large, foramina actually at the waist (Fig 24.22). Injection studies of fresh amputation specimens[28] have demonstrated that the main blood supply to the bone is from a vessel which enters its waist on the antero-lateral aspect, with a smaller independent artery supplying the tubercle alone. These facts explain the unequal rate of union of fractures of the tubercle, the waist and the proximal pole and the variation in the incidence of avascular necrosis (Figs 24.23 to 24.31).

Fractures of the distal pole. Sometimes, and particularly in children, a compression injury occurs at the distal pole. The distal articular surface is flattened and sometimes broadened, suggesting that the injury is the result of direct compression. In other words, if the fall occurs in radial deviation of the wrist the scaphoid lies flexed within the carpus and the thrust of the injury is along its long axis. Non-union of the scaphoid in children is best managed by bone grafting through an anterior approach.[29]

In fractures of the waist both fragments usually have a free blood supply but there is no natural fixation of the fracture and union is secured only if the wrist joint is completely immobilised in a plaster cast or the fracture stabilised with a screw. If the fracture is recent it usually unites within six to ten weeks.

Fractures of the proximal pole. About two-thirds of fractures of the proximal pole are similar to fractures of the waist; each fragment has an adequate blood supply, and if the wrist is immobilised adequately union is complete within eight weeks. In one-third of proximal pole fractures there may be impairment of the blood supply of the proximal fragment with slow repair by 'creeping substitution' and prolonged immobilisation may be necessary if bone union is to be achieved.

The fractured scaphoid and carpal instability.[1] Most soft tissue injuries of the wrist are caused by a fall on the outstretched hand, and it is in dorsiflexion that the carpus is at its most vulnerable. The *transverse carpal ligament* may be avulsed from its attachment, and in this respect acts as a shock absorber although it adds nothing to the stability of the carpus. A thickened band of the volar radio-carpal ligament runs across the concavity of the scaphoid and this structure, along with the tendon of flexor carpi radialis, helps to maintain stability of the scaphoid within the carpus. If carpal instability is associated with distal detachment of the radial collateral ligament and the capsule between the scaphoid and the trapezium, the bone is now free to move within the carpus and this leads to recurrent intracarpal dislocation of the scaphoid (rotatory subluxation).

The degree of carpal instability associated with the fractured carpal scaphoid is the key to prognosis and its further management. There are two simple tests which will indicate whether instability of the wrist is present or not; namely, a lateral radiograph of the wrist in the neutral position and secondly, an estimate of the antero-posterior excursion of the carpus compared with the uninjured wrist.

Treatment of fractures of the scaphoid

Treatment may thus be rationalised as follows:

1. Recent fractures. If the fracture of the scaphoid is undisplaced and there is no carpal instability, the wrist should be immobilised in a plaster cast or close-fitting enveloping splint with the wrist held in radial flexion and some twenty degrees of dorsiflexion (Fig 24.11). The cast should be taken to the elbow joint and extend distally as far as the palmar crease on the volar aspect and the metacarpal heads on the dorsum. The thumb should be placed opposed to the middle finger and the plaster taken to the base of the proximal phalanx. In this way the trapezium and the trapezoscaphoid joint will be immobilised. Other positions have been advocated[30] (and any extreme position will immobilise the carpus) but the dorsal-radial flexion position impacts the scaphoid fragments and minimises the shearing effects which are exerted upon the fracture with movement of the hand and forearm. The patient must be instructed to protect the plaster and prevent it getting broken and wet. If the plaster becomes loose it should be quickly renewed. Immobilisation is maintained from six to eight weeks. Although it has been recommended in the past that the cast should be retained for nine months or even longer to make sure that the fracture is totally consolidated, the economic effects on a young working man and the disuse atrophy that follows prolonged immobilisation may outweigh the possible beneficial results.[31]

2. Screw fixation. If at the end of two months the fracture remains painful or appears ununited on a radiograph the fracture should be fixed by means of a lag screw,[32] as described by McLaughlin[33] and Maudsley (Fig 24.32).[34] If however the proximal fragment has become avascular, immobilisation should continue until at least the fracture has united by creeping substitution and the bone revascularised.

Screw fixation may be required immediately or after some delay. Where there is any displacement of the fracture, evidence of associated carpal instability or carpal dislocation, the scaphoid should be fixed internally as soon as the displacement has been reduced since the unstable carpus will be splinted by the rigid fixation of the scaphoid (Fig 24.33).

The screw can be inserted by closed or open methods.

In the *closed method* an incision is made at the base of the thumb centred over the tuberosity of the scaphoid. A fine Kirschner wire is inserted down the long axis of the scaphoid under the control of the image intensifier, a cannulated crown drill is passed over the Kirschner wire and the scaphoid drilled as far as the scapho-lunate joint. The drill is withdrawn and the wire retained. A cannulated screw of appropriate length is slipped over the wire and is screwed home using a cannulated screw driver (Fig 24.34). Impaction of the fracture is achieved during the last few turns and it is important to be sure of a firm grip upon the proximal fragment. The wire is then withdrawn. Immobilisation of the wrist is not essential if good fixation and impaction has been achieved.

In *open reduction* a lateral incision is made and removal of the radial styloid allows inspection of the fracture site. A Kirschner wire can be inserted under direct vision and a similar procedure adopted as outlined in the closed method (Figs 24.35 to 24.37). The open method is technically easier and it has the advantage of allowing the fracture site to be curetted

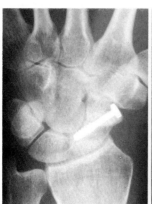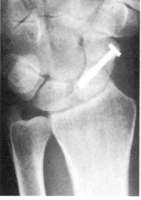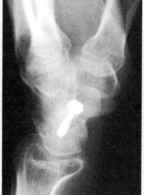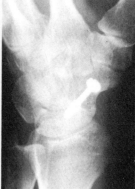

Fig 24.32 Screw fixation by open method with removal of the styloid process of the radius.

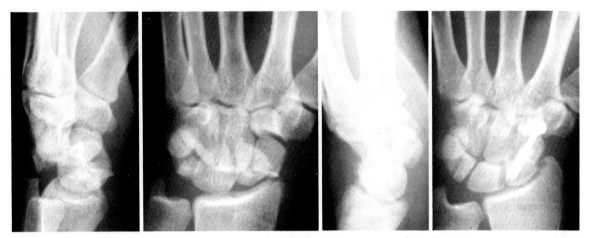

Fig 24.33 Trans-scaphoid trans-triquetral perilunar dislocation of the carpus treated by manipulative reduction and primary closed screw fixation of the fractured scaphoid.

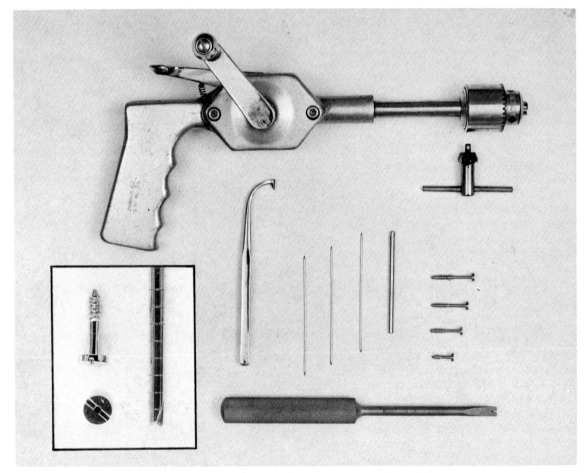

Fig 24.34 Instruments for screw fixation of the scaphoid. (a) Hand drill. (b) Maudsley scaphoid hook. (c) Kirshner wires. (d) Cannulated calibrated crown drill. (e) Set of cannulated lag screws. (f) Cannulated screw driver. (Reproduced by kind permission of the publishers from *Operative Surgery*, 3rd edn Orthopaedics. Surgery of the Wrist. Butterworths, London.)

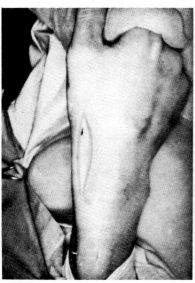

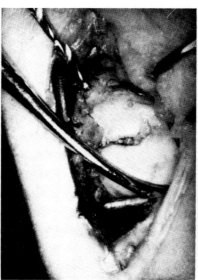

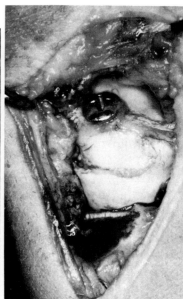

Fig 24.35   **Fig 24.36**   **Fig 24.37**

Figs 24.35 to 24.37 The fracture is exposed by an incision from the base of the first metacarpal to the radial styloid process (Fig 24.35). The proximal fragment is held reduced by a small bone hook while the bone is drilled at a very oblique angle backwards and the ulnar side. It will be noted how close to the upper part of the incision the drill is lying (Fig 24.36). When the lag screw is finally driven home the fracture line should be compressed (Fig 24.37). (Reproduced by kind permission of the *Journal of Bone and Joint Surgery* and of Mr R H Maudsley and Mr S C Chen from their article (1972) Screw fixation in the management of the carpal scaphoid. *Journal of Bone and Joint Surgery*, 54-B, 432).

and chip-grafted at the same time. Even in the presence of avascular necrosis internal fixation is to be encouraged since it ensures prolonged and firm immobilisation of the dead bone. Some authorities recommend routine internal fixation of all fractures of the scaphoid but as more than 90 per cent of them will unite by conservative means its routine use is hardly justified.[31] After internal fixation in carpal instability it is wise to immobilise the wrist in plaster for three to six weeks to allow the ruptured ligaments to heal.

3. Symptomless non-union. If the scaphoid is ununited and symptom free it is likely that the carpus is stable. The patient may suffer only negligible disability and treatment is not indicated. If, however, the patient has suffered a second injury the wrist should be immobilised in a plaster cast for three to six weeks not to achieve union of the scaphoid but in order to overcome the effect of the second sprain.

4. Styloidectomy for radiocarpal arthritis. If carpal instability or the injury to the scaphoid has resulted in radio-carpal arthritis, excision of the radial styloid will often bring about considerable

relief of discomfort and restore radial flexion to the wrist. This operation however should *not* be performed if the scaphoid is ununited, since there is the danger of the distal fragment prolapsing over the cut end of the radius (Fig 24.38).

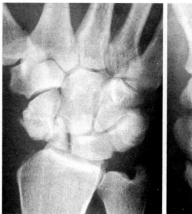

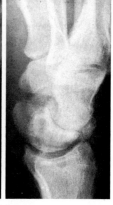

Fig 24.38 Unwise excision of the radial styloid in the presence of an ununited fractured scaphoid with carpal instability has exaggerated the deformity and allowed the distal half of the scaphoid to impinge against the cut surface of the radius.

5. Wedge grafting for non-union associated with instability. If the fractured scaphoid remains ununited as a result of the carpal instability the anterior margins of the fracture will have resorbed, giving rise to the hump-backed scaphoid. Reduction of the concertina deformity of the carpus will open up a wedge-shaped defect in the scaphoid based laterally and forwards. In these circumstances the scaphoid should be grafted. In previous editions it has been recommended that a peg-shaped bone graft[35,36] should be inserted down the long axis of the scaphoid to obtain both union and fixation of the scaphoid, but this places an excessive demand upon a bone peg which needs to be strong enough not only to support the weak wrist but at the same time enhance bony union. An alternative method is to graft the scaphoid from the front as advocated by Matti[37] and Russe.[38,39] This operation consists of exposing the scaphoid through an anterior incision, curetting out the fracture and packing this with one large graft and filling in the interstices with bone crumbs. This is a very successful method of producing bone union but it does not overcome the inherent deformity. Wedge-grafting[40] allows correction of the deformity and is best achieved by exposing the scaphoid through a lateral bayonet incision, removing the radial styloid and preserving it for later use (Fig 24.39). The fracture site is curetted free of fibrous tissue and each fragment drilled with a fine $\frac{3}{64}''$ drill. The defect in the scaphoid can be displayed by displacing the carpus volarwards which reduces the concertina deformity. A pyramidal graft is now cut from the excised radial styloid and gently tapped into position. This restores the length of the scaphoid and takes up the slack of the ruptured ligaments so that the wrist becomes immediately stable (Fig 24.40). The graft is held in position by the resilience of the soft structures

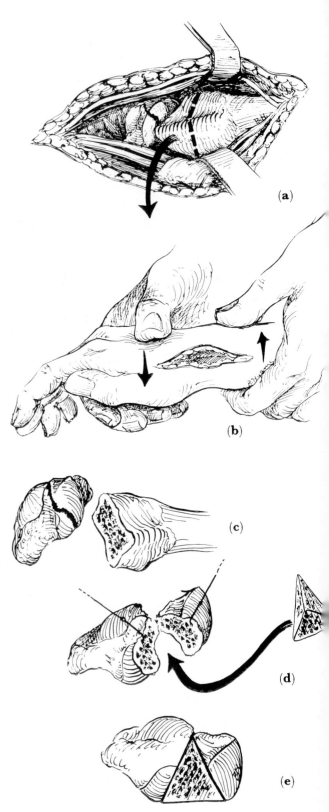

(a)

(b)

(c)

(d)

(e)

Fig 24.39 Wedge grafting of the ununited fractured scaphoid. (a) The radial styloid process is removed through the incision outlined above, but the excised bone is carefully preserved. (b) The fracture is identified and cleared of fibrous tissue. If the concertina deformity is now corrected by traction and anterior displacement of the carpus, the defect in the scaphoid is disclosed as wedge-shaped, based anterolaterally. (c, d and e) The fractured surfaces are curetted and if they are excessively sclerosed multiple fine drill holes are made in both fragments. The carpus is then manually realigned by an assistant and a wedge of appropriate size and shape is cut from the radial styloid process, fitted into the defect and tapped home with a bone punch. When the traction is released the resilience of the soft tissues holds the graft firmly in position and it is not necessary to transfix it by wire or screw. (Reproduced by kind permission of the publishers from *Operative Surgery*, 3rd edn. Orthopaedics. Surgery of the Wrist. Butterworths, London.)

and it is usually not necessary to use internal fixation. After grafting by any method the wrist should be immobilised for about eight to twelve weeks. A powerful painless wrist can be usually achieved but at some expense of extremes of movement.

6. Bentzon's operation.[41] This operation accepts non-union of the scaphoid and attempts to render this painless by the insertion of a fibro-fatty pad taken from the surrounding soft tissues. The operation contributes nothing to the stability of the carpus which is the underlying cause of the non-union but there might be an occasional indication for its use.

7. Excision of the proximal pole. Where the proximal part of the scaphoid is small or has undergone avascular necrosis with fragmentation of the proximal pole a useful result may be obtained by excising this proximal fragment (Figs 24.41 to 24.44). Indeed excision of the whole proximal row of the carpus has been recommended[42,43,44] where there is a radiocarpal arthritis in addition to the non-union. This certainly results in a painless pseudarthrosis with restoration of mobility but some loss of power.

8. Acrylic or silicone prosthetic replacement[45] of the scaphoid is fashionable at present but in view of the complex nature of scaphoid movement it can at its best act only as a space-filler.

9. Established non-union of the scaphoid with generalised carpal arthritis is best treated by arthrodesis of the wrist extending from the base of the third metacarpal to the radius. The wrist should be fused in a little dorsiflexion and ulnar flexion, and it is most conveniently achieved from a dorsal approach using an iliac crest graft. Arthrodesis of the wrist produces an excellent functional result with a powerful painless grip. Loss of carpal movement is only a disability where the subject requires to put the supinated hand underneath or behind objects.

10. Preiser's disease.[46] This condition, which is diagnosed more commonly on the Continent, corresponds to Kienböck's disease of the lunate (Fig 24.45). The whole scaphoid or, more commonly, its proximal part, fragments, resorbs and heals in a deformed position. Most authorities believe that this process follows an undiagnosed fractured scaphoid in which the proximal part has undergone avascular necrosis, but it is sometimes difficult to identify the fracture.

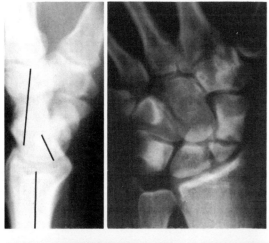
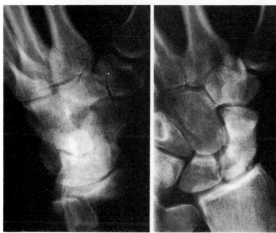
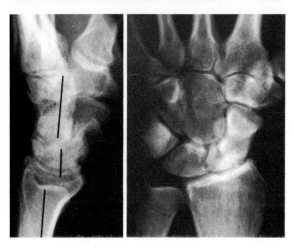

Fig 24.40 Wedge-grafting of an ununited fracture through the proximal pole of the scaphoid has promoted bone union and corrected the concertina deformity.

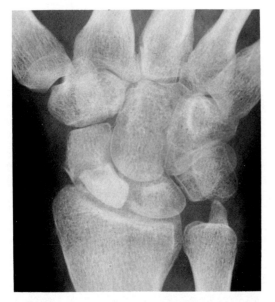

Fig 24.41

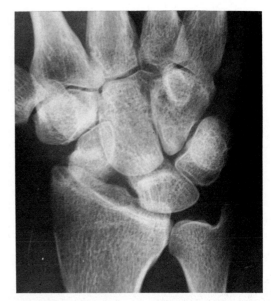

Fig 24.42

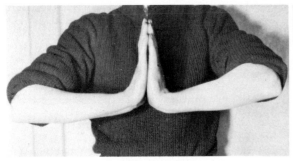

Fig 24.43

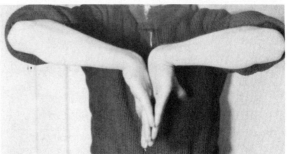

Fig 24.44

Figs 24.41 to 24.44 A skilled mechanic sustained a fracture of the carpal scaphoid bone and a few months later there was evidence of avascularity of the proximal half (Fig 24.41). To avoid a long period of treatment the avascular half was excised without delay (Fig 24.42). He returned to his trade three months after operation. The range of wrist joint movement after six months is shown in Figures 24.43 and 24.44. He could lift weights up to 100 lb (45 kg) and even after a heavy day's work he had no further symptoms. Such excellent function is usually secured only after *early* excision.

DISLOCATIONS OF THE CARPUS

The variety of dislocations and fracture-dislocations of the carpus is almost infinite.[47] Success in the treatment of carpal dislocations must depend on accurate diagnosis. This is often difficult and requires experience and careful study of the radiographs. It is only too easy for the young surgeon or the radiologist to fail to notice the altered alignment of the carpal bones, or indeed fail altogether to observe a displaced carpal bone, particularly the lunate. It is tempting to dismiss the condition entirely as 'a jumble of bones' or attribute the abnormal appearances to incorrect positioning of the wrist by the radiographer. Nearly every carpal dislocation includes disruption of the lunocapitate joint, and a study of the lateral radiographs often gives a key to the injury and suggests how the injury should be reduced. Most carpal injuries when first seen are easy to reduce by traction and manipulation, but if this proves unsuccessful early surgery is essential if the carpal function is to be retained and the chances of avascular necrosis minimised. Some classifications differentiate between those injuries in which the carpus is dislocated leaving one or more bones in place, as for instance perilunar dislocation of the carpus, and those in which these

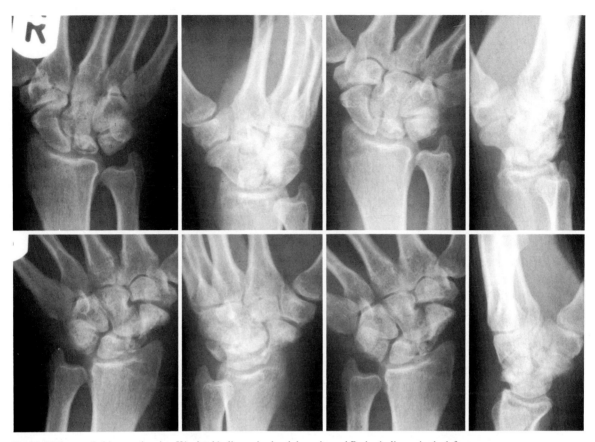

Fig 24.45 A remarkable case showing Kienböck's disease in the right wrist and Preiser's disease in the left.

bones have been displaced from the carpus. However, no good purpose is served by this division since perilunar dislocation of the carpus is the first stage of an injury which proceeds to dislocation of the lunate at the second stage when the resilience of the soft structures allows the carpus to spring back into its normal alignment. Indeed, understanding these two stages is essential if a dislocation is to be successfully reduced. Carpal bones are not squeezed out of position like orange pips between the finger and thumb, and cannot simply be pushed back into place without possible damage to the median nerve and other structures, with the added danger of producing a mal-alignment of surrounding articulations.

The mechanism of carpal dislocation always includes application of a transverse force exerted at the midcarpal joint, and antero-posterior movement of the carpus is always increased because of the associated ligament rupture. The various combinations of carpal dislocation are illustrated diagrammatically in Figure 24.46.

Trans-styloid radio-carpal dislocation (Figs 24.46a and 24.47a). In this injury the carpus is sheared off its articulation with the radius, taking with it the radial and ulnar styloid processes. It is often associated with injury to the radial articular surface. The deformity may be easily reduced but is often unstable and cannot be easily controlled by plaster fixation alone. It may be necessary to resort to open reduction with internal fixation of the radial styloid. Radiocarpal fusion may be required when the fracture has consolidated and where the articular surfaces have been damaged beyond repair.

Perilunar injury and dislocated lunate (Fig 24.46c). In perilunar dislocation the carpus is displaced backwards by dorsiflexion and compression forces. The capitate is dislocated from the cup of the lunate and comes to lie behind it (Fig 24.47b). Extensive ligamentous injury must have occurred but the volar radial attachments of the lunate will remain intact. Reduction is usually easily achieved in the

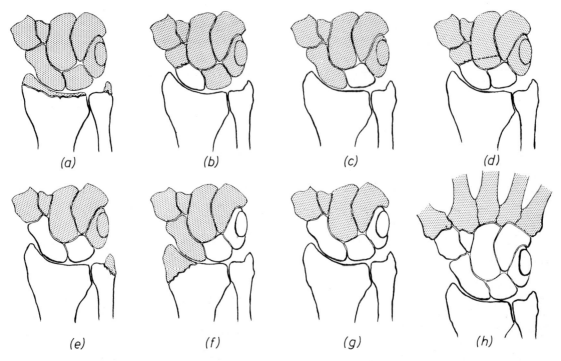

Fig 24.46 Diagram of carpal dislocations (the shaded bones are those which are displaced.) (a) Trans-styloid radiocarpal dislocation; (b) periscaphoid dislocation; (c) perilunar dislocation; (d) trans-scaphoid perilunar dislocation; (e) perilunar periscaphoid dislocation; (f) perilunar peritriquetral dislocation; (g) mid-carpal dislocation; (h) carpometacarpal dislocation. (Reproduced by kind permission of Butterworths from *Clinical Surgery*. The Hand. Fig 66, p. 103.)

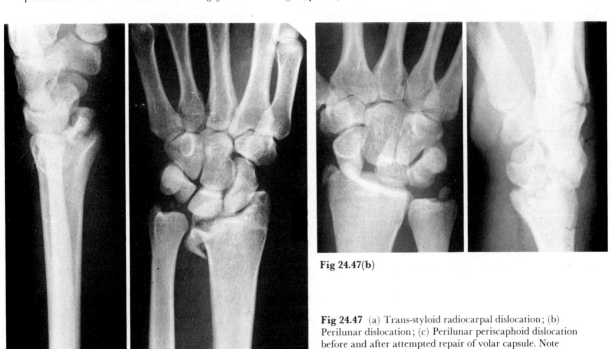

Fig 24.47(b)

Fig 24.47(a)

Fig 24.47 (a) Trans-styloid radiocarpal dislocation; (b) Perilunar dislocation; (c) Perilunar periscaphoid dislocation before and after attempted repair of volar capsule. Note avascular necrosis of the lunate.

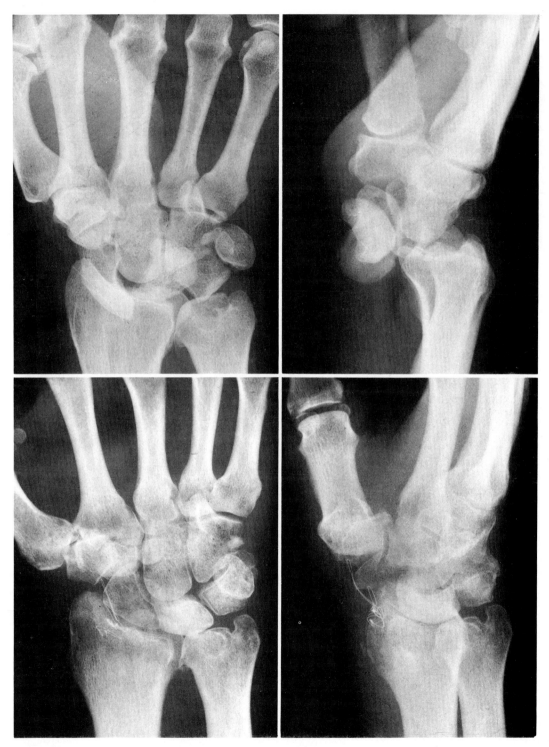

Fig 24.47(c)

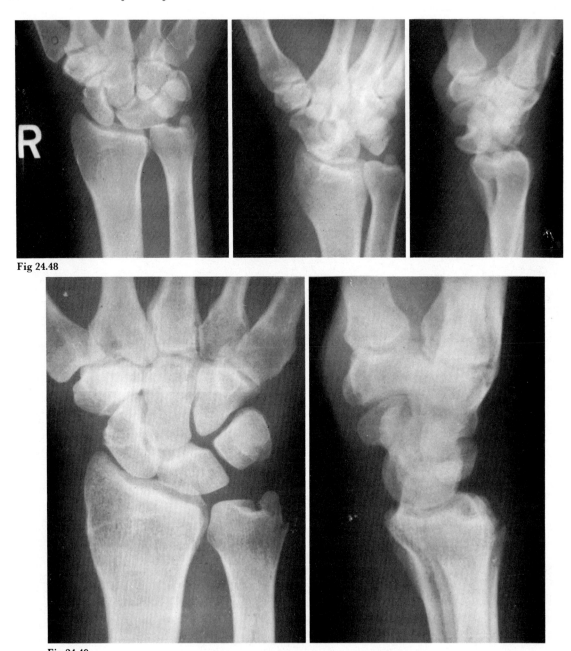

Fig 24.48

Fig 24.49

Figs 24.48 and 24.49 Forward dislocation of the lunate, obvious in the lateral projection because the cup is tilted forwards and unoccupied by the head of the capitate behind it. In antero-posterior projection the lunate is sector-shaped, like a piece of cheese (Fig 24.48). After reduction the head of the capitate is within the cup of the lunate and quadrilateral in shape (Fig 24.49).

early stages by traction, retention of the lunate upon the radial articular surface and then flexion of the wrist joint. *Dislocated lunate* occurs when rebound takes the carpus back into position but rolls the lunate forwards (Figs 24.48 to 24.50). These injuries almost invariably involve the median nerve and attempts to push the lunate back into position simply damages the nerve still further; and in any case collapse of the carpus, blood clot and oedema so diminishes the gap as to make it well nigh impossible to persuade the

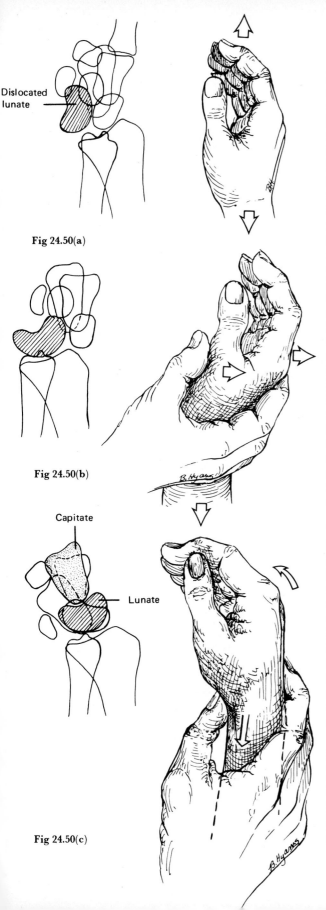

Fig 24.50(a)

Dislocated lunate

Fig 24.50(b)

Fig 24.50(c)

Capitate

Lunate

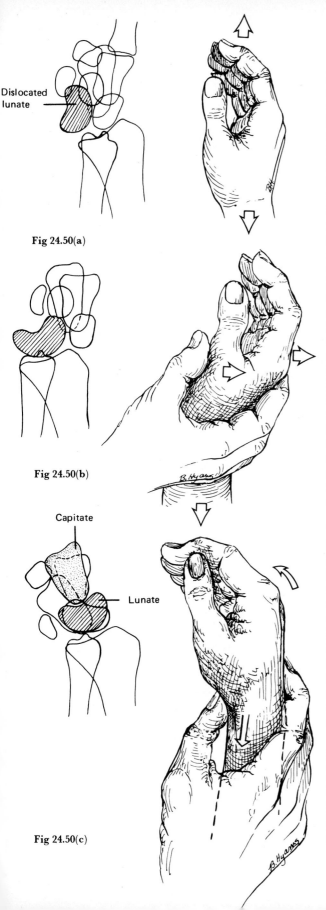

lunate to return to its normal alignment. Reduction should be achieved by dislocating the carpus backwards from its articulation with the radius (Fig 24.50a and b). The lunate is then rolled back into its correct position, held gently with the thumb (Fig 24.50b) and then by traction and flexion of the wrist by the other hand, the carpus is brought back into its normal position (Fig 24.50c). Where delay in diagnosis and swelling prevent manipulative correction, open reduction[48] may be attempted from the front and possibly through the dorsum as well by a transverse incision at the chaplet crease of the wrist. After reduction the wrist should be supported in a well-padded plaster cast in a little flexion and the limb kept elevated until all oedema is gone. If signs of median nerve compression have supervened, it is sometimes wise to incise the transverse carpal ligament or not repair it again at the end of the operation. In the late case open reduction may be achieved only at the expense of extensive damage to the articular surfaces of the lunate and neighbouring bones. In these cases the lunate may have lost its blood supply and it is wiser to remove it. Lunectomy results in a very satisfactory function of the wrist with some loss of power but retention of movement. There is at present a tendency to replace the lunate by a metal, acrylic or silicone prosthesis. However, unless such an artificial substitute is carefully aligned and combined with meticulous capsular repair it may dislocate, and will need to be removed.

The 'horizontal' scaphoid. Dislocation of the lunate is usually associated with rupture of the ligaments surrounding the scaphoid. When the lunate is reduced, particularly after delay, the proximal pole of the scaphoid may be pushed over the dorsal lip of the radius so that it remains horizontally placed within the carpus. A dorsal capsular flap may lie between the scaphoid and capitate and although the lunate appears satisfactorily reduced the patient may find dorsiflexion limited and painful and have the sensation of a bony block when he attempts this movement (Figs 24.51 to 24.53). Open reduction is then necessary by approaching the carpus from the dorsal aspect. The operation may be successful even

Fig 24.50 *Reduction of a dislocated lunate.* Traction is applied to the wrist and the carpus is dislocated posteriorly from its articulation with the radius, while pressure with the thumb rolls the lunate into its correct position (Fig 24.50 a and b). The rest of the carpus is restored to its anatomical position by traction and flexion (Fig 24.50 c). (Reproduced by the kind permission of Butterworths from *Operative Surgery*, 3rd edn., Orthopaedics. Surgery of the wrist, p 542).

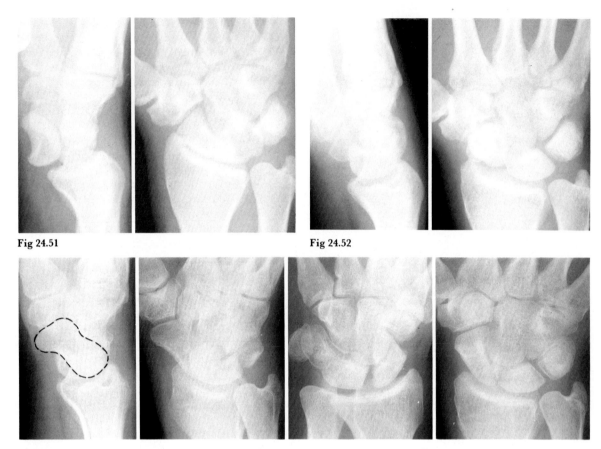

Fig 24.51   Fig 24.52

Fig 24.53

Figs 24.51 to 24.53 This deep-sea diver sustained a dislocated lunate in a motor cycle accident (Fig 24.51). Open reduction was necessary but the scaphoid assumed a horizontal position in the carpus preventing dorsiflexion of the wrist (Fig 24.52). Open reduction of the scaphoid through a dorsal approach restored its position and wrist movement allowing him to return to his hazardous occupation (Fig 24.53).

after some months' delay. The scaphoid is carefully freed from adhesions, interposed soft parts are removed and the proximal pole of the scaphoid may be repositioned under direct vision. If this proves to be impossible an osteotomy of the dorsal lip of the radius allows the scaphoid to slip back into place and the divided bone left to heal itself. Careful repair of the dorsal ligaments should be performed to prevent recurrence of the deformity and the wrist immobilised in some dorsiflexion in a padded plaster cast.

Dislocation of the scaphoid[49,50] (Figs 24.54 and 24.55). This is an uncommon injury. The mechanism of displacement resembles that of the carpal lunate, resulting from a forced dorsiflexion-supination force upon the hand. The proximal pole of the scaphoid comes to lie over the radial styloid which is commonly

fractured and depressed. Reduction is difficult to achieve by manipulation and open reduction is usually necessary, because of infolding of volar capsule. At the same time the radial articular surface may be reduced and fixed by one or more fine Kirschner wires.

Isolated dislocation of the scaphoid implies not only a rupture of the volar radio-carpal ligament but its capsular attachments to the lunate, the capitate and the trapezium, and the whole scaphoid may undergo avascular necrosis.

Recurrent intracarpal dislocation of the scaphoid[5] (Figs 24.56 and 24.57). If the capsular attachments of the scaphoid are ruptured without its dislocation from the radius the scaphoid may undergo recurrent intracarpal dislocation. The scaphoid will

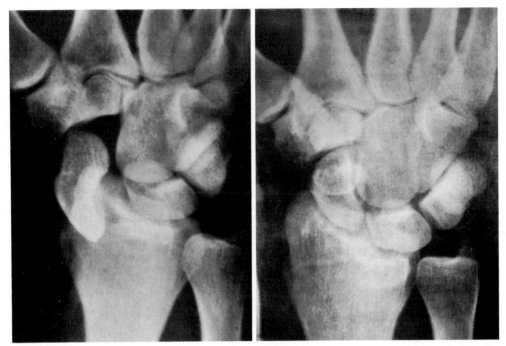

Fig 24.54   Fig 24.55

Figs 24.54 and 24.55 Dislocation of the carpal scaphoid bone. The proximal pole is displaced over the radial styloid process (Fig 24.54). It can usually be reduced by manipulation, but an interposed curtain of capsule may make operative reduction necessary.

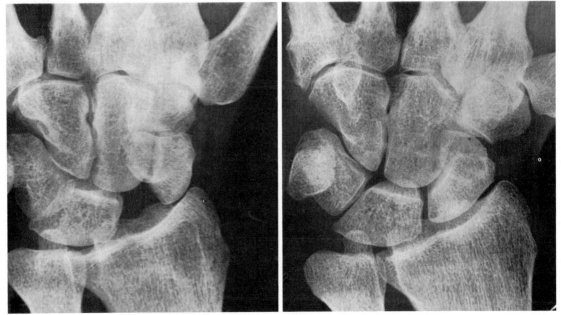

Fig 24.56   Fig 24.57

Figs 24.56 and 24.57 Recurrent dislocation of the carpal scaphoid bone. As with other dislocations, if the first injury is not suitably immobilised the dislocation will recur. In this patient, who was seen at the London Hospital and recorded by Vaughan-Jackson, the bone dislocated every time he threw a dart. The disability can sometimes be relieved by capsular reefing behind the proximal pole of the bone. (Reproduced by kind permission of the *Journal of Bone and Joint Surgery* and of Mr Vaughan-Jackson, from his article (1949) A care of recurrent subluxation of the carpal scaphoid. *Journal of Bone and Joint Surgery*, 31-B, 532).

jump into a horizontal position, sometimes with an audible snap, when a compression force is exerted upon the carpus as for instance in gripping. Indeed, the patient may learn a trick movement in which he is able to dislocate the scaphoid at will. Surgical stabilisation is often difficult to achieve and may involve reefing the dorsal capsule and repairing the volar radio-carpal ligament through separate incisions. Scapho-lunate fusion has been advocated but this has the disadvantage of seriously limiting carpal movement, since this joint is essential in midcarpal movement and radial flexion.

Trans-scaphoid perilunar dislocation (Figs 24.33 and 24.46d). This is a serious injury to the carpus and its appearance on the X-ray is often confusing. The proximal pole of the scaphoid and lunate remain upon the end of the radius or are displaced forwards by the rest of the carpus. It is easy to mistake the proximal pole of the scaphoid for the lunate since that bone comes to overlie the hamate. This injury in the author's experience almost invariably leads to avascular necrosis of the proximal pole of the scaphoid. After reduction of the fracture-dislocation by manipulation the scaphoid fragments may remain displaced from one another indicating the instability of the carpus. Primary internal fixation of the scaphoid should be performed but there is now an indication for prolonged immobilisation in a plaster cast, since the avascular proximal pole may disintegrate despite its fixation.

Perilunar periscaphoid dislocation (see Figs 24.46e and 24.47c). Both bones may be displaced completely and come to lie in front of the radius. Open reduction is usually necessary.[48] The dislocation is however sometimes associated with a fracture through the proximal pole of the capitate and attempts to reduce the dislocation results in this fragment being turned upside down. In these circumstances it is better either to remove the fragment entirely or after reduction impale it for a few weeks with a Kirschner wire.

Midcarpal dislocation (see Fig 24.46g). Owing to the complex outline of this joint it is virtually impossible to sustain a midcarpal dislocation without associated fractures. Dislocation of the hamate and capitate bones accompanied by the ulnar three metacarpals has been seen.

Carpo-metacarpal dislocation (see Fig 24.46h). This injury with or without fracture is sustained by forced dorsiflexion of the hand, as for instance in a motor cycle injury when the handlebars displace dorsally all four metacarpals. Dislocation may surprisingly enough not be recognised because of the extreme swelling. It is usually unstable and reduction may only be maintained if the hand is splinted in full palmar flexion, and internal fixation by a number of Kirschner wires may be necessary (see Chapter 25). However, even if the dislocation is not recognised, the carpo-metacarpal joints usually ankylose leaving an ugly swelling on the dorsum of the wrist and a shortened palm but a high degree of function.

Unusual injuries of the carpus. Subluxations and dislocations of every single one of the carpal bones have been reported. Furthermore, chip fractures which are not of any particular significance are quite common[51]—they need only protection in a dorsal plaster cast for two or three weeks. Dislocations of the trapezium,[52] trapezoid[53] or hamate[54] are more important because they sometimes need open reduction.

INJURIES OF THE RADIO-ULNAR ARTICULAR DISC

The space between the ulnar margin of the radius and the tip of the ulnar styloid is filled by the triangular fibro-cartilage with which the lunate and triquetral bones articulate. This disc is occasionally damaged in Colles' fracture and any disruption of the inferior radio-ulnar joint may avulse one of its bony attachments—nearly always at the radius. Coleman[55] suggested that the mechanism of injury is forced dorsiflexion and pronation. The injury gives rise to pain over the inferior radio-ulnar joint, weakness of grip and a painful clicking. The symptoms are aggravated by resisted pronation and supination as in using a wrench or screwdriver. The diagnosis is established by injection of 'hypaque' into the ulnar side of the wrist joint when the fluid may be seen running into the inferior radio-ulnar joint through a perforation or defect in the triangular cartilage. If symptoms warrant it the disc may be excised through an incision placed over the dorsum and ulnar aspect of the wrist joint.

KIENBÖCK'S DISEASE

Lunatomalacia was first described by Kienböck in 1910[56] (see Fig 24.45). This condition remains a mystery and there is no immediately effective treatment. Kienböck felt the condition was caused by ischaemia of the lunate from damage to the blood supply at its ligamentous attachments. Alternatively it has been suggested that Kienböck's disease arises from a fissure fracture of the lunate resulting from trauma, the fracture failing to unite because it is not recognised and the separate fragments proceed to resorption and non-union. It is rare for the sufferers to recollect a specific injury to the wrist but many of them recall a period of unusual or intensive active use of the hand. The condition is characterised by intermittent aching in the wrist with swelling, tenderness and limitation of movement. X-ray examination will show patchy sclerosis of the lunate followed later by collapse and healing in a deformed condition which must affect the function of its surrounding articulations. The whole process may take two years to develop and heal. In the severest cases the lunate may remain fragmented, ununited and flattened.

Several predisposing causes have been suggested, one of them being 'ulnar variance'.[57] This postulates that relative shortening of the ulnar predisposes patients to lunatomalacia and that the lunate is compressed excessively because of the loss of support by the ulna. Moberg[58] and others have reported relief of symptoms by lengthening the lower ulna by a step osteotomy. Lee[59] demonstrated the different patterns of blood supply to the lunate in cadavers. Two-thirds of them had palmar and dorsal vessels which anastomosed. A quarter had either a single palmar or dorsal vessel and the rest had two vessels which did not anastomose.

An interesting association of Kienböck's disease with cerebral palsy has been demonstrated by Rooker and Goodfellow.[60] Of 53 residents in a home for adult spastics, twelve were found to be suffering from pain in one or both wrists and five of the twelve were found to be suffering from Kienböck's disease. There appeared to be a close relationship between the flexed and pronated posture of the hand at rest and the presence of lunatomalacia, suggesting that the blood supply to the lunate might be jeopardised.

Many patients, perhaps up to 50 per cent, particularly in the younger age groups, are rendered comfortable by immobilisation of the wrist in a plaster cast for two or three months, followed by provision of a moulded polythene wrist support, which is worn during working hours for perhaps as long as two years after the onset of the symptoms. However in older age groups and in particular those in which there has been some distortion of the articulation of the carpus, simple excision of the lunate relieves the pain, but with some loss of power.

Where there are associated degenerative changes in the rest of the carpal bones proximal carpectomy has been recommended. This will restore movement but with some permanent loss of stability and power.[43]

Prosthetic replacement of the lunate by metal, acrylic or silicone substitute has its advocates. Lichtman and others[61] reporting a series of patients whose lunates had been replaced by silicone prostheses felt that this operation is to be preferred to prolonged immobilisation. The results were better if the lunate was replaced before collapse had taken place with its accompanying diastasis at the scapholunate joint and the proximal migration of the capitate. The prosthesis may be inserted by either anterior or posterior approach, preferably the latter, excising the fragmented lunate piecemeal and carefully preserving the ligamentous attachments. The implant has a stem which is inserted into a drill hole in the triquetrum.[62] Unfortunately these prostheses are apt to displace unless the size is carefully selected and the dorsal capsule meticulously repaired.

NERVE PALSY IN WRIST INJURIES

Although the cutaneous branches of the radial nerve can sometimes be damaged by direct injury over the radial styloid and give rise to a tiresome paraesthesia, the important nerve lesions associated with wrist fractures and dislocations are those of the median and ulnar nerves. Usually these nerve palsies are the result of compression by haematoma, or displaced bone fragments, within the tunnels through which the nerves pass; but occasionally they are due to direct contusion, interneural fibrosis, and even ischaemic changes.

Paralysis of the median nerve from carpal tunnel compression. The carpal tunnel of the wrist joint, with the carpal bones in its floor and the transverse carpal ligaments as its roof, is occupied fully by the flexor tendons and the median nerve—there is no room for anything else. Spontaneous onset of median nerve compression symptoms without injury, due to swelling of the soft tissues within the tunnel, was fully described over 30 years ago[63] and is now a well known condition. Acute compression of the median nerve under the carpal ligament may arise occasionally after a Colles' fracture, and more rarely after recent fractures of the scaphoid; but by far the most frequent cause of acute median nerve compression in wrist injury is a dislocation of the lunate, or one of the varieties of perilunar dislocations.

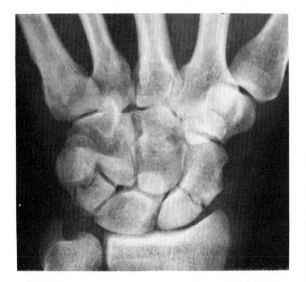

Fig 24.58 An apparent recent fracture of the carpal scaphoid with acute median nerve compression. Study of the films shows that there was also a fracture of the cuneiform, and this was, in fact, a trans-scapho-perilunar-trans-cuneiform fracture-subluxation. Within 48 hours there was agonising pain the median nerve distribution with paralysis which was relieved promptly by division of the anterior carpal ligament. The nerve had been compressed by haemorrhage and effusion within the carpal tunnel. The patient was a distinguished violinist—and the injury was to his left hand, but he is now leading his orchestra once again.

Figure 24.58 shows the wrist joint of a distinguished musician. As well as the fracture of the carpal scaphoid there was a fracture of the cuneiform, and this was, in fact, a trans-scaphoperilunar-trans-cuneiform fracture-subluxation of the joint. Within 48 hours he developed excruciating pain in the median distribution of the hand with impairment of touch sensation and evidence of incomplete median paralysis. As an emergency procedure the anterior carpal ligament was divided. The symptoms were relieved at once. It was nearly four months before recovery from the median palsy was complete, but after that he resumed duty as the leader of his orchestra.

Tardy median nerve palsy after old fracture of the scaphoid. Median neuritis is very rare indeed in recent fractures of the scaphoid, but after many years of non-union, with secondary arthritis and the formation of osteophytes which crowd the carpal tunnel with new bone formation, paralysis of the median nerve arises not uncommonly. Zachary reported one case of bilateral un-united scaphoid fracture which presented with median nerve palsy on both sides 40 years later.[64] The patient whose X-rays

and operative findings are shown in Figures 24.59 and 24.60 developed evidence of nerve compression 20 years after the fracture. In such injuries complete relief is gained by division or excision of the transverse carpal ligament. It is interesting to note that tardy median palsy of this type is often predominantly motor in presentation, which was attributed by Zachary to the larger motor fibres of the nerve being

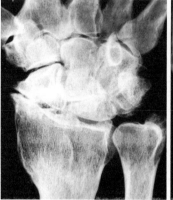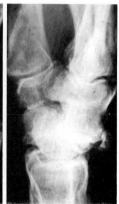

Fig 24.59

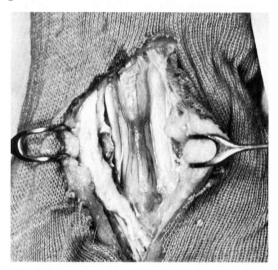

Fig 24.60

Figs 24.59 and 24.60 Twenty-year-old ununited fracture of the carpal scaphoid bone, possible associated with peri-semilunar dislocation of the wrist, in which secondary arthritis with osteophyte formation caused crowding and compression within the carpal tunnel so that tardy median palsy developed (Fig 24.59). Note at operation when the anterior carpal ligament was divided how seriously the trunk of the median nerve was compressed (Fig 24.60). Division of the ligament was all that was needed to cure the median nerve paralysis. (Photograph by Mr Ruddick at the Orthopaedic and Accident Department of the London Hospital.)

more vulnerable to pressure. Acute median nerve compression, on the other hand, is nearly always sensory in its mode of onset.

Ulnar nerve palsy in wrist injuries. This is commonly the result of injuries to the hamate, and the bones in the immediate vicinity;[65] but cases resulting from severely displaced Colles' fractures have also been reported.[66] The motor branch of the nerve is particularly susceptible as it passes around the hook of the hamate and in one series five out of six cases reported presented with a motor paralysis alone.[65] The one case with additional sensory deficit was associated with a fracture of the pisiform—an injury which could be expected to affect the whole nerve trunk. In nerve palsies occurring as part of an acute injury expectant conservative management should be followed in the first instance, but decompression must be carried out if there is no recovery by six to eight weeks.

Delayed ulnar palsy after fracture of the hamate bone has already been reported.[67] In this patient there was both motor and sensory paralysis, and at operation the nerve was found to be densely bound down in fibrous tissue at the level of the bifurcation into its motor and sensory branches. A good recovery in sensation followed the neurolysis. Exploration of the nerve is clearly indicated in such cases.

REFERENCES

1. Fisk G R 1970 Carpal instability and the fractured scaphoid. Annals of the Royal College of Surgeons of England 46 : 63
2. Linscheid R L, Dobyns J H, Beabout J W and Bryan R S 1972 Traumatic instability of the wrist. Diagnosis, classification and pathomechanics. Journal of Bone and Joint Surgery 54-A: 1612
3. Landsmeer J M F 1960 Studies in the anatomy of articulation. Acta Morph. Neerl-Scand 3 : 304
4. Taliesnik J 1976 The ligaments of the wrist. Journal of Hand Surgery 1 : 110
5. Vaughan-Jackson O J 1949 A case of recurrent subluxation of the carpal scaphoid. Journal of Bone and Joint Surgery 31-B: 532
6. Palmer A K, Dobyns J H, Linscheid R L 1978 Management of post-traumatic instability of the wrist secondary to ligament rupture. Journal of Hand Surgery 3 : 507
7. Blood W 1942 Tenosynovitis in industrial workers. British Medical Journal ii : 468
8. Flowerdew R E, Bode O B 1942 Tenosynovitis in untrained farm workers. British Medical Journal ii : 367
9. Taylor-Jones T H E 1942 Tenosynovitis in untrained farm workers. British Medical Journal ii : 440
10. Williams J G P 1977 Surgical management of traumatic non-infective tenosynovitis of the wrist extensors. Journal of Bone and Joint Surgery 59-B: 408
11. Drury B J 1955 Tendovaginitis of extensor digiti quinti proprius. Journal of Bone and Joint Surgery 37-A: 407
12. Dickson D D, Luckey C A 1948 Tenosynovitis of the extensor carpi ulnaris tendon sheath. Journal of Bone and Joint Surgery 30-A: 903
13. Fitton J M, Shea F W, Goldie W 1968 Lesions of the flexor carpi radialis tendon and its sheath causing pain at the wrist. Journal of Bone and Joint Surgery 50-B: 359
14. de Quervain F 1895 Uber eine form von chronischer tendovaginitis. Korrespondenz-Blatt für Schweizer Arzte 25 : 389
15. Finkelstein H 1930 Stenosing tendovaginitis at the radial styloid process. Journal of Bone and Joint Surgery 12 : 509
16. Giles K W 1960 Anatomical variations affecting the surgery of de Quervain's disease. Journal of Bone and Joint Surgery 42-B: 352
17. Bunnell S 1944 Surgery of the hand. Lippincott, Philadelphia
18. Ritter M A, Inglis A E 1969 The extensor indicis syndrome. Journal of Bone and Joint Surgery 51-A: 1645
19. Secrétan H 1901 Oedema dur et hyperplasie traumatique du métacarpe dorsal. Rev Méd de la Suisse Romande 21 : 409
20. Vander Elst E 1961 The thick hand. The Second Hand Club 110. British Society for Surgery of the Hand
21. Milch H, Green H H 1938 Calcification about the flexor carpi ulnaris tendon. Archives of Surgery 36 : 660
22. Weber E R, Chao E Y 1978 An experimental approach to scaphoid wrist fractures. Journal of Hand Surgery 3 : 142
23. Graziani A 1940 L'esaine radiologico del carpo. La Radiologia Medica Torino 27 : 382
24. Boyd G I 1933 Bipartite carpal navicular bone. British Journal of Surgery 20 : 455
25. Faulkner D M 1928 Bipartite carpal scaphoid. Journal of Bone and Joint Surgery 10 : 284
26. Childress H M 1943 Fractures of a bipartite carpal navicular. Report of a Case. Journal of Bone and Joint Surgery 25 : 448
27. Obletz B E, Halbstein B M 1938 Non-union of fractures of the carpal navicular. Journal of Bone and Joint Surgery 20 : 424
28. Taleisnik J, Kelly P J 1966 The extra osseous and intra osseous blood supply of the scaphoid bone. Journal of Bone and Joint Surgery 48-A: 1125
29. Southcott R, Rozman M A 1977 Non-union of carpal scaphoid fractures in children. Journal of Bone and Joint Surgery 59-B: 20
30. Squire M 1959 Carpal mechanics and trauma. Journal of Bone and Joint Surgery 41-B: 210
31. London P S 1961 The broken scaphoid bone. The case against pessimism. Journal of Bone and Joint Surgery 43-B: 237
32. Gasser H 1965 Delayed union and pseudarthrosis of the carpal navicular; treatment by compression screw osteosynthesis. A preliminary report on twenty cases. Journal of Bone and Joint Surgery 47-A: 249
33. McLaughlin H L 1954 Fracture of the carpal navicular (scaphoid) bone. Some observations based on treatment by open reduction and internal fixation. Journal of Bone and Joint Surgery 36-A: 765
34. Maudsley R H, Chen S C 1972 Screw fixation in the

management of the fractured carpal scaphoid. Journal of Bone and Joint Surgery 54-B: 432

35. Armstrong J R 1941 Closed technique for fixation of fractured carpal scaphoid. Lancet i: 537

36. Butler A A 1942 Bone pegging of the carpal scaphoid. Proceedings of the Royal Society of Medicine 35: 760

37. Matti H 1937 Über die Behandlung der Navicularefraktur und der Refractura patella Plombierung mit spongiosa. Zeutralbl. für Chirurgie 64: 2353

38. Russe O 1960 Fracture of the carpal navicular—diagnosis, non-operative treatment and operative treatment. Journal of Bone and Joint Surgery 42-A: 759

39. Trojan E 1974 Grafting of ununited fractures of the scaphoid. Proceedings of the Royal Society of Medicine 67: 1078

40. Fisk G R 1978 Surgery of the Wrist. In: Bentley G (ed) Orthopaedic surgery 540. Operative surgery. Butterworths, London.

41. Bentzon P Gr K 1946 On fracture of the carpal scaphoid. A method for operative treatment of inveterate fractures. Acta Orthopaedica Scandinavica 16: 30

42. Stamm T T 1944 Excision of the proximal row of the carpus. Proceedings of the Royal Society of Medicine 38: 74

43. Crabbe W A 1964 Excision of the proximal row of the carpus. Journal of Bone and Joint Surgery 46-B: 708

44. Jorgensen E C 1969 Proximal row carpectomy—An end-result of twenty-two cases. Journal of Bone and Joint Surgery 51-A: 1104

45. Barber H M 1974 Acrylic scaphoid prostheses: A long term follow-up. Proceedings of the Royal Society of Medicine 67: 1075

46. Preiser G K F 1911 Zur Frage der typischen traumatischen Ernährungstörungen der kurzen Hand- und Fusswurzelknochen. Fortschritte a.d. Gebiete der Röntgenstrahlen, vol. 17, 360–362

47. Russell T B 1949 Intercarpal dislocations and fracture-dislocations. A review of fifty-nine cases. Journal of Bone and Joint Surgery 31-B: 524

48. Campbell R D, Thompson T C, Lance E M, Adler J B 1965 Indications for open reduction of lunate and perilunar dislocations of the carpal bones. Journal of Bone and Joint Surgery 47-A: 915

49. Buzby B F 1934 Isolated radial dislocation of the carpal scaphoid. Annals of Surgery 100: 553

50. Woodd Walker G B 1943 Dislocation of the carpal scaphoid reduced by open operation. British Journal of Surgery 30: 380

51. Fairbank T J 1942 Chip fractures of the os triquetrum (carpal cuneiform). British Medical Journal ii: 310

52. Siegel M W, Hertzberg H 1969 Complete dislocation of the greater multangular (trapezium). A case report. Journal of Bone and Joint Surgery 51-A: 769

53. Stein A H 1971 Dorsal dislocation of the lesser multangular bone. Journal of Bone and Joint Surgery 53-A: 377

54. Geist D C 1939 Dislocation of the hamate bone. Report of a case. Journal of Bone and Joint Surgery 21: 215

55. Coleman H M 1960 Injuries of the articular disc at the wrist. Journal of Bone and Joint Surgery 42-B: 522

56. Kienböck R 1910 Ueber traumatische Malazie des Mondbeins und ihre Folgezustände. Fortsch. Geb. Roentgen 16: 77

57. Gelberman R H, Salomon P B, Jurist J M, Posch J L 1975 Ulnar variance in Kienböck's disease. Journal of Bone and Joint Surgery 57-A: 674

58. Moberg E 1970 Discussion. Journal of Bone and Joint Surgery 52-A: 251

59. Lee M L H 1963 The interosseous arterial pattern of the carpal lunate bone and its relation to avascular necrosis. Acta Orthopaedica Scandinavica 33: 43

60. Rooker G D, Goodfellow J W 1977 Kienböck's disease in cerebral palsy. Journal of Bone and Joint Surgery 59-B: 363

61. Lichtman D M, Mack G R, MacDonald R I, Gunther S F, Wilson J N 1977 Kienböck's disease. The role of silicone replacement arthroplasty. Journal of Bone and Joint Surgery 59-A: 899

62. Swanson A B 1970 Silicone rubber implants for the replacement of carpal scaphoid and lunate bones. Orthopaedic Clinics of North America 1: 299

63. Brain W R, Wright A D, Wilkinson M 1947 Spontaneous compression of both median nerves in the carpal tunnel—Six cases treated surgically. Lancet i: 277

64. Zachary R B 1945 Thenar palsy due to compression of the median nerve in the carpal tunnel. Surgery, Gynecology and Obstetrics 81: 213

65. Howard F M 1961 Ulnar-nerve palsy in wrist fractures. Journal of Bone and Joint Surgery 43-A: 1197

66. Watson-Jones R 1929 Carpal semilunar dislocations and other wrist dislocations with associated nerve lesions. Proceedings of the Royal Society of Medicine 22: 1071

67. Baird D B, Freidenberg Z B 1968 Delayed ulnar-nerve palsy following a fracture of the hamate. Journal of Bone and Joint Surgery 50-A: 570

25

Fractures and Joint Injuries of the Hand

N. J. Barton

'Too often these fractures are treated as minor injuries, and major disability results' P. R. Lipscomb*

FRACTURES

Why have fractures of the hand been so neglected? Innumerable papers have been published on fractures of the femur or tibia, but hand fractures have received scant attention in the literature and all too often in the fracture clinic as well. They are among the most frequent of all fractures, so the explanation for this neglect must be that they have been considered unimportant and unworthy of much thought and study. However, Sir Reginald Watson-Jones, in the early editions of this book, pointed out that 'An open fracture of a phalanx is no less worthy of the skill of an expert than an open fracture of the femur. There is often little difference in the economic value of surgical treatment'. Similarly, Sir John Charnley has said: 'The reputation of a surgeon may stand as much in jeopardy from a fracture of the proximal phalanx of the finger as from any fracture of the femur'.[1]

The essential steps in treating any fracture are:

1. Define the aim of treatment.
2. Identify the type of fracture.
3. Apply the principles of fracture treatment.

AIM OF TREATMENT

In fractures of the lower limb, whose prime requirement is stability, the aim is to secure bony union in an acceptable position as soon as possible; other considerations are of secondary importance. In the upper limb, and especially in the hand, the need is for mobility. When a hand injury is followed by a bad result, the badness is usually stiffness. Unfortunately the stiffness is often a consequence of poor treatment. Non-union occurs so rarely that it is not a factor in planning treatment, but mal-union is a significant

problem after certain types of hand fracture and it is important to pick these out and distinguish them from the majority which can be treated by early movements.

Dr Alfred B. Swanson has put it very well: 'Hand fractures can be complicated by deformity from no treatment, stiffness from over-treatment, and both deformity and stiffness from poor treatment'.[2] This suggests that we must choose the treatment which is most appropriate to each particular fracture, bearing in mind that many hand fractures would obtain a better result with no treatment at all than with bad treatment. Poor results are seldom due to lack of knowledge or technical skill: the cause is usually failure to *think* about the problem.

TYPE OF FRACTURE

Adequate radiographs are essential and should include antero-posterior oblique, and *lateral* views. You should train your X-ray department to take lateral views routinely, as without them it is impossible to assess the amount of angulation and therefore to know whether reduction is necessary.

A fracture may be confused with a nutrient artery, an overlying soft-tissue shadow, or an epiphyseal line:

1. Nutrient arteries pass obliquely through the cortex of the phalanx, usually at the junction of the middle and distal thirds.
2. The shadow of the soft tissues of the web or of a neighbouring finger may at first glance look like a fracture: make sure that the 'fracture-line' is confined to bone.
3. The epiphyses in the hand appear at the age of two or three and fuse to the diaphysis at puberty. Unlike the larger long bones, the metacarpals and phalanges have an epiphysis *at one end only*. In the

*Lipscomb P R 1963 Management of fractures of the hand. The American Surgeon 29: 277.

phalanges it is at the proximal end, but in the metacarpals it is at the distal end, except for the first metacarpal which (like the first metatarsal) has its epiphysis at the proximal end (Fig 25.1). Sometimes, however, a pseudo-epiphysis is seen at the distal end of the first metacarpal (Fig 25.2) and this is often mistaken for a fracture. For practical purposes in treating hand fractures this is all one needs to know, though the exact sequence and timing of the appearance and fusion of the epiphyses has been worked out in great detail and is the basis for estimating skeletal age.

If in doubt, relate the radiographic appearances to the clinical findings: if it is not tender, it is not a recent fracture. In addition, a radiograph can be taken of the other hand for comparison, though this is seldom necessary.

Classification

Having established that a fracture is present, one must decide what sort of fracture it is. Here, again, comparison with the femur is instructive. An orthopaedic surgeon, faced with a fractured femur, will first determine whether it is subcapital, trochanteric, subtrochanteric, mid-shaft, supracondylar or whatever, because treatment and prognosis depend upon the type of fracture. The same surgeon, confronted by a fractured finger, seldom applies the same procedure, though it is just as necessary to classify fractures in the hand as elsewhere.

The most obvious classification of phalangeal fractures is whether they affect the proximal, middle or distal phalanx. However, a transverse fracture of the mid-shaft of the proximal phalanx is similar to a transverse fracture of the mid-shaft of the middle phalanx, but quite different to an avulsion fracture

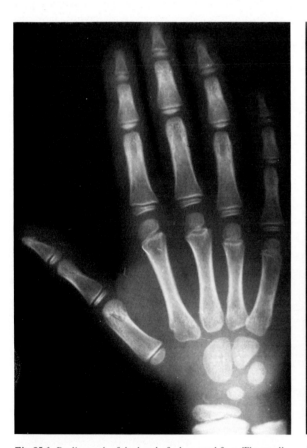

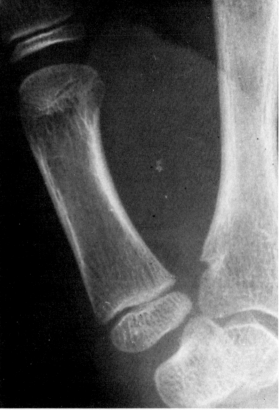

Fig 25.1 Radiograph of the hand of a boy aged four. The small long bones in the hand have an epiphysis at only one end: the proximal end of the phalanges and first metacarpal, and the distal end of the finger metacarpals.

Fig 25.2 Sometimes a pseudo-epiphysis is seen at the distal end of the first metacarpal. This may be wrongly diagnosed and treated as a fracture.

from the side of the base of the proximal phalanx. It is therefore more helpful to use a classification based upon the pattern of fracture. The same applies to the metacarpals, though each individual metacarpal is prone to certain types of fracture, such as the fractured neck of the fifth metacarpal and the fractured base of the first metacarpal. The following classification has been found useful:

1. Phalangeal fractures
   a. Fingertip
   b. Epiphyseal
   c. Shaft
   d. Comminuted
   e. Articular
2. Metacarpal fractures
   a. Base
   b. Shaft
   c. Neck
   d. Head
3. Special types of fracture
   a. Compound fractures
   b. Multiple fractures
   c. Pathological fractures.

Most of these have subdivisions which will be described below.

PRINCIPLES OF TREATMENT

The basic principles of fracture treatment must be applied in the hand as much as anywhere else. All too often an aluminium splint is applied instead.

Reduction

The surgeon must first decide whether reduction is necessary.

Angulation may be in three planes: antero-posterior, lateral or rotational. In the phalanges, angulation is usually concave dorsally (Fig 25.3). In the metacarpals it is almost always concave towards the palm (Fig 25.4). This difference is usually explained in terms of muscle pull[3] but may really be due to the direction of the force which caused the fracture: most phalangeal fractures are caused by a fall on the outstretched hand or by something falling onto the back of the outstretched hand, whereas metacarpal fractures are usually sustained with the fingers flexed, either in fighting or falling.

Most phalangeal fractures have little or no displacement and therefore do not need reduction, but this must not lead to a carefree attitude that reduction is unimportant in all finger fractures. Displaced fractures of the proximal phalanx (Fig 25.3) always involve the floor of the fibrous flexor tendon sheath

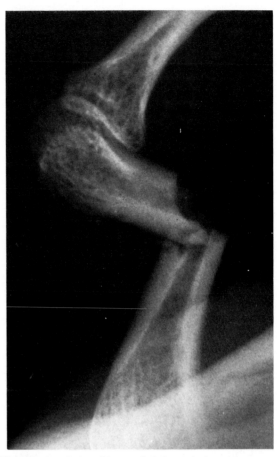

Fig 25.3 Angulation of fractured phalanges is almost always concave dorsally. A fracture like this must involve the sheath of the flexor tendon, which rests on the front of the phalanx, and the tendon is therefore likely to become adherent at the fracture site. (Reproduced by permission of the editor of *The Hand*).

and precise alignment is essential to ensure a good result.[4] In the shafts of the phalanges it is *more* important to obtain and maintain good reduction than in the shafts of long bones in the arm or leg, because the phalanges are so close to tendons which have a large excursion that even slight displacement interferes with function.[5,6] Similarly, articular fractures with large fragments must be accurately reduced.

In the metacarpals the situation is different. Moderate angulation of a fracture of the neck of the fifth metacarpal is accepted because, although it could be reduced, the methods necessary to maintain reduction are undesirable and are more likely to cause lasting disability than the angulation itself. Moreover the intact neighbouring metacarpal limits to some extent the possible angulation.

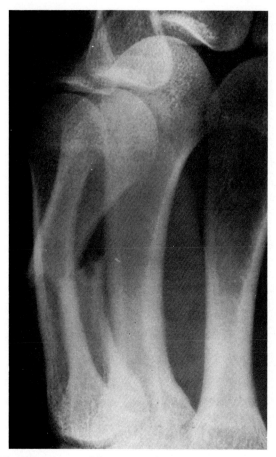

Fig 25.4 Fractures of the metacarpals angulate in the opposite direction: concave anteriorly.

In both metacarpals and phalanges, however, it is absolutely necessary to detect and correct any *rotational* deformity. Failure to do so results in the situation shown in Figure 25.5: in extension the deformity is not obvious but in flexion the affected finger crosses over its neighbour. Such a finger is, at best, of little use and, at worst, a hindrance to the function of the intact fingers, and needs correction by rotational osteotomy. This is a difficult procedure in the hand, and it is much easier and better to correct any rotation at the time of the fracture. Such deformity may not be obvious on the radiograph or on a hasty examination of the hand itself, as the fracture limits flexion of the finger. You must therefore examine the fingers end-on and check the plane of the finger-nails by comparison with the other hand.

The method of reduction is usually by manipulation under local or general anaesthetic. Fractures of the

proximal phalanx can be most easily reduced if the proximal phalanx is stabilised by flexing the M.P. joint[7] (which is also the position in which the fracture should be immobilised). An abducted fracture at the base of the little finger can sometimes be reduced by using a pen in the web of the finger as a fulcrum. In open injuries, the fracture can be reduced under direct vision; when closed fractures are exposed for operative treatment, open reduction is usually followed by internal fixation.

Retention

In the early editions of this book it was taught that hand fractures should be immobilised like any other. Time has shown that this is neither necessary nor desirable. Broken bones in the hand are not normally subjected to the stresses of weight-bearing*, and the muscles acting on them are less powerful than the large muscles in the leg. Like the clavicle, they will nearly always unite despite movement, and slight deformity is preferable to stiffness. Borgeskov, after reviewing 267 phalangeal and metacarpal fractures treated conservatively and followed up for five years, found good functional results in 68 per cent: only 4 per cent complained of discomfort and only 2.9 per cent had significant permanent disability. He concluded that it is important to avoid over-treatment of fractures in the hand.[8] Wright, having reviewed 809 patients with fractures of the metacarpals or phalanges treated in Edinburgh, found that the hand must be mobilised early if normal function is to be maintained.[9]

Stable phalangeal fractures need only be strapped to the adjoining finger (Fig 25.6) or treated in a Bedford type of support (Fig 25.7), which achieves the same purpose. This reminds the patient and other people that the finger is injured, but allows flexion and extension while limiting side-to-side movements. It can be regarded as a dynamic splint, the intact finger being used as a motor to move the injured one.

Which fractures are stable and which are not? The distinction must be based upon experience of different types of fracture and to some extent upon trial and error. Undisplaced fractures are probably always stable, and most fractures of the second, third, fourth and fifth metacarpals are stable, being adequately supported by the intact metacarpal alongside. Figure 25.8 shows on the left the types of fracture which are usually stable and therefore do not need immobilisation, and on the right those which are unstable and

*This is not frivolity: patients with severe arthritis or neurological disease affecting the lower limbs may have to take a lot of weight on their hands when walking with crutches or rising from a chair.

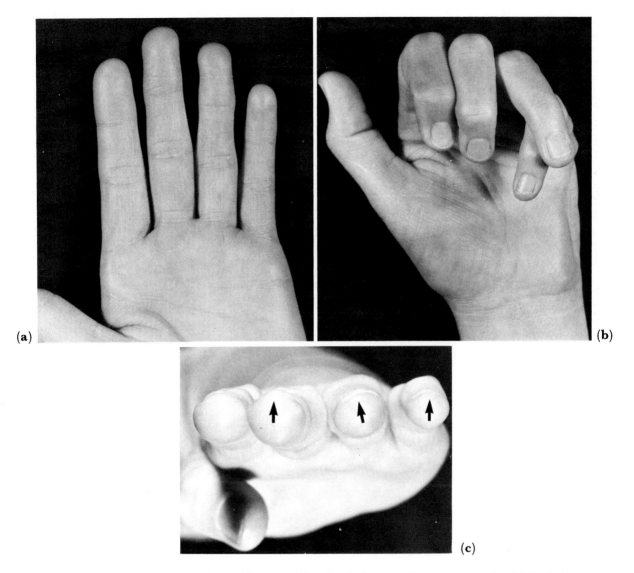

Fig 25.5 (a) In this position, there is no obvious deformity. (b) But when the fingers are flexed, a severe rotational deformity is revealed: this will seriously interfere with the use of the hand. (c) If it is not possible to flex the injured finger, it must be examined end-on to detect any mal-rotation: the pronation of the ring finger can be detected by comparing the plane of its fingernail with that of the other fingers.

do need splintage. In general, any fracture which needs reduction also needs retention.

The malleable padded aluminium splint is a simple, versatile and useful device, but it must be applied correctly. Sumner Koch pointed out as long ago as 1934 in a lecture to the American Medical Association that there is a definite pattern of stiffness after hand injuries: the M.P. joints are prone to extension contractures but the P.I.P. joints develop flexion contractures.[10] It follows (though it did not actually follow till twenty years later) that the best position in which to immobilise the finger is with the metacarpo-phalangeal joints flexed and the inter-phalangeal joints extended, because this is the position least likely to result in permanent stiffness.[11] The widespread adoption of this position has greatly reduced the frequency of joint contractures after hand injuries, and is due to the work of Professor James of

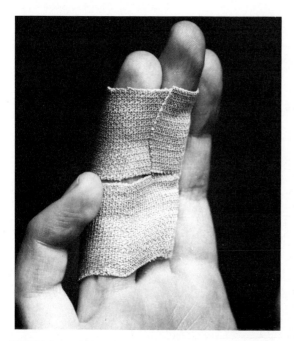

Fig 25.6 Most phalangeal fractures should be treated simply by fastening the finger loosely to the adjoining finger with adhesive strapping, using a minimum of strapping to avoid impeding movements.

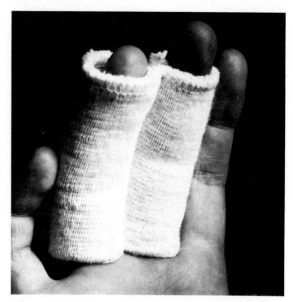

Fig 25.7 An alternative method of supporting a fractured finger is by using a cloth Bedford support. These are available commercially, or can be made in the sewing-room at your hospital.

Edinburgh; both names have been applied to this position of the hand.

The flexion crease for the M.P. joint is that formed by the transverse palmar creases, as you can see by looking at your own hand from the side. The flexion crease at the base of the finger is halfway down the proximal phalanx. The aluminium splint should be bent to 90° in the middle and strapped to the palm with the angle just proximal to the transverse proximal *palmar* crease for the index and middle

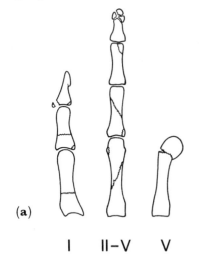

(a)

I   II–V   V

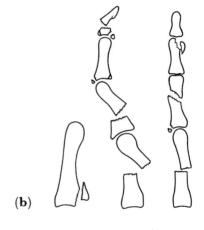

(b)

Fig 25.8 (a) *Stable fractures*. These fractures, most of which are undisplaced, are usually stable and can be treated by active movement in strapping or a Bedford support. (b) *Unstable fractures*. These displaced fractures are unstable. Those involving large fragments may need splintage or internal fixation. (Modified from *A Practical Guide to the Care of the Injured* by London, P. S. 1967. Livingstone, Edinburgh)

fingers, or distal *palmar* crease for the ring and little fingers. The fracture is then reduced and the finger laid onto the distal part of the splint so that the M.P. joint is flexed to a right angle and the I.P. joints are straight (Fig 25.9). The splint need not cross the wrist joint. It is unnecessary to double the splint back along the dorsum of the finger, and undesirable because it prevents inspection of the finger end-on to check that any rotational deformity has been reduced. The flexibility which enables the surgeon to adjust these splints also makes it too easy for the patient to alter the position of immobilisation or even remove the splint altogether: a malleable splint should therefore only be used if the patients can be trusted to leave it alone. For this reason, the method is unsuitable for use in treating primitive or uneducated peoples.

Plaster casts are seldom used for a fractured finger but provide good immobilisation for a fractured thumb, the fingers being left free. Plaster may also be used when dealing with multiple fractures in the hand, the best method being to use two plaster slabs. First, apply a volar slab with the M.P. joints flexed and I.P. joints straight, as described above, and when it has set, add a dorsal slab to maintain the position of the fingers against the volar slab (Fig 25.10). Longitudinal ridges may be added to the slabs to give them greater rigidity. The thumb should be left free if possible, but if included must be in palmar abduction at the carpo-metacarpal joint: I have seen

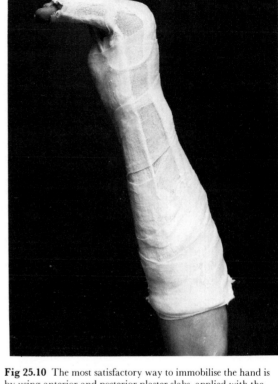

Fig 25.10 The most satisfactory way to immobilise the hand is by using anterior and posterior plaster slabs, applied with the joints in the safe position.

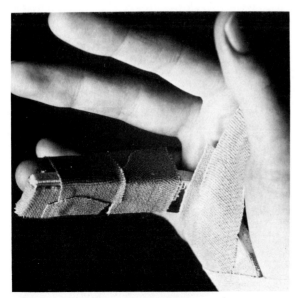

Fig 25.9 Finger splinted correctly. The M.P. joint is flexed, the I.P. joints are extended, and the finger can be examined end-on to check rotation.

adduction contractures of the thumb in hands in which the thumb has not been injured but was included in the dressing in such a way as to produce a flat tidy package. Unlike the fingers, the thumb should be immobilised with both the M.P. and I.P. joints in extension. A hand which has been properly immobilised is bulky, but the term 'boxing-glove dressing' ought to be avoided because it suggests flexion of the interphalangeal joints.

Immobilisation should, with few exceptions (see below), be limited to three weeks, because splintage for longer than this usually results in some permanent stiffness. Callus is seldom seen in finger fractures, so nothing is gained by taking further radiographs; it is reasonable and practical to assume that there is clinical union after three weeks.

Traction has been largely superseded by internal fixation, because it was clumsy and liable to result in stiffness, especially if applied by a pin through the bone or soft tissue.

Internal fixation of hand fractures was first described by Vom Saal of New York in the *Journal of*

Bone and Joint Surgery in 1953.[12] He had in fact submitted the paper earlier, when it was brusquely rejected as a dangerous and unacceptable form of treatment. Later he read the paper at a meeting when the editor of the journal was present, and was invited to submit it for publication. It is now established as a valuable method of treating certain types of fracture:

1. Displaced fractures of the shafts of the phalanges, if closed treatment has failed to achieve satisfactory position.
2. Displaced fractures close to or involving a joint.
3. Major hand injuries with loss of skeletal stability.[13]

Internal fixation, however, also has its problems and is not a panacea. Theoretically, it should allow early movement and so avoid stiffness: in practice, fingers treated by internal fixation are often stiffer than if they had been treated conservatively. The technique is more difficult than in larger bones, with very little margin for error, and even its most enthusiastic proponents conclude that the 'final results of post-operative treatment can be unsatisfactory and the operation itself can be very difficult'.[14] The improvements which have been made over the last twenty years in technique and equipment for fixing small fragments have not altered the indications but have made it possible to do the job better when it is indicated, which is probably in less than 5 per cent of all hand fractures.

Kirschner wires are the simplest, cheapest and most versatile method of fixation and have the advantage that they can sometimes be introduced percutaneously without exposing the fracture,[15, 16, 17] which is particularly useful for maintaining reduction of the joint in fracture-dislocations. However the point of the wire can easily slip on the sharply curved surface of the phalanges and it need only slip one or two millimetres to break the dorsal or volar cortex so that it is impossible to complete the fixation. It is particularly difficult to introduce a Kirschner wire obliquely by hand: either it skids off and runs outside the cortex or it is passed too transversely. A power tool is essential for this purpose: it should be small enough to hold steady with one hand (while your other hand holds the fracture) and should provide a high-speed rotation. The 3M mini-driver is recommended. The wire should be about three inches (7.5 cm) long and pointed at both ends so that it can be introduced by the retrograde method if necessary. It probably does not make much difference what metal the wire is made of or what kind of point it has, but to avoid distraction it is best to use a wire with a bevelled end slightly *wider* than the rest of the wire

which will in effect over-drill the fragment through which it first passes. It seldom does any harm to transfix a joint temporarily with a wire, if this is the only way you can hold the fracture. Opinions differ as to whether it is necessary to cut off the end of the wire and bury it subcutaneously; this reduces the risk of infection but removing the wire may become even more difficult than putting it in. The cut end of the wire often extrudes through the skin in a week or two anyway, and if the plan is to remove the wire at three weeks it is probably safe to leave the end sticking out.

Experimental work by Fyfe[18] in Nottingham using cadaveric bone has shown that in transverse fractures a single longitudinal wire gives poor resistance to angulatory forces, and of course no resistance to rotation. Crossed oblique Kirschner wires (Fig 25.11) give rigid fixation but may cause distraction at the fracture site. It may be possible to avoid this by first stabilising the fracture with a temporary longitudinal wire, then inserting the crossed oblique wires, and finally removing the longitudinal wire. Lister's intra-osseous wiring,[19] with one oblique Kirschner wire and a wire loop, through transverse drill-holes on either side of the fracture (Fig 25.12), allows compression and also gives rigid fixation but requires considerable skill. You should practise on cadaveric phalanges before using these methods on patients. Another method of internal fixation, called semicircular wiring, is to drill a hole in the cortex on either side of the fracture line, pass a length of flexible wire through the two adjacent cortices and twist it into a loop; another smilar loop can be inserted on the other side of the bone,

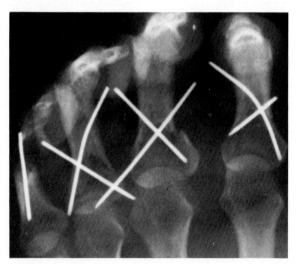

Fig 25.11 Multiple fractured phalanges immobilised by crossed oblique Kirschner wires.

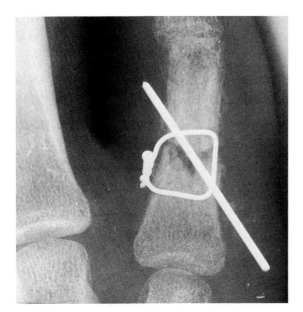

Fig 25.12 Intra-osseous wiring. The wire loop provides compression, or at least prevents distraction. (Reproduced by permission of the editor of *The Hand*.)

Small screws and plates are now available, very good ones being made to the specifications of the A.S.I.F. group of Swiss surgeons. The screws may be useful for fixing large articular fragments. Plates are valuable in some unstable fractures of the metacarpals but should not be used in the fingers because the extensive exposure is certain to result in adherence of tendons. The fixation achieved is in any case less rigid than that given by crossed Kirschner wires or Lister's intra-osseous wiring, because it is impossible to put the plate on the flexor aspect of the phalanx where it would be most effective as a tension band.

Operating on a hand fracture will itself cause stiffness. If, at the end of the operation, you have not fixed the fracture well enough to allow early movement, then all you have done is to add another cause of stiffness. Bad internal fixation is much worse than no internal fixation. If in doubt, remember Mr. Punch's advice to persons about to marry: Don't![20]

A completely different approach, described recently, is to use external fixation. No special equipment is needed. Two parallel Kirschner wires are passed transversely through the proximal fragment and two more through the distal fragment. Another two stout Kirschner wires are then used to form a longitudinal external frame, and are fixed to the transverse wires by small blobs of acrylic cement.[21, 22] This method has not yet been used enough to assess its value, but may be helpful when there is skin damage.

Rehabilitation

Rehabilitation, or the restoration of the best possible movement and function, is *always* needed. It is not an optional extra tacked on at the end of treatment, but is the very essence and purpose of the treatment. In unstable fractures it may be necessary to defer the actual process of rehabilitation for a few weeks until splintage has been discontinued, but rehabilitation should be in the mind of the surgeon from the moment he first sees the patient, and especially when he is planning the programme of treatment.

In most cases rehabilitation can start immediately, because most hand fractures do not require immobilisation and those which have been internally fixed should also be able to begin movements within a day or two.

The patient finds that when he moves his finger it hurts and he naturally thinks that this means he should not move it, which indeed is true of most fractures. It is up to us to explain to the patient that he must move the finger even if it hurts. Deeds speak louder than words, and the most effective method is first to demonstrate with your own hand the movement which you wish the patient to make, and then get him to do the same with his injured hand. When he has reached his limit of active movement, use your hand to move his finger further, through as full a range as he can tolerate. Then instruct him how to do these passive movements on himself, using his uninjured hand. Finally, make him do this too under your supervision. Having shown him what he can do, you must convince him that these movements should be carried out for at least five minutes in every waking hour—preferably more—and re-assure him again that although such exercises may be hurtful they are not harmful: indeed failure to do them is harmful because it will allow the finger to stiffen.

All this may seem very humdrum, but a minute or two spent in this way is the most valuable thing you can do in most cases and achieves more than much longer periods spent in elaborate forms of treatment or operation (Fig 25.13).

Most reasonably intelligent adult patients can do these movements on their own. Children usually recover so quickly that they do them without being told. Treatment in a physiotherapy department is therefore only needed for very nervous or unintelligent patients and for fractures which are particularly likely to cause stiffness. Those patients who do need physiotherapy should attend for treatment every day: attendance two or three times a week is of little use, and the valuable but limited resources of the physiotherapy department are better spent treating

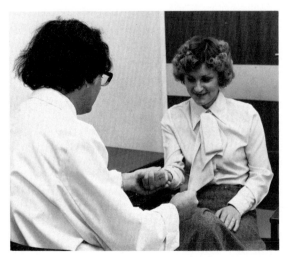

Fig 25.13 The most important part of treatment: explaining to the patient the need to practise active movements of the injured finger.

a few patients intensively than many patients occasionally.

The actual physiotherapy is simple; so simple that the physiotherapist may find it boring and resort to gadgets which achieve little but distract from the real purpose, which is to regain a full range of active movements. Treatment consists of practising over and over again the sequence of events described above as carried out by the surgeon at the patient's first attendance. Gentle passive assistance of this sort is helpful; passive manipulation in any vigorous sense does more harm than good and is prohibited. If it is necessary to concentrate on a particular inter-phal-angeal joint, it is legitimate to use a small piece of wood to block flexion of more proximal joints, though it is also necessary to practise movement of the whole finger because this is what is needed in the long run. (It is worth knowing that an injury which one would expect to produce stiffness of either the P.I.P. or the D.I.P. joint usually in practice causes stiffness of both I.P. joints amd may therefore result in more disability than was originally anticipated.) Squeezing a rubber ball or a bit of putty should be forbidden as it prevents the full range of flexion which is the goal of treatment, and flexion against resistance may lead to displace-ment or re-displacement of a fracture. A *full range* of movement is the target; the restoration of full power can and should wait till later and usually happens on its own with normal use of the hand. Occupational therapy is not helpful in the short but intensive programme of rehabilitation needed for most hand fractures.

Hand fractures are common in working men, and may cause loss of income to the patient and his family, and loss of production for his employers and his country. Fortunately, an early return to work is generally the best treatment for the fracture as well as the patient: once enough movement has been obtained for him to carry out his job, further progress can be expected with use.[23] Office workers seldom need to stay away from work at all, and only patients with very heavy or rough jobs or with multiple injuries need be off work longer than three or four weeks. A few companies in the United Kingdom have special workshops where a machine can be adapted so that it requires a particular movement, such as flexion of the thumb, to work it. This provides effective treatment and also enables the patient to start producing and earning again as soon as possible.

Amputation
With some fractures, particularly severe crushing injuries involving joints, even prolonged physiother-apy is unlikely to restore a useful range of movement, so the best and quickest way to get the patient back to work is to amputate the injured finger at the time the patient is first seen. It is essential to have good quality skin and subcutaneous fat on the end of the stump, even if this means further shortening of bone. The digital nerves should be diathermied and cut as far proximally as possible, so that the cut ends are deeply buried beneath a thick pad of soft tissue. The tendons should also be cut as short as possible, and their ends should *not* be sutured together over the end of the stump.

FRACTURES OF THE PHALANGES
James, in 1962, reviewed the results of 196 fractures of the proximal and middle phalanges. 96 were judged to be stable, and 76 of these regained full function; of the others 16 had slight loss of movement and only four had serious loss of movement. In contrast, only 19 of the 100 unstable fractures regained full function: 17 of the 75 unstable fractures treated in plaster casts and two of the 25 treated by open reduction of internal fixation, most being left with some permanent flexion contracture at the P.I.P. joint. If the fracture was compound, or involved a joint or tendon, some loss of function was all but certain.[24].

Fourteen years later a review was made of all the phalangeal fractures occurring in Nottingham in a one-year period. There were 657 patients: 360 children and 297 adults, from a population of about 750 000. (These figures divided by three should give the incidence of phalangeal fractures in an average district general hospital serving 250 000 people: about 220 patients a year). These are therefore very common injuries, and James has shown that they are serious ones.

In the Nottingham series, I was able to follow up 403 patients with 454 fractures. The detailed results have been reported elsewhere.[25, 26] It is on this study, and on the published literature, that the opinions which follow are based.

Fingertip fractures

The tips of the three longest fingers, the index, middle and ring, are more exposed to injury than any other part of the body. If they are crushed, a radiograph will often show a fracture of the distal phalanx, but this should usually be ignored and the lesion treated as a soft-tissue injury. No splintage is needed and active movements of the D.I.P. joint should be encouraged from the start even, or perhaps especially, if the fracture runs proximally into that joint. A painful sub-ungual haematoma should be released by trephining with the tip of a pointed scalpel blade or by burning through it with the red-hot end of a straightened paper clip. If, as is often the case, the fracture is compound, the wound should be sutured, but the small distal fragment of bone should not be excised as this leaves a floppy ineffective finger-tip.

Smith and Rider showed that these fractures nearly always unite and the fragments seem to contract to re-form the normal contour of the finger, though this process takes five months or more.[27] Clinical recovery takes longer than one might think, tenderness preventing full use of the finger for an average of six weeks.

Epiphyseal fractures

Phalangeal fractures are especially common between the ages of ten and fifteen. This peak is due to fractures involving or close to the growth plate, which in the phalanges is at the proximal or basal end. Epiphyseal fractures are usually caused by a fall on the outstretched hand or the finger being struck by a ball.

The Salter-Harris Type 2 epiphyseal fracture is the commonest type in the hand as elsewhere.[28] This is a fracture-separation with the line of injury passing along the growth plate and then distally through the metaphysis so that a triangular metaphyseal fragment displaces with the epiphysis from the rest of the metaphysis (Fig 25.14). Another common type of fracture runs transversely through the metaphysis, a few millimetres distal to the growth plate (Fig 25.15): this is not, strictly speaking, an epiphyseal fracture but in practice can be classed with them for it is similar in incidence and prognosis to the Type 2

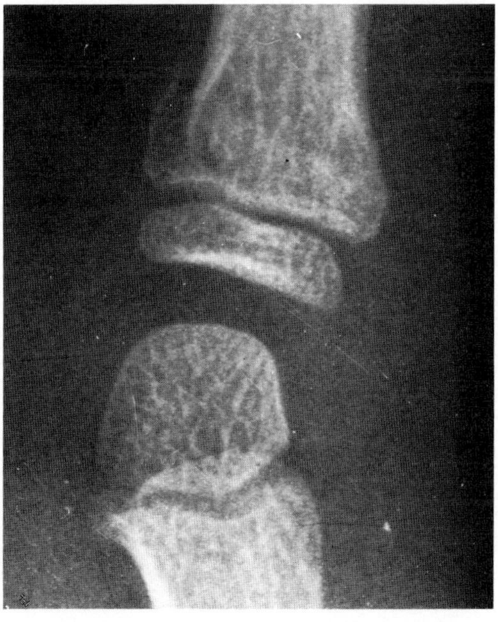

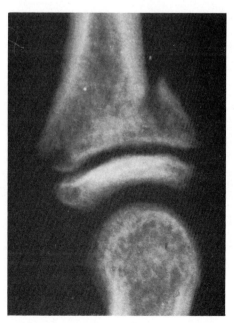

Fig 25.14 Salter-Harris Type 2 fracture-separation at the base of the proximal phalanx of the little finger. This is the commonest type of epiphyseal injury.

Fig 25.15 Metaphyseal fracture. In this type of injury, the fracture line runs across the metaphysis, close to but not involving the growth plate.

injury and it may be difficult on the original radiographs to distinguish between them. Type 2 and metaphyseal fractures both have a good prognosis because, even if the fracture is not reduced, remodelling will occur. However, if there is much displacement it seems reasonable to reduce the fracture to restore normality sooner, although in a child this usually needs a general anaesthetic. A few cases have been reported in which the fracture was irreducible due to interposition of soft tissues such as the flexor tendon, and open reduction was necessary, but this must be very rare.[29] Internal fixation is never justified in these types of fracture. If reduction is needed then retention is also needed, usually with an aluminium splint, though sometimes a child sustains similar epiphyseal fractures in two, three or four fingers simultaneously, for which plaster slabs are the best method of immobilisation.

Other types of epiphyseal fracture are rare in the hand and fortunately tend to occur in children approaching maturity who have little growth left and therefore little potential for increasing deformity.

Eighty per cent of epiphyseal fractures in the hand occur in the proximal phalanges, close to the M.P. joint, which is not a hinge but allows side-to-side movement as well. Such fractures usually re-model fully in both planes, leaving no deformity (Fig 25.16). The I.P. joints are true hinges and it seems that epiphyseal fractures in the middle and distal phalanges, which are much less common, re-model in the plane of flexion and extension but lateral and rotational deformities are not corrected (Fig 25.17). Accurate reduction is therefore necessary.

Epiphyseal fractures in the distal phalanx may displace dorsally forcing the distal fragment out through the nail-bed (Fig 25.18), as described by Seymour.[30] These are the most difficult type of epiphyseal fracture in the hand and if poorly treated result in mallet deformity and occasionally, since they are compound fractures, in chronic infection. Seymour advises that the nail should not be removed but the fracture should be openly reduced and the proximal edge of the nail replaced deep to the nail fold where it will act as a splint. In addition the D.I.P. joint should be splinted in extension (like a mallet finger) for two weeks.

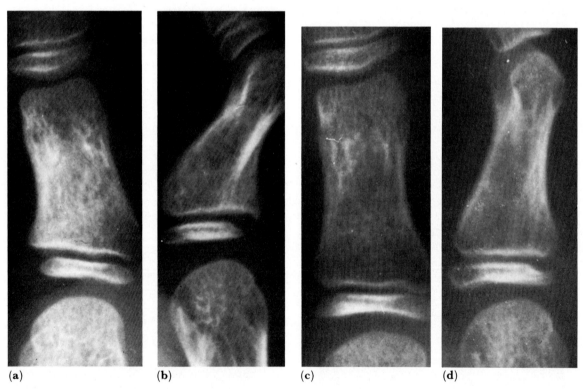

(a)   (b)   (c)   (d)

Fig 25.16 Remodelling in both planes of Salter-Harris type 2 epiphyseal fracture-separation at the base of the proximal phalanx of the thumb. (a) and (b) Three months after fracture. (c) and (d) Twenty months after fracture. (Reproduced by permission of the editor of *The Hand*.)

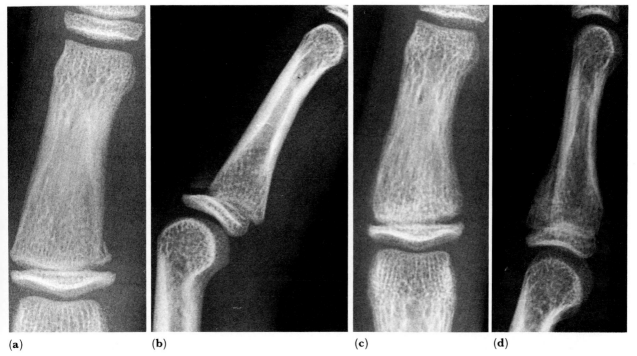

(a)   (b)   (c)   (d)

Fig 25.17 Remodelling in the sagittal but not in the coronal plane of Salter-Harris Type 2 epiphyseal fracture at the base of the middle phalanx. (a) and (b) At the time of the fracture. (c) and (d) Six months later. (Reproduced by permission of the editor of *The Hand*.)

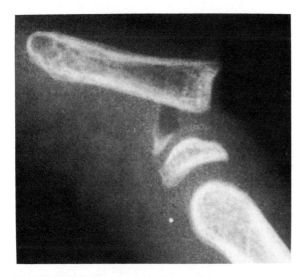

Fig 25.18 Salter-Harris Type 2 epiphyseal fracture at the base of the distal phalanx, as described by Seymour. These fractures are usually compound, the distal fragment coming out through the nail bed. Persistent deformity is common if the injury is not treated properly. (Reproduced by permission of the editor of *The Hand*.)

Shaft fractures

Patients with fractures of the shafts of the phalanges, in contrast to those with epiphyseal fractures, often do badly, with a long time off work and an unsatisfactory final result. Undisplaced shaft fractures may be regarded as stable and treated by neighbour strapping, but displaced fractures must be anatomically reduced to give the least possible disturbance of tendon function.

Spiral fractures (Fig 25.19) are produced by rotational forces and in such fractures it is particularly important to look for and correct any rotational deformity. After reduction, the fracture is usually stable and can be treated by strapping it to the neighbouring finger in such a way as to maintain the correct rotation.

Oblique fractures (Fig 25.20) are inherently unstable. It is worth trying manipulative reduction onto an aluminium splint but if, as is likely, this fails to achieve really good position then internal fixation is indicated. Stabilisation of this type of fracture is

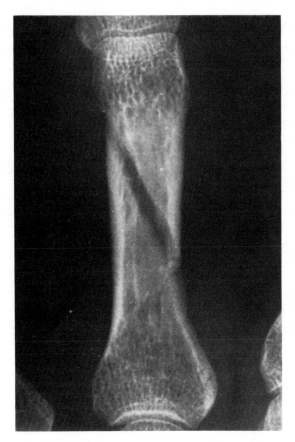

Fig 25.19 Spiral fracture of the shaft of the proximal phalanx. This is the radiograph of the patient whose hand is shown in Fig 25.5.

relatively easy using a Kirschner wire perpendicular to the fracture, but this does not give rigid fixation and three weeks of external splintage is advisable.

Transverse fractures at the base of the phalanx (Fig 25.21), unlike other types of hand fracture, often occur in elderly ladies. Coonrad and Pohlman have shown how easy it is to overlook marked angulation in these fractures, because clinically the angulation is mistaken for hyperextension at the M.P. joint and radiologically it is obscured by the other phalanges on the lateral X-ray[31] (which is the view which would show the angulation). Failure to reduce such fractures leaves an extension deformity with permanent loss of flexion, but also results in loss of extension at the I.P. joints because the extensor tendon becomes adherent: the resulting deformity looks like the clawing of an ulnar nerve lesion. This need not happen if the angulation is recognised and

reduced, and the finger splinted for three weeks with the M.P. joint flexed and the I.P. joints extended.

Transverse fractures of the mid-shaft of the phalanx (Fig 25.3) may be very severely angulated and since the anterior surface of the proximal and middle phalanges is the floor of the flexor tendon sheath, some degree of tendon adherence is almost inevitable. This would argue for internal fixation and early mobilisation, but rigid internal fixation of transverse fractures is difficult and may in itself cause tendons to adhere. It is wisest first to carry out manipulative reduction under X-ray control and apply a splint. If perfect reduction is obtained the splint is retained for three weeks (Fig 25.22).

If reduction is not perfect, then open reduction is indicated: occasionally this will give a stable reduction which can be maintained by external splintage but usually internal fixation should be carried out. The best exposure is through a dorsal lazy-S incision, splitting the extensor tendon in the mid-line.[32] Kirschner wires can be introduced either by the retrograde method or percutaneously but under direct vision. Lister uses the same approach for his intra-osseous wiring.[19] After fixation, the tendon edges are approximated with a few interrupted

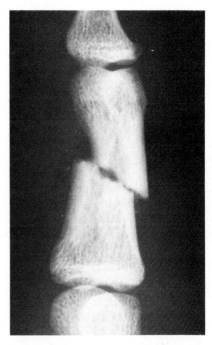

Fig 25.20 Oblique fracture of the shaft of the phalanx. These are unstable fractures. (Reproduced by permission of the editor of *The Hand.*)

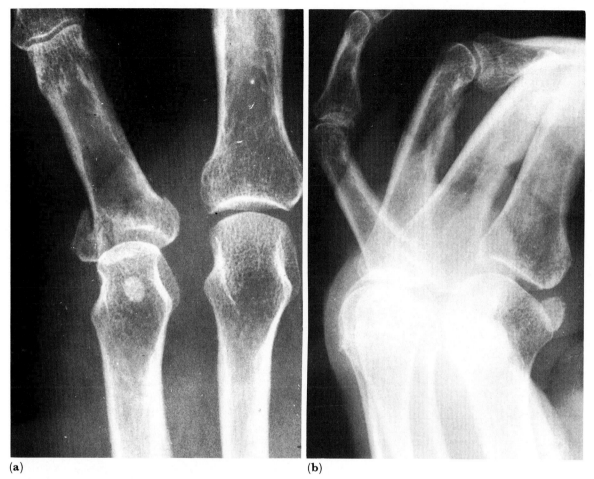

(a)　　　　　　　　　　　　　　　　　(b)

Fig 25.21 Transverse fracture of the base of the shaft of the proximal phalanx of an elderly lady who fell on her outstretched hand. (a) The anterior-posterior view showing slight abduction deformity. (b) The lateral view shows that there is some 40° of angulation concave dorsally, though this is not immediately obvious because the other fingers are superimposed. (Reproduced by permission of the editor of *The Hand*.)

sutures but immobilisation is unnecessary and, provided the internal fixation is adequate, active movements can be started next day.

Transverse fractures of the neck of the phalanx (Fig 25.23), at the other end of the phalanx from basal transverse fractures, are also at the other end of the age-group, as they occur most often in children. The tendency is to assume that growth will correct any deformity, as it does so remarkably in most children's fractures. This is an illogical assumption. There is no growth plate at the distal end of phalanges and therefore no mechanism for re-modelling: in practice *little or no re-modelling occurs after this type of fracture* (Fig 25.24) and permanent loss of

flexion may result.[33] These fractures must therefore be fully reduced, though this is difficult because of the very small size of the distal fragment. If conservative methods fail, open reduction and Kirschner wire fixation are needed: this may necessitate temporarily transfixing the joint as well as the fracture, though Leonard has described a method of fixing the fracture while leaving the joint free.[34]

Comminuted fractures

In Britain, these are commonly due to crushing injuries and are often compound, though usually stable because the periosteal sheath remains in continuity. The fracture may or may not enter a joint (Fig 25.25) but, either way, the best results are

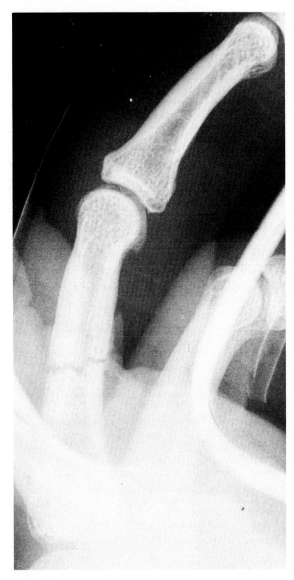

Fig 25.22 Good reduction of a transverse fracture of the midshaft of the proximal phalanx, immobilised on an aluminium splint. If the reduction is not as good as this, it is not good enough.

generally achieved by early mobilisation. This functional treatment can give surprisingly good results even in badly comminuted fractures; in fact the results are no worse than in shaft fractures which are not comminuted.

Sometimes the fracture is demonstrably unstable and splintage is required. Fractures of the thumb are often comminuted and for these immobilisation is

usually the best treatment, because in the thumb stability is as important as mobility and it is easy to apply a dorsal aluminium splint or a scaphoid type of plaster to the thumb without restricting movement of the fingers.

In children crushing injuries sometimes cause a longitudinal splitting fracture (Fig 25.26) of a type seldom seen in adults. Fortunately the split does not run into the epiphysis. These may be classified as comminuted fractures and should be treated by early mobilisation which will probably result in a normal finger.

Articular fractures

The risk of stiffness plagues all hand injuries but is likely to become endemic if the injury directly involves a joint, unless preventive measures are taken. Here, even more than with other types of fracture in the hand, it is necessary to distinguish between the many fractures which should be ignored to allow

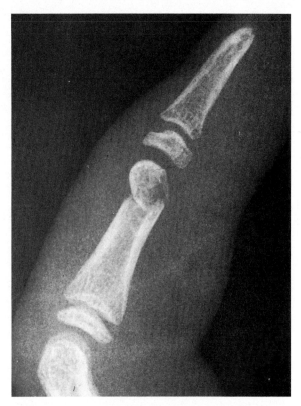

Fig 25.23 Fracture of the neck of the phalanx, an injury most often seen in children. Reduction must be achieved, because remodelling does not occur at the distal end of the phalanx, even in young children. (Reproduced by permission of the editor of *The Hand.*)

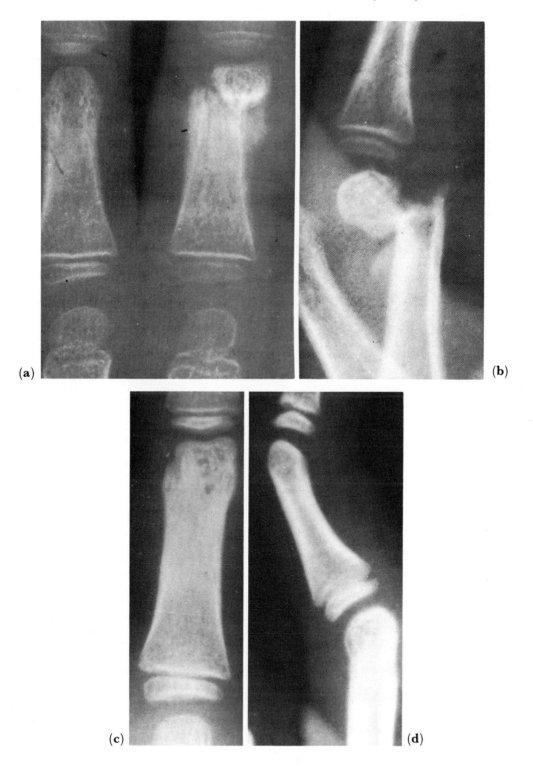

Fig 25.24 Absence of remodelling following fracture of the neck of the phalanx in a boy aged five. (a) and (b) Two weeks after the fracture. (c) and (d) Five years later. Deformity persists in both planes. (Reproduced by permission of the editor of *The Hand.*)

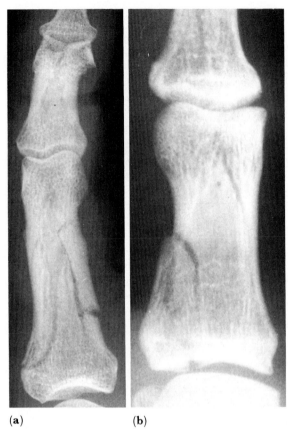

(a)   **(b)**

Fig 25.25 Comminuted fractures of proximal phalanx: (a) Not involving either joint (though there is also an articular fracture of the head of the middle phalanx, entering the D.I.P. joint). (b) Extending into M.P. joint. (Reproduced by permission of the editor of *The Hand.*)

enough for internal fixation, then it is not: trying to pass a Kirschner wire or screw across it is likely to produce several even smaller fragments and no fixation.

Subluxation of the main joint surfaces, as opposed to displacement of a small fragment of the articular surface, is not compatible with normal function of the joint, and though the resulting loss of movement may be tolerable in the D.I.P., M.P., and carpo-metacarpal joints it is never desirable and in the P.I.P. joint is never acceptable.

Steel reviewed 139 articular fractures of the phalanges of the hand to determine the types of fracture and their response to treatment.[35]

Sprain fractures. These are tiny flakes of bone pulled off by the ligament, capsule, or volar plate

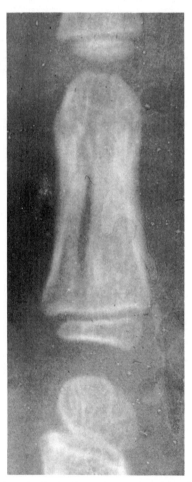

Fig 25.26 Longitudinal splitting fracture in a child whose finger has been crushed. (Reproduced by permission of the editor of *The Hand.*)

early mobilisation and the few which require some form of retention.

Classification is complicated, as so many different varieties may occur, but there are two key questions. Is the bony fragment a large one? Is the joint subluxed? If the answer to either of these questions is 'yes', the injury is a serious one and must be treated seriously. If the answer to both questions is no, the injury is probably less serious, though there are a few exceptions when a small fragment of bone is avulsed by tendon or ligament.

The distinction between large and small fragments is a practical one: a small fragment is one which is too small for internal fixation. However, this does not mean that a large fragment in which internal fixation is technically possible should necessarily be treated in that way. If you are not sure if the fragment is big

which is attached to them (Fig 25.27). They should not be called chip fractures as this suggests that they are due to an impact on the bone, which is seldom the case with these very small bony fragments, though it may be true of the slightly larger fragments discussed below.

They are best ignored as the injury is essentially to the soft tissues and should be treated as such (see below—Joint injuries). They are particularly common around the P.I.P. joint, where they may accompany dislocation: indeed they may not be noticed until the post-reduction radiograph is taken.

Provided there is no instability or subluxation, sprain fractures should be treated by early mobilisation which will usually produce a good result.

Basal fractures. *a. Undisplaced marginal fractures.* These are not a problem and should be treated by early movement.

b. Displaced marginal fractures with the possibility of joint subluxation or dislocation. These may result from an end-on blow, the base of the phalanx being split by impact on the head of its proximal neighbour, or from avulsion of the attachment of a tendon, ligament or volar plate.

Fractures of the dorsal lip of the base of the distal phalanx (Fig 25.28) are the bony equivalent of a tendinous mallet finger injury, and provided there is no subluxation, may be treated in a mallet finger

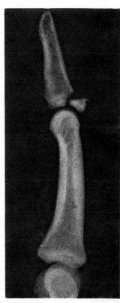

Fig 25.28 Mallet finger fracture, without subluxation. The bony fragment has been pulled off by the extensor tendon which is inserted into it. Despite the displacement, this will unite by bone.

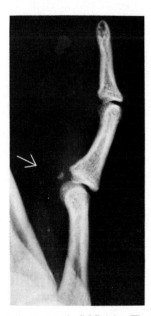

Fig 25.27 Sprain fracture at the P.I.P. joint. The flake of bone has been pulled off by the distal attachment of the strong volar plate (the thickened anterior capsule of the joint).

splint. Lee, in a valuable study of the late results of articular fractures, found that even displaced fractures of this type ultimately unite by bone with a good functional result.[36] Subluxation is uncommon, but if it is present, then a mallet finger splint makes it worse: reduction is easily achieved by manipulation, but the only satisfactory way to maintain it is by transfixing the joint in the reduced position with a wire or needle. (This was in fact the type of injury in which internal fixation was first used in the hand).[37] A rarer injury is detachment of the volar lip of the distal phalanx, which should be regarded and treated as avulsion of the insertion of the profundus tendon.[38]

Fractures of the anterior lip of the base of the middle phalanx are fairly common in the cricket season, when a ball strikes a fielder's hand on the end of one of the fingers. They are also common in Australian-rules football. They are serious injuries because they are often accompanied by subluxation (Fig 25.29). These must *not* be treated by unrestricted movements: it is essential to reduce the subluxation and keep it reduced, or the P.I.P. joint will be permanently stiff and painful. Many methods of varying complexity have been described, but the simpler ones are to be preferred. The unstable position is extension, and Dobyns' ingenious method of extension block splinting (Fig 25.30) prevents full

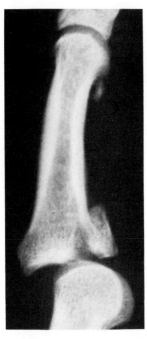

Fig 25.29 Fracture-subluxation of the P.I.P. joint in a professional cricketer who was hit on the end of the finger while trying to catch a fiercely driven cricket ball. As in Fig 25.27, there is a fracture of the anterior lip of the middle phalanx, but, far more important, in this case there is also subluxation of the main joint surfaces.

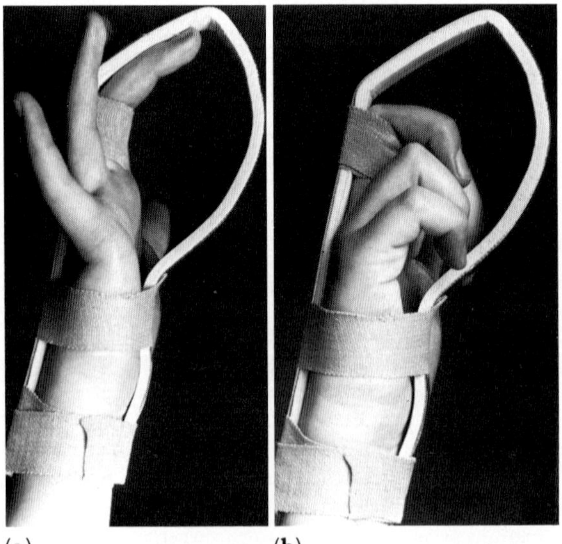

extension while allowing flexion.[39] This would seem to be the first choice, but if X-rays taken in the splint show any persistent subluxation, this should be reduced and held by a Kirschner wire transfixing the joint (Fig 25.31). The wire is introduced under X-ray control through the bare area on the dorsum of the proximal end of the middle phalanx, distal to the insertion of the central slip and between the two lateral bands of the extensor tendon. The wire is removed after three weeks and most patients regain a good range of movement surprisingly quickly.

Fractures of the base of the proximal phalanx of the fingers, involving the M.P. joint, give surprisingly good results with early active mobilisation, although a large displaced fragment may need internal fixation with a Kirschner wire or very small screw. It is necessary to incise the transverse fibres of the extensor hood to gain access to the fragment.

In the thumb, avulsion of the ulnar corner of the base of the proximal phalanx (Fig 25.32) is the bony version of rupture of the ulnar collateral ligament, both of which have been described by Stener.[40] In

(a)   (b)

Fig 25.30 Extension block splint. An aluminium splint is carefully shaped and strapped to the hand and proximal phalanx (a) to prevent extension of the P.I.P. joint (b) while allowing flexion.

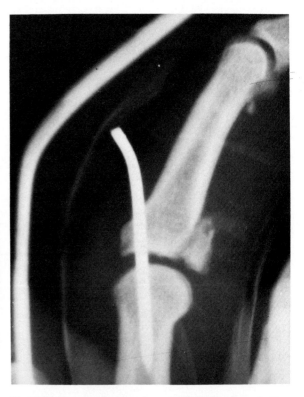

Fig 25.31 The same finger as shown in Fig 25.29, after reduction of the subluxation and percutaneous wiring to maintain the reduction. The wire was removed after three weeks, and a few weeks later the patient scored 170 runs for his county 2nd eleven.

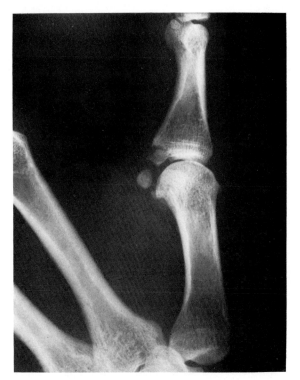

Fig 25.32 Stener fracture of the M.P. joint of the thumb. A small fragment of the base of the proximal phalanx has been pulled off by the ulnar collateral ligament which is attached to it.

London[41] classifies them into three groups:

a. Stable because the proximal part of the fracture line is transverse: these should be treated by protected activity.

b. Injuries in which the fracture line is oblique and the fracture is therefore unstable, allowing longitudinal displacement of the fragment (Fig 25.33a). These are commonest and most important in the head of the proximal phalanx involving the P.I.P. joint. Occasionally the fracture is undisplaced and may be treated by splintage, but usually there is displacement, and in few fractures is there a greater difference between the results of conservative treatment and operative treatment. I have never succeeded in controlling a displaced fracture of this type by conservative means, and have found the results of conservative treatment to be uniformly bad: the finger is not only stiff and painful but is also crooked, with lateral angulation to the side of the fracture. Accurate open reduction and internal fixation are indicated.[42] London recommends a dorsal longitudinal incision: I prefer a short mid-lateral incision over the proximal end of the fracture, but not entering the P.I.P. joint. If the proximal part of the fracture is anatomically reduced, then the distal intra-articular part should also be anatomically reduced, which is what is required. Fixation may be with one or two transverse Kirschner wires, depending on the size of the fragment, or with a very small screw (Fig 25.33b).

both, the distal end of the ligament usually comes to lie superficial to the extensor hood and therefore cannot heal properly. If the bony fragment is big enough it should be pinned back: if not, it should be excised and the distal end of the ligament reattached to the proximal phalanx.

c. Comminuted articular fractures in which the articular surface is driven into the phalanx.

Steel[35] found that the results depended largely on the degree of soft-tissue damage: in sporting injuries (usually blows on the end of the finger, with the force transmitted axially) good results were the rule, but not so if crushing was a factor. Neither rigid splinting nor operative treatment are recommended, the best management being early active exercises.

Condylar fractures. Tiny flakes avulsed from the head or neck of a phalanx can be ignored provided there is no ligamentous instability, but large fragments carrying a significant part of the articular surface require more precise treatment, especially if they involve the P.I.P. joint.

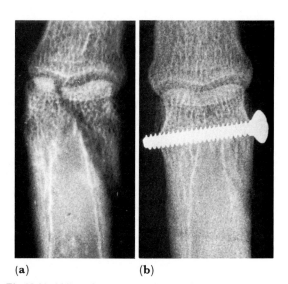

(a)　　　　　　**(b)**

Fig 25.33 Oblique fracture of the head of the proximal phalanx. (a) These are unstable fractures and allow the fractured condyle to displace proximally. (b) Accurate open reduction and internal fixation are indicated.

The operation is fiddly and difficult: the fracture surfaces need to be cleaned to allow hair-line reduction, and one must take care not to damage the soft-tissues around the joint. The fixation must be right first time, because the fragment is usually not big enough to allow a second try. The wire is cut off as short as possible. Next day the bandages are removed and active exercises started, with only a very small dressing which will not restrict movement.

Condylar fractures into the D.I.P. joint (Fig 25.25a, top) are less amenable to surgical treatment: they are often due to crushing injuries at work and the fragment is even smaller. Some stiffness and lateral angulation at the D.I.P. joint are less troublesome than in the P.I.P. joint and early active movement may be the best treatment.

c. Comminuted fractures, including T-shaped ones, have a bad prognosis and may be best treated by immediate arthrodesis or even amputation.

FRACTURES OF THE METACARPALS

Whereas Colles' fracture of the radius usually occurs in women, fractures of the metacarpals, only a few inches away, occur nine times out of ten in men. By far the most common sites of injury are the base of the first metacarpal and the neck of the fifth metacarpal, as shown in Roberts' series of 1200 fractures of the fingers and hands treated in Sir Reginald Watson Jones' fracture clinic at the Liverpool Royal Infirmary[43] (Fig 25.34).

Fractures of the first metacarpal are usually at its proximal end, fractures of the middle metacarpals in their mid-shafts, and fractures of the fifth metacarpal at its distal end.

Basal fractures of the metacarpals

Fractures at the base of the thumb. The first metacarpal is more freely moveable than the other metacarpals and is more like a phalanx (the thumb has only two actual phalanges). It is desirable to maintain this mobility, but not essential for satisfactory function of the hand: arthrodesis of the trapezio-metacarpal joint is an acceptable form of treatment for some disorders of this joint. The real need is to prevent an adduction contracture, which, if severe, can render the thumb almost useless. It is especially important to maintain *palmar* abduction, i.e. abduction in an anterior direction, as produced by abductor pollicis brevis. Radial abduction (in a lateral direction) of the thumb is not quite so important.

A patient with a fracture of the first metacarpal is likely to be off work for twice as long as a patient with

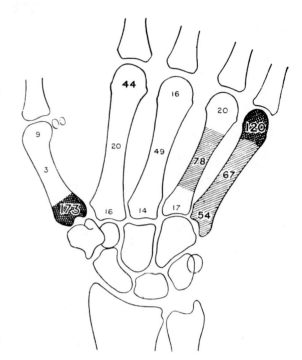

Fig 25.34 Distribution of fractures of the metacarpals, in the series of Mr. N. W. Roberts. Nowadays fractures of the neck of the fifth metacarpal are probably commoner than fractures of the base of the first metacarpal.

a fracture of one of the other metcarpals.[44] Fractures of the first metacarpal must therefore be taken seriously. They nearly always occur at the proximal end, and may or may not involve the carpometacarpal joint.

Transverse fractures across the shaft of the bone near its base but distal to the carpometacarpal joint (Fig 25.35) are the commonest type of fracture of the first metacarpal and present no great difficulty. They are often angulated into adduction, but this can be corrected by manipulative reduction. The thumb is then immobilised in a plaster cast, similar to that conventionally used for a scaphoid fracture, keeping the first metacarpal abducted. The cast should be retained for three weeks.

Bennett's fracture. In 1881 Edward Bennett, Professor of Surgery at Trinity College, Dublin, who had earlier worked in the Anatomy Department where he was able to collect many specimens of bone pathology, reported to the Dublin Pathological Society a type of fracture which he had observed in specimens of human bones, involving the base of the first metacarpal and detaching 'part of the articular

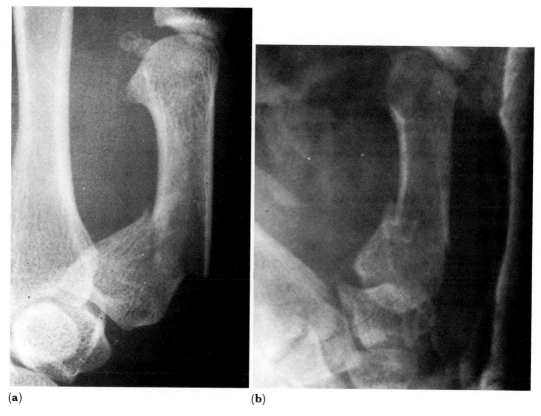

(a)   **(b)**

Fig 25.35 (a) Transverse fracture near the base of the first metacarpal, with angulation into flexion. These are twice as common as fractures entering the carpo-metacarpal joint. (b) After reduction and plaster fixation.

facette with that piece of bone supporting it which projects into the palm'.[45] He had deduced that this fracture must be accompanied by subluxation of the joint, and had later seen a patient in whom he was able to confirm this. In 1885 he published a further report in which he said that he had now 'seen a great number of examples both of the recent injury and of the united fracture. Most remarkable is the fact that in every case the accident has been on the right side of the body'.[46] This illustrates the danger of drawing conclusions from too small a series, but to his credit Bennett published a third paper to say that he had now encountered an example in the left hand. This patient was one of his medical students whose horse fell at a water-jump 'so that the point of his thumb was dashed with great violence against the pommel of the saddle'. Bennett adds, 'a year later I called on this young gentleman to amputate a limb through the hip-joint. During the operation I noticed him to wince, and asked the reason, when he said 'My left thumb never failed me until now'—a fair proof of the

long-lasting ill effects of the injury allowed to go without treatment'.[47]

The key point about this injury is that the fracture allows the base of the metacarpal to displace in a radial direction (Fig 25.36). Such injuries had been recognised before Bennett's time, but had been thought to be pure dislocations. Bennett, by correlating his clinical finding of crepitus when reducing the injury with his observations of anatomical specimens, concluded correctly that it is a fracture-dislocation or, more usually, a fracture-subluxation. He, and others following him, stated that the small fracture fragment included a volar hook of bone which normally prevents dorsal dislocation, but Gedda, in a study of 34 anatomical preparations, found that most had little or no bony hook and concluded that the real importance of the small fragment is that it carries the attachment of the strong volar ligament and that it is this ligament which normally prevents dislocation.[48] The injury is in fact analogous to the Stener fracture seen one joint distally on the same

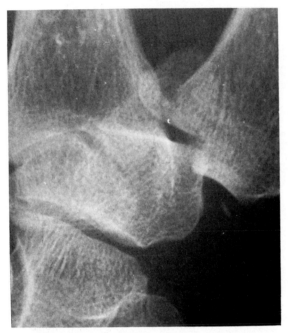

Fig 25.36 Conventional view of a Bennett's fracture-subluxation of the base of the first metacarpal. Note the subluxation of the joint, the base of the metacarpal being displaced radially in relation to the trapezium (similar in principle to the injury shown in Fig 25.29).

side of the thumb: it is a similar avulsion of the bony attachment of a ligament, though the displacement is in a different direction because of the differing attachments of muscles and ligaments.

Bennett's fracture is an uncommon injury, but has provoked a surprising number of publications, the most comprehensive being the thesis by Gedda in 1954.[48] He reviewed 105 cases treated in Moberg's department at Gothenburg in Sweden, and found that the injury usually occurred in men, between the ages of 20 and 45, and in the dominant hand (hence Bennett's original error). He also found that conventional radiographic projections often do not show how much displacement is present and recommended that the lateral view (lateral of the thumb, but approximately A.P. of the hand) should be taken with the palm of the hand downwards on the film, the hand and wrist then pronated about 20°, and the beam inclined downwards but tilted proximally about 20°. The frontal view of the thumb (lateral of the hand) is taken with the hand pronated as much as possible, so that it rests on the first and second metacarpals: the beam is aimed downwards but tilted proximally about 10°. The difference between the

radiographs obtained in this way and by conventional views is striking (Fig 25.37), and explains much of the uncertainty and confusion in the usual methods of assessment of displacement and reduction.

Conventional conservative treatment has been well described by Charnley.[1] A small pad of orthopaedic felt is placed on the extensor surface of the base of the first metacarpal and another on the flexor surface of the metacarpal head, after which a plaster cast of scaphoid type is applied and moulded by firm pressure over the two felt pads to reduce the subluxation and abduct the first metacarpal (Fig 25.38). The felt pads prevent pressure sores developing beneath the plaster where it has been impressed by the moulding fingers, It cannot be over-emphasised that this is a precise and exacting technique: merely putting on a plaster which includes the abducted thumb is useless. It is important that abduction is maintained by pressure on the head of the metacarpal, not on the thumb itself, as some people can hyperextend the M.P. joint of the thumb, so that the thumb looks extended though actually the first metacarpal is still adducted.

In 1976 Harvey and Bye showed, rather surprisingly, that reduction can also be maintained with the first metacarpal in line with the radius, in a very carefully applied and moulded plaster cast.[49] However, treatment in abduction seems preferable to minimise the risk of an adduction contracture.

In practice it is sometimes difficult to maintain reduction by plaster fixation alone, and in 1944 Johnson described a simple method of maintaining reduction by fixing the first metacarpal to the second using one or more Kirschner wires.[50] Wagner modified this, passing the wire into the trapezium, which is more logical as the wire is then at right angles to the direction of displacement, but more difficult because the entry into the metacarpal shaft must be very oblique. The subluxation is first reduced by manipulation and is held in the corrected position while, with a power drill, a stout Kirschner wire is passed into the first metacarpal and then proximally into the trapezium to maintain these bones in their correct relationship (Fig 25.39). No attempt is made to pass the wire through the small bony fragment, which is usually undisplaced, as reduction and fixation of the subluxation also reduces and holds the fracture.[51] If the wire goes rather too transversely it may enter the base of the second metacarpal instead of the trapezium, but this holds the reduction almost as well and is in fact preferred by some surgeons.

A method of open reduction of the fracture itself was devised by Moberg and is described and recommended by Gedda, but this is a more difficult

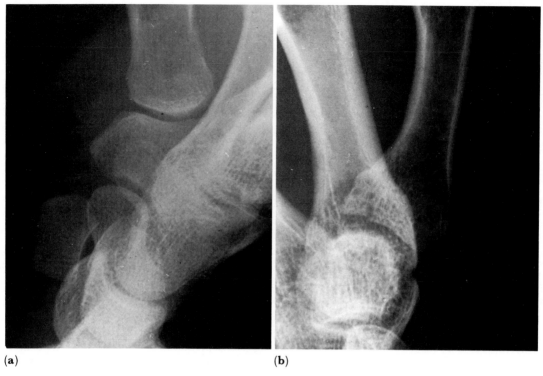

(a)   **(b)**

Fig 25.37 Gedda's radiographic projections give a much clearer view of the saddle-shaped trapezio-metacarpal joint and the displacement of the fractured fragment. (a) The antero-posterior view of the joint, in which the joint appears concave distally. (b) True lateral view of the joint, in which the joint looks concave proximally.

procedure. The argument for it is based upon the proposition that this is an intra-articular fracture and must be anatomically reduced or secondary osteoarthritis will develop. No really long-term studies of the results of Bennett's fracture are available, but of the 54 patients treated conservatively and reviewed by Gedda 1 to 14 years later (average 7 years) all were managing their work and only five were experiencing symptoms, though radiologically most cases had evidence of osteoarthritis. All the 29 patients treated

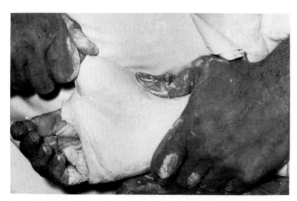

Fig 25.38 After manipulation of a Bennett's fracture-dislocation it is important to maintain the position by moulding the plaster while still maintaining traction and abduction of the thumb.

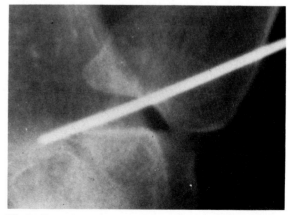

Fig 25.39 Radiograph of the Bennett's fracture shown in Fig 25.36 after reduction and percutaneous wire transfixion of the joint by Wagner's method.

by open reduction and internal fixation were working normally, and they regained function more quickly than those treated conservatively. Griffiths reviewed 38 patients from 2 to 30 years after the fracture and found that, although in many patients the fracture had not been well reduced, they had few symptoms and osteoarthritis rarely developed. There was usually some loss of movement but this caused little disability, and he concluded that 'it seems doubtful whether the use of complex methods of treatment is justifiable'. Nevertheless, those patients with undisplaced or fully reduced fractures had the best results.[52] A study of 45 patients treated in Malmo, Sweden, and reviewed 1 to 14 years later (average six years), found that a modification of Wagner's technique using two wires produced a pain-free joint in 21 out of 24 cases, the other three having only slight discomfort and being able to work normally. However, 63 per cent had radiological osteoarthritis.[53]

The satisfactory results of conservative treatment in these series is surprising, as it seems to have been poor conservative treatment. However, Pollen has shown that conservative treatment carried out with care and attention to detail, following the method described by Charnley, can achieve and maintain excellent reduction.[54]

The best programme would therefore appear to be:

1. Manipulation and plaster.
2. Check X-ray in plaster.
3. (a) If X-ray shows good reduction, maintain plaster.
   (b) If X-ray shows poor position, percutaneous pinning.
   The immobilisation should be maintained for six weeks, for if the plaster or wires are removed too soon, redisplacement may occur. There is seldom a problem in regaining movement afterwards.
4. Open reduction and fixation of the fracture itself should be reserved for those cases in which simpler methods have failed, full movements are essential for the patient, the fragment is reasonably large, and a surgeon experienced in hand surgery is available. It is also appropriate for the rare cases in which the small bony fragment is itself displaced in relation to the trapezium.

Other types of fracture at the base of the first metacarpal are uncommon. They include the epiphyseal fracture which corresponds to a Bennett's fracture (a Salter-Harris Type 3 or 4 injury) and various comminuted fractures involving the joint, such as T-shaped fractures, Rolando's Y-fracture, and Kuss' H-fracture.

Fractures at the base of the fifth metacarpal. As in the first metacarpal, these may be transverse fractures through the proximal part of the shaft of the metacarpal, or fracture-subluxations of the carpo-metacarpal joint similar to a Bennett's fracture. This second type, sometimes called an "Ulnar Bennett's fracture", has been said to give troublesome symptoms if unreduced. However, Petrie and Lamb, who reviewed 14 patients treated conservatively by unrestricted mobilisation and followed up for an average of $4\frac{1}{2}$ years, found that although most patients had radiological deformity, few had significant symptoms and none had pain increasing with time. They considered that the case for pin fixation was not strong.[55]

Fractures at the base of the second, third or fourth metacarpal. These bones, being closely attached to each other, have a more restricted range of movement. Displaced fractures of one of them are therefore unusual, but fracture-dislocations of two or three of these middle metacarpals do sometimes occur and may be overlooked if the lateral X-ray is not studied carefully.

Reduction is secured by an assistant applying traction to the fingers while the surgeon presses with the base of the thenar eminence over the back of the metacarpals against the counter-pressure of his other hand over the front of the carpus. Even a closely moulded plaster cast often fails to maintain reduction, and it is therefore better to secure the reduction when it is first achieved by running Kirschner wires obliquely through the metacarpals into the carpus. The wires may be removed after four weeks, during which a protective plaster cast should be worn.

Fractures of the shafts of the metacarpals
The only frequent disability after fracture of the shafts of the metacarpals is stiffness of the fingers from excessive immobilisation. The lateral support and fixation of the metacarpal bones by the muscles and fascial tissues between them minimises displacement and controls mobility of the fractured fragments, so that mal-union and non-union are no more frequent than in fractures of the ribs which are similarly anchored.

Spiral fractures (Fig 25.40.) Here, as in spiral fractures in other parts of the body, it is especially important to check whether there is any rotational

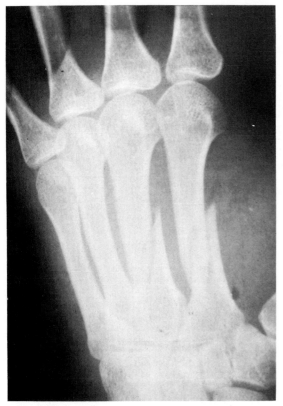

Fig 25.40 Spiral fractures of the second and third metacarpals. These fractures are stable and, provided that any rotational deformity has been corrected, they need little or no immobilisation.

deformity, by looking at the fingers end-on, If so, it can often be corrected by manipulation, after which the finger attached to the metacarpal is fastened by adhesive strapping to the neighbouring finger. The strapping must be applied in such a way as to rotate the affected finger towards its neighbour to restore correct rotation.

Very occasionally, if conservative methods fail, open reduction and internal fixation with Kirschner wires or small screws may be needed.

Transverse fractures (Fig 25.4). These are less stable and may give rise to more difficulty. There is angulation concave anteriorly but this is often concealed by swelling and may not be appreciated unless a lateral X-ray is taken and studied carefully. Radiographers do not like this view because the four metacarpals are superimposed, but no other view shows the real angulation. There may also be rotational deformity.

Angulation of up to 30° is acceptable, but if there is more than this correction should be attempted as it could cause both disability and deformity. 60 per cent of such fractures occur in the fifth metacarpal. If this is the only bone broken, then reduction can be maintained by placing adhesive felt pads on the kyphos of the fracture dorsally and on the base and head of the metacarpal anteriorly, putting 3-inch elastoplast over these around the metacarpal region and wrist, applying 3-inch plaster of Paris bandage over the elastoplast, and moulding the plaster over the felt pads to provide three-point fixation (Fig 25.41). The elastoplast sticks to the skin and the plaster sticks to the elastoplast and is thus held in place.

If this fails, reduction can be maintained by the use of transverse Kirschner wires, as described below for the treatment of metacarpal neck fractures. Plating is very seldom necessary for a fracture of a single metacarpal bone, but may be the best treatment for multiple metacarpal fractures (which are discussed below), to allow early flexion of the M.P. joints.

Fractures of metacarpal necks

Fracture of the neck of the fifth metacarpal is one of the commonest fractures in the hand and, indeed, among the commonest of all fractures. It is 'an injury which owes its origin to the disparity between an individual's pugnacity and his pugilistic technique'*: the patient is often inebriated and as a result his fist strikes awkwardly against some part of an opponent or against a wall (the less inebriated opponent having dodged the blow). The fifth metacarpal is fractured through its neck and the metacarpal head further flexed towards the palm to create a deformity with a volar concavity. Less frequently, the fracture is caused by a fall onto the clenched fist. There is often slight comminution but, surprisingly, there is seldom damage to the overlying skin. The juvenile version of this injury, a Salter-Harris Type 2 fracture, is also common.

In such patients, cosmetic aspects are of little importance: the aim of treatment is to restore full function, and especially a strong grip, as soon as possible. Treatment should be judged on the restoration of function, not on the restoration of normal bony anatomy as displayed by radiographs.

The history of treatment of these fractures shows how the pendulum of orthopaedic fashion has swung

---

*As Blum said of Bennett's fracture,[56] though in more recent European series fighting has been an uncommon cause. However, the phrase is too good to waste and can be more appropriately applied to fractures of the neck of the fifth metacarpal.

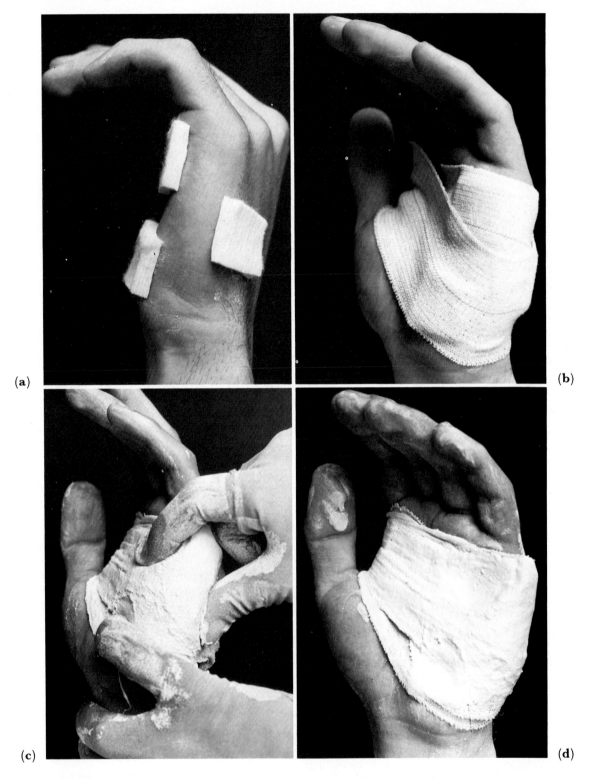

Fig 25.41 Application of hand plaster to maintain reduction of a transverse fracture of the metacarpal shaft. (The method is not intended for use on fractures of the metacarpal neck). (a) Three small pads of adhesive orthopaedic felt are applied in preparation for three-point pressure. (b) Adhesive strapping is applied to the hand, over the felt pads. (c) A three-inch plaster bandage is applied over the adhesive strapping and moulded by firm pressure over the felt pads to provide three-point fixation. (d) The completed plaster.

to and fro. For many years they were treated by bandaging over a roller bandage with the finger flexed, but no real attempt was made to reduce the fracture. In 1932 McNealy and Lichtenstein[3] recommended that the deformity be corrected by using a straight dorsal splint.* Following this, treatment in extension became common, sometimes using traction or a banjo splint, but this tended to produce extension contractures at the M.P. joint. In 1938 Jahss[57] advised reduction by flexing the M.P. joint to tighten its collateral ligaments so that the small distal metacarpal fragment was held firmly to the proximal phalanx. The P.I.P. joint was also flexed, and reduction achieved by pushing dorsally along the line of the proximal phalanx which in turn pushed the metacarpal head back into place. The finger was then immobilised in this flexed position for two and a half weeks. This ingenious method was recommended in earlier editions of this book, and it did reduce the fracture, but it transferred the problem to the P.I.P. joint which was prone to develop a flexion contracture, as Jahss himself found. For this reason, the technique is now rightly condemned.

Since any disability following these injuries is more likely to be the result of treatment than of the fracture itself, we have now reverted to the earlier practice of accepting the deformity, provided that angulation (as judged on a *lateral* radiograph) is not extreme, and concentrating on regaining a full range of movement of all the joints. It has been shown, in policemen and firemen from Philadelphia, that treatment by a simple supportive plaster slab in a functional position for ten days allows most patients to return to work in about four weeks even though they were receiving full pay while off work.[58] Angulation of less then 40 degrees was accepted: if it was more than 40 degrees an attempt was made to reduce it under local or regional anaesthesia. After ten days, the slab was removed twice a day to allow active exercises in warm water, and after two and a half weeks it was discarded completely. Many patients had residual angulation at the fracture site, sometimes as much as 70 degrees, but this did not prevent an early return to work because the mobility of the fifth carpo-metacarpal joint allows the fifth metacarpal to be dorsiflexed enough to prevent the palmar-flexed fifth metacarpal head from creating a prominence in the palm. None of the patients complained of deformity of the hand. A few had an extension lag at the P.I.P. or M.P. joint at the time they returned to work, but this corrected

*This appears, incidentally, to be the first mention in the literature of the malleable splint now so widely used: it is attributed to one Zuppinger but no reference is given.

itself with normal use and the passage of time in all but one patient. It is questionable whether even such limited immobilisation is necessary, and in Britain treatment is often even more nihilistic, consisting only of elastoplast strapping or a crepe bandage, with equally satisfactory results. The most foolish of all treatments, though regrettably it is sometimes used by inexperienced casualty officers, is a Colles type of plaster cast, which, of course, does not even include the fracture!

Less commonly, fractures of the metacarpal neck affect the *second metacarpal* which, in the clenched fist, forms the other border of the hand. Here it is more important to correct angular deformity, because the lack of mobility at the second carpo-metacarpal joint does not allow compensatory extension.[59] The simplest and safest way to maintain reduction is by a transverse Kirschner wire introduced percutaneously, a method described in simultaneous papers from the U.S. Marine Hospital[60] and the U.S. Army Medical Corps[61] in 1943, when it was necessary to get injured men back to full duties as soon as possible. Reduction is achieved by pushing the *proximal* fragment forwards, and wires then passed transversely through the fractured metacarpal and on into its intact neighbour. (It is now recommended that there should be at least one wire through each fragment.[62]) The wires are cut off subcutaneously, but removed three weeks later. No external support is needed.

This treatment may also be justified occasionally in fractures of the neck of the fifth metacarpal in patients to whom any deformity in the hand might cause real distress or difficulty.

It is hard to see any justification for the routine fixation of metacarpal neck fractures with small plates, as advocated by some surgeons.[13]

Fractures of the metacarpal heads
These are not very common, but are sometimes encountered in the border metacarpals, especially the second (Fig 25.42). Although the fracture is intra-articular, surprisingly good results are obtained by functional treatment with early active exercises. Operative treatment is not recommended, as the internal fixation must usually transgress the articular cartilage of the distal fragment.

SPECIAL TYPES OF FRACTURE

Open fractures
Open fractures in the hand may be compound from within, but are usually due to crushing injuries and therefore accompanied by more widespread damage

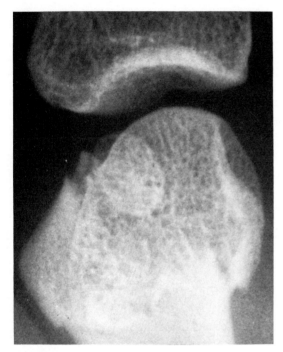

Fig 25.42 Fracture of the metacarpal head. These are commonest in the second metacarpal and should be treated by early movements.

to soft tissues than the laceration itself. Such fractures obviously carry a risk of infection and the risk of stiffness is greater.

There is little skin to spare in the hand and it is wisest not to excise the skin edges unless they are actually damaged. They must, however, be very thoroughly cleaned, especially if the hand has been crushed by dirty machinery. The surrounding intact skin should be cleaned first, with a scrubbing brush and Savlon, and the open wound then cleaned more gently with a wet swab. Solutions containing spirit should not be used on open wounds. This cleaning should be continued for five minutes by the clock.

If the wound *comes together easily*, it should be sutured: if there is the slightest tension or difficulty, it is best to leave it open for secondary suture, or to apply a split skin graft. Primary suture should also be avoided in patients who are first seen more than about twelve hours after the injury, though the acceptable delay depends upon the nature of the wound and the extent of contamination.

Splintage in the presence of soft tissue damage may present particular difficulty, and there is often a good case for internal fixation with Kirschner wires, since the fracture is exposed and visible anyway and the

risk of infection is probably little increased by such a procedure. Fixation of the bone will also protect the soft tissues from further damage and give them the best chance of healing.[63] External fixation is an alternative solution.[21]

Multiple fractures
Multiple fractures in the hand present particularly difficult problems in treatment, but have hardly been studied at all. Butt, in a review of 390 patients with hand fractures selected at random from the files of the Workmen's Compensation Board of Ontario,[64] found that 35 had multiple fractures, the distribution being: thumb 4, index 4, middle 16, ring 24, little 18.

In a retrospective review of 100 patients with multiple fractures in the hand treated in Nottingham and at Harlow Wood Orthopaedic Hospital, there were 50 injuries to the left hand, 45 to the right hand, and five injuries involving both hands; (as there were 100 patients in the series, these and subsequent figures are also percentages.) Most of the patients were young men: 55 had multiple phalangeal fractures, 31 had multiple metacarpal fractures and 14 had fractures of phalanges and metacarpals.

Of the 55 patients with multiple phalangeal fractures, 34 had fractures of two phalanges and 14 had fractured three phalanges, either in the same or different fingers. There were four patients who had fractures across the board: that is to say fractures at similar levels in all four fingers. One man fractured six phalanges in one hand, and a five year old boy on whose hand a paving-stone had fallen, sustained seven phalangeal fractures, mostly of a longitudinal splitting type, though interestingly the epiphyses were not split (Fig 25.43). The greatest number of phalangeal fractures in one patient was nine, in a man who had both hands crushed in a machine press.

Among the patients with multiple metacarpal fractures, 20 fractured only two metacarpals, often the fourth and fifth, though there were seven patients who broke three metacarpals, and four patients who broke all four finger metacarpals.

14 patients had fractures of metacarpals and phalanges: in seven there were more metacarpal than phalangeal fractures, in three more phalanges than metacarpals, and in four patients the numbers were equal.

Problems. The multiplicity of the fractures creates problems in management which do not apply to solitary fractures.

First, it is more important to get a good result. One stiff finger can be tolerated if it is not too bad, or

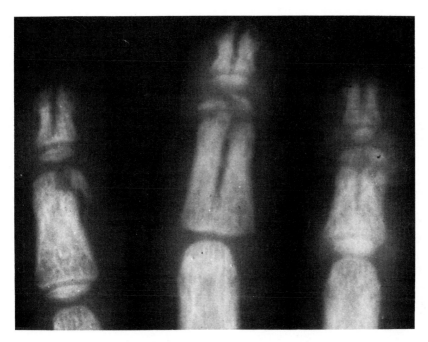

Fig 25.43 Multiple split phalanges in a boy aged five on whose hand a paving stone had fallen. There was also a similar fracture of the distal phalanx of the thumb. The epiphyses are not split, even though there are fractures of the phalanges proximal and distal to them. Note also (though the doctors who were treating him failed to do so) that the epiphysis at the base of the middle phalanx is displaced: it was in fact lying in front of the head of the proximal phalanx. (Reproduced by permission of the editor of *The Hand*.)

amputated if necessary, but two stiff fingers cause considerable disability and three or four constitute a major handicap.

Second, it is more difficult to obtain a good result: a patient with multiple metacarpal fractures has much more swelling than with a single fracture, and swelling leads to stiffness. It is therefore especially important to elevate the hand. This can be done on an out-patient basis, using a sling adjusted to keep the hand high, (Fig 25.44), but when dealing with severe hand injuries, it is best to admit the patient to hospital where the hand can be elevated more fully (Fig

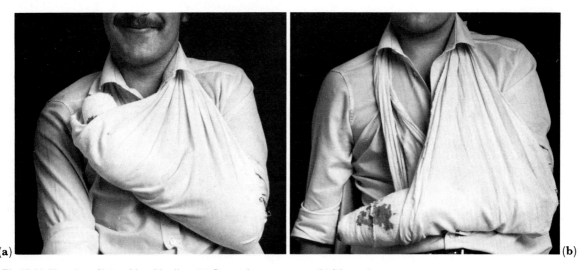

(a)   (b)

Fig 25.44 Elevation of injured hand in sling: (a) Correct but uncommon. (b) Wrong, but common.

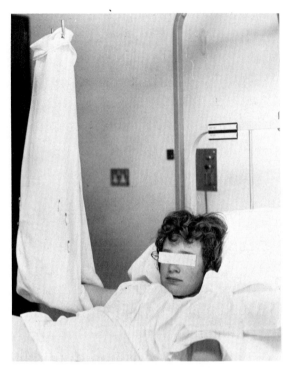

Fig 25.45 The hand can only be really effectively elevated with the patient in hospital. The hand is held up in a simple roller towel attached to a drip stand. The edge of the roller towel should be padded to avoid pressure on the ulnar nerve, though a pillow can also be used to take the weight of the upper arm.

25.45). Moreover, it is especially desirable to start movements as soon as possible, which may need internal fixation and will certainly need intensive physiotherapy many times each day, for both of which the patient must be in hospital.

Third, some of the methods used in treating a single hand fracture are inappropriate for multiple fractures, especially of the fingers. Most single-finger fractures are best treated simply by strapping the injured fingers together. If there are fractures of the middle and ring fingers, each can be strapped to an intact neighbour, and in some cases it may be satisfactory to strap three fingers together, but often it is necessary to support the hand in plaster slabs (as described on p. 745), even though this prevents early movement.

Fourth, one must conserve as much as possible. For a single badly damaged finger, immediate amputation may be the best treatment, but if several fingers are damaged one must think very carefully before amputating, not only because the disability and deformity from the loss of several fingers is greater,

but also because it may be possible to use some of the tissues from a badly damaged finger for reconstruction elsewhere in the hand, either in primary treatment or later on. Sometimes, if a digit is too badly crushed and damaged to survive, there is no choice but to amputate, but in multiple hand fractures this decision should be postponed as long as possible. However, if there are multiple fractures in one digit but the other digits are undamaged or little damaged, one should be *more* willing to consider amputation as the prognosis for function in a doubly injured finger is worse.

Multiple hand fractures differ from single ones in quality as well as quantity. Figure 25.46 shows the hand of a young man of sixteen, a keen exponent of grasstrack racing, whose car went out of control as shown in Figure 25.47. This dramatic picture shows why multiple hand fractures tend to be worse, fracture for fracture, than solitary ones: they are often due to much more violent forces. Thus the fractures are more likely to be comminuted or severely displaced and, worse still, are *often associated with soft tissue damage* which, as Green and Rowland vividly express it, 'inevitably calls forth a tremendous

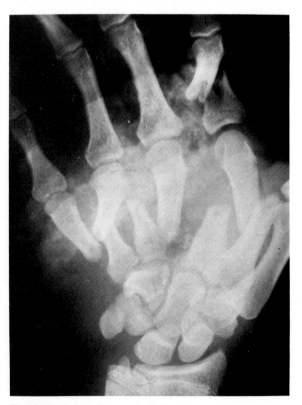

Fig 25.46 Multiple fractures in the hand.

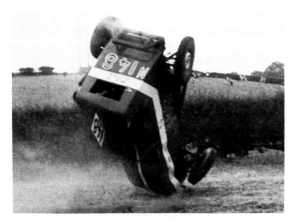

Fig 25.47 This is the accident which caused the fractures shown in Fig 25.46. The hand injury probably happened a second or two later when the car rolled over onto its side and the patient's hand, which was gripping the door frame, was crushed between the sliding car and the ground.

accumulation of oedema fluid. Tendons, ligaments, and intrinsic muscles become bathed in this protein-rich fluid, which gradually becomes transformed into tough unyielding fibrous tissue'.[65] The permanent crippling of the hand which may result is usually due more to the soft tissue damage than to the fractures, though, of course, both act together and in particular they adhere together, the soft tissues becoming stuck down at the fracture site.

When multiple hand fractures are due to high-speed accidents or violent forces, *they are often associated with other injuries*, which must not be missed and must be specifically looked for. In these circumstances the hand is not the most urgent part to treat. The first priority is to keep the patient alive and to deal with the most immediately threatening injuries, which may take a long time, so that possible internal fixation of the hand fractures may have to be deferred. However, treatment of the hand must not be delayed for more than a day or two, as it can become stiff very quickly, and it is embarrassing if, when you finally get round to reducing the hand fractures, you find that they have already united or perhaps malunited.

There may, in addition, be other injuries in the upper limb proximal to the injured hand. Just as a severe head injury may be accompanied by damage to the neck, and a fracture of the femur by dislocation of the hip, a patient who has done something really violent to his hand may also have broken his arm. You must not only look for this, but must take account of it in planning treatment; the arm injury alone could interfere with hand function and, acting in

conjunction with multiple fractures in the hand itself, can result in a really stiff hand.

Conversely, fractures in the hands may be overlooked altogether on the first assessment when more dangerous injuries dominate the situation, and patients with multiple injuries must always be re-examined from top to toe next day, to find any injuries which may have been missed at the time of admission when the patient was too ill to complain of pain or tenderness and when swelling or bruising had not yet appeared.

Those are the problems. The solutions are not so easy to define; in fact sometimes there is no entirely satisfactory solution and you just have to do the best you can.

Management of multiple fractures. The fundamental decision is whether to immobilise the hand or to mobilise it. 'Multiple displaced fractures may create marked instability of the entire hand skeleton and yet prolonged immobilisation can be disastrous.'[65]. In our series the patients fell into four groups: 32 patients were injured in crushing injuries of various types, 30 in road traffic accidents, 23 by falling onto the hand, and 15 in other ways.

Falls. It is well known that a fall on the outstretched hand can produce a variety of injuries in the upper limb, from a broken wrist to a dislocated shoulder, but one of the commonest injuries to result from a fall on the hand is a fractured finger: in fact this is much the most frequent cause of single-finger fractures. A fall may also produce multiple fractures in the hand, and it is interesting that 16 out of the 23 patients in this group had fractures at the base of the proximal phalanx. Nine were multiple epiphyseal or metaphyseal fractures in children, and the seven adult patients with multiple fractures at the bases of the proximal phalanges were all women, who seem particularly prone to this type of fracture.

In general, multiple hand fractures due to falls can be treated as though the fractures were single ones, and the problems are not too great.

Crushing injuries. Here the situation is very different. 28 out of the 32 in this series occurred at work, affecting the left hand in 17 patients, the right hand in 13 patients, and both hands in two patients. 25 had compound fractures. They were all men and none had other injuries elsewhere—that is to say these were purely hand problems in working men. The injuries varied from the trivial, such as one patient who sustained two fingertip fractures, to the very severe such as a fitter whose hand was squashed for fifteen minutes by a load of about 30 cwt. with the result that three fingers became gangrenous a few days later and had to be amputated.

In crushing injuries there is always soft-tissue damage and one should regard them, in Rank and Wakefield's classification,[66] as untidy injuries in which primary repair of the major damaged structures is contra-indicated: to put it another way, internal fixation of crushing fractures is very hazardous because the overlying skin may die even if it appeared to have survived the original injury. Moreover, the fractures are usually comminuted and satisfactory internal fixation therefore difficult. The best treatment is elevation on a volar slab with the M.D. joints flexed and the I.P. joints straight, ice-packs, and mobilization after four or five days, but retaining the volar slab between exercises for a further two or three weeks. At a later stage, say six months, it is occasionally helpful to do a tenolysis, though of course there must be good enough skin cover to allow such an operation.

Road traffic accidents. These provide some of the most difficult problems. There were 30 in this series: six in children who fell off their bicycles, 20 in motor cyclists involved in collisions, and only four in people in cars. The dominance of motor cycle accidents is not surprising since the hand is near the front of the machine, is relatively unprotected, and may crash into something at very high speed. Of the 30 patients with multiple hand fractures due to road traffic accidents, 16 had other injuries, often severe. In general, and if other circumstances permit, internal fixation of the multiple hand fractures is often the best treatment, particularly in the metacarpals. Howard says that 'the more fractures present, the greater the necessity for exact anatomical alignment. Internal fixation, therefore, becomes the method of choice'.[5]

Internal fixation of fractured phalanges, even by experts, is usually more difficult and less satisfactory than the surgeon had hoped. In dealing with multiple

Fig 25.48 Fractures of the second, third, fourth and fifth metacarpals (a) Marked ulnar deviation. (b) Treatment by skin traction with correction of deformity.

(b)

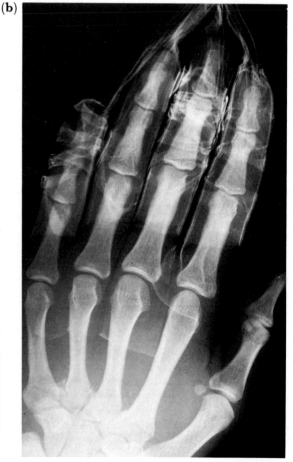

(a)

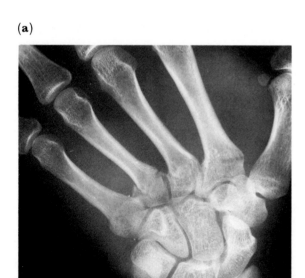

finger fractures (Fig 25.11) one must take each on its merits; operate on it if you are sure it is needed and, if in doubt, don't. With multiple displaced metacarpal fractures, however, there is a stronger case for open reduction and internal fixation. One is dealing here with a group of parallel bones forming one unit; the situation may be compared to multiple rib fractures causing an unstable segment, which must somehow be stabilised. Fractures in the proximal half of the metacarpals (Fig 25.40) can be treated conservatively, usually by means of a plaster cast, though the patient shown in Figure 25.48, a motor cyclist who fractured the bases of four metacarpals with very marked ulnar deviation deformity, was treated by skin traction on each finger which produced a much improved position. However, distal metacarpal fractures cannot be externally splinted without splinting the M.P. joint and to correct angulation, which is concave anteriorly, one would have to immobilise the M.P. joints in extension, the very position in which they are likely to become stiff, especially in multiple hand fractures. Immobilising the finger with I.P. joints flexed is, of course, even worse. However, ignoring the metacarpal fractures, and starting early movements is not satisfactory either: in the phalanges this works well but when the patient with multiple fractured metacarpals tries to flex the M.P. joints he flexes the fractures instead, which helps neither the fractures nor the joints. Conservative treatment of multiple metacarpal fractures is therefore more difficult than in the phalanges, but operative treatment is easier: the bones are bigger and they are more easily accessible without creating soft tissue damage which will result in crippling adhesions.

Longitudinal or oblique Kirschner wires are the simplest though the least rigid method of fixation. Alternatively, Kirschner wires may be passed transversely through the proximal and distal fragments and on into the next intact metacarpal.[62] Semi-circular wiring is another possibility, but when dealing with spiral fractures, very good and rigid fixation can be achieved by transverse screws. Transverse fractures of the metacarpals can only be rigidly fixed by plating: this is probably the only indication for the use of plates in treating hand fractures. Often the best solution is a combination of these methods (Fig 25.49).

Dickson applied external fixation to multiple metacarpal fractures, using transverse Kirschner wires, bonded with acrylic resin to an external longitudinal wire to create an improvised external fixator. His patient, who had fractures of the third, fourth and fifth metacarpals, was able to begin using

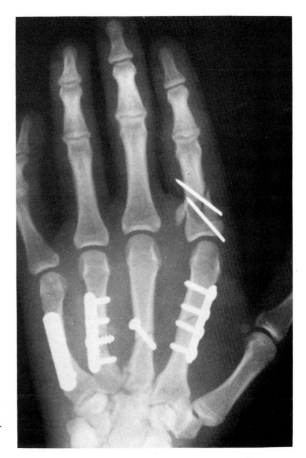

Fig 25.49 The hand shown in Fig 25.46, after open reduction and internal fixation. The third metacarpal, the only one which was not plated, developed non-union and required bone grafting.

the hand after 24 hours and regained full function in three weeks.[22]

Pathological fractures

Much the commonest pathology is an enchondroma. The frequency of these lesions is uncertain, as they may cause no symptoms and be discovered only by chance: in the hand, two out of three which present with symptoms do so because of a fracture, following injury which may be very minor.

Noble and Lamb reviewed 25 patients with fractures through enchondromata.[67] All those fractures left to heal spontaneously did so. The enchondroma did not heal but usually became smaller and less obvious on the radiograph. Surgical treatment, whether by curettage alone or by curettage and bone grafting did not help: in fact in one grafted case the fracture went on to non-union!

COMPLICATIONS OF HAND FRACTURES

The various complications of hand fractures have already been mentioned, but it may be helpful to review them briefly.

1. Stiffness

Prevention is easy, but cure difficult. Whenever possible, early movement should be encouraged, i.e. active steps taken to ensure that the movements are practised frequently in the critical early weeks. If immobilisation is essential, it must be in the correct position.

2. Infection

This is seldom a problem except when there are open wounds caused by crushing. Primary closure of such wounds is usually a mistake.

3. Mal-union

Here again, prevention is better than cure. Rotational deformities are the most common problem, because they are easily overlooked at the time of the injury when they could be easily corrected. Rotational and lateral angulatory deformities both cause the affected finger to cross over its neighbour when the fingers are flexed. This may render the injured finger almost useless and may need correction by osteotomy,[68] which is a tricky operation.

4. Delayed union

In most hand fractures, rapid clinical union is the rule, and one should not wait for radiological union, which may take months. However fractures of the middle phalanx (Fig 25.50), particularly at the junction of the middle and distal thirds, may take 10 or even 16 weeks to unite.[69] In these fractures, therefore, external splintage or internal fixation should not be removed at the usual three weeks because the fracture will probably slip. Immobilisation for a longer period may result in some stiffness of the D.I.P. joint, but fortunately this is not as great a disability as stiffness of the M.P. or P.I.P. joints.

5. Non-union

This is a rare complication. I have only seen it following attempted internal fixation (Fig 25.49). There is no entirely satisfactory solution: union can be achieved by miniature Phemister bone-grafting, but a stiff finger usually results.

JOINT INJURIES

Injuries to the soft tissues of joints require more skill in diagnosis than fractures because the lesion is not

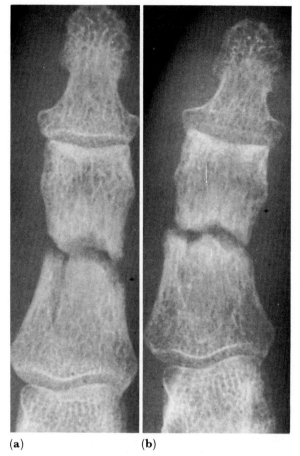

(a)   **(b)**

Fig 25.50 (a) Transverse fracture of middle phalanx. These are slow to unite. (b) Seven weeks later. There is little evidence of union, and slight angulation has developed.

evident on the radiographs, but the risk of stiffness is even greater. The key to management of these injuries is therefore a careful *clinical* assessment, based upon an understanding of the anatomy and pathology of the joint concerned.

ANATOMY

Metacarpo-phalangeal and interphalangeal joints. The three joints of the fingers are similar in their main anatomical features, although there are important differences in detail between the M.P. and the I.P. joints. The descriptions in standard text-books of anatomy are inadequate, but good accounts are available in specialist journals[70, 71] and in Eaton's excellent monograph on *Joint Injuries of the Hand* which is the most comprehensive work on this subject.[72]

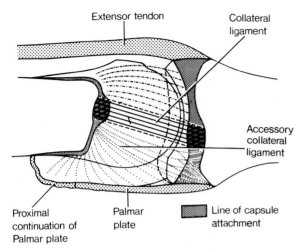

Fig 25.51 Anatomy of the proximal interphalangeal joint. The components of the lateral capsule are: (1) The dorsal portion. (2) The collateral ligament. (3) The accessory collateral ligament. (Reproduced by permission of the Editor of *The Journal of Bone and Joint Surgery*, and Dr K. Kuczynski, from his paper 'The proximal interphalangeal joint, modified. *Journal of Bone and Joint Surgery* 50-B, 656.

The two bones which form each joint are held together by capsule, which is thickened on its anterior (or palmar, or volar) aspect, and on each side to form a sort of open box (see Figs 25.51 and 25.52). The

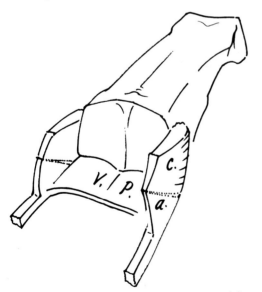

Fig 25.52 The thickened ligamentous structures around the P.I.P. joint form an open-topped box in which rests the head of the proximal phalanx. VP = volar plate. C = collateral ligament. A = accessory collateral ligament. (Reproduced by the kind permission of Dr R. G. Eaton from his monograph *Joint Injuries of the Hand*. The drawing is by Dr William Littler.)

anterior capsule is modified to form a separate and distinct structure of great importance: the volar or palmar plate, whose distal part is several millimetres thick and lined on its deep surface with fibrocartilage. Its superficial surface forms part of the floor of the fibrous sheath of the flexor tendons. Proximally the volar plate is much thinner and tapers down to a thin areolar sheet which can wrinkle up to allow flexion of the joint.

On both sides of the joint are collateral ligaments. Their distal attachment is close to the base of the distal bone, but proximally they are attached further back from the joint, on each side of the head of the proximal bone, from which the collateral ligaments swing around the head of the bone like the arms of an acrobat hanging from a bar. In the interphalangeal joints the proximal attachment of the collateral ligaments is at the axis of rotation of the joint so the tension in the ligaments remains constant throughout the range of rotation, but in the M.P. joints the ligaments are attached dorsal to the axis of rotation, creating a cam mechanism which tightens the ligaments as the joint flexes. This is why the M.P. joints allow considerable lateral movement in extension, but none in flexion, and why they must be immobilised in flexion to prevent contracture of the ligaments.

The volar plate is suspended from the collateral ligaments by thinner but important fan-shaped accessory collateral ligaments, which fill the gap between the volar plate and collateral ligaments and complete the open box in which rests the head of the proximal bone. The box is not, of course, literally open, but on the dorsal aspect of the joint is thin and elastic to allow full flexion, though it is reinforced to some extent by the insertion of the extensor tendon into the base of the distal bone. When treating injuries of these joints, you must have a clear mental picture of the ligamentous structures and must make a precise diagnosis as to which is injured. Strictly speaking, there is seldom injury to one element in isolation; for example a tear of the collateral ligament is likely to be accompanied by a tear of the accessory collateral ligament and of that side of the volar plate (in fact abnormal lateral movement is not possible unless these other structures are also damaged) but in practice there is usually one element whose injury predominates and it is this which must be defined.

Carpo-metacarpal joints. The anatomy of the carpo-metacarpal joints is different. That of the thumb allows movement in all directions, by means of saddle-shaped surfaces,[73] and its most important ligamentous thickening is on the ulnar aspect, as discussed above in connection with Bennett's fracture.[48] The bases of the second and third metacarpals interlock with the carpus and allow hardly any movement, but the carpo-metacarpal joint of the ring finger permits 15 degrees and that of the little finger 25 to 30 degrees of flexion and extension, enabling hand to be cupped when grasping a round object. The dorsal ligaments are the strongest, and in addition there are strong ligamentous attachments between the bases of adjacent metacarpals.[74]

PATHOLOGY

Injuries to the joints in the hand which involve a fracture of the articular surface have already been described. Injuries to the soft tissues alone may be grouped under four headings:

1. Contusions and cuts.
2. Sprains.
3. Complete tears of the soft tissues on one aspect of the joint:
    a. collateral ligament.
    b. volar plate.
    c. tendon.
4. Dislocation.

Contusions and cuts. The hand is more exposed to minor injury than any other part of the body, so contusions and cuts around the finger joints are very common. Contusions may be due to something falling onto the hand, to crushing injuries, or to fighting. They cause pain and swelling which may last for several weeks. The importance of cuts is that there may be damage to tendons, ligaments or nerves. Cuts over the back of the finger joints have sometimes been sustained on somebody's tooth, though the patient may conceal this, especially if the fracas was a domestic affair. Such injuries, like others due to human bites, are liable to become infected by a variety of organisms which live in the mouth (see Chapter 17).

Sprains. A lateral force may tear some of the fibres of the collateral ligament, producing pain and swelling but no instability or laxity provided that part of the ligament remains intact. In pathological terms these sprains are the least severe type of joint injury, but in clinical practice they often cause surprisingly persistent and troublesome symptoms.

Torn collateral ligaments. If the ligament is completely torn (together with the other capsular structures on that side of the joint), abnormal lateral

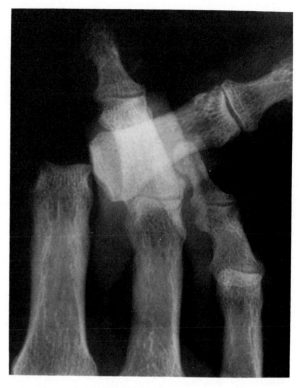

Fig 25.53 Lateral angulation of the joint tears the collateral ligament.

angulation is possible; though to look at it another way, abnormal lateral movement must occur if the collateral ligament is to be torn (Fig 25.53). This sort of injury may therefore be associated with momentary lateral subluxation or even dislocation, but the finger returns spontaneously to its normal alignment or is pulled back into a straight position by the patient or a bystander. Thus the joint is usually not dislocated at the time the doctor sees the patient, and from a practical point of view the need is to detect whether it is possible to produce again the abnormal lateral movement.

Ligaments usually tear at one end rather than in the middle. They may pull off a flake of the bone to which they are attached: such injuries, although technically fractures, should be regarded and treated as ligamentous disruptions. Occasionally the torn end of the ligament becomes turned into the joint, preventing complete reduction; conversely, at the M.P. joint of the thumb the ligament is usually displaced so that it lies superficial to the adductor aponeurosis.

An untreated complete ligamentous tear heals but

with lengthening which may cause weakness, especially if it affects the ulnar side of the thumb or the radial side of the index finger, which are pressed together in pinch-grip and depend upon the stability provided by their collateral ligaments (Fig 25.54).

Volar plate injuries. The volar plate is strong, and avulsion of its distal bony attachment is more common than a tear through the thick ligamentous substance of the plate. Fractures of this type may allow dorsal subluxation of the distal bone, but injuries to the volar plate itself can produce either of two opposite effects: the bleeding and subsequent fibrosis and contracture may cause a flexion contracture, or the volar plate may heal in a lengthened position allowing hyperextension of the joint.

Tendon injuries. Detachment of the insertion of a tendon is not really a joint injury, but mallet finger is so common and the boutonnière injury so frequently missed that they will be discussed under the appropriate joint. Flexor tendon injuries remain one of the most difficult problems in the hand, despite much research and experiments with many different methods of treatment which are beyond the scope of this book. Injured flexor tendons should if possible be treated by an experienced hand surgeon, most of whom now carry out primary tendon suture provided the wound is clean-cut and suitable conditions and equipment are available. An inexperienced surgeon

should not attempt this, as he will create internal scarring which can never be removed and will probably cause permanent limitation of movement. He should suture the skin only and refer the patient to the nearest hand surgeon as soon as possible, having arranged for passive movements to be practised in the meantime to prevent stiffening of the joints.

Dislocations. Dislocation is not a momentary event after which the joint can be restored to normality by reducing the dislocation. It implies rupture of at least one and often two of the ligamentous structures which normally hold the joint together. The skin also may be damaged: compound dislocations occur particularly in sporting injuries and around the D.I.P. joint of the fingers and the I.P. joint of the thumb, where the skin is attached to bone by fibrous septa.

In the hand the dislocation is usually in a dorsal direction (i.e. of the distal bone in relation to the proximal one) and the volar plate is torn or detached at one end. In most cases, reduction is simple, but occasionally the torn volar plate or other soft tissues become interposed between the joint surfaces and prevent reduction. These are sometimes called 'complex dislocations' or 'irreducible dislocations', but the most appropriate and accurate antonym to simple dislocation is 'difficult dislocation'. Closed manipulative reduction is impossible, but reduction can—and must—be achieved by open operation to extract the interposed soft tissues which are obstructing reduction. Anterior dislocations are less common but more likely to require open reduction.

After reduction of a dislocation, whether by closed or open methods, the joint should be tested for lateral stability. The collateral ligaments may be intact, having swung round dorsally in the same manner but the opposite direction to their normal movement in flexion. If so, reduction is stable. If one of the collateral ligaments has been torn, then testing after reduction will reveal abnormal lateral movement.

The late results of dislocations in the hand are usually good; as in the knee, they often cause less disability than injuries in which the damage is not so extensive.

Diagnosis

A careful clinical assessment is essential in all injuries of the finger joints in order to distinguish those which need immobilisation or operative treatment from those which may be treated by early movements, and in this respect the history may be helpful in determining whether the force which injured the finger was applied in a lateral direction, end-on, or in

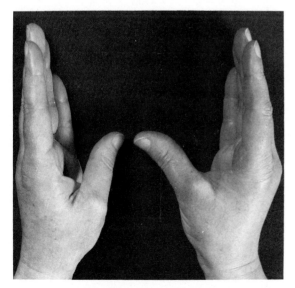

Fig 25.54 Rupture of the ulnar collateral ligament of the M.P. joint of the right thumb allowing abnormal radial deviation compared to the normal thumb.

some other way. The key points in the examination are:

1. Localisation of tenderness and swelling.
2. The test of active motion. Eaton particularly emphasises the value of getting the patient to put the joint through a full range of active movement, from *full* extension to *full* flexion.[72] If this is not possible, a significant injury must be suspected.
3. Lateral stress test. If the collateral ligament is only sprained or partly torn, stressing it will be painful but will produce little or no abnormal lateral mobility. If the collateral ligament is completely torn, lateral mobility is usually obvious, especially if compared with the corresponding joint in the uninjured hand (Fig 25.54). If in doubt, a ring block can be introduced to allow more vigorous stressing. Stress radiographs seldom add anything to what can be learned from clinical testing, and are therefore only of academic value.

It is important to remember that there may be more than one injury in the same finger, especially if the cause was an end-on blow: dislocation of two joints in the same finger has been reported. You must examine the whole finger and indeed the whole hand since there may also be an injury to another finger which is less painful and which the patient has not mentioned. For this screening, the test of active motion is especially valuable.

Radiographs should be taken to detect any associated fracture, or any slight incongruity of the joint surfaces which is the clue to soft tissue interposition. A.P. and true lateral views are essential.

After reduction of the dislocated joint, it must be tested for lateral stability, and further radiographs taken to check that a perfectly congruous reduction has been achieved.

DISTAL INTERPHALANGEAL JOINT OF FINGERS AND INTERPHALANGEAL JOINT OF THUMB

Sprains, collateral ligament injuries and volar plate injuries are uncommon at the distal joints because of the short lever arm available to produce such an injury, and because the object applying the displacing force tends to slip off the end of the finger. In contrast, crushing injuries to the distal part of the fingers and thumb are very common and may involve the periarticular tissues of the distal joint. Pain and swelling sometimes persist for several months, but early movement should be encouraged.

Mallet finger is also a very common injury. It is due

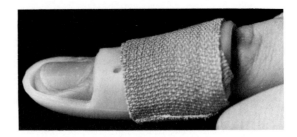

Fig 25.55 Stack type of mallet finger splint.

to a flexion force on the tip of the extended finger, classically in a housewife who is making a bed and, while trying to tuck in the bedclothes, catches the tip of her finger on some projection. Less commonly, the injury is due to a laceration on the back of the finger. The extensor tendon is torn or cut over the back of the D.I.P. joint, producing an extension lag which does not usually exceed 45 degrees because Landsmeer's retinacular ligaments are intact.[75] The patient retains full active flexion of the finger so there is little disability; the problem is essentially a cosmetic one. Surgical repair of the tendon is not indicated because it is likely to result in some loss of flexion, which is worse than the original mallet deformity. Treatment is therefore conservative and consists of splinting the D.I.P. joint for six or eight weeks uninterruptedly. This is simple in theory but not so straightforward in practice.

Various types of splint are available and it does not matter which is used provided that it maintains the D.I.P. joint in full extension and does not cause pressure on any part of the skin under the splint. The P.I.P. joint need not be immobilised. A moulded polythene splint, as designed by Stack, (Fig 25.55) is probably the most satisfactory: it is made in a variety of sizes* to fit different sized fingers.[75] If mallet-finger splints are not available, any short strip of wood or metal, suitably padded, can be used.

This condition has a bad reputation, because its treatment is often badly done. The commonest errors are:

1. Incorrect application of the splint. It may fail to prevent flexion; alternatively it may hyper-extend the joint, which is painful, unnecessary, and exsanguinates the skin on the dorsum. It is not good enough just to order a mallet finger splint to be applied: you must either apply it yourself or see the patient again to check the splint after it has been put on.

*Available from Pryor and Howard, Willow Lane, Mitcham, Surrey, England.

2. Failure to maintain uninterrupted extension of the joint. Many patients remove the splint periodically because it has become dirty or to see how the finger is getting on. If the D.I.P. joint is allowed to flex while the splint is off, all the benefit of the treatment is lost. The patient must be told not to remove the splint unless it is absolutely essential and then to hold the fingertip in extension until the splint is reapplied.

3. Splintage for too short a period. For most hand injuries immobilisation, when indicated, should not be maintained for longer than three weeks. Mallet finger is an exception to this rule and requires at least six and preferably eight weeks of splintage, and even then continue using the splint at night for another two or three weeks.

Dislocations are not common in these distal joints. When they do occur they are usually in a dorsal direction (Fig 25.56), and may be compound because the skin over the distal phalanx is tethered to bone to prevent it slipping about while the fingertip is being used to hold things: the skin may therefore be torn when the joint is dislocated. The distal phalanx is easily reduced by longitudinal traction, and is stable after reduction. Rarely, the volar plate may be interposed, requiring open reduction.[76]

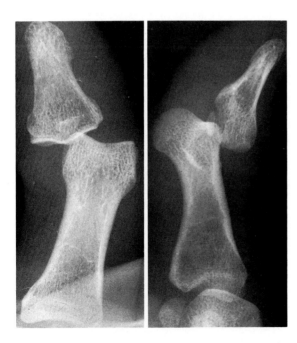

Fig 25.56 Dislocation of the I.P. joint of the thumb.

PROXIMAL INTERPHALANGEAL JOINT

Sprains. These are common and notoriously troublesome. The patient is frequently sent back to hospital by his general practitioner two or three months after the injury because, understandably, they both feel that it should be better by then. Unfortunately, it may continue to be painful for six months or more, and swollen for up to two years. At this stage, the only treatment which helps is reassurance that slow recovery is normal and that it will get better in the end. If the patient is seen soon after the injury, it may shorten the period of disability if the joint is splinted in extension for ten days.

Collateral ligament tears. These injuries occur on the radial side of the joint six times more often than on the ulnar side. Several authors have claimed, and Redler and Williams[77] have documented, good results following surgical repair. But are the results after surgery any better than after conservative treatment? Coonrad studied 43 patients treated by splintage and found a stable joint in all but two of those treated in plaster for three or four weeks, but poor results after no treatment, strapping, or splintage for less than three weeks.[78] Such experienced surgeons as Moberg[79], Milford[80] and Eaton[72] also recommend conservative treatment. In the light of this, and of the fact that operation may itself cause loss of movement at the P.I.P. joint, it seems wisest to treat such injuries by splintage for three weeks, provided that radiographs taken after reduction show *perfect* congruity of the joint surfaces. If there is any incongruity (Fig 25.57), than the joint should be explored to extract the interposed ligament, which is then sutured back in place, after which protective splintage for three weeks is still necessary.

Volar plate injuries. Most patients who suffer a hyperextension injury need neither splintage nor operation and regain fairly normal function and movements within six months.[81] In some, however, deformity develops, and it is one of the unsolved mysteries of life that extension injuries to the P.I.P. joint sometimes result in a flexion contracture and sometimes in a hyperextension deformity. There is a suggestion that avulsion of the distal end of the volar plate may be followed by hyperextension, which may in turn cause a swan-neck deformity, whereas tearing of the proximal end of the volar plate may result in a flexion deformity with secondary hyperextension of the D.I.P. joint, which has been described as the pseudo-Boutonnière injury.[42] Kaplan showed that, in

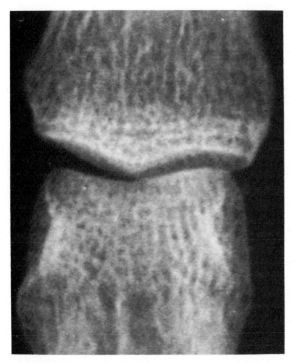

Fig 25.57 This is the radiograph taken after reduction of the injury shown in Fig 25.53. The surfaces of the P.I.P. joint are not exactly parallel: the joint appears slightly opened up on the radial side. At operation the torn end of the radial collateral ligament was found to be turned in between the joint surfaces.

normal cadavers, division of the volar plate alone does not allow significant hyperextension of the P.I.P. joint: it is necessary to cut the collateral ligaments as well.[82] It is hard to understand why the volar plate

should ever tear at its distal end, which is so much stronger than the proximal end, but undoubtedly this does sometimes happen. Very little work has been done on these injuries but it is possible that those patients who develop significant hyperextension in the joint, so that they have difficulty in actively flexing it over top dead centre, are those with a constitutional tendency towards hyperextension, as judged by examination of the corresponding joint in the other hand. Immobilisation in flexion is logical but seldom effective, and if the hyperextension proves troublesome, an operation to advance and resuture the volar plate is required and can produce an excellent result.

Boutonnière injury. Avulsion of the central slip of the extensor mechanism from its attachment to the dorsum of the base of the middle phalanx is less common and less obvious than the mallet finger injury. The central slip is not only detached from the bone distally, but is separated from the lateral bands by rupture of the fine transverse fibres which normally tether the central slip to the lateral bands (Fig 25.58). At first, active extension of the injured joint is still possible because the lateral bands still lie dorsal to the axis of movement of the joint, but as the days go by they gradually migrate forwards along the side of the P.I.P joint until they can no longer extend it. As the days pass into weeks the lateral bands move so far forwards that they become flexors of the P.I.P. joint, which prolapses dorsally between them, like a button through a buttonhole, to produce the deformity known in the English-speaking world as the boutonnière deformity but called by the French 'le button-

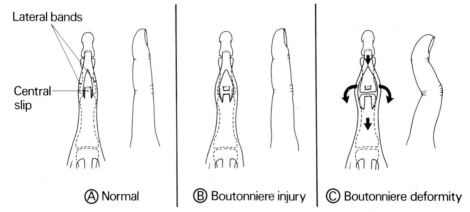

Ⓐ Normal　　Ⓑ Boutonniere injury　　Ⓒ Boutonniere deformity

Fig 25.58 (a) Normal anatomy of extensor mechanism of finger. (b) The central slip, which extends the P.I.P. joint, has been torn, as have its attachments to the lateral bands. At this stage active extension of the P.I.P. joint is still possible, by means of the lateral bands. The significance of the injury is, therefore, often overlooked. (c) The lateral bands have migrated forwards on either side of the P.I.P. joint and the whole extensor mechanism has moved proximally. The boutonnière deformity is now established, with loss of extension at the P.I.P. joint and loss of flexion at the D.I.P. joint.

hole'! In addition, the detachment of the central slip allows the whole extensor mechanism to be drawn proximally by the extensor muscles so that the D.I.P. joint becomes hyperextended and cannot be flexed fully: this may trouble the patient as much as the loss of extension at the P.I.P. joint.

If treatment is started early, satisfactory results are achieved in 75 per cent of cases by splinting the M.P. and P.I.P. joints in full extension (but leaving the D.I.P. joint free) for four weeks, after which a Capener spring splint is worn for another two weeks or more to allow some flexion of the P.I.P joint but return it to an extended position most of the time. This programme can be successful even if started several weeks after the injury, provided that full passive extension of the joint is still possible. Surgical treatment gives worse results than splintage, due to loss of flexion, and is therefore not recommended.[83]

Unfortunately, the patient (and sometimes even his doctor) does not realise that this is a potentially serious injury, and often does not seek expert advice until later, by which time a flexion contracture has developed. It is then necessary to use a dynamic splint to stretch the joint gradually back into full extension, before the programme of splintage described above can be started.

Dislocations. Dorsal dislocation of the P.I.P. joint is a fairly common injury (Fig 25.59). In experiments

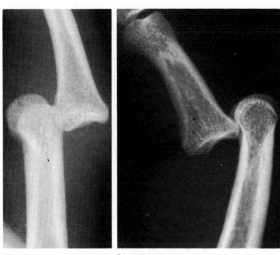

Fig 25.59   **Fig 25.60**

Fig 25.59 Dislocation of the P.I.P. joint is usually in a dorsal direction and is easily reducible.

Fig 25.60 Volar dislocation of the P.I.P. joint is less common but there may be soft tissue interposition which makes closed reduction impossible.

on cadavers it was found that a combination of extension and lateral stress is needed to produce this dislocation. The volar plate was always completely disrupted and there was always some damage to the accessory collateral ligaments. In about half the cases, both collateral ligaments remained intact; in the other half, one collateral ligament was wholly or partly disrupted, but in no case did it obstruct reduction. The central slip of the extensor tendon and the bifid insertion of flexor digitorum superficialis were never damaged.[81]

Reduction by manipulation is usually simple. It can be achieved without anaesthetic, but it is kinder to carry out a ring block first, which has the added advantage that after reduction the joint can be properly tested for lateral stability. If it is stable, no immobilisation is needed. If there is abnormal lateral movement, then the collateral ligament has been damaged and should be splinted (unless there is any clinical or radiological evidence of soft tissue interposition, in which case operation is necessary). Similarly, if the joint redislocates easily, it should be splinted in slight flexion or with an extension-block splint. In this way it should be possible to prevent recurrent dislocation of the joint.[84] A post-reduction radiograph must be taken to exclude interposition of the volar plate or other soft tissues.

Volar dislocation (Fig 25.60) is much less common and more likely to be irreducible by closed methods. The head of the proximal phalanx may button-hole between the central slip and the lateral bands of the extensor mechanism so that they grasp it around the neck and prevent reduction. In this situation open operation is needed.[85]

METACARPO-PHALANGEAL JOINT OF THE THUMB

Anatomically, this is intermediate in structure between the P.I.P. joints and the M.P. joints of the fingers. In some people the metacarpal head is well-rounded, allowing much flexion, but in others it is flatter and the range of flexion is small. Clinically, this joint is particularly exposed to injury because the thumb sticks out from the rest of the hand and the M.P. joint is where the two parts meet. In consequence, the M.P. joint of the thumb is much more often injured than those of the fingers, and dislocations of this joint are five times more common than in all four M.P. joints of the fingers put together.

Sprains. If neglected, these remain painful and interfere with grasp for many months. The M.P. joint of the thumb should therefore be immobilised in a scaphoid type of plaster cast, leaving the I.P. joint free, for four weeks.[86]

Tears of the collateral ligaments. The ulnar collateral ligament is torn ten times more often than the radial one (Fig 25.54). This injury is sometimes wrongly referred to as gamekeeper's thumb, but the condition which occurs in gamekeepers is a *gradual* stretching of the ulnar collateral ligament from repeated strains while breaking the necks of rabbits, without any specific injury.[87]

The classic account of the injury is by Stener,[88] who found that the ulnar collateral ligament is usually avulsed at its distal end, which then becomes folded back in a proximal direction. This occurs because at the time of the injury the joint is momentarily subluxed, and as it returns to a normal position the adductor expansion catches under the torn end of the ligament and pushes it back proximally (Fig 25.61). Normal healing is impossible because the adductor expansion is interposed between the ligament and its site of attachment, and open surgical repair is therefore indicated, the main purpose being to incise the adductor expansion and replace the ligament deep to it. The distal end of the ligament can be sutured to the periosteum or fastened to bone with a pull-out suture; the adductor aponeurosis is also sutured and the M.P. joint is immobilised in plaster for four weeks afterwards. (In the thumb, as opposed to the fingers, the correct position for immobilisation of the M.P. joint is in extension.) The I.P. joint should be left free for active movements.

On the Pentland Hills outside Edinburgh is an artificial ski-slope which provides ideal conditions to produce this injury: fast-moving skiers fall down and catch their thumbs in one of the holes in the openwork matting surface. A review of 50 patients treated in Edinburgh confirmed that the results of operative treatment were indeed better than those of conservative management.[86]

Tears of the radial collateral ligament, which are uncommon, heal satisfactorily with splintage, because on the radial side there is no adductor expansion to become interposed.[89]

Dislocations. Forcible extension or an impact on the end of the thumb may produce dorsal dislocation of the M.P. joint, with tearing of the volar plate. In this particular joint the position of the plate can be seen on the radiograph because the sesamoid bones are embedded in the thick distal part of the volar plate.* Adductor pollicis is inserted into the ulnar sesamoid and flexor pollicis brevis into the radial sesamoid, and these muscular attachments usually prevent the torn volar plate from being drawn into the joint, so the dislocation can usually be reduced by simple manipulation: traction should be avoided as it is thought that this can convert a simple dislocation into a difficult one.

If the dislocation proves irreducible, open reduction is necessary:[90] this can be satisfactorily achieved through a longitudinal mid-lateral incision along the distal half of the radial side of the metacarpal, with an extension medially from its distal end, running in the flexion crease at the base of thumb. The interposed volar plate which is blocking reduction is either pushed back into place with a smooth blunt elevator or pulled back with a sharp skin hook. After reduction, the joint should not be immobilised for more than a day or two as this often leads to permanent stiffness. Late cases, where the dislocation has been present for two weeks or more, do badly and are best treated by immediate arthrodesis.

METACARPO-PHALANGEAL JOINTS OF THE FINGERS

Sprains of these joints are uncommon because they are designed to allow some sideways movement.

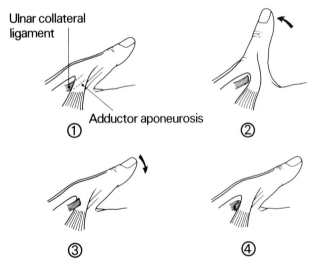

Ulnar collateral ligament

Adductor aponeurosis

① ② ③ ④

Fig 25.61 (1) Normal anatomy of the ulnar side of the M.P. joint of the thumb. (2) Forcible radial deviation of the thumb tears the ulnar collateral ligament at its distal end. (3) As the thumb returns to its normal alignment, the adductor expansion pushes the torn ligament proximally. (4) The torn ligament has been folded right back so that its torn distal end overlies its intact proximal end. In this position, the ligament cannot be expected to heal.

*Sesamoids are also sometimes seen in the volar plate of the M.P. joints of the fingers, especially the little finger.

When sprains do occur they are, like other injuries involving the M.P. joint of the fingers, less likely to produce lasting symptoms than the corresponding injury to the P.I.P. joint.

Collateral ligament tears are similarly infrequent, and can usually be treated conservatively. The least uncommon is a torn radial collateral ligament of the M.P. joint of the little finger, due to forcible abduction, and therefore corresponding to the torn ulnar collateral ligament in the thumb. In the little finger there may be damage not only to the collateral ligament, but to the radial side of the extensor hood, allowing the long extensor tendon to displace to the ulnar side and the abductor digiti minimi to draw the finger into marked ulnar deviation. Effective splintage is necessary to allow healing, and may be best done by transfixing the joint with a Kirschner wire in an over-corrected position for four weeks.[72]

Dislocations. These are much less common in the metacarpo-phalangeal joints of fingers than in the thumb and are almost confined to those on the border of the hand—the index and little finger. Dislocation is usually in a dorsal direction (Fig 25.62) and can be overlooked in a hasty examination. Radiographically, the diagnosis may also be missed, particularly in a child and if there is no good lateral view, though even the A.P. view shows an apparent narrowing of the joint space.

'Reduction by closed manipulation is either easy or impossible'.[91] It should be carried out by first hyperextending the proximal phalanx to about 90 degrees and then pushing the dorsum of the base of the phalanx distally and forwards. After reduction, stability is checked; usually the joint is stable and no immobilisation is needed.

A difficult dislocation should be suspected when the joint surfaces are widely separated, suggesting soft-tissue interposition: this occurs in 50 per cent of dislocations of the M.P. joint of the index finger. The classic paper by Kaplan[92] describes how the second metacarpal head buttonholes forwards between the lumbrical radially, the flexor tendons to the ulnar side, the superficial transverse metacarpal ligament proximally, and the torn volar plate distally. The metacarpal neck is, as Eaton strikingly describes it, 'grasped by these structures like a sphincter'. Closed reduction proves impossible and exploration is needed, as in the patient whose radiograph is shown in Figure 25.62. The key structure is the volar plate, which has been detached at its proximal end and is tightly wedged between the joint surfaces, from which

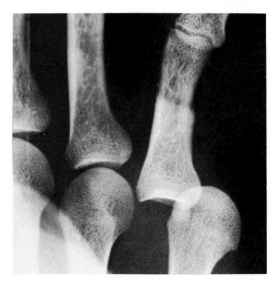

Fig 25.62 Dorsal dislocation of the M.P. joint of the index finger with button-holing of the capsule needing operative reduction.

position it must be pulled out with a fine hook. Once this has been done, reduction is easy and usually stable.[93] The joint should not be immobilised as this usually leads to permanent limitation of movement.

Locking. Most doctors are familiar with the locking of the interphalangeal joints in flexion which occurs in a trigger finger or thumb. Locking of the M.P. joint in flexion is less common and, although not really an injury, worth mentioning because it may puzzle anyone who is not familiar with it. It is seen most often in the index finger, and there are usually degenerative changes in the M.P. joint. Many different mechanisms have been described,[94] of which the most frequent seems to be that the volar plate is caught on a volar osteophyte, like a fish on a hook.[95] Alternatively the collateral ligaments, which as the M.P. joint flexes normally move anteriorly along the side of the metacarpal head, may pass over large lateral osteophytes and become stuck in the anterior position.[96] Open reduction is usually needed and should be planned to allow access to the volar plate if necessary: it is therefore preferable to approach the joint from the palmar aspect, retracting the flexor tendons, and splitting the volar plate longitudinally.

CARPO-METACARPAL JOINTS

These are infrequently injured, because the joints distal to them take most of the deforming force and thus protect the carpo-metacarpal joints, which are inherently more stable in any case. Sprains and collateral ligament injuries are therefore very rare, but sufficiently violent forces can cause dislocation. Usually this is a fracture-dislocation, but pure dislocations can occur.

Dislocation of the carpo-metacarpal joint of the thumb (Fig 25.63) is nearly always in the same direction as in a Bennett's fracture-dislocation and it is logical to treat it in the same way. If it proves impossible to achieve or maintain perfect reduction, an open surgical procedure is required. The ulnar ligament of the joint, which has been torn, is so short that direct suture is impossible, and Eaton has described a tenodesis using half of the flexor carpi radialis to replace the torn ligament.[72]

The carpo-metacarpal joint of the little finger may dislocate in a similar way, with the base of the fifth metacarpal displacing away from the other metacarpals, though in this case in an ulnar direction. Percutaneous pinning may be needed to maintain reduction. Dislocation may also occur in the other direction, the base of the fifth metacarpal being displaced radially across the palm in front of the base of the fourth metacarpal, as the result of a direct blow on the ulnar border of the hand (Fig 25.64). Bruising may conceal the deformity when the finger is

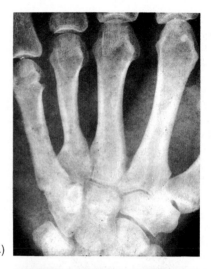

(a)

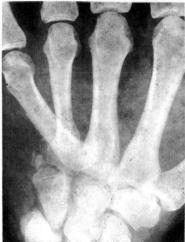

(b)

Fig 25.64 (a) Unreduced dislocation (with a tiny fracture) of the carpo-metacarpal joint of the little finger, in a policeman who had fallen on the ulnar side of the wrist seven weeks earlier. (b) After open reduction. An incision was made over the ulnar border of the hand and the displaced metacarpal pulled back into position by a hook. The operation presented no difficulty but there was such erosion of the articular surfaces that it was decided to arthrodese the joint.

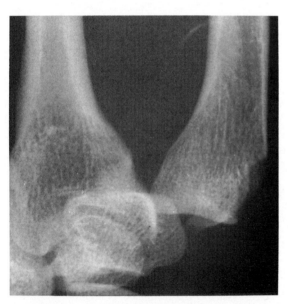

Fig 25.63 Dislocation of the carpo-metacarpal joint of the thumb, in this case accompanied by a small fracture on the radial side of the metacarpal. This contrasts with Bennett's fracture-dislocation, where the fracture is on the ulnar side (see Fig 25.36), but in both cases the displacement of the joint is in a radial direction.

extended, but if the patient is asked to bend the little finger, it flexes down towards the *distal* end of the first metacarpal instead of in the normal direction towards the tuberosity of the scaphoid. Open reduction is usually necessary.[97]

The bases of the finger metacarpals are held together by strong ligaments and may dislocate together as one unit, comprising two, three, four or even five metacarpals, usually in a dorsal direction (Fig 25.65).[98] Soft tissue swelling obscures the abnormal

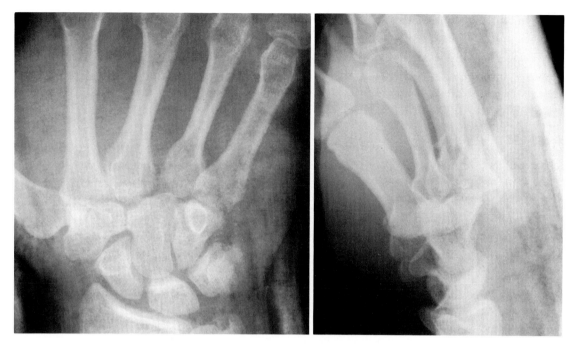

Fig 25.65 Dorsal dislocation of the second, third and fourth carpo-metacarpal joints. The displacement is best seen in the lateral view, but the overlapping of the joints is visible on the antero-posterior view. It was easily reduced by manipulation.

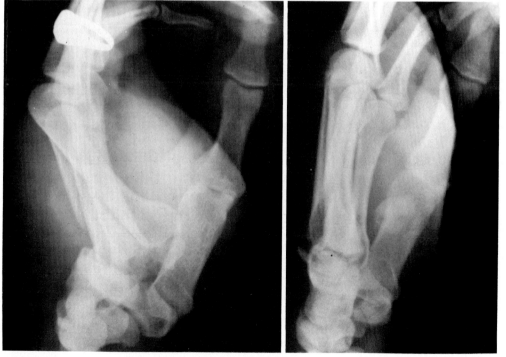

(a)   **(b)**

Fig 25.66 (a) In this unusual carpo-metacarpal dislocation, the bases of all four metacarpals were displaced forwards into the palm. (b) The displacement was reduced by manipulation by Miss Pearson at Raigmore Hospital, Inverness, Scotland. A fragment from the base of the index metacarpal remained displaced in the palm, but function was good.

bony prominence and the diagnosis may be missed if a lateral radiograph is not taken, particularly as the patient is often a motor cyclist with multiple injuries. In one such patient, who died from his other injuries, post-mortem showed longitudinal splits in the dorsal capsule of the carpo-metacarpal joints, with the soft tissues stripped back for an inch.[99] It used to be thought that reduction was unimportant, and it is true that the displacement does not cause loss of stability of the skeleton of the hand, but it does cause pain and interference with the actions of the extensor tendons, so the dislocation should be reduced. This is usually easy but unstable, and redisplacement is likely if the hand is treated in plaster: transfixion with Kirschner wires for six weeks is therefore advisable.[100]

Rarely, the bases of the metacarpals dislocate forwards into the palm (Fig 25.66) where they may compress the deep motor branch of the ulnar nerve.[101] Closed reduction is usually possible, by traction and direct pressure in the base of the palm, but wire transfixion is again advisable. The M.P. joint should be flexed to draw the extensor hood distally, and the wire introduced into the ulnar or radial side of the metacarpal head, through the recess beneath the origin of the collateral ligament, and then passed up the shaft of the metacarpal and on into the carpus. In this way the wire does not pass through the extensor tendon and early movements are possible.[100]

CONCLUSION

There are many different types of fracture and joint injury in the hand. Detailed assessment of the clinical and radiological findings and careful thought are necessary before deciding on the best method of treatment for each injury. The aim is early restoration of function; this is sometimes best achieved by anatomical reduction, and sometimes by ignoring the anatomy and concentrating on early mobilisation of the injured part. Rigid fixation is seldom helpful; rigid thinking never. The fractures most likely to produce lasting disability are those between the metacarpal head and the neck of the middle phalanx.

REFERENCES

1. Charnley J 1961 The closed treatment of common fractures, 3rd edn. Churchill-Livingstone, Edinburgh
2. Swanson A B 1970 Fractures involving the digits of the hand. Orthopaedic Clinics of North America 1 : 261
3. McNealy R W, Lichtenstein M E 1932 Fractures of the metacarpals and phalanges. Surgery, Gynecology and Obstetrics 55, 758
4. Lamphier T A 1957 Improper reduction of fractures of the proximal phalanges of fingers. American Journal of Surgery 94 : 926
5. Howard L D, Niebauer J J, Pratt J J, Brown R L (undated) Fractures of the small bones of the hand. Published privately. (Obtainable from Dr Niebauer, 516 Sutter St. San Francisco)
6. Kilbourne B C 1968 Management of complicated hand fractures. Surgical Clinics of North America 48, 201
7. Mansoor I A 1969 Fractures of the proximal phalanx of fingers: A method of reduction. Journal of Bone and Joint Surgery 51-A, 196
8. Borgeskov S 1967 Conservative therapy for fractures of the phalanges and metacarpals. Acta Chirurgica Scandinavica 133, 123
9. Wright T A 1968 Early mobilisation in fractures of the metacarpals and phalanges. Canadian Journal of Surgery 11, 491
10. Koch S L 1935 Disabilities of hand resulting from loss of joint function. Journal of the American Medical Association 104, 30
11. James J I P 1970 The assessment and management of the injured hand. The Hand 2, 97
12. Vom Saal F H 1953 Intramedullary fixation in fractures of the hand and fingers. Journal of Bone and Joint Surgery 35-A, 5
13. Robins R H C 1961 Injuries and infection of the hand. Arnold, London
14. Heim U, Pfeiffer K M 1974 Small fragment set manual: technique recommended by the A.S.I.F. group. Springer Verlag, Berlin, Heidelberg, New York
15. Green D P, Anderson J R 1973 Closed reduction and percutaneous pin fixation of fractured phalanges. Journal of Bone and Joint Surgery 55-A, 1651
16. Blalock H S, Pearce H L, Kleinert H, Kutz J 1975 An instrument designed to help reduce and percutaneously pin fractured phalanges. Journal of Bone and Joint Surgery 57-A, 792
17. Joshi B B 1976 Percutaneous internal fixation of fractures of the proximal phalanges. The Hand 8, 86
18. Fyfe I S, Mason S 1979 The mechanical stability of internal fixation of fractured phalanges. The Hand 11, 50
19. Lister G 1978 Intraosseous wiring of the digital skeleton. Journal of Hand Surgery 3, 427
20. Punch 1845 8:1
21. Crockett D J 1974 Rigid fixation of bones of the hand using K-wires bonded with acrylic resin. The Hand 6, 106
22. Dickson R A 1975 Rigid fixation of unstable metacarpal fractures using transverse K-wires bonded with acrylic resin. The Hand 7, 284
23. Wynn Parry C B 1966 Rehabilitation of the hand, 2nd edn. Butterworths, London
24. James J I P 1962 Fractures of the proximal and middle phalanges of the fingers. Acta Orthopaedica Scandinavica 32, 401
25. Barton N J 1979 Fractures of the shafts of the phalanges of the hand. The Hand 11, 119
26. Barton N J 1979 Fractures of the phalanges of the hand in children. The Hand 11, 34

27. Smith F L, Rider D L 1935 A study of the healing of one hundred conservative phalangeal fractures. Journal of Bone and Joint Surgery 17, 91

28. Salter R B, Harris W R 1963 Injuries involving the epiphyseal plate. Journal of Bone and Joint Surgery 45-A, 587

29. Von Raffler W 1964 Irreducible juxta-epiphysial fracture of a finger. Journal of Bone and Joint Surgery 46-B, 229

30. Seymour N 1966 Juxta-epiphyseal fracture of the terminal phalanx of the finger. Journal of Bone and Joint Surgery 48-B, 347

31. Coonrad R W, Pohlman M H 1969 Impacted fractures in the proximal portion of the proximal phalanx of the finger. Journal of Bone and Joint Surgery 51-A, 1291

32. Pratt D R 1959 Exposing fractures of the proximal phalanx of the finger longitudinally through the dorsal extensor apparatus. Clinical Orthopaedics 15, 22

33. Leonard M H, Dubravcik P 1970 Management of fractured fingers in the child. Clinical Orthopaedics 73, 160

34. Leonard M H 1976 Open reduction of fractures of the neck of the proximal phalanx in children. Clinical Orthopaedics 116, 176

35. Steel W M 1979 Articular fractures in the hand. Paper read to the British Society for Surgery of the Hand at Sheffield on 13 May 1978

36. Lee M L H 1963 Intra-articular and peri-articular fractures of the phalanges. Journal of Bone and Joint Surgery 45-B, 103

37. Pratt D R 1952 Internal splint for closed and open treatment of injuries of the extensor tendon at the distal joint of the finger. Journal of Bone and Joint Surgery 34-A, 785

38. Robins P R, Dobyns J H 1975 Avulsion of the insertion of the flexor digitorum profundus tendon associated with fracture of the distal phalanx: a brief review. American Academy of Orthopaedic Surgeons Symposium on Tendon Surgery in the Hand. Mosby, St. Louis, p 151

39. McElfresh E C, Dobyns J H, O'Brien E T 1972 Management of fracture-dislocation of the proximal interphalangeal joints by extension-block splinting. Journal of Bone and Joint Surgery 54-A, 1705

40. Stener B, Stener I 1969 Shearing fractures associated with rupture of ulnar collateral ligament of metacarpophalangeal joint of thumb. Injury 1, 12

41. London P S 1971 Sprains and fractures involving the interphalangeal joints. The Hand 3, 155

42. McCue F C, Honner R, Johnson M C, Gieck J H 1970 Athletic injuries of the proximal interphalangeal joint requiring surgical treatment. Journal of Bone and Joint Surgery 52-A, 937

43. Roberts N 1938 Fractures of the phalanges of the hand and metacarpals. Proceedings of the Royal Society of Medicine 31, 793

44. Goodwill C J, Bridges P K, Gardner D C 1969 The causes and costs of absence from work after injury. Annals of Physical Medicine 10, 180

45. Bennett E H 1882 Dublin Journal of Medical Science 73: 72. Quoted in part in Rang M 1966 Anthology of orthopaedics. Livingstone, Edinburgh

46. Bennett E H 1885 Injuries of the skeleton: value of accumulation of specimens. British Medical Journal, 199

47. Bennett E H 1886 On fracture of the metacarpal bone of the thumb. British Medical Journal, 12

48. Gedda K O 1954 Studies of Bennett's fracture: anatomy, roentgenology and therapy. Acta Chirurgica Scandinavica, Supplementum 193

49. Harvey F J, Bye W D 1976 Bennett's fracture. The Hand 8, 48

50. Johnson E C 1944 Fracture of the base of the thumb. A new method of fixation. Journal of the American Medical Association 126, 27

51. Wagner C J 1950 Method of treatment of Bennett's fracture-dislocation. American Journal of Surgery 80, 230

52. Griffiths J C 1964 Fractures at the base of the first metacarpal bone. Journal of Bone and Joint Surgery 46-B, 712

53. Salgeback S, Eiken O, Carstam N, Ohlsson N M 1971 A study of Bennett's fracture—special reference to percutaneous pinning. Scandinavian Journal of Plastic and Reconstructive Surgery 5, 142

54. Pollen A G 1968 The conservative treatment of Bennett's fracture-subluxation of the thumb metacarpal. Journal of Bone and Joint Surgery 50-B, 91

55. Petrie P W R, Lamb D W 1974 Fracture-subluxation of base of fifth metacarpal. The Hand 6, 82

56. Blum L 1941 The treatment of Bennett's fracture-dislocation of the first metacarpal bone. Journal of Bone and Joint Surgery 23, 578

57. Jahss S A 1938 Fractures of the metacarpals: a new method of reduction and immobilisation. Journal of Bone and Joint Surgery 20, 178

58. Hunter J W, Cowen N J 1970 Fifth metacarpal fractures in a compensation clinic population. Journal of Bone and Joint Surgery 52-A, 1159

59. Holst-Nielsen F 1976 Subcapital fractures of the four ulnar metacarpal bones. The Hand 8, 290

60. Waugh R L, Ferrazzano G P 1943 Fractures of the metacarpals exclusive of the thumb. A new method of treatment. American Journal of Surgery 59, 186

61. Berkman E F, Miles G H 1943 Internal fixation of metacarpal fractures exclusive of the thumb. Journal of Bone and Joint Surgery 25, 816

62. Lamb D W, Abernethy P A, Raine P A M 1973 Unstable fractures of the metacarpals. A method of treatment by transverse wire fixation to intact metacarpals. The Hand 5, 43

63. London P S 1964 Open fractures in the hand. Postgraduate Medical Journal 40, 253

64. Butt W D 1962 Fractures of the hand. Canadian Medical Association Journal 86, 731, 775 and 815

65. Green D P, Rowland S A 1975 Fractures and dislocations in the hand. In: Rockwood L A, Green D P (eds) Fractures. Lippincott, Philadelphia and Toronto

66. Rank B K, Wakefield A R, Hueston J T 1968 Surgery of repair as applied to hand injuries 3rd edn. Livingstone, Edinburgh

67. Noble J, Lamb D W 1974 Enchondromata of bones of the hand. A review of 40 cases. The Hand 6, 275

68. Campbell Reid D A 1974 Corrective osteotomy in the hand. The Hand 6, 50

69. Moberg E 1950 The use of traction treatment for fractures of phalanges and metacarpals. Acta Chirurgica Scandinavica 99, 341

70. Kuczynski K 1968 The proximal interphalangeal joint. Anatomy and causes of stiffness in the fingers. Journal of Bone and Joint Surgery 50-B, 656

71. Wise K S 1975 The anatomy of the metacarpo-phalangeal joints, with observations of the aetiology of ulnar drift. Journal of Bone and Joint Surgery 57-B, 485

72. Eaton R G 1971 Joint injuries of the hand. Thomas, Springfield, Illinois
73. Kuczynski K 1975 The thumb and the saddle. The Hand 7, 120
74. Harwin S F, Fox J M, Sedlin E D 1975 Volar dislocation of the bases of the second and third metacarpals. Journal of Bone and Joint Surgery 57-A, 849
75. Stack H G 1969 Mallet finger. The Hand 1, 83
76. Palmer A K, Linscheid R L 1977 Irreducible dorsal dislocation of the distal interphalangeal joint of the finger. Journal of Hand Surgery 2, 406
77. Redler I, Williams J T 1967 Rupture of a collateral ligament of the proximal interphalangeal joint of the fingers. Journal of Bone and Joint Surgery 49-A, 322
78. Coonrad R W 1970 In the discussion after the paper by McCue et al. Journal of Bone and Joint Surgery 52-A, 956
79. Moberg E 1960 Fractures and ligamentous injuries of the thumb and fingers. Surgical Clinics of North America 40, 297
80. Milford L W 1968 Retaining ligaments of the digits of the hand. W. B. Saunders Co, Philadelphia
81. Benke G D, Stableforth P G 1979 Injuries of the proximal interphalangeal joint of the fingers. The Hand 11 : 263–268
82. Kaplan E B 1936 Extension deformities of the proximal interphalangeal joints of the fingers. An anatomical study. Journal of Bone and Joint Surgery 18, 781
83. Souter W A 1967 The Boutonnière deformity. Journal of Bone and Joint Surgery 49-B, 710
84. Palmer A K, Linscheid R L 1978 Chronic recurrent dislocation of the proximal interphalangeal joint of the finger. Journal of Hand Surgery 3, 95
85. Murakami Y 1974 Irreducible volar dislocation of the proximal interphalangeal joint of the finger. The Hand 6, 87
86. Lamb D W, Abernethy P J, Fragiadakis E 1971 Injuries of the metacarpophalangeal joint of the thumb. The Hand 3, 164
87. Campbell C S 1955 Gamekeeper's thumb. Journal of Bone and Joint Surgery 37-B, 148

88. Stener B 1962 Displacement of the ruptured ulnar collateral ligament of the metacarpo-phalangeal joint of the thumb. Journal of Bone and Joint Surgery 44-B, 869
89. Coonrad R W, Goldner J L 1968 A study of the pathological findings and treatment in soft-tissue injury of the thumb metacarpo-phalangeal joint. Journal of Bone and Joint Surgery 50-A, 439
90. MacLaughlin H L 1965 Complex 'locked' dislocations of the metacarpophalangeal joints. Journal of Trauma 5, 683
91. Robins R H C 1971 Injuries of the metacarpo-phalangeal joints. The Hand 3, 159
92. Kaplan E B 1957 Dorsal dislocation of the metacarpo-phalangeal joint of the index finger. Journal of Bone and Joint Surgery 39-A, 1081
93. Green D P, Terry G C 1973 Complex dislocation of the metacarpo-phalangeal joint. Journal of Bone and Joint Surgery 55-A, 1480
94. Dibbell D G, Field J H 1967 Locking metacarpal phalangeal joint. Plastic and Reconstructive Surgery 40, 562
95. Goodfellow J W, Weaver J P A 1961 Locking of the metacarpo-phalangeal joints. Journal of Bone and Joint Surgery 43-B, 772
96. Aston J N 1960 Locked middle finger. Journal of Bone and Joint Surgery 42-B, 75
97. Ker H R 1955 Dislocation of the fifth carpo-metacarpal joint. Journal of Bone and Joint Surgery 37-B, 254
98. Waugh R L, Yancey A G 1948 Carpo-metacarpal dislocations. Journal of Bone and Joint Surgery 30-A, 397
99. Shephard E, Solomon D J 1960 Carpo-metacarpal dislocation. Report of four cases. Journal of Bone and Joint Surgery 42-B, 772
100. Kleinman W B, Grantham S A 1978 Multiple volar carpo-metacarpal joint dislocation. Journal of Hand Surgery 3, 377
101. Gore D R 1971 Carpo-metacarpal dislocation producing compression of the deep branch of the ulnar nerve. Journal of Bone and Joint Surgery 53-A, 1387

26

Injuries of the Spine

Sir George Bedbrook

Surgical anatomy

The articulation between two vertebral bodies has immense strength and depends on the interbody synarthrosis and the posterior ligamentous complex consisting of the ligamentum nuchae, the interspinous ligaments and the capsules of the articular facets. Such capsular ligaments are continuous with the single tent shaped ligamentum nuchae at each space. The synarthrosis is formed by the disc which has two parts, the annulus fibrosus and the nucleus pulposus. The fibres of the annulus fibrosus are criss-cross in a number of directions to make an immensely strong articulation. Posterior to the spinal canal, articulation occurs between adjacent vertebrae by ordinary synovial articular facet joints which have the usual structure of any other synovial joint, whilst between the laminae there is the ligamentum flavum. This is also a remarkably strong elastic ligament, capable of stretching with a surprising degree of tensile strength which, however, is reduced by age. Stability of this articulation is therefore only interfered with when major trauma occurs. In the cervical spine the articulation is similar with the exception of the atlas and axis where special arrangements suffice.

In the thoracic spine stability is increased by the rib cage which forms a protective splint to this part of the spine unless there are fractures both anteriorly in the manubrio-sternal area as well as in the spine posteriorly (see Figs 26.22 and 26.23), and in high thoracic fractures the sternum is regularly buckled or fractured. Thoracic fractures can also be associated with symptoms caused by mediastinal haematoma in conjunction with both the respiratory tract and oesophagus. These symptoms of dysphagia, substernal pain and tracheal irritation should be regularly looked for. Therefore, stability in the cervical and lumbar spine is not so great as in the thoracic spine.

In the cervical region the lateral articulations are small, flat and face upwards and backwards in the lower vertebrae, whilst downwards and forwards in the upper so that the postero-lateral joint consists of two small flat oval surfaces at an oblique angle, whilst in the coronal plane the upper articular facet lies in front and above the lower.

In the thoracic spine the postero-lateral facet still lies in the coronal plane whilst the line of the joint is more vertical than in the cervical. The articular surfaces face almost directly antero-posteriorly.

In the lumbar spine the facets are large and strong, those of the upper vertebrae now point directly laterally and have a marked convex curve, those of the lower vertebrae point directly medially and have a synchronising concave curve. Thus the postero-lateral joints in the lumbar spine embrace one another; the spinous processes here are large and heavy and the posterior ligament is extremely strong re-inforced by powerful muscles.

The stability of the spine is a matter of great importance when considering the fractures which may occur. It is true to say that if all of the anterior structures, that is the longitudinal ligament and the disc plus one of the posterior structures are ruptured, then clinical instability is inevitable. Vice-a-versa if all of the posterior structures are damaged plus one of the anterior structures then again instability can occur. In many fractures however, e.g. the flexion/rotation injuries, the anterior longitudinal ligament often remains intact and thus will act as a stabiliser once the fracture has been properly clinically reduced.

SOFT TISSUE AND JOINT INJURIES WITHOUT BONE INJURIES

The intervertebral disc, the intervertebral canal, facet joint and interspinous ligaments must be considered as a mobile complex joint (Fig 26.1).[1] Injuries of such can lead to severe and sometimes permanent handicap without gross physical characteristics; such are commonly seen in motor vehicle,

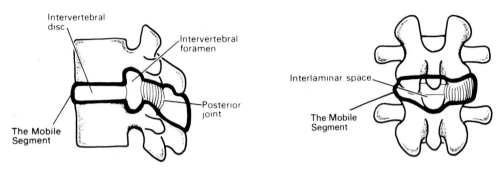

Fig 26.1 The mobile segment. (From: Macnab, I., (1977) *Backache.* Courtesy of The Williams and Wilkins Co., Baltimore)

sports and particularly compensatable accidents. These are much more common than bony injuries and cause much morbidity both emotional and physical. It is impossible to consider such injuries without considering the psychosomatic as well as the physical.

Together with such major factors it must be regularly recognised that pain from such injuries will not always be local but referred to distant structures via neural pathways.

Degenerative changes commonly seen radiologically in the lower cervical and lumbar spine add to the difficulties of diagnosis. The etiology of such changes may be chemical or hormonal whilst the importance of stress or trauma cannot be excluded.[2] In cases clinically aggravated by trauma there is no doubt that radiologically permanent aggravation occasionally follows but clinically this also follows in the emotionally unstable group as defined by Macnab.[1] Experimental models produced by Farfan[2] now help us to understand that macroscopic changes do

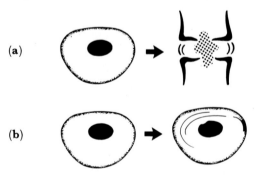

Fig 26.2 (a) Compression failure is due to fracture of the endplates and leads to the formation of Schmorl's nodes. Loss of internal support from annulus may increase its susceptibility to injury. (b) Torsional strains result in peripheral annular separations and distortions of the peripheral annulus at point of maximum stress. (From: Farfan, H. F. (1973) *Mechanical Disorders of the Low Back*—Courtesy of Lea & Febiger, Philadelphia)

occur confirming the early studies of Harris in Toronto.[3] For example, Farfan's experimental models in compression studies include appearances of Schmorl's nodes close to end plate fractures (Fig 26.2).

The mobile segment in the experimental models stood up to torsional rotational forces poorly and such may be an initial cause of degenerative changes.[2] The normal capacity for such to be without effect is apparently only within a range of 5 degrees.

Most accidents or even incidents are a combination of a number of forces, bending, torsion and compression. As we know in more severe injuries bending and torsion acting together are by far the worst combination (Fig 26.3).

Extension is a force to avoid if possible as it may damage not only ligamentous structures but also the osteochondral surfaces of the facet articulations particularly if:

1. rotation or torsion is added.
2. if asymmetrical loads are used, or
3. when asymmetrical boney articulations exist.

The smaller the number of such articulations, e.g. in the lumbar spine with only four vertebrae, the greater the possibility of that spine being subjected to injury.

The rectus abdominis and oblique abdominal muscles have an important role in preventing and minimising such stresses and thus a great role in therapy.

Injury or indeed incident to the mobile segments of the vertebral column occur very commonly indeed, particularly in the mobile areas of lower cervical, lumbo-dorsal and lumbo-sacral. In dealing with such conditions the surgeon must remember not only the stress itself but the pre-existing normal or abnormal conditions such as degenerative changes, fused segments congenitally, 'abnormal' congenital articula-

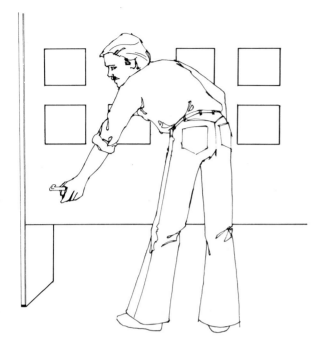

Fig 26.3 Asymmetric loading applying bending and torsion simultaneously. A male or female with a 50 lb load 10 inches from the midline may generate torque sufficient to cause injury. (From: Farfan, H F. (1973) *Mechanical Disorders of the Low Back.* Courtesy of Lea & Febiger, Philadelphia.)

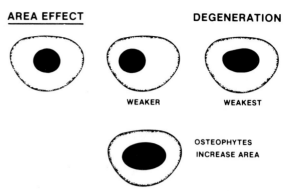

Fig 26.4 The transverse sectional area of the annulus, particularly its outermost 25%, is very important for torque strength. (From: Farfan, H. F. (1973) *Mechanical Disorders of the Low Back.* Courtesy of Lea & Febiger, Philadelphia.)

tions and abnormal areas of spine fixation after surgery (Figs 26.4 and 5).

The conditions associated with injury and encountered clinically may be one or even more of the following:

1. Ligamentous strains—the sprung back of Newman—true strains are seen in young people with a good prognosis; like other stresses of ligamentous tissues re-use before healing prolongs the condition[1] (Fig 26.6).
2. Minor fractures of osteophytes can be easily missed unless looked for particularly in those who have had 'unstable' backs for some time.[3]
3. Osteochondral injuries of the articular facets may lead to locking episodes or unexplained facet syndromes after torsion-extension stress, in work accidents. Whilst not difficult to view in mortuary specimens such are not easy to diagnose.
4. Adhesions or fringes within the articular facets with pedunculated loose bodies can occur as Harris

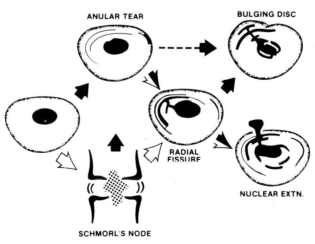

Fig 26.5 The natural history of the degenerative process towards the two surgical 'end points'. Schmorl's Node and Nuclear Extrusion (Ext.[n]). Solid and open arrows denote respectively torsion and compression strains. (From: Farfan, H.F. (1973) *Mechanical Disorders of the Low Back.* Courtesy of Lea & Febiger, Philadelphia.)

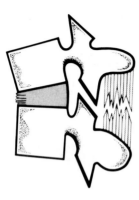

Fig 26.6 Diagram illustrating ligamentous tear. (From: Macnab, I (1977) *Backache.* Courtesy of The Williams and Wilkins Co, Baltimore.)

and Macnab[3] showed. They, like similar conditions elsewhere, have more pain at the end of the day with spinal instability.

5. Subluxations, joint play or dysfunction as Mennel[4] described (Fig 26.7) can occur after incident or injury with a similar syndrome of pain as in (4) above and occasional radiological evidence in stress films. Rarely the sacro-iliac joint may show such dysfunction but should be searched for.

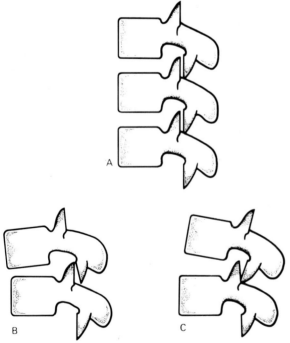

Fig 26.7 Facet subluxations associated with disc changes due to degenerative disease. (From: Macnab, I. (1977) *Backache.* Courtesy of The Williams and Wilkins Co., Baltimore.)

6. To all of these we must add muscle strain, minor or moderate. When the strain heals spasm of reflex origin may replace it.

7. Rarely in the early stages will there be intervertebral canal radiculopathy with dermatome pain. Any of many pathological states occurring in tissues around the intervertebral canal can give rise to similar symptoms particularly when there are pre-existing pathological changes in facets, pedicle or disc.

8. Rarely, but definitely, a well documented stress will cause pre-existing disc bulges to extrude disc material causing the acute disc prolapse so well known. This condition has received more emphasis in trying to explain back pain after stress than its occurrence deserves (Fig 26.5).

ACCELERATION, DE-ACCELERATION INJURY OF THE CERVICAL SPINE OR WHIPLASH INJURY

This is a very common injury caused usually by rear end collisions where muscles have no chance of preventing damage and occurring in all age groups. Its pathology varies from a muscle strain only to fracture dislocation of extension origin with tetraplegia usually in the cervical column (see Fig 27.1b); it rarely affects the lumbo-dorsal column.

The pathology includes—from minor to major changes.

1. Anterior longitudinal ligament strain continuing to rupture at single or multiple levels.
2. Disc disruption at the epiphyseal plate.
3. Minor posterior longitudinal strain.
4. Varying degress of extradural haemorrhage.
5. Posterior joint strain or osteochondral damage.
6. Fracture of spinous processes.
7. Occasionally petechial haemorrhages in the spinal cord.

These soft tissue or articular injuries of the cervical spine need early rest and isometric activities—without physical therapy—mobilisation should be slow and very well supervised. Late in management discography is valuable with myelography to localise the major movement segment involved. Fusion of single or even double levels is valuable; fusion of more than two levels does not give good relief whilst pre-existing disc degeneration makes treatment difficult. Collars, gentle mobility, analgesics and antirheumatic drugs are also to be used.

GENERAL MANAGEMENT OF SOFT TISSUE LESIONS

There is no doubt that most of these lesions in either cervico-dorsal or lumbo-sacral spine and even in the degenerative spine heal, but the healing may leave extra anxiety symptoms. Inflammation proceeds to scar which reduces elasticity of the disc or mobility of the joint. The area remains at risk, 'normal' healing proceeds by scar, osteophytosis, contracture and/or ligamentous thickening, all of which processes are proportional to the original stress. Joint dysfunction[4] may then result—although instability is rarely established. Most of the healing processes are completed within six weeks.

Psychological factors

To all of these processes we must add the emotional-pre-existing and following. We can prevent some of these by early explanation, others can be reduced by ensuring income maintenance at survival levels at least. The problems that occur when social security swamps the individual are many, for motivation and natural challenge are lost causing 'neurosis' and long term handicap without great physical disability.

Physical examination

Patients deserve careful interrogation; history taking must be perfect so that the amount of stress and its type be determined.

Physical examination must be detailed; accurately the level of the damage must be determined and the effect on the mobile segment noted. Local detailed palpation (repeated if needed) will determine the level and the tissue which is affected. Local anaesthetic for diagnostic purposes can help pin point ligament, joint or muscle. X-ray will exclude gross bony trauma so that a physical diagnosis can be made accurate to detail; a strained back is not sufficient. Full and detailed diagnosis together with a prognosis must be given to patient.

Management

Treatment depends on the lesion. In general, early rest in good posture with isometric muscle activity, heat and analgesics. When pain eases then mobilisation with increasing isometric activity within the limit of pain. Manipulations do not usually help in the first weeks in fact, will help make some conditions worse.

As mobility increases physically graded rehabilitation should be used in suitable areas for increasing periods of time. War-time lessons need relearning in this group, where early class activities and graded physical restoration gave better results.

If lesions diagnosed as strains, muscle tears, joint strains have not been fully relieved at six weeks—a new history and examination is required to detect further conditions which may be arising.

1. Emotional instability.
2. Joint dysfunction and locking.
3. Adhesions and joint scarring giving night pain.
4. Further disc protrusion or disc bulging

Such late manifestations may need only a few days of manipulation, as in joint dysfunction but rarely surgery. As the disc narrows further irritative or compression signs may arise. After all definitive physical care has been used psychotherapy could be needed to assist the emotionally unstable; back education classes as detailed by Hall in Toronto (consisting of four classes to include lectures on anatomy, psychology, physical activity and examples) will help to give better results. Epidural local anaesthetics and depomedrol facet injections have a place whilst skin and epidural stimulators of varying types may occasionally be used in chronic unremitting pain.

Of most importance, however, is further rehabilitative effort either vocational, social or educational.

Morbidity can be reduced by early admission to orthopaedic services with special expertise. Long delays, legal argument, high compensation rates, poor diagnostic efforts and treatment are common factors in delaying or preventing full medical recovery whilst inadequate explanation and advice to patients can cause much morbidity.

BONY INJURIES OF THE SPINAL COLUMN

Pathology of fractures and fracture dislocations of the spine. Fractures and fracture dislocations are now being experienced from a large number of causes, but generally they break up into the following groups:

1. Sports injuries.
2. Industrial injuries.
3. Motor vehicle injuries.
4. Occasional domestic injuries.

It matters not which of these causes is aetiological except perhaps in relationship to income maintenance for the problems of pathology remain similar physically (but not socio-economically and emotionally).

Pathologically the fractures and fracture-dislocations of the vertebral column can be described in a number of ways.[5] A simple classification is:

1. The simple forced flexion with slight compression of the vertebral body (Figs 26.8 and 26.9).
2. Flexion and rotational injury disrupting the posterior longitudinal ligaments (Fig 26.10).
3. The violent vertical compression injury (Fig 26.11).
4. The hyperextension or retro-flexion injury (Fig 26.12).

The flexion injury or flexion/compression injury

These occur most commonly as the result of forced flexion of the spine when the individual is least prepared for it or least able to resist it, e.g. in coal-mining accidents or ejection injuries of motor vehicle trauma.

If the posterior ligament complex remains intact then the violence is expended on the vertebral bodies so that one or more of the bodies are forced into their own substance, producing a wedge-like deformity of the anterior halves. The anterior vertical depth is reduced by up to a half but the posterior vertical depth remains unchanged. This type of fracture can occur in any region below C.2. It is particularly common in the thoracic spine (Fig 26.9). In normal persons it is caused by a force which must be considerable. In association with osteoporosis this is a common fracture and is produced by very little force. Since the articular processes and posterior ligaments

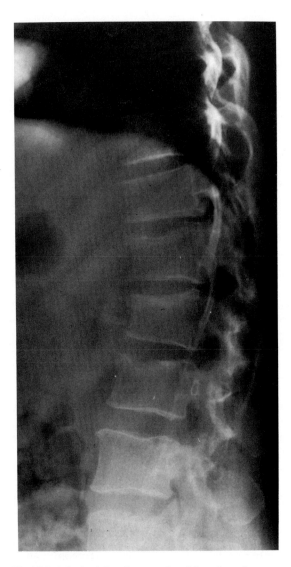

Fig 26.9 A flexion injury has caused wedging of vertebrae T_{12}–L_2. This injury is stable.

are intact the injury is stable. Further displacement will not occur unless the spine is subjected to greater violence than that which caused the fracture.

Flexion and rotation injuries (Figs 26.13, 26.14, 26.15, 26.16 and 26.20)

In the cervical spine these are caused by a blow to the back or side of the head as in a car accident when the head strikes the roof or side of the car. In the thoracic and lumbar spine the cause may be a fall from a height on to heels, buttocks or shoulders (Fig 26.15).

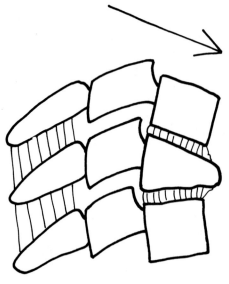

Fig 26.8 Flexion injury causing wedging of vertebral body.

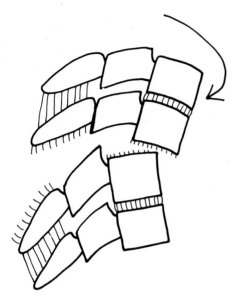

Fig 26.10 Flexion-rotational injury causing tearing of posterior ligaments and intervertebral joint dislocation. (Note: Intact anterior ligament).

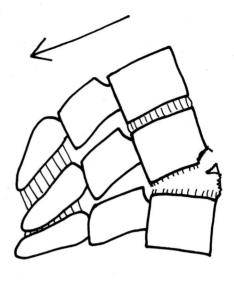

Fig 26.12 Extension injury with rupture of anterior intervertebral ligament and disc substance.

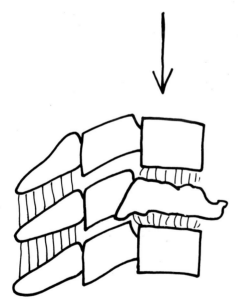

Fig 26.11 Compression injury.

The spine is flexed and twisted on impact. Sometimes the cause may be impact from a heavy object falling across the back of the trunk.

In this group of injuries the first structure to break is the ligament between the spinous processes. The posterior joints are disrupted so that the vertebrae may be dislocated—visible on first X-ray. (see Fig 26.20) It may be a pure dislocation or one associated with fracture of the articular facets and adjacent laminae. Joint disruption may be unilateral (Fig 26.16) or bilateral (Fig 26.20).[6] The vertebral bodies cannot be compressed because there is no fulcrum for the lever. The dislocation is by a rotatory movement and as the upper vertebral body slides round and forwards over the lower one, it may take with it a slice off the upper surface of the lower vertebra (Fig 26.14).

Spinal fracture dislocations can therefore be divided into: Type I, Unilateral facet dislocation (Figs 26.16 to 26.19); and Type II, bilateral facet dislocation (Figs 26.20 and 26.21). Whilst in the latter instability is inherent, in the former some stability is present because the injury retains a hinge on the intact side. Therefore Type II, fractures are usually well stabilised six weeks after adequate reduction.

Pathological anatomy. The pattern of these two types of injury vary in the different regions. In the cervical region the forces required to disrupt the posterior joints are lower than elsewhere but pure dislocations are uncommon. As already stated the dislocation may be unilateral or bilateral. When the dislocation is unilateral the lateral radiograph will show only a minor degree of forward displacement of the upper vertebral body (Figs 26.16 to 26.19). The explanation is simple. The injury is a rotatory one and a lateral radiograph does not demonstrate rotation, though a

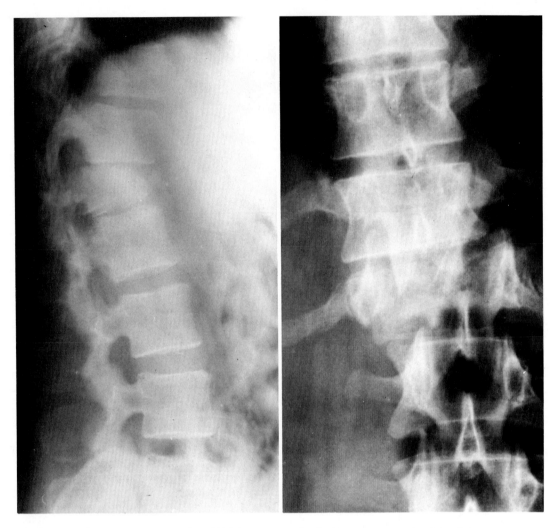

Fig 26.13 Rotational fracture dislocation T_{11}–T_{12}. This injury was associated with permanent cord and root damage.

correctly centred antero-posterior film will show the spinous process rotated (Fig 26.17). In an anatomical specimen it is possible to demonstrate that with one facet completely locked and the other one in normal position the maximal forward displacement of a vertebral body is not more than one-third of the antero-posterior diameter of the body and the spinal canal area (and capacity) is not seriously reduced. If the forward displacement of the vertebral body is more than one half then both posterior joints are involved (Figs 26.20 and 26.21) and the canal area (and capacity) is considerably reduced. In the thoracic spine this injury is uncommon because the thoracic cage provides some stability. However, when

it does occur it is associated with fractured articular facets, gross displacement of vertebral body, fractured ribs and severe spinal cord damage because the cord canal ratio is low. (Figs 26.22 and 26.23).

The thoraco-lumbar junction is the most common site for a fracture-dislocation. It is (in 96 per cent of all injuries) at this level that a slicing injury of the lower vertebral body is common. This injury is commonly associated with serious cord and nerve root damage. Pure dislocation is very uncommon in the lumbar spine (Figs 26.24 and 26.25).

Common pathological features of the flexion and rotation injuries include a paravertebral haematoma, gross muscle damage, extra dural mediastinal and

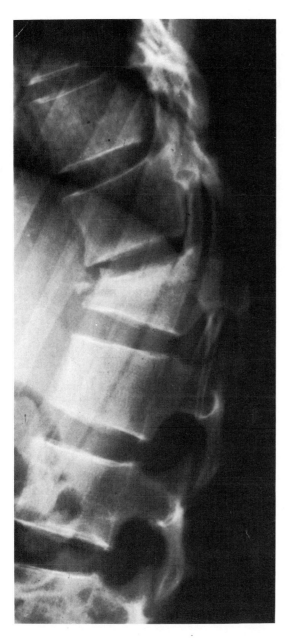

Fig 26.14 Acute flexion injury to T.12 with marked wedging of the vertebral bodies.

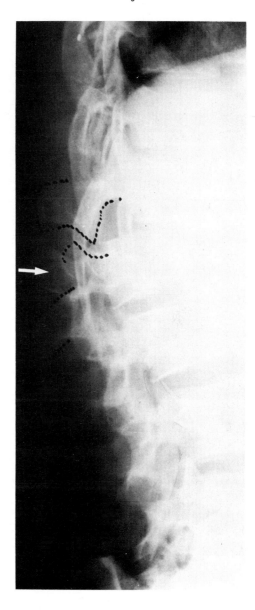

Fig 26.15 A special radiograph is required to demonstrate the separation of the spinous processes and posterior joint dislocation. This is important as it indicates that this injury is not stable.

extra peritoneal haematomatas, all of which will heal with scar but which may even in the non paraplegic injuries result in dural adherence and dural pain (see Chapter 27).

Axial compression injuries (Figs 26.26 and 26.27)

These result from a force delivered either from above,

such as one from diving into a swimming pool and striking the vertex of the head on the bottom, or from below, such as from a fall on to the buttocks. The force causes an injury to the section of the spine that can be held quite straight, namely the cervical or lumbar regions. One vertebra is shattered by the force and squashed in all directions. In the cervical region forward protrusion of bone fragments can be

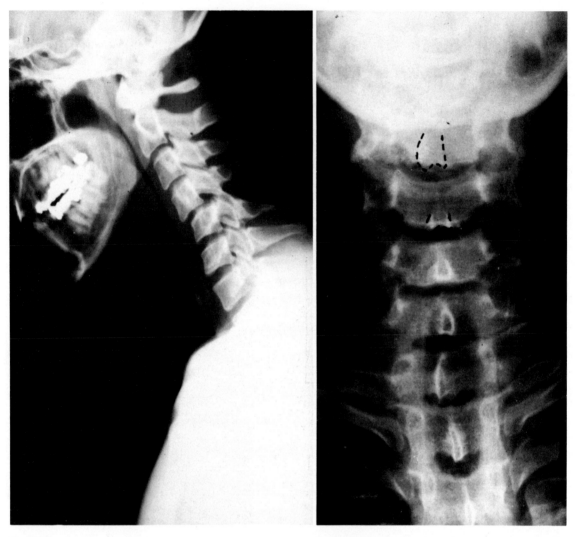

Fig 26.16   Fig 26.17

a cause of transient dysphagia, while at any level backward protrusion may cause cord or root contusion with oedema. Sagittal and coronal fractures are common at two levels. The anterior and posterior ligaments are not involved so that the fracture is stable. Cord damage in lumbo-dorsal injuries is usually incomplete, but in cervicodorsal injuries is often complete due to cord compression, cord buckling and distortion.

Hyperextension injuries[7]
These injuries were thought to be uncommon but this

is not so. They are common in the cervical spine (26 per cent of the total) and are seen occasionally in the lumbar region. In road accidents the neck can be dangerously hyper-extended during sudden rapid forward acceleration of the body, or by the head striking the car roof or windscreen when the injury leaves a tell-tale abrasion on the forehead. Another common source of these injuries is a fall headlong downstairs, particularly by elderly persons stumbling at night to find the bathroom (see Fig 27.1b).

There is a variable degree of stretching of the muscles and soft tissue in the front of the neck, but the main effect is on the anterior longitudinal ligament,

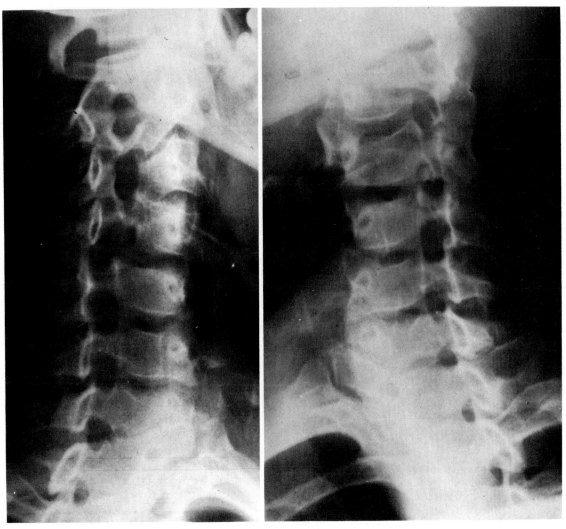

Fig 26.18   **Fig 26.19**

Figs 26.16 to 26.19 Unilateral rotatory dislocation of cervical spine. Fig 26.16: Flexion rotation dislocation with slight forward body displacement. Fig 26.17: Antero-posterior radiograph shows spinous process of C.4 is out of line with C.5. This suggests that one pair of facets only are dislocated. Figs 26.18 and 26.19: Oblique radiographs show that the right side facets are locked in dislocated position (Fig 26.18). Those on the left side are normal (Fig 26.19).

which is stretched. In the presence of cervical spondylosis and disc degeneration one disc can be torn open by the force of extension, allowing two vertebral bodies to separate to such an extent that there can be extensive damage to the cord. Then the vertebral bodies snap back into position and the only radiological sign of injury is a tiny avulsed osteophyte from the front of one of the vertebral bodies. This indicates the level of rupture of the anterior longitu-

dinal ligament (Fig 26.28 and 27.1b). If the anterior ligament does not rupture the extension force may cause fractures of laminae and spinous processes, or tear open a vertebral body.[7] Spinal cord damage is not uncommon in the presence of degenerative changes. It is very uncommon in their absence. In these injuries the posterior ligament complex is always intact. They are stable injuries in all usual positions of head, neck or trunk.

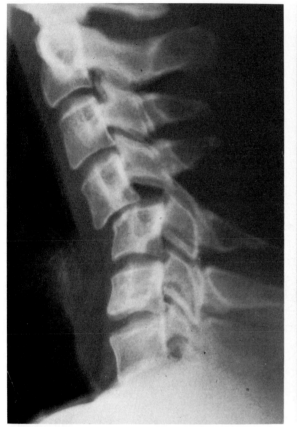

Fig 26.20

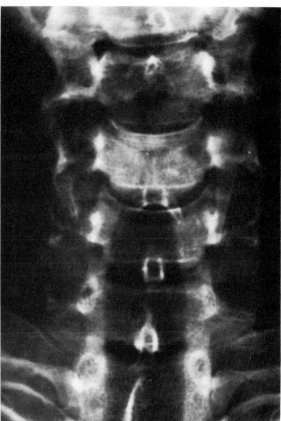

Fig 26.21

Figs 26.20 and 26.21 Complete dislocation of cervical spine. Fig 26.20: Flexion rotation dislocation with half forward body displacement indicating instability of both right and left facet joints. Fig 26.21: Antero-posterior radiograph shows spinous processes are in line.

Chance's fracture (Figs 26.29 and 26.30). This fracture has appeared in modern injuries of the spinal column usually lumbar injuries, associated with lap seat belts.[8] It is possible that Chance's fractures may be a pure tension injury rather than having any horizontal shear for the characteristics of such a fracture are:

1. Longitudinal separation of disrupted posterior elements—bony or ligamentous.
2. A minimum decrease in anterior-vertical height of the involved vertebral body.
3. Little or no forward displacement.
4. Usually occurring in the first and third lumbar vertebrae.

Most of these injuries have been recorded as being associated with seat belt injuries. The displacement posteriorly varies from being minor to being quite disruptive and may occur as a bony injury or a major ligamentous injury at the disc space (Figs 26.29 and 26.30). As the injuries retain the anterior longitudinal ligament and at least part of the disc, even in the major motion segment injuries, they are basically stable, and hyperextension will usually bring them into a satisfactory position, if necessary under deep analgesia. Some surgeons advise internal fixation of such injuries but this is generally unnecessary. Although a few of these injuries may be associated with paraplegia, it must be remembered that without seat belts most people sustaining this type of fractured spine would probably have not survived the severity of the collision responsible for such severe trauma.

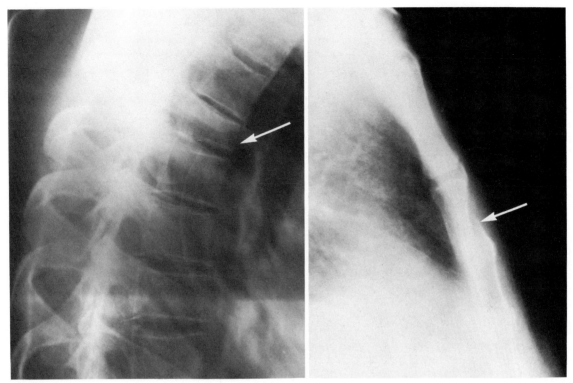

Fig 26.22

Fig 26.23

Fig 26.22 and 26.23 A compression fracture of an upper thoracic vertebral body (Fig 26.22) is not uncommonly associated with a buckle fracture of the sternum (Fig 26.23).

FRACTURES OF TRANSVERSE AND SPINOUS PROCESSES

Fractures of the transverse processes and of the spinous processes may be individual injuries and therefore trivial but they may be associated with any of the other fractures and fracture dislocations of the spine as the forces extend further than was originally thought.

Fractures of the lumbar transverse processes (Fig 26.31). These can be associated with severe flexion rotation injuries or compression injuries but are usually caused by sudden contraction of the quadratus lumborum muscle against resistance which causes avulsion of its insertion into the transverse processes, rather the same as when the pull of the quadriceps muscle against body resistance fractures the patella, or the pull of the triceps muscle avulses the olecranon process. The quadratus lumborum

muscle is an extremely powerful muscle with two sheets one behind the other, the anterior extending from the crest of the ilium to the lumbar transverse processes whilst the posterior extends from the crest of the ilium to the lower border of the 12th rib, both layers however attach to the transverse processes. Thus the injuries that occur are quite comparable to other traction injuries and they may be multiple. They heal poorly, usually because of the traction process so that healing is usually by fibrosis. Particular problems occur at the musculo tendinous insertions, which give rise to quite a lot of pain. As the quadratus lumborum may occasionally fibrose, continuous pain over a long period of time can be experienced. The extent of the violence may be even greater. The line of injury may be traced from a fracture of ilium, through to fractures of all five lumbar transverse processes (Fig. 26.31) with evidence of extensive tearing of muscle and aponeuroses. Retroperitoneal

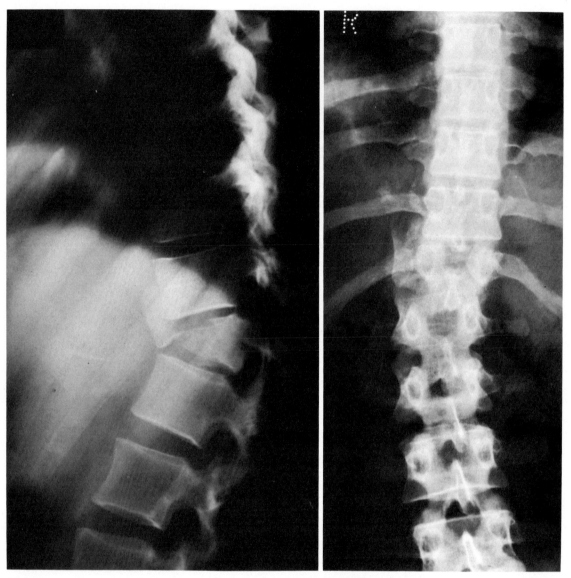

Fig 26.24

Fig 26.25

Figs 26.24 and 26.25 Severe rotational fracture dislocation of T.12. This unstable injury was not associated with neurological damage and fused in the position of displacement.

haemorrhage will cause abdominal pain and rigidity whilst blood loss with profound shock may occur. A large haematoma in the lumbar angle is not to be unexpected. Such a severe injury must be regarded as one of the whole posterior abdominal wall and not just the transverse processes. The resorption of haemorrhage can be slow and quite often a drain must be put into the haematoma. Isometric muscle activity must be commenced as soon as the patient is

comfortable to assist in the restoration of function of the quadratus lumborum.

Fractures of the thoracic spinous processes.
Whilst fractures of the lumbar spinous processes are common and even indeed in the cervical column, fractures of the thoracic spinous processes have been described as the 'clay shovellers' fracture. It was first

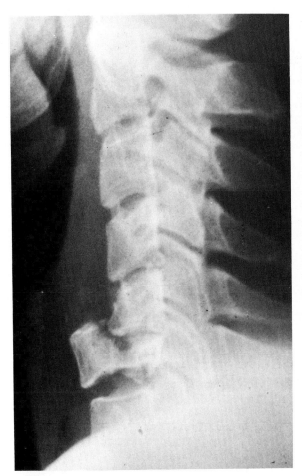

Fig 26.26

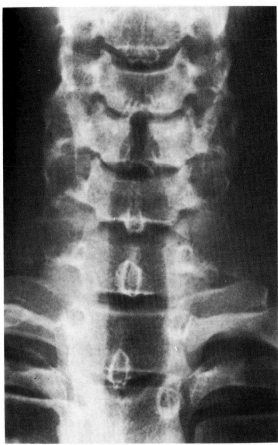

Fig 26.27

Figs 26.26 and 26.27 A compression fracture of C.6. Fragments may be displaced into the neural canal.

described after the unusual use of a shovel during the 1932 recession in Australia. It was often sustained when these men drove a spade into heavy soil whereupon they received sharp pain on thrusting the spade up, the pain occurring between the shoulder blades. Careful radiographic examination will show the avulsion of the tip of the spinous process usually at the 7th cervical and 1st thoracic. Such a muscle avulsion with a fragment of bone usually needs no more treatment other than a few weeks rest and the aid of local injection of Novocain and particular attention to isometric muscle restoration. The injury is not seen so commonly these days as the labourers do not appear to have so much stress on their lumbar spine particularly perhaps in these days of adequate social security and workers' compensation.

DIAGNOSIS OF FRACTURES AND FRACTURE DISLOCATIONS OF THE SPINE

When a patient is brought to a casualty department suspected of suffering from a fracture of the spine he or she will usually have had some sort of first aid or pre-hospital, post-accident treatment and is thus presented to the surgeon with a diagnosis having been already made. However, this does not absolve the receiving surgeon from taking a careful history of the accident, making a full clinical examination and concluding with proper radiological investigations. The history of the accident and any pre-existing diseases may easily give the guidelines to more adequate treatment, for the treatment is not completely dependent on the type of injury; in fact quite

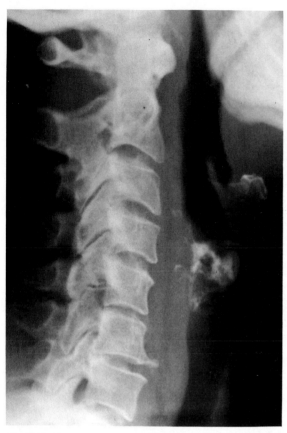

Fig 26.28 Hyperextension injury to cervical spine with avulsion of tiny osteophyte from the front of lower border C_6. Note the retro-tracheal bulge due to haemorrhage.

common today than it ever was because of the social habits of many people. Bladder conditions may pre-exist the accident and an over distended bladder if not relieved quickly may inevitably give the patient a type of neurogenic bladder for many months to come (see Chapter 27).

Neurological examination is essential, even in patients who can apparently move legs and arms, for incomplete tetraparesis or incomplete paraparesis may easily not be diagnosed; for example, a woman aged 40, injured in a motor accident where her mother was even more seriously injured refused early medical care because of anxiety for her parent, but noted that her left upper extremity felt heavy and weak. Twenty-four hours later she found that she had not passed urine (and this in a person who normally voided every hour and a half). After careful clinical examination, incomplete tetraparesis (of a Brown Sequard type) due to fracture dislocation C2 on C3 was diagnosed. This recovered but inevitably the bladder did not recover and went on to a long term major disability.

Radiological examination should only be commenced after accurate clinical examination, for once the level of the injury has been determined by physical examination of palpation and tenderness then radiological examination will be more meaningful. A definite order must be put for proper X-ray plates. The normal standard X-ray examination will be made, antero-posterior, lateral and oblique, of the damaged area of the vertebral column, whilst tomography should only be asked for if the original plates do not give all the adequate information. With the use of these three standard views and tomograms most injuries can be diagnosed when the details of the fracture dislocation can be built up into a three dimensional picture. Rarely flexion and extension lateral X-ray plates will be required to further elucidate the injury. It should be noted that tomography has assisted greatly in defining the multiplicity of these injuries. Rarely is the injury just at one level. The maximum level will be a single one but minimal fractures may easily occur above and below the maximal level. The use of the computer scanning techniques has yet to be evaluated although it seems that in some fractures it will give considerable assistance in defining the exact detail of the injury, particularly as small fragments of bone may be displaced sometimes into the neural canal. Adequate radiological examination must be undertaken at the end of the physical examination and not at the beginning, for levels of the fracture cannot be defined until after clinical examination has been made. When

often the treatment depends on the patient's pre-existing diseases, or the history of the accident; for example; small aircraft accidents are well known to cause fractures of the spine, they also cause multiple long bone fractures. A surgeon should be wary of a patient who has been involved in such an accident, even where pain is not complained of in the lumbo-dorsal or lumbo-sacral spine. The history is also relevant as to the pre-existing activities of the previous hours; for example, whether the patient was at a social function, or whether the injury occurred is in the course of his ordinary work activity. This will inevitably assist in the rehabilitative efforts that will be essential later. Physical examination of the patient should be careful and painstaking, all systems should be examined.[9] Frequently thoracic injuries will cause mediastinal complaints such as dysphagia or respiratory difficulties. Pre-existing respiratory disease can then be picked up, obstructive lung disease is more

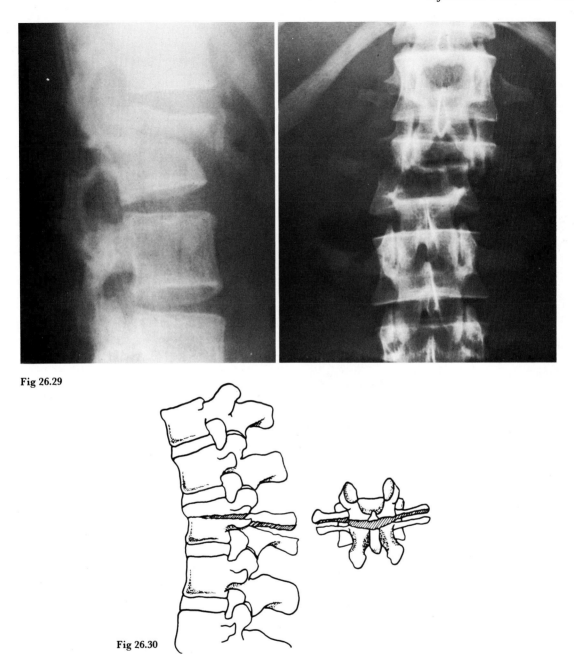

Fig 26.29

Fig 26.30

Figs 26.29 and 26.30 Chance's fracture.

the diagnosis has been completed and the radiological pictures have been shown then, and then only, can definitive treatment be undertaken. Whilst the investigations are being completed however the first aid measures of proper posture, emptying the bladder and transport to a suitable centre for management can be undertaken.

TREATMENT OF SPINAL INJURIES

All injuries of the spinal column should be adequately diagnosed both from the point of view of the clinical problem involved as well as the pathological basis of change which will of course give the basis of all methods of treatment. Injuries are generally divided

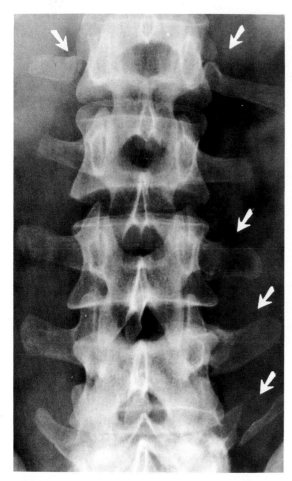

Fig 26.31 Fractures of the third, fourth and fifth lumbar transverse processes on the right side, with subperiosteal ossification in the origin of the quadratus lumborum from the ilium.

into those which are stable and those which may be unstable;[9, 10] in fact the majority of injuries that are thought to be unstable rapidly stabilise after adequate conservative care. A stable injury is one in which further deformity of significance does not normally occur even if mobilisation has occurred.[5] The so-called unstable injuries may deform but in fact very few of them do if properly prevented by treatment.

Recovery of function and particularly the restoration of muscle function is the prime aim of treatment when most injuries will heal by satisfactory callus and bony restoration.[9,11] However, many of the injuries, particularly the hyperextension injury, will heal usually by soft tissue repair.

The process of treatment is usually a graded one so that early management will normally be conservative whilst later management may occasionally be more active.[12]

METHODS OF CONSERVATIVE TREATMENT

Cervical injuries

Cervical collar. A collar may be used to support the neck during the phase of acute pain following a strain of the cervical spine. Strains may occur in car accidents, in the rugby scrum or in a forward roll in the gymnasium and are characterised by local pain and guarding of movement by muscle spasm. Such spasms must be carefully differentiated from a more serious injury by complete radiographic examination. The radiographs must consist of an anteroposterior view which includes a through mouth view of C.1 and C.2, a lateral view which must extend down to C.7 (Figs 26.32 and 26.33) right and left oblique views properly labelled, and if necessary lateral views in the positions of flexion and extension.

If the radiographs show no bone or joint damage the neck can be protected in a collar of Sorbo rubber or plasterzote, if the clinical picture warrants treatment (Fig 26.34).

Continuous cervical traction. Continuous traction is employed either to reduce a dislocation or to maintain an unstable injury in a stable position. It is essential to employ it when cervical spine movements could cause or increase cervical cord damage. It is desirable that such traction be easy to apply, comfortable to the patient, effective in use and permit a change of position of the patient with safety. Halter traction with slings under the chin and occiput is not recommended except as a temporary first aid measure. When it is effective in treatment it is uncomfortable to wear and liable to produce pressure sores.

Skull traction is the method of choice and the calipers of the Crutchfield or Cone variety are recommended (Figs 26.35, 26.36). These can be applied using local anaesthesia through two stab incisions in the scalp over the parietal region in a line joining each external auditory meatus. The stabs should be equidistant from the mid-line. A hole is drilled by hand in the outer table of the skull using a special drill which has a guard to prevent penetration of the inner table. Each caliper point is inserted into a hole and after the caliper has been tightened the required weight is attached to the caliper. It is necessary to check the caliper daily to ascertain that it is of sufficient tightness. With the caliper in position

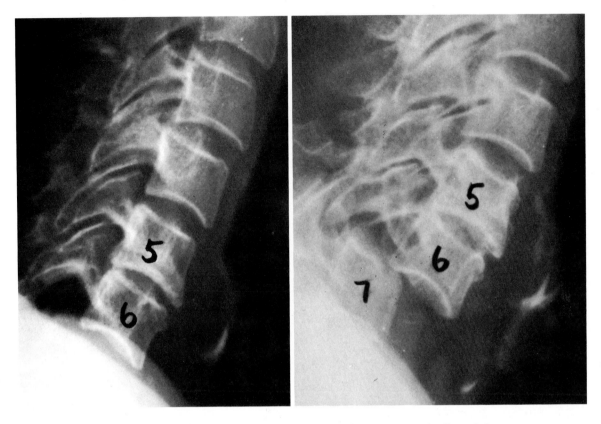

Fig 26.32 An inadequate lateral radiograph of the cervical spine because C.7 is not seen.

Fig 26.33 A correct lateral radiograph demonstrates a gross dislocation the facets are locked on each side. There were no neurological signs.

it is possible for the patient to change position and turn on to side of face. Slow reduction of fracture dislocations by traction first in flexion to unlock and then in retro-flexion to maintain is the most common method of care.

If there is any doubt as to whether or not traction is needed the method should be used. Traction should be applied before transferring a patient with an unstable injury from one hospital to another, or even from one department to another in the same hospital.

Minerva plaster (Fig 26.37). This is a body cast of plaster extending from occiput and frontal region to the iliac crests used to immobilise the cervical spine. The patient can be ambulant. There are some important points to remember about this cast. It requires skill to produce a comfortable fit. It will not hold an unstable dislocation. Despite its critics it has a place in immobilising the cervical spine in certain injuries while consolidation is taking place.

Lumbo-dorsal injuries

The conservative management of lumbo-dorsal injuries involves the surgeon in postural care so that the normal curves of the body are maintained, usually with the aid of suitable pillows or pads (see Figs 27.5 and 27.6). This method of care must be undertaken immediately after the fracture and as soon as possible after the patient's admission to hospital. Suitable posturing on suitable beds, e.g. the ordinary traction bed or the Stoke Mandeville bed will quickly bring the patient comfort (Fig 26.38a and b; and see Figs 27.5 and 27.7). As the age of the patient increases the size of the pillow must decrease as the lumbar lordosis diminishes over a period of time (Figs 27.5 and 27.6).

Plaster jacket or exoskeleton. This is a body cast extending from sternum to the symphysis pubis allowing room in the axilla and permitting hip flexion of 90 degrees. It is applied with the patient standing or sitting in a normal erect posture. Halter

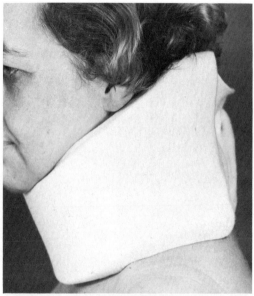

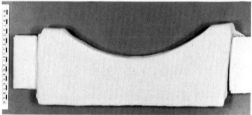

Fig 26.34 Sorbo rubber collar used for acute neck strain. The rubber used should be shaped low under the chin and high over the occiput. The collar is made from 1 inch (2.5 cm) thick Sorbo rubber and covered with stockinette.

traction may assist in steadying a patient during the application. The position of hyper-extension is no longer recommended during application.

Common methods of management. Whichever area of the human spine is damaged by a fracture or fracture dislocation there are a few common methods of management.

1. *Isometric muscle activity.* It is important that isometric muscle activity be started as soon as possible by the physical therapists so that muscle power be maintained and even increased if necessary. This is a tedious and sometimes time consuming operation but the results are so beneficial as to make it essential. Unfortunately many fractures are not given the benefit of such isometric activity.
2. *Respiratory management.* It is important to maintain respiratory function as normal as possible. Thus the physical therapist has the important task of seeing that all areas of the lung and pleura are expanded adequately on a regular basis.
3. *Dietetic management.* This is very important—the obese should have a reducing diet, the asthenic should be well looked after to see that high protein, high carbohydrate diet will quickly overcome any negative metabolic balance that may occur.
4. *Other methods of management* must be planned depending on whether or not the patient had other medical or surgical conditions.

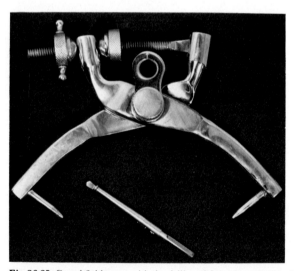

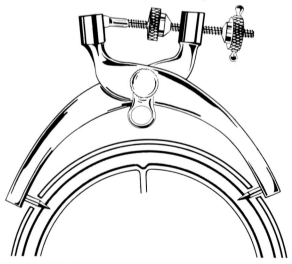

Fig 26.35 Crutchfield tongs with the drill used for penetrating the bone of the skull. Note the shoulder on the drill preventing penetration into the brain.

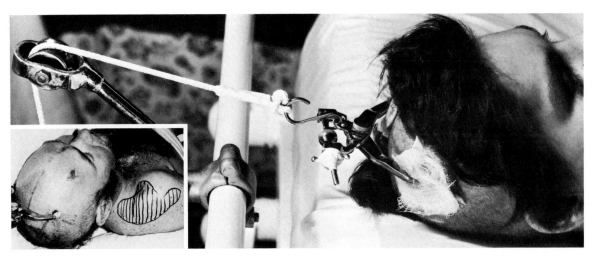

Fig 26.36 Crutchfield skull traction in situ. The tongs are placed much higher on the vertex than the Blackburn calipers. They are inserted in line with the external auditory meati, (see inset).

MANAGEMENT OF VARIOUS GROUPS INCLUDING SURGICAL METHODS

Flexion compression injuries

A wedge compression injury of a vertebral body without tearing of interspinous ligaments is a stable injury. The wedging is of slight degree and does not require reduction or immobilisation. In the cervical region the amount of pain is variable, but a few days of bed rest may be needed and this is wise as it gives time to confirm stability. Thereafter a Sorbo-rubber or plasterzote collar can be worn and the patient mobilised (Fig 26.39).

In the thoracic region it is not uncommon for more than one vertebra to be wedged. This does not affect treatment. Bed rest need not be for more than a few days and thereafter the spine can be mobilised with confidence by extension and flexion exercises.

In the thoraco-lumbar and lumbar region the same form of treatment applies, provided the wedging is of a minor degree. Sometimes, however, in this region the deformity of the vertebral body is marked, with separation of the spinous processes and some subluxation of the facets. In these conditions a more cautious approach is needed, and bed rest is advised for three or four weeks followed by a plaster jacket for a further four to eight weeks (Figs 26.13, 26.14). Also, in the thoraco-lumbar region, a vertebral body may be wedged on a lateral side, the so-called lateral wedge fracture described by Nicoll.[10] Such lateral wedging must be associated with some distortion of the posterior joint on the opposite side and good quality oblique radiographs are needed to assess the damage and hence the stability. These lateral wedge fractures cannot be reduced. Most of the injuries are stable and can be treated as such, but pain at the fracture site

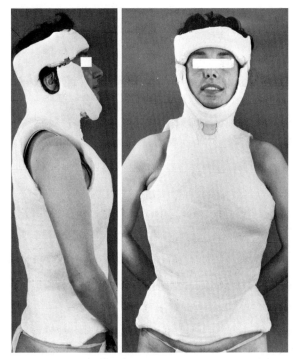

Fig 26.37 Photographs of a patient in a Minerva jacket after fracture of the spine. Note the moulding onto the iliac crests and the cut-away portion over the 'Adam's apple'.

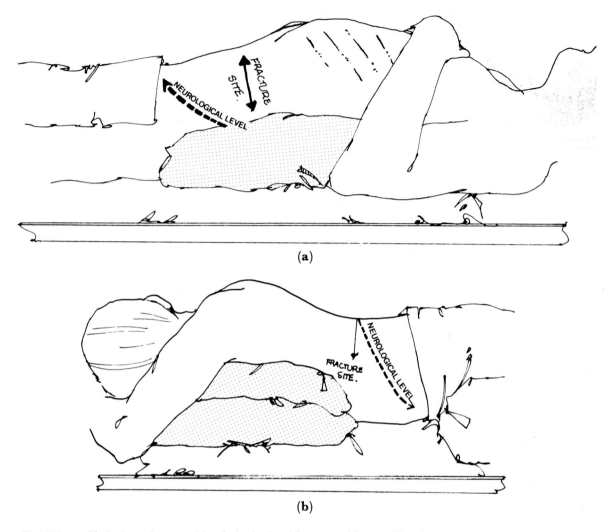

(a)

(b)

Fig 26.38 a and b Supine and prone positions for lumbo-dorsal fractures and fracture dislocations. Note: Both fracture site and neurological levels (if any) are clearly marked.

persists longer than with the more usual anteriorly wedged fracture (Fig 26.40).

Flexion-rotation injuries

These injuries may be unstable, particularly grade 2 (bilateral fracture dislocation or dislocations), and the purpose of treatment is to secure stability. This is produced by ankylosis (usually bony) between the affected vertebrae. In the lumbar region where the injury is usually a fracture-dislocation, bony ankylosis will very often occur spontaneously. In the cervical region, however, a significant fracture is not so common. The injury is mainly a rupture of the posterior ligament complex which may not heal

sufficiently strongly to produce stability, although osteogenesis under the intact anterior longitudinal ligament is commonly seen. With adequate conservative care, traction and posture, 90 per cent of these cervical injuries achieve firm ankylosis. Ten per cent remain unstable until vertebral bodies are fused by operative methods (Figs 26.20, 26.21, 26.41, 26.42 and 26.43). Open surgical methods have a very limited use and are discussed in the chapter on paraplegia.

Cervical spine. The injury must be accurately diagnosed by radiographs, and good quality oblique

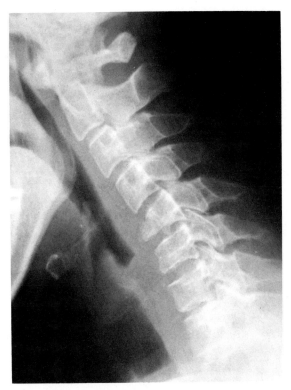

Fig 26.39 A simple wedge fracture of one cervical vertebra. This is a stable flexion injury.

pictures are required (Figs 26.16, 26.17, 26.18 and 26.19).

Reduction by traction. Displacement must be reduced. Skull traction is applied, (Figs 26.35, 26.36) first in flexion, using a weight of 10 to 12 lb (4.5 to 5.4 kg). A proportion of injuries will be reduced within 12 hours. In those unreduced, a careful increase in weight is used, with radiographic control, gradually up to approximately 30 lb (13.6 kg) may be needed. Two or more times each day radiographic examination is needed to guard against unwise distraction. In some centres all cervical dislocations with or without paresis are manipulated under anaesthesia on the day of admission as the treatment of choice, and then skull traction is applied.[13] This dramatic approach is not essential. There is no possible harm in adopting the more simple method of skull traction alone as an initial procedure. It is the treatment of choice which is nearly always effective, and within 48 hours the majority of dislocations will be reduced. Manipulation should be reserved for those dislocations which are unreduced in 24 to 48 hours which may then be reduced under general anaesthesia with relaxation.[13]

Manipulative reduction (Figs 26.44a, b, c, and d, and 26.45a, b, c, and d). It is mandatory that the side of the dislocated facets be localised by oblique radiographs before manipulation of such a spine. If the facets on each side are locked, straight traction is needed. If the facets are locked on one side, the manipulation technique is manual straight traction followed by side flexion away from the locked facet followed by rotation. If the dislocation is not reduced by manipulation then open reduction may be used (see Chapter 27).

Management—following reduction. However the dislocation is treated the reduction must be seen to be complete in lateral and oblique radiographs, and after reduction skull traction must be maintained with a reduced weight of about 7 lb (3.2 kg) as all these injuries are unstable. Two courses of subsequent management are then available. Traction can be maintained, waiting to see whether or not any new bone forms anteriorly between the two vertebral bodies at about six weeks. If this happens, stability is occurring and mobilisation of the patient in a rigid collar or a Minerva plaster can be permitted until stabilisation is complete. The second method is early spinal fusion. This is not to be regularly recommended as there are increased morbidity problems. Selection of its use is necessary and most centres use fusion as a late method of care.

Open reduction of locked facets. It may be impossible to unlock facets and reduce the dislocations by traction or manipulation. This may be due to distortion of a facet by the fracture. In such cases assessment in regard to fitness for surgery is necessary. In a few an open operation is undertaken using a posterior approach. The facets are gently unlocked usually requiring partial facetectomy. Subsequently the spinous processes are held together by suitable clamps or wire whilst slivers of iliac graft are laid across the laminae of the affected vertebrae. It must be noted that no form of collar or plaster fixation will hold a flexion rotation injury in a reduced position unless there is evidence of spontaneous or operative fusion occurring. Such support is therefore useless in the early management of such injuries.

Management of late cases. A dislocated cervical spine may be seen for the first time some weeks after injury. The treatment of unrecognised dislocations varies. Some of those cases in which only one facet is locked are remarkably free of symptoms and can be left alone but watched by regular radiographs until stabilisation is confirmed. Unrecognised bilateral facet injuries and single facet injuries associated with root pains or other neurological symptoms should be

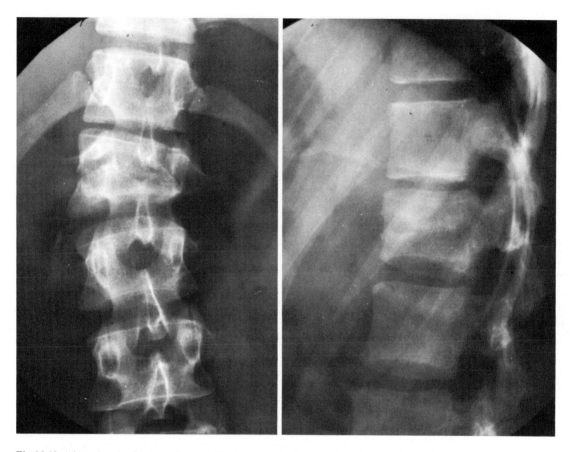

Fig 26.40 A lateral wedge fracture of L₁. This fracture is stable. It cannot be reduced by manipulation.

treated. It is possible to reduce some dislocations that are up to four or even eight weeks old by skull traction. After reduction anterior strut grafting is a well recognised method to reinforce the damaged anterior tissues where the osteogenesis is poor and even avascular necrosis may have occurred. Those injuries which cannot be reduced completely by traction may require open reduction by a facetectomy (Figs 26.46, 26.47, 26.48, 26.49, 26.50, 26.51, 26.52, 26.53). However, such cases can be difficult to reduce even at surgery and post operative traction reduction after facetectomy may then succeed. Whether or not the dislocation is completely reduced by these means the dislocated level must be fused by a bone graft; for instability is a far more serious problem than the initial distortion of the neural canal, and can lead to further narrowing of the canal and occasionally to delayed vascular changes in the spinal cord.

Fracture dislocations of the cervical spine particularly in the older age group must always be watched extremely carefully. Instability is always to be suspected and careful conservative management may not necessarily give a good result. However, by waiting up to three months surgery can usually be reserved for only those few cases where gross instability occurs. Less than 6 per cent of all fracture dislocations of the cervical spine, particularly the bilateral lesions, will be unstable.

Thoraco-lumbar region (Fig 26.15). These flexion rotation injuries are regarded by many surgeons as unstable; stability will however rapidly occur reduced or unreduced. Fracture-dislocation with pedicle fractures will reduce merely by laying the patient supine (Figs 26.38 a and b) when the lesions will stabilise spontaneously with good nursing and/or exoskeletons. It is not necessary to accurately reduce them or to fix them internally with plates and bolts. Some of those so fixed do not consolidate until the bolts have cut out from the spinous processes, allowing

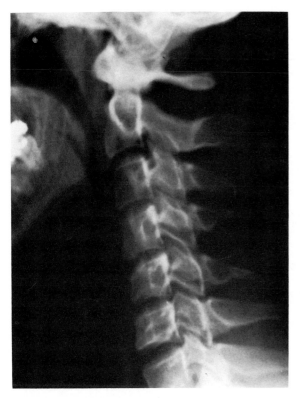

Fig 26.41 Dislocation easily reduced by traction.

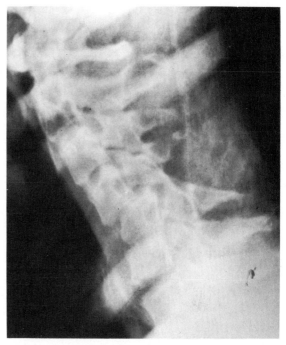

Fig 26.42 This unstable injury was immobilised in a Minerva plaster. It redislocated quietly in the plaster. At this stage with such instability either re-reduction with further rest, or spinal fusion is indicated.

the vertebral bodies to collapse together. It is also unnecessary to bone graft these injuries. Nicoll[11] has shown this to be true in miners, who are heavy workers and require a mobile spine, and who can return to work after proper conservative management. Long fusions are to be avoided.[12] New methods of fixation e.g. Harrington Rods may occasionally be needed in grossly unstable injuries.[14] (See also Chapter 27).

The patient is treated lying supine with a pillow behind the fracture on a firm mattress and careful turning from side to side every two hours is instituted. (See Chapter 27). At seven to ten days a plaster jacket can be applied and active physical rehabilitation proceeds whilst in plaster.[11] A plaster bed is not necessary. At about eight to ten weeks the injury will be sufficiently stable to either remove the exoskeleton, or to continue ambulation in a plaster jacket which should be maintained until there is consolidation of the injury in about a further four to six weeks. Active mobilisation is then commenced to produce a strong mobile spine.

In the case of the rare true dislocation or unilateral fracture dislocation in the thoraco-lumbar region, the facets are locked and will not unlock with simple change of position; hyperextension can be dangerous. If reduction by manipulation (Figs 26.56a, b, c, d, and e) fails it may be necessary to unlock the injury by open operation (Figs 26.54a and b and 26.55). Depending on the clinical state, local fusion only should be advised.

Open methods have been largely advocated for paraplegia—very occasionally they are useful in non paraplegics (see Chapter 27).

Vertical compression injuries. Such injuries are stable in whatever position they occur in the vertebral column, but it must be carefully defined that they are not associated with a flexion-rotation injury at the segment above for these injuries can then be very unstable. Flexion and extension lateral X-rays may be needed. Most of such injuries are perfectly stable because of the integrity of both the anterior and the posterior ligamentous complex. However, the vertebral bodies are extensively comminuted and may invade the retro-pharyngeal or retro-peritoneal space

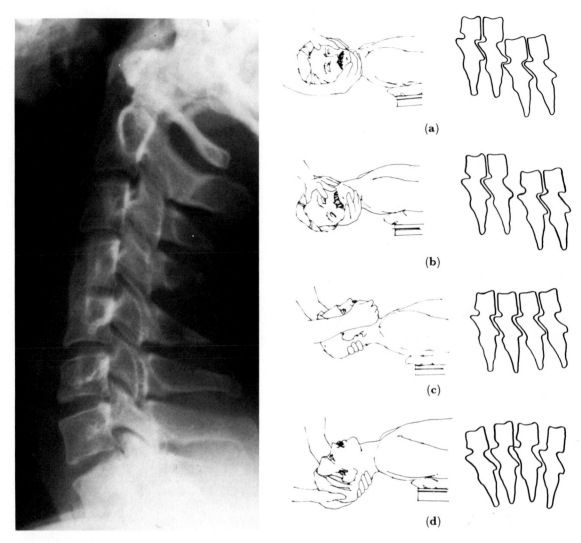

Fig 26.43 Anterior interbody spinal fusion has been undertaken however even after such instability dislocation can recur. Some surgeons prefer posterior wiring and graft. Redisplacement as seen may take place six to eight weeks after injury even when the position appears to have been satisfactorily held by an apparently adequate plaster, or by traction.

Fig 26.44 Manual reduction of the unilateral fracture dislocation. (a) Traction and rotation away from the dislocated side. (b) Lateral flexion and rotation away from the dislocated side. (c) Reduction. (d) Hyperextension to maintain.

as well as the neural canal. Rarely does the invasion of fragments into the neural canal call for any operative procedure and in fact traction may effectively reduce many of these fractures. However, normally they do not need reduction, and certainly they never require open reduction or internal fixation. Even if the vertebral bodies are reconstituted by technical methods. They must inevitably collapse as Nicoll[10] showed long ago, for the reduced vertebra

certainly has a central core of blood clot. Bed rest is needed for a period of time, usually four to five weeks, followed by some type of exoskeleton and the usual restorative activity of muscle function.

Extension injuries. These injuries are stable in the normal position of recumbency. As has already been indicated most occur in the cervical spine and can be safely treated in a Sorbo collar. It is unnecessary to

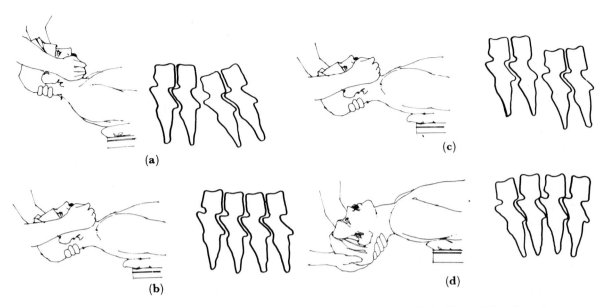

Fig 26.45 Manual reduction of the bilateral cervical dislocation. (a) Traction and flexion to unlock. (b) and (c) Traction and extension to reduction. (d) Hyperextension to maintain.

confine the patient to bed for longer than a few days, even in the presence of neurological damage. For extension and compression injuries in the lumbar region it may be necessary to use a plaster jacket for approximately eight weeks to allow consolidation of the vertebral body injury (Fig 26.57).

FRACTURES AND FRACTURE-DISLOCATIONS OF THE ATLANTO AXIAL AREA[15]

Studies of autopsy material including X-ray examinations reveal that injuries of the cranio cervical area

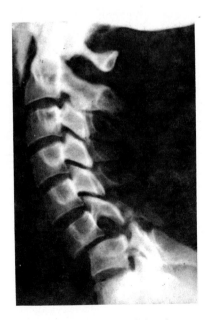

Fig 26.46 Two month-old unreduced dislocation.

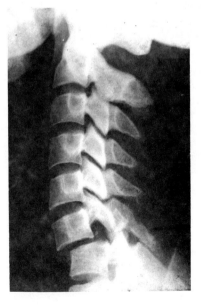

Fig 26.47 First day: 20 lb (9 kg) skull traction.

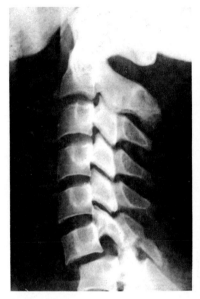

Fig 26.48 Second day: 25 lb (11.3 kg) skull traction.

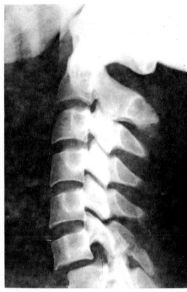

Fig 26.49 Third day: 30 lb (13.5 kg) skull traction.

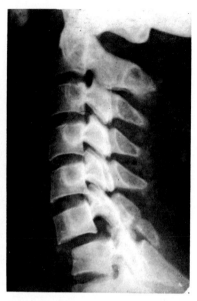

Fig 26.50 Fourth day: 35 lb (15.6 kg) skull traction.

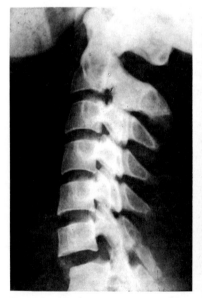

Fig 26.51 Fifth day: 40 lb (18 kg) skull traction.

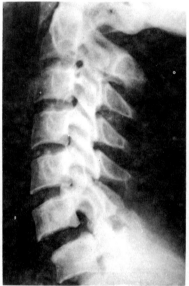

Fig 26.52 Sixth day: 40 lb (18 kg) skull traction with oblique pull.

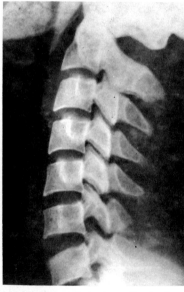

Fig 26.53 Seventh day immediately after facetectomy: 12 lb (5.4 kg) skull traction.

are largely caused by the major forces of flexion, extension rotation and axial compression as in the lower cervical spine. Atlanto occipital injuries nearly always occur in pedestrians and are flexion lesions associated with rotation, giving severe brain stem injuries and causing instant death. Occasionally however unilateral injuries survive without neural damage, some with fracture dislocation, and a few with unilateral subluxation at the cranio occipital or atlanto axial area. It must always be remembered

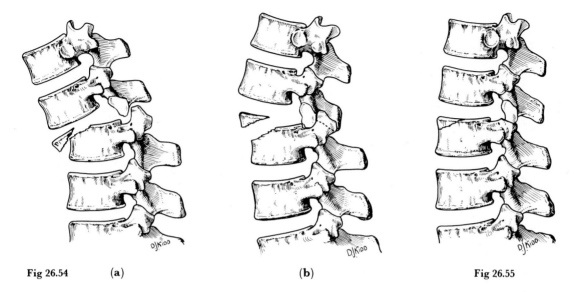

Fig 26.54   **(a)**   **(b)**   **Fig 26.55**

Figs 26.54 a and b and 26.55 Pure dislocation of the posterior facets is rare in the thoraco-lumbar spine (Fig 26.54 a). If the spine is simply hyperextended the upper facets cannot slide back and further damage to the cord can occur (Fig 26.54 b). These injuries can be reduced (Fig 26.55) by traction under general anaesthetic see Fig 26.56, or if such fails open operation may be indicated with local fusion only. Rods and fixation instruments are not absolutely indicated.

that cervical spine injuries are well known to be associated with head injuries and post-mortem studies of fatal cases show the association to be about 10 per cent, whilst neurosurgical services show similar figures. At C.1–2 rotation is an important pathogenic cause of ligamentous, bony and chondral injuries, while at C.2–3 hyperextension is more important so that the 'hangman' type injury is most common. Locking of injuries by facetal inter-digitation is rare. Late articular changes of some consequence can be seen after so called minor neck injury in motor vehicle accidents (Figs 26.60, 26.65, 26.66 and 26.67). Virtually all injuries of this area are at one or two adjacent levels. Beware, the patient who indicates clinically his head feels like 'falling off'. Present seat belts and head restraints in vehicles have done little as yet to restrict or prevent injuries at the upper cervical spine.

Fracture of the atlas. The usual cause of fracture of the atlas is a fall on the head from a height or a mass falling on to the head. It is therefore an axial compression injury. The blow is transmitted from the skull through the two lateral masses of the atlas which are forced apart so that the bone fractures at one or more of the weaker points, the anterior and/or more commonly the posterior arch (Figs 26.58, 26.59,

26.60). There is usually no cord lesion and the injury is by no means necessarily fatal.[15, 16]

Clinical features. There is spasm of the neck muscles and the patient holds himself rigidly as if balancing a weight upon his head. When getting up from recumbency or with any other change of position, the patient usually supports his head with his hands. Nodding and rotatory movements are limited. There may be pain and sometimes anaesthesia in the area supplied by the great occipital nerve.

Treatment. Skeletal skull traction may realign the displaced fragments and should be used for several weeks. If there is no complication such as tetraparesis (very rare) the neck can be immobilised in plaster with the head in the mid-position for three months. As this injury is stable and simple collars can be safely used for maintaining position, e.g. Sterno Occipital Mandibular Immobiliser (S.O.M.I. Collar).

Fractures of the odontoid process. These are usually caused by severe flexion or extension forces, and their incidence has been increasing in recent years. That many patients die from such injuries is demonstrated by autopsy studies, but the numbers are now on the decline. Non-union poses a threat to neurological function, but less now than in previous years when this hazard was not well recognised. The

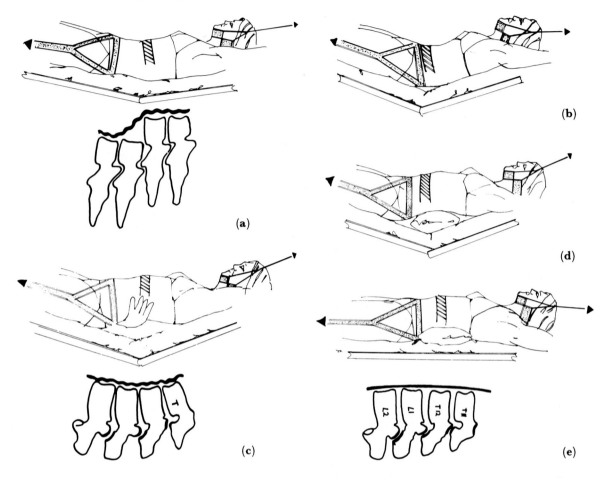

Fig 26.56 Manual reduction of lumbo dorsal fracture dislocations under general anaesthetic. (a) Initial posture with traction. (b) Flexion and traction. (c) The reduction by the operator. (d) Insertion of pillows. (e) Maintenance.

most severe complication is that of instability associated with varying degrees of atlanto axial subluxation or dislocation[17] (see later).

After a study of odontoid blood supply Anderson and D'Alonzo[18] described three types of fracture:

Type I: Fracture of the extreme tip. As they have a good blood supply these fractures unite without difficulty, but may be confused with a 'os odontoide'.

Type II: These are situated at the 'waisted' base which is the site of attachment of the accessory ligaments (and therefore blood supply). They are slow to unite—frequently show non union and need more rigid fixation, firstly by traction and then by exoskeletal assistance. In some cases a late Gallie type fusion is required (Figs 26.61, 26.62).

Type III: This is really a fracture of the body of C.2 and as the area is liberally supplied with blood vessels it unites well and with minimum trouble.

Fractures of the cervical spine in children.[15]
Fractures of the dens and subluxations of this area account for a high percentage, over 75 per cent, of such injuries in children below the age of eight years. In adults and older children they account for only 10 per cent of cervical injuries. The odontoid by virtue of its synchondrosis and thus cartilaginous plate at the base is vulnerable from the time of delivery (by forceps) until the plate fuses at first circumferentially at puberty into adult years. Fractures thus tend to occur through this plate and to disrupt the ligamentous structures. Diagnosis is difficult; clinically high cervical tenderness is usual with occasional torticollis. Some are dismissed as strains. Radiology is not always helpful unless careful lateral flexion and extension views are taken under sedation. Union is regularly achieved with adequate immobilisation by plaster and collar.

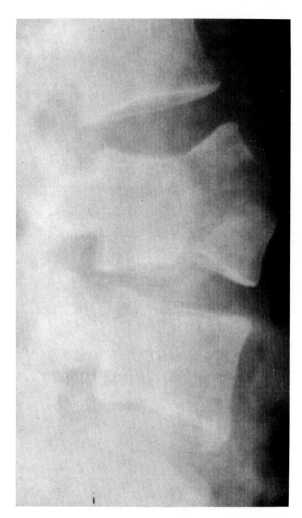

Fig 26.57 Comminuted fracture of the lumbar spine due to hyperextension. It is usually necessary to support the spine in a plaster jacket for a period of about eight weeks to allow consolidation of the vertebral body injury.

Fractures of the remainder of the cervical spine in children occur rarely but are becoming more frequent with the increase in motor vehicle accidents. Before making the diagnosis it should be remembered that at C.2–3 there is normally movement up to three to 4 mm on flexion and extension. After careful clinical examination radiology to diagnose subluxation or dislocation by oblique views and tomography is essential. Rarely is the dislocation severe enough to warrant skeletal traction, but, if required, a halo is the wisest choice. Careful realignment of spinous processes and lateral articulations is needed if late deformity is to be minimised.

In children epiphyseal injuries must not be overlooked particularly with spinal paralysis. Since some injuries are multiple in level late severe kyphos is possible. If it is considered that this is likely to occur early anterior fusion at end of six to eight weeks will be useful to prevent both deformity and aggravation of spinal paralysis.

Dislocation of the atlas. The stability of the atlas depends upon the transverse ligament, which lies between the lateral masses and braces the odontoid process to its anterior arch. If the ligament is torn the atlas can dislocate forwards. Similarly, if the base of the odontoid process is fractured the atlas and the odontoid fragment may be displaced together. The usual mechanism is a complicated succession of

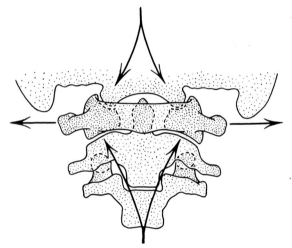

Fig 26.58

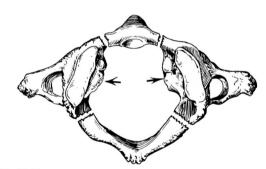

Fig 26.59

Figs 26.58 and 26.59 Fracture of the atlas due to a fall on the head. The force is transmitted through the lateral masses which are driven apart so that the arch fractures at its weakest point. (Diagrams adapted from those first published by Jefferson (1920) *British Journal of Surgery*, 7 : 407.)

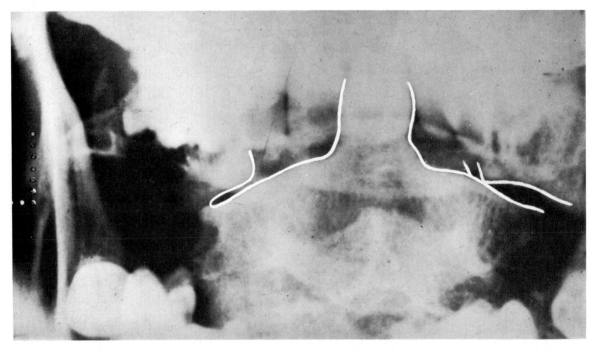

Fig 26.60 A bursting fracture-dislocation of the atlas with lateral separation of each side.

torsion and flexion forces. Dislocation is more serious than fracture-dislocation because if the odontoid is intact the spinal cord is in danger of being crushed against it (Figs 26.63, 26.64).

When there is a minimal displacement the cord escapes injury and the clinical picture resembles that of a fracture of the atlas, but importantly, as a rule, there is also rotatory displacement of the head.

The dislocation must be replaced, with care to protect the spinal cord by preventing flexion or rotation of the patient's head during induction of anaesthesia. The usual method will be by skeletal traction using a Crutchfield caliper or Halo to help effect reduction. Traction over 5 lb (2.2 kg) must not be maintained as it causes non union. Later, after three to four weeks, a plaster cast can be applied with the neck and head in the neutral position, the cast taking a purchase across the front of the forehead and also being moulded under the chin. A halo vest technique may also be used. Immobilisation is continued for three months. It is then safe to begin active exercises and within a few weeks to encourage more energetic rehabilitation by which to restore the patient's confidence in his recovery. If lateral radiographs taken whilst in traction show that there is still a forward shift of the atlas, further extension may be needed.

Internal fixation by wiring the posterior arch of the atlas to the spinous process of the axis with onlay cancellous grafts may be undertaken to reduce and fix difficult cases (Figs 26.61, 26.62, 26.65, 26.66). After surgery further traction may be required to prevent displacement.

It is important to remember that in children under the age of 14 a slight forward shift of the atlas on the axis in flexion is a normal appearance and that after injury it is not to be mistaken for atlanto-axial dislocation.

Flexion fracture-dislocation of atlas and odontoid. It is often said that the gravity of dislocation of the atlas is increased if there is also a fracture of the odontoid process. Precisely the opposite is the case. A fracture of the odontoid process improves the chances of survival, and with suitable treatment the patient makes a complete recovery; there should be no permanent disability. The atlas and the odontoid process are displaced together; as a rule there is both forward and rotatory displacement. Under traction the head is turned to the neutral position, the cervical spine is extended as already indicated. Minimal skeletal traction should be used initially for three to four weeks (as discussed) although a closely moulded plaster has been used. Immobilis-

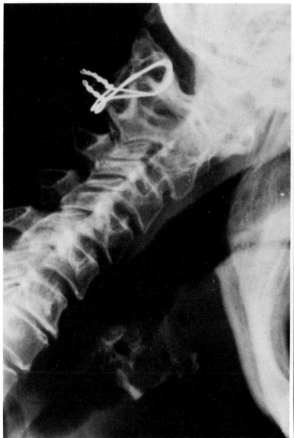
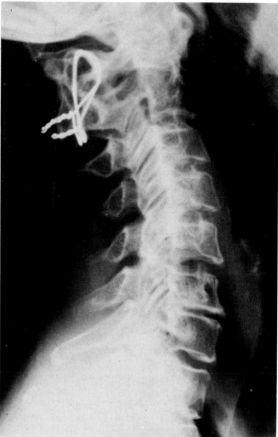

Fig 26.61

Fig 26.62

Figs 26.61 and 26.62 Flexion and extension radiographs after
cancellous bone graft and wiring of atlas and axis showing
restoration of stability. Surgery was required because of the
length of history before recognition.

ation is continued for three months. If reduction of
the displacement is accurate the odontoid fracture
unites by bone or by a fibrous ankylosis, but if left
untreated late instability may necessitate posterior
atlanto-axial fusion (Figs 26.61, 26.62, 26.65, 26.66).

**Hyperextension fracture-dislocation of atlas
and odontoid.** Sometimes the displacement is in the
opposite direction and the atlas, together with the
odontoid process is displaced backwards. Such a
displacement is shown in Figure 26.67.

The antero-posterior radiographs taken through
the open mouth show the fracture of the base of the
odontoid process and slight lateral displacement of
the interarticular joints. In this case the displacement
was reduced by flexion of the head and a plaster
jacket was applied, but the patient was elderly and

querulous, and within a few days it was necessary to
replace the plaster with a moulded block-leather
collar (Fig 26.68). Plasterzote collars reinforced with
polypropylene can also be used.

**Unreduced dislocation or fracture dislocation
at C.1–2.** If a dislocation of the atlanto axial joint is
overlooked considerable displacement may be observed months or years after injury. Sometimes a
perilous degree of displacement becomes firmly
stabilised by scar tissue; in other cases the transverse
ligament is weak and attenuated, displacement is
progressive, and paraplegia may develop from late
compression of the cord. If there is radiographic
evidence of increasing deformity or neurological
evidence of pressure on the cord, skeletal traction

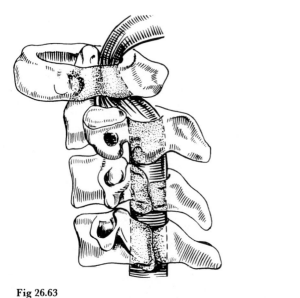

Fig 26.63

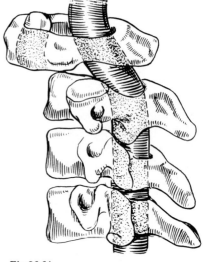

Fig 26.64

Figs 26.63 and 26.64 Forward dislocation (Fig 26.63) and fracture-dislocation (Fig 26.64) of atlas. If the odontoid is displaced forwards there is less danger of cord compression.

may effect some reduction prior to spinal fusion (Figs 26.61, 26.62, 26.65, 26.66).

Spontaneous dislocation at the atlanto axial joint. Spontaneous dislocation of the atlas causing sudden death is very rare, but spontaneous subluxation with 'acquired torticollis' is more frequent. It nearly always occurs in children aged from six to 12 years, and may complicate any infection in the upper part of the neck. Such displacements have occurred after tonsillitis and some after nasopharyngitis, retropharyngeal abscess, tuberculous adenitis, acute mastoid infection and osteomyelitis of the occipital bone. About a week after the onset of infection the

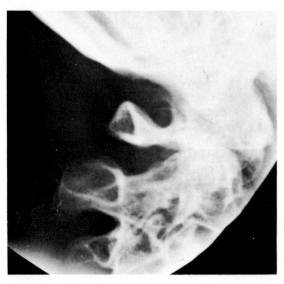

Fig 26.65 Radiograph of a fractured odontoid process which occurred 45 years ago.

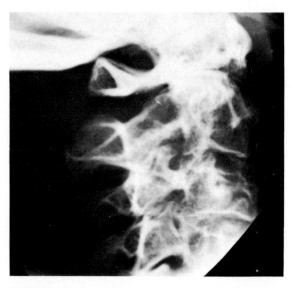

Fig 26.66 Extension produces reduction of the dislocation.

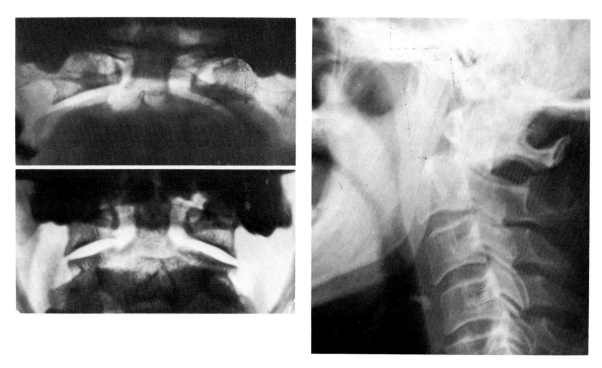

Fig 26.67 Hyperextension fracture-dislocation of the atlas and odontoid. Compare the antero-posterior view through the open mouth with the normal below.

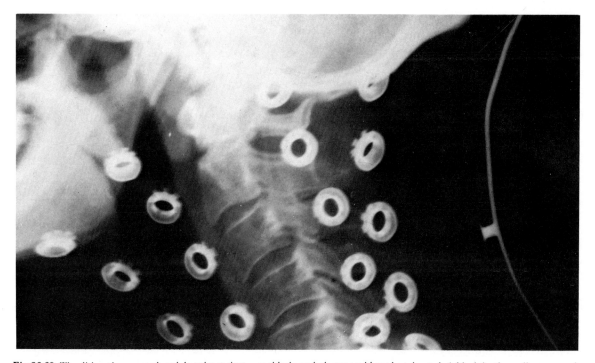

Fig 26.68 The dislocation was reduced, but the patient was elderly and plaster could not be tolerated. A block-leather collar was used.

child complains of a 'crick in the neck'. The head is held rigidly in the position of torticollis but there is no contracture or spasm of the sternomastoid; the rigidity and deformity are due to spasm of the deep cervical muscles.

Radiographs show forward rotatory displacement of the atlas. The displacement should be reduced by skull traction using a Halo and slow traction. After reduction and maintenance a close fitting plaster is applied with the head in neutral rotation and extension. After the primary focus of infection has healed immobilisation is continued for 10 weeks. Then a removable collar is best used for two to three weeks longer until a full range of painless movement is regained.

Some 'spontaneous' displacements are really related to missed trauma in motor vehicle accidents where other injuries dominate the clinical picture. Thus the need for full and repeated examination of all ages in multiple injuries should be emphasised. In adults spontaneous dislocations may occur in upper cervical spine cases of rheumatoid disease. Reduction may not be possible but stabilisation is occasionally needed.

Hyperextension fracture-dislocation of atlas and axis. This is a variant of the 'hangman's fracture' and is a variation of traumatic spondylolithesis of the axis[17, 19] and is usually caused by first hyperextension when the longitudinal ligament is ruptured, followed by flexion (Fig 26.71). Here the line of injury passes between the second and third cervical vertebral bodies and through the weak part of the neural arches of both vertebrae (Fig 26.69). The bodies of both atlas and axis are tilted backwards. Occasionally the spinal cord is contused or extradural haemorrhage causes paralysis and death. If the spinal cord escapes injury the treatment is the same as in hyperextension fracture-dislocation of C.2–3. Fusion occurs in nearly 100 per cent.

Hyperextension fracture-dislocation C.2 on C.3 (Figs 26.70 and 26.71). This is the other variant of spondylolithesis of the axis[19] sometimes known as the injury between cervico-cranium and the rest of the cervical spine (because of its association with judicial execution this lesion is sometimes referred to as 'the hangman's fracture'). The fracture lines in this injury can be variable in position (Fig 26.71). They may run across the neural arch of the axis or into the vertebral body. The injury on each side of the vertebra may be a different location. The body of the axis may appear tilted forwards or backwards. Any

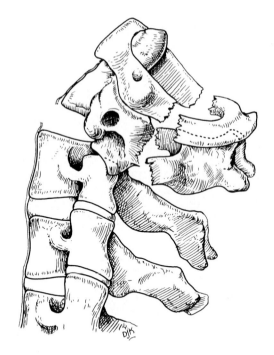

Fig 26.69 Hyperextension fracture-dislocation of the atlas and axis.

displacement in alignment can be corrected with straight skull traction. Later a Minerva plaster can be applied. It will hold this injury. Commonly new bone formation occurs between the front of the vertebra C.2–3 and this stabilises the vertebral column. It is not necessary to treat this injury surgically as union always occurs even in the displaced flexed position (Fig 26.71) giving an attenuated new pars interarticularis.

The real difference between these injuries seen after present day motor vehicle accidents and those seen as 'hangman fractures' is that the latter were caused by hyperextension and distraction and had a high incidence of neurological involvement whilst the former (now more common) are caused by hyperextension and axial compression with a low incidence of neurological involvement.

CHANGES IN FRACTURES AND FRACTURE-DISLOCATION OF THE SPINE

Whilst the basic fracture patterns have not changed over many years, nevertheless the emphasis on some injuries is not so great. For example, hyperextension injuries of the cervical spine have become much

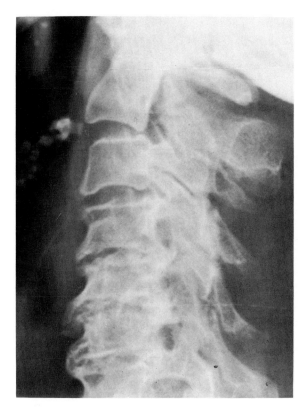

Fig 26.70 Hyperextension fracture-dislocation of C.2 on C.3.

better known and are more common, mainly as a result of the motor vehicle epidemic of injuries that we are now experiencing. The severity of these hyperextension and axial compression injuries of the cervical spine can be deceptive for on X-ray an apparently minimal fracture of the anterior-superior margin of the body of the vertebra may be associated with severe and unremitting tetraplegia.

An unusual fracture of the spine possibly related to a seat belt injury is the Chance fracture which has already been discussed. This is probably a hyperflexion injury passing through the vertebral body and the vertebral pedicles or even the discal mobile segment 'pivoting' on the anterior abdominal wall. Its characteristics are obvious from discussion and plates already shown. Severe rotatory fracture dislocations of the lumbo-sacral junction or traumatic spondylolithesis are very uncommon, but occasionally are seen in paraplegic services. No doubt as time goes by the emphasis will change once again and further changes with new fractures and fracture-dislocations will be seen for in many different ways the human spine is being exposed to much greater trauma.

Another interesting and more common manifestation is the multiplicity of injuries in the spinal column. Some 5 per cent of injuries to the column will damage multiple vertebral levels and at all stages surgeons should watch for such multiple injuries, even with some five to six level skipping of the associated injuries.

Most vertebral fractures and dislocations heal well with good results. Functional restoration should be started early, and Nicoll[10] has shown extraordinary good results where, although reductions were not perfect, functional restoration was excellent. Early operations to restore perfect alignment carry risks in most centres, whilst early efforts at physical rehabi-

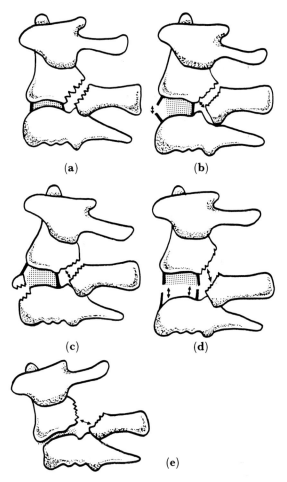

Fig 26.71 Progression of fracture in axis. (a) Fracture interarticularis. (b) Hyperextension with ligament and disc rupture. (c) Avulsion of bone anteriorly. (d) Disruption of C.2–3 space. (e) Forward migration C.2 on C.3 follows the injury. (By courtesy of Francis, W. R. & Fielding, J. W. (1978) *Orthopaedic Clinics of North America*, 9 (4): 1011.

litation do not. Prognosis is good in well over 85 per cent of cases. Residual lumbar pain can be kept to a minimum. With more social security and workers' compensation, as well as third party compensation, the psychological factor is greater than ever. To prevent social difficulties early attention to isometric muscle activity is paramount whilst vocational assistance is desirable.

REFERENCES

1. Macnab I 1977 Backache. Williams & Wilkins, Baltimore
2. Farfan H F 1973 Mechanical disorders of the low back. Lea & Febiger, Philadelphia
3. Macnab I, Harris R I 1952 Structural changes in lumbo-sacral region and their significance as causes of low back pain and sciatica. Journal of Bone and Joint Surgery 34-A: 1006
4. Mennell J 1952 The science and art of joint manipulation. Churchill, London, vols 1 & 2
5. Holdsworth F W 1963 Fractures, dislocations and fracture dislocations of the spine. Journal of Bone and Joint Surgery 45-B: 6
6. Beatson T R 1963 Fractures and dislocations of the cervical spine. Journal of Bone and Joint Surgery 45-B: 21
7. Marar B C 1974 Hyperextension injuries of cervical spine. Journal of Bone and Joint Surgery 56-A: 1655
8. Smith W S, Kaufer H 1969 Patterns and mechanisms of lumbar injuries associated with lap seat belts. Journal of Bone and Joint Surgery 51-A: 239
9. Holdsworth F W, and Hardy A G 1953 Early treatment of paraplegia from fractures of the thoraco-lumbar spine. Journal of Bone and Joint Surgery 35-B: 540
10. Nicoll E A 1949 Fractures of the dorsilumbar spine. Journal of Bone and Joint Surgery 31-B: 376
11. Nicoll E A 1948 Redevelopment of muscle function. Surgeons conference of the miner's welfare commission of 1947. Journal of Bone and Joint Surgery 30-B: 392
12. Southwick W O, Robinson R A 1957 Surgical approaches to vertebral bodies in cervical and lumbar area. Journal of Bone and Joint Surgery 39-A: 631
13. Evans D K 1961 Reduction of cervical dislocation. Journal of Bone and Joint Surgery 43-B: 552
14. Dickson J H, Harrington P R, Erwin W D 1978 Results of reduction and stabilisation of the severely fractured thoracic and lumbar spine. Journal of Bone and Joint Surgery 68-A: 799
15. Symposium of Upper Cervical Spine 1978 Orthopaedic Clinics of North America 9 (4)
16. Grogono B J S 1954 Injuries of atlas and axis. Journal of Bone and Joint Surgery 36-B: 397
17. Cornish B L 1968 Traumatic spondylolithesis of the axis. Journal of Bone and Joint Surgery 50-B: 31
18. Anderson L D, D'Alonzo R T 1974 Fractures of the odontoid process of the axis. Journal of Bone and Joint Surgery 56-A: 1663
19. Francis W R, Fielding J W 1978 Traumatic spondylolithesis of the axis. Orthopaedic Clinics of North America 9 (4): 1011

27

Injuries of the Spine with Paralysis complete or incomplete

Sir George Bedbrook

Spinal injury associated with complete or incomplete paralysis has been recorded for thousands of years. The hopelessness and helplessness experienced by patient and doctor until the present time was expressed by the writer of the Edwin Smith Surgical Papyrus in 1700 BC when he indicated that it was 'an ailment not to be treated'. Despite sporadic records, as that in the second book of Samuel where Mephibosheth (Saul's grandson) having sustained a spinal injury was rehabilitated, the air of despondency, complacency and misery, with universal complications persisted until about four decades ago. The outcome was death in 85 per cent of cases usually the result of urinary infection, septicaemia and bedsores, whilst a few lingered in institutions from which as many medical personnel as possible kept away.

Pioneers such as Munro in Boston, Botterell in Toronto and particularly Guttmann in England then showed that pessimism was unfounded. Gowland[1] from the Star and Garter Home for Paraplegics expressed this pessimism when he wrote 'Enough sedatives must be given to counteract the shock which is intensified by contemplating years of inaction and invalidism; more morphine, atropine and hyoscine is used in this place than in any other place of the same size'. The present position is exactly the opposite, optimism, little sedatives, complications reduced and a healthy and productive future.

Munro of Boston,[2] one of the great pioneers, said: 'If they have good upper limbs and are intelligent they can be assured of an ability to walk though perhaps with appliances; they will gain complete 24-hour control of the bladder and bowel; and they will earn their own livings and lead an almost normal life'. Surely this is an amazing reversal of attitude; a reversal now generally accepted and acknowledged. Unlike the sole survivor of traumatic paraplegia from the First World War, of the 4000 American soldiers paralysed from spinal injury in the Second World War, more than 2000 survived and of these, 80 per cent became able to walk and to hold down jobs. In Toronto, Botterell and his colleagues resettled paraplegics, many of them driving their own cars to the city and getting about not only with wheelchairs but with such crutch walking as is needed for an active life.[3] Even more remarkable results have been gained by Guttmann[4] at the Stoke Mandeville Hospital near London. Not only did he restore neglected decubitus ulcers, contractures of joints and spasm of the lower limbs in patients with traumatic paraplegia of long standing, but above all he inspired them with a new faith and new hope. Guttmann's major advance was to advocate early admission to comprehensive units under management of well trained physicians or surgeons. He was followed by Holdsworth and Hardy and now in most parts of the World the atmosphere of new hope engendered by these great pioneers has spread and continues to do so.

The incidence of spinal cord injury is estimated at between 35 and 80 per million of population per year in most nations and as yet shows no signs of reduction. Prevention of this incidence is a goal to be strived for, since most cases are caused by motor vehicle trauma, sports injuries and home accidents as well as industrial trauma. The proportion varies as does the character of the community. For example, in mining communities industrial accidents are a common cause, whilst in other areas motor vehicle trauma can be dominant. In most countries during the last two decades lumbo-dorsal injury has waned whilst cervico-dorsal injuries have increased—and this is directly related to the mounting epidemic of road traffic accidents, and to the increased incidences and severity of sports injuries.

COMPREHENSIVE UNITS FOR THE TREATMENT OF SPINAL INJURY

Whilst these units were advocated prior to 1940 by Riddoch in the United Kingdom and Gallie and Munro in North America it was not until Guttmann[4] was invited by the British Ministry of Pensions to open such a unit in Britain that the first really comprehensive spinal injury centre in England was opened at Stoke Mandeville. Whilst spinal units had previously been opened before 1940 they were not truly comprehensive as they did not admit patients immediately after injury, and were therefore not responsible for their complete management. In a comprehensive unit early admission is essential, and not so to admit a spinal paralytic must be regarded as less than adequate care.

Such management must be multidisciplinary since the paraplegic patient needs the expertise of many specialities in medicine. A symposium on spinal units in 1967[5] stressed the importance of such care and also stressed how some specialists will be required to concentrate all or much of their time on this care. Thus Guttmann and Botterell emphasised the development of a new specialty either as an entirely independent entity, or as a super specialty superimposed on some other specialisation in medicine. The results of this type of management can be quite extraordinary when compared to no comprehensive care, and the results are comparable to other areas of great disability—70 per cent back to work, 75 per cent at home, 70 to 75 per cent at least without complications, an almost normal life span, reduction in hospital time from years to a few months, invalidism reduced and a life worth living. Not only is early admission essential but specialised long term extended care is needed to maintain the good health and physical fitness now possible. Organisations such as paraplegic associations have contributed greatly to this 'final responsibility to emergency' (Bedbrook),[6] whilst Guttmann[7] has emphasised both acute and extended care in his essay 'Total Responsibility of the Surgeon in the Rehabilitation of the Spinal Paralysed and other Severely Disabled' given to the Royal Australasian College of Surgeons Jubilee Seminar on Rehabilitation. Piecemeal and dichotomised care between consultants can no longer be accepted as satisfactory.

PATHOLOGY AND NEUROLOGY

The clear exposition of pathological change and its relation to neurological change in spinal injuries remains the basis of all care. Kakulas and Bedbrook[8] and Jellinger[9] have shown that in the first 24 hours after injury, necropsy has not infrequently shown little or no neural damage, clinically, some of these will account for the syndrome of concussion with good recovery. Spinal injury with neurological involvement shows a galaxy of pathological changes, ranging from extradural haemorrhage with petechial haemorrhages within the cord in 'minor cases', to gross dehiscense of the neural tube and dura with evidence of cord crushing, central necrosis, subarachnoid haemorrhage, shredding of nerve roots both in the area normally occupied by the cord as well as in the cauda equina. The lesion has always a longitudinal as well as a sagittal and coronal dimension (see Fig 27.1a and b), and it is important that the three dimensional macroscopic nature of the spinal cord injury should be 'visualised' by the physician. Rarely in cases at postmortem is continuing cord compression observed, and the amount of neural damage has no relationship to the X-ray appearances of the injury and cannot be estimated accurately by the X-ray findings. Factors to be considered in the clinico-pathological estimation include:

1. The degree of trauma.
2. The patho-dynamics of the injury.
3. The observed state of associated injuries.
4. The classification of the injury—whether the force has been expended across a disc space (flexion and extension injuries) or absorbed in a vertebral body (compression injury).
5. An accurate neurological examination.

Factors not easily estimated are the normal anatomical relationship between canal and cord whereby a big cord in a small canal is much more vulnerable, such as in the aged patients where cervical spondylosis has reduced the canal size.

The pathological and clinical classification, simple yet clinically useful that has evolved from Holdsworths early definition of stable and unstable injuries is thus.

	Bony	*Neural*
Stable {	Compression or depression	Haemorrhage necrosis Stretching increasing to
	Extension and rotation	Disruption
	Flexion and rotation	Crushing

Unstable injuries usually only occur in the flexion-rotation group and then only in those with greater than one third displacement in either sagittal or coronal planes. The unilateral fracture dislocation is stable with no great reduction in neural canal capacity.

Bilateral fracture dislocations will be unstable in 10 per cent of cases (after good initial reduction without recourse to surgery). In such cases the neural canal capacity is very reduced until reduction is effected.

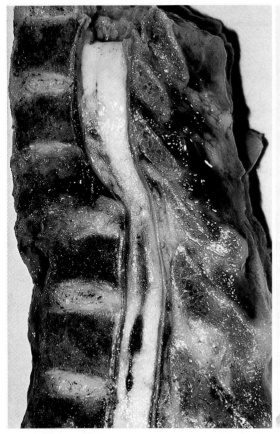 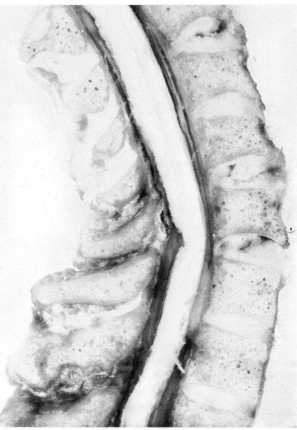

Fig 27.1a. Acute flexion compression injury of cervical spine shows that the anterior ligamentous structures are intact. There is gross extradural haemorrhage, longitudinal cord damage, cord necrosis and multiple level injuries.

Fig 27.1b. Acute hyperextension injury emphasising the multiplicity of level as well as other features already stressed

Pathological changes are progressive for a period of days after the injury as the chemical and toxic factors are cumulative. Experimentally, anoxia, hypotension and hormonal chemicals have been proven as being the cause of such progression. As yet these factors are not proven in the human injury but the following progressive changes have been shown to occur:

1. Extension of haemorrhagic necrosis.
2. Colliquative necrosis.
3. Early cyst formation.
4. Microscopic and macroscopic Wallerian changes.
5. Nerve root regeneration in areas of axonotmesis.

In the cervico-dorsal area intact neural fibres of C8, T1 passing through the damaged area can recover whilst in the lumbo-dorsal area three theoretical groups exist as illustrated in Figure 27.2 accounting for the neural differences in some fractures and fracture dislocations with apparently, similar radiological appearances.

In cervical and thoracic injuries upper motor neurone manifestations with increased tendon reflex spasm and reflex visceral responses will be manifest, whilst lumbar injuries will show lower the motor neuron changes of flaccidity with paralysis and a flaccid bladder. In a few cervico-dorsal and most lumbo-dorsal injuries both upper motor neuron and lower motor neuron manifestations will occur (see Fig 27.2). This is a feature of the three dimensional state.

Neurological conditions after spinal cord injury must always

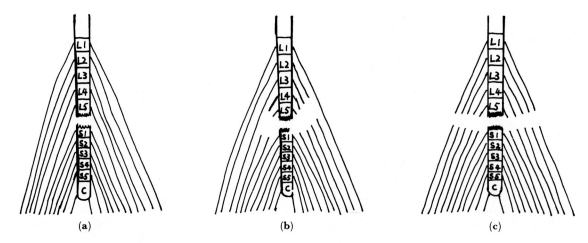

Fig 27.2 The possible effects on the spinal cord and nerve roots of a fracture-dislocation at the thoraco-lumbar junction. (a) Complete cord division. Nerves intact. (b) Complete cord division. Partial nerve division. (c) Complete cord division. Complete nerve division.

be assessed remembering the three dimensions of the pathological state.

Any neurological sparing on admission is a manifestation of incompleteness, e.g. sparing in the saddle area of the perineum means that excellent visceral return of function will occur. But patients with an injury in any area of the spine, particularly at the lumbo-dorsal level, where paralysis (both sensory and motor below an intact neurological segment) is still complete six to eight hours after admission will usually remain so. However, in the cervico-dorsal area caution must be expressed, as very soon after injury sensory or motor sparing may disappear and this can mean that the examiner at 12 to 16 hours can miss initial sparing and thus be misled in the prognosis. Some 10 to 15 per cent of such cases may show neurological recovery (see Tables 27.1 and 27.2).

The clinical classification (see Fig 27.3) now used is:

A. Complete paralysis.
B. Sensory paralysis only.
C. Motor paralysis useless (less than 2—Medical Research Council).
D. Motor paralysis useful (greater than 2).
E. Recovery.

Using such criteria the lesions can be determined as:

1. Complete
2. Incomplete; and the incomplete paralysis can be

Table 27.1 Review of spinal injuries with paraplegia. Neurological state on admission and discharge

	Admission		Discharge	
	Incomplete	Complete	Incomplete	Complete
A. Cervical	65%	35%	78%	22%
B. Dorsal	22%	78%	30%	70%
C. Lumbo-dorsal	35%	65%	43%	57%

Table 27.2 Neurological sequelae of spinal cord injury

Cervical cases	
Useful recovery	41%
Useful recovery in incomplete cases	48%
Useful recovery in complete cases	18%
Lumbo-dorsal cases	
Useful recovery overall	36%
Useful recovery in incomplete cases	80%
Useful recovery in complete cases	11%

further subdivided (see Table 27.3) into:
a. Central cord.
b. Anterior cord.
c. Posterior cord.
d. Hemi-cord (Brown Sequard).

Careful repeated clinical neurological examination enables the examiner to follow the pathological changes. Such evaluation when correlated to methods of care have shown that no specific procedure or operation yet devised has altered the natural history of this pathological sequence. When non operative methods are used there is indeed a little evidence that

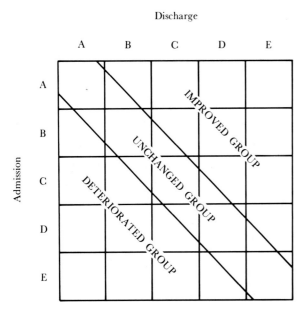

Discharge

Fig 27.3 The grid method of Frankel to evaluate neurological status in spinal cord injury. A = complete paralysis; B = sensory paralysis only; C = motor paralysis useless; D = motor paralysis useful; E = Recovery. (Reproduced by kind permission of the Editor of the *Journal of Bone and Joint Surgery* (1979) 61-B, 369).

Guttmann's[10] and Young and Dexter's[11] conservative methods give slightly better results.

Because the nervous system is plastic and compensatory time shows great adaptation even after complete paralysis. The incomplete cases change neurologically over one to two years, whilst even complete cases via compensatory neuromuscular mechanisms (e.g. in Latissimus Dorsi), or by the autonomic nervous pathways, may show useful return of sensory response to conscious stimuli.

FUNCTIONAL DISABILITIES AND EXPECTATIONS

Clearly the neurological level of the lesion in spinal cord injuries will determine the physical limitation. Impairment of some (or all) of the activities of daily living can be expected. These will include:

1. Personal hygiene, including visceral function.
2. Ambulation (walking with or without crutches and orthoses, or by wheelchair).
3. Transfers (e.g. movement on and off beds, chairs and toilets, in and out of cars).
4. Dressing.
5. Eating.
6. Communicating (either by writing, typewriter or telephone).

Table 27.3 Summary of clinico-pathological correlation in spinal cord injuries. (From *Paraplegia* 4:54 (1967). Reproduced by kind permission of the editor of *Paraplegia*.)

Pathological		Clinical	Treatment
Neuro	Bony		
Haematomyelia or central necrosis	Vertical compression	Anterior cord syndrome Central cord syndrome Lateral cord syndrome Post. cord syndrome Complete syndrome	Conservative (rarely open reduction)
Crushing of cord	Flexion rotation — Extension rotation		
Longitudinal changes (a) Necrosis (b) Extra-dural Haemorrhage (c) Early cysts	3 or more variable vertebral fractures of all above types	Complete lumbar syndrome Incomplete cervical syndromes Extensive L.M.N. lesion with U.M.N. signs in lower limbs	Conservative
Continuing compression by: (a) Haemorrhage (b) Bony	without above as above	Paresis becoming complete	Open decompression Closed reduction
Nil	Unstable after 3 months non-union	Varies greatly	Reduction Grafting
Thrombosis of cord vessels Arterial insufficiency	Any of the bony problems	Paraplegia late onset without block	Conservative

In the rehabilitation process, many of the disabilities originally present can be completely or partially restored through adaptive techniques, devices and training, and the final level of performance will be characterised by: (i) Complete independence; (ii) Requiring standby assistance; (iii) Requiring physical assistance; (iv) Total dependence.

Common disabilities. At all injury levels genital functions are impaired. Adjustments in sexual activity will therefore be required, particularly in the male. Ability to achieve and sustain an erection depends on the viability of the portion of the cord distal to the injury. In upper motor neuron lesions reflex genital activity can be achieved but in lower motor neuron lesions, this is lost.

Sacral lesions (S.2 to S.4). Only bowel and bladder function is initially impaired. With appropriate treatment, control of the bowel can be achieved and the bladder can be satisfactorily emptied by the methods of strain and manual expression (crede*). Incontinence may still be a problem particularly if bladder neck surgery is required to effect satisfactory residual volumes. The male may have to wear an external appliance.

Lumbo-sacral lesions (L.4 to S.1). Control of bowel and bladder can usually be obtained in the same fashion as described above. Independence in walking is also restored with the assistance of two canes or two crutches and often with the use of short leg braces (ankle-foot orthoses). Prolonged standing may remain impaired but no wheelchair is necessary.

Lumbar lesions (L.1 to L.3). Bowel and bladder function can likewise be controlled. If sacral reflexes are present, these may be employed to assist with evacuation. The bladder may be emptied by stimulating these reflexes such as by tapping or anal dilatation. If resistance at the external urethral sphincter impedes adequate bladder emptying and urethral sphincter/detrusor dyssynergia exists, sphincterotomy may be required. Walking in long leg braces (knee–ankle–foot orthoses) and with crutches is possible for short distances. Wheelchairs are also used in which the patient can be expected to become completely independent.

Thoracic lesions (T.7 to T.12). The bowel and bladder are usually always of an upper motor neuron type and evacuation is as described above. Complete independence in bowel and bladder function is

achieved and independence in walking in long-leg braces can usually be achieved unless deformities in the lower extremities are present. While possible, walking is none the less very strenuous and patients fatigue quickly. Therefore for complete independence a wheelchair is necessary. With training, transfers, dressing and driving also become independent.

Thoracic lesions (T.2 to T.6). Bowel and bladder are managed as described above. Patients in this category require a wheelchair as their main means of ambulation. With extensive treatment, they can become independent in all activities of daily living.

Cervical lesions (C.7 to T.1). Bowel and bladder evacuation is achieved as above. The bladder in quadriplegics is likely to be more reflexly active and therefore incontinence is virtually always a problem. While males may well require external collection devices at lower levels, they are a virtual necessity in all patients at this level or above. Female patients present a difficult problem since satisfactory external collection devices are not available at present. In some instances, it is necessary to resort to an indwelling catheter, albeit with much reluctance. The patients rely on a wheelchair for their primary means of transportation and almost all can become completely independent in all activities of daily living consistent with the ability to live alone. Some however, either because of deformities weakness, obesity or other medical problems, may require partial physical assistance.

Cervical lesions (C.6). Only a small number of patients achieve complete independence in all functions. Living alone is not practical as the majority require partial physical assistance for all their activities of daily living with the exception of eating and communicating (and in some instances—driving). While patients in this class are able to propel a manual wheelchair with modified handrims, it is very difficult and tiresome. For this reason, if ramps and grades are routinely encountered in their environment, an electric wheelchair may also be required.

Cervical lesion (C.5). All patients in this category will require assistance for all activities of daily living and living alone again is not possible. Once transferred to their electric wheelchair, they should be independent in wheelchair ambulation.

Cervical lesions (above C.5). Total dependence is also to be expected and in addition, breathing function is impaired, and the use of special respiratory equipment is required. Propulsion in an electric wheelchair is possible for some patients with appropriate chin or mouth pieces.

---

*After Credé (Karl Siegmund Franz)—a Leipzig gynaecologist of the last century, who described a manoeuvre to express the placenta by pressure on the abdomen.

FIRST AID AND EMERGENCY CARE

The earliest responsibility for the management of a patient immediately after an accident usually falls to a person trained in first aid or occasionally to a doctor. The first duty of the doctor or first-aider is to preserve life by controlling haemorrhage and maintaining an airway. The second responsibility is to remove the patient from continuing harmful effects of the accident, such as surf, drowning and injury by falling masonry or, in the case of road traffic accidents, injury by other vehicles (often preventable by the proper use of bystanders in directing traffic). If the patient has to be moved quickly before diagnosis has been completed an attempt should be made to maintain spinal rigidity. With great gentleness the patient is moved to a safe area and postured supine with neck traction, the head kept low to allow fluid (usually water or stomach contents) to drain out of the respiratory tract.

Diagnosis by the first attendant should be careful and thorough in elucidating the spinal injury, the paralysis and the associated injuries. Having completed this then the initial medical attendant must consider two matters. First, he must arrange immediate admission within a few hours to a comprehensive unit, even if this means use of aircraft. Such admission is urgent and much better than going to the local hospital, except in transit to await suitable transport. In many areas of the world suitable evacuation systems already exist and are well known to accident authorities. It is wrong to admit, except very temporarily, a seriously injured person with spinal injuries to a hospital—albeit the nearest—which has not a comprehensive unit. The early days of management will determine urinary complications, pressure problems and even the possibility of neural recovery. Remoteness is no excuse as communications are now possible for thousands of miles where advice and help can be sought. The flying doctor service in Australia and commercial flights can bring patients 1500 miles (2400 kilometres) to the spinal units in less than eight hours. Secondly, he must appreciate that the correct arrangement for transport and movement are vital as there is now evidence from Dublin and Chicago that prompt efficient evacuation results in a greater number of incomplete cases with better prognosis.

In moving a patient with spinal injury and paralysis from where he lies to a stretcher, ambulance or aeroplane, the essential principle of first aid treatment is to keep the spine in the neutral position, neither flexed nor extended. It is dangerous to lift a patient who is lying on his back by the shoulders and hips because the spine then sags between the points of support and the forced flexion that results may further crush the spinal cord. If the patient is in a prone or face-down position, such lifting is relatively harmless because the spinal column is extended, and in some fracture-dislocations extension of the spine reduces the displacement and relieves the possibility of compression of the cord. Many years ago transportation prone was advised of all patients with suspected spinal injury. This is clearly, not regularly advisable. There is sometimes danger if the spine is forcibly extended, especially in lumbar fracture-dislocation with interlocked facets, and also in cervical injuries. Thus the first aid worker should do all he can to keep the spine straight, neither flexed nor extended simply padding the normal curves. If possible a flat board or stretcher should be placed alongside the patient, who is lifted onto it by male assistants taking support of the head, neck, thoracic, lumbar pelvis and thigh regions, keeping the spine in the neutral position throughout the lifting as laid down in the St. John Ambulance First Aid Manual. Once the patient is on the stretcher he should not again be lifted from it until surgical and radiographic examination has disclosed the exact site of injury and the type of displacement.

When early admission to a comprehensive unit within a few hours is possible no further treatment may be needed but beware (a) the distended bladder and (b) the problem of pressure. During diagnosis the first aider and doctor must record bladder fullness by percussion. If empty then defer emptying by catheter as oliguria has or will occur but if full and percussible, empty by simple sterile catheterisation at nearest hospital with facilities. *An overdistended bladder—made worse if a parental intravenous infusion is started—can result in bladder atony that may not recover.* If an intravenous drip is to be continued a catheter must be inserted using careful sterile techniques. But remember that a catheter which has been left indwelling because of the use of intravenous resuscitation will only remain sterile for up to 48 hours and must then be changed.

Four hours in any one position may allow skin necrosis. Therefore after two hours the patient must be turned onto the side posture, moving in one piece and maintaining a neutral position of spine and limbs by using pillows. *No plaster of paris should be used*; if transport is delayed for some hours then two-hourly changes of posture must be immediately organised. It is also important to properly cleanse and completely undress the patient at this stage because other injuries may become apparent.

CLINICAL ASSESSMENT

All spinal injuries with neural involvement need a very accurate clinical examination after admission to the emergency room or to the comprehensive unit. Frequently records show that this is not done, nor are the results well recorded. Such an omission can have serious consequences—an incomplete lesion can be missed, or associated injuries overlooked.

First, a thorough general examination. If hypotension and anoxia are discovered these should be corrected after estimating the blood gases, by extra nasal oxygen therapy and by the use of blood substitutes in intravenous fluids. All paraplegics and tetraplegics lose vasomotor tone temporarily, having a normal blood volume in an enlarged vascular compartment. Bandaging legs and an abdominal binder are useful procedures in combatting this vascular disorder.

Neurological examination. Remembering the detailed myotome and dermatome segmental distribution a detailed neural examination by an experienced clinician is essential. It is not enough to just ask the patient to move voluntarily or to roughly test sensory levels. Each muscle group must be tested and each dermatome checked for all sensory modalities, particularly the sacral segments (see Figs 27.4a, b and c). All reflexes must be tested carefully—the slightest voluntary movement or sensation below the level of cord lesion is certain evidence of cord continuity with better prognosis. If the paralysis is complete after eight hours together with symmetrical returning reflexes and priapism in the male—an unfavourable prognosis is to be expected, particularly in lumbo-dorsal injuries.

Reflex activity. The return of any reflex activity below the level of the lesion is certain evidence that spinal shock has passed in those segments and therefore any remaining paralysis and anaesthesia may be due to damage to long tracts or cauda equina. If there is total sensory and motor paralysis of the trunk and lower limbs persistent for more then eight hours, the reappearance of reflex activity in the trunk or legs is evidence that the distal part of the spinal cord has been separated from cerebral control by severance of the cord. Of these reflexes the three most important are:

1. The anal reflex—a stimulus to the perineum causes contraction of the external anal sphincter.
2. The bulbo cavernosus reflex—compression of the glans penis or labia causes contraction of the pubo rectalis muscle, and

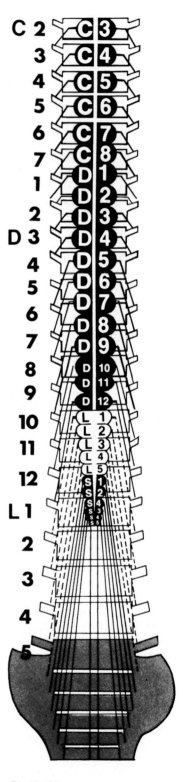

Fig 27.4(a)

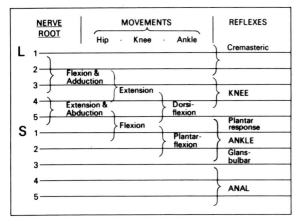

NERVE ROOT	MOVEMENTS			REFLEXES
	Hip · Knee · Ankle			
L 1				Cremasteric
2	Flexion & Adduction			
3		Extension		KNEE
4	Extension & Abduction		Dorsi-flexion	
5		Flexion		Plantar response
S 1			Plantar-flexion	ANKLE
2				Glans-bulbar
3				
4				ANAL
5				

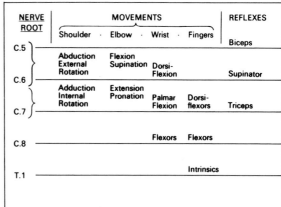

NERVE ROOT	MOVEMENTS				REFLEXES
	Shoulder ·	Elbow ·	Wrist ·	Fingers	
C.5					Biceps
	Abduction External Rotation	Flexion Supination	Dorsi-Flexion		
C.6					Supinator
	Adduction Internal Rotation	Extension Pronation	Palmar Flexion	Dorsi-flexors	Triceps
C.7					
C.8			Flexors	Flexors	
T.1				Intrinsics	

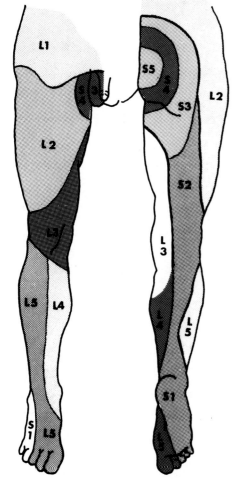

Fig 27.4(b)

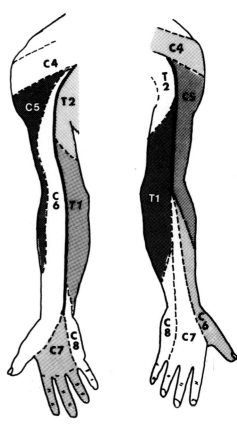

Fig 27.4(c)

Fig 27.4 Relation of segments of the spinal cord and nerve-roots to the vertebral bodies. (a) This diagram shows the relationship of segments of the spinal cord and the emerging nerve roots to the vertebral bodies. Note that all the lumbar segments of the spinal cord are concentrated at the level of the tenth dorsal to the first lumbar vertebrae. (Acknowledgement to the late Sir Frank Holdsworth and Dr A. G. Hardy.) (b) Sensory and motor distribution of the lumbo-sacral nerve roots. (c) Sensory and motor distribution of the brachial plexus nerve roots.

The tables show the motor distribution of corresponding nerve roots and the reflexes associated with them.

3. The plantar response, either extensor or flexor—
a stimulus to the sole of the foot causes movement
of the great toe.

After transection of the cord, despite spinal shock,
one or more of these reflexes may re-appear quite
early, or indeed they may never disappear at all. It is,
therefore, usually possible to know within a few
hours, from the association of a complete motor and
sensory paralysis with such reflexes, that the spinal
cord has been divided.

Radiology. Having checked the clinical bony lesion
by careful palpation and looked for multiplicity in
levels (5 to 10 per cent of cases), accurate radiology
is essential to help build up for the examiner a three
dimensional picture of the bony lesion.

Radiographs should include *at first* antero-posterior,
lateral and obliques of the injured area. When these
are checked remember such views demonstrate a
partly reduced condition. Particular attention must
be paid to C.1–2 and C.7, T.1 because visualisation of
these sites is sometimes inadequate. The interspinous
spaces should be examined carefully for ligament
damage. Occasionally sagittal and coronal tomography may be undertaken to obtain more detail of bony
damage, and later axial tomography may be useful to
give details if loose fragments of bone are suspected.

Myelography has not proved of value in assisting
with early diagnosis as subarachnoid and extra dural
oedema and haemorrhage are usually present. Pathologically, after adequate reduction and also in those
cases not needing reduction, the presence of a space-
occupying lesion (such as a disc prolapse, or protrusion
of a loose bone fragment) is extremely rare in the
series described. Routine myelography results vary,
for the spinal block fluctuates and is rarely caused by
remediable pathology.

Using normal anatomical knowledge (see Fig 27.4)
radiological and clinical correlation must then be
carefully undertaken, remembering that rarely are
both sides symmetrical in either cervico-dorsal or
lumbo-dorsal injuries (Table 27.3). In fracture
dislocations of the thoracic spine (above the tenth
thoracic vertebra) the level of bone injury of the
vertebra as determined by radiographic examination
corresponds accurately with the level of spinal cord
injury as shown by neurological examination. In
fracture dislocations between the tenth dorsal and
first lumbar vertebrae there is usually disparity in the
level of bone injury, as shown radiologically, and by
the clinical signs of a two finger gap in interspinous
ligaments, and the level of nerve injury, as shown by

neurological examination. When this is so it is an
indication that in addition to damage to the spinal
cord there has also been damage to the nerve roots.

Let us take two simple examples;
1. If there is a fracture dislocation of the spine as
shown by radiographs between the 12th thoracic and
first lumbar vertebra, and if the neurological examination reveals a complete motor and sensory paraplegia from the 'first' lumbar neurological segment
downwards, then the nerve damage is from transection of the cord at the first sacral segment together
with injury to all the lumbar nerve roots. The first
sacral segment of the cord is opposite the fracture
dislocation, as are all the lumbar nerve roots (see Fig
27.4).
2. If there is a similar fracture dislocation of the 12th
thoracic vertebra and neurological examination
reveals a complete paraplegia from the first sacral
segment downwards, then again there has been
division of the cord at the first sacral segment, but in
this instance all the lumbar roots have escaped
damage. Figures 27.2a and c illustrate the two lesions.
The former shows complete root escape, and the latter
complete root division.

Many variations of root escape can occur and may
be detected with care. For example, neurological
examination of a patient with the lesion illustrated in
Figure 27.2b would reveal a greater loss of sensation
and motor power on the right side than on the left,
corresponding to the greater number of damaged
roots on the right side. Complete paraplegia at and
below the first sacral segment is due to injury to the
cord. Thus it is possible to distinguish between cord
and root damage.

The lumbar nerve roots are of great importance
for they control hip flexion, knee extension and much
of the sensation of the leg (Fig 27.4). Root escape or
recovery from injury may make all the difference
between a permanent wheelchair existence and a
more vigorous life of standing and walking, and
therefore every endeavour must be made to protect
the nerve roots from further injury. Very rarely relief
from further neural compression is needed, but
usually careful postural nursing suffices. Surgery was
introduced in an attempt to help recovery, however
in practice such surgery has not proved useful. It
must be declared as forcefully as possible that
operations involving internal fixation of the fracture
dislocation of the spine can never be a substitute for
good nursing. The first and most essential part of the
treatment of a paraplegic patient is to nurse him in
such a way that good posture is maintained and no
pressure sores or contractures occur and no urinary

infection develops. It is unfortunate that recently progress should have been retarded by some surgeons[15] who have thought that no problem of nursing would arise if operations were performed for internal fixation of the fractured spine.

Summary of neurological and radiographic investigation

1. Spinal concussion causes motor and sensory paralysis below the level of injury, but the motor and sensory disturbance is nearly always incomplete and usually there are signs of recovery within a few hours.

2. Injury to the cord and nerve roots at the low cervical level. At the cervico-dorsal junction there are usually combined injuries of the cord and nerve roots.

Injury below the 5th cervical level. If there is injury leaving C.5 intact (usually C.4 on C.5) the arms exhibit complete motor and sensory paralysis rarely symmetrical. Trunk and lower limbs are paralysed whilst respiration is by diaphragm only.

Injury below the 6th cervical level. With an intact C.6 (usually C.5 on C.6) deltoid, biceps and radial wrist extensors are intact with sensation laterally to thumb and index. Whilst C.6 is usually spared in C.6 on C.7 dislocation, C.7 may also be partially spared thus some triceps action may be present.

Injury below 7th cervical level. With C.7 intact only the long flexors and intrinsics are paralysed, long extensors are intact giving a man en griffe hand. Sensation is deficient in ulna side of arm only.

Injury below 8th cervical level leaves a good hand with only intrinsic paralysis and a claw hand.

3. Complete damage of the thoracic cord. This causes complete sensory, motor and visceral paralysis. At first isolated cord function is overshadowed by spinal shock, with suppression of reflex activity in the distal separated part of the cord so that paralysis is flaccid, reflexes are suppressed, and the flaccid bladder spontaneously functions only by overflow incontinence. But within a few hours reflex activity, as in the spinal or decerebrate animal, becomes apparent in the reappearance of anal and glans-bulbar reflexes associated with motor and sensory loss beyond the level of injury. Within a few days or weeks, full reflex activity in the separated part of the cord is established perhaps with spasticity of muscles and a tendency to contracture, and with reflex emptying of the bladder.

4. Complete damage of the lumbar nerve roots of the cauda equina. In the lumbar spine this causes loss of sensation and flaccid paralysis with an isolated lower motor neuron bladder, at first with overflow incontinence and then imperfect emptying of the bladder by crede and myoneural reflex activity. Whereas recovery is impossible after transection of the spinal cord, complete recovery may occur from injury to the nerve roots of the cauda equina if axontomesis exists.

5. Crushing of the thoraco-lumbar cord, as well as the nerve roots alongside at the tenth thoracic to the second lumbar level. This is perhaps the greatest problem because it is sustained at the site where fracture dislocations occur most frequently—the thoraco lumbar junction of the spine. Disparity in the level of the nerve lesion as between the radiographic and neurological study will distinguish between the cord and root damage. Persistent total loss of power and sensation below the level of cord damage, especially with return of reflex activity in these segments, indicates transection of the cord, (an irrecoverable injury), but the root paralysis and anaesthesia may recover. Sensory sparing is more common immediately. Whether or not the roots have been damaged they must be protected by careful posturing after fracture dislocation, because they make the difference between a wheelchair life and a life of reasonable walking with crutches. Bladder function may be expected to be restored by training.

Having carefully correlated the clinical features with the radiological features the surgeon should then be able to make a specific clinico pathological diagnosis as described by Michaelis[12] (see Table 27.3 for example).

'The patient has a flexion rotation unilateral fracture dislocation of C.5 on C.6 with complete paralysis below C.6' (meaning C.6 is the lowest intact neural segment) or 'the patient has a compression fracture of T.10 with incomplete paralysis below T.10' (meaning that T.10 is the lowest totally intact neural segment).

Further details can be added as the three-dimensional cord picture is built up, whilst description of the bony lesion can include whether the spine is likely to be stable or unstable clinically, according to whether the ligamentous and facetal bony dislocation are together great enough to suspect this (see Fig 27.5a and b).

Spinal cord injuries in children show that 50 per cent do not have bony injuries on original examination—beware the flaccid neonate—particularly after breech delivery—some are spinal column and cord injuries.

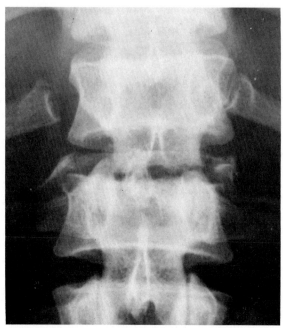

Fig 27.5a Fracture-dislocation of the thoraco-lumbar spine produced by rotational force with a 'slice fracture' of the vertebra associated with injury to the apophysial joints. Evidence that the injury was produced by rotational violence is shown in the dislocation of the twelfth rib on the left side. This type of fracture-dislocation can be unstable. (Reproduced by courtesy of the late Sir Frank Holdsworth.)

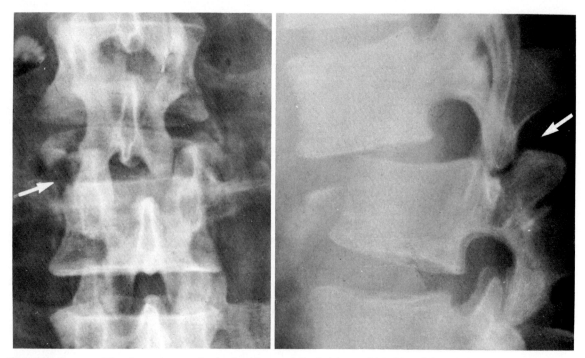

Fig. 27.5b Fracture-dislocation at the upper lumbar level from rotational violence with locking of the articular processes. Such fracture dislocation cannot be reduced by simple posture unless the pedicles are also fractured and may need (a) closed reduction (b) occasionally open reduction.

Associated injuries to trunk and limbs are not uncommon and can only be diagnosed by careful clinical examination, particularly palpation of bony and joint margins and careful assessment of residual voluntary movement and passive mobility.

EARLY MANAGEMENT

The literature on early management of spinal injuries with paraplegia is dominated by an argument, now over 100 years old, as to whether early surgery is of value. As yet no one has shown that early surgical endeavours have helped either in greater neurological recovery, or that spinal function and mobility is definitely improved by such procedures. On the contrary, many, particularly Guttmann[10], Morgan et al[13], Bedbrook[14] and Sussman[15] have shown that ill-advised, but even adequate surgery can cause extra complications to occur. These include greater spinal deformity, increased neurological damage, rigid spines and increased general complications such as urinary infection and thrombosis. The key word for management when a patient is admitted should be *prevention*. Prevention of deformity, prevention of urinary infection, prevention of pressure areas, prevention of debilitation, prevention of loss of further muscle power, prevention of respiratory and thrombotic episodes. Each method of care must coordinate with the others, and dominance of one method must be avoided.

MANAGEMENT OF THE SPINE

Stable injuries such as compression fracture–subluxations and hyperextension injuries need only treatment by the postural methods discussed under nursing care (see Figs 27.6 to 27.8). Flexion rotation injuries with displacement should be managed in a progressive manner always and there is no hurry to advise a surgical procedure. Gross dislocations clearly need reduction urgently.

Positioning in bed. The patient is first put into a normal postural supine position and later the lateral position with the aid of pillows (see Figs 27.6 and 27.7). Even if the dislocation is to be reduced later using other methods, postural methods must be introduced first, for *they are the basis of all care.* Turning two hourly must be started immediately.

Reduction of displacement. Gross fracture dislocations may be reduced by either of two methods.

Firstly, rapid reduction using re-positioning and manipulation under general anaesthesia, and in the cervical column such a procedure is perfectly safe in the hands of experienced surgeons[16] (see Chapter 26). Under full relaxation anaesthesia and intubation a suitable cranial caliper (Crutchfield forceps) is applied usually anterior to the inter mastoid line. When this has been fixed an appropriate manipulation is carried out as described by Walton many years ago. In bilateral facet dislocations this is achieved by traction and gentle flexion at 35° to 45° to unlock the dislocation and then extension to complete the reduction. In unilateral facet dislocations traction with lateral and forward flexion away from the dislocated side followed by extension will reduce the displacement. By these means the neural canal will be restored almost to normality and the cord, which rarely occupies more than 50 per cent of the canal capacity, will be given adequate room to expand with oedema. These methods are also applicable to the lumbo-dorsal spine by using trunk-pelvis distraction under anaesthesia in flexion and then unlocking by extension.[16] No experienced clinician has reported permanent neural deterioration as a result of this treatment, although in lumbo-dorsal injuries there may be a temporary, two-segment deterioration.

The alternative method is by slow reduction and is the one commonly used after 24 to 48 hours and in patients for whom anaesthesia is contraindicated. In cervico-dorsal injuries calipers are applied to the skull under local anaesthetic, and in lumbo-dorsal injuries pelvic traction as for the application of a corrective scoliosis jacket. Traction in flexion up to 35° is maintained using sedation and increasing weights, with half to one hour X-ray controls, until the fracture dislocation has been distracted and unlocked. Then, carefully maintaining traction, the posture is changed to extension to 'relock' and maintain the reduction (see Chapter 26).

Those patients with gross fracture dislocations of either cervico-dorsal or lumbo-dorsal area who have fractures through the pedicles and vertebral body, usually reduce without traction when sedation and adequate posture is instituted, and need only (in cervico-dorsal injuries), cervical traction and extension to be maintained. However, the surgeon must always treat each condition individually, and the method chosen will depend upon careful assessment and accurate diagnosis. It will not necessarily be similar in all cases.

Thoracic fracture dislocations between T.2 and T.10 are normally stable and cannot be reduced conservatively because of the stabilising influence of

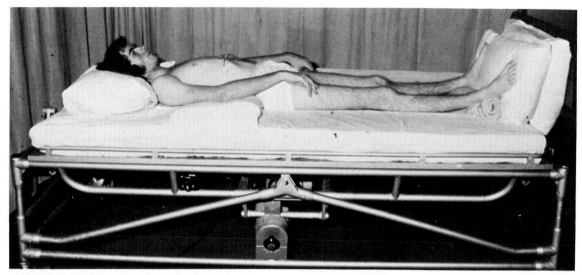

Fig 27.6

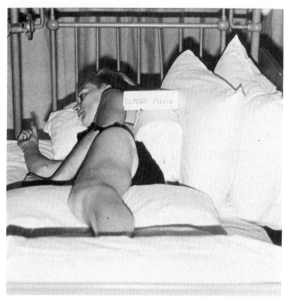

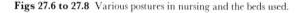

Fig 27.7

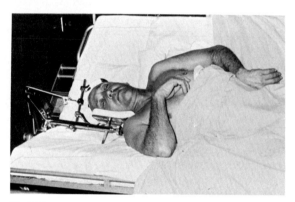

Fig 27.8

Figs 27.6 to 27.8 Various postures in nursing and the beds used.

the chest cage, although occasionally a fractured sternum may make such injuries more mobile. However postural reduction maintenance should always be attempted.

Having reduced the deformity postural care must be maintained with strict discipline (see Figs 27.6 to 27.9). But if the fracture dislocation can not be reduced the surgeon must finally consider the use of the operative methods of reduction.

Open reduction with or without fixation. Laminectomy in the treatment of spinal injury has long since been abandoned as having little or no use unless in the rare case of laminal fractures causing compression. The factors to be considered before the use of open reduction are:

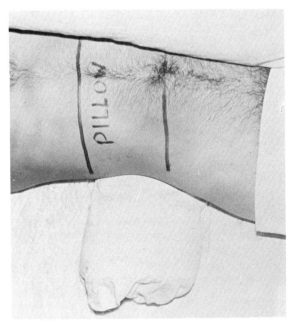

Fig 27.9 It is important to mark on the skin the position where the posterior pillow should be placed under lumbo dorsal spine.

1. The general condition.
2. The extent of dislocation (whether unilateral or bilateral).
3. The involvement of other systems e.g. urinary infection, skin sepsis.
4. Other injuries.
5. The neurological prognosis.
6. The length of time after the accident.
7. The suitability of facilities for surgery.
8. The availability of the necessary expertise.

When all these factors have been considered a few cases (less than 5 per cent of lumbo-dorsal fracture dislocations) may benefit by open reduction. In cervico-dorsal fracture dislocations early open surgery is generally contra-indicated and rarely necessary for good results. There are no absolute indications for surgical intervention, but some of the conditions which may require it are included in the following:

1. Gross irreducible fracture dislocations, particularly at lumbo-dorsal spine, when complete spinal disruption has occurred.
2. When major neurological deterioration occurs surgical exploration must be considered but the value of this has not yet been proven.
3. In gunshot injuries general debridement of the wound and reduction of any dislocation present must be carried out.

Plate fixation, previously considered satisfactory by Holdsworth and Hardy, should be abandoned as mechanically inefficient. If internal fixation is considered necessary, Harrington rod stabilisation carried out by an expert conversant with the method used in scoliosis is the method of choice. If traumatic scoliosis in complete disruptions is suspected both anterior fixation by the Dwyer anterior instrumentation and Harrington posterior instrumentation may be required. The details of the operative techniques involved are beyond the scope of this chapter and have been described elsewhere[16].

Finally, surgeons must always remember that no operative technique is an alternative for good nursing. Operation should never be indicated merely to supplement the nursing care, for it neither makes the nursing easier or significantly relieves the patient's pain.

NURSING

Expert nursing of the acute paraplegic or tetraplegic patient is of greatest importance in establishing the patient's hope in the future and in prevention of unnecessary complications. The postural nursing techniques employed, some of which are illustrated in Figures 27.6 to 27.10, will:

1. Prevent bed sores.
2. Maintain normal posture.
3. Improve the care of the neurogenic bladder and bowel.
4. Maintain reduction.
5. Prevent contractures.
6. Allow the development of extension reflexes in the case with upper motor neuron manifestations.
7. Care for the neurogenic bowel.
8. Correct by diet protein and calcium loss.
9. Help prevent deep vein thrombosis with stockings.

In a comprehensive unit a special turning team of a trained nurse and two orderlies (see Fig 27.10) maintain around the clock two hourly turns. Each patient has a turning chart; with the aid of pillows, rolls and packs normal posture is maintained. Special beds such as the Stoke Mandeville bed are useful and even essential in the early stages (see Fig 27.6 and 27.8). All excessive strains at the fracture site must be prevented—great gentleness is needed. A few centres who make early use of exoskeletons of plaster and polythenes prevent bed sores by regular turning. With such regular care diligently and accurately carried out no acute paraplegic should have skin

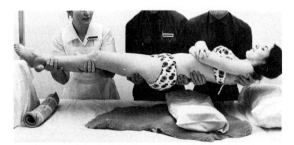

Fig 27.10 Figure shows method of lifting patient supine off the bed giving good support to lumbo dorsal area.

problems in the paralysed desensitised areas. Pressure sores must be prevented by

1. Nursing.
2. Changing posture.
3. Inspection.
4. Varying routine if any skin blemish occurs.

CARE OF THE PARALYSED BLADDER AND BOWEL

Until 1949 most spinal paralytics developed urinary infection from organisms introduced from the exterior by various means. All patients usually have a flaccid bladder paralysis in the early weeks. Those who have a true cord lesion will ultimately develop a reflex upper motor neuron bladder, while those with a cauda equina lesion have an atonic lower motor neuron bladder (see Fig 27.11). There will be a few in the lumbo-dorsal area where a mixed bladder can be expected.

In the first few days prevention of distension and infection is of paramount importance. If an indwelling intravenous infusion is needed to combat ileus then a temporary indwelling catheter changed meticulously each 48 hours is the best method to prevent distension and infection. Preventing infection is not just related

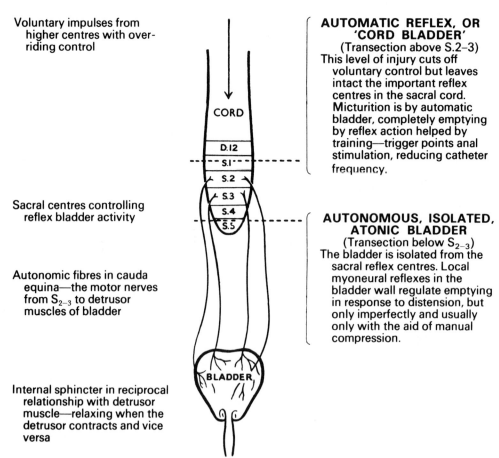

Voluntary impulses from higher centres with over-riding control

CORD

D.12
S.1
S.2
S.3
S.4
S.5

AUTOMATIC REFLEX, OR 'CORD BLADDER'
(Transection above S.2–3)
This level of injury cuts off voluntary control but leaves intact the important reflex centres in the sacral cord. Micturition is by automatic bladder, completely emptying by reflex action helped by training—trigger points anal stimulation, reducing catheter frequency.

Sacral centres controlling reflex bladder activity

AUTONOMOUS, ISOLATED, ATONIC BLADDER
(Transection below S_{2-3})
The bladder is isolated from the sacral reflex centres. Local myoneural reflexes in the bladder wall regulate emptying in response to distension, but only imperfectly and usually only with the aid of manual compression.

Autonomic fibres in cauda equina—the motor nerves from S_{2-3} to detrusor muscles of bladder

BLADDER

Internal sphincter in reciprocal relationship with detrusor muscle—relaxing when the detrusor contracts and vice versa

Fig 27.11 Diagram to show sacral centres controlling reflex bladder activity, and the distinction between the automatic, reflex or 'cord bladder', and the atonic, autonomous or isolated bladder.

to better methods of catheterisation. Other factors include:

1. Meticulous ward cleaning which should be checked microbiologically.
2. Every member of staff washing hands between cases.
3. Adequate supply of sterile equipment.
4. Meticulous aseptic techniques of catheterisation.
5. Good methods of bowel control and perineum cleansing.

In comprehensive units the nursing staff should provide a catheter and cross infection team, consisting of nurses, urology technicians, medical students and doctors. Once the intravenous line has been removed intermittent catheterisation can be commenced within eight hours, usually associated with reduction of fluid intake to prevent risk of distension. Sir Ludwig Guttmann[17] and more recently Pearman and England[18] have shown that such a technique reduces late urinary complications to a minimum. Those units who use a continuous indwelling catheter technique in the early stages experience a later return of bladder function, early urinary infection, and even genito urinary infection (urethritis and early pyelonephritis). For those who must use an indwelling catheter the McGibbon catheter is useful, or a small self retaining Foley's catheter can be used. These should have all connections well sealed to prevent contamination, plus a urodrain bag having an outlet where antiseptic can be introduced.

Having had experience of both methods the author has no doubt that regular intermittent bladder evacuation and, equally important, regular intermittent perineum toilet after stool, together with *all* of the other basic principles, will allow an uninfected neurogenic bladder to commence functioning sometimes within a week or ten days of injury. Antibiotics should be used sparingly when the bacteriuria is greater than 10 000/ml in a mid-stream specimen. Pearman and England's[18] criteria are strict but effective. Meticulous detail is essential and will result in a saving of time, beds and antibiotics, and will produce fitter patients as well as an enthusiastic staff. Daily microbiological surveys are made on every specimen until catheters are suspended.

Early bowel care depends on whether one expects an upper motor neuron or lower motor neuron bowel. For the latter, digital evacuation gently using softeners and careful technique is effective. In the former after early manual evacuation reflex function must be stimulated by the use of suppositories, aperients and physiologically stimulating bowel reflexes such as the gastro-colic.

EARLY PHYSICAL REHABILITATION

Immediately after admission attention should be directed firstly to maintaining adequate respiratory function by regular treatment (including postural drainage), care of the tracheostomy in high tetraplegics, assisted respiration and developing voluntary muscles of respiration; secondly, preventing stiffness and contractures by gentle passive movements, thus assisting venous return; and thirdly, developing all muscles surviving the injury.

Development of the trunk and erector spinae. It is not generally remembered that the erector spinae muscles have a surviving nerve supply at least two segments below the lesion by communications via the posterior primary rami. There are also muscles which regularly span the bony and neural lesions, e.g. trapezius, latissimus dorsi and levator scapulae. Developing such muscles will help not only voluntary power but also the sensations of stereognosis.

Development of the upper limb muscles. Here early provision of simple measures to maintain and develop by isometric means all surviving muscles will give good results and stimulate independences early. Simple weights and pulley systems to beds and using a graded system is excellent (see Figs 27.12a, b and c).

Too often such activity is provided only after a period of immobilisation of six to eight weeks. The physical therapist must work hard to stimulate the patient and maintain motivation.

Occupational therapy. The occupational therapist must first provide adequate static hand splints to protect contractures and then quickly provide dynamic arm orthoses such as a tenodesis dynamic splint of the Enger type. With such, tetraplegics can quickly become better motivated as they attempt small activities of daily living. At the same time as power is developed so sensation remaining should be developed by touching, feeling and contacting. All staff must be aware of this important sensory restoration through their nursing and physical therapy activities.

SOCIAL REHABILITATION

The social worker should be involved early to offer help and advice to patient and family about the initial problems concerned with spinal paralysis. In this early stage maintaining adequate financial support

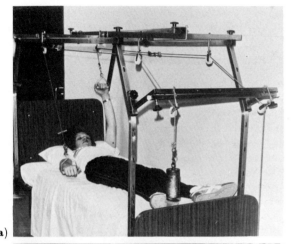

(a)

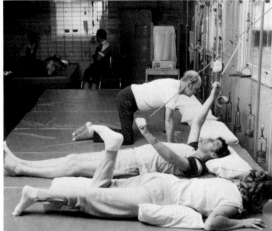

(b)

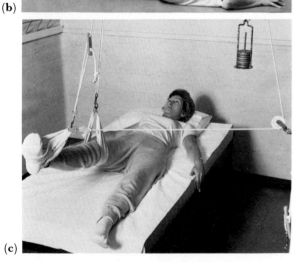

(c)

Figs 27.12a, b, c Developing and maintaining voluntary muscles should be started immediately on admission by a bed pulley weight system. In time such a principle can be then continued in the gymnasium or even at home.

by pension or allowance, sorting out domestic difficulties and arranging for legal advice will be an important and essential part of rehabilitation. Later, as the patient improves a psycho-social history should be taken and made available for adequate team discussion.

Within a few days of admission the medical officer in charge must discuss all aspects of care with the members of the ward team and with other consultants who are involved. The latter discussion can usually be best achieved by a once weekly grand round with all consultants—radiologist, microbiologist, orthopaedist, neurosurgeon, urologist, plastic surgeon, psychiatrist and rehabilitation consultant, and where opinions can be offered and decisions made.

LATER MANAGEMENT

Most patients with spinal injuries and paralysis will be immobilised in bed for six to eight weeks on the routine care already detailed, although a few may be mobilised earlier with exoskeletons (cervical or lumbo-dorsal). Some of the fracture dislocations at the end of six to eight weeks will show movement on stress X-rays, but the vast majority are stable (see Tables 27.4 and 27.5).

Over the same period neurological advancement will be made in the incomplete cases and must be followed by the regular and meticulous clinical examination and recordings. It is only by such careful follow-up examination that the clinician can be dogmatic as to further progress. Rapid improvement in the first week after admission will mean a good final recovery, but if any improvement lags for a few weeks the degree of recovery will be doubtful. By the end of six weeks 6 to 10 per cent of cases, particularly cervical dislocations, may need anterior or posterior spinal fusion because of their instability, followed by the use of exoskeleton supports during mobility. However, the vast majority of cases, having had adequate bed physical therapy (see Figs 27.12a, b and c), can now be mobilised out of bed, possibly using exoskeletons. Most of the patients will have already been in the erect or near erect position by using a tilting table, thus having by practice overcome the vaso vagal attacks of getting erect. Slowly stereognosis returns as the patient learns to sit and then transfers to a wheelchair. By three months the majority of spinal fractures are well healed and stable with minimal deformity, provided the postural method has been well practised and maintained throughout the period.

Table 27.4 Collected figures of cervical fracture dislocation with tetraparesis

		Dall	Frankel	Cheshire	Bedbrook	Total	Percentage
Compression	stable	22	48	63	63	196	26%
	unstable	1	0	0	0		
Flexion rotation 1	stable	25	129	60	75	289	38%
	unstable	9	0	6	8		
Flexion rotation 11	stable	22	25	35	45	127	17%
	unstable	3	2	6	8		
Extension	stable	6	16	66	53	141	19%
	unstable	0	0	0	1		
Total number of stable injuries		75	218	224	236	753	100%
Total number of unstable injuries		13	2	12	17	44	5.8%

Table 27.5 Review of cervical fractures and fracture dislocations, Perth, Western Australia. Neurological state on admission and discharge

		Admission	Discharge	Complete—Incomplete
Compression	Complete	30 = 47.5%	20 = 32%	10 = 16%
	Incomplete	33 = 52.5%	43 = 68%	
		63	63	
Flexion rotation 1	Complete	17 = 23%	11 = 15%	6 = 8%
	Incomplete	58 = 77%	64 = 85%	
		75	75	
Flexion rotation 11	Complete	25 = 55%	14 = 31%	9 = 20%
	Incomplete	20 = 45%	31 = 69%	
		45	45	
Extension	Complete	9 = 17%	6 = 11%	.3 = 6%
	Incomplete	44 = 83%	47 = 89%	
		53	53	Average 12%

LATE MANAGEMENT OF THE BOWEL AND BLADDER

With the patient out of bed bowel training can proceed according to the neurological state. Those with reflex evacuation can learn to empty their bowel by using suppositories given after an aperient and fluids and finally dilatating the anal canal by digital insertion. The latter manoeuvre will also stimulate reflex micturition. Those with flaccid lesions must learn to evacuate manually.

As soon as the initial few weeks are over bladder retraining commences. In the patient with a flaccid bladder and no return of bulbo-cavernosus anal response or reflex priapism, suprapubic crede or first expression before the six to eight hourly catheterisation will help to establish a routine, but usually a large residual urine persists and this must not be allowed to accumulate. Values over 10 per cent of bladder capacity are not acceptable and ultimately

surgical release of sphincter or bladder neck will be required. Those patients with upper motor neurone reflexes and thus early reflex emptying have a trigger point around the perineum and genitalia which must be found by the regular, repeated practice of stimulation. As the residual urine diminishes catheterisation frequency can be reduced until daily or bi-daily residuals only are used.

The return of neurogenic bladder function is irregular and slow, related to previous individual micturition function, and the surgeon, nurse, technician and principally the patient must be tolerant and strict in discipline of care—sometimes over many weeks. Those who have been treated by continuous catheterisation are slower to return such function, and persistent infection will delay not only bladder recovery but also neurological recovery. In a reported study of 99 cases by Pearman[19] using the intermittent catheterisation method already described, the 75 males had no calculi, no hydronephrosis, no epididymo-orchitis, one pyelonephritis, and no strictures or diverticuli. All were catheter free (although one had an ileal diversion for persistent bladder and kidney infection). Such are the results possible with this method of bladder management.

The introduction of studies in bladder physiology using profiles and recordings of urethral, sphincter and bladder pressures to study the dyssynergy will help the urologist to decide on those few males who need either sphincterotomy or transurethral neck resection.

In both male and female the use of drugs such as probanthine, dibenyline and urecholine can greatly assist in bladder retraining so that one can agree with Guttmann and Munro when they stated that all such cases can have an adequately social bladder. The male can be fitted with condom type urinals meticulously applied with cement usually to the erect penis and a suitable bag. Simple sterilisation of the bag by immersion in water off the boil for five minutes until cold or at 36°C for 20 minutes has been shown by Pearman[18] to be quite satisfactory. Provided these methods are followed closely, 50 per cent of cases will remain sterile indefinitely, 40 per cent will have one to four episodes of bacteriuria yearly and in only 10 per cent will there be recurrent infections. However, clean surroundings, the washing of hands, clean clothes, adequate bowel toilet and good personal hygiene cannot be overstressed.

Nursing care in the later stages remains a dominant essential function, but as well as regular care already described, postural care must continue almost indefinitely. The nurse now has an important role in patient education. Patients are only able to take care individually if they are fully instructed in every aspect—the nurse thus has an important role in restoration by educational methods. The prevention of urinary sepsis is a constant responsibility of the nurse over the remaining months of hospitalisation and even later, as well as the prevention of pressure sores. Immediately the patient is out of bed a wheelchair must be supplied properly made to fit the patient. The pressure clinic—run by nurses and engineers supply these essentials together with tailored cushions to also help prevent any decubiti. The chair manufacturer must have a regular contact with the nurse and engineer so that sore prevention is continued.

SEXUAL REHABILITATION

All paralysed patients, and particularly young people, are concerned with regard to their future sexual responses and functions and they should be reassured on admission that help is available. Meanwhile, the non-physical side of sexuality must be encouraged and stimulated through the real affection and love the patient has for his or her partner.

After the neurological state has become finalised a careful assessment will reveal that in the female intercourse and conception is possible, and sexual orgasm may be obtained from other erotogenic areas, even if perineum sensation is lost. Indeed, in the course of time and with practice some women patients may recover cervical-vaginal orgasm via sympathetic pathways. In the male, reflex erection in those with spinal cord isolation becomes more intense the more proximal the lesion, and thus intercourse is possible with help from their partner. Normal orgasm is not experienced, but an abnormal orgasm may occur. Reflex ejaculation is rare. The flaccid lesion has only a small chance of psychogenic erection and thus coitus may not be possible. However in disabled couples other sexual techniques involving self-stimulation, other erotogenic methods and prolonged foreplay will help. Each case must be treated individually.

PHYSICAL REHABILITATION

Once the patient is out of bed the tempo of therapy increases and all the principles and practices of physical rehabilitation as discussed in other chapters on rehabilitation are used. The isometric method must be improved whilst sensory perception is also taken care of through occupational therapy. The slow process of vocational care is aided as needed by external agencies and people such as vocational counsellors. Enthusiastic work by all therapists will result in excellent results—goals can be laid down by a knowledge of the neurological levels possible. Regular weekly discussion monitors all progress made by the physical therapists as they encourage practice to improve function (see Figs 27.13a, b, and c, 27.14 and 27.15).

Sport as a therapeutic measure should be introduced as soon as possible after, or even before, getting up. As part of physical restoration sport plays a big part in general patient care. Sir Ludwig Guttmann's early experiments in such care has led to interesting and enthusiastic methods, including weightlifting, dartchery, archery, billiards, field events and basketball. Guttmann's textbook on *Sport for the Disabled*[20] emphasises the many aspects of this variety of therapy, both inside and outside comprehensive units. For the purpose of competing the athletes are classified neurologically into six classes (see Fig 27.16). Partic-

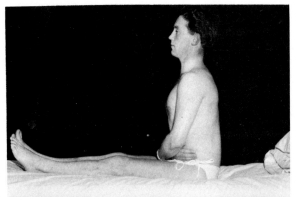

Fig 27.13 (a) Teaching the paraplegic patient to sit upright. This is more difficult than it would seem. (b) and (c) In traumatic paraplegia balance may depend solely on the trunk muscles innervated from a level higher than the fracture. In dorsal fractures the latissimus dorsi is often the only muscle which can stabilise the trunk and allow the patient to sit, stand and later to walk. The first and most important treatment is to teach the patient to sit (Fig 27.13a), then to sit with arms outstretched (Fig 27.13b), and then to acquire balance despite sudden strains; such exercises as throwing a ball to a physiotherapist and then catching it back are excellent (Fig 27.13c).

(a)

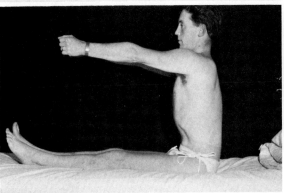

(b)

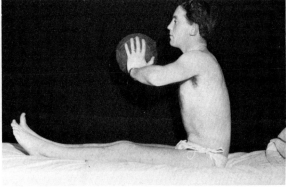

(c)

ipation encourages individualism, competition and ability to live in a community; for such activities reduce disability and increase functional ability. Whilst within the comprehensive unit the patient must be introduced to the world wide Stoke Mandeville Games activities both at club, state, interstate, national and international levels. The ramifications are many, particularly at world level each fourth year the International Stoke Mandeville Games are held, usually in the same country as the Olympics. In Arnhem in 1980 1055 paraplegic athletes took part.

Social restoration continues until the patient has been adequately resettled into the community. The social worker must look into the patients personality, his ability to cope, intelligence and the problem solving methods as well as his ability to tolerate frustration. Principally however, domestic resettlement must be dominant. Those that are independent and fit usually go home, or to suitable hostels. Those that are dependent may go home with adequate support, or be discharged to dependent nursing areas run by voluntary bodies (see Fig 27.17). Paraplegic Associations, churches or Government hospital

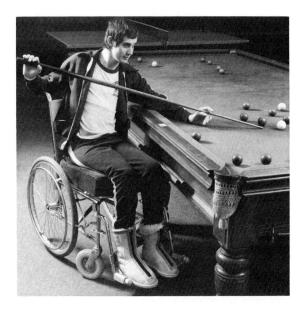

Fig 27.14 Quadriplegic using snooker as a method of physical rehabilitation (a) in upper extremities (b) as a method of improving stereognosis of the trunk.

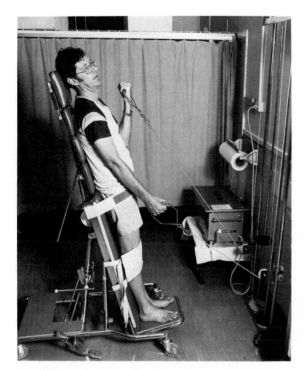

Fig 27.15 Physical rehabilitation in incomplete quadriplegic using weight resisting exercises for upper extremities.

authorities, realising that the provision of extended care facilities are essential to restoration of function and that such will lead to earlier discharge, will become involved in their provision either directly or indirectly.

COMPLICATIONS

There are some patients who, however adequately rehabilitated in a comprehensive unit, will develop complications. These include urinary infections, bedsores, contractures and spasm (upper motor neuron), psychological and social problems. When such occur urgent readmission is needed in some cases, or adequate outpatient care in others. Whatever the problem a careful diagnosis must be made and appropriate treatment given. Prevention has already been discussed—treatment must be definite, aggressive and complete. Only too often paraplegics still lack such care for their complications.

Urinary infection. Diagnosis of bacilluria in some patients, or real pyelonephritis in others, calls for urgent microbiological checks and appropriate antibiotics. Catheters should be avoided unless used intermittently for retention and residual urine. Having treated the episode, continuous use of urinary antiseptics such as Mandelamine and Ammonium chloride should be introduced again. Renal investigations, intravenous pyelogram, ureteric catheters, cystogram, micturating cystograms and pressure studies must all be used to investigate persistent re-infections. The source of the organism must be sought even in the most unlikely places—for example, in the domestic washing machine.

Decubiti or pressure sores. These can only be treated by relieving pressure. Minor ones heal at home, major ones need admission. Early debridement of necrotic tissue, regular four hourly use of Milton solution, and regular microbiological checks—superficial and deep—will result in sterile ulcers and wounds. If necessary, osteomyelitis must be surgically excised and treated with carefully chosen antibiotics. Serum analysis allows adequate dosage. Reparative surgery by an expert plastic surgeon, combined by good nursing and posture worked out prior to surgery, has given good results. By such techniques 50 per cent saving in hospital time will occur and 50 per cent cost reduction. Occasionally special beds—water, sand mud or air, can be of great use. After healing careful attention to the wheelchair and its cushioning on a regular repetitive basis, combined with patient education, will result in a fall in hospital admission by 50 per cent and an improvement of general health. Since pressure sores can be a manifestation of social problems these must be searched out, eradicated or relieved.

Contractures and spasm. Over the years these have reduced greatly as comprehensive units increase and early prevention is practised. If they do occur however and are seriously impeding activities of daily living treatment must be instigated. This can be by medical measures, such as the use of valium and baclofen; or by surgical measures—tenotomies, myotomy, nerve crushes and neurotomies. Following correction, rehabilitative treatment will be essential once again.

The paralysed hand offers a special challenge. The spastic paralysed hand may be a useful hand if spasm can be 'trained'. Reconstructive methods in such hands do not succeed. In the flaccid hand dynamic orthoses, training and practice will usually result in adaptations and different ways of conducting daily activities. In a few patients, largely those paralysed below C.6 and C.7, surgical procedures in the form of tendon transfers are useful. For example, in C.7

MEDICAL CLASSIFICATION

PARAPLEGIC AND TETRAPLEGIC SPORT

CORD LEVEL	CLASS	CLASS CHARACTERISTICS

		1A	TRICEPS 0 – 3
C4			
C5	1A	1B	TRICEPS 4 – 5 WRIST FLEXION & EXTENSION
C6	1B 1C	1C	TRICEPS 4 – 5 WRIST FLEXION & EXTENSION
C7			FINGER FLEXION & EXTENSION
C8			
T1			NO USEFUL BALANCE
T2			NO USEFUL ABDOMINALS
T3	11		NO LOWER INTERCOSTALS
T4			
T5			
T6			SOME BALANCE
T7			UPPER ABDOMINALS
T8	111		
T9			
T10			
T11			GOOD BALANCE
T12			GOOD ABDOMINALS & SPINAL EXTENSORS
L1	1 V		SOME HIP FLEXORS AND ADDUCTORS
L2			POINTS: 1 – 20 TRAUMATIC
L3			POINTS: 1 – 15 POLIO
L4			POINTS 21 – 40 TRAUMATIC
L5	V		POINTS: 16 – 35 POLIO
S1	V1		POINTS: 41 – 60 TRAUMATIC
S2			POINTS 36 – 50 POLIO

NOT ELIGIBLE

TRAUMATIC 61 POINTS AND ABOVE

POLIO 51 POINTS AND ABOVE

Fig 27.16 Medical classification of paraplegic and tetraplegic sport, showing neurological levels and points. (Reproduced by kind permission of Editor of the *Journal of Bone and Joint Surgery* (1979) 61-B, 277.)

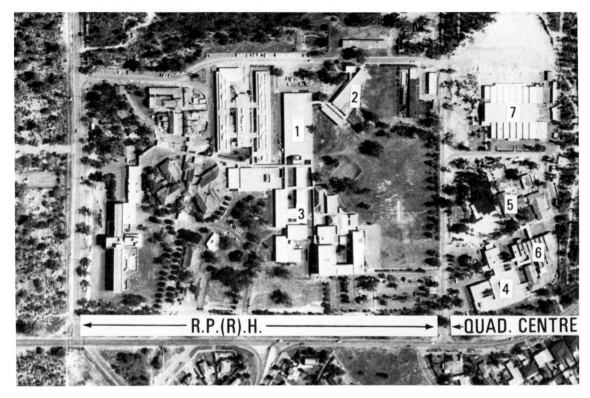

Fig 27.17 The comprehensive unit. (1) The ward. (2) Physical therapy and outpatients. (3) Laboratory. (4) Long-term nursing unit. (5) Hostel. (6) Activity therapy. (7) Workshop. The comprehensive unit thus handles all aspects of care from acute to extended care. (Reproduced by the kind permission of the Editor of the *Journal of Bone and Joint Surgery* (1979) 61-B, 261).

paralysis Brachio-radialis to flexor pollicis longus, flexor carpi radialis to long finger flexors and pronator teres elongated as a thumb opposer will give a better hand function.

Social complications. These abound and must be prevented by the introduction of an extended care service to each comprehensive unit. Acute care without extended care only produces complications that could have been prevented.

EXTENDED CARE

Expert multidisciplinary acute care for patients with spinal cord injuries treated in comprehensive units is now generally accepted. Equally expert multidisciplinary after-care is sometimes not generally pursued with enthusiasm, and rehabilitation is often considered complete when the patient is discharged. A sophisticated acute care environment can only be justified in terms of a similar comprehensive after-care programme. Discharge planning should be seen

only as the initial stage in the after-care programme and not as the final stage in the rehabilitation programme.

Follow up. The value of continuous follow-up of the paralytic patient whose disability is irreversible but not static, lies in the prevention, early detection, and relatively inexpensive treatment of the complications. Continuous follow-up helps to maintain a high level of health, prevents social and economic disruption, and releases hospital beds for the care of the acute sick.

Results from Western Australia confirm this. Specialist clinics for people with spinal cord injury have been available there since 1970. Routine follow-up for all patients is scheduled at spinal clinics, urology clinics and tissue trauma clinics, with provision for referral to psychiatric, medical and pain clinics. In addition, the assistance of a social worker, vocational counsellor, orthotist, physiotherapist and occupational therapist is available as needed. This service, combined with a hospital-based domiciliary nursing service and residential accommodation for those people not able to be cared for at home, has resulted in fewer re-admissions to the Spinal Unit. In 1971, 55 new (traumatic and non-traumatic) patients were admitted to the spinal unit and 232 patients, previously discharged were readmitted. In 1977, the number of new admissions totalled 83 but the readmissions numbered only 143. Patients on the whole respond well to routine scheduling. With very little extra care, appointments can be arranged to prevent disruption to domestic life, work, or leisure activities.

Community living. Spinal cord injured patients, upon discharge, will invariably want to return to their former life style, to live in their own home, to work at a meaningful occupation and to be able to get about in the community. This requires, in nearly every instance, some alteration to their house, some aids, suitable means of transport and often adaptation of work facilities. Even so, there are people with severe disability for whom living in the community will not necessarily provide the optimum life. In the past, those who could not be cared for at home were placed into institutions for the chronically sick, where their bodily needs were provided for without recourse to community stimulation. This is no longer generally accepted. Great Britain after the Second World War, provided hostels, such as the Thistle Foundation in Scotland and Lyme Green in Macclesfield, for disabled servicemen. More recently a hostel at Stoke Mandeville has been built to provide dependent living for people with spinal cord injuries (Guttmann 1973).

In Holland, experiment in design for disabled living has produced the village at Het Dorp. Architectural devices are used to simplify living, and assistance upon request is available to each apartment. In Sweden, Fokus Flats for disabled people are integrated into normal housing areas all over the country and provide a readily available support service to residents. Denmark with its collective house system offers a similar service. Following the Swedish experiment, the Habinteg Housing Association in Britain offered about a quarter of its homes in any one scheme to the disabled. There is provision for help on call and easy access throughout.

Any system for housing the disabled must be seen to be offering a flexible choice. For those who wish to live in the community, and a majority will choose to do so, aid and support must be given so that they can remain a part of that community. For those who choose instead—institutional care, the choice should include the achieving of an optimum life style rather than the need for absolute dependence.

In Australia, residential accommodation provided by Paraplegic and Tetraplegic Associations does not pretend to be integrated in the sense that the able and disabled live side by side. A total-care section is provided as well as self-care single room accommodation. Some residents work in the community and some work in the sheltered workshop, where those who live in the community may also choose to work. For those who are too disabled to participate in the workshop, an Activity Therapy Centre offers an alternate occupation, not only for residents but for those who live in the community. A recreational area provides the venue for both residential and community activities.

It is sometimes questioned whether living together in a residential environment offering opportunities and facilities for optimum independence segregates the disabled from the mainstream of life. The severely disabled can be more segregated from society living in their own home than the disabled living together in a residential community. If it is recognised that segregation occurs naturally at all levels of society, the question then becomes one of quality of life. For some, residential living will offer greater enrichment.

No community can afford to have only a comprehensive Spinal Unit important though it is. Outside the hospital there must exist a community facility for their welfare. This may be made up of separate groups, but ideally should be co-ordinated by an association such as the Paraplegic and Tetraplegic Association (see Fig 27.17). Its functions will include:

1. Provision of independent hostel.
2. Provision of dependent nursing home using all the nursing methods of the acute unit.
3. Provision of recreational areas.
4. Support a sports club.
5. Provision of a sheltered workshop for all disabled.
6. Provision of an activity therapy centre (diversional area) for the very severely handicapped.
7. Active liaison with the acute comprehensive unit.

Such associations need professional medical support at many levels.

This is just as important as the early medical care by a comprehensive unit. Challenge and stimulation for medical and nursing personnel exist in these areas as the multidisciplinary approach is maintained. Education of staff and patient is vital to prevention of those complications—urinary and pressure—that lurk in the background ever ready to appear if medical and nursing discipline should fail. During the long term extended care period of years new talents are discovered, old diseases are treated as they appear modified by paralysis and neurological adaptation continues as these people live lives of some contentment and fulfilment.

The care of the patient with a spinal cord injury should be seen as a continuum, beginning with expert initial and rehabilitation care, and followed by a comprehensive specialist long-term after-care. Without this foundation the concept of an individual choice of life style is hardly valid.

REFERENCES

1. Gowland E L 1934 Medical Press 188: 81
2. Munro D 1948 Rehabilitation of veterans paralysed as a result of injury to the spinal cord and cauda equina. American Journal of Surgery 75: 3
3. Botterell E H, Jousse A T, Aberhart C, Cluff J W 1946 Paraplegia following war. Canadian Medical Association Journal 55: 249
4. Guttmann L 1973 Spinal cord injury, comprehensive management and research. Blackwell, Oxford
5. Organisation of spinal units symposium 1967 Paraplegia 5: 115–187
6. Bedbrook G M 1976 The final responsibility of emergency. Medical Journal of Australia 1: 107–110
7. Guttmann L 1977 Total responsibility of surgeon in the rehabilitation of the spinal paralysed and other severely disabled. In: Royal Australasian College of Surgeons. Proceedings of Rehabilitation Workshop, Perth, Western Australia. *Also in:* Guttmann L 1978 Total responsibility of the surgeon in the management of traumatic spinal paraplegics and tetraplegics. Paraplegia 15: 285–299
8. Kakulas B, Bedbrook G M 1976 Pathology of injuries of the vertebral column. In: Vinken P J, Bruyn G W (eds) Handbook of Clinical Neurology 25: 27–42, New Holland Publishing Co Amsterdam
9. Jellinger K 1976 Neuropathology of cord injuries. In: Vinken P J, Bruyn G W (eds) Handbook of clinical neurology 25: 43–121, New Holland Publishing Co, Amsterdam
10. Guttmann L 1976 The conservative management of closed injuries of the vertebral column resulting in damage to the spinal cord and spinal roots. In: Vinken P J, Bruyn G W (eds) Handbook of clinical neurology 26: 285–306, New Holland Publishing Co, Amsterdam
11. Young J S, Dexter W R 1978 Neurological recovery distal to the zone of injury in 172 cases of closed, traumatic spinal cord injury. Paraplegia 16: 39–49
12. Michaelis L S 1976 Prognosis of spinal cord injury. In: Vinken P J, Bruyn G W (eds) Handbook of clinical neurology 26: 307–312, North Holland Publishing Co, Amsterdam
13. Morgan T H, Wharton G W, Austin G N 1971 The results of laminectomy in patients with incomplete spinal cord injuries. Paraplegia 9: 14–23
14. Bedbrook G M 1969 The use and disuse of surgery in lumbo dorsal fractures. Journal of Western Pacific Orthopaedic Association 6: 5–26
15. Sussman B J 1978 Fracture dislocations of the cervical spine. A critique of current management in United States. Paraplegia 16: 15–38
16. Bedbrook G M 1979 Spinal injuries. Operative surgery— orthopaedics. Butterworths, London
17. Guttmann L, Frankel H 1966 The value of intermittent catheterisation in the early management of traumatic paraplegia and tetraplegia. Paraplegia 4: 63–83
18. Pearman J W, England E J 1973 The urological management of the patient following spinal cord injury. Charles C Thomas, Springfield, Illinois
19. Pearman J W 1976 Urological follow-up of 99 spinal cord injured patients initially managed by intermittent catheterisation. British Journal of Urology 48: 297–310
20. Guttmann L 1976 Textbook of sport for the disabled. H. M. & M., Aylesbury, UK

28

Injuries of the Pelvis

All papers written in recent years on pelvic fractures have emphasised that the incidence of these injuries is steadily on the increase and that their severity should not be underrated. Very broadly the fractures may be divided into stable and unstable injuries: the stable variety being of little consequence and produced by relatively minor trauma; whereas the unstable fracture may have far reaching consequences and is produced by very severe trauma.

For the purpose of this chapter, which sets out to list the individual types of injury and their management, the fractures of the pelvic ring will be considered under six headings:

1. Avulsion fractures due to muscular violence (stable fractures).
2. Isolated fractures of the pelvic ring due to direct violence without loss of integrity of the ring (stable fractures).
3. Double fractures, or fracture-dislocation, due to disruptive or compression forces, and with loss of integrity of the pelvic ring (unstable fractures).
4. Complications of pelvic fractures.
5. Compound injuries.
6. Fractures of the sacrum and coccyx.

Fractures of the acetabulum producing central dislocation of the hip are discussed with other hip dislocations in Chapter 29.

Avulsion injuries and isolated fractures of the pelvic ring are usually single injuries, unassociated with the complications of other fractures, and therefore simple to treat. Fracture-dislocations, on the other hand, are only too often part of a serious multiple injury, with the choice of treatment dictated by other priorities. Fracture of the pelvis in these circumstances can be a killing lesion, and in one survey of over 600 pelvic injuries there was an overall death rate of 14 per cent; elderly pedestrians were particularly vulnerable, and shock was the main contributory factor as the cause of death.[1] But it is also important to appreciate that a severe pelvic injury, at any age, can sometimes result in a devastating haemorrhage, and that this in itself may produce a major problem of resuscitation.[2,3] In one survey of the mortality from pelvic fractures it was estimated that in the 26 deaths primarily due to pelvic injury 93 per cent of patients were in hypovolaemic shock and 69 per cent exsanguinated themselves in the first nine hours.[4]

AVULSION OF MUSCLE INSERTIONS

Sudden and uncontrolled effort may detach any of the muscles arising from the pelvis and avulse fragments from their sites of origin. The powerful, long-bellied muscles of the thigh are most commonly involved.

Anterior inferior iliac spine—avulsion of the rectus femoris. A boy playing Rugby football whose enthusiasm is greater than his strength is determined to convert a try however difficult the angle and however distant the posts; at the moment of kicking the ball he feels sharp pain in the groin and falls to the ground; active flexion of the hip is found to be painful and limited. Radiographs show slight downward displacement of a fragment of bone from the anterior inferior iliac spine just above the margin of the acetabulum. The bone has been avulsed by the rectus femoris muscle (Fig 28.1). This fracture is to be distinguished from the epiphyseal line of a separate ossicle of bone which may develop normally in this situation. There is no need for operative suture. Recumbency for a few weeks with the hip flexed to a comfortable position is the only treatment required. Myositis ossificans,[5] and even exostosis formation,[6] has been reported as a late complication interfering with hip movement. Such cases should be treated by excision of the spur of bone when it is mature. This usually means a delay of about 12 months.

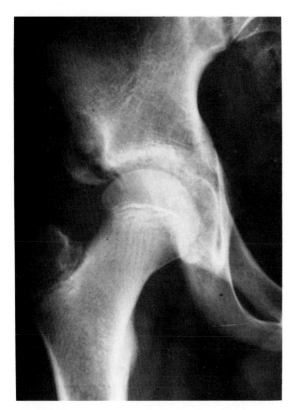

Fig 28.1 Avulsion of the anterior inferior iliac spine by the rectus femoris muscle sustained by a schoolboy playing Rugby football.

Anterior superior iliac spine—avulsion of the sartorius. Forcible contraction of the sartorius muscle may avulse bone from the anterior superior iliac spine resulting in localised pain over the anterior part of the iliac crest, a feeling of weakness in the hip, and pain on active flexion and straight leg raising. The fragment is slightly displaced but again there is no indication for operation. The pain is relieved by flexion of the hip. Even if the displacement is not perfectly corrected, the fragment often unites in a slightly lower position and functional recovery is usually complete within a few months (Figs 28.2 and 28.3).

Epiphysis of the ischium—avulsion of the hamstrings. The hamstring muscles arise from the tuberosity of the ischium, and a bone fragment may be avulsed by sudden muscular contraction especially in youths whose epiphyses are not united. In the acute phase the patient may have a marked limp and complain of severe pain in the ischial tuberosity on passive straight leg raising. There is always local tenderness over the hamstring origin and sometimes superficial bruising and swelling. Figure 28.4 shows the typical X-ray appearance of an avulsion sustained by a track-runner during a 100 yard sprint. The track surface was imperfect, and the injury was sustained at the moment that a slight hollow in the ground called for an increased and unexpected muscular effort. Although the X-rays are diagnostic of the injury cases presenting late with an incomplete history can be easily missed if the X-ray examination is confined to the hip joint alone (Figs 28.5 and 28.6). There is always complete recovery and the epiphysis unites firmly with considerable new bone formation. Many of these injuries have been seen in young athletes. The lunge forward in fencing is a movement particularly prone to be complicated by this injury, and some cases have been reported as resulting from a fall on to the buttocks. There is nothing unusual about it, and of course there is no need at all for surgical intervention.

Incomplete avulsion of the iliac epiphysis. This rare form of avulsion injury has been reported in immature athletes as a result of overaction of the abdominal muscles with sudden directional changes while running.[7] Severe pain is experienced in the anterior part of the iliac crest and X-rays show elevation of the anterior 2 to 3 cm of the epiphysis. Crutch walking for one to two weeks followed by restricted athletic activities for six weeks is the only treatment required.

ISOLATED INJURIES OF THE PELVIC RING (STABLE FRACTURES)

The two innominate bones, by their articulation with the sacrum posteriorly and with each other at the symphysis pubis, form an intact pelvic ring. If a fracture breaks the continuity of this ring at only one place, significant displacement of the fragments cannot arise and the fracture is stable. In this respect the pelvis can be likened to a wooden hoop which will bowl along quite well when only broken in one place. If, however, there is a second injury to another part of the ring or hoop its integrity is lost, the structure becomes unstable, and considerable displacement may occur. Isolated injuries of the ring include fractures of the pubic rami (Fig 28.7), fracture of the body of the ilium (Fig 28.8), slight separation of the symphysis pubis (Fig 28.9) and subluxation of the sacro-iliac joint (Fig 28.10).

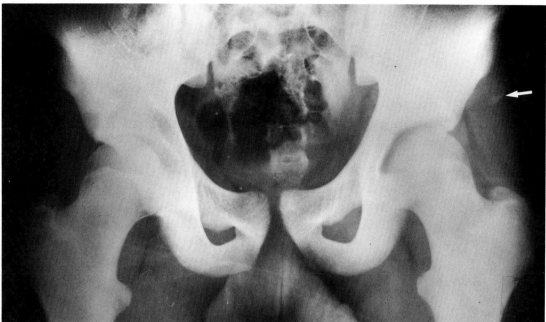

Fig 28.2

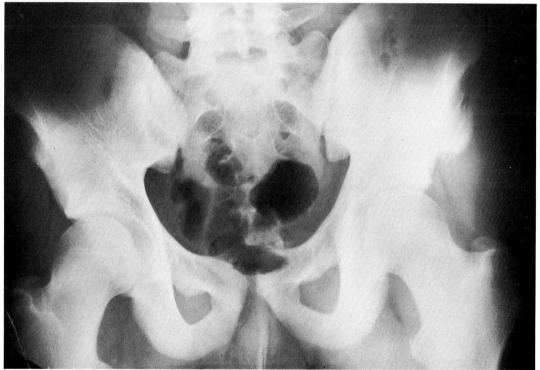

Fig 28.3

Figs 28.2 and 28.3 Avulsion of the anterior superior iliac spine on the left side sustained in a 16-year-old schoolboy who was kicking a hockey ball clear while keeping goal (Fig 28.2). Within one month his pain had disappeared and in seven months the displaced fragment of bone had united in a slightly lower position, but with no residual disability (Fig 28.3).

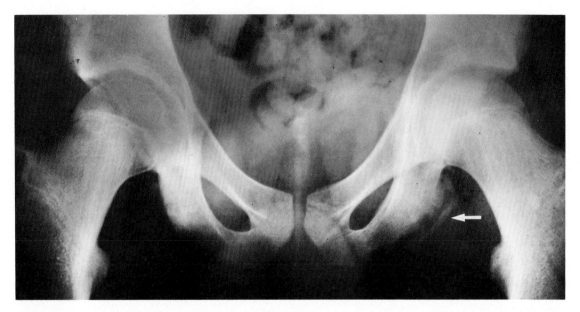

Fig 28.4 Avulsion of ischium by hamstrings sustained by a track runner.

Fractures of the pubic rami. The most common injury is unilateral fracture of one or both pubic rami. Elderly patients may be referred with the provisional diagnosis of an impacted fracture of the femoral neck, but the localised tenderness and the X-ray appearance will make the diagnosis clear. Movement of the fragments is very slight and immobilisation is therefore unnecessary. Bed rest is usually needed for a week or so for symptomatic relief, but during this time trunk, hip and leg movement should be practised in so far as the patient's comfort will allow in order to prevent muscle wasting and the possibility of venous thrombosis. Ambulation is usually possible after this and recovery is complete within two months. Stress fractures of the pubic and ischial rami can occur in the elderly and the discomfort resulting from these injuries can persist for many months (Fig 28.11). These fractures are probably the result of very low grade osteomalacia, but the typical biochemical changes in the serum are rarely found.

Isolated fractures of the ilium and minor separations of the symphysis pubis also recover fully without treatment. The surgeon must, however, satisfy himself that separation of the symphysis pubis is in fact an isolated injury. If there is wide displacement of the pubic bones there is very probably an associated injury in the sacro-iliac region which may easily be overlooked and often accounts for

persistent disability. Very occasionally isolated fractures of the ilium may be widely separated and give rise to persistent pain on respiration. If such a fracture has not become stable by three to four weeks, open reduction and internal fixation with Kirschner wires is indicated.[8]

Strain of the symphysis pubis. Athletes, and in particular professional footballers, may develop a painful instability of the symphysis pubis.[9] This usually takes the form of pain on exercise in the region of the symphysis, radiating into the groin and lower abdomen, and is sometimes associated with clicking in the joint. X-rays of the symphysis taken weight-bearing on one or the other limb may demonstrate slight upward displacement of one side. The condition usually settles after prolonged rest, but bone graft is occasionally necessary.

Sacro-iliac subluxation even without much displacement can cause persistent pain and incapacity. The injury is to be recognised clinically by the local pain, tenderness over the joint and typical displacement. The ilium is pushed slightly backwards and towards the mid-line. The posterior superior iliac spine is therefore more superficial than the corresponding bony prominence of the opposite side, and it lies nearer to the spinous processes (Figs 28.10 and 28.12). Manipulative reduction consisting of direct

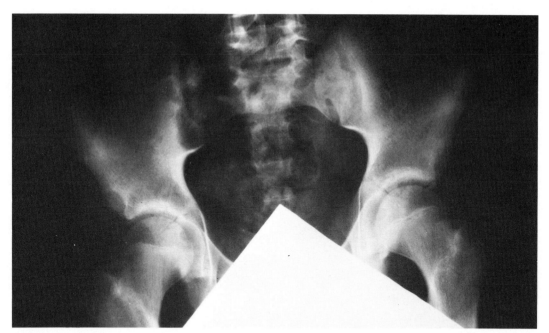

Fig 28.5

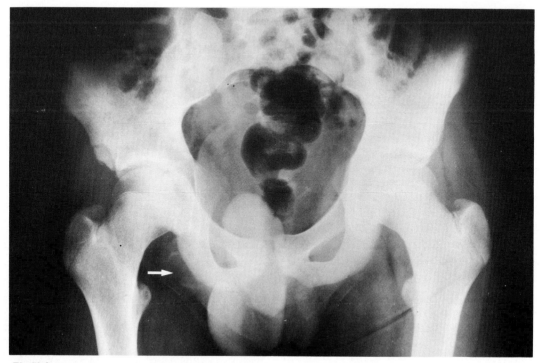

Fig 28.6

Figs 28.5 to 28.6 This patient presented two months after a 'hip strain' playing football. His hip X-rays were normal but his ischial tuberosities were obscured by a protective lead shield (Fig 28.5). Late films of the ischium revealed a typical avulsion injury (Fig 28.6). Beware of lead shields in pelvic X-rays!

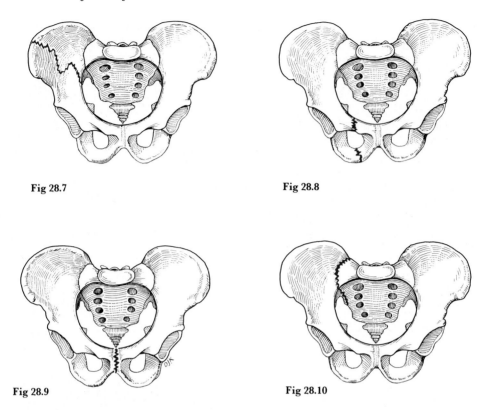

Fig 28.7

Fig 28.8

Fig 28.9

Fig 28.10

Figs 28.7 to 28.10 Isolated injuries of the pelvic ring. There is no marked displacement and no special treatment is indicated.

pressure over the sacro-iliac joint and rotation forwards sometimes produces dramatic relief; but usually bed rest for two or three weeks is all that is necessary. Discomfort, especially on forward bending, is likely to persist for several months, but providing full mobilising exercises of the spine and hip are regularly practised recovery should be complete within approximately three months.

DOUBLE FRACTURE CAUSING DISRUPTION OF THE PELVIC RING (UNSTABLE FRACTURES)

The pelvic ring is made up of the anterior pubic segments, which are developed for the protection of the pelvic viscera and for the attachment of muscles, and the postero-lateral iliac segments, which also serve the function of weight-bearing. Combined fractures of the pelvic ring are of two types. In the first, both fractures lie in the pubic segments; in the second, one fracture is in the pubic segment and one in the weight-bearing iliac segment.

Combined injuries of pubic segment of pelvic ring. Double fractures of the pubic part of the pelvis are the result of lateral crushing. The victim may be a pedestrian crushed by a motor vehicle which strikes the opposite side of the pelvis or a miner trapped by

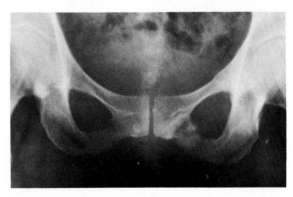

Fig 28.11 This patient developed a vague and unexplained pain in the left buttock. X-rays of the pelvis showed a stress fracture at the junction of the ischial and pubic rami, and also in the superior pubic ramus.

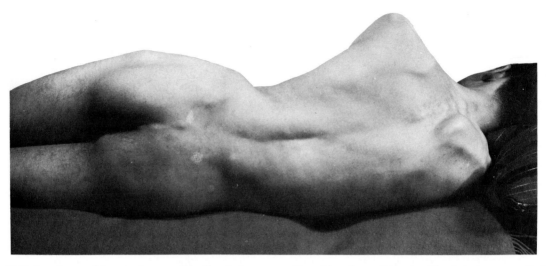

Fig 28.12 Prominence of the posterior part of the ilium indicates sacro-iliac subluxation or dislocation. The displacement is easily felt and, as in this case on the left side, it may be obvious on inspection.

a fall of roof. The injury may be a bilateral fracture of both pubic rami (the 'straddle' fracture), or a unilateral fracture of both rami with separation of the symphysis pubis (Figs 28.13 and 28.14). The detached fragment of bone is relatively small. Its displacement is limited by the attachments of many muscles, and whatever the degree of displacement there is no shortening of either limb and no alteration in the alignment of weight-bearing joints. There is always extensive bruising in the perineum giving an indication of the degree of haemorrhage which occurs in all pelvic fractures. The only treatment necessary for the fractures is rest in bed. None the less, tearing of the perineal membrane and the membranous urethra may occur in these injuries, and a soft rubber catheter should always be passed to verify integrity of the urinary tract if the patient cannot pass water. For the management of urinary tract injuries complicating pelvic fractures see Chapter 10.

Combined injuries of iliac and pubic segments of pelvic ring. The most common combined injury causing complete disruption of the pelvis is a dislocation of the symphysis with a dislocation of the sacro-iliac joint (Fig 28.15). Less frequently there is a dislocation of the symphysis with a fracture of the ilium near the sacro-iliac joint (Fig 28.16), or a fracture of both pubic rami with a dislocation of the sacro-iliac joint (Fig 28.17).* When the fractures of the pubic rami are on the opposite side to the sacro-

*This is the Malgaigné fracture first described in 1847.[10]

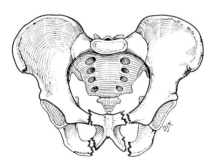

Fig 28.13

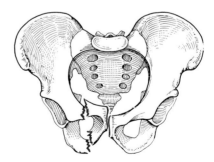

Fig 28.14

Figs 28.13 and 28.14 Combined injuries of the pubic segment of the pelvic ring produced by lateral compression of the pelvis. There is only slight displacement. Patients can be nursed on their backs. (Reproduced by courtesy of the *British Journal of Surgery* from R.W.-J.'s article (1938) Dislocations and fracture-dislocations of the pelvis. *British Journal of Surgery*, 25, 773.)

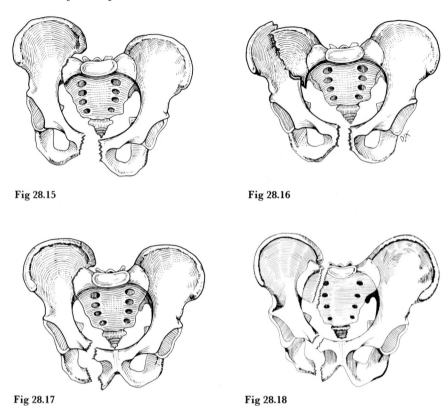

Fig 28.15

Fig 28.16

Fig 28.17

Fig 28.18

Figs 28.15 to 28.18 Combined injuries of the pubic and iliac segments of the pelvic ring produced by antero-posterior compression. There may be severe displacement. Patients can be nursed on their sides or in a sling. (Reproduced by courtesy of the *British Journal of Surgery* from R.W.-J.'s article (1938) Dislocations and fracture-dislocations of the pelvis. *British Journal of Surgery*, 25, 773.

iliac dislocation the fracture is referred to as a 'bucket handle' injury. Sometimes the fracture line passes vertically through the ala of the sacrum producing an unstable sacral fracture which may be associated with damage to the upper three sacral nerves[11] (Fig 28.18). In all these combinations of fractures one half of the pelvic girdle is widely displaced, carrying with it the lower limb, so that there is deformity and shortening. The clinical signs may be grossly distorted by other injuries to the trunk and lower limbs, but provided there are no long bone fractures careful examination should detect that the leg is externally rotated on the side of the fracture, and the leg length measurement (made from the umbilicus) is shorter on the injured side. This is, of course, a measurement of 'apparent' shortening resulting from one side of the pelvis moving proximally. A difference in 'real' length of the limbs would be an indication that there is also a fracture of the long bones, or a dislocation of the hip. Finally, with very severe compression and disruption force a complete dislocation of the pelvis

can occur with wide separation of the pubic symphysis and dislocation or fracture around both sacro-iliac joints. This injury and the hemipelvic dislocation are the most frequent pelvic fractures to be complicated by urethral and bladder damage.

Unlike the first type of combined injury, which is produced by lateral compression of the pelvis, these injuries are produced by antero-posterior compression: a patient is standing with his back to the wall when he is crushed by a motor vehicle, or he is lying on the roadway and the wheel of the vehicle mounts one side of the pelvis; in some cases head-on collisions are responsible; and again the injury can occur in mining accidents as the result of a fall of a roof. The mechanism of injury is important because it gives a clue to the technique of manipulative reduction.

Mechanism of displacement in dislocation of the pelvis. Radiographic examination shows obvious separation of the two pubic bones but often with only slight displacement of the sacro-iliac joint, which may be overlooked. Only careful examination shows that the ilium overlaps the back of the sacrum more than on the normal side and that the iliac joint surface is slightly higher than the sacral joint surface. Similarly, on clinical examination, it may also be possible to put a fist between the displaced pubic bones and yet there is only a trace of undue prominence of the posterior superior iliac spine. This is because the displaced innominate bone is rotated round a longitudinal axis near the sacro-iliac joint. The dislocated half of the pelvis is swung outwards, and only secondarily in more severe injuries is it displaced upwards into the loin. This outward rotation is shown in radiographs by the outwardly rotated position of the femur, the unusual prominence of the ischial spine, and the disappearance of the obturator foramen (Fig 28.19). It is a displacement maintained by the weight of the limb.

Overlapping displacement of the symphysis pubis.[12] This is a rare injury which results from side to side compression such as can occur when a person is trapped between moving vehicles. Sometimes it develops from over-reduction of divarication of the pelvis using slings.[8] On clinical examination there may be accentuation of the lateral hollows of the upper thigh, with bruising or abrasions over the trochanteric area, and the urethra may be damaged. X-rays will show marked overlap of the symphysis pubis and some disruption of the sacro-iliac joint (Figs 28.20 and 28.21). Although it is sometimes possible to reduce the displacement by thrusting the iliac crests laterally[13] this manipulation often fails. Fortunately open reduction through a transverse incision is not difficult provided it is done without delay. The reduction is stable and rarely requires internal fixation, but a double hip spica should be used for two months.

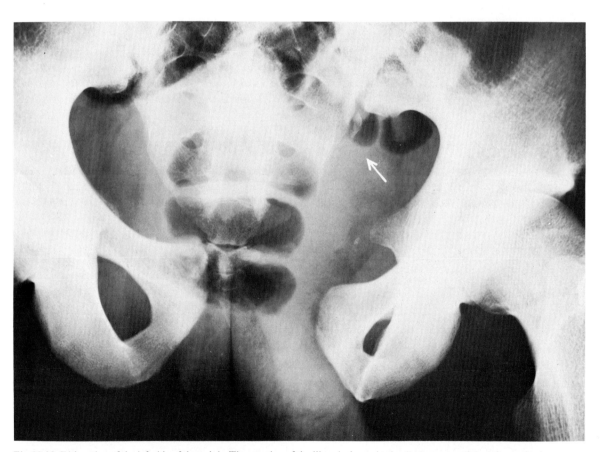

Fig 28.19 Dislocation of the left side of the pelvis. The rotation of the ilium is shown in the displacement of the left symphysis away from the mid-line, the prominence of the ischial spine, the disappearance of the obturator foramen and the abnormal overlap of iliac and sacral shadows. The arrow points to the lower margin of the sacral articular surface.

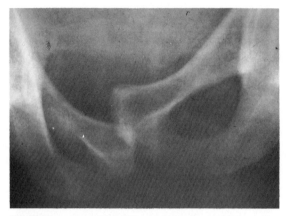

Fig 28.20

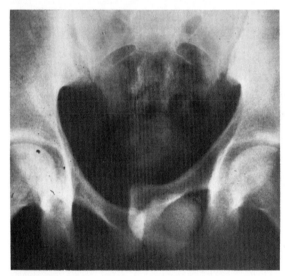

Fig 28.21

Figs 28.20 and 28.21 Side to side compression injury of the pelvis with overlap of the symphysis pubis (Fig 28.20). Attempts to reduce the displacement by manipulation were unsuccessful. Through a transverse incision disimpaction was easily carried out and a very stable reduction was obtained. Note the displacement at the left sacro-iliac joint (Fig 28.21). (Treated by Mr E. L. Trickey at Edgware General Hospital.)

TREATMENT OF DISRUPTIONS OF THE PELVIC RING

Many types of treatment have been devised to correct pelvic displacement, but basically they all depend upon a clear understanding of the pathological anatomy of the injury. The dislocated pelvis is like a partly opened bivalve shell—an oyster or a mussel—

where the hinge posteriorly has also been partially damaged by strain along its long axis. Treatment requires action to restore the hinge to its rightful position and rotation with compression to close the lid. This can be achieved by a variety of methods of which the most useful are:

1. Reduction by traction and pelvic suspension.
2. Postural reduction in lateral recumbency and plaster fixation.
3. Internal fixation of the symphysis pubis.
4. External skeletal fixation.

Reduction by traction and pelvic suspension.
Both external rotation deformity and upward displacement of the fractured hindquarter can be corrected by suspension in a pelvic sling combined with traction on the affected leg. The importance of early closure of the two halves of the pelvis in order to control and prevent further haemorrhage cannot be overemphasised. Peltier has said: 'Too frequently preoccupation with associated injuries results in total neglect of the pelvic fractures. Yet with every breath, cough, or movement, the unstabilised fracture fragments shift and promote further bleeding'.[14] Although perfect reduction is not always obtained the method is simple and is the treatment of choice in most pelvic injuries with displacement, particularly when the fracture is complicated by urethral or bladder damage, or when there are other major injuries to be treated; it has the advantage that it can be applied immediately and without anaesthetic. The pelvic sling must be made of stout material, such as sailcloth, and should have the upper margins strengthened with a wooden rod sewn into a seam (Fig 28.22). Sufficient weights are used which will just counterbalance the patient's own trunk weight, the upper edges of the slings being directed to the opposite side to give an internal rotation thrust to the displaced hemi-pelvis. Traction is applied to the limb on the affected side. Observations on the cadaver have shown that hyperextension of the hips increases the diastasis after rupture of the symphysis pubis,[15] and a more satisfactory reduction is obtained if the hips are flexed about 20 degrees.[16, 17] A convenient way to do this is to rest the legs on Braun frames or put them up in Hamilton Russell traction with the hip and knee bent to 20 degrees (Fig 28.22). The pelvic sling must be well padded with felt to avoid skin sores, particularly over the trochanter and buttock areas. This method of treatment requires careful nursing attention, but provided this is available the patient will tolerate the fixation remarkably well and the

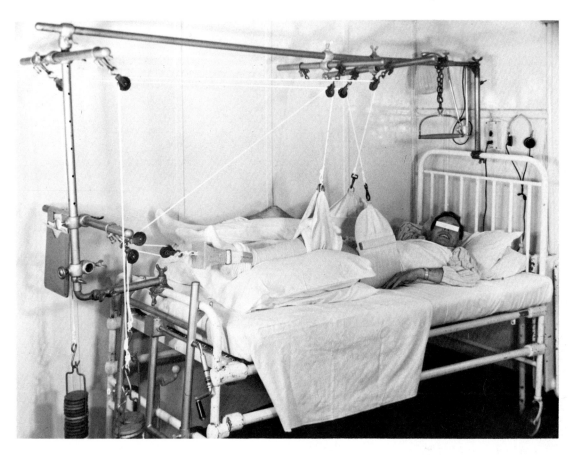

Fig 28.22 Treatment of a fracture-dislocation of the left side of the pelvis by traction and pelvic suspension. Note that the top of the sling has been strengthened with a wooden strut to prevent rucking by the pull of the suspension. The cords of the pelvic suspension are crossed to produce compression and internal rotation, and the hips are both flexed to assist this correction. Upward displacement of the hemi-pelvis has been corrected by Hamilton Russell traction to the left leg.

position can be maintained without difficulty for six weeks. By then the fracture should be sufficiently solid to allow the patient to lie free in bed, and after two or three weeks to get up walking with crutches. A sacro-iliac belt should be worn for a few months after the patient becomes ambulant and crutches used for the first month or so.

Fractures which should not be treated by pelvic slings. A cautionary note must be added about using a pelvic sling in cases where there are comminuted fractures of the acetabuli due to a compression injury. The effect of the sling may cause inward bowing of the pelvic wall, resulting in a triradiate pelvis (Figs 28.23 to 28.25). The same advice applies to hemi-pelvic fracture dislocation where on rare occasions the displacement is towards

the mid-line with overlapping of the symphysis pubis (see Figs 28.20 and 28.21). These injuries are produced by lateral compression and can only be further displaced by pelvic slings.

Postural reduction and plaster fixation.[18] In an uncomplicated fracture-dislocation of the pelvis, particularly when transport elsewhere is necessary, postural reduction and the application of a double hip spica still has a place in treatment of displaced fractures. Slight separations of the symphysis pubis with subluxation of the sacro-iliac joint may be reduced without anaesthesia. If there is greater displacement a general anaesthetic should be given. A plaster table or any form of pelvic rest is used with the perineal post removed. The patient is placed on his uninjured side with the ilium and trochanter lying

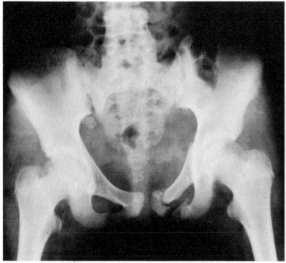

Fig 28.23

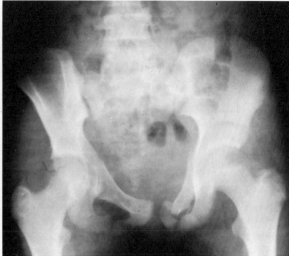

Fig 28.24

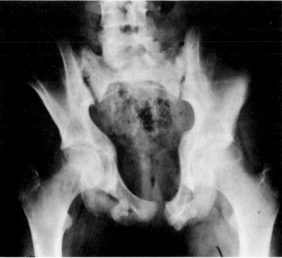

Fig 28.25

Figs 28.23 to 28.25 Pelvic slings should not be used in the treatment of compression injuries of the pelvis. Figure 28.23 shows a comminuted fracture involving the floor of the acetabuli and the pubic rami. The application of a pelvic sling increased the deformity (Fig 28.24), finally resulting in a triradiate pelvis (Fig 28.25).

on the pelvic rest and the two lower limbs held one above the other by an assistant. In many cases the dislocation is already reduced by the time the patient is in this position. If the pubic bones are not perfectly approximated and the posterior superior spine of the ilium is still unduly prominent, pressure should be applied over the crest of the dislocated ilium, pushing and rotating it downwards and forwards towards the normal half of the pelvis. Accuracy of reduction may be confirmed by taking radiographs before the plaster is applied (Figs 28.19 and 28.26). If necessary the patient can be laid on the injured side so that lateral compression is increased by the addition of body weight.

It must be remembered that during the first 48 to 72 hours patients with severe pelvic injuries can develop paralytic ileus and this may require gastric suction, intravenous fluids and even bivalve of the plaster spica. After this stage and throughout the period of recumbency the patient is encouraged to lie on one side. After eight weeks the plaster is removed and the patient allowed to mobilise in bed for two weeks before starting to walk with the aid of crutches. A sacro-iliac belt should be worn for several months.

Internal fixation of the symphysis pubis. Where there has been a complete disruption of the ligaments around the symphysis pubic the integrity

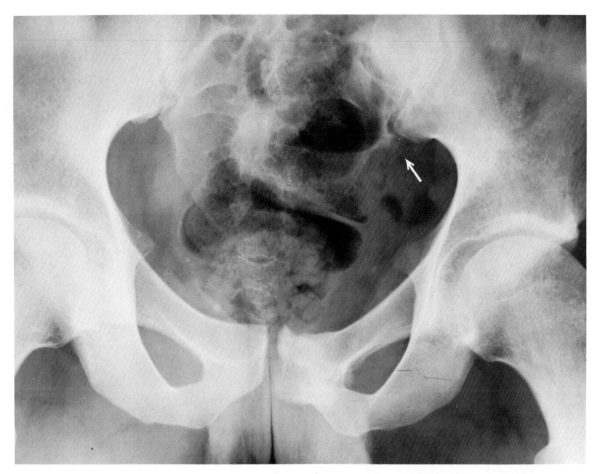

Fig 28.26 Same case as that of Figure 28.19, 12 months after reduction by simple lateral recumbency with the application of a double plaster spica. The separation of the asymphysis is corrected and the sacro-iliac displacement is reduced.

of the pelvic ring can sometimes be completely restored by efficient internal fixation. Usually this will only be achieved by plating the superior pubic rami (Figs 28.27 and 28.28). It can be a difficult operation and should not be undertaken unless conservative measures fail or cannot be used. Previously attempts to repair the pelvis by wiring together the symphysis pubis have met with only a variable measure of success, and the poor results from this method have been largely responsible for the bad reputation of internal fixation at this site. It is claimed that fixation of the symphysis by using two crossed Kirschner wires is a simple and effective way to establish pelvic stability,[8] but it is difficult to believe that such a fragile arrangement can be expected to prevent further displacement. The plating operation is carried out through a transverse Pfannenstiel's

incision centred about 1 inch (2.5 cm) superior to the symphysis and may form part of the procedure to repair a bladder or urethral injury. In order to allow adequate fixation of the plate with either screws or bolts at least 2 inches (5.1 cm) of the superior pubic ramus on both sides must be exposed.[19]

External skeletal fixation.[20] Although suspension in a sling, combined with lower limb traction, will usually establish an acceptable reduction of a pelvic dislocation, it is not always practicable, particularly in compound fractures and in paraplegia, to maintain this type of fixation and in some cases it may not be possible to obtain adequate stability with plaster or wire. In these circumstances external skeletal fixation using the Hoffmann apparatus, or one of its variants, can prove a very useful method of stabilising the

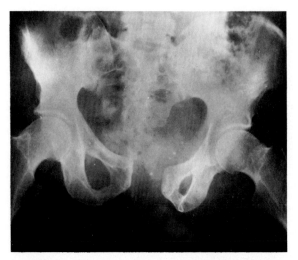

Fig 28.27

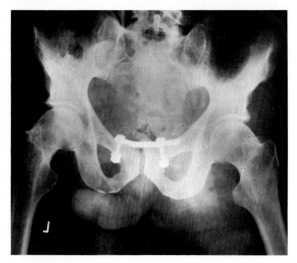

Fig 28.28

Figs 28.27 and 28.28 Divarication of the symphysis pubis stabilised by plating. (Treated by Mr A. Rushforth at St Albans City Hospital).

fracture. The method has been reported as being particularly useful in cases of total disruption of the pelvic ring with dislocation of both sacro-iliac joints.[20a] Three of the threaded half pins are inserted into the anterior third of the iliac crest on either side. Care must be taken to ensure that the section chosen for the pins is a stable fragment. The fracture is reduced manually and the pins clamped together using universal joints and cross bars (Fig 28.29). This fixation gives immediate stability and allows the

patient to be moved about in safety. Traction for the pelvic fracture is not required with this appliance, but it can, of course, be used if needed for the treatment of the lower limb fractures; compound fractures of the pelvis and lower limbs can be dealt with more easily once the pelvic fracture is stable, and if there are signs of paraplegia the patient can be turned from side to side without detriment to the pelvic fractures.

COMPLICATIONS OF FRACTURES OF THE PELVIS

Vascular problems. Intrapelvic haemorrhage is by far the most serious complication of fractures of the pelvis,[4, 14] and in one series these injuries ranked as the third most common cause of death in road traffic accidents.[2] Bleeding originates partly from the fracture surfaces but mainly from laceration of large vessels on the pelvic wall, and when there is an associated urethral or bladder injury severe bleeding can occur from the prostatic plexus. One case has been recorded of intramural damage to the external iliac artery with ischaemia of the lower limb.[21] Ecchymosis of the scrotum, spreading to the inguinal ligaments and the buttocks, is an important sign of severe intrapelvic bleeding.[22, 23]

It has been pointed out that there has often been a relatively long survival time in patients who have died from intrapelvic bleeding,[23] and that this should allow time for an effective resuscitation programme. It must be emphasised, however, that these cases may need transfusion of very large quantities of blood. It is not uncommon for the amount of blood transfused to be in excess of the patient's total blood volume, and precautions must be taken to deal with the metabolic effects of such a large transfusion.

Signs of intraperitoneal bleeding, visceral perforation or urinary tract injury are certain indications for laparotomy. The value of surgery in severe retroperitoneal bleeding, however, is more uncertain. In the face of a rapidly expanding palpable haematoma or in compound fractures with severe bleeding, it may be necessary to ligate one or even both internal iliac arteries.[2] The very fact that it is possible to ligate both these vessels without causing damage to the viscera is a clear indication of the very wide anastomosis between the pelvic vessels and explains why this radical approach may not always arrest the bleeding. Whenever possible, therefore, a conservative regime should be followed and arterial ligation reserved for only the most desparate situations.[14] Arterial embolisation has been suggested as a method

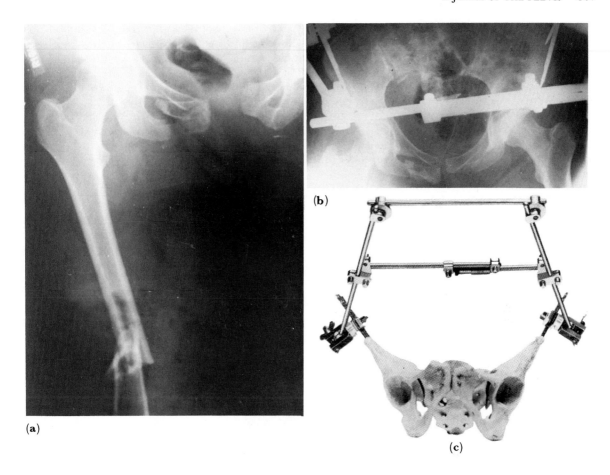

(a)

(b)

(c)

Fig 28.29 This patient was in a severe motor accident sustaining a widely displaced fracture-dislocation of the pelvis, an extensive compound fracture of the femoral shaft (a) and a compound double fracture of the tibial shaft. Temporary pelvic sling fixation was applied but this could not be adequately maintained because of problems with the compound wounds. External skeletal fixation produced excellent stabilisation (b). Model of fixation is shown in (c).

of controlling haemorrhage, but unfortunately it is an impracticable technique except in the more sophisticated centres.

Injuries of the bladder and urethra. Every displaced pelvic fracture which in any way involves the pubic rami or the symphysis pubic must be carefully checked to exclude damage to the lower genito-urinary tract. In several large series of cases the overall incidence of urinary tract complications has been 10 to 12 per cent,[14, 24] rising to 40 per cent in cases where there were bilateral fractures of the pubic rami.[25] Bruising in the perineum, retention of urine and particularly fresh blood at the tip of the urethra are important signs pointing to a possible urinary tract injury. If the patient is unable to pass urine, catheterisation with a small soft catheter should be attempted very gently (a rough technique can be responsible for further damage in partial rupture of the urethra). If urine is not easily obtained a retrograde cystogram should be carried out without delay. (For details of technique and definitive treatment see Chapter 10).

Bowel complications. Paralytic ileus has already been mentioned as a complication when treating the acute case in plaster. It may also be troublesome even when treating fractures in pelvic slings. It is treated by gastric suction and an intravenous drip of saline. Rectal injuries rarely complicate fractures of the pelvis unless there is a compound injury involving the perineum: they demand an immediate defunctioning colostomy and regular irrigation of the distal loop with an antibiotic. It has been said: 'Blunt and penetrating injuries to the pelvis with deep perineal lacerations cause great morbidity and frequently result in death'.[26] Lunt has drawn attention to a rare but important complication of bowel entrapment within the pelvic fracture itself.[27] In three of the four cases described the diagnosis was made only after an interval of time when the patient presented as a case of intestinal obstruction. In several of the injuries there was a long, oblique fracture of the acetabular floor of the type seen in central dislocation of the hip (Fig 28.30).

Rupture of the diaphragm. An abdominal complication of pelvic fractures which is commonly overlooked is traumatic rupture of the diaphragm. Both injuries are produced by severe antero-posterior compression of the trunk and therefore it is not surprising that they occur together. In one series of pelvic fractures the diagnosis was made late in three cases, and in one case it was an unexpected finding at exploratory laparotomy;[14] in another series of abdominal injuries associated with fracture of the pelvis

four out of six diaphragmatic ruptures were associated with pelvic fractures.[28] The complication is of sufficient importance to make routine antero-posterior chest X-rays mandatory in all cases of severely displaced pelvic fractures, and vice versa.

Nerve injuries. Nerve injuries complicated pelvic fractures probably occur more commonly than is generally appreciated. The reported overall incidence for all pelvic fractures varies from 1.2 per cent to 10 per cent.[29, 30] But the figure becomes much higher when only double vertical pelvic fractures involving the sacrum are considered, and one paper reports an incidence of 46 per cent.[30] However, this includes every minor neurological abnormality, and probably a more true estimate is that of Räf who suggests 18 per cent.[31] This is more in keeping with the 16 per cent incidence of sciatic nerve palsy in fracture-dislocation of the hip. Bonnin in a classic paper in 1945 described a fracture of the sacro-iliac part of the sacrum which passed through a zone of weakness formed by the anterior foramina of the first and second sacral nerves.[32] An obstetric X-ray view of the pelvic inlet may show the anterior displacement

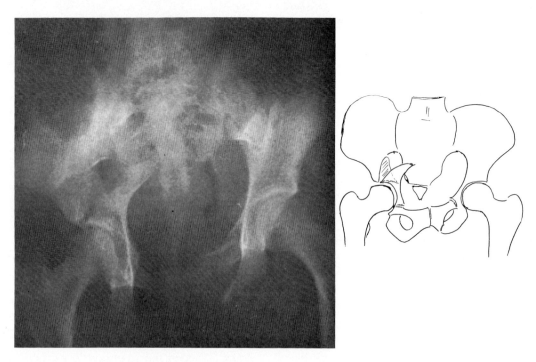

Fig 28.30 This fracture of the ilium just above the acetabulum produced a central dislocation of the hip and entrapped a complete segment of the ilium between the fracture surfaces. This resulted in a late intestinal obstruction 15 days after the accident. Both the use of traction and pelvic slings can increase the effects of entrapment and the fracture must be opened up to release the bowel. (Reproduced by the kind permission of the Editor in *Injury* and H. Randle W. Lunt from his paper in *Injury* (1970) 2, 121.)

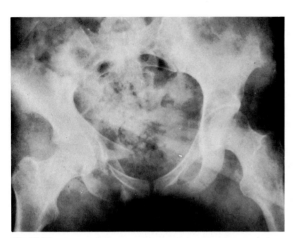

Fig 28.31

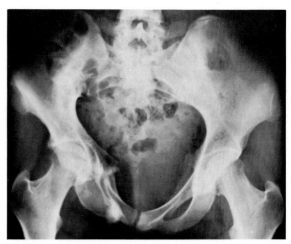

Fig 28.32

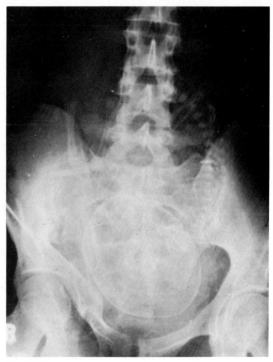

Fig 28.33

of the sacral fragment. The effects of nerve injury complicating pelvic fractures are widespread and point to injury at plexus level rather than to one nerve trunk, as in sciatic nerve palsy after hip dislocation. In addition to the first two sacral roots being involved the lumbo-sacral trunk is particularly vulnerable as it passes across the ilio-lumbar ligament and upper part of the sacro-iliac joint,[33] and it was found to be the most common lesion in post-mortem studies.[11] A few cases of damage to the nerve roots at spinal level have been reported in association with pelvic fractures,[34] and myelography has shown avulsion diverticuli due to rupture of the dural root sleeves. However, these diverticuli do not carry the same grave prognosis as in traction lesions of the cervical roots and a number of the lumbar traction injuries have recovered almost completely.[35] Muscle weakness may be apparent in the buttock, hamstrings and calf muscles, and paraesthesia with sensory loss may affect the whole of the back of the leg and the outer side of the foot. The prognosis is good in the cases of lesser degree, with an expected recovery within a year. Severe cases have a poor prognosis.

Effect of fracture of the pelvis upon childbirth.
Women patients who have had pelvic fractures are often concerned about the possible effect upon any future confinement, and the medico-legal aspects of this are sometimes of considerable importance. In one survey of pelvic fractures[36] it was found that obstetric complications were extremely rare, and on enquiry at a large women's hospital only two cases of obstetric problems after pelvic fracture could be recalled. Even major deformities of the pelvic inlet are not incompatible with natural childbirth as is shown in Figures 28.31 to 28.33

Figs 28.31 to 28.33 This displaced fracture of the right side of the pelvis occurred in a young married woman (Fig 28.31). It was not possible to reduce the deformity by manipulation, and union resulted with considerable distortion of the pelvic inlet (Fig 28.32). X-rays taken two years later while in the last weeks of pregnancy showed that the foetal head was engaging the pelvic rim (Fig 28.33). A trial labour was allowed and normal confinement followed. However, although fractures of the pelvis rarely cause difficulties in childbirth facilities for Caesarian section must always be readily at hand.

However, it is possible that the absence of reported cases of obstetric complications after pelvic fractures may reflect more upon the efficiency of the midwifery services in the civilised countries than give a true indication of the possible problems; and perhaps those who work among the less fortunate in the underdeveloped countries would be wise to keep in mind Malgaigné's words written 130 years ago concerning a woman in labour two years after a severe pelvic fracture:[37] 'The woman came back to the Hospital Saint Louis two years afterwards, pregnant, and near her full term. She had previously had five successful accouchments, but this one was terrible; she was only delivered at the fourth day, by means of forceps, and after such violent tractions that, to say nothing of other extremely grave injuries, she had a fracture of the ischium on the right side. Death ensued at the end of two days'.

Total dislocation of the ilium—an unusual fracture of childhood.

Apart from avulsion injuries fractures of the pelvis in childhood are rare. An unusual injury of total dislocation of the ilium in a 13 year old child has been described by MacKinnon and Lansdowne.[38] In this case there was a fracture-dislocation of the sacro-iliac joint and the entire ilium had separated through the triradiate cartilage and rotated posteriorly and laterally (Figs 28.34 and 28.35). It is probable that this injury could only occur in the immature skeleton. Manipulation failed to reduce the displacement and open reduction was performed at four days. After reflection of the muscles from both sides of the iliac crest it was possible to reduce the sacro-iliac dislocation by swinging the ilium forwards and medially, thereby also restoring the triradiate cartilage to normal. The pelvis was then stabilised by two screws inserted through the

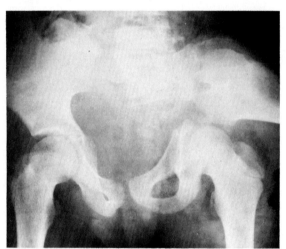

Fig 28.34

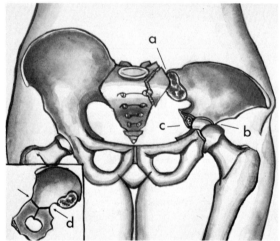

Fig 28.35

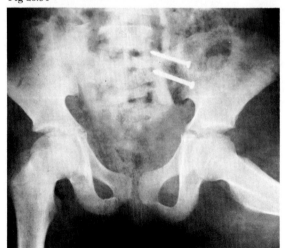

Fig 28.36

Figs 28.34 to 28.36 A 13 year old girl slipped, fell down a hill and was crushed by falling rock. She sustained a complete dislocation of the ilium through the sacro-iliac joint and the triradiate cartilage (Fig 28.34). The drawing shows the lines of separation (Fig 28.35). The displacement was reduced by open operation and the sacro-iliac joint stabilised by two screws (Fig 28.36). Reproduced by the kind permission of the Editor of the *Journal of Bone and Joint Surgery* and Mrs W. M. MacKinnon for the late Dr W. B. MacKinnon and Dr E. L. Lansdown from their paper in the *Journal of Bone and Joint Surgery* (1972) 54–B, 720.

posterior part of the ilium into the sacrum (Fig 28.36).

Impotence after pelvic fractures. In 1975 King reviewed 90 men under the age of 60 who had suffered a fracture of the pelvis.[39] He found that 43 per cent of those with a urethral injury suffered from impotence. There were three patients with impotence who had had no injury to the urethra, but in only one of these was the impotence complete, and in that patient the pelvic fracture had been complicated by damage to the rectum and considerable disturbance to the sacral outflow. The incidence was also found to be higher in those patients who had sustained a divarication of the symphysis pubis. There is no indication from these figures that impotence was more common in litigation cases, and there seems little doubt that its incidence is directly related to the severity of the injury, particularly when the urethra is involved.

Compound injuries. The same principles of treatment apply to the management of compound fractures of the pelvis as apply to any other compound injury. But it must be remembered that a compound injury at this site is more likely to be complicated by intrapelvic or intra-abdominal soft tissue injury which may require urgent laparotomy. The perineum is also particularly vulnerable to impalement injuries such as may be sustained when climbing over spiked railings or, more commonly nowadays, as a result of being thrown from a motor car involved in a collision. This type of injury demands wide surgical exploration, although sometimes it is surprising how the pelvic contents miraculously escape damage (Fig 28.37).

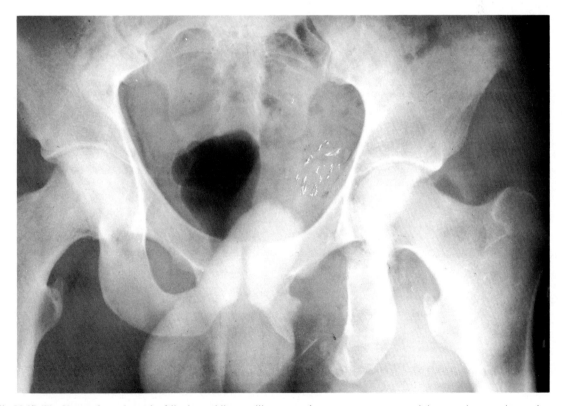

Fig 28.37 The X-ray of a patient who fell asleep while travelling at speed on a motorway, mounted the central reservation, and awoke to find himself impaled on a stake which had penetrated the floor of the car. The stake entered the left ischio-pubic region, crossed the inner wall of the pelvis, and made an exit wound in the left buttock. Despite the obvious fragments of bone within the pelvis (outlined by the white spots) at laparotomy there was no evidence of injury to the pelvic contents. Very severe bleeding, however, was encountered from the depths of the wound—presumably from the gluteal vessels as they passed through the sciatic notch. Ligation of the internal iliac artery had little effect on this bleeding but eventually it was successfully controlled by packing both ends of the wound.

Compound wounds may result from direct trauma to the lower abdomen as a result of 'runover' injuries causing destruction of skin, muscle and pelvic wall, and when severe, disembowelment may follow such as injury.[34] Compound fractures of this type, with a destructive fracture of the ilium, are very commonly associated with bowel rupture and necrosis. They demand a full intraperitoneal inspection of the adjacent abdominal contents (Figs 28.38 and 28.39).

The more common open fracture of the pelvis is one associated with a perineal wound, produced either by impalement or by blunt trauma splitting open the perineum. In a recent review of 12 perineal injuries only one was the result of impalement. The injury is therefore nearly always due to blunt trauma which forces the two halves of the pelvis apart, often resulting in a hemipelvic dislocation with considerable divarication. It is also not uncommon for there to be a complete avulsion of the coccygeal segments, and possibly the lower end of the sacrum (Fig 28.40). Isolated wounds of the anus and perineum may be

repaired primarily; the wound must be thoroughly debrided, lightly packed and finally closed by delayed primary suture within a few days. In many compound pelvic wounds bleeding can be difficult to stop because the natural tamponade of a closed fracture is lost through the open wound. Sometimes control can only be established by packing for several days, repeating this if necessary. When there is a tear of the rectum or lower colon a defunctioning colostomy followed by cleansing of the distal bowel by disempaction and antibiotic irrigation of the distal loop become mandatory. The bladder and urethra must be checked for injury by gentle catheterisation, possibly with retrograde cystography. Whenever possible the bladder, urethra and bowel should be repaired at the same time when the wound is explored. In desperate circumstances, however, when long reparative surgery is not possible, or the necessary expertise is not available, a suprapubic catheter alone is permissible. But restoration of continuity of the urinary tract must be established as soon as possible.

Fracture-dislocations of the hemipelvis can usually

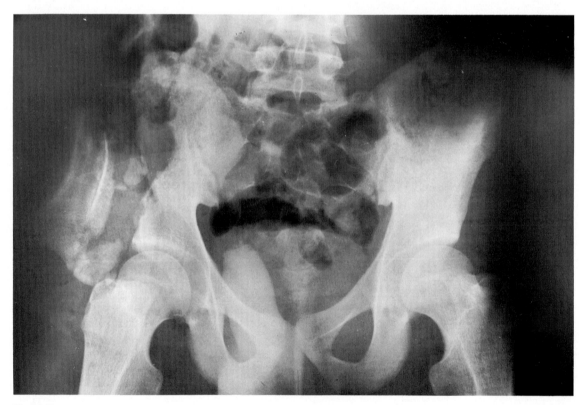

Fig 28.38

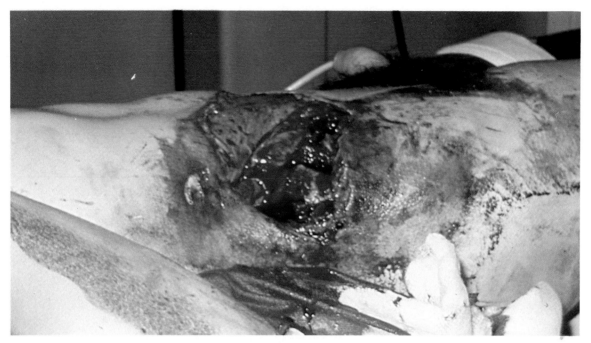

Fig 28.39

Figs 28.38 and 28.39 This young man was thrown from a motorcycle and then partially run over by a car. He sustained a severely comminuted fracture of the wing of the ilium (Fig 28.38) with exposed colon (Fig 28.39). Such injuries demand a wide exploration of the adjacent abdominal contents.

be controlled by a pelvic sling and traction on the lower limbs, but if the soft tissue injuries are extensive fixation by the Hoffmann method of external skeletal fixation may simplify the nursing management. Sometimes stabilisation of the symphysis pubis with a plate or wire may be carried out, but in compound fractures of the pelvis, where there is a high risk of infection, internal fixation with metallic implants should be avoided if possible.

INJURIES OF THE SACRUM AND COCCYX

Fractures of the sacrum. Extensive crushing injuries of the pelvis are often accompanied by fractures of the sacrum. These usually involve the ala of the bone, the fracture passing through a line of weakness formed by the anterior foramina of the first, second and sometimes third sacral nerves.[32] There may be associated nerve injury. These injuries can be easily missed and the fracture illustrated in Figure 28.41 was not diagnosed until the patient presented

again with weakness of the gluteus maximus muscle on the side of the fracture. This type of fracture may be more easily recognised by comparing the bony arches of the sacral foramina on both sides.[34] Sometimes an obstetric view of the pelvic inlet will reveal an anterior segmental displacement of the ala of the sacrum.[40] Isolated fractures are rare, and when they are due to direct trauma to the back of the sacrum the injury is usually a crack fracture without displacement, recovering rapidly and completely. Occasionally the lower half of the sacrum is displaced forwards into the pelvic cavity, and there may be injury to the distal sacral nerves with saddle anaesthesia of the gluteal regions and incontinence of urine. Bonnin describes an interesting fracture of the lower lateral margin of the bone which he considers to be an avulsion injury of the sacrotuberous ligament.[40] An unusual fracture of the upper segment of the sacrum due to compression in the long axis of the body is shown in Figure 28.42. There was temporary incontinence of urine and permanent saddle anaesthesia. There was a marked anterior tilt of the upper fragment and the patient lost 1½ inches

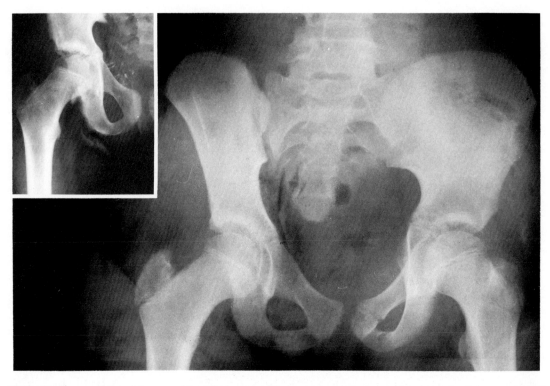

Fig 28.40 This fracture of the pelvis occurred in an 8 year old child who was knocked over crossing the road and thrown astride the bonnet of a car. The pelvis was fractured without gross displacement (Fig 28.40), but there was an extensive perineal laceration which involved the vagina and ano-rectal junction indicating that the pelvis had been split open. The soft tissue laceration extended to the back of the sacrum and the coccyx was completely detached (inset).

(3.8 cm) in height. A number of these injuries have now been described.[41, 42, 43] The mechanism of the injury has been the same in nearly every case. A force has been applied to the back of the lower lumbar spine while the hips were flexed and the knees extended with the feet in a fixed position, such as might occur while sitting in a low car seat with the feet against the bulkhead or foot pedals, or while bending over a machine carrying out repairs. The fracture follows the segmental anatomy of the sacro-iliac joint, the first sacral segment along with the entire vertebral column is forced forward on the pelvis. Bucknill and Blackburne[42] have pointed out that the transverse processes of the fifth lumbar vertebra are always fractured, indicating a rupture of the strong ilio-lumbar ligaments which stabilise the upper sacrum. Neurological signs have usually resolved spontaneously and a sacral laminectomy advised by some authors[43] is rarely indicated. Some improvement in the position has been obtained by pelvic traction, but it is impossible to obtain an accurate reduction. Manipulation per rectum is quite useless.

Injuries of the coccyx. A fall in the sitting position may cause contusion, fracture or dislocation of the coccyx. If the distal fragment is completely separated it is pulled forwards by the ano-coccygeal and levator ani muscles. The injury always causes considerable pain and may persist for several months. There is difficulty in sitting and the only comfortable positions are standing and lying. Movement of the coccyx during examination per rectum will always reproduce the pain and may reveal deformity at the sacro-coccygeal junction. No special treatment is needed except to minimise pain by protecting the bone from further injury. It is wise to give a warning from the beginning that recovery from this injury may not be complete for many weeks or months, otherwise disappointed patients are liable to preserve their pain. These patients are sometimes improved by manipulation of the sacro-coccygeal joint under

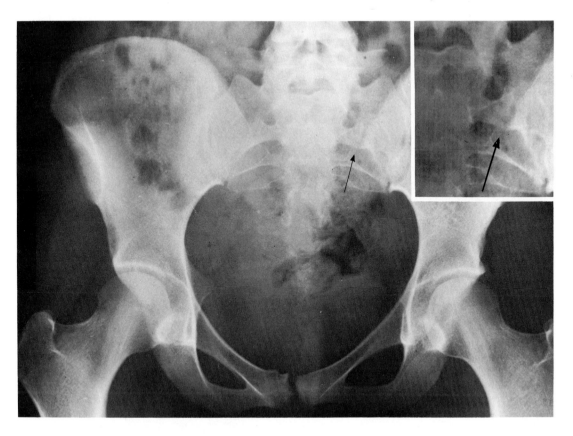

Fig 28.41 This patient was known to have had undisplaced fractures of the pubic rami following a road traffic accident, but it was not until she presented with pain in the left sacro-iliac region, and wasting with loss of tone in the gluteus maximus, that the fracture through the upper third of the ala of the sacrum was observed (see arrow and inset).

anaesthetic associated with an injection into the joint of 2 to 3 ml of a mixture of cortisone (25 mg), hyalase (1500 units) and 1 per cent lignocaine. In chronic cases it is important to exclude any predisposing cause for persistent symptoms. A pilonidal cyst may sometimes flare up after a local injury and be a cause of disabling coccygeal pain. A tell-tale dimple in the midline over the sacro-coccygeal area should alert the surgeon to the possibility of this diagnosis.

Operative treatment. The slowness of repair of coccygeal injuries is explained by the pull of many muscles inserted into the bone. If there is non-union or mal-union the symptoms are relieved when the coccyx is excised. Even where no bony injury can be demonstrated 90 per cent of patients will be relieved by excision.[44, 45] If the operation is done with care and the stump of the sacrum is rounded, the results are entirely satisfactory.

Coccydynia associated with disorders of the lumbo-sacral disc. It has been recognised for many years that even when there has been no actual fracture or displacement of the bones of the coccyx there may be persistent pain in the coccygeal area accompanying lumbo-sacral disc disease. Richards in a study of 102 patients with coccydynia found a history of injury in less than 50 per cent of cases and that nearly half the patients who had coccydynia also complained of low back symptoms or sciatica. Many of the patients in this study had gained relief of the coccygeal pain by immobilisation in a plaster jacket.[46] It is probable that the nerve supply of the coccyx and sacro-coccygeal joint is derived from the first sacral root.[47] It is possible, therefore, that a lesion affecting the root may refer pain to the coccygeal area, and that in certain cases the pain may even be the result of a flexion injury to the lumbo-sacral disc provoked by a fall into the sitting position.

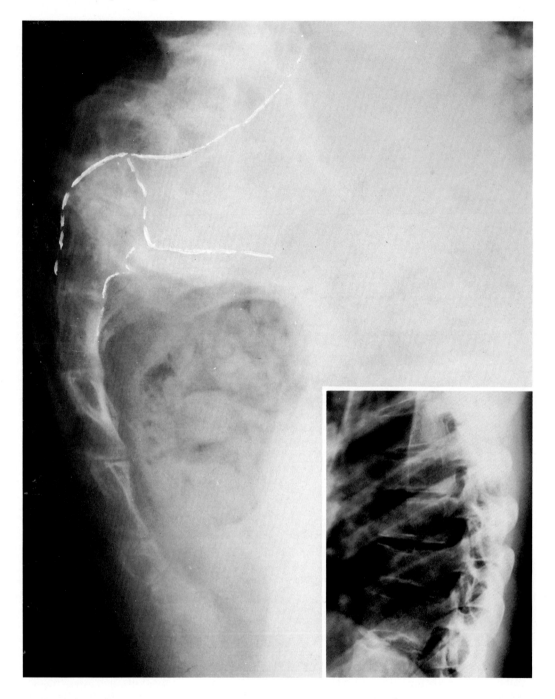

Fig 28.42 The patient who sustained this fracture of the sacrum was asleep on the reclining front seat of a motor car when it collided with another vehicle. His urinary incontinence was regarded as hysterical until an X-ray showed up this fracture. The compression strain also caused a 'concertina' fracture of the bodies of two thoracic vertebrae (inset). He recovered bladder control but he lost 1½ inches (3.8 cm) of his height.

REFERENCES

1. Patterson F P, Morton K S 1973 On the cause of death in fractures of pelvis. Journal of Bone and Joint Surgery 55-B: 660

2. Perry J F, McClellan R J 1964 Autopsy findings in 127 patients following fatal road traffic accidents. Surgery, Gynecology and Obstetrics 119: 586

3. Hamilton S G I 1973 Blood in pelvic fractures. Symposium on pelvic fractures and their complications. Proceedings of the Royal Society of Medicine 66: 629

4. Rothenberger D A, Fischer R P, Strate R G, Velasco R, Perry J F 1978 The mortality associated with pelvic fractures. Surgery 84: 356

5. Goodwin M A 1959 Myositis ossificans in the region of the hip joint. British Journal of Surgery 46: 547

6. Irving M H 1964 Exostosis formation after traumatic avulsion of the anterior inferior iliac spine. Report of two cases. Journal of Bone and Joint Surgery 46-B: 720

7. Godshall R W, Hansen C A 1973 Incomplete avulsion of a portion of the iliac epiphysis. An injury of young athletes. Journal of Bone and Joint Surgery 55-A: 1301

8. Whiston G 1953 Internal fixation for fractures and dislocations of the pelvis. Journal of Bone and Joint Surgery 35-A: 701

9. Harris N H, Murray R O 1974 Lesions of the symphysis pubis in adults. Journal of Bone and Joint Surgery 56-B: 563

10. Malgaigné J F 1847 Traité des fractures et des luxations. Chez J-B Baillière Paris vol 1 p 650–656

11. Huittmen V-M 1976 Lumbosacral nerve injuries. In Vinken P J, Bruyn G W (eds). Handbook of clinical neurology. North Holland Publishing Company, Amsterdam and Oxford, vol 25, p 475–476

12. Shanmugasundarem T K 1970 Unusual dislocation of symphysis pubis with locking. A case report. Journal of Bone and Joint Surgery 52-A: 1669

13. Webb P 1977 Overlapping dislocation of the symphysis pubis. Journal of Bone and Joint Surgery 59-A: 839

14. Peltier L F 1965 Complications associated with fractures of the pelvis. Journal of Bone and Joint Surgery 47-A: 1060

15. Domisse G F 1960 Diametric fractures of the pelvis. Journal of Bone and Joint Surgery 42-B: 432

16. Holdsworth F 1948 Dislocation and fracture-dislocation of the pelvis. Journal of Bone and Joint Surgery 30-B: 461

17. Holdsworth F 1963 Injuries to genito-urinary tract associated with fractures of the pelvis. Proceedings of the Royal Society of Medicine 56, 1044

18. Watson-Jones R 1938 Dislocations and fracture-dislocations of the pelvis. British Journal of Surgery 25: 773

19. Sharp K 1973 Plate fixation of disrupted symphysis pubis. Journal of Bone and Joint Surgery 55-B: 618

20. Müller J, Bachmann B 1978 Behandlung von instabilen Beckenringfracturen mit dem äusser Spanner nach Wagner. Helvetia Chirurgica Acta 45: 59

20a. Sahlstrand T 1979 Disruption of the pelvic ring treated by external skeletal fixation. A case report. Journal of Bone and Joint Surgery 61-A: 433

21. Wilson J N 1952 Fracture of the pelvis complicated by ischaemia of the lower limb. Journal of Bone and Joint Surgery 34-B: 68

22. Braunstein P W, Cooper W, Helpern M, Seremetis W, Wade P A, Weinberg S B 1964 Concealed haemorrhage due to pelvic fracture. Journal of Trauma 4: 832

23. McCarroll J R, Braunstein P W, Cooper W, Helpern M, Seremetis M, Wade P A, Weinberg S B 1962 Fatal pedestrian automotive accidents. Journal of the American Medical Association 180: 127

24. Zorn G 1960 Beckenbruche mit Harnröhrenverletzungen: ihre Behandlung und Ergebnisse. Beiträge zur Klinischen Chirurgie 201: 147

25. Hartmann K 1955 Blasen- und Harnröhrenverletzungen bei Beckenbrüchen. Archiv fur Klinischen Chirurgie 282: 943

26. Maull K I, Sachatello C R, Ernst C B 1977 The deep perineal laceration—an injury frequently associated with open pelvic fractures: a need for aggressive surgical management. Journal of Trauma 17: 685

27. Lunt H R W 1970 Entrapment of the bowel within fractures of the pelvis. Injury 2: 121

28. Levine J I, Crampton R G 1963 Major abdominal injuries associated with pelvic fractures. Surgery, Gynecology and Obstetrics 116: 223

29. Patterson F P, Morton K S 1961 Neurological complications of fractures and dislocations of the pelvis. Surgery, Gynecology and Obstetrics 112: 702

30. Huittmen V-M, Slätis P 1972 Nerve injury in double vertical pelvic fractures. Acta Chirurgica Scandinavica 138: 571

31. Raf L 1966 Double vertical fractures of the pelvis. Acta Chirurgica Scandinavica 131: 298

32. Bonnin J G 1945 Sacral fractures and injuries of the cauda equina. Journal of Bone and Joint Surgery 27: 112

33. Urist M R 1953 Obstetric fracture-dislocation of the pelvis. Report of a case with injury to the lumbo-sacral trunk and first sacral nerve root. Journal of the American Medical Association 152: 127

34. Froman C, Stein A 1967 Complicated crushing injuries of the pelvis. Journal of Bone and Joint Surgery 49-B: 24

35. Harris W R, Rathbun J B, Wortzman G, Humphrey J G 1973 Avulsion of lumbar roots complicating fracture of the pelvis. Journal of Bone and Joint Surgery 55-A: 1436

36. Lowe L W 1965 Personal communication

37. Malgaigne J F 1847 Traité des fractures et des luxations. Translated from the French by John H Packard)1859). Lippincott, Philadelphia, p 526

38. MacKinnon W B, Lansdown E L 1972 Total dislocation of the ilium. Report of a case. Journal of Bone and Joint Surgery 54-B: 720

39. King J 1975 Impotence after fractures of the pelvis. Journal of Bone and Joint Surgery 57-A: 1107

40. Bonnin J G 1957 A textbook of fractures. Related injuries. William Heinemann, London, p 456–457

41. Purser D W 1969 Displaced fracture of the sacrum. Report of a case. Journal of Bone and Joint Surgery 51-B: 346

42. Bucknill T M, Blackburne J S 1976 Fracture-dislocation of the sacrum. Report of three cases. Journal of Bone and Joint Surgery 58-B: 467

43. Fountain S S, Hamilton R D, Jameson R M 1977 Transverse fractures of the sacrum. A report of six cases. Journal of Bone and Joint Surgery 59-A: 486

44. Pyper J B 1957 Excision of the coccyx for coccydynia. A study of the results in 28 cases. Journal of Bone and Joint Surgery 39-B: 733

45. Torok G 1974 Coccygodynia. Journal of Bone and Joint Surgery 56-B: 386

46. Richards H J 1954 Causes of coccydynia. Journal of Bone and Joint Surgery 36-B: 142

47. Dittrich R J 1951 Coccygodynia as referred pain. Journal of Bone and Joint Surgery 33-A: 715

29

Injuries of the Hip

The ball-and-socket shape of the hip joint, together with the thickness of the capsule and the arrangement of bone lamellae in the line of stress of the femoral neck, account for its strength and stability. Nevertheless the joint is usually susceptible to injury at three stages of life. In adolescence, before the epiphyseal lines have fused, there may be avulsion of the trochanteric epiphyses or displacement of the upper femoral epiphysis. In old age when there is senile osteoporosis the femoral neck may be fractured by simple stumbles or trivial strains. Even in middle life, when the defences seem most sound, there is one position in which the joint is vulnerable to injury—if the femur is flexed to the right angle and adducted it is held in position only by capsule, and a forcible thrust along the line of the femur may dislocate the joint. Thus there are three main groups of injury in the region of the hip joint to be considered and these can be further subdivided as given below:

1. Avulsions and displacements of the epiphyses at the upper end of the femur.
   a. Avulsions of trochanteric epiphyses.
   b. Displacement of the upper femoral epiphysis.
2. Traumatic dislocation of the hip.
   a. Simple anterior and posterior dislocation.
   b. Fracture dislocations.
   c. Central dislocation.
3. Fractures of the neck of the femur
   a. Intra-capsular fractures. (Transcervical or subcapital.)
   b. Extra-capsular fractures. (Pertrochanteric or intertrochanteric.)
   c. Ununited fractures.

It is doubtful whether injuries to any other part of the body have been responsible for generating more surgical argument and in consequence, more provocative writing, than those involving the hip. There is disagreement on the causation and management, on the statistical results of treatment, on the reasons for complications, and a host of other topics. What is more, almost a seasonal change of clinical opinion exists. For what is fashionable one year may be quite the reverse the next. It is important, therefore, that any textbook which is to be used as a working handbook should give a balanced view of the subject and not be over-enthusiastic about new methods which in a few years may have been rejected. Thus in dealing with the injuries around the hip a middle of the road policy has been adopted with the emphasis on well tried methods of treatment, rather than highlighting the more esoteric, and possibly short-lived, techniques. In general, surgical procedures which demand a very high degree of technical skill should always be approached with caution, for not all of us are surgical wizards. Simplicity of technique is often the hallmark of success.

AVULSIONS AND DISPLACEMENTS OF THE EPIPHYSES AT THE UPPER END OF FEMUR

Avulsion of trochanteric epiphyses

Avulsion of the lesser trochanter. The epiphysis of the lesser trochanter is sometimes avulsed by the powerful iliopsoas muscle (Fig 29.1). Like other tendon ruptures and avulsions the injury occurs from the active contraction of the muscle against the resistance of a strain in the opposite direction. The usual cause is a tackle at Rugby football or an attempt to stop suddenly when running at speed. The psoas tendon is attached to the epiphysis itself, but the iliacus is inserted into a broader area of the femoral shaft and this often limits the degree of displacement. Moreover, the epiphysis fuses to the femur at the age of 18 years, and avulsion of the iliopsoas after that age is exceptional, although one case has been recorded of an avulsion fracture of the lesser

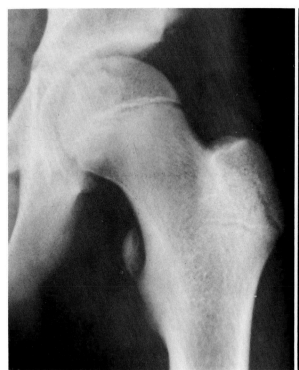

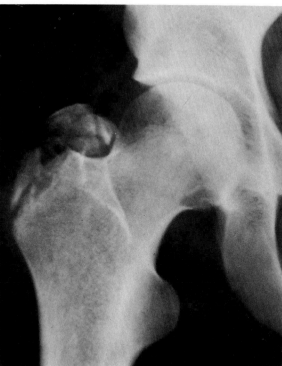

Fig 29.1 Avulsion of the epiphysis of the lesser trochanter by the iliopsoas muscle.

Fig 29.2 Avulsion of the greater trochanter by the abductor muscles of the hip.

trochanter sustained by an adult during a wrestling match. On clinical examination there will be local tenderness in the groin and some bruising; but the diagnostic sign, however, is an inability to actively lift the thigh when the patient is in the sitting position (*Ludloff's sign*).[1] Operative treatment is not indicated. If the hip is flexed through 90 degrees the raw bone surface of the femur is brought up to the retracted fragment and the position can be maintained by a simple arrangement of pillows. There is no need for complete immobilisation in splints or plaster, but the patient should stay in bed for about two weeks.

Avulsion of the greater trochanter.[2] A direct blow over the greater trochanter may cause an isolated fracture, but complete separation and displacement of the trochanteric epiphyses, although a rare injury, can occur from muscular violence, the abductor and lateral rotator muscles avulsing the bone fragment which is retracted so that it lies above the neck of the femur. In the child or adolescent when the injury occurs through the epiphysis, treatment is usually conservative. When the hip is abducted the

upper shaft of the femur is brought into accurate apposition with the avulsed trochanter, and firm union is secured if the position is maintained by means of a plaster spica for about six weeks. This injury can also occur in young adults and in the elderly (Fig 29.2) due to direct trauma. If the fragment is widely displaced it should be repaired using a simple wire loop suture.

DISPLACEMENT OF THE UPPER FEMORAL EPIPHYSIS—ADOLESCENT EPIPHYSEAL COXA VARA—EPIPHYSIO-LYSIS CAPITIS FEMORIS

Several features distinguish slipping of the upper femoral epiphysis from the displacements caused by injury to other epiphyses at the ends of long bones. This epiphyseal displacement occurs much more commonly in boys in adolescent years, some showing evidence of hypopituitarism or hypogonadism with obesity and sexual immaturity while others give a history of recent rapid growth so that the child is tall and slender.[3] Burrows, in a careful survey of 100 cases found that a quarter of the boys and two-thirds of the girls showed evidence of some endocrine defect, quite apart from those who were unusually fat.[4] Moreover, although the line of separation is at the usual level of the junction of the metaphysis with the epiphyseal cartilage, the epiphysis in its backward and downward displacement does not carry with it a triangular fragment from the margin of the diaphysis over which it is displaced as it does in other epiphyseal injuries.[5] This is because the displacement is not simply one of movement in one or two planes, but is due to a torsional slip around an axis lying in the intertrochanteric region.[6] The frequency of simultaneous involvement of both hip joints, often without history of injury to either, indicates that the lesion is not a simple traumatic displacement. About 50 per cent of the displacements arise without recognised injury,[4] and even in other cases there is seldom severe injury causing immediate and complete displacement. More often the onset is insidious with slowly increasing pain and limp and with radiological evidence of progressive epiphyseal slipping. Indeed, it is sometimes found that while one hip has been treated for epiphyseal displacement by immobilisation and traction, the epiphysis on the opposite hip, which has not been immobilised, has been slipping gradually and unobserved. One case is even recorded of severe displacement developing while the affected hip was immobilised on an abduction frame.[7] Clearly there must be predisposing factors causing such a degree of epiphyseal separation. The predisposition is observed between the ages of 12 and 17 years, although cases have been reported in adult men suffering from Simmond's disease,[8] or from hypopituitarism resulting from intracranial tumour.[9] The longest interval in bilateral cases between the onset of slipping on one side and on the other is about 18 months. The underlying factor is not always evident, but sometimes it is quite obvious. The link with abnormal sexual development is inescapable. Affected boys may be excessively fat and have delayed sexual maturity with undeveloped testicles and absence of pubic and axillary hair—hypopituitarism of the French type, or hypogonadism described as adipose gynandrism. In girls it is exceptional to find epiphyseal slipping once they have started to menstruate.[4] Displacement has also been described resulting from failure of epiphyseal calcification in renal rickets.[10]

Aetiology. The aetiological factors may therefore be summarised under three headings.

1. An endocrine disorder with deficiency of sex hormone or perhaps excess of growth hormone predisposing to slipping of the epiphysis during a period of two or three years in adolescence. Harris showed that sex hormone increases the shearing strength of the epiphyseal plate and growth hormone reduces it.[11] Growth hormone increases the width of the hypertrophying cartilage cells and it is always through this layer that the epiphysis fails, and more recent studies of the ultra-structure of the growth plate in patients with slipped epiphysis has shown that the cartilage matrix in the hypertrophic zone differs markedly from normal, with the collagen arranged in irregularly orientated fibres.[12] Harris considered that hormonal changes might be significant in displacements of the upper femoral epiphysis, which occur so often in association with the adipose-genital syndrome or with rapid adolescent growth and in which there is relative lack of sex hormone and relative excess of growth hormone. Also, a case has been reported of a slip occurring while an adolescent girl was under treatment with growth hormone for retardation of growth.[13]

2. The validity of Harris's hypothesis has been seriously challenged by the findings in patients with hypopituitarism secondary to an intracranial tumour. No evidence of an increase in growth hormone was found, even though there were clear signs of hypogonadism.[9] It has been suggested that the relationship of excessive body weight to delayed skeletal maturation may be a more important factor. Under these circumstances muscle retraction could produce gradual and insiduous displacement without injury and without weight-bearing.

3. Occasionally an injury such as a severe wrench or stumble precipitates the displacement acutely.

Pathological anatomy. The primary and important displacement of the epiphysis is not downwards but backwards, and epiphyseal coxa vara is a less accurate anatomical description than epiphyseal coxa anteverta.[14] Griffiths[6] describes the shape of the metaphyseal side of the upper femoral epiphysis as virtually straight in the coronal plane, but curved into roughly a quarter circle in the sagittal plane. The separated femoral head epiphysis rotates easily in a posterior and downward direction following the sagittal curve of the metaphysis. Any pressure on the separated epiphysis will move it in this direction until it eventually comes to rest abutting against the back of the neck of the femur, with its long axis at right angles to the axis of the femoral neck. This rotatory deformity of the head and neck of the femur was described as far back as 1905 by Schlesinger[15] who spoke of a 'torsion of the head' in which 'the head assumed a position of flexion while the femur moved in a direction of extension'.

As the deformity increases the limb rotates laterally in order to maintain a more or less central position of the epiphysis in the acetabulum and the more the epiphysis displaces the greater is the development of lateral rotation deformity. At the same time, because the epiphysis is slipping in rotation, the shaft of the femur becomes extended in relationship to the head. Ultimately the epiphysis can slip no more, because its lower margin locks in the digital fossa and the lateral rotation deformity then amounts to 80 degrees. Thus the final deformity of the lower limb is one of extreme external rotation, extension and, because of the downward displacement, an adduction deformity is nearly always present.

Clinical diagnosis. The clinical signs of a severely displaced upper femoral epiphysis are easily recognised. An adolescent boy, either obese with sexual immaturity or unusually tall and slender, has limitation of all hip movements with slight shortening of the limb, but there is no flexion-adduction deformity, whereas there is from 40 to 80 degrees of lateral rotation deformity with 20 to 30 degrees of extension deformity. These signs are unmistakable. But they should never have arisen; the diagnosis has been made too late. If the epiphysis is already displaced and fixed in its deformed position a perfect result is difficult to achieve no matter what the treatment may be. A provisional clinical diagnosis can always be made before there is fixed lateral rotation deformity, and only then is there any chance of avoiding residual disability.

Early clinical diagnosis. It is in the early stage that an epiphyseal slip is frequently missed, and often this is because the practitioner fails to *think of the diagnosis.* If a boy, or sometimes a girl, aged from 12 to 17 years, develops intermittent limp and complains of occasional stiffness in the thigh, slipping of the upper femoral epiphysis should be suspected. Pain in the thigh and knee is even more frequent than pain in the hip. The symptoms can be intermittent, and in the intervals the patient may run, jump and pursue normal recreations. The important clinical sign is the limitation of medial rotation movement of the hip joint. The range must be estimated accurately in degrees; the common practice of perfunctorily rolling the extended limb is useless. The hip and knee joints should be flexed to the right angle, the leg from knee to ankle being used as the arm of a protractor, and it is then easy to demonstrate that medial rotation

movement is less than the normal 30 to 40 degrees. The range of lateral rotation may be somewhat greater than the normal 50 to 60 degrees. Moreover, it is impossible to flex the hip joint fully in a normal manner so that the knee touches the front of the chest. Backward and downward rotation of the femoral head has imposed a new axis of flexion movement on the joint, and the more it is flexed the more the knee moves away from the mid-line. In full flexion of the hip joint, the knee lies at the side of the chest near the axilla and the limb is laterally rotated. All these clinical signs may not be present. It is enough that an adolescent has complained of intermittent limping or stiffness and that medial rotation movement of the hip is restricted. On these grounds alone complete radiographic examination is imperative.

Radiographic diagnosis of displacement of the upper femoral epiphysis. Look at the radiograph in Figure 29.3. Is this a normal hip joint? In isolation it could be mistaken as normal. But look at the comparison with a normal femoral head in Figure 29.4. The capital epiphysis on the suspected side is now seen to be more crescentic than the normal, and if a line is drawn upwards from the superior margin of the femoral neck it does not cut off

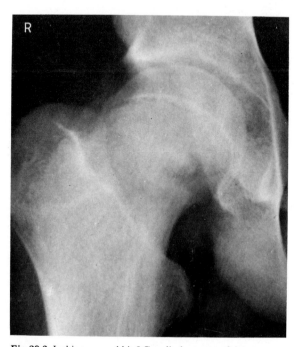

Fig 29.3 Is this a normal hip? Can displacement of the upper femoral epiphysis be excluded in this radiograph? See Figures 29.4 and 29.5.

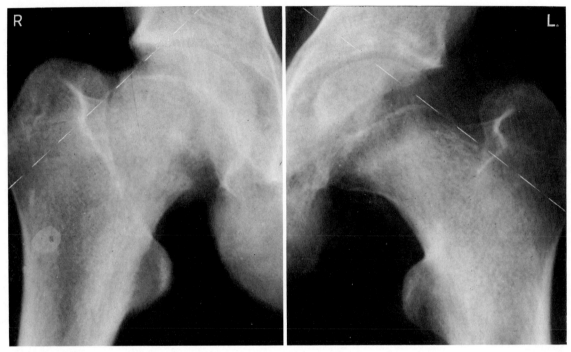

Fig 29.4

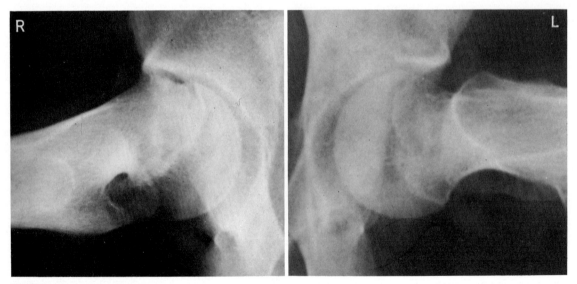

Fig 29.5

Figs 29.4 and 29.5 Same case as that shown in Figure 29.3. (Antero-posterior projection Fig 29.4; lateral projection, Fig 29.5.) Comparison with the normal left hip, which in this particular case is not displaced at all, shows in the antero-posterior projection that the depth of the epiphysis seems to be less than on the normal side; the important point is that the line of the upper margin of the femoral neck projected proximally lies clear of the upper part of the epiphysis, whereas normally it cuts off an appreciable sector. In the lateral projection, backward rotation of the epiphysis so that its lower part lies in the digital fossa is even more obvious.

a sector of the epiphysis but passes outside it. A lateral radiograph taken on the same day shows an advanced degree of slipping of the epiphysis which has reached almost the final stage of displacement beyond which it can slip no more (Fig 29.5). If displacement of such severity can be masked in an antero-posterior view how much more easily can it be concealed when slipping has just begun. A lateral radiograph should always be taken, and without such projection suspected displacement of the upper femoral epiphysis has not been excluded (Figs 29.4 and 29.5). In the days before the technique of lateral radiography was perfected a 'pre-slipping' was described. There is no such stage; if lateral radiographs had been taken at the time it would have been obvious that the epiphysis was already displaced.

Failure to take lateral radiographs during treatment may cause still more trouble. An upper femoral epiphysis with gross displacement can be made to appear to be reduced by taking antero-posterior radiographs with the limb in medial rotation (Figs 29.6 to 29.9). The position of the epiphysis in relation to the femoral neck has not changed at all, and yet 30 degrees of medial rotation gives an appearance of reduction, and with still more medial rotation the displacement may even appear to be over-reduced. This illusion has caused the destruction of many hip joints. Years ago hips were manipulated under general anaesthesia and a plaster spica applied with the hip internally rotated as much as possible; only to find after removal of the plaster, that the original displacement was shown once more. Throughout, the position of the epiphysis remained unchanged, and the only effect of the manipulations, and of immobilisation in a strained position of full medial rotation, was to stretch the blood vessels of the capsule and ligamentum teres, thus causing avascular necrosis with disintegration of the epiphysis and degeneration of the articular cartilage.

Technique of lateral radiography. The limb should be flexed, abducted and laterally rotated.[16] With the X-ray tube centred in the ordinary way and a cassette behind the hip, a lateral projection of the femoral head and neck is secured. It is usually wise to put the patient in the lithotomy position so that the upper ends of both femora are seen in lateral projection on one film. An accurate measurement of the amount of epiphyseal slip can be obtained by taking Billings' lateral view of the hip[16a] (Fig 29.10).

Early radiographic signs (Fig 29.11). The first sign is the evidence in the lateral view that the cup-shaped epiphysis is no longer fitting accurately on the curved surface of the metaphysis; part of the metaphysis is uncovered in front and a break of the epiphysis projects behind. In antero-posterior projections the depth of the epiphysis seems to be less than in the normal hip. The downward displacement is shown in the antero-posterior view if a line is drawn along the upper margin of the femoral neck and projected beyond the epiphysis. Normally this line cuts off a fairly large sector of the upper part of the epiphysis and, if the whole of the epiphysis lies below it, considerable displacement has already occurred (Fig 29.4).

A number of observers[17, 18, 19] have noted that the normal caput femoris (the part of the femur which is contained within the acetabulum) includes part of the inferior diaphysis (Fig 29.12). When there is even a minimal slip of the capital epiphysis inferiorly the diaphyseal portion of the caput femoris is pushed out of the acetabulum and the lower margin of the epiphysis becomes beak-shaped. Finally, it has been observed that the margin of the proximal metaphysis of the normal femur shows a series of sharp intersecting lines. When a slip has occurred the margins become blurred.[20] All these four points can be appreciated in the antero-posterior X-ray at a very early stage (Figs 29.11 and 29.13).

Late radiographic signs. In later stages the displacement is obvious even in antero-posterior radiographs. The epiphysis lies well below its normal level and is so much rotated backwards that it is no longer in profile. The whole circle of the epiphyseal surface is outlined clearly (Figs 29.14 to 29.15).

Treatment of displacements of the upper femoral epiphysis

The treatment of displacements of the upper femoral epiphysis is not a very happy chapter in the history of orthopaedic surgery. In former years many hip joints were destroyed by forcible manipulations which were thought to have corrected the displacements but had not corrected them at all (the illusion being sustained by the incorrect interpretation of X-rays taken in different positions of rotation (see Figs 29.6 to 29.9). Indeed, such manipulations have been considered directly responsible for the onset of avascular necrosis with permanent stiffness of the joint and late arthritis.[6] Robert Jones used to say: 'Leave them alone; just put them to bed; you will get into less trouble that way'. But we have learned much since then and certain principles of treatment have now been defined.

Principles of treatment. The principles of treat-

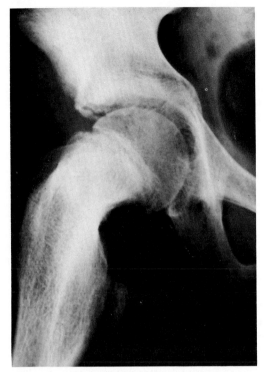

Fig 29.6 Antero-posterior projection in lateral rotation.

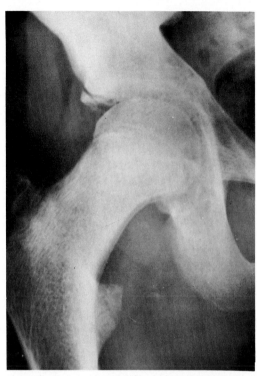

Fig 29.7 Antero-posterior projection in medial rotation.

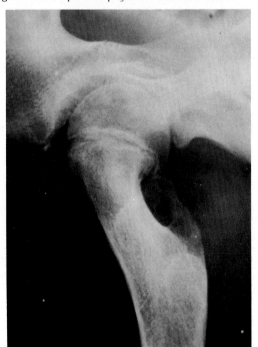

Fig 29.8 Lateral projection in lateral rotation.

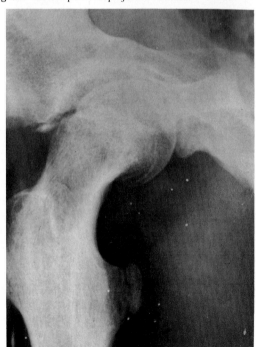

Fig 29.9 Lateral projection in medial rotation.

Figs 29.6 to 29.9 Concealment of epiphyseal displacement by medial rotation of the hip joint giving a false appearance of reduction. Fig 29.6 shows an obviously displaced upper femoral epiphysis. After medial rotation of the hip joint the displacement appears to have been reduced (Fig 29.7). Actually the position has not changed; the displacement is simply concealed in the antero-posterior view; but it has appeared in the lateral view (Fig 29.9), whereas previously it was partly concealed in the lateral view (in lateral rotation) (Fig 29.8).

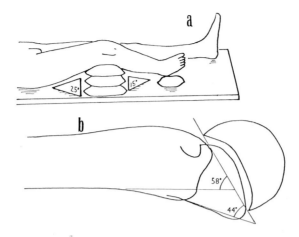

Fig 29.10 Billing's lateral view of the upper end of the femur. (a) Technique. With the patient lying supine on the X-ray table and the knee maintained in 90° flexion the hip is allowed to fall into a position of external rotation and abduction. The knee is supported to bring the shaft of the femur to a position of 25° of elevation while the height of the lateral malleolus is adjusted so that the shin subtends an angle of 15° to the table. If hip movements are restricted it may be necessary to tilt the pelvis by placing a support under the opposite buttock. A vertical beam is centred over the femoral head and the X-ray plate is placed to include the upper third of the shaft of the femur. (b) Interpretation. The neck axis is indicated by the relatively straight anterior border of the distal half of the femoral neck and the shaft axis by the anterior border of the upper third of the femoral shaft. The line connecting the anterior and posterior margins of the epiphysis defines the epiphysial plane. The true angle between the diaphysis and the epiphyseal plane, the epiphyseal plane angle, is the mean of two angles, the epiphyseal-neck and the epiphyseal-shaft angles. In the case above these are 44° and 58° respectively, giving an epiphyseal plane angle of 51°. If a normal value of 90° is assumed the amount of slipping is 90 − 51 = 39°. (Reproduced by the kind permission of Mr John Angel.)

ment of displacements of the upper femoral epiphysis are:

1. If the epiphysis has begun to displace there can be no safety until the epiphyseal line has fused—premature fusion causes little or no disability and moreover it is inevitable.
2. When there is minor displacement the epiphysis should be fused at once, by pinning, in the position in which it lies.
3. When there is an acute major slip it may be possible to reduce the deformity gently by traction, or under an anaesthetic, into a position which can be fixed with pins (although there are some who hold the view that there is no such thing as a 'gentle manipulation', and that even traction may predispose to avascular necrosis of the femoral head[6]).
4. When the displacement cannot be reduced easily and where the displacement is too great to allow pinning in situ, open reduction by cervical osteotomy must be considered.
5. Older fixed displacements in which the epiphysis has already fused by bone should be treated by

corrective osteotomy at intertrochanteric or subtrochanteric level.

There is no safety until the epiphyseal line has fused. The predisposition to displacement of the upper femoral epiphysis is so strong that it is not enough to correct the displacement; it will almost certainly recur if treatment is abandoned at any time before fusion of the epiphysis is complete. Premature fusion of the epiphyseal line is of course inevitable, and it is clearly better to make sure that it fuses in the correct position. Such fusion should be secured by the simple procedure of inserting stabilising pins across the epiphyseal line (Figs 29.15 and 29.16)*. At least two pins, and preferably three or four, should be used (Figs 29.17 and 29.18). They are preferred to the Smith-Petersen nail fixation for two reasons: (1) The pins can often

* There are a variety of suitable pins for this purpose. Moore pins have a screwed end over which a knurled nut can be applied to prevent migration. These pins are very slender. Newman pins are the size of a Steinmann's pin and stronger, but have no screwed end and can easily migrate. Adams pins have a threaded base to engage the cortex of the trochanteric area and are probably the best of the three.

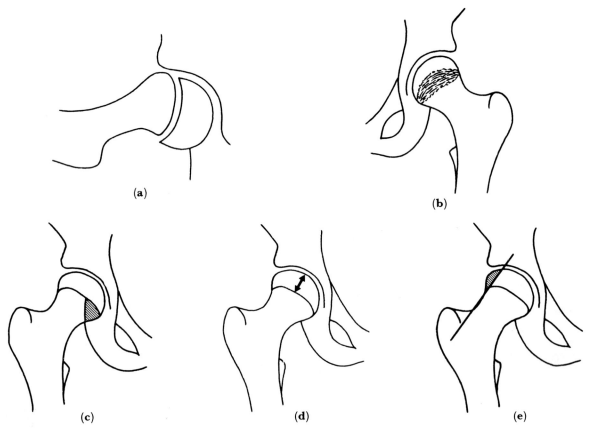

Fig 29.11 Diagrams of early radiographic signs in slipped upper femoral epiphysis. (a) The lateral radiograph will show a step between the metaphysis and the epiphysis; (b) Marginal blurring of the proximal metaphysis; (c) In the normal hip the lower margin of the metaphysis is included within the acetabulum but excluded in early epiphyseal slip; (d) In the normal a line drawn along the superior margin of the femoral neck transects the epiphysis, but will be above it if there has been a slip; (e) The depth of the epiphysis can be measured and compared with normal. The measurement is smaller on the displaced side. (Reproduced by the kind permission of the Editor of *Clinical Radiology* and Dr T. J. Bloomberg *et al* (1978) from their paper Radiology in early slipped femoral capital epiphysis. *Clinical Radiology*, 29, 657.

be inserted when there is too much residual deformity to allow a nail to be used; (2) There is less chance of the segmental avascular necrosis which is sometimes seen after Smith-Petersen nail fixation (Figs 29.19 and 29.20).

Treatment of minor displacements of the upper femoral epiphysis. If there is clinical and radiographic evidence of early displacement of the upper femoral epiphysis with no more than about 20 degrees limitation of medial rotation movement, it is wise to act in advance of the serious displacement that will almost certainly arise and fuse the epiphysis by the insertion of pins. Very commonly this treatment is needed for what might at first seem to be the 'normal hip' in a patient who is being treated for severe displacement of the

upper femoral epiphysis of the other hip. Although there may have been no symptoms on this side, the epiphysis should be pinned if radiographs show early slipping (Figs 29.15 and 29.16, left hip).

Forcible correction by manipulation under anaesthesia is indefensible. Major displacements have sometimes been reduced by forcible medial rotation and abduction of the limb under anaesthesia—but this is a dangerous manoeuvre for the incidence of avascular necrosis is high. If the displacement has been occurring gradually over several months, such manipulation stretches the posterior capsular vessels upon which the vascularity of the epiphyseal fragment depends.[21, 22] Even in recent acute slips manipulation under anaesthesia can be responsible for avascular necrosis. For in this

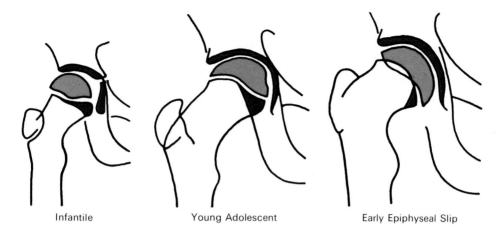

Infantile   Young Adolescent   Early Epiphyseal Slip

Fig 29.12 Diagram showing how the diaphysis extends medially under the epiphysis forming part of the articular femoral head in the infant and young adolescent. The exclusion from the acetabulum of the articular portion of the diaphysis by the downward and backward thrust of the epiphysis is one of the earliest radiological signs of adolescent slipping of the upper femoral epiphysis.[13] The downard pointing epiphyseal beak is apparent even when the displacement is less than shown in the drawing. (Reproduced by kind permission of the *Journal of Bone and Joint Surgery* and of F. C. Durbin, from his paper (1960) Treatment of slipped upper femoral epiphysis. *Journal of Bone and Joint Surgery*, 42–B, 289.)

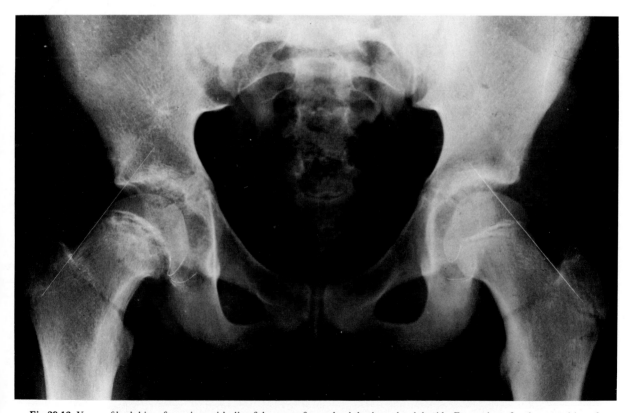

Fig 29.13 X-ray of both hips of a patient with slip of the upper femoral epiphysis on the right side. Four points of early recognition of a minor slip of the epiphysis can be seen in this antero-posterior view of both hips: (1) the height of the epiphysis is diminished; (2) the upper femoral neck line does not include a segment of the capital epiphysis; (3) the inferior diaphysis of the neck is not included in the acetabulum; and (4) the metaphyseal side of the epiphysis is ill defined.

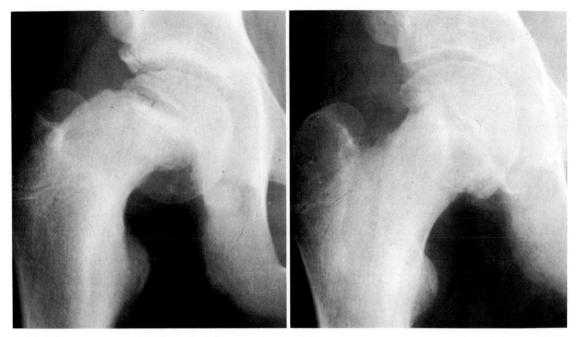

Fig 29.14 Displacement of the upper femoral epiphysis before and after reduction by gradual traction on a frame. Note the premature fusion of the epiphysis which in this case occurred even without surgical intervention. Such early fusion is inevitable and should be promoted when the displacement has been corrected by pinning (see Figs 29.15 and 29.16).

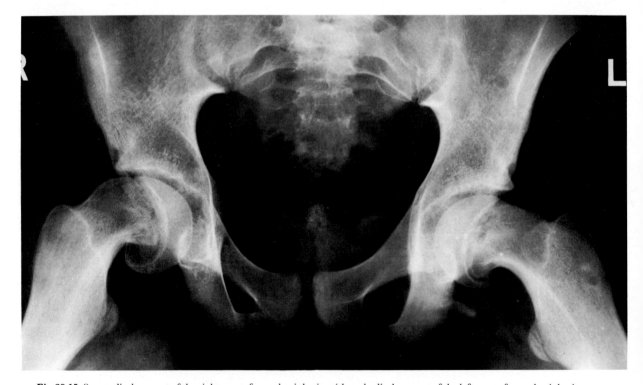

Fig 29.15 Severe displacement of the right upper femoral epiphysis, with early displacement of the left upper femoral epiphysis.

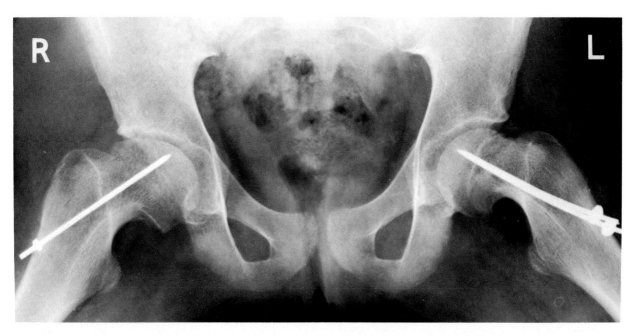

Fig 29.16 Same case as Figure 29.15. The epiphysis on the left side was pinned in its slightly displaced position with two Moore pins, external fixation not being used. The displacement on the right side could not be reduced by traction, and it was corrected by a curved osteotomy at the epiphyseal level, with fixation by one Moore pin and the support of a plaster spica for two months. (Mr Philip Newman's case.)

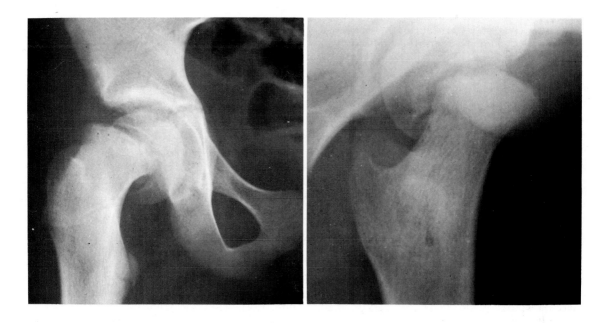

Fig 29.17 An acute slip of the right upper femoral epiphysis, reduced by gently putting the leg into neutral position on the Hawley table, and successfully fixed with four Moore pins.

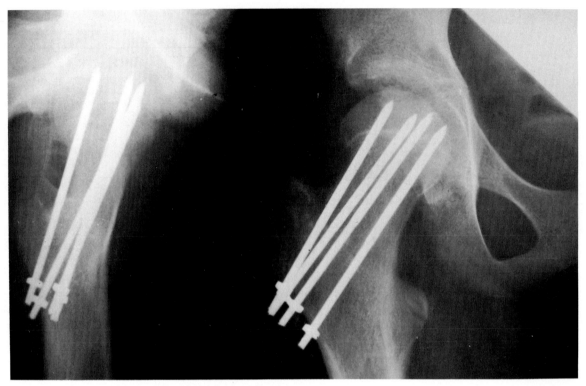

Fig 29.18 The second X-ray was taken six months after operation.

variety of injury it is possible to over-reduce the epiphysis—a manoeuvre particularly likely to be followed by avascular change.[23] It is exactly this treatment by forcible correction or over-reduction that has been responsible for establishing the bad reputation of all forms of manipulation and has resulted in much conflicting advice on the management of the acute slip.[6, 24, 25] In recent displacements forcible manipulative reduction is no better than gentler methods; in older displacements it is positively harmful. Why then perpetuate it? Let us abandon forcible manipulation in the treatment of displacements of the upper femoral epiphysis.

Treatment of major displacements of the upper femoral epiphysis—the acute on chronic slip. Just because the results of forcible manipulation are so bad does not mean that gentle inturning of the hip, either while on traction or under anaesthetic, should not be used in an attempt to reduce the displacement to a position where the epiphysis can be pinned (Figs 29.17 and 29.18). It must be emphasised, however, that this treatment is only applicable in recent severe slips. It cannot be successful if the history of acute pain is of

more than three weeks' duration, or if there are already signs of new bone formation at the posterior or inferior margins of the epiphysis. Moreover, it carries with it a much higher risk of avascular necrosis. Skin traction from adhesive tapes is all that is needed to obtain an adequate pull on the hip with a rotatory bandage at the knee to correct external rotation deformity; it matters not whether there is balanced traction with weights, traction on a frame, or Pugh's traction from the foot of the bed. *What is important is that it should be gentle.* There is no need to force the position or to insist on wide abduction; even traction in the adducted position will often succeed.[26] Indeed, powerful traction can be harmful, and cases of subluxation of the hip have been reported;[19] the use of sliding bed traction should never be needed. It will be evident in a week or two whether or not an acceptable position has been achieved; if it has, the reduction should be stabilised by inserting Moore pins. Even when the acute slip is thought to have occurred within a very short period (up to about a week), examination under anaesthesia and pinning should be preceded by a few days of traction in

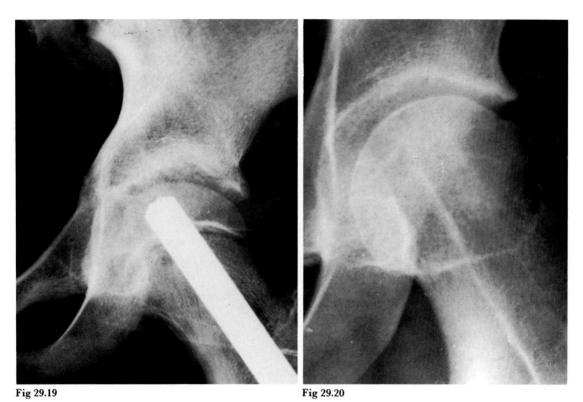

Fig 29.19   **Fig 29.20**

Figs 29.19 and 29.20 Figure 29.19 shows an X-ray of a slipped upper femoral epiphysis fixed with a Smith-Petersen nail. Note the segmental avascular change three years later in close proximity to the nail track (Fig 29.20).

internal rotation. Casey et al reported no incidence of avascular necrosis in acute slips manipulated after a few days of traction, whereas almost half those treated by manipulation alone became avascular.[23] It must be made clear that this examination is by no means a manipulation; it consists of no more than internally rotating the hip and applying gentle traction on the orthopaedic table. Opponents of this procedure draw attention to the vital importance of the posterior vascular pedicle in maintaining the viability of the displaced epiphysis.[21] They (quite rightly) point out that this pedicle is put on stretch by any manipulation of internal rotation. But the manoeuvre is not a manipulation, it is an examination under anaesthesia, and as such it is less likely to cause any more trouble than has already occurred as a result of the original displacement.

The reason for using preliminary traction and any subsequent examination under anaesthetic is to discover whether an acutely displaced epiphysis can be gently replaced into a position in which it can be pinned. But even if the position can not be improved pinning may still be possible. Boyd has suggested that

provided the hip can be flexed to 90 degrees *without* an accompanying external rotation of the thigh it should be possible to pin the epiphysis *in situ*.[27] But even more deformity than this can often be stabilised by the careful insertion of pins, which may sometimes have to pass out of the posterior cortex of the femoral neck before they can engage the displaced epiphysis. The important deformity to measure is the lateral neck shaft angle which is an indication of the amount of posterior epiphyseal displacement (Fig 29.21).[28] In the normal hip this angle measures about 10 degrees, but in a case of slipped upper femoral epiphysis the angle can exceed 60 or 70 degrees. Previously it has always been considered that pinning in situ was impossible if the increase in the lateral neck shaft angle was greater than 30 degrees, but more recent work has shown that pinning is still a possibility with differences as high as 60 degrees, and provided the deformity can be stabilised excellent remodelling can occur with results comparable with the best obtained from corrective osteotomy.[29]

Technique of pinning in situ. If there is only a small increase in the lateral neck shaft angle the patient

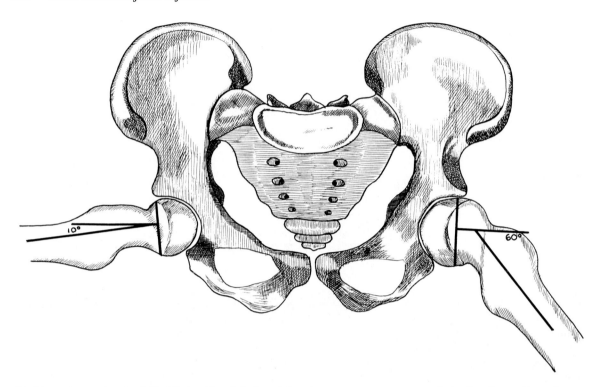

Fig 29.21 (after Southwick ref 28). The lateral neck shaft angle is an important measurement to make in slipped upper femoral epiphysis and is an indication of the degree of backward displacement of the femoral head. It is useful in deciding whether pinning in situ is possible, and in estimating the wedges required in any corrective osteotomy. To obtain a good comparison with the opposite side 'frog-leg' laterals should be taken with the hips abducted and externally rotated to the maximum.

may be put upon an orthopaedic table in the orthodox way; but where there is a marked backward deformity which cannot be improved the usual lateral X-ray taken with the lower limbs fixed can be difficult to obtain and it is wise to drape the affected leg free of fixation so that a frog-leg lateral can be obtained. Two or three pins should be used and if there is marked displacement they should be started well over to the antero-lateral surface of the femur and directed posteriorly towards the displaced epiphysis. It matters not whether the pins escape from the back of the femoral neck so long as they finally engage the main bulk of the epiphysis. Accurate measurement of length is critical if good fixation is to be obtained. Following operation the patient should be allowed up with crutches within a few days, but should not take unprotected weight on the limb for three months.

Severe chronic slip. These are the cases where the displacement has occurred some time before and when a period on traction has not resulted in sufficient improvement to allow pinning. Manipulation under anaesthesia is absolutely contraindicated in this type—it will inevitably precipitate avascular necrosis. The choice of treatment lies between open reduction by cervical osteotomy and corrective intertrochanteric osteotomy.

Cervical osteotomy. The opinions of orthopaedic surgeons vary greatly on the value of this operation. Early enthusiasts of the method carried out an arthrotomy and open reduction rather than osteotomy,[30] and there was a high incidence of avascular necrosis after this procedure. In 1950 Compere described a wedge osteotomy of the superior surface of the femoral neck which had been carried out in 20 hips with only one case of avascular necrosis.[31] Just under 20 years ago Dunn[21] described a technique of cervical osteotomy in which he emphasised the importance of removing a trapezoid fragment of bone from the femoral neck in order to relieve strain on the posterior vessels (Figs 29.22 and 29.23). The operation is indicated for slips of one-third or more of the epiphysis, and is contraindicated if there is evidence of bony fusion between the femoral neck

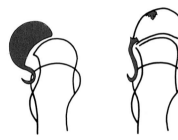

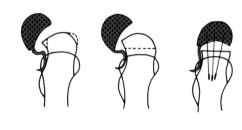

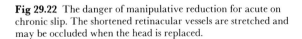

Fig 29.22 The danger of manipulative reduction for acute on chronic slip. The shortened retinacular vessels are stretched and may be occluded when the head is replaced.

Fig 29.23 Trapezoid osteotomy for acute on chronic slip. Note the shortening of the neck and the consequent relaxation of the retinacular vessels when the head is replaced. (Figures 29.22 and 29.23 are reproduced by kind permission of the *Journal of Bone and Joint Surgery* and D. M. Dunn from his article (1964). The treatment of adolescent slipping of the upper femoral epiphysis. *Journal of Bone and Joint Surgery*, 46–B, 621.)

and the displaced epiphysis.[22] The operation is carried out through a lateral approach, detaching the trochanter at its growth plate to gain good access; the capsule is opened through a T-shaped incision, the vertical limb of the T extending along the line of the neck towards the trochanter. The posterior vascular pedicle can be easily distinguished by its red, velvety appearance in contrast to the relatively pale and avascular looking anterior margin of the femoral neck. It should be eased away from the back of the neck very gently, great care being taken to avoid damage to the vessels where they enter the epiphysis. Diathermy must not be used. The epiphysis can be lifted off the metaphysis by inserting a gouge into the epiphyseal plate and using it as a lever. The first cut of the osteotomy is to remove the posterior beak of bone and this is followed by the removal of a few millimetres of the femoral neck and epiphysis. The remains of the growth plate in the femoral head must also be removed if rapid bone union is to be achieved. Three Adams pins are driven up the neck of the femur just penetrating the surface of the metaphysis. The epiphysis is reduced on to the pins which are then driven on to gain a good fixation of the epiphysis. Dunn emphasises the importance of fixing the epiphysis in about 20 degrees of valgus in order to maintain stability and encourage early union. The patient is nursed in traction for four weeks and then remains non-weight-bearing until there is evidence of union of the epiphysis (usually in three to six months).

This is not an easy operation. In the hands of the originator it has given excellent results, and there is little doubt that close attention to operative detail is vital to its success. The occasional operator on slipped epiphysis is less likely to obtain consistently good results and would be wiser to use a corrective subtrochanteric osteotomy for the treatment of a slip which cannot be reduced.

Subtrochanteric osteotomy. The deformities produced by slipping of the upper femoral epiphysis are adduction, external rotation and hyperextension. The osteotomy to correct these has been referred to as a cuneiform triplane osteotomy.[28, 32, 33] It is made just distal to the transverse trochanteric line with a wedge based laterally and anteriorly: de-rotation to correct the external rotation deformity accentuates the effect of the antero-lateral wedge in correcting the extension deformity. The size of the wedge can be determined before operation by measuring the lateral neck shaft angle (See Fig 29.21). The osteotomy is fixed with a pin and plate (Figs 29.24 and 29.25).

Griffiths[6] describes a geometric flexion osteotomy which is carried out in the intertrochanteric region. It is considered that this is the true plane of the axis around which the epiphysis rotates and lies at an angle of 65 degrees with the femoral shaft. An anterior wedge equal to the angle of rotation of the epiphysis is removed from the front of the intertrochanteric area. It is claimed that closure of the osteotomy corrects all three components of the deformity. This is not an easy operation to understand and seems to have little to recommend it over the standard subtrochanteric procedure.

Chronic slip with fused epiphyseal line. Cervical osteotomy has no part to play in the treatment of this deformity.[22] Vessels are already passing up the neck into the femoral head and destruction of these endangers its blood supply. The deformity should be corrected by subtrochanteric osteotomy.

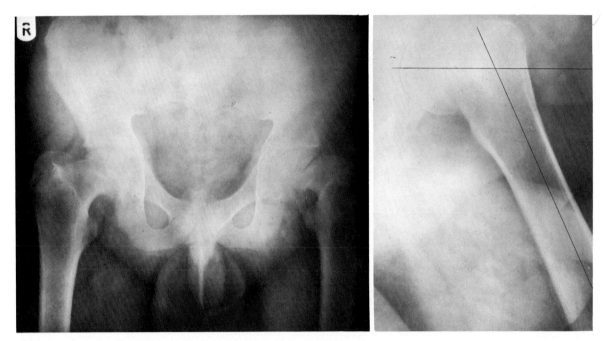

Fig 29.24 This 17-year-old boy of 17 stone (108.2 kg) presented with a gross slip of both upper femoral epiphyses causing a complete loss of abduction and an external rotation deformity of 45 degrees on the right and 60 degrees on the left. Note also the extension deformity which has been marked on the lateral X-ray. These hips were treated by a triplane subtrochanteric osteotomy, removing a bone wedge to correct the adduction and extension deformity, and at the same time internally rotating the femoral shaft (see Fig 29.25).

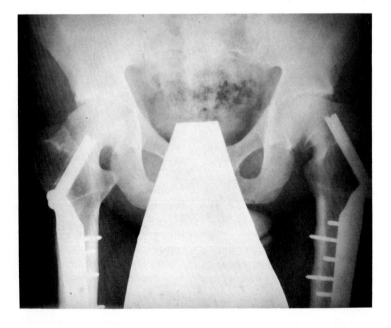

Fig 29.25 Same case as Figure 29.24. This is an X-ray of the hips five years later. The patient had no pain and there was over 90 degrees of flexion and 20 degrees of abduction in both hips.

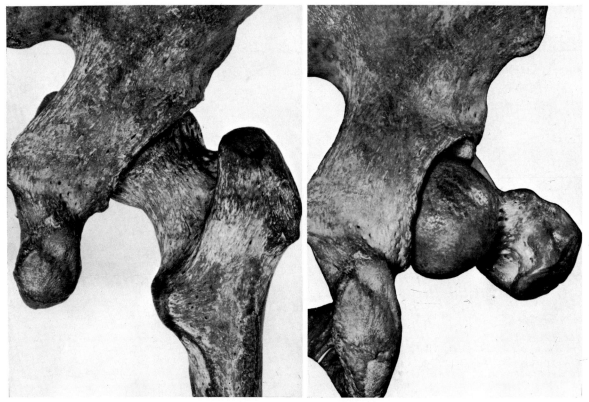

Fig 29.26   **Fig 29.27**

Figs 29.26 and 29.27 Posterior view of the hip joint with the femur in the neutral position (Fig 29.26) and in the flexed-adducted position (Fig 29.27). It is obvious that the stability of the 'ball and socket' joint applies only when the limb is in the neutral position. When the limb is flexed and adducted the support from the acetabular rim is much reduced and the head of the femur is kept in position mainly by capsule. In this position the joint is vulnerable to posterior dislocation—to paralytic dislocation if there is over-traction of the flexor adductor muscles, to pathological dislocation if the flexor adductor muscles are in spasm, and to traumatic dislocation from longitudinal thrusts on the flexed and adducted femur.

Summary of treatment of slipped upper femoral epiphysis

1. Epiphysis displaced but still in acceptable position. Pin in situ without any attempt to alter position. A good result can be expected in 90 per cent of cases.

2. Severe acute slip, or acute on chronic slip. Restore to a position which can be pinned by examination under anaesthetic or by a period of traction. Sixty per cent good results can be expected.

3. Irreducible slip (epiphyseal line still open). Correct by cervical or subtrochanteric osteotomy—outcome uncertain.

4. Slip with fused epiphyseal line. Subtrochanteric osteotomy.

TRAUMATIC DISLOCATION OF THE HIP JOINT

Dislocation of the hip may be conveniently discussed under three headings:

1. Simple dislocation—usually posterior, but more rarely anterior displacements.
2. Fracture dislocations.
3. Central dislocation with acetabular fracture.

Although these three conditions are being considered as separate entities it will be appreciated that each is closely interrelated, often with a common injury pattern and a traumatic anatomy of a very similar type. In fracture-dislocations in particular a clear

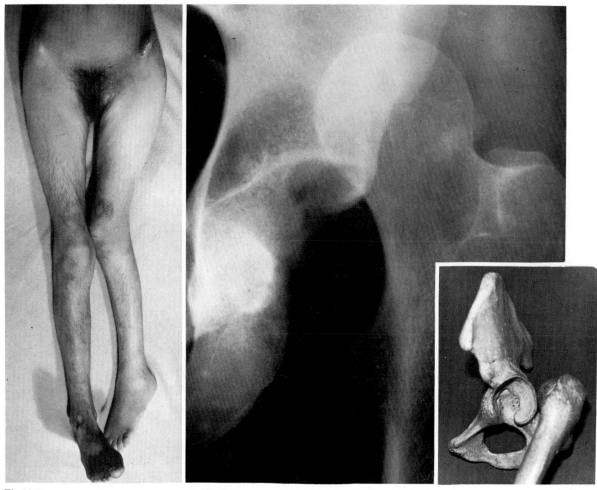

Fig 29.28   **Fig 29.29**

Fig 29.28 Posterior dislocation of the hip joint showing the typical deformity.

Fig 29.29 Radiograph of posterior dislocation of the hip joint—the femoral head is on the dorsum ilii.

understanding of the mechanisms and fracture patterns of the dislocation are an essential prequisite to choosing the correct treatment.

Simple dislocation of the hip

Mechanism. When the femur is flexed and adducted the hip joint is in its least stable position, for the femoral head is less well supported by the acetabulum and is more dependant upon the capsule for stability of the joint (Figs 29.26 and 29.27). It is for this reason that spontaneous dislocation can occur in poliomyelitis, spina bifida, spastic palsy, and infective arthritis of the hip joint.[34] Paralytic dislocation is not uncommon in poliomyelitis and spina bifida if the

flexor and adductor muscles remain active while the extensor and abductor muscles are paralysed—there need be no injury; unopposed action of the flexor-adductor group of muscles is enough to dislocate the joint. Similarly, in cerebral palsy over-action of the spastic flexor-adductor muscles may cause dislocation. Infective or tuberculous arthritis with uncontrolled flexor-adductor spasm and a stretched and softened capsule causes pathological dislocation. In all these conditions the flexed adducted position of the hip joint allows the muscles to drive the femoral head slowly but surely against the capsule until it is displaced.

Similarly a normal hip joint is vulnerable to traumatic dislocation if the femur is driven back

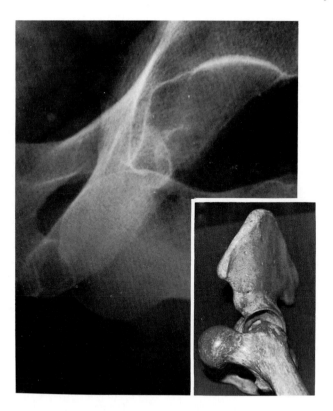

Fig. 29.30 Anterior dislocation of the hip joint with the head of the femur lying on the obturator foramen and the limb fixed in a typical position of deformity with fixed abduction and therefore relative lengthening.

The inset photographs show the effect of the 'watershed' formed by the anterior superior spine, the acetabulum and the tuber ischii. The dorsum of the ilium slope away on one side and the ischio-pubic rami on the other. A displaced head of femur must pass to one or other side. If it passes backwards it must lie adducted and internally rotated; if it passes anterior it must come to lie in abduction and internal rotation.

while the thigh is flexed and adducted. In this position a powerful thrust in the long axis of the limb forces the femoral head through the capsule onto the dorsum of the ilium. The injury often occurs in head-on motor collisions and has been described as the 'dashboard dislocation' because the usual victim is the front seat passenger who is sitting with hips flexed and knees crossed so that the knee which lies nearest the dashboard and sustains the impact is that of the flexed adducted hip.[35]

Although most dislocations of the hip joint are sustained from a backward drive on the femur in its adducted position there may also be dislocation when the flexed joint is not fully adducted as, for example, from a fall of roof on the back of a stooping miner. In this position the femoral head is at least partly protected by the acetabulum, and when it is driven backwards the posterior lip of the acetabulum is usually fractured and displaced with it.[36] If the thigh

is not adducted at all, or is even very slightly abducted at the moment of impact, a central fracture-dislocation may be produced with comminution of the floor of the acetabulum. Furthermore, a fall of roof on the back of a miner whose hip joints are widely abducted may cause anterior dislocation.[37,38] Similar anterior dislocations may result from severe injuries from the rear, such as when a pedestrian is hit in the back by a car.[39] The head of the femur then lies over the obturator foramen or on the pubic crest. Falls of roof may produce bilateral anterior dislocations of the hip joints, and many such cases have been recorded.[40,41] Indeed one dislocation of the hip has been reported where the femoral head was driven into the scrotum.[42] Sometimes there has been 'button-holing' needing open reduction.[38,43]

It is thus evident that the more completely the hip joint is adducted at the moment of injury the more certainly will the joint be dislocated backwards without fracture. With lesser degrees of adduction the backward dislocation will often be accompanied by fracture of the margin of the acetabulum. If the thigh is not abducted at the moment of impact there may be a central fracture-dislocation of the hip joint. If the hip joint is widely abducted at the time of injury it may be dislocated forwards. Look at a pelvis from the side and you will see that the anterior-superior spine, acetabulum and tuber ischii form a watershed, with the dorsum of the ilium sloping away on one side and the ischio-pubic rami on the other. When the head of the femur is displaced it must fall to one or other side of this shed; and moreover, if it is displaced backwards the femur must be rotated medially and adducted; whereas if it is displaced forwards the femur must be rotated laterally and abducted (Figs 29.28 to 29.30). Try it with a pelvis and femur.

In modern times the severe injuries associated with high velocity road traffic accidents have greatly increased the frequency of traumatic dislocation. The violence caused by these accidents is in striking contrast with the milder perils of previous generations when every writer emphasised the rarity of this injury. (One paper published just after the First World War commented upon the infrequency of traumatic dislocation compared with pathological dislocation[34]). On the highway, in industry and in competitive sport we must now live in a world of speed and increasing endeavour which result in the most complex and bizarre injuries of which dislocation of the hip is but one. It is now one of the more common injuries and series of more than 200 dislocations have been reported by individual surgeons.[44, 45] Even in children this dislocation is no longer an unusual injury.[46, 47, 48]

Posterior dislocation of the hip joint. *Clinical diagnosis.* The deformity is obvious (Fig 29.28). Since the head of the femur lies on the dorsum ilii the limb must be in adduction with medial rotation and true shortening, with of course restriction of all movements. There should be no difficulty in establishing the diagnosis. But although the clinical signs are obvious there remains the important decision as to whether or not the acetabulum is fractured, and this can be established only by X-ray examination.

Radiographic diagnosis. There may be detachment of a small fragment from the posterior-superior margin of the acetabulum, which remains held to the neck of the femur by the joint capsule and is replaced accurately when the dislocation is reduced by manipulation. On the other hand there may be a fracture of a much larger fragment from the back of the acetabulum, which tilts out of position and demands operative reduction. Furthermore, this fracture is sometimes complicated by paralysis of the sciatic nerve, and operative replacement is then needed urgently.

It is often difficult to assess the displacement and size of the acetabular fragment by the routine antero-posterior and lateral X-rays of this hip. Stereoscopic radiography can be used on occasions, but this method assumes more importance when it is used to assess displacement in central dislocation. An oblique view taken with the affected hip tilted 45 degrees towards the X-ray tube brings the posterior margin of the acetabulum into profile;[49, 50] it should be taken routinely whenever an acetabular fracture is suspected.

Anterior dislocation. There are two types of anterior dislocation: the low type where the femoral head comes to lie near the obturator foramen (Fig 29.30); and the high type where the head comes to rest in front of the horizontal ramus of the pelvis opposite the ilio-pectineal eminence. Hogarth Pringle carried out experiments on cadavers and established that the low type of dislocation was produced by forced external rotation and abduction in flexion. While the high type was the result of the same forces in extension.[51] The first injury may result from a head-on collision while driving a motor cycle, severe anterior trauma being applied to the thigh with the hip flexed, abducted and externally rotated. The second variety is nearly always the result of a severe blow from behind, such as when a pedestrian is struck by a passing car. The anterior dislocation is considerably less common than posterior dislocation the ratio being approximately 1:20.[52, 53] The clinical deformity is classical; in the low type the limb is fixed in up to 60 degrees of abduction, full external rotation and some flexion; while in the high type there will be marked external rotation in full extension and some abduction.

Reduction of dislocation of the hip. The classical method of reduction of dislocation of the hip joint was first described by Jacob Bigelow of Boston. When he was still a young man at the Massachusetts General Hospital he established his reputation for skill in the correction of this displacement. On one occasion he reduced a dislocation in the Casualty Department and, shortly thereafter, having been reproved for side-tracking his chief's cases, he obligingly re-dislocated the joint and sent the patient up to the wards, only to be called upon later to reduce it once again because his chief had failed. His method depended on circumducting the limb through the opposite position of deformity into the neutral position. In a posterior dislocation in which the hip was adducted and medially rotated the limb was flexed, abducted, laterally rotated and then brought down into extension and neutral rotation. Anterior dislocations were reduced in the opposite direction; the abducted, laterally rotated limb was flexed, adducted, medially rotated and finally extended. By this procedure it is just possible that an anterior dislocation is converted to a posterior dislocation, or a posterior dislocation into an anterior dislocation. This has been shown to occur in cadaveric experiments and reported also in real life.[51] Examination of the 'watershed' from the anterior iliac spine to the tuber ischii makes it obvious how this can happen (Figs 29.28 to 29.30 (insets)). In posterior dislocations, circumduction of the limb from its position of medial rotation to that of lateral rotation may swing the femoral head from behind the joint, right past the notch below the acetabulum, to the front of the joint. Similarly in anterior dislocations circumduction in the opposite direction may rotate the head from the front of the joint, again past the acetabular notch, to the back.

There is a much easier method of manipulative reduction, and it applies equally to posterior and anterior displacements. With the patient lying on blankets on the floor the flexed hip is turned into the neutral position and the femur is then lifted into the acetabulum (Fig 29.31). No matter whether the

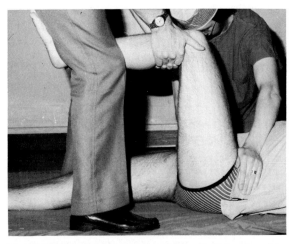

Fig 29.31 Manipulative reduction of traumatic dislocation of the hip. The limb is turned into neutral rotation and the femoral head is then quite gently lifted into the acetabulum.

femur is adducted and medially rotated from a dorsal dislocation, or abducted and laterally rotated from the anterior dislocation, when the hip is turned into the normal position the head of the femur lies below the acetabulum and is quite gently lifted into it. There is no need for forcible traction or violent manipulation.

This manipulation is, of course, carried out under general anaesthesia, and provided there is good muscular relaxation, the reduction is usually easy to perform. Indeed, if the reduction is difficult and the head of the femur does not return to the acetabulum with a satisfying 'clunk' a fracture-dislocation with an obstructing fragment of bone should be suspected and further X-ray views taken to exclude this complication.

If, under particularly adverse conditions, general anaesthesia is not available or cannot be used, it is sometimes possible to reduce the hip by Stimson's manoeuvre:[54] the patient is laid prone with the lower limbs hanging over the end of the table so that the femoral head can be pushed down into the acetabulum (Fig 29.32).

Management after reduction. In the uncomplicated dislocation, provided the reduction is stable (and this should always be tested while the patient is still anaesthetised), the only immobilisation necessary is in Hamilton Russell traction using skin extensions. This would be maintained for three weeks, followed by three weeks' partially weight-bearing with crutches. Full weight-bearing is allowed six weeks from the time of dislocation. However, it has been pointed out by Amihood[53] that 'this time-honoured schedule has no clinical rationale' and provided there are no complications and the joint is painless there is probably no reason why weight-bearing should not be recommended within two to three weeks, or even less. In this respect, however, it is useful to remember that a simple dislocation after successful reduction should rapidly become pain free, and if it does not do so cartilage necrosis is sometimes the cause. In these cases weight-bearing should be delayed until painless movements are restored.

Inability to reduce a hip dislocation by manipulation is commonly the result of obstruction, either by bone fragments or by the soft tissues (labrum and capsule). Sometimes it can result from the 'locking' together of the adjacent fracture surfaces on the femoral head and acetabular rim. One case of irreducible anterior dislocation was caused by a 'button holing' of the femoral head between the limbs of Bigelow's ligament. Instability after reduction always indicates that there has been a fracture of the

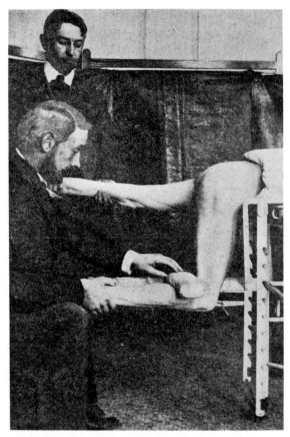

Fig 29.32 Stimson's method of reduction of a dislocated hip. The affected limb is held flexed over the end of a table and traction applied, while an assistant applies downward pressure to the displaced femoral head. (From Stimson, L. A. (1908) *A Treatise on Fractures and Dislocations.* New York: Lea & Febiger.)

acetabular margin. If the fragment is very large or the instability very easy to demonstrate, open reduction and fixation of the acetabular fracture should be considered. If the acetabular rim is grossly comminuted fixation can be very difficult, if not impossible, and there is grave risk of myositis ossificans developing. Unless it is impossible to hold the hip reduced treatment in such cases should be conservative with a period of traction for six weeks followed by immobilisation in a short hip plaster spica for another six weeks.

Errors from misinterpretation of the post-reduction radiograph. Errors often arise in the treatment of dislocations of the hip joint from misinterpretation of radiographs. After manipulation of a dorsal dislocation in which the femoral head was obviously riding up on the ilium well above the hip joint it may appear that replacement has been effected with the femoral head at its normal level—and yet the joint may still be held in a position of complete backward dislocation. Figure 29.33 is one of many examples. This was accepted as a satisfactory reduction, but of course the dislocation was never adequately reduced: agreed the head of the femur is no longer on the dorsum ilii; agreed that it is at the joint level and the outline of femoral head and acetabulum coincide more or less; but the fact is that the head of the femur is lying entirely behind the acetabulum and the appearance of successful reduction arises only from fairly accurate superimposition of the shadows of the dislocated head and the acetabulum. In this particular case even the superimposition is not quite accurate. Shenton's line is broken—that is to say, the continuation of the curved line of the lower margin of the superior ramus of the pubis lies well below the curved line of the lower end of the neck of the femur with which it should be continuous. This in itself is enough to say that the dislocation is not reduced. Sometimes the shadows coincide even more accurately, and there may be little or no break in the continuity of Shenton's line. But there is still clear radiographic evidence, even in antero-posterior projections, in the disappearance of the lesser trochanter. The shadow of the trochanter becomes smaller as the hip joint is rotated inwards, but, within the normal range of medial rotation of the joint, rarely disappears entirely. If it has disappeared it means that the hip joint is rotated inwards so fully that the femoral head is probably behind the acetabulum. Failure of reduction may of course be confirmed with even greater certainty by taking lateral or stereoscopic radiographs of the joint, but it should be obvious from the clinical evidence of persistent medial rotation deformity with restriction of all movements.

FRACTURE-DISLOCATIONS OF THE HIP JOINT

Dislocation of the hip may be associated with fractures of the acetabular rim, fractures of the femoral head, fractures of the femoral neck, and sometimes fractures of the femoral shaft. Nearly always in these circumstances the dislocation is posterior, and on occasions more than one fracture may be present. The so-called central dislocation of the hip has an entirely different mechanism and is really a fracture of the floor of the acetabulum with complete disorganisation of its articular surface. This will be discussed later in a separate section.

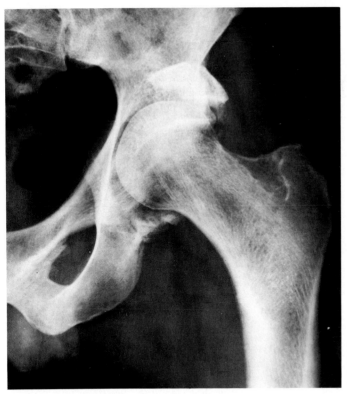

Fig 29.33 Dislocation of the hip joint with marginal fracture of the acetabulum after manipulation. (Of course, it is not reduced—the femoral head is behind the acetabulum.)

Dislocation with fracture of acetabular rim

When dorsal dislocation of the hip joint is associated with a posterior marginal fracture of the acetabulum, the fragment is usually held close to the head of the femur by fibres of joint capsule so that it is replaced accurately when the dislocation is reduced. Occasionally a larger fragment is detached from the acetabular margin and tilted outwards so that operative reduction may be needed. In the absence of sciatic nerve signs the decision to operate depends upon whether the hip is unstable in flexion, adduction and internal rotation. Not all large fragments require open reduction and surprisingly large and widely displaced acetabular rim fractures may be completely stable (Fig 29.34). When in doubt the hip should be re-examined under anaesthetic a few days after the injury. It has been reported in some cases of fracture of the acetabulum that the sciatic nerve has been impaled by the sharp margin of the acetabular fragment; prompt removal of the pressure may save the nerve from permanent paralysis. Thus the treatment of dislocations of the hip joint with fracture of the margin of the acetabulum resolves itself into three groups of cases:

1. In most fracture-dislocations the acetabular fragment is replaced when the dislocated joint is reduced by manipulation, and if this is confirmed by radiographic examination and the joint is stable the treatment should be the same as for uncomplicated dislocations.

2. If a large acetabular fragment is not replaced by manipulation and the hip is unstable in flexion, adduction and external rotation, the joint should be exposed through a posterior incision, the fragment

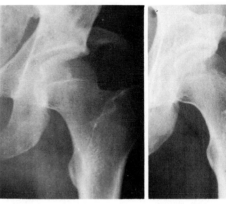

Fig 29.34(a)   **Fig 29.34(b)**

Fig 29.34 Despite the large and widely displaced acetabular rim fracture associated with this hip dislocation (Fig 29.34(a)) the reduction was completely stable and no operative stabilisation was required. Fig 29.34(b) shows the appearance 2 years later. When in doubt about whether to fix an acetabular rim fracture the hip should be examined under anaesthesia and the stability assessed.

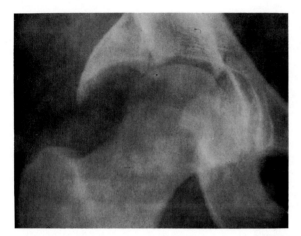

Fig 29.35 Dorsal dislocation of the hip joint. After manipulative reduction it is obvious from radiographic examination (through plaster) that a large acetabular fragment is tilted outwards. Four weeks had elapsed since injury before the patient was first seen.

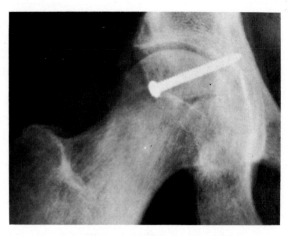

Fig 29.36 The displaced fragment of the acetabulum was replaced through a postero-lateral incision and fixed with a screw. In this case there was no paralysis of the sciatic nerve.

being replaced and fixed in position by a single screw (Figs 29.35 and 29.36).

3. If there is a fracture-dislocation with sciatic palsy and the acetabular fragment remains tilted after manipulative reduction, the back of the joint and the sciatic nerve trunk should be explored as an emergency procedure—certainly within 24 hours—the nerve being gently freed from the bone fragment, which is then replaced and fixed with a screw.

The operation is carried out through a posterior approach which should extend proximally as far as the sciatic notch. On splitting the gluteus maximus muscle the fracture of the acetabular rim usually becomes readily visible, very often with the cartilage of the posterior part of the femoral head already exposed. The sciatic nerve must be thoroughly explored from well below the hip to the sciatic notch and any impingement by bone fragments removed. It is a wise precaution to inspect the inside of the acetabulum for small fragments of bone however sure one may be that reduction is complete. The acetabular fragment always involves the postero-medial rim and it may be difficult to achieve a satisfactory reduction without either dividing part of the gluteal insertion or by osteotomy of the greater trochanter. When reduction has been accomplished the detached acetabular fragment should be fixed by one or two screws.

Immobilisation after open reduction and screwing of an acetabular fragment should take the form of traction until the wound is satisfactorily healed, followed by a short hip spica for six weeks.

Fractures of the ipsilateral femur

We must now go on to discuss dislocation associated with fractures of the femur on the same side, remembering that these may be quite often accompanied by acetabular rim fractures. The injuries to be considered are: fractures of the femoral head, fractures of the femoral neck, separations of the upper femoral epiphysis, and fractures of the shaft of the femur. As long ago as 1934 these fracture-dislocations were reviewed by Henry and Bayumi.[55] At that time there were case reports in the literature of 13 dislocations with marginal fracture of the femoral head, 16 dislocations with fracture of the neck of the femur and 16 dislocations with fracture of the shaft of the femur; but very many more have been dealt with since then,[45, 52] and we now have better methods of treatment for these difficult injuries.

Dislocation of the hip joint with fracture of the femoral head. As the head of the femur is driven out of the acetabulum a marginal sector may be sliced from it. These fractures can be missed very easily if X-rays of indifferent quality, or in one plane only, are accepted. Figure 29.37 shows the antero-posterior X-ray of such a case; a large anterior fragment is clearly seen in the lateral view only (Fig 29.38). If the dislocation can be treated by manipulative reduction in the usual way it will sometimes be found that the detached fragment has come to lie in the reduced position; but if this is not so the hip joint must be opened and the fragment excised. If the dislocation is still unreduced the operation is more

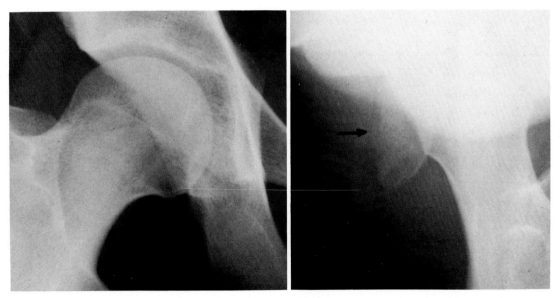

Fig 29.37   **Fig 29.38**

Figs 29.37 and 29.38 Figure 29.37 shows the antero-posterior X-ray after reduction of a dislocation of the right hip. All looked well, but the hip was painful to move. The lateral projection (Fig 29.38) showed that a large fragment had been sliced off the femoral head and was lying anteriorly within the joint.

easily carried out through a posterior approach, detaching the greater trochanter, but if the hip has already been reduced by manipulation the approach which gives the easiest access to the fragment is used. However, as has already been stated this type of fracture-dislocation may be impossible to reduce by manipulation. The reason is usually because the loose fragment obstructs the reduction (Fig 29.39), but sometimes it is caused by the raw fracture surface under the femoral head impacting against a damaged posterior rim of acetabulum. The prognosis for this injury of the hip, occurring as it does in a weight-bearing joint, can never be good. Even uncomplicated dislocations of the hip cause late traumatic arthritis, so that if the articular surface of the femoral head is roughened by a fracture of one sector, the risk of arthritis must be considerably increased.[56] Brav[57] reported a 70 per cent incidence of traumatic arthritis in dislocation associated with femoral head fractures, compared with just over 20 per cent in uncomplicated dislocations; Epstein[45] had 11 poor results out of 17 treated conservatively. There seems little doubt that the high incidence is directly related to the severity of the local injury. Unlike marginal fractures of the acetabulum, fragments of the femoral head cannot be easily replaced and internally fixed, although this has

been carried out successfully in a few exceptional cases (Figs 29.43 and 29.44). Therefore, if manipulative reduction fails to replace the fragment accurately the surgeon should be prepared to excise it, thus preparing the way for any later reconstructive surgery that may be needed. Only large fragments (one-third or more of the femoral head) should be considered for internal fixation.

Dislocation of the hip joint with fracture of the femoral neck. Traumatic dislocation of the hip joint complicated by fracture of the femoral neck is a rare occurrence. In elderly patients it is wise to accept the inevitability of avascular necrosis of the separated head with resulting degenerative arthritis of the hip joint and treat by prosthetic replacement of the femoral head. Where the injury occurs in a young adult, open reduction with Smith-Petersen nailing of the femoral neck fracture is the operation of choice. It should be performed through a postero-lateral approach with detachment of the greater trochanter. The incidence of avascular necrosis is high.[58] If there is comminution of the dislocated femoral head primary prosthetic replacement should be carried out (Fig 29.45).

Pertrochanteric fracture complicating dislocation

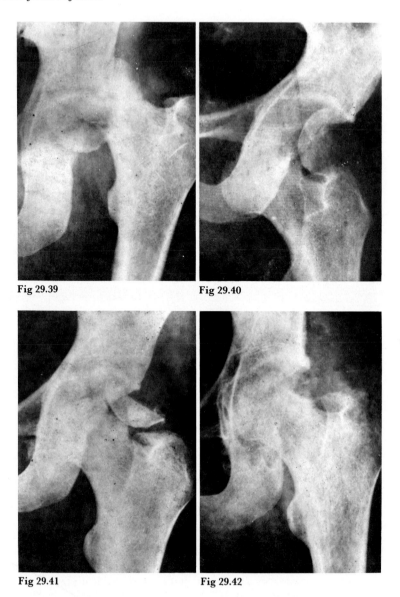

Fig 29.39   Fig 29.40

Fig 29.41   Fig 29.42

Figs 29.39 to 29.42 Dislocation of the hip joint with fracture of the head of the femur. Originally it was a posterior dislocation with the fragment displaced below the head (Fig 29.39), but attempted manipulative reduction converted it into an anterior dislocation with the marginal fragment above the head (Fig 29.40). A second manipulation reduced the dislocation, but with the fragment upside down in the joint (Fig 29.41). The fragment was excised, but the joint remained stiff and painful (Fig 29.42).

presents a different problem. It is always the result of severe trauma and may often be part of a multiple injury.[58] In these cases it is essential to reduce the hip as soon as is practicable and stabilise the fracture with internal fixation. If the fracture line passes distal to the psoas attachment there may be considerable deformity of the upper fragment as a result of

unopposed psoas action—the whole fragment being markedly flexed and adducted.[59] The displacement can make reduction very difficult; it is essential to have access to both sides of the joint and this can only be achieved by a lateral approach with osteotomy of the greater trochanter. Choice of the wrong approach may result in complete failure to reduce

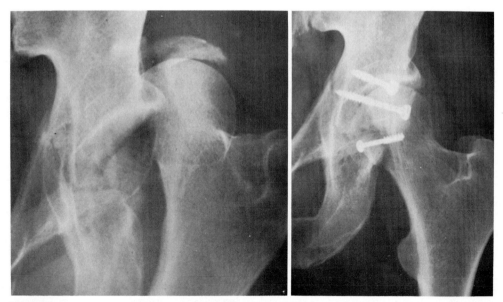

Fig 29.43

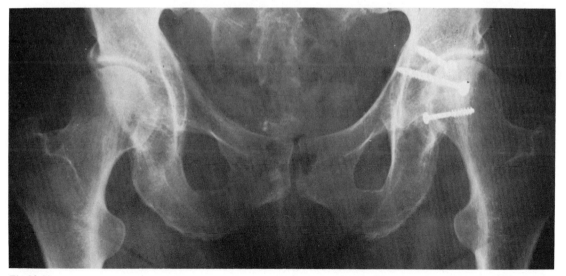

Fig 29.44

Figs 29.43 and 29.44 This patient sustained a severe fracture-dislocation of the left hip, with both a fracture of the inferior aspect of the femoral head and of the acetabular rim. The femoral fragment was reduced by open reduction and fixed with a small intra-articular screw, while the fracture of the acetabular rim was stabilised with two screws. Figure 29.43 shows the initial X-ray and the position a few weeks after operation, and Figure 29.44 is an X-ray at two-and-a-half years. Apart from slight limitation of full rotation this hip is indistinguishable from normal. (The initial operation in this case was performed by Dr P. Elzenga, St. Geertruden, Ziekenhuis, Deventer, Holland.)

either the dislocation or the fracture (Figs 29.46 and 29.47).

Dislocation of the hip joint with displacement of the upper femoral epiphysis. In the corresponding injury of the child, which is a dislocation of the hip joint with separation of the upper femoral epiphysis, the displaced epiphysis should not be excised even though there is again a risk of vascular embarrassment and

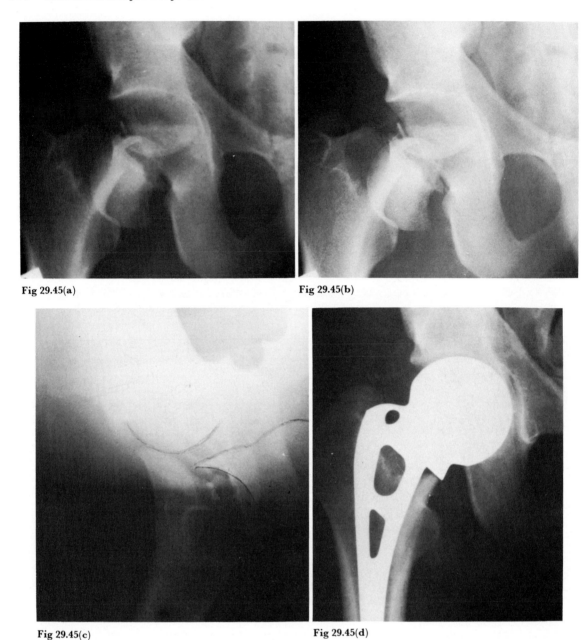

Fig 29.45(a)

Fig 29.45(b)

Fig 29.45(c)

Fig 29.45(d)

Fig 29.45 This 20-year-old youth sustained a dislocation of the right hip with fracture of the neck of the femur. The femoral head was split into two large fragments which were completely devoid of blood supply. It was replaced by an Austin Moore prosthesis.

possibly late traumatic arthritis. One such case is illustrated in Figures 29.48 and 29.49. The epiphysis was replaced through a short incision, and the early functional result was satisfactory. In two other reported cases treated by open reduction and multiple pin fixation good joint function was present nine and

18 years later despite flattening of the femoral head from avascular change.[58] However, even without dislocation this is a serious injury and is commonly followed by avascular necrosis. In one series of nine cases only three could be classified as good clinical, and radiological results.[60]

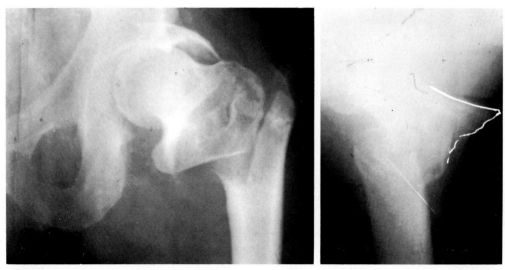

Fig 29.46

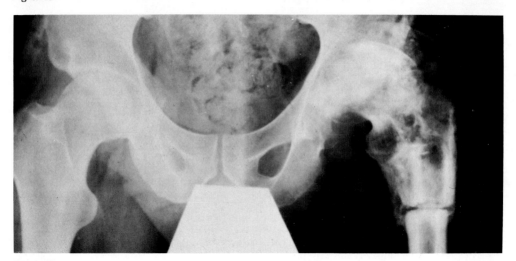

Fig 29.47

Figs 29.46 and 29.47 Antero-posterior and lateral X-rays of a dislocation of the hip complicated by a pertrochanteric fracture of the neck of the femur and a fracture of the acetabular rim. Note the marked anterior and adduction tilt of the upper fragment due to unopposed psoas action. The first attempt to reduce the dislocation was by a posterior approach—this was unsuccessful. A further attempt 10 days later was made through a Smith-Petersen approach which was equally unsuccessful. The hip was never reduced and required ilio-femoral arthrodesis and corrective osteotomy some months later (Fig 29.47). It is possible that success might have been achieved if both sides of the joint had been exposed through a lateral approach, detaching the greater trochanter. (Reproduced by the kind permission of Mr K. I. Nissen.)

Dislocation of the hip joint with fracture of the shaft of the femur. This rare combination of injuries was first described by Sir Astley Cooper in 1823.[61] Papers reviewing the problem emphasise that in the literature over half the cases were diagnosed late or not at all.[62, 63] To avoid missing the diagnosis

there should be a routine check of the hip for bony deformity and bruising in every fracture of the shaft of the femur. Careful examination of the displacement at the fracture site in the femoral shaft may arouse suspicions that all is not right in the hip joint. Helal and Skevis[63] observed that in all their cases X-rays

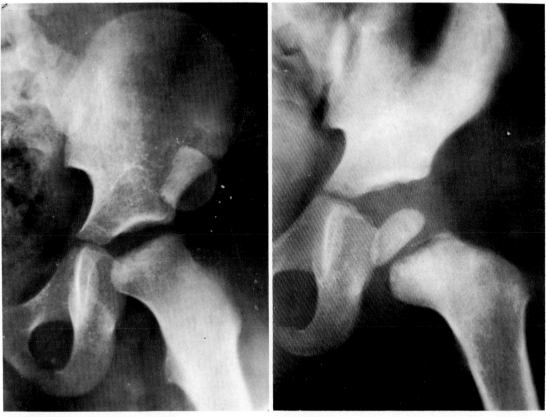

Fig 29.48   **Fig 29.49**

Figs 29.48 and 29.49 Posterior dislocation of a hip joint in a child with separation and displacement of the upper femoral epiphysis, which was replaced after operative exposure (Fig 29.49). After protection of the joint for several months the early functional result was satisfactory.

showed a transverse fracture with adduction of the upper fragment (Fig 29.50), whereas in most uncomplicated fractures of the femoral shaft the upper fragment is abducted; if it is adducted the fracture line is never transverse but directed obliquely downwards and medially.

Treatment. The manipulative reduction of traumatic dislocation of the hip joint depends essentially on applying traction to the shaft of the femur in various positions of rotation so that by circumduction of the limb the femoral head may be guided into the acetabulum. This is obviously impossible if there is also a fracture of the mid-shaft of the femur. Even the Stimson method [54] (see Fig 29.32) is uncertain in its results, although the most likely technique to be successful. It is very probable therefore that an open reduction and internal fixation of the fracture will be necessary before the dislocation can be manipulated.

If possible, open reduction of the dislocation should be avoided because this procedure greatly increases the incidence of unsatisfactory results. [63] Moreover, the injuries are commonly only part of a multiple injury occurring in a patient who is unfit for an immediate major joint surgery. Provided the combined injury is recognised immediately no harm can come from an attempt to reduce the dislocation and the fracture by closed methods, and an excellent result of manipulative reduction of the combined injury in a child has been described by Wadsworth. [64] Closed reduction has been successfully achieved with the aid of a Scudari traction screw inserted into the greater trochanter—a useful technique to remember in multiple injury cases. [65] A good example of management of a dislocated hip with fracture of the shaft of the same femur is in the patient illustrated in Figures 29.51 and 29.52, who had also sustained a

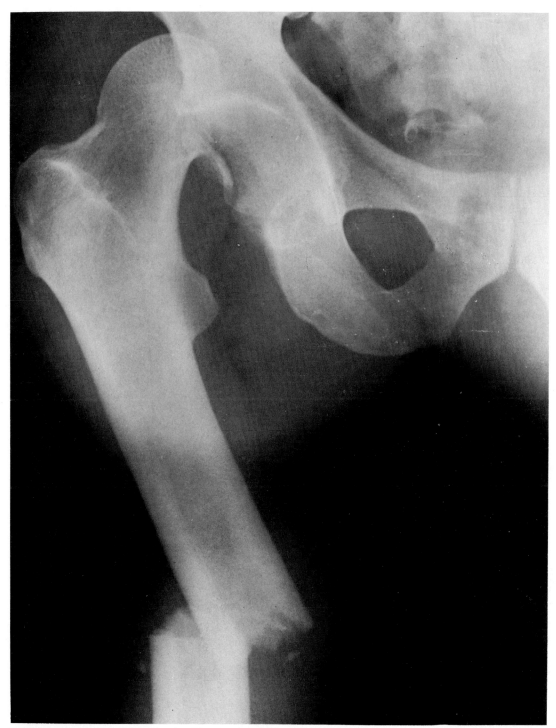

Fig 29.50 Fracture-dislocation of the hip joint. There is a dorsal dislocation of the hip joint with fracture of the upper shaft of the femur; but in addition there is a marginal fracture of the head of the femur, the detached fragment lying on the posterior lip of the acetabulum. This unusual case, therefore, demonstrates two of the three rare types of fracture-dislocation. Note particularly the adducted upper femoral shaft associated with a transverse fracture. Any fracture of the femoral shaft with this combination of deformity should have the hip included in the X-ray picture.

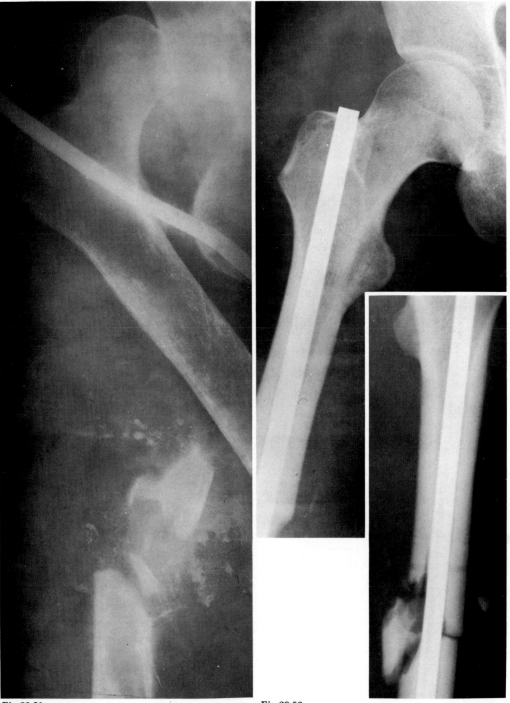

Fig 29.51   Fig 29.52

Figs 29.51 and 29.52 Posterior dislocation of the hip joint with comminuted fracture of the shaft of the same femur treated by open reduction and intramedullary nailing of the fractured shaft of the femur; after that, reduction of the dislocated hip and the management thereafter presented relatively little difficulty. (Reproduced by kind permission of Dr Preston Wade and Dr Harrison McLaughlin of New York.)

difficult comminuted fracture of the shaft of the other femur. On one side of the fracture-dislocation the comminuted fracture of the femoral shaft was first reduced by open operation, and after the reduced fracture had been immobilised by intramedullary nailing, the dislocation of the hip joint was reduced by closed manipulation. The comminuted fracture of the shaft of the femur on the opposite side was then also reduced by open operation and immobilised by intramedullary nailing. Nailing the adducted shaft of the upper fragment may prove difficult or impossible, and having exposed the bone closed reduction of the dislocation should always be attempted by grasping the upper fragment with bone holders and applying traction and circumduction in the usual way.

COMPLICATIONS OF ANTERIOR OR POSTERIOR DISLOCATION OF THE HIP JOINT

Several of the complications of traumatic dislocation of the hip have already been mentioned. The following must now be considered in more detail:

1. Myositis ossificans.
2. Sciatic nerve paralysis.
3. Traumatic arthritis and avascular necrosis.
4. Recurrent dislocation.
5. Unreduced dislocation.
6. Irreducible dislocation.

1. Myositis ossificans. This is almost unknown in a simple uncomplicated dislocation of the hip. It is said to be more common after repeated manipulation;[66] but the very fact that repeated manipulation is necessary indicates that the dislocation is complicated, either by obstruction or instability, and is almost certainly associated with an acetabular rim fracture. However, myositis ossificans is not an uncommon complication following open reduction,[67] either for removal of a femoral head fragment or for screw fixation of an acetabular rim fracture (Figs 29.53 to 29.56). After operations of this type it is important to avoid early movement, and although in the first post-operative week traction is sufficient immobilisation, this must be followed by a period of immobilisation in a short hip spica for six weeks. It should also be remembered that myositis ossificans can occur (without operative trauma) as a complication of hip dislocation associated with severe head injury (Figs 29.57 and 29.58). It is interesting to note that the only case of myositis recorded in a series of

dislocations in children occurred in a head injury patient.[68]

2. Sciatic nerve palsy. The incidence of sciatic nerve palsy in all types of dislocation of the hip varies from 10 to 13 per cent.[67, 68, 69] It is three times more common after fracture-dislocation than after simple dislocation, and in four out of five cases the lesion is incomplete, usually affecting the peroneal division.[70] The prognosis for recovery is variable, and in one series only 3 cases out of 17 recovered completely,[67] although there was partial recovery in about half the patients. In another series there was a 60 per cent overall recovery rate.[45]

Much importance has been paid in the past to damage from impalement of the nerve by fragments of bone. This is probably an unusual cause of paralysis, and in the majority of cases the damage is done by the nerve being stretched at the time of dislocation. Thompson and Epstein[69] record two instances where the sciatic nerve was found damaged by acetabular fragments, but without palsy; Stewart and Milford[67] mention one such case in a series of 17 nerve palsies. But even though in most cases the paralysis is probably due to traction the indentation of the nerve by bone fragments may well be responsible for some of the permanent paralyses, and in some the bone fragments may be the cause of a troublesome causalgia in the limb. Therefore, although there is little place for exploration of the nerve in a sciatic palsy following dislocation without fracture, nerve injuries associated with fractures, particularly of the acetabulum, may require surgical intervention. Small rim fractures without wide displacements can be disregarded, but when the nerve lesion is associated with a large, and possibly comminuted fragment detached from the acetabulum, it should be explored to exclude local pressure from displaced bone fragments and at the same time the rim of the acetabulum repaired.

3. Traumatic arthritis from avascular necrosis after dislocation of the hip. The nutrient vessels of the shaft of the femur extend no higher than the femoral neck, and the head of the femur is supplied with blood vessels entering from the capsule and to a lesser extent from the ligamentum teres. In dislocations of the hip joint both these structures are damaged, and if all the blood vessels within them are torn or thrombosed, avascular necrosis is inevitable. The incidence of avascular necrosis in uncomplicated dislocations is about 10 per cent,[71] and this is equally true of dislocation of the hip in children.[72, 73] There

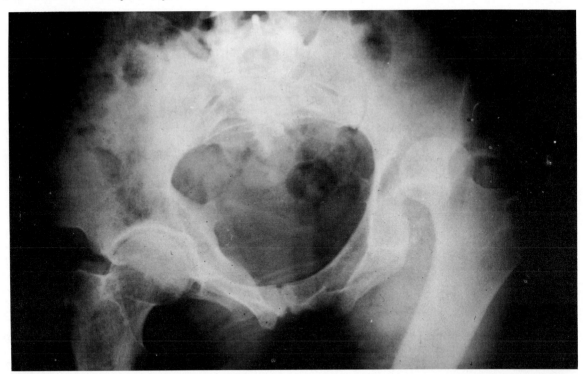

Fig 29.53

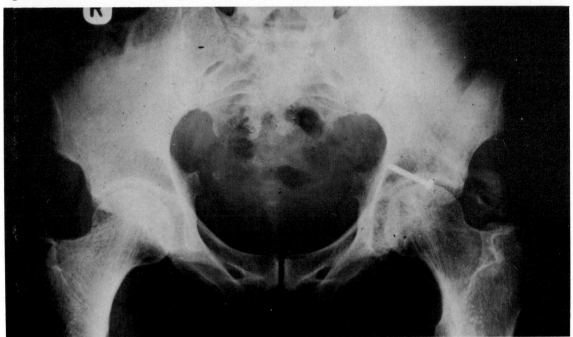

Fig 29.54

Figs 29.53 and 29.54 This miner sustained a dislocation of the hip with a large acetabular rim fracture (Fig 29.53). Manipulation reduced the dislocation easily, but because of possible instability open reduction and screwing of the acetabular fracture was carried out some days later. X-rays five months later (Fig 29.54) show myositis ossificans in the typical site between the superior capsule and the small gluteal muscles.

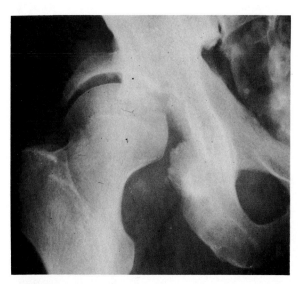

Fig 29.55

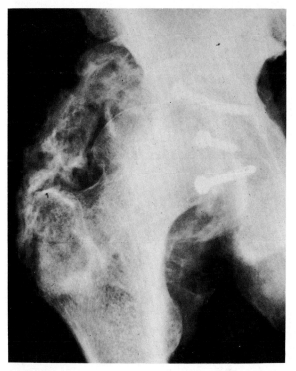

Fig 29.56

Figs 29.55 and 29.56 Gross comminution of the acetabular rim causes major instability and is difficult to correct by operation (Fig 29.55). A long period of immobilisation in a plaster spica is essential if the degree of myositis ossificans shown in Figure 29.56 is to be avoided.

is no evidence to suggest that a prolonged period of non-weight-bearing will prevent the onset of avascular change in any age group.[68,72] In children avascular necrosis presents the radiological appearance of Perthes' disease, and as soon as this is diagnosed the child should be non-weight-bearing in a pattern-ended caliper until the femoral head is revascularised. The prognosis in traumatic avascular necrosis is much better than in Perthes' disease.[74]

In considering avascular necrosis in adult dislocations distinction must be made between it and degenerative arthritis. It is quite possible that the former may be the precursor of the latter; but frank avascular change appears within 12 months, whereas the onset of degenerative arthritis may be delayed for several years (Figs 29.59 and 29.60). A very early sign of both avascular change and degenerative change is a cystic irregularity at the junction of superior articular surface of the femoral head with the neck (Figs 29.61 and 29.62). The incidence of traumatic degenerative arthritis increases rapidly when there is an associated fracture of the acetabulum or femoral head; Armstrong[74a] reported 15 per cent incidence in dislocations without fracture; 25 per cent in cases where there was fracture of the acetabular rim; and 50 per cent if there was a fracture of the femoral head. A similar incidence has been found by other authors.[69] Avascular change and late traumatic arthritis are usually considered to be the result of damage to the capsular vessels, but there is also well documented experimental evidence to show that direct impact can seriously impair the integrity of articular cartilage, and it has been shown that the axial force sufficient to fracture a femur when applied to the hip produces chondrocyte death and fissuring.[75]

It is clear, therefore, that although the incidence of avascular necrosis may be relatively small, a sizeable proportion of patients who have a had a dislocation of the hip will develop degenerative arthritis and will probably require surgical treatment. Most of the patients faced with this problem will be young and will have only one hip involved: the salvage operation of choice is therefore an arthrodesis although it must be appreciated that where there is avascular necrosis of the femoral head bony fusion of the hip can be difficult to achieve. In the early stages of degenerative arthritis it is always worthwhile carrying out an osteotomy, provided there is still good mobility. A good result is shown in Figures 29.63 and 29.64 but the results are unpredictable. Arthroplasty should be reserved for the elderly patient or for those patients with both hips diseased. It remains to be seen whether limited resection total hip replacement by re-surfac-

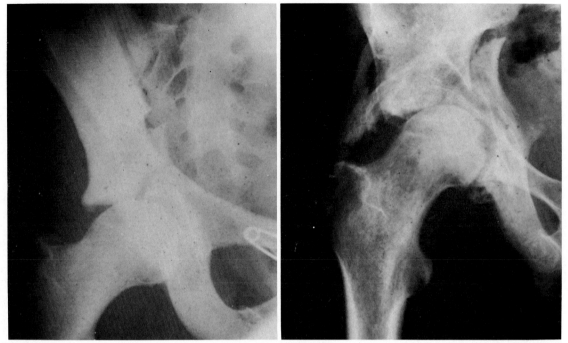

Fig 29.57   **Fig 29.58**

Figs 29.57 and 29.58 Myositis ossificans is a very rare complication after conservative treatment for dislocation of the hip, but it can occur in association with severe head injury as a general manifestation of excessive calcification. Figure 29.57 shows the initial manipulative reduction of a central fracture-dislocation of the hip, and Figure 29.58 shows the soft tissue ossification which has taken place after six months.

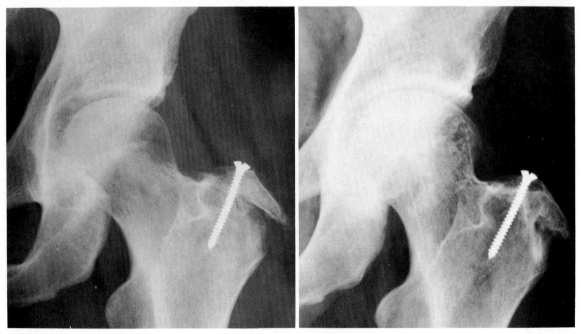

Fig 29.59   **Fig 29.60**

Figs 29.59 and 29.60 This patient sustained a fracture-dislocation of the hip which required operative intervention to reduce the hip and remove an intra-articular fragment sheared off the femoral head. Figure 29.59 shows the hip about 12 months after operation when the patient was symptom-free. Figure 29.60 shows the degree of degenerative change which appeared six years later.

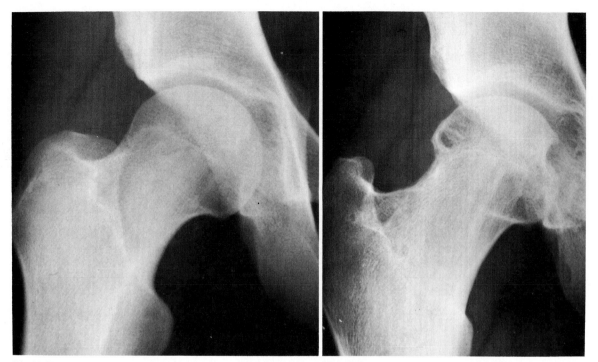

Fig 29.61   Fig 29.62

Figs 29.61 and 29.62 Figure 29.61 shows the hip of a patient shortly after reduction of a fracture-dislocation. Figure 29.62 is an X-ray two years later showing subcortical cyst formation at the superior articular surface preceding avascular changes in the femoral head.

ing has a sufficiently long life to make it safe to recommend as a primary form of treatment.

4. Recurrent dislocation. Provided there has been no fracture of the acetabulum traumatic dislocations of the hip should be completely stable after reduction. Even where there are minor injuries to the acetabular rim it is rare for them to be the cause of redislocation, although, in these cases, the stability of the hip should always be tested immediately after reduction. Although some cases have been reported of recurrent dislocation occurring without a fracture,[76, 76a] there is usually a large posterior acetabular defect which is sometimes not fully appreciated if only the routine antero-posterior and lateral X-rays are taken; an oblique view (antero-posterior projection with hip tilted 45 degrees towards the tube) can be very helpful (Figs 29.65 and 29.66). Figures 29.67 and 29.68 show the hip joint of a young man aged 28 years. Within two weeks of reduction of the dislocation of the joint he was allowed to stand and walk, and during the next fortnight the hip gave way and he fell to the ground on six separate occasions. There was recurrent dislocation; every time that the limb was rotated medially the femur slipped on to the dorsum ilii (Fig 29.67); every time that it was rotated laterally the dislocation was spontaneously reduced (Fig 29.68). In this case the disability was relieved by immobilising the joint in a plaster spica for 10 weeks; the marginal fracture united and the dislocation did not recur afterwards. But, of course, the recurrence should never have been allowed to take place in the beginning. An unstable dislocation of this type should be explored by a posterior incision, the acetabular fragments replaced and fixed by bone screws. This operation must be followed by immobilisation in a plaster spica for six to eight weeks.

It has already been said that a small number of cases have been recorded in the literature of recurrent dislocation without a fracture.[76] A rent in gluteus minimus and the superior aspect of the capsule was

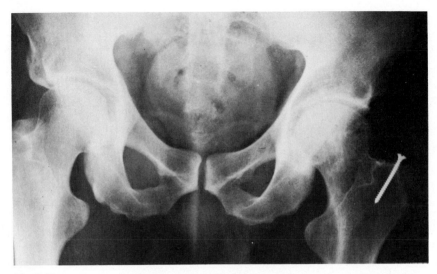

Fig 29.63

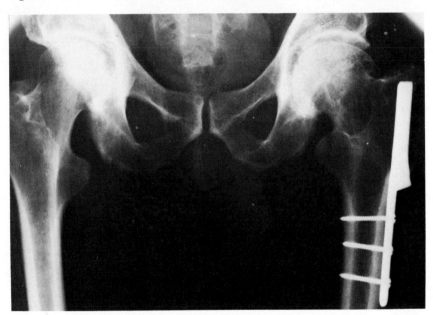

Fig 29.64

Figs 29.63 and 29.64 The later X-rays of the same patient whose early X-rays were shown in Figures 29.59 and 29.60. Figure 29.63 shows the extent of degenerative change just prior to osteotomy. Figure 29.64 shows the hip 15 years after osteotomy. The joint remains pain free, with 90 degrees of flexion, and without flexion deformity.

successfully repaired by posterior bone block in one case,[77] and in other cases a large posterior capsular pouch was successfully obliterated by 'double breasting' the capsule[78], or repairing a defect between the short rotators.[76a]

Delayed posterior dislocation of the hip.[79] Two cases have been reported of a delayed dislocation at two days and six weeks after injury. In neither case was

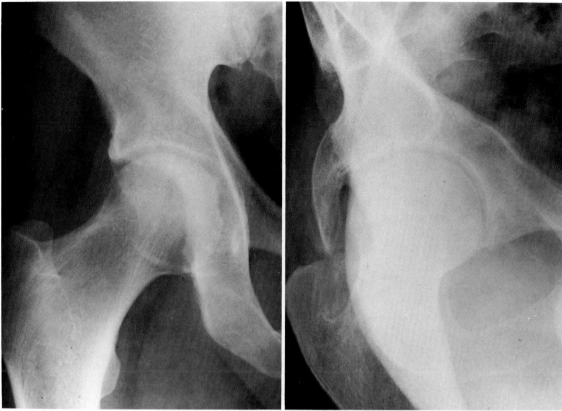

Fig 29.65   **Fig 29.66**

Figs 29.65 and 29.66 Figure 29.65 is an antero-posterior X-ray of a patient who sustained a dislocation of the right hip three years earlier. He complained of pain in the hip after sitting. Figure 29.66 is an oblique X-ray showing a large acetabular fragment projecting backwards. This view was taken by antero-posterior projection with the affected hip tilted 45 degrees towards the tube.

there evidence of a dislocation at the initial examination, although clearly injury (and probably a spontaneously reduced dislocation) must have occurred because in both cases there was an acetabular rim fracture. An early reduction was achieved, although open reduction was necessary in one because of obstruction. The final result in both cases was excellent.

5. Unreduced dislocation of the hip joint. If a dislocated hip joint is left unreduced for several months the difficulties of treatment are very great and probably arthrodesis if acceptable, is the best treatment that can be offered to the patient. Although it is tempting to advise total hip replacement the

technical difficulties of insertion of a prosthetic joint and the young age group of most of the patients are firm contra-indications to this form of surgery. Manipulative reduction is more often than not impossible, and operative reduction involves hazards and perils. The femoral head is firmly bound in its displaced position by thick scar tissue. It may be tightly wedged in the sciatic notch, and the problem of exposing and dislodging it is increased by the proximity of the sciatic nerve, which is seldom in a normal position. There is always difficulty in identifying and clearing the acetabulum; it is full of scarred capsule and distorted soft tissues, with the femoral vessels sometimes unusually close on the inner side. Haemorrhage from exposure of the femur, resection of the capsule and clearing the acetabulum is

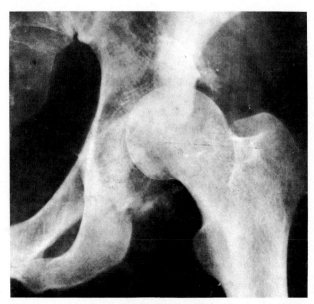

Fig 29.67

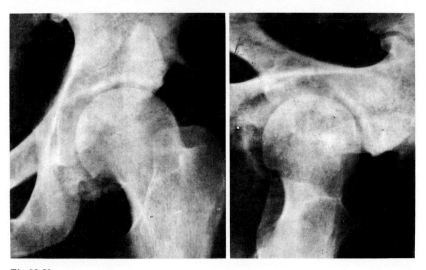

Fig 29.68

Figs 29.67 and 29.68 Recurrent dislocation of the hip joint due to immobilisation at the time of injury for not more than 10 days. Whenever the limb was medially rotated the head of the femur dislocated (Fig 29.67), and when the limb was laterally rotated the dislocation was reduced (Fig 29.68). The disability was relieved by immobilisation in a plaster spica.

considerable, and there may be severe shock. Moreover, even after successful reduction, degenerative arthritis very commonly develops. The troubles are still not over, because the femoral head is nearly always avascular and dead so that arthrodesis by the usual technique of denuding the joint surface and

driving in a three-flanged nail will very possibly fail. In one case a second attempt at fusion by ischiofemoral arthrodesis also failed. In these exceedingly difficult cases the treatment of choice is to perform an operative reduction through a Smith-Petersen or posterior-lateral approach and fuse the joint, either at

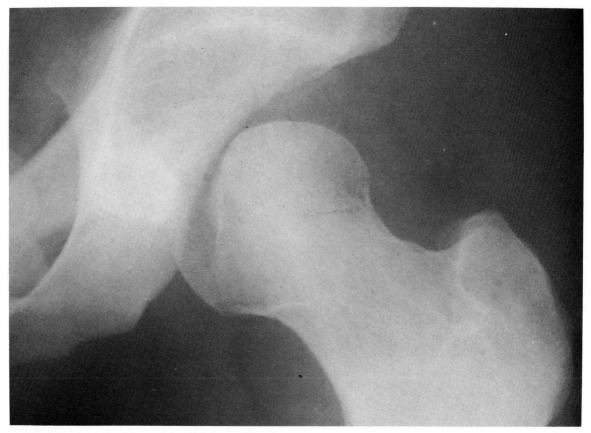

Fig 29.69 X-ray taken during attempted manipulation of a dislocated hip showing obstruction to reduction by a bone fragment detached from the femoral head.

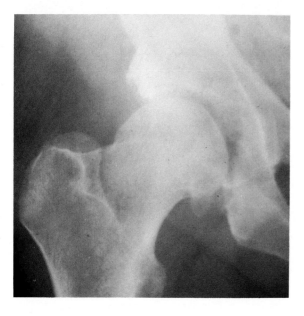

Fig 29.70 Antero-posterior X-ray after reduction of a hip dislocation with a comminuted fracture of the acetabular rim. The head of the femur is not concentrically placed in the acetabulum. The hip was explored and several small fragments of bone removed from within the joint. (Mr A. Benjamin's case.)

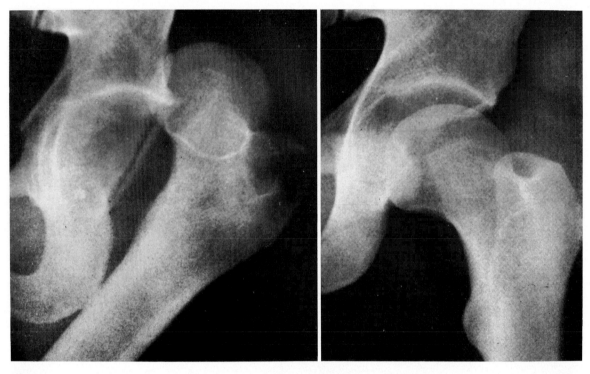

Fig 29.71   Fig 29.72

Fig 29.73

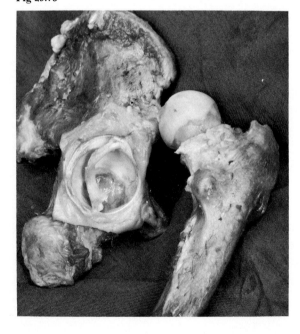

Figs 29.71 to 29.73 Figure 29.71 shows the X-ray of a simple posterior dislocation with a linear acetabular rim fracture. Figure 29.72 is an antero-posterior X-ray after closed reduction—the head of the femur is not concentrically placed in the acetabulum due to soft tissue obstruction. Figure 29.73 shows a prepared specimen illustrating the bucket handle tear and displacement of the acetabular rim which was found at open reduction. (Reproduced by kind permission of the *Journal of Bone and Joint Surgery* and of I. Paterson from his article (1957) The torn acetabular labrum. *Journal of Bone and Joint Surgery*, 39–B, 306.)

the same time or at a second-stage operation, with a strong buttress of iliac bone wedged tightly into the pelvis and fixed to the neck and base of the greater trochanter with a single screw, together with many iliac bone chips impacted firmly in the joint space and around the main graft. The limb must be immobilised in a double plaster spica for not less than four months and sometimes longer. It is only if there is already serious stiffness of the knee joint that early arthroplasty is advisable.

Unfortunately arthrodesis of the hip is not acceptable in many undeveloped countries where people are accustomed to squatting, and it is in these very countries that late dislocations of the hip are encountered most frequently; and where total prosthetic replacement cannot safely be undertaken. Huckstep, in a series of 37 patients from East Africa, found that it was possible to reduce the dislocation by closed manipulation in 11 patients, including one case a year-and-a-half after dislocation. In hips where there was a useful range of painless movement, a corrective osteotomy gave a useful joint, but in painful, stiff joints a Girdlestone excision arthroplasty was necessary.[80] More recently Gupta and Shravat have reported experience in seven patients where reduction was achieved by the application of heavy traction for up to 17 days.[81] This method failed in only one case, and in this instance the hip had been dislocated for nine months. The other cases restored a very satisfactory range of movement by two years and showed no signs of avascular necrosis. Traction of 7–18 kilograms was applied through a tibial pin, using heavy sedation (meperidine) and muscle relaxants (mephenesin). When the head was opposite or below the acetabulum the leg was abducted to reduce the hip, and reduced traction maintained for a further five weeks.

6. Irreducible dislocations. It is rare for the closed reduction of a dislocated hip to be difficult. If there has been a struggle to achieve reduction, or if despite a proper manipulative technique and satisfactory anaesthesia it has still not been possible to reduce the femoral head into the acetabulum, look for obstruction by a bone fragment which is usually separated from the under surface of the femoral articular surface (Fig 29.69). If open reduction becomes necessary the fragment should be removed (see below).

Occasionally a dislocation is apparently reduced fairly easily, but the post-operative X-ray shows that the femoral head is not concentrically placed in the acetabulum. This complication is nearly always the result of obstruction within the acetabulum by bone fragments broken off from the femoral head or acetabular rim (Fig 29.70); but it can sometimes be brought about by the labrum acetabulare becoming turned into the acetabulum as a bucket handle tear[82, 83] (figs 29.71 to 29.73).

CENTRAL FRACTURE-DISLOCATION OF THE HIP JOINT

'There is great confusion in the literature about the treatment of central-fracture-dislocations'.[87]

The views on the management of central dislocations have altered considerably in the last 20 years. They are no longer lumped together as one injury, treatable only by conservative means, but have been classified into a number of varieties, some of which can be improved by operative measures.

Classification. Although several classifications have been suggested,[84, 85, 86, 87] basically two distinct fractures of the acetabulum can be recognised: *Group 1* with an intact weight-bearing articular surface (Fig 29.74) and *Group 2* in which the acetabulum has been reduced to a bag of bones (Fig 29.75). The mechanism of production of these two fractures is probably quite different. Group 2 fractures are the result of a direct injury to the side of the greater trochanter and pelvis, such as seen when a pedestrian crossing the road is knocked over by a car, or is sustained by the occupant of a car stove in from the side (Fig 29.76). Indeed this type of fracture has been produced experimentally by applying a direct force to the greater trochanter.[88] Group 1 fractures, on the other hand, are the result of a more complex system of forces applied to the trochanter and also along the shaft of the femur from the knee; this is the combination of forces which commonly prevail in a high-speed motor accident, the dashboard injury to the knees providing the femoral thrust, while a side swipe blow on the car produces the direct injury to the greater trochanter (Fig 29.77). In these Group 1 fractures the displacement of the femur is rarely central. True, it is displaced medially, but usually there is an accompanying posterior, or more rarely anterior, dislocation. The injury can be considered as fracture-dislocation of the hip in which there is a large acetabular fragment.

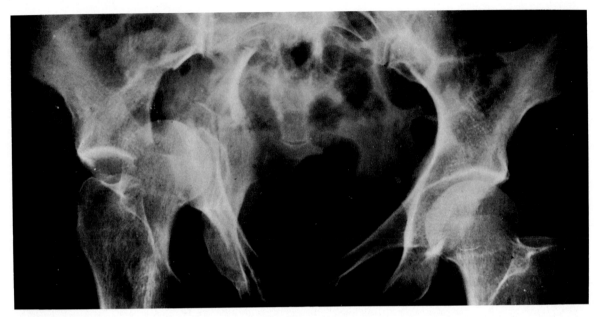

Fig 29.74 Group 1 central dislocation of the hip with intact acetabular roof, but postero-medial displacement of the femoral head.

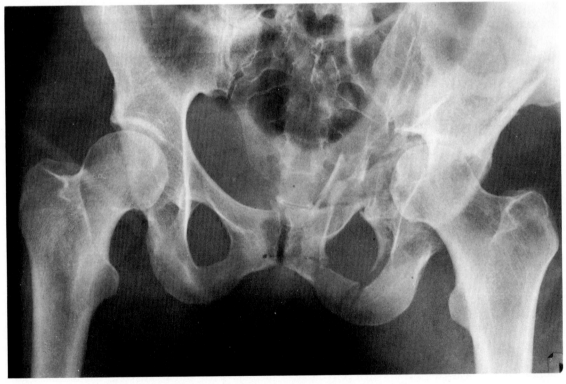

Fig 29.75 Group 2 central dislocation of the hip with comminution of the acetabular roof. (*Proceedings of the Royal Society of Medicine,* 1960, 53, 944. By kind permission of the Editor.)

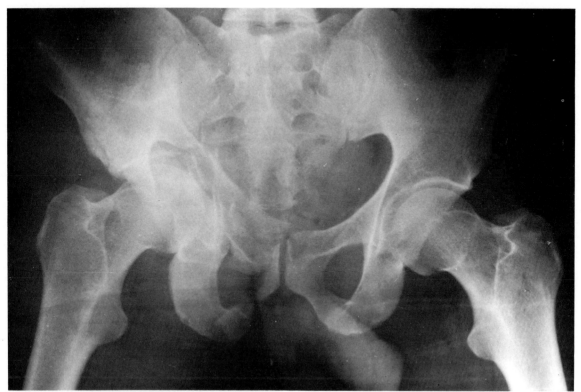

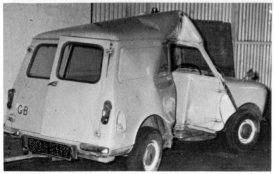

Fig 29.76 The patient who sustained this Group 2 central dislocation of the hip was driving a van which skidded and struck a lamp standard sideways on (inset). The head of the femur was forcibly driven against the floor of the acetabulum, causing a disruption of the floor and direct medial displacement of the femoral head. The same injury can occur when a pedestrian is struck on the hip by a car.

Clinical appearance. In a displaced acetabular fracture with central dislocation there is usually ample evidence of local injury to the hip. The Group 2 injury is always associated with signs of trauma directly over the trochanteric area. This may be only swelling, tenderness and bruising, but on occasions the blow to the lateral aspect of the hip responsible for the acetabular fracture will also produce a deep laceration over the trochanteric fat pad. Sometimes,

in women, the soft tissue injury may produce a split in the capsule of this fat pad (without breaking the skin), causing the pad to displace inferiorly and interfering with the normal trochanteric contour (Fig 29.78). It has been described as the 'battered buttock syndrome' and is often mistaken for a resolving haematoma.[89] It should always be suspected, however, if there is extensive bruising initially (Fig 29.78 inset). The deformity can be corrected surgi-

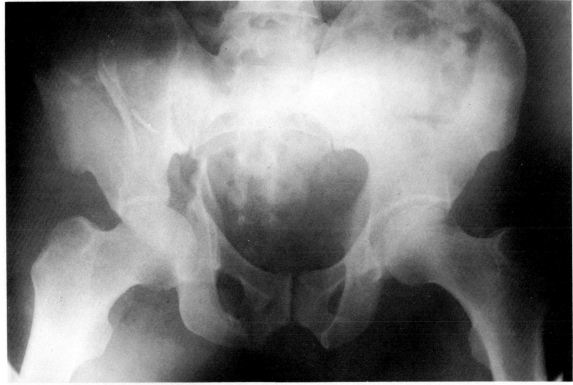

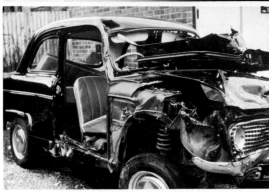

Fig 29.77 X-ray of a Group 1 central dislocation of the right hip occurring in a patient who was the driver of the car shown in the inset. Note that the damage to the front and side of the car indicates that the forces on the right hip could be resolved into two components, that is, along the femoral shaft and at right angles to it.

cally, but if left untreated results in a permanent cosmetic disability.

In Group 1 central dislocations there may be some real shortening, but this can be difficult to detect: in Group 2 injuries there is no shortening. Active hip movement is often too painful to test, but passive movements, although not necessarily grossly restricted, are usually limited in abduction and in rotation. These injuries are, of course, severe fractures of the pelvis and as such are often accompanied with considerable blood loss (see Chapter 28). Occasionally

there is associated damage to the genito-urinary tract, and catheterisation, and sometimes a cystogram may be required to exclude urethral or bladder damage. Despite the extent of the acetabular injury, central dislocation can often be missed initially because, more often than not, it forms only part of a severe multiple injury. It is well to bear this in mind when treating the severely injured; particularly if the extent of the other injuries is inconsistent with a poor response in a patient being treated for shock. Under these conditions a straight X-ray of the pelvis may reveal

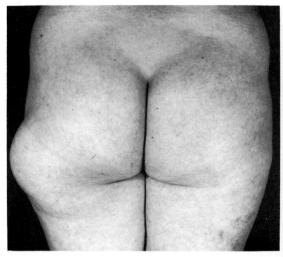 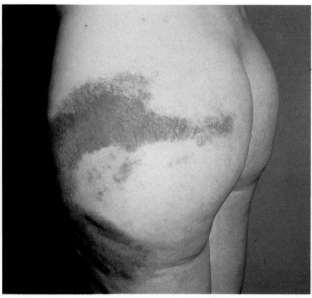

Fig 29.78 The 'Battered Buttock' syndrome. A direct blow over the trochanter may cause a central dislocation of the hip and in the same process split the trochanteric fat capsule with displacement of the fat pad inferiorly. This is often mistaken for an unresolved haematoma. The clue to the injury is the severe bruising which occurs initially (right).

the true cause of the deterioration. Finally, linear fractures of the floor of the acetabulum can occur without dislocation and be responsible for unexplained pain in the hip. These fractures are often seen only in the oblique X-ray (Figs 29.79 and 29.80).

Radiological diagnosis. Before any decision is made to carry out an open reduction and fixation of an acetabular fracture it is essential to have a very detailed radiological examination. First, the fracture-dislocation must be classified with one of the two main groups. This can be simple, such as in the case of the two examples shown in Figures 29.74 and 29.75. In the one case the acetabulum is clearly totally disorganised (Fig 29.75), whereas in the other (Fig 29.74) there are two distinct fragments dividing the acetabulum into two parts. Unfortunately, it is not always so easy to classify the fractures, yet it is essential that the distinction should be made, because the treatment of the two types is quite different. Three extra radiographs are necessary in addition to the routine antero-posterior and lateral views; these are: stereographic studies, internal oblique and external oblique views.[84] Stereographic views are of the utmost value in determining the nature of the fracture and the displacement of fragments, but their use does demand some practice and ability of interpretation

on the part of the viewer, and any surgeon who is intending to carry out an open reduction of these injuries is urged to become conversant with stereographic X-ray technique. The three-quarter internal oblique view (Fig 29.81) profiles the whole of the anterior ilio-pubic component of the acetabulum, while also displaying the posterior lip of the acetabulum; the three-quarter external oblique view (Fig 29.82) shows up the posterior edge of the iliac bone and will demonstrate a fracture which passes up towards the sciatic notch; it also allows study of the anterior lip of the acetabulum. Figures 29.83 to 29.85 illustrate the value of the oblique views in assessing the degree of comminution and give some indication of the wide variation in the two basic groups of acetabular fracture.

Treatment. It is important to emphasise again that a central dislocation of the hip is usually associated with severe comminution of the acetabulum and is always accompanied by profound shock due to the extensive intrapelvic haemorrhage. It has been estimated that up to 2 litres or more of blood may be lost with this type of injury, and remembering that the fracture is not uncommonly one of multiple fractures, early treatment must be directed towards resuscitation and any operative procedures deferred

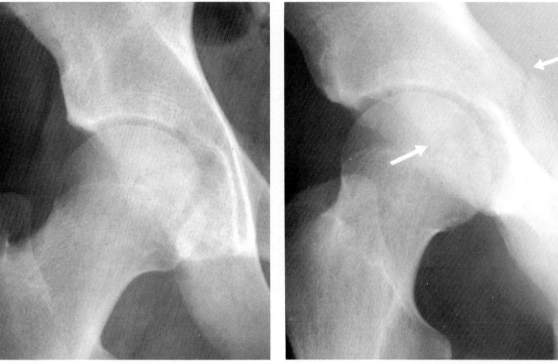

Fig 29.79   **Fig 29.80**

Fig 29.79 to 29.80 The X-ray shown in Fig 29.79 was reported as normal. The patient however complained of severe pain and the clinical signs suggested an intra-articular injury. The external rotation oblique view (Fig 29.80) showed a linear fracture across the floor of the acetabulum. If this had displaced it would have resulted in a Group 1 central dislocation of the hip.

until the patient has fully recovered from the initial effects of the injury. While awaiting a decision on definitive treatment the affected limb should be put up in Hamilton-Russell traction.

There is a great deal of controversy over the question of conservative treatment versus operation in the management of these injuries and open reduction has been described as 'not only difficult, but also ineffective in improving the end result'.[90] Those in favour of conservative measures point out that 75 per cent of patients with central acetabular fractures can achieve good results with conservative treatment,[85] whereas the advocates of operative treatment emphasise that even though the femoral head can be reduced only operative measures can hope to restore the acetabular fragments to normal position, and recommend open reduction in all cases, except when there is no displacement. Both protagonists in this argument have failed to appreciate the two basic principles in the treatment of fracture-dislocation. The first principle is that a joint which is totally disorganised because of multiple fractures

cannot possibly be restored to normality. It therefore requires no reduction and treatment should be conservative—the so-called 'bag of bones' method aiming to restore function from the very first moment. The second principle is that fracture-dislocations with displacement of a large single fragment should be reduced as accurately as possible, and to do this will often require open reduction and internal fixation. It is the neglect of these two principles in treatment of fracture-dislocations that has led to the confusion in the interpretation of results of both conservative and operative measures and has resulted in much unnecessary complication in the classification of these injuries. Let it be said again two groups only need recognition: Group 1 (intact acetabular roof with a large displaced fragment), which require accurate reduction, and Group 2 (completely disorganised acetabulum), which do very well without reduction and with early restoration of function. Excluding cases where there has been damage to the femoral head it has been observed that a favourable outcome is dependent on two factors: an intact superior

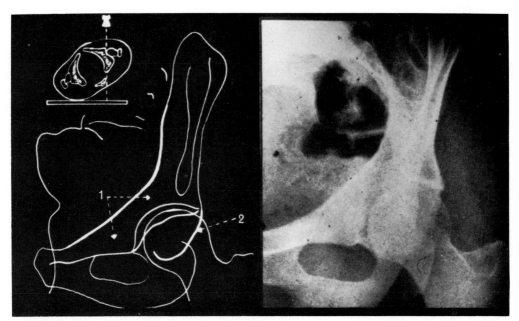

Fig 29.81

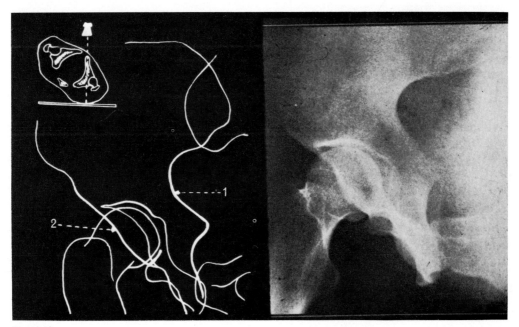

Fig 29.82

Figs 29.81 and 29.82 Figure 29.81 (top) shows a three-quarter internal oblique view of the hip (patient supine and rotated 45 degrees away from the injured side). (1) Iliopubic column. (2) Posterior lip of the acetabulum.

Figure 29.82 (bottom) shows a three-quarter external oblique view of the hip (patient supine and rotated 45 degrees toward the injured side). (1) Posterior lip of the ilium. (2) Anterior lip of the acetabulum. (Reproduced by kind permission of the *Journal of Bone and Joint Surgery* and of the late Professor Robert Judet from a paper by Judet, R., Judet, J. & Letournel, E. (1964) Fractures of the acetabulum; classification and surgical approaches for open reduction. *Journal of Bone and Joint Surgery*, 46–A, 1615.)

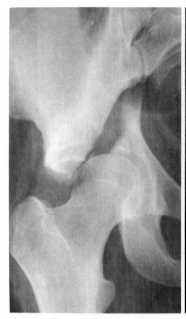

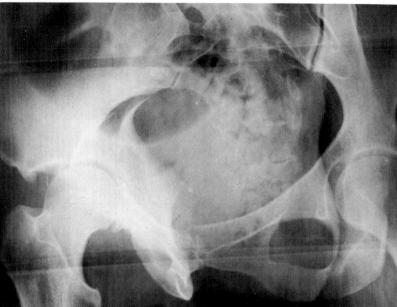

Fig 29.83   **Fig 29.84**

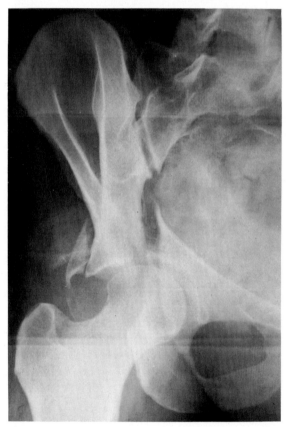

Fig 29.85

acetabular dome, and a good relationship between it and the femoral head.[91] Good results can be expected if these conditions are achieved by either closed or open methods.

Conservative treatment. Traction is applied to the leg by the Hamilton-Russell method using a tibial Steinmann's pin, and active and assisted flexion exercises are encouraged immediately. It has been pointed out that the central displacement of the femoral head can only be corrected by lateral traction.[90] This is of importance only if all types of central dislocation are to be treated conservatively. Group 2 fractures are better left in the displaced position, or only pulled out as far as longitudinal traction will permit. This allows the femoral head to mould a new acetabulum from the many shattered pieces which remain medially displaced and closely related to the femoral head. It is unlikely that the femoral head could be completely reduced to its normal position; indeed, it is better that it should not,

Figs 29.83 to 29.85 Figure 29.83 shows the antero-posterior X-ray of a Group 1 central dislocation of the hip. The weight-bearing portion of the acetabulum is intact, but the head of the femur has moved medially with the lower fragment. Figure 29.84 (external oblique view) shows the fracture of the ischial part of the acetabulum extending superiorly towards the sacro-iliac joint. Figure 29.85 (internal oblique view) shows the additional comminution of the posterior acetabular rim. (Reproduced by kind permission of Mr A. Benjamin.)

because the acetabular floor will certainly not follow suit and an inconguity will result (Figs 29.86 to 29.88). Therefore in this type of central dislocation the principle of conservative treatment is to mould a new socket within the framework of the medially displaced and shattered acetabulum. Figure 29.89 shows the result which will be obtained by this method. Over 90 degrees of flexion is not uncommon as the end result, but very little movement in other directions can be expected. Traction should be retained for not less than six weeks, and following this the patient must walk only with crutches, taking minimal weight until three months from the time of injury. There is some evidence to suggest that there is a higher incidence of good results in patients who have not given up their crutches too early.

Open reduction. The careful selection of cases and the correct choice of operative approach are both of great importance in the success of any open reduction.

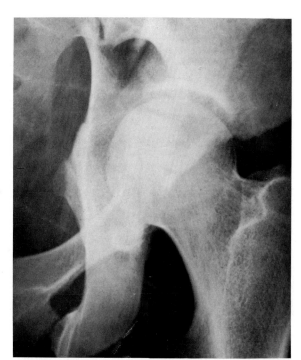

Fig 29.86 Group 2 central dislocation of the hip. The whole of the weight-bearing part of the acetabulum has displaced with the femoral head, indicating that gross comminution has occurred.

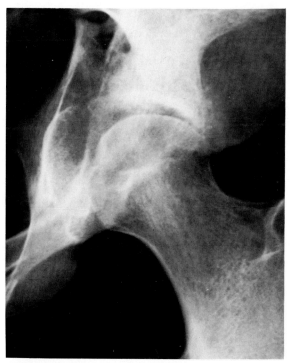

Fig 29.87

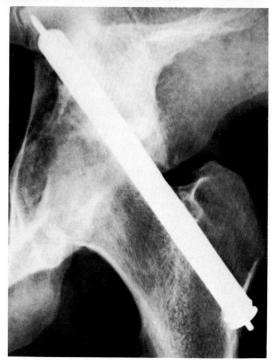

Fig 29.88

Figs 29.87 and 29.88 The head of the femur has been pulled out of the pelvis by skeletal traction but, as often happens, the floor of the acetabulum has failed to follow and is still displaced inwards. The irregularity of the acetabulum caused arthritis necessitating arthrodesis. 'Reduction' in this case resulted in the inconguity of joint surfaces. A more satisfactory result would be expected if the displacement had been left undisturbed.

Only a small proportion of Group 1 central dislocations require operation. Provided the femoral head
remains in its normal relationship to the weight-
bearing surface of the acetabulum and is stable,
fixation of a displaced acetabular fragment is not
indicated. Figure 29.90 is the X-ray of such a case.
This hip was treated conservatively with restoration
of function almost indistinguishable from normal at
two years (Fig 29.91). Some fractures can masquerade
as Group 1 injuries if the routine antero-posterior
view only is taken (Fig 29.92). An irregular shadow
in the wing of the ilium should arouse suspicions that
there is comminution of this segment of the acetabulum; the internal oblique view will confirm if this is
present (Fig 29.93). An injury of this type will not
benefit from open reduction and should be treated
conservatively.

The ideal case for open reduction is the type of
Group 1 fracture shown in Figures 29.94 and 29.74.
In both these injuries there are two distinct bone
fragments with the femoral head completely dislocated from under an intact weight-bearing articular
surface. With less displacement the femoral head may
come to lie partially under the weight-bearing
articular surface and partially in contact with the
displaced fragment, the 'double dome' deformity of
Knight and Smith.[86] This displacement should be
corrected whenever possible, otherwise it will cause
rapid deterioration in joint function (Figs 29.95 and
29.96). Unfortunately, there is usually no way in
which the displacement can be stabilised by operation
and prolonged traction both longitudinally and
laterally for 12 weeks is the best form of management.

Operative technique. In most of the cases suitable for
open reduction the operation can be carried out
through the posterior approach, and only very
occasionally, when the femoral head has displaced
with an anterior fragment of acetabulum, is an
approach from the front indicated. The southern
approach is used (see operative exposures), but with
rather more extensive splitting of the gluteus maximus
posteriorly than is usual for a simple exposure of the
hip joint. If more exposure of the anterior part of the
acetabulum is necessary the approach can be converted to a 'goblet' incision by extending it forwards
towards the anterior superior iliac spine and detaching the greater trochanter. The sciatic nerve should
be isolated and traced up to the sciatic notch where it
may be in intimate contact with the fracture. At this
stage it should be possible to distinguish the two main
components of the fracture, and the femoral head
will be found displaced posteriorly and medially with
the inferior fragment of the acetabulum: traction on

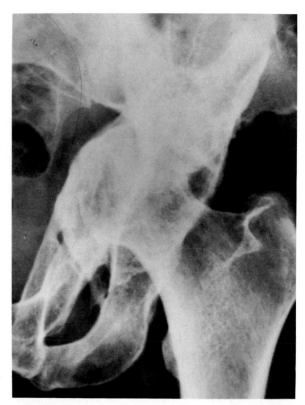

Fig 29.89 An X-ray taken 18 months after a Group 2 central
dislocation of the hip which was treated conservatively by six
weeks in Hamilton-Russell traction. The patient regained 90
degrees of painless flexion. The initial X-ray of this fracture is
shown in Figure 29.75.

this fragment with a bone hook in the sciatic notch
will slowly draw the fragments together and restore
the femoral head to its rightful place under the iliac
part of the acetabulum. Sometimes manipulating the
lower limb will help in reduction. Where the fracture
line is more vertical than horizontal the lower
fragments may extend well up towards the sacroiliac
joint (Fig 29.74) and produce a spike of bone which
is difficult to reduce. This needs gentle treatment if an
awkward haemorrhage from the superior gluteal
vessels is to be avoided. Careful dissection with a
periosteal elevator will probably free it, but if
necessary the sharp tip of the bone can be osteotomised. Reduction is maintained with a small, four-hole
plate screwed into the adjacent parts of the iliac and
ischial components. If there is difficulty in exposing
the iliac side of the fracture the surgeon should have
no hesitation in osteotomising the greater trochanter
to gain better access (Fig 29.97).

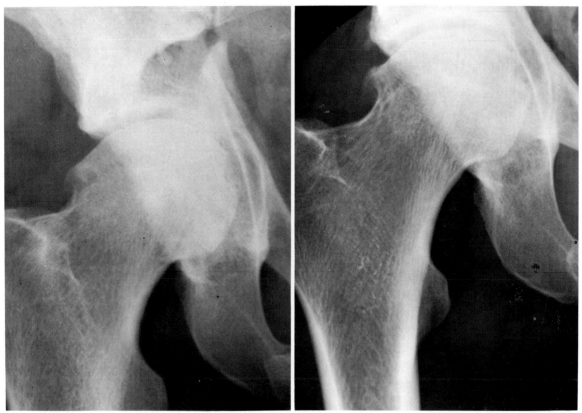

Fig 29.90   **Fig 29.91**

Figs 29.90 and 29.91 A Group 1 fracture of the acetabulum where the femoral head has not displaced with the loose fragment (Fig 29.90). This hip was examined under anaesthesia at two weeks and found to be completely stable. Conservative treatment of traction for six weeks and non-weight-bearing for three months restored function almost to normal. Figure 29.91 shows the X-ray appearance two years later.

Anterior exposure of a central acetabular fracture is carried out through a Smith-Petersen approach, but with the intermuscular dissection on the pelvic side of the iliac crest, separating iliacus from the inside wall of the ilium to expose the whole of the ilio-pubic column. Internal fixation with a small plate or screws can be achieved via this approach.

Following operation, the hip should be immobilised on traction until the wound is healed, and then a single hip spica for six weeks. There should be no weight-bearing for three months.

Complications and prognosis. Sciatic nerve palsy is not a common complication in central fractures of the acetabulum, and in a personal series of 40 cases the incidence of permanent paralysis was 10 per cent. Other series have shown a much higher figure, but this included over 50 per cent of temporary palsies.[91] Degenerative arthritis, with or without avascular change, occurs frequently in cases where there is incongruity between the femoral head and the superior acetabulum—the so-called 'double dome' deformity. Associated injury to the femoral head, although an uncommon complication, is nearly always followed by degenerative change and has a very poor prognosis.

Stewart and Milford have suggested that cellular damage to the femoral head at the time of injury may be responsible for some cases of late degenerative arthritis,[67] and in vitro experiments have shown that the chondrocytes and the structural integrity of articular cartilage are compromised if a critical impact load is exceeded[75] (see page 913). Poor

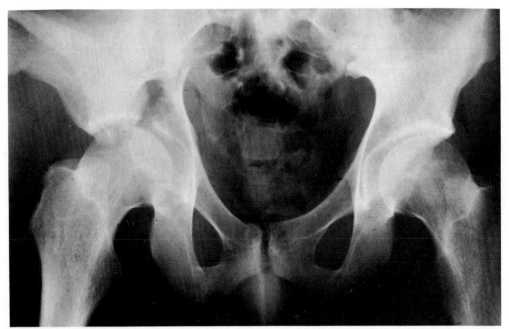

Fig 29.92

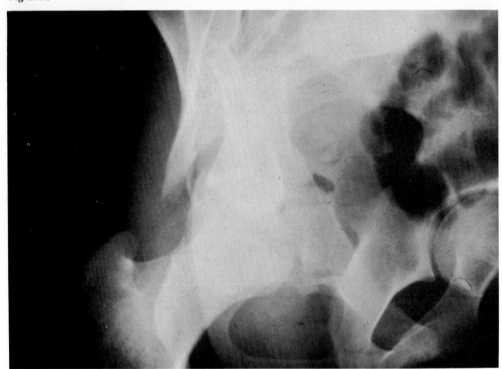

Fig 29.93

Figs 29.92 and 29.93 The antero-posterior X-ray of this acetabular fracture shows an apparently intact weight-bearing component (Fig 29.92); but the irregularity of the wing of the ilium should arouse the suspicion that there is a fracture through this part. The internal oblique view (Fig 29.93) confirms the gross comminution of the acetabular roof. (Reproduced by kind permission of Mr A. Benjamin.)

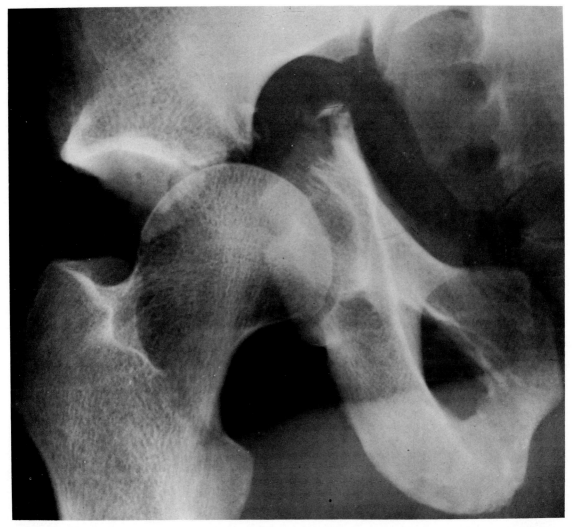

Fig 29.94 Group 1 central dislocation of the hip. The acetabulum is broken into two major fragments and the femoral head has displaced from under the weight-bearing area of the acetabular roof. Unless a stable reduction can be obtained by manipulation this injury should be treated by open reduction and internal fixation.

clinical function at six months carries a poor prognosis. On the other hand, if there is good function at one year the hip is unlikely to deteriorate.[91, 92]

Myositis ossificans rarely occurs except as a complication of operative treatment,[87] and its incidence is much less if the hip is immobilised in a plaster spica for at least six weeks after open reduction. Some authors have related this complication to the timing of the operation after injury,[91, 93] but the evidence for this is not conclusive.

In summary, there seems little doubt that the grossly disorganised fractures of the acetabulum do well if treated conservatively by methods which aim at early restoration of function; this also applies to the treatment of cases where the femoral head remains in good relationship with the superior acetabulum. Where, however, an incongruous articulation exists between the femoral head and the acetabular roof every effort should be made to restore it to normal; these are the cases which after very careful evaluation of X-rays may be considered suitable for open reduction and internal fixation.

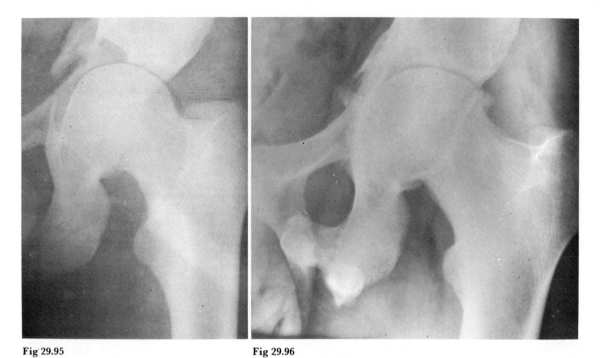

Fig 29.95   **Fig 29.96**

Figs 29.95 and 29.96 Figure 29.95 shows Group 1 central dislocation of the hip with the formation of a 'double dome' deformity of the superior articular surface of the acetabulum outlined on the X-ray. This resulted in marked degenerative change in the femoral head within one year of the injury (Fig 29.96).

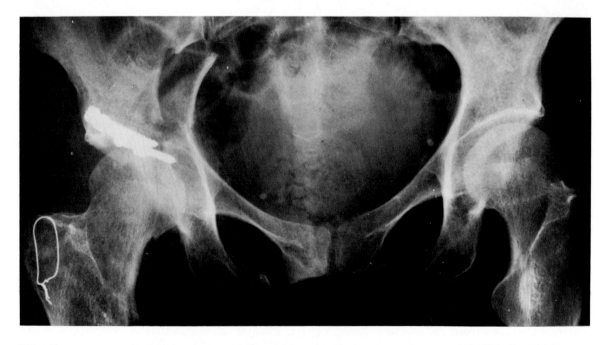

Fig 29.97 Open reduction and internal fixation of the Group 1 central dislocation illustrated in Figure 29.74. Note that it has been necessary to osteotomise the sacro-iliac spike.

FRACTURES OF THE NECK OF THE FEMUR

Fractures of the neck of the femur are usually sustained by old people from trivial strains such as tripping on a stair or stumbling on a carpet; but they may occur at any age in patients of either sex although elderly women predominate. The injuries may be *intracapsular*, where the fracture line can vary from the middle of the neck to the subcapital region (Fig 29.98); or *extracapsular*, where the fracture can be at the very base of the neck or through the pertrochanteric line (Fig 29.99). In the extracapsular fractures there is usually gross deformity and loss of function, but in the undisplaced intracapsular fracture it is sometimes possible for the patient to move the hip or even to walk despite the injury, and such ordinary signs of fractures as shortening of the limb seldom develop until after several days or weeks. Quite often with minor displacement the only clinical sign that is obvious is slight lateral rotation deformity, and a provisional diagnosis should be made on this evidence alone (Fig 29.100). Every elderly patient who, after injury, complains of pain in the region of the hip and lies with the limb in lateral rotation should be assumed to have sustained a fracture of the femoral neck until radiographs taken in two planes prove otherwise.

Many years ago this fracture was often a terminal event in the lives of feeble and fragile individuals who died from cardiac, pulmonary or renal complications, aggravated by the recumbency and immobility that was attendant upon the conservative regime advised at that time. This state of affairs no longer prevails because it has long been recognised that the treatment of these fractures is essentially surgical, and that operative measures should not be withheld except under the most exceptional circumstances. In the past active treatment was often delayed for as long as three or four weeks because it was believed that attempts to fix the fracture by operative internal fixation would in themselves prove fatal. Nothing could be further from the truth. Internal fixation of the fracture, or prosthetic replacement of the femoral head, carried out as soon as possible after injury is vitally important in order to permit early mobilisation and thus avoid the dangers of prolonged recumbency and immobility in elderly patients.[94] Even in the very elderly, operative treatment usually succeeds in avoiding fatal complications and in restoring a useful and painless hip. A short expectation of life does not justify the miseries of an ununited fracture—the old have as much right to live in

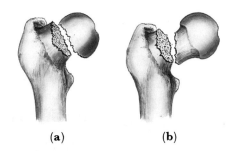

(a)   **(b)**

Fig 29.98 Intracapsular fracture. (a) Subcapital. (b) Transcervical.

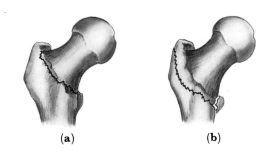

(a)   **(b)**

Fig 29.99 Extracapsular fracture. (a) Intertrochanteric. (b) Pertrochanteric.

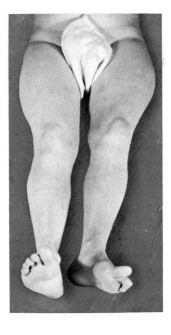

Fig 29.100 Intracapsular fracture of the neck of the femur with typical lateral rotation deformity.

comfort as the young—and the fact is that old people tolerate modern anaesthesia and surgical intervention extremely well.[95]

When considering treatment intracapsular fractures through the neck of the femur must be clearly differentiated from extracapsular fractures in the trochanteric region. An external rotation deformity of the limb gives the clue to the general diagnosis, but only good antero-posterior and lateral X-rays can differentiate between the two types, for which the plan of treatment as well as the prognosis differs widely. However, one factor common to both is that treatment should be surgical, the method only varying with the type of fracture, its displacement and to some extent, the age of the patient. The management of the acute fractures will therefore be considered under two main headings—intracapsular and extracapsular fractures, with a third section devoted to the treatment of ununited fractures.

Intracapsular fractures of the femoral neck

Classification. At one time femoral neck fractures were divided into abduction and adduction fractures (Fig 29.101). The former were said to be impacted and therefore stable, while the latter were mobile and potentially unstable.[96] This classification is, of course, nonsense, for all the fractures are degrees of the same basic injury and produced by the same mechanism. Per Linton was probably the first person to show there was no foundation for making the distinction between the so-called abduction and adduction fractures.[97, 98] In each group of fractures the cause of

injury is the same; both arise from lateral rotation strains, and the only real distinction to be made is in the degree of displacement. When a lateral rotational strain is applied to the lower limb and transmitted to the femoral neck, the bone is broken by a rotational force at or near the subcapital level. The plane of fracture is not strictly transverse—it is more nearly spiral, the proximal fragment including the femoral head together with a large beak of bone from the back of the femoral head. Figure 29.102 shows a femoral head excised from a patient with a recent fracture of the femoral neck; there can be no doubt that it was a spiral fracture (see also Per Linton's case in Figure 29.103). In the first degree of displacement the fragments are impacted and the plane of fracture seems to be horizontal; but as the rotational force continues the impaction is broken up, the fragments separate, and the plane of fracture seems more vertical. But, in fact, the plane of fracture has been the same from the beginning.

Thus apparently different planes in fractures of the neck of the femur represent no more than the radiographic appearances of varying degrees of displacement of the same rotational injury. Moreover, the term 'impacted fracture' implies only that injury has stopped short after the first stage of displacement in response to a force which if continued would have produced a displaced fracture.* It is true that the first stage of displacement, represented by an impacted fracture of the femoral neck, is relatively stable and

* Incidentally we must recognise that this applies not only to fractures of the neck of the femur but to all so-called impacted fractures wherever they may occur.

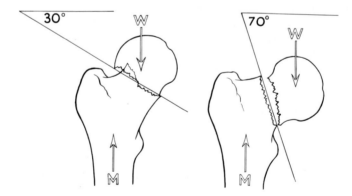

Fig 29.101 At one time fractures of the neck of the femur were classified as abduction or adduction fractures according to the angle of the fracture line. Body weight in the one produced further impaction, while in the other it was responsible for introducing a shearing strain. They are, of course, all one of the same type and mechanism and are merely degrees of displacement produced by the same rotational strain. What is more, the so-called impacted abduction fracture can disimpact and become an 'adducted' unstable injury (see Figs 29.104 and 29.105).

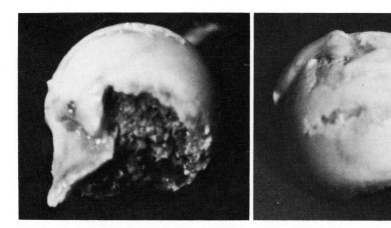

Fig 29.102 Head of the femur excised and replaced by a prosthesis after a fresh subcapital fracture of the femoral head. Note that the plane of fracture is not transverse; it is much more nearly spiral.

may remain so without the addition of internal fixation; but there is no absolute safety. Per Linton reported one such fracture, treated by recumbency in bed, in which complete displacement developed while the patient was under observation (Figs 29.104 and 29.105). Note in these radiographs how the apparently horizontal plane of fracture in the first stage of displacement became an obviously vertical plane of fracture in the second stage of displacement. It is a good example of a radiographic illusion which can be so misleading.

Garden's classification. By far the most valuable contribution of recent years on the mechanism and classification of transcervical fractures is that of Garden.[99, 100] Developing the work of Per Linton, Garden has shown that subcapital fractures tend to follow the same basic pattern and that it is only on rare occasions that there is a true variation in the obliquity of the fracture. The Pauwels classification[101] into horizontal and vertical fractures is less satisfactory and is only meaningful if applied to the fracture *after* reduction when it is a reliable indication of the degree of posterior cortical collapse. Garden's classification distinguishes four types of fracture and

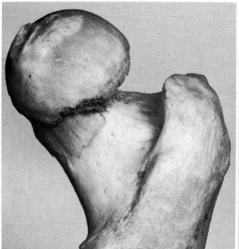
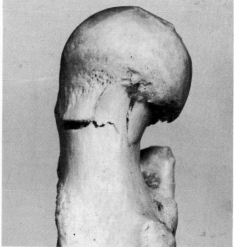

Fig 29.103 This is an 'impacted abduction fracture'. Note that it is a rotational spiral injury. In some radiographic projections the plane of fracture appears to be horizontal but in others it appears to be vertical. (Reproduced by kind permission of the *Journal of Bone and Joint Surgery* and of G. Per Linton from his article (1949) Types of displacement in fractures of the femoral neck. *Journal of Bone and Joint Surgery*, 31–B, 184.)

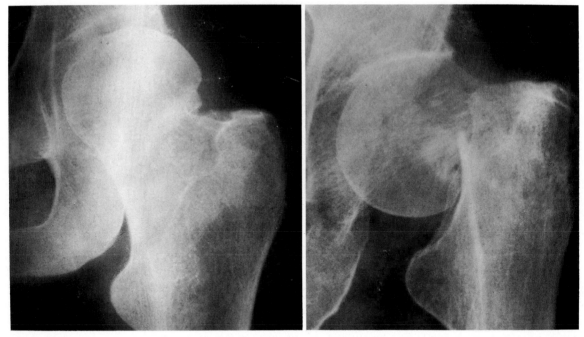

Fig. 29.104   Fig 29.105

Figs 29.104 and 29.105 A fracture of the femoral neck which appeared to be impacted in 'abduction' (Fig 29.104) was treated by simple bed rest. It soon became a typical 'adduction' fracture with displacement, and an apparently vertical plane of fracture (Fig 29.105). (Reproduced by kind permission of the *Journal of Bone and Joint Surgery* and of G. Per Linton from his article (1949) Types of displacement in fractures of the femoral neck. *Journal of Bone and Joint Surgery*, 31–B, 184.)

recognises the significance of radiographic appearances in various stages of displacement *before* reduction. The four Garden types are as follows:

1. Incomplete fracture. The so-called 'abducted' or 'impacted' injury in which the inferior cortex has not been completely breached (Fig 29.106).

2. Complete fracture without displacement. The inferior cortex of the neck has broken but no tilting of the head has occurred (Fig 29.107).

3. Complete fracture with partial displacement. Full lateral rotation of the distal fragment has not occurred, and the distal hinges on the proximal fragment tilting it into abduction and medial rotation (Fig 29.108).

4. Complete fracture with full displacement. The distal fragment has now fully rotated in a lateral direction. Intimate contact between the two fragments has been lost, allowing the proximal fragment to resume its natural position in the acetabulum (Fig 29.109).

It must be admitted, however, that it can be very difficult to distinguish between types 1 and 2, and between types 3 and 4. As far as treatment is concerned, and for simplicity, the Garden types 1 and 2 can be considered as one variety and types 3 and 4 as another.

Treatment of intracapsular fractures

In discussing the management of intracapsular fractures of the femoral neck the patients can be arbitrarily divided into three age groups in which the treatment required, the complications likely to occur, and the prognosis will vary considerably. These groups are:

1. Fractures in the elderly (over 70 years of age).
2. Fractures in the young and middle-aged.
3. Fractures in children.

Each group has its own problems, but it must be remembered that there is one factor common to them all—the danger of injury to the retinacular vessels with avascular necrosis of the femoral head. This can sometimes be the cause of non-union of the fracture whatever method is used for immobilisation and even in cases where union has occurred late avascular

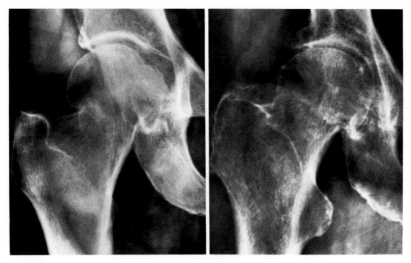

Fig 29.106   **Fig 29.107**

Figs 29.106 and 29.107 Stage 1 (Fig 29.106): *Incomplete subcapital fracture* was commonly known as the 'abducted' or 'impacted' fracture. As in a greenstick fracture, the medial trabeculae at the junction of the head and neck often appear to be bent rather than broken. Stage 2 (Fig 29.107): *Complete subcapital fracture without displacement.* The alignment of the medial trabeculae in the two fragments is undisturbed.

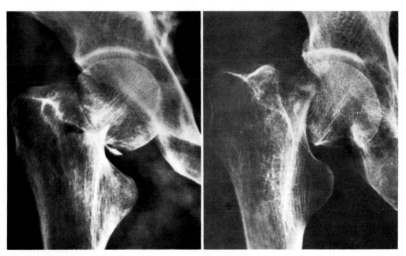

Fig 29.108   **Fig 29.109**

Figs 29.108 and 29.109 Stage 3 (Fig 29.108): *Complete subcapital fracture with partial displacement.* The capital fragment is rotated medially as shown by the direction of its medial trabecular group, and full lateral rotation of the distal fragment has not yet occurred. Stage 4 (Fig 29.109): *Complete subcapital fracture with full displacement.* The distal fragment is in full lateral rotation, and end-to-end contact between the two fragments has been lost. The capital fragment is now free to resume its natural position in the acetabulum, and its medial trabeculae lie in normal alignment with their fellows in the pelvis. (Figures 29.106 to 29.109 are reproduced by kind permission of the *Journal of Bone and Joint Surgery* and of R. S. Garden from his paper (1964) Stability and union in subcapital fractures of the femur. *Journal of Bone and Joint Surgery*, 46–B, 630.)

change in the weight-bearing segment of the femoral head can result in a stiff and painful joint. It is not without reason that the injury has been labelled 'the unsolved fracture'.[102]

However, it is important not to be persuaded by some enthusiasts that specific forms of treatment are applicable only to certain age groups. This is particularly relevant when considering the merits of internal fixation against those of prosthetic replacement and is well summed up in Nicoll's colourful words: 'decapitation by age groups is about as scientific as tossing a coin'.[102] There must be no rigid lines of demarcation, each fracture and each patient must be carefully and individually assessed; then, and only then, can a decision on the most appropriate treatment be taken.

Historical background to treatment. Up until the advent of prosthetic replacement of the femoral head treatment of intracapsular fractures was directed towards obtaining an adequate reduction and maintaining it until union ensued. Whitman believed he could do this by immobilisation in a plaster spica, but persistently refused to publish his results. Of the patients who survived the ordeal of plaster it is thought that about one third obtained union of the fracture.

Many surgeons therefore turned their attention towards internal fixation,[103, 104, 105] but it was not until Smith-Petersen[106] introduced his triflanged nail made of non-electrolytic metal that the results from internal fixation became more acceptable. These nails were first introduced under direct vision after open reduction of the fracture, but this technique was rapidly overtaken by the introduction of closed nailing under X-ray control, using a cannulated nail and guide wire.[107] This method forms the basis of all modern internal fixation of femoral neck fractures, and although many variants of the fixation have been devised[108–115] the Smith-Petersen nail is still widely used throughout the world.

Developments in fixation have been directed towards producing a more efficient device which will rigidly fix the fracture. Twenty-five years ago Charnley[116] introduced a spring loaded compression screw with a lateral plate fixation. But this was a cumbersome apparatus and results from its use were disappointing. A number of sliding nail plates have been devised[117, 118] but they have not produced any appreciable increase in the percentage of fractures united. Smythe[119] popularised the use of an ingenious combination of two screws joined by a plate to form a triangular fixation; this, he claimed followed the

natural trabecular columns which support the femoral neck. Garden[120] described a rather similar arrangement using two crossed screws. These latter two methods of fixation in the hands of the originators are probably the most efficient at our disposal to date.[121] However, the technique of introduction of crossed screws is more difficult, and their position more critical, than the simple insertion of a Smith-Petersen nail, and in other surgeons' hands the fixation obtained is certainly not immune to failure (Figs 29.110 and 29.111). It still remains to be *proved by more general use of the method* whether the results are an improvement on the less sophisticated measures.

Principles of treatment—internal fixation versus prosthetic replacement. Every one of the procedures already described are of course simple variants of the same principle of reducing the displacement by manipulation and then securing firm internal fixation to avoid the hazards of prolonged immobilisation. All those who favour internal fixation of femoral neck fractures emphasise the importance of accuracy in reduction, just as much as they emphasise the need for secure fixation. In a comparative review of internal fixation versus prosthetic replacement Bracey[122] commented that 'those fractures accurately reduced definitely did better'; but despite this his overall union rate was only 47 per cent. Garden considered that accuracy of reduction in the lateral view 'as the best mirror of reduction and the best guide to prognosis'.[123] Also, Garden was of the opinion that a fracture with a perfect reduction was less likely to be complicated by avascular necrosis, and hence the prognosis was largely determined by the position accepted for the internal fixation.

Undoubtedly there is a very good chance of obtaining successful union in a reasonably high proportion of these fractures—certainly over 50 per cent. But there still remains the unknown quantity— the damage done to the vascular supply of the femoral head *as a result of the injury itself*, and the consequences of this are quite out of the control of the surgeon. The blood supply to the femoral head from capsular vessels running in retinaculae close to the bone is often cut off by the fracture. If this happens some avascular necrosis of the femoral head is inevitable, causing delayed or non-union, and often giving rise to a painful degenerative arthritis within a few years. Thus, despite all operative skills, a perfect functional result from the nailing operation cannot always be secured and occurs in only about two-thirds of the cases, whichever appliance is used.

The uncertainty of union after properly applied

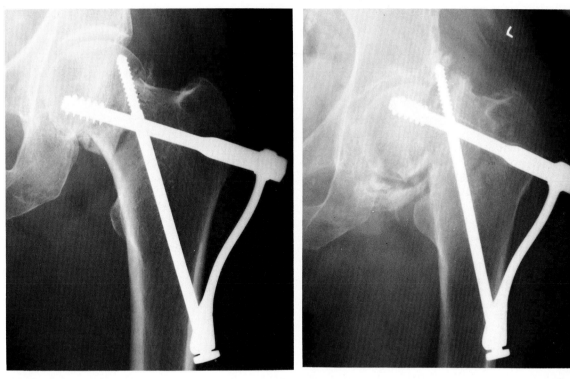

Fig 29.110   Fig 29.111

Figs 29.110 and 29.111 Crossed screws are not immune from complications! A fractured neck of femur was apparently well fixed with crossed Smyth screws (Fig 29.110). Two months later the screws had cut out of the head and the fracture had redisplaced (Fig 29.111).

internal fixation and the possibility of late avascular necrosis even in those fractures which have united have led a large number of surgeons to abandon the nailing procedure for displaced fractures and to use prosthetic replacement of the femoral head as a primary treatment. In some centres this operation has become the treatment of choice in elderly patients who have a displaced subcapital fracture. Indeed, in one paper it is advised that 'Thompson arthroplasty is the routine treatment for all these fractures', presumably displaced or undisplaced.[124] The evidence, however, does not support these views. Boyd and Salvatore[125] in a review of over 500 patients found that nearly 60 per cent of fractures united without avascular necrosis, and by no means all of those who developed avascular change or non-union required further operative treatment. Also, the results of prosthetic replacement as a primary treatment for femoral neck fracture leave much to be desired when compared with simple pinning.[126, 127] The mortality

is higher, post-operative infection is more common, and there is the added risk of dislocation. As the numbers of prosthetic replacement have increased other problems associated with the operation have become more apparent, such as acetabular erosion and loosening.[124] However, the arguments for and against prosthetic replacement still rage, and will probably continue to do so for as long as there are enthusiasts adamantly supporting one or other method. But, at last, a more rational attitude towards the problem does seem to be appearing. Each case must, of course, be considered on its own merits and circumstances which prevail in the unit responsible for the treatment, but it is becoming clear that the femoral head should not be sacrificed lightly in 'every fracture', particularly when the fracture is undisplaced, or can be reduced accurately. Primary prosthetic replacement should be reserved for the very old or infirm, and for pathological, irreducible, or grossly comminuted fractures.

Treatment by age groups. Although it is accepted that 'to decide the fate of the femoral head against a yardstick of age alone is to offer an unworthy clinical judgement',[123] there must be some arbitary division into age groups when considering treatment and these are outlined below.

1. Fractures of the femoral neck in the elderly (over 70). Those fractures with minimal displacement, and the so-called 'abduction' fractures are undoubtedly best treated by internal fixation with a Smith-Petersen nail or one of its variants; these fractures unite freely, and avascular necrosis is rare. But in displaced fractures the story is different; it is often difficult to obtain union, and avascular change is common. However, despite these problems a united femoral neck fracture with an intact head is better than any prosthesis, and where there is a reasonable chance of good internal fixation, and accurate reduction can be obtained, nailing should still be the operation of choice.

2. Fractures in middle age and in young adults. It is fortunate that these fractures are rare before the age of 50, but there are appreciable numbers in the 50 to 60 age group, and these often give rise to problems in treatment. Union of the fracture can usually be achieved, but avascular necrosis is not uncommon. A primary prosthetic replacement at this age is clearly not to be desired, for it would be required to remain satisfactory for 20 to 30 years and perhaps even longer. It is wiser, therefore, to reduce and nail even the most widely displaced and comminuted fractures, bearing in mind that a second operation of either osteotomy or even prosthetic replacement may be necessary later. Very occasionally, in young adults, the fractures may be irreducible by manipulation, and in these cases open reduction and nailing should be performed.

3. Fractures of the femoral neck in children. These are always more basal than the adult fractures and are usually displaced. Union can be achieved by internal fixation with a Smith-Petersen nail or multiple pins, but avascular necrosis is common. Even the undisplaced fracture is not immune from this complication.[128] Sometimes the femoral head may be displaced and the fracture distracted as the nail is driven home,[129] and because of this it is wiser to use the multiple pin method of Austin Moore for the fixation and supplement it by immobilisation in a single hip spica for three months. Every possible precaution should be taken to avoid avascular change which, if it occurs, will almost certainly result finally in an osteotomy or arthrodesis.

TECHNIQUE FOR NAILING FEMORAL NECK FRACTURES

The following description is of the technique used for the insertion of a Smith-Petersen nail. Although this method has been modified in many centres to allow the use of more sophisticated fixation devices, the basic technique is the same for all operations.

The fracture must first be reduced and the reduction must be accurate. In earlier editions of this book it was said that 'the bad results of nailing were the results of bad nailing'. This, of course, is true, but perhaps the emphasis was put too much on the importance of technique rather than the accuracy of reduction. It is not enough simply to produce a position where it is possible to insert a nail or screws to stabilise the fracture. That is easy to achieve. To obtain accurate fracture reduction can be difficult and time consuming, but there is ample evidence to show that it is important. Sometimes all that is needed is to take the foot of the injured limb, apply gentle traction, turn it to the position of neutral rotation, and abduct it about 20 degrees. But often it is not so easy to reduce the fracture satisfactorily and several attempts may be required before the surgeon is satisfied that an acceptable position has been obtained. The time honoured Leadbetter manoeuvre,[130] which used traction in 90 degrees flexion followed by internal rotation to reduce the fracture has been modified by Flynn.[131] Instead of applying traction in the long axis of the thigh, with the hip flexed to 90 degrees the traction is applied laterally in the axis of the femoral neck. The limb is then extended and internally rotated by an assistant while the lateral traction is maintained (Figs 29.112 to 29.115). Thus the 'loosely packed' position of the hip in flexion is used to facilitate reduction, while the 'closely packed' position[132] of extension, slight abduction and internal rotation helps to maintain it. This method of manipulation has been shown to be superior to both the Leadbetter manoeuvre and to the straight traction and internal rotation advocated by Whitman.[133] Not only does it produce a higher percentage of accurate reduction but it has never been responsible for the over-reduction into valgus and anteversion a position commonly associated with iatrogenic avascular necrosis.[99]

Although it is possible to nail a fractured neck of femur on an ordinary operating table using a special cassette holder and perineal post, whenever possible a special orthopaedic table should be used; there are now many varieties of these (Fig 29.116), allowing easy access both for radiographer and surgeon. Unless

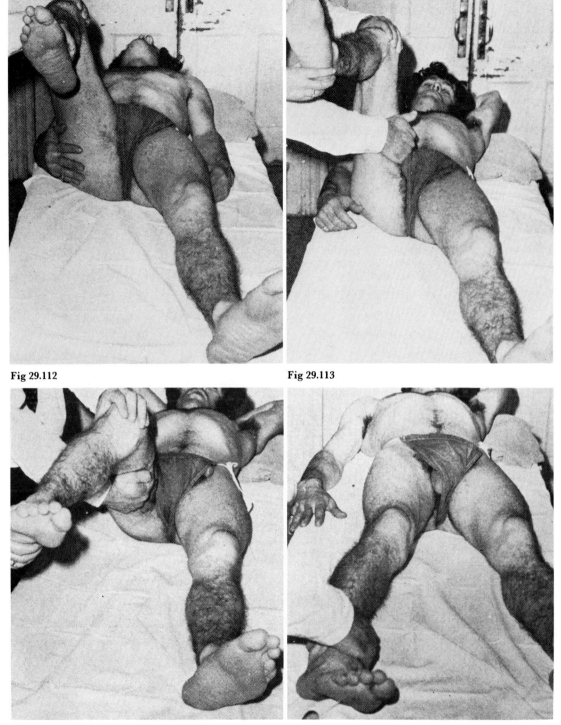

Fig 29.112

Fig 29.113

Fig 29.114

Fig 29.115

Figs 29.112 to 29.115 Flynn's method of reduction of an intracapsular fracture of the femoral neck. The affected hip is first flexed to 90 degrees in slight abduction (Fig 29.112). Traction is applied in the long axis of the femoral neck with the one hand while the other is used to steady the knee. An assistant supports the heel (Fig 29.113). The hip is extended by the assistant while traction on the femoral neck is maintained (Fig 29.114). The reduced position is in extension and medial rotation (Fig 29.115). (Reproduced by the kind permission of the Editor of *Injury* and Mr M. Flynn from his paper in *Injury* (1974) 5, 309.)

an image intensifier with a C arm is available two X-ray tubes are required set up for a lateral and antero-posterior projection (see inset Fig 29.116). Since the introduction of the mobile X-ray image intensifier units even more elaborate tables have come into being (Fig 29.117), because, unfortunately, the C arms of the intensifier cannot operate around the leg pieces of an ordinary traction table such as shown in Figure 29.116. One might speculate whether the additional benefit and convenience of these machines justifies their expense. The patient is placed on the pelvic rest and shoulder support. The uninjured limb is secured to the foot support on that side and fixed in neutral rotation and about 40 degrees of abduction. After manipulation the surgeon then applies gentle traction to the injured limb, turns it into neutral rotation, and fixes it on the table in about 20 degrees of abduction with just sufficient traction to keep it taut. At this stage there is danger of over-reduction if too much traction is used, especially if combined with abducting the limb too widely. It has been shown by several workers that an abduction deformity of the capital fragment can jeopardise the blood supply from the round ligament,[99, 134] and nailing in this position has a high incidence of avascular necrosis. Radiographs in antero-posterior and lateral projections should then be taken, and the position of the limb is adjusted until the fragments lie in a perfect position. Garden[99] has observed that in the antero-posterior view of the normal hip the trabeculae of the head make an angle of 160 degrees with the medial cortex of the femoral shaft, while the trabeculae in the lateral view should be in line with the axis of the femoral neck. Increase in the antero-posterior trabeculae angle to 180 degrees and over indicates considerable over-reduction into valgus and is associated with a high incidence of avascular necrosis; so also is an alteration of more than 25 degrees in the lateral trabecular angle.

After preparing and towelling off the patient's trochanteric area a 4 or 5 inch (10.2 or 12.7 cm) incision is made over the lateral aspect of the thigh, centred on the upper shaft of the femur just below the lower margin of the greater trochanter. The incision is deepened to bone, and the exact lower limit of the greater trochanter is identified by seeing the level at which the upper fibres of vastus lateralis disappear and merge with it. About ⅝ inch (1.5 cm) distal to the trochanteric margin is the point on the femoral cortex that coincides with the centre of the femoral neck. Here a small hole, ½ inch (1.3 cm) in diameter, is gouged or drilled in the cortex. This is a most important step because without it the guide wire

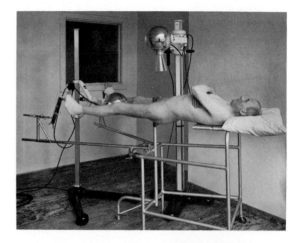

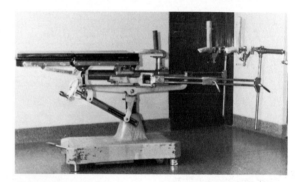

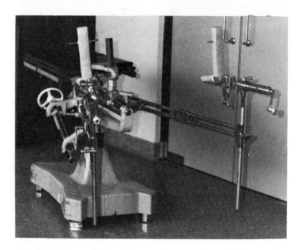

Fig 29.116 An orthopaedic operating table should be as simple as possible allowing easy access both for the surgeon and for the X-ray apparatus. The top illustration shows the original Watson-Jones traction table which is easily made up from tubular steel. It is inexpensive, robust and efficient. It still has a very useful part to play in orthopaedics, particularly in underdeveloped countries where expensive equipment is at a premium.

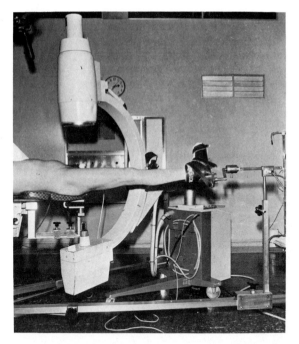

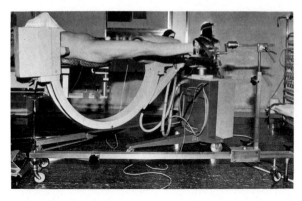

Fig 29.117 If an image intensifier C arm is to be used for nailing femoral neck fractures a special orthopaedic table must be used to allow the C arm to be swung into two planes at right angles.

cannot be introduced by sense of touch. If a hole is not first made the cortical bone grips the guide wire and, after the point and first part of it is engaged, the direction cannot be altered. With a cortical hole which allows the position of the guide wire to be slightly altered the surgeon can 'feel the way' up the middle of the femoral neck. He feels resistance if he strikes the cortex of the femoral neck below or above,

or behind or in front. There is very slight resistance as he passes the line of fracture, and much more firm resistance when the point of the guide reaches the subchondral bone of the femoral articular surface, usually at a depth of penetration of about $3\frac{1}{2}$ to $3\frac{3}{4}$ inches (8.5 to 9.5 cm). As a rule, a guide wire that is passed parallel with the floor at an angle with the long axis of the thigh of about 40 degrees, will go up the middle of the neck. A useful landmark to aim for is the anterior superior iliac spine on the opposite side.

Innumerable mechanical guides have been invented—they all have their deficiences and none is better than the surgeon's own sense of direction.

Radiographs are then taken in both antero-posterior and lateral planes. If the guide wire does not lie in an acceptable position a second wire should be introduced at such an angle to the first as the radiographs indicate. For the introduction of a single nail or screw the ideal position of the guide wire should allow the appliance to lie along the line of the neck in its lower half and approximately mid-way between the anterior and posterior cortices. A proximal and anterior placement of the nail should be avoided because this position is associated with a high failure rate.[122]

When a final and accurate position of the wire is confirmed, the required length of nail is estimated by measuring the length of wire outside the bone and substracting it from the known total length; the length should be estimated to allow the point of the nail to lie within about half a centimetre from the subchondral bone of the head after impaction of the fracture. The chosen nail is held in a cannulated punch and driven over the wire until it is home. But between every second or third stroke of the mallet the projecting wire should be measured by an assistant to exclude the possibility of its being caught in the cannula of the nail and thus being driven in with it. The steps of the operation are shown in radiographs taken in the operating theatre (Figs 29.118 to 29.121).

When the nail has been gently driven in until its head lies flush with the cortex an impactor punch should be hammered cautiously on the trochanter (the punch having a central hole larger than the head of the nail so that the force is applied only to the bone) in order to close any gap that may have arisen at the site of fracture as the nail was driven across it. In the early days of nailing a cross pin was inserted through the head of the nail to prevent extrusion. This is no longer recommended as it prevents the small amount of extrusion which can occur in the first few weeks due to absorption of bone at the

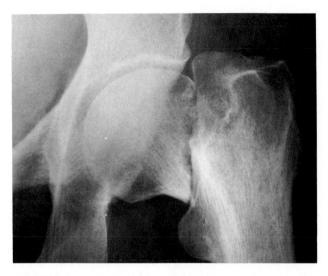

Fig 29.118

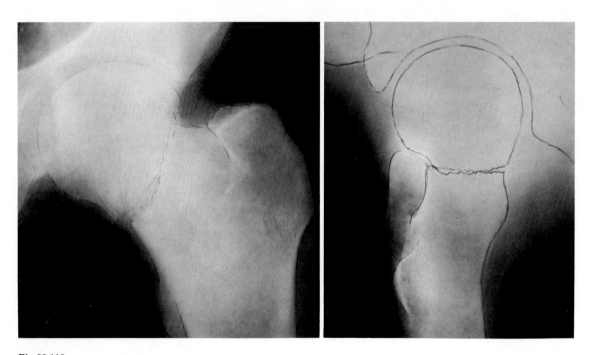

Fig 29.119

Figs 29.118 to 29.121 Three stages of extra-articular operation for nailing fractured neck of femur. Fig 29.118: Subcapital fracture neck of femur with typical displacement before operation. Fig 29.119: First stage. After manipulative reduction and fixation of both lower limbs on a traction table, radiographs show accurate reduction of the fracture. Fig 29.120: Second stage. Two guide wires have been inserted. Radiographs show that the lower and least penetrated guide wire lies correctly. The other is withdrawn. The length of nail is measured by subtracting the length of wire outside the bone from the known total length. Fig 29.121: Third stage. The nail has been threaded over the guide wire and punched home; the fragments have been cautiously impacted. *Note:* this nail is a little too short, it should reach to within ½ cm of the subcortical bone.

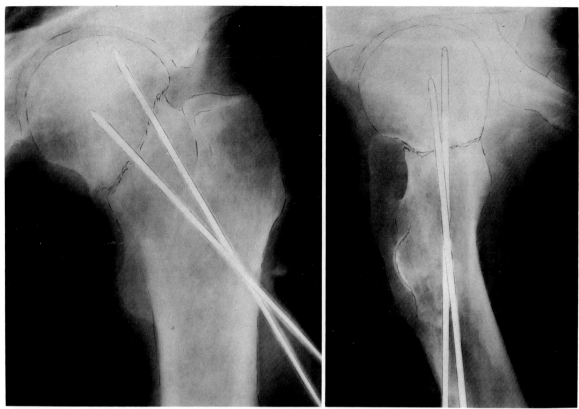

Fig 29.120

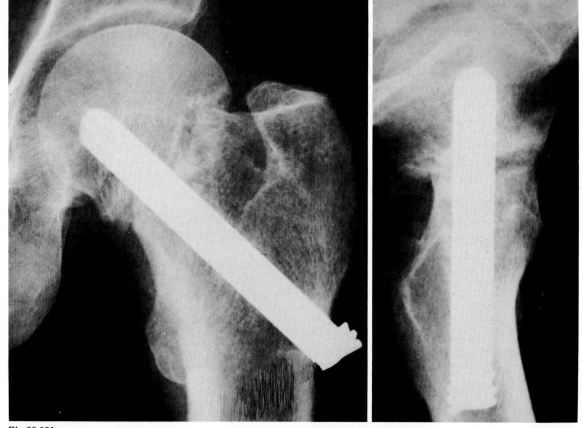

Fig 29.121

fracture site. If the nail is not allowed to extrude at this stage it will either penetrate the head, cut out of the head, or result in a gap at the fracture line.

The wound is closed in layers with suction drainage, and the patient is returned to bed. There should be no need for traction or any form of splint to prevent rotation; indeed, the horizontal bar on a slipper or plaster previously recommended to prevent external rotation can never exclude this strain completely; it may even increase the strain by fixing the foot while allowing free movement of the rest of the body, and it has a bad reputation for producing pressure sores over the tendo Achillis region. A cradle to support the bed clothes on the affected side is all that is required.

Post-operative treatment after nailing. The day after operation the patients should sit up in bed and move about freely. If they are of fairly light build and easily moved they should be allowed to sit out in a chair; otherwise they should be encouraged to sit on the side of the bed during bed making. Deep breathing exercises are ordered. The knee joint of the injured limb must be moved as much as possible from the first day. At first the patient may find this difficult, but unless initial fear is overcome and movements are practised despite cramp there will be much more difficulty in mobilising the stiff joint at a later stage. From 24 hours after operation the patient should be given assisted hip and knee flexion exercises, but attempts to produce active leg raising of the limb are forbidden as this movement produces a considerable strain upon the femoral fracture. At about 12 days (when the operation wound is healed), the patient is allowed up partially weight-bearing with axillary crutches or a walking frame. To make an old person walk strictly non-weight-bearing with crutches is almost impossible and probably a little dangerous, but some form of walking aid is essential until the fracture is radiographically healed.

The timing of operation. There is considerable difference of opinion on whether femoral neck fractures should be treated as an emergency or whether the patients do better if there is a delay of 24 to 48 hours to allow them to be properly assessed. It must be admitted that in many centres the timing of the operation depends upon other factors such as the availability of the theatre and the commitments of the staff. It is tempting to suppose that delay in operating may increase the risk of avascular necrosis but there is no firm evidence to support this.[122] There is, however, proven evidence that the death rate is much higher in patients who are operated on when they still have a depressed pulmonary function, as measured by a respiratory peak flow of less than 100 litres per minute.[135] Many old people admitted with a femoral neck fracture do require a careful medical assessment pre-operatively and may benefit from a short period of chest physiotherapy before being submitted to an anaesthetic. On balance these patients should not be rushed to theatre as an emergency and there is no positive evidence to support the view that the worse the general condition the greater the urgency for surgery.

VARIANTS OF THE BASIC NAILING TECHNIQUE

Many variations of the original nailing procedure have been introduced since the method was first described nearly 50 years ago. These variations have arisen because surgeons became disatisfied with the results obtained from the use of the Smith-Petersen nail alone, and in the M.R.C. trial reported by Barnes *et al*[121] just over 50 per cent of displaced fractures united after Smith-Petersen nailing, compared with a 70 per cent union rate if a sliding nail plate or crossed screws were used. The message is clear: if the simpler Smith-Petersen nailing technique is to be used it must be supplemented by additional fixation, with a screw or multiple pins. Brief details of some of the other techniques are given below.

1. Low angle nailing (Fig 29.122). This method is mentioned only to be condemned. It was first advised in this country by Brittain[136] and popularised by a number of other writers.[99, 137] The buttressing effect of the nail upon the calcar femorale, the three point fixation obtained and the early weight-bearing allowed have all been stressed as advantages of the technique. But against these must be weighed the difficulty in placing the nail, the increased possibility of it backing out and the risk of pathological fracture through the cortex of the femoral shaft at the site of entry. In one series[99] of subcapital fractures nailed by this method the overall union rate for displaced fractures (stage 3 and 4) was 75 per cent and dropped to 57 per cent when stage 4 injuries alone were considered. These figures show no improvement over the average union rate of about 60 to 70 per cent using the standard technique and understandably the reporter of this series has abandoned this method of fixation. The other advantage of direct weight-bearing over partial weight-bearing using crutches has little to recommend it; most of these old people are very unsteady on their feet after the fracture and

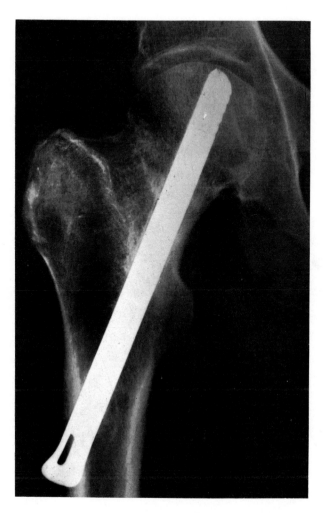

Fig 29.122 Subcapital fracture of the femur treated by low-angle Kuntscher nail. Although claimed to give rigid three point fixation of the fracture it is difficult to insert and has been associated with pathological fractures at the site of insertion. (Reproduced by kind permission of the *Journal of Bone and Joint Surgery* and Mr R. S. Garden from his paper (1961) Low-angle fixation in fractures of the femoral neck. *Journal of Bone and Joint Surgery*, 43–B, 647.)

require several months of protection with crutches while walking.

2. The use of pin and plate. This has been advocated by a large number of surgeons and very many devices have been made. The ordinary pin and plate used for fixation of trochanteric fractures is not satisfactory, because it does not allow for the inevitable absorption which occurs at the fracture line. Sliding and compression nail plates overcome this problem, and a reduction in the incidence of non-union by 20 per cent has been claimed by some workers,[138, 139] but others have found the overall number of patients with bony union to be much the same as when a single nail is used.[117] It is doubtful whether it has much

advantage over Smith-Petersen nail fixation augmented by two or three Newman pins. The addition of a plate can be useful, however, when a secondary operation becomes necessary because of extrusion of the nail before the fracture has united. The shortening of the neck due to fracture line absorption has taken place by this time, so that it is quite safe to change the simple nail for a nail and plate device (Figs 29.123 and 29.124), or even to reinsert the original nail and prevent its extrusion by applying a plate over its lower end (Fig 29.127).

3. Transarticular nailing. This method has been used by Jarry in 44 cases with an 85 per cent union rate in 21 patients who were followed up for more than one

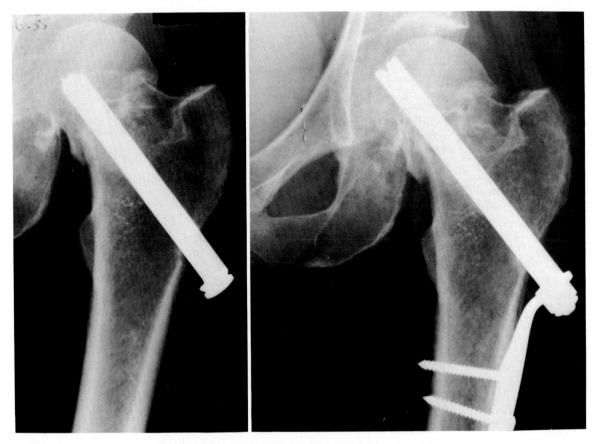

Fig 29.123 Early extrusion of Smith-Petersen nail one month after fracture.

Fig 29.124 The result three months after changing the fixation to a nail plate.

year.[140] It is claimed that by transfixing the acetabulum the proximal fragment is squeezed between the neck and the acetabulum, producing rigid fixation of the fracture. However, the very long period of bed rest and wheelchair life (up to 90 days) necessary in this technique is a grave disadvantage, and when this is combined with damage to the acetabular joint space the disadvantages far outweigh the gain from the possible increase in fixation.

4. The use of nail and hip pins (Fig 29.125). This simple additional fixation to the Smith-Petersen nail using Newman pins can be useful in two ways: (1) it increases the hold on the femoral head and (2) if the nail extrudes it is unlikely that all the pins will come out at the same time, so that the fracture is held until the nail can be reinserted (Figs 29.126 and 29.127). The technique which is no more difficult than that for simple Smith-Petersen nailing considerably increases the fixation of the single nail. Care must be

taken, however, to avoid penetrating the femoral head with the pins, because if this occurs it may result in their medial migration across the acetabulum. The use of Crawford Adams' pins, which are threaded laterally to engage the femoral cortex, should avoid this complication, and also that of backing out from the femoral head. This method of Smith-Petersen nailing and additional pinning is recommended as a simple and effective way of fixing an intracapsular fracture.

5. Cross screw fixation. There are two variants of this method of fixation—the cross screws advocated by Garden[120] (Fig 29.128) and the 'triangular' pinning of Smyth[119] (Fig 29.129). Both present a high torque resistance by forming a rigid double lever system with a common fulcrum at their point of crossing; and as a result they are probably the most rigid type of fixation for femoral neck fractures. In both techniques the upper screw is inserted first, passing

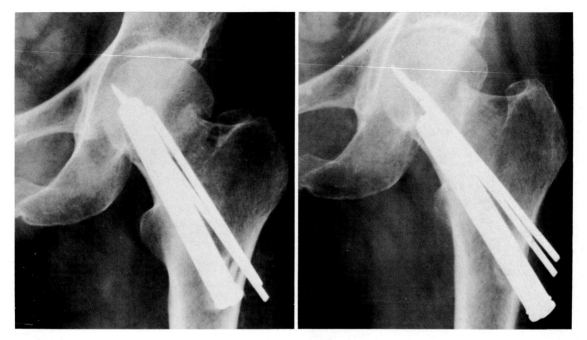

Fig 29.125   **Fig 29.126**

Figs 29.125 and 29.126 Smith-Petersen nail fixation supplemented by Newman hip pins used for primary fixation of femoral neck fracture. Despite the backing out of the nail the pins have prevented the fracture from displacing and time is allowed to reinsert the Smith-Petersen nail (Fig 29.126).

almost transversely from the anterior part of the trochanter into the inferior part of the femoral head. Using either a special guide, or the triangle connecting plate, the direction of the low oblique screw is determined so that it passes up the calcar from an entry position in the posterior femoral cortex until the point comes to lie in the centre of the femoral head. Ideally, the two screws should be in contact at the point of crossing. To obtain the maximum effective fixation the screws must cross, and therefore the position of the Garden screws shown in Figure 29.130 is incorrect. The crossed screw method of fixation is not an easy technique to master and any surgeon embarking on these operations for the first time would be well advised to read the original papers outlining the operation technique.[119, 120]

The best choice of internal fixation methods.
In summarising the points for and against the various methods of fixing an intracapsular fracture of the femoral neck one fact stands out clearly, and that is the relative inefficiency of the fixation afforded by a Smith-Petersen nail alone. However, this disadvantage must be weighed against the advantages of

simplicity of technique when compared with other methods of fixation. That the Smith-Petersen must be supplemented by additional fixation is without doubt. The obvious compromise which does not complicate the technique is to insert Newman or Crawford Adams pins above the nail. Time alone will tell if this very simple addition to the operation is as effective as some of the more complicated techniques.

Complications of the operation. The success of any surgical operation depends upon many factors, but above all it depends upon the skill and perseverance of the surgeon. This is certainly true of the operation of nailing a fracture of the neck of the femur. Although it also is true that many perfectly executed nailing operations come to a disastrous end because of local conditions at the fracture site, nevertheless a shoddy operative technique, a poorly reduced fracture, or a badly placed nail can lead to a non-union which might not otherwise have happened.

It seems unprofitable to discuss every complication that has occurred from errors of technique, but at the same time it must be emphasised that simple as the operation may appear to be from its description it is

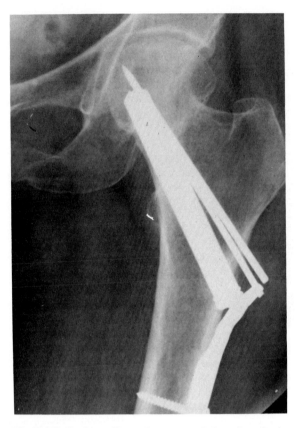

Fig 29.127 Further nail extrusion prevented after reinsertion by applying (but not attaching) a plate to the lower end of the nail.

indeed charged with every possibility of disaster. First, there must be perfect asepsis; many hip joints have been destroyed by infection. Secondly, there must be good radiography in the lateral as well as the antero-posterior plane; no surgeon should begin to try to nail the neck of the femur unless he can rely on lateral radiographs. Thirdly, there must be attention to every detail of the technique described. No longer should there be failures because the guide wire was not accurately inserted, because the nail entered the lateral and not the central part of the head, or because the nail was too long and penetrated the joint, or too short and failed to hold the fragments (Figs 29.131 and 29.132). No longer should the vascularity of the femoral head be further endangered by tilting it into a valgus position by a malplaced nail (Figs 29.133 and 29.134). No longer should there be failures because imperfect steel was used so that the nail loosened or broke. No longer should a guide wire be driven ahead of the nail into the pelvis because it

caught in the cannula (Fig 29.135). These are complications that should be avoided if attention is paid to every detail of technique. But there will still remain failures from vascular complications which are beyond the control of the surgeon.

Complications arising from avascular necrosis of the femoral head. No matter how successful the nailing operation may have been it is always possible that, at the moment of fracture, the blood vessels to the femoral head, where they lie in retinaculae running from the capsule to the bone, were destroyed by the injury. In these circumstances avascular necrosis of the femoral head will develop, with consequent degenerative changes. If the destruction of blood supply is complete the whole of the proximal half of the femoral head will die—that is, all that part of the head supplied by capsular vessels, which corresponds roughly with the original epiphysis. A line of separation between dead bone and living bone develops. This has often been misinterpreted as non-union of the fracture itself, whereas the fracture has in fact united and the new pathological line of separation is more proximal, at about the level of the earlier epiphyseal line. No surgeon should ever be blamed for the pathological separation of dead and living bone that occurs from the avascular necrosis at a level so proximal to the line of fracture that has already united so successfully. In confirmation, the same avascular necrosis can occur in impacted abduction fractures which have never been operated upon at all, and in which the fragments have united spontaneously (Figs 29.136 and 29.137). It has been shown by Smith, from observations made during arthroplasty of the hip,[134] that the valgus position of the femoral head completely shuts off the blood supply from the round ligament. Garden[99] has devised an alignment index of reduction based on the angle between the medial group of trabeculae in the capital fragment and the line of the medial femoral cortex, and shows convincingly that when the head is left in severe valgus deformity the rate of avascular necrosis is high.

Local sectors of necrosis of the femoral head perhaps caused by heavy nails. Though surgeons may be exonerated from responsibility for those cases of avascular necrosis in which the whole proximal part of the femoral head undergoes death, it must be pointed out that in many other cases only one sector of the bone dies, in the upper third, and no clinical observer can escape the fact that the apex of this cone-shaped area of dead bone is nearly always at the point of the nail. It is tempting to speculate whether the nail itself has

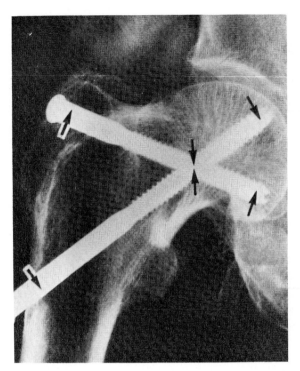

Fig 29.128 The cross screw fixation advocated by Garden. The screws lie in contact at their point of crossing and the arrows indicate the thrust and counterthrust by which they maintain stability. (Reproduced by the kind permission of the Editor of the *Journal of bone and Joint Surgery* and Mr R. S. Garden from his paper in the *Journal of Bone and Joint Surgery* (1964) 46–B, 630.)

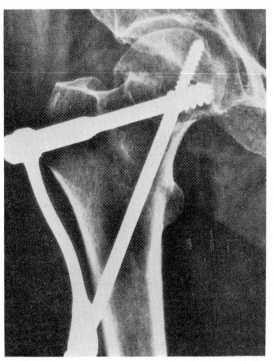

Fig 29.129 The triangular pinning of Smyth. This is a crossed screw fixation which has been strengthened by completing the lateral side of the triangle formed by the two screws. (Reproduced by the kind permission of the Editor of the *Journal of Bone and Joint Surgery* and Mr E. H. J. Smyth from his paper in the *Journal of Bone and Joint Surgery* (1964) 46–B, 664.)

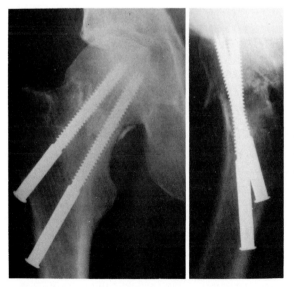

Fig 29.130 The Garden screws used in the fixation of this fracture have been used incorrectly. They must cross in the neck of the femur to give maximum fixation.

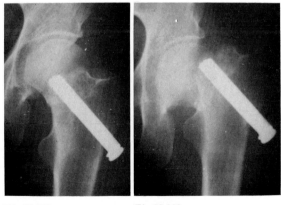

Fig 29.131   **Fig 29.132**

Figs 29.131 and 29.132 An immediate post-operative X-ray showing a nail which, although in good alignment, is far too short. Figure 29.132 shows the inevitable disengagement of the fracture which occurred a few weeks later.

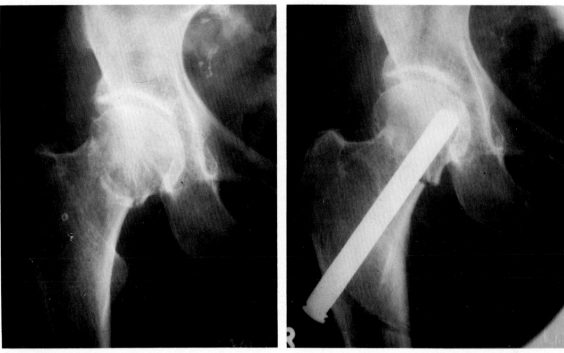

Fig 29.133   **Fig 29.134**

Figs 29.133 and 29.134 Figure 29.133 is the antero-posterior X-ray of a transcervical fracture of the neck of the femur just before nailing. Figure 29.134 shows the valgus tilt produced by the point of the nail entering the lowermost part of the head. This deformity can endanger the blood supply to the femoral head.

not destroyed the blood vessels to this sector, and the studies of Trueta[141] on the distribution of blood vessels within the bone, showing how great a concentration there is in this region, spreading to supply a particular sector of the femoral head, suggests that this may be so. On the other hand, Mary Catto's careful histological studies of femoral heads removed for segmental collapse indicate that the blood vessels in the ligamentum teres play little part in revascularisation, which seems to depend upon vessels crossing the fracture site.[142] And so we must keep an open mind on the possible dangers of using heavy nails for the internal fixation of fractures of the femoral neck—certainly if these are used to fix an undisplaced fracture, the standard type of nail can tilt the head into valgus while it is being driven across the fracture line (Fig 29.134), thereby increasing the possibility of avascular necrosis. It is wiser to use the multiple pin fixation of Austin Moore for this type of fracture. St. Clair Strange and other workers[143, 127] have advised multiple pin fixation, even in displaced fractures, claiming a percentage union equal to that of the standard nailing operation but with a significant lowering of the incidence of avascular necrosis.

They also stress the minimal operative trauma inflicted by this technique, which can be carried out under local anaesthesia, and the low infection rate.

PROSTHETIC REPLACEMENT OF THE FEMORAL HEAD FOR INTRACAPSULAR FRACTURES

'Thompson arthroplasty is the routine treatment of these fractures'.[124] *'This is a dangerous operation—it is too easy to do'*.[125]

The two directly contrary views quoted above are typical examples of the arguments heard between surgeons who are enthusiasts for one or other treatment. Clearly there must be a compromise. It has been recommended by some surgeons that the majority of patients over the age of 65 with displaced transcervical fractures of the neck of the femur should be treated by prosthetic replacement. While others emphasise that the union rate produced by any of the standard nailing procedures is in the order of 70 to 80 per cent, with up to 90 per cent union claimed by the exponents of the sliding nail fixation,[139] and although

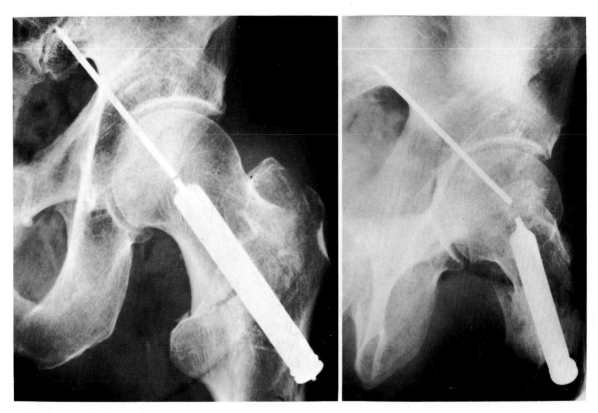

Fig 29.135 Guide wire caught in cannula of nail and inadvertently driven through the hip joint. The difficulties were increased by fracture of the wire, the central part of which had to be removed by an abdominal approach. There are two further mistakes illustrated in these X-rays: (1) the nail is too short, and (2) the fracture is too basal to be fixed with a nail alone; a nail plate should have been used. (Reproduced by kind permission of the *British Journal of Surgery* from R. W.-J's article (1936) Fractures of the neck of the femur. *British Journal of Surgery*, 23, 787.)

in those which unite there is still a very real danger that late avascular necrosis of the femoral neck will result in painful limitation of movement, it can be urged that a prosthetic replacement should be reserved for the treatment at this stage rather than as a primary operation. However, protagonists for prosthetic replacement point out that early replacement of the femoral head has certain advantages; firstly, full weight-bearing can be applied as soon as the wound is healed;[144] and secondly, an elderly patient is spared the trauma and danger of another operation. Recent studies have shown that re-operation is appreciably higher in the internally fixed cases, and that the results at one year show a decided bias in favour of prosthetic replacement.[144a] Unfortunately, other studies of the results of primary prosthetic replacement show that the mortality rate and morbidity from the operation are appreciably higher than in simple nailing.[126] In one comparable series of cases,[122] the clinically satisfactory results at six months of internal fixation and prosthetic replacement were almost identical at just over 60 per cent, but the mortality in the prosthetic cases at the same stage was 30 per cent compared with 21 per cent in those internally fixed. These mortality figures became even more significant when considered for the under 70 age group where the difference was between 7 per cent for the internal fixation cases and 20 per cent for the prostheses. It is therefore important that patients for primary replacement should be carefully selected. The immediate result from the insertion of a prosthesis is usually excellent, but there is a danger of sepsis and dislocation, and it is wise to recommend that the operation is never done as an emergency procedure, thus giving an opportunity to operate under optimum conditions and with an antibiotic cover started preoperatively. While awaiting operation the patient can be made comfortable with the leg in traction.

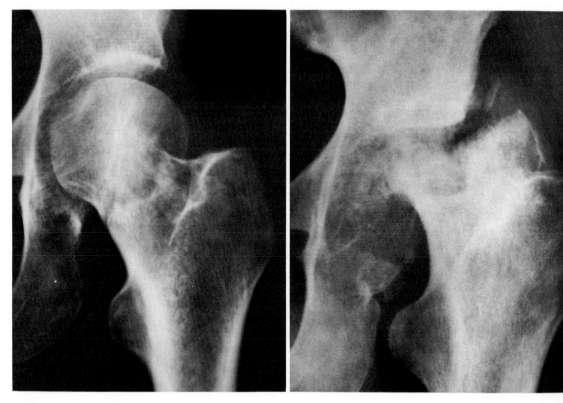

Fig 29.136 Subcapital fracture of the neck of the femur with impaction treated by simple bed rest. No operation was performed, and no splints or plaster were used. The fracture united.

Fig 29.137 Same case as Figure 29.136. After five years there was obvious evidence of avascular necrosis of the femoral head with destruction and crushing of bone causing degenerative arthritis with pathological subluxation.

Operative technique. The first dose of the prophylactic antibiotic can be given with the premedication and continued twice daily for 24 to 48 hours.* Whether prophylactic anticoagulants are also used will depend upon the views of the surgeon, but probably the safest effective regime is to give subcutaneous calcium heparin in a dose of 5000 units 8-hourly until the patient is fully ambulant, or mobilised in a wheel chair. The operation may be performed through an anterior or posterior approach (see Chapter 15), the latter giving a rather easier access, but with a slightly greater risk of dislocation. The hip joint having been entered the detached femoral head should be controlled by inserting a corkscrew into its cut surface and extracted from the acetabulum. The extraction of the head is sometimes made easier by splitting it with an osteotome and

removing it in two halves. If there is any suspicion that the fracture may have occurred through pathological tissue a specimen of bone should be sent for examination. One of the femoral stem prostheses of the Austin Moore or Thompson pattern should be used. Measurement of the removed head gives the size of the prosthesis required, which can then be tested for stability by a trial fit before the stem is inserted into the femur; a good suction fit should be obtained. The broken edges of the distal part of the femoral neck are trimmed to allow the flange of the femoral prosthesis to abut as accurately as possible against the calcar femorale. The medullary cavity of the upper part of the femur must be prepared for the insertion of the stem of the prosthesis; this is usually done by use of a special rasp which corresponds to the shape and length of the prosthesis stem. When using an Austin Moore prosthesis care must be taken to avoid splitting the calcar when the broad base of the stem is driven home. This is much less likely to

* Cephradine (one of the Cephalosporins) is a broad spectrum antibiotic and can be given as a loading dose of 1 gm with the premedication and followed by 1 gm 12 hourly for two doses.

happen if the narrower standard Thompson appliance is used, but this has the disadvantage of having less solid fixation in the bone and usually requires embedding in acrylic cement;* whereas the Austin Moore appliance, which is referred to as a 'self-locking' device, has a firm hold in the bone which can be reinforced by packing cancellous bone into the two large holes provided in the base of the neck of the prosthesis. No cement is required for the fixation of this appliance.

After reduction of the prosthesis into the acetabulum the hip should be stable, and if the fit is good there should be no evidence of dislocation or subluxation at the extremes of rotation. It is rarely possible to repair the small rotator muscles when the posterior approach has been used, but this does not seem to predispose to instability. Suction drainage should always be used post-operatively, and sometimes in a fat patient two drains are necessary. No traction or other form of splintage is used, but the patient should remain in bed, or allowed only to sit in a chair, until the stitches are removed. Full weight-bearing is then permitted, at first with the aid of elbow crutches but rapidly progressing to two walking sticks. Although immediate walking (within 24 hours of the operation) is advocated by some,[124] many of these elderly patients are quite incapable of following this regime and do better with the more gentle form of rehabilitation.

Late complications. These are: loosening of the femoral stem, distal migration of the prosthesis and intrusion of the head of the prosthesis into the pelvis.[147] Loosening and migration of the stem is less common with the Austin Moore prosthesis than with the uncemented Thompson appliance,[147] although if cement is used with the Thompson prosthesis this becomes marginally superior.[148] The use of cement, however, carries with it the increased hazard of infection and the possible danger of circulatory collapse during operation: it also adds to the difficulties of extraction and replacement should this be demanded by late complications. Intrusion of the head of the prosthesis towards the inner wall of the pelvis has been found to vary from 11 to 15 per cent of patients[147] and it can be expected to increase with longer survival rates. In one series it was found that

this complication was considerably higher in the younger age groups (60 to 70), which led to the salutary advice that 'it seems prudent to withhold primary Thompson arthroplasty from younger patients except when other infirmities make prolonged survival uncertain'.[124] Some cases have been thought to be due to excessive pressure being developed in the hip joint as a result of using too large a prosthesis or one with too long a femoral neck.[124] Intrusion is invariably associated with pain and an overall bad result and, if the patient is sufficiently fit, should be treated by the insertion of a total hip prosthesis.

Two component prostheses. In an attempt to overcome the complication of acetabular erosion a number of captive two component appliances have been developed.[149, 150] The principle behind all these devices is the same, that is that there is a small captive femoral head articulating with a high density polyethylene cup, which is itself free to move within the normal acetabulum. The late results from these prostheses have yet to be evaluated but the immediate results are promising. However, there is one grave warning to be heeded. High density polyethylene cups, if not cemented into the acetabulum, must be backed by metal. Bare polyethylene articulating with articular cartilage can result in a serious wear problem, the products of which can stimulate an alarming degree of fibrous tissue reaction (Fig 29.138).

EXTRACAPSULAR OR TROCHANTERIC FRACTURES OF THE FEMUR

Fractures through the intertrochanteric line of the upper end of the femur, and pertrochanteric fractures at a slightly more distal level, unite readily no matter what treatment is used because the broad fractured surfaces are richly supplied with blood and there is seldom wide displacement. Unlike transcervical fractures, firm union can usually be relied upon, and on the very few occasions when non-union occurs it is always due to interposition of soft tissues. But at the same time, unless suitable precautions are taken, the fracture may unite in a position of coxa vara with shortening of the limb and limitation of hip movements. Moreover, this fracture occurs in elderly patients even more than fractures of the femoral neck itself and the same risks from prolonged immobility and recumbency arise. Thus treatment should be so planned as to encourage union without deformity, and at the same time allow early mobilisation. Thus

---

* In the past few years there have been a number of reports of circulatory collapse following the insertion of acrylic cement into the femur. The majority of these cases have occurred in association with the insertion of a Thompson prosthesis for fractured neck of femur,[145, 146] and in one series there was a 3 per cent incidence of death in theatre.[122] There is also an added disadvantage to the use of cement in that its removal can be difficult if a total hip replacement is required later.

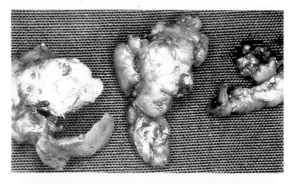

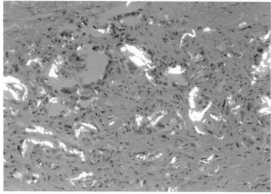

Fig 29.138 Fibrous tissue reaction which occurred around a two component captive prosthesis used without acetabular cement. Lower illustration shows the numerous giant cells and wear particles (white spaces) within the fibrous reaction, resulting from the polyethylene rubbing against the bare acetabulum (polarised light preparation). High density polyethylene cups, if not cemented in place must be backed by metal. (Reproduced by the kind permission of Professor J. T. Scales of the Biomedical Engineering Department, Institute of Orthopaedics, Stanmore. Slides prepared by Miss Mary Waite.)

the treatment of choice should be operative, employing some form of internal fixation.

Classification of trochanteric fractures. In former days extracapsular fractures of the femoral neck were either labelled basal, intertrochanteric, or pertrochanteric, according to where the fracture line was situated. But these were only indications of the level of the injury and made no attempt to analyse the fracture anatomy, or assess the stability. As far as treatment was concerned all fractures were lumped together as 'trochanteric fractures' and treated by internal fixation or traction, according to the whim of the surgeon. All this has now changed. It has been recognised for some time that the fractures can be divided into stable and unstable injuries and that the

operative technique of internal fixation is different for the two varieties.[151, 152]

Stable fractures. These can be displaced or undisplaced. The undisplaced fractures are of no importance and sometimes can be left untreated, although it is wise in most cases, as in intracapsular fractures, to err on the side of safety and fix them with a pin and plate, rather than risk the embarrassment of dissolution later. Whether displaced or undisplaced these fractures have the same basic configuration—they are two fragment injuries. The type of displacement depends upon whether the greater trochanter remains attached to the proximal or distal fragment.[153] If it is attached distally the upper fragment will remain in neutral rotation and the fracture can be reduced accurately by internally rotating the leg; while if the trochanter is still attached to the proximal fragment this will be externally rotated by the attached muscles and therefore the fracture can only be reduced by external rotation of the leg (Figs 29.139 to 29.142). Both injuries, however, are stable when reduced and can be fixed in the normal anatomical position.

Unstable fractures. An unstable fracture has been defined by Dimon and Hughston as one where the fracture 'lacks continuity of bone cortex on the opposing surfaces of the proximal and distal fragments'.[152] This is due either to comminution on the medial aspect of the neck in the region of the calcar, or to complete separation of a posterior trochanteric segment. At the worst this may end up as a four fragment injury, the two main components being the shaft and the head and neck, with the lesser and greater trochanters lying free as the third and fourth fragments (Fig 29.143). These injuries are difficult to stabilise by conventional pin and plate fixation with the fracture anatomically reduced (Fig 29.144). That this position can sometimes be successful is shown in Figures 29.145 and 29.146, but in a high proportion of cases this sort of excellence is not achieved and the patient ends up with a broken or detached pin and plate, and with a fracture which unites in considerable varus (Fig 29.147). These failures led Mervyn Evans to advise that unstable fractures should be fixed in the position of deformity,[154] while Clawson advocated a return to radical conservatism, with continuous traction as the treatment of choice.[155] Certainly if treated by conventional pinning the results are poor and a complication rate of up to 50 per cent can be expected.[152] These fractures need medial displacement of the distal fragment to stabilise them, followed by pin and plate fixation. Dimon and Hughston found that by using this technique their complication rate dropped from 51 per cent to 8 per cent.

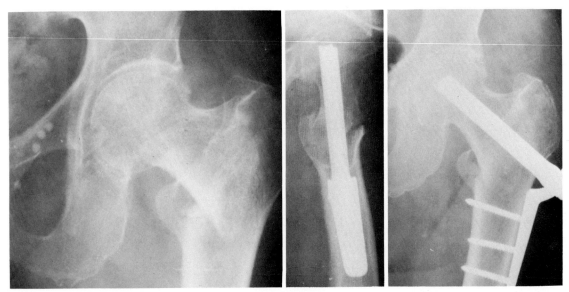

Fig 29.139   Fig 29.140

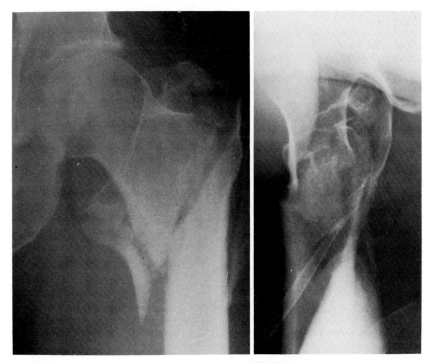

Fig 29.141   Fig 29.142

Figs 29.139 to 29.142 Figure 29.139 is an antero-posterior view of a trochanteric fracture in which the trochanter is attached to the distal fragment. The head and neck are therefore not externally rotated. The fracture is reduced accurately by internal rotation of the leg (Fig 29.140). Figure 29.141 is the antero-posterior view of a fracture where the greater trochanter has moved with the femoral neck, which is therefore *externally* rotated (as seen by the more foreshortened appearance of the neck and the lateral view (Fig 29.142). This fracture can only be reduced by external rotation.

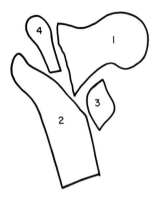

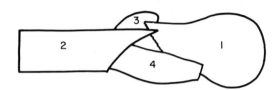

Fig 29.143

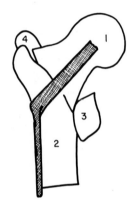

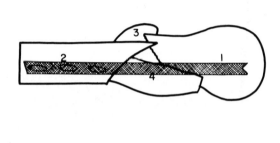

Fig 29.144

Figs 29.143 and 29.144 Figure 29.143 shows a drawing of the major components of a four fragment unstable trochanteric fracture. The two main fragments are shown as 1 and 2 on the drawing. 3 and 4 are those of the lesser and greater trochanter. Figure 29.144 emphasises that a conventional pin and plate fixation, although apparently satisfactory in the antero-posterior projection, gives very little support when seen in the lateral view. (Reproduced by the kind permission of the Editor of the *Journal of Bone and Joint Surgery* and Drs Dimon and Hughston from their paper in the *Journal of Bone and Joint Surgery* (1967) 49–A, 440.)

Undoubtedly, where there is gross comminution and instability this is the operation of choice.

Treatment by operation. Internal fixation, using one of the many varieties of articulated or fixed pin and plate, is used almost universally nowadays in the treatment of trochanteric fractures. With modern anaesthesia and resuscitation there are very few patients who are not considered fit enough to undergo the procedure; in fact, most of these patients will withstand an operation better than the long period of immobilisation necessary for the alternative treatment by conservative measures. At one time it was recommended that internal fixation should be carried out as an emergency procedure, but this is unneces-

sary: old people are usually considerably shocked by this injury, and the journey to hospital may cause further deterioration in their condition; a period of 12 to 24 hours of rest in bed with traction on the leg allows time to recover from the initial effects of the injury and gives time for the patient to be assessed; a chest X-ray can be taken, a haemoglobin estimation carried out and blood cross-matched.

Orthodox internal fixation for stable fractures. After a preliminary manipulation to reduce the fracture (usually all that is necessary is to rotate into either internal or external rotation according to the type of fracture), the patient is set up on a fracture table. The operative procedure differs very little from

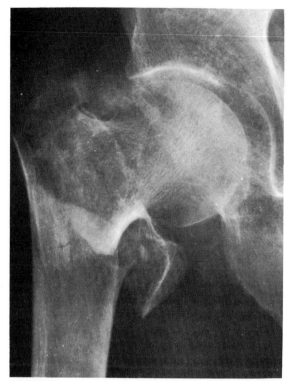

Fig 29.145

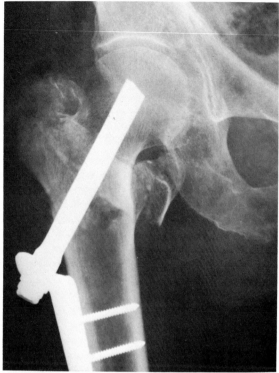

Fig 29.146

Figs 29.145 and 29.146 Figure 29.145 shows an unstable four fragment trochanteric fracture with commencing adduction deformity. This was successfully fixed with an orthodox pin and plate and united with only minor deformity. Not all unstable fractures require medial displacement.

that already described for Smith-Petersen nailing of transcervical fractures, except for the addition of a plate. This is, of course, necessary in order to extend the grip of the nail in the trochanter to the shaft of the bone, for without a plate the fixation of the outer end of the nail could not withstand the angulating varus force of the proximal fragment. There are many varieties of appliance which can be used, and the choice largely depends upon the preference of the surgeon rather than the nature of the fracture; but in general a two-piece nail plate is rather easier to insert than the fixed angle, one-piece variety; and of the two-piece nail plates, the stainless steel type designed by McKee of Norwich (which allows simple adjustment of angle by bending the plate) is a little less complicated than its counterpart made in cobalt-chrome alloy (which has the added disadvantage of difficulty in removal, should it be necessary later on).

There are one or two technical points about the operation which must be stressed. Firstly, the nail should be inserted in the lower half of the neck and follow the line of the inferior cortex (Fig 29.146); this

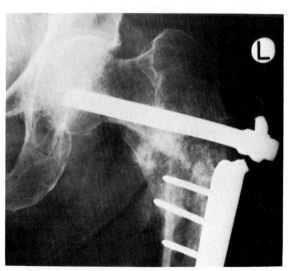

Fig 29.147 This patient's unstable four fragment trochanteric fracture was pinned in an anatomical position. The inevitable varus occurred and the shaft moved medially after the plate and nail became detached. Union occurred but with considerable deformity.

allows for some upward movement in the head if the fracture deforms into the varus position after operation. Secondly, the length of the nail should be calculated to leave at least $\frac{3}{4}$ inch (1 cm) between its tip and the articular surface of the femoral head; again this allows for movement of the nail within the head if the fracture angulates.[154] In deciding upon a nail length the lateral part which lies outside the bone between cortex and plate must be taken into consideration. Thirdly, as already mentioned, Mer-vyn Evans[154] has pointed out the importance of maintaining the limb in external rotation to obtain a good position in the lateral plane—internal rotation tending to angulate the fracture and cause separation of bone surfaces. Lastly, the choice of plate will depend upon the extent of the fracture. Usually a four- or five-hole plate is sufficient, but where there is a spiral extension of the fracture into the upper shaft, a seven-hole, or even twelve-hole, plate may be required (Figs 29.148 and 29.149).

Figs 29.148 and 29.149 A severely comminuted trochanteric fracture of the femur with a spiral extension into the upper third of the bone (Fig 29.148). It required a 12-hole McLaughlin pin and plate to stabilise this fracture (Fig 29.149).

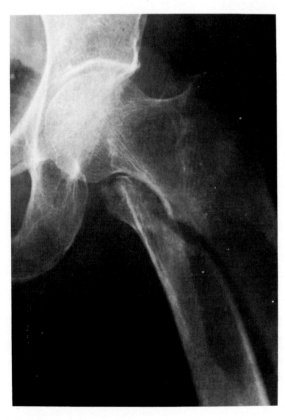

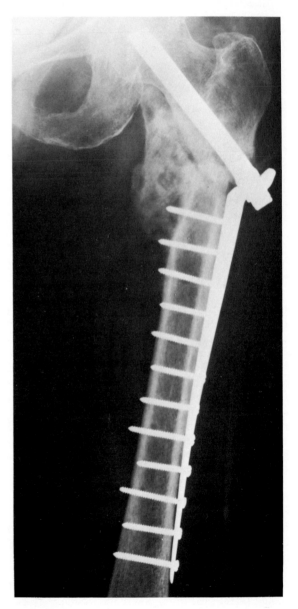

Fig 29.148

Fig 29.149

Internal fixation for unstable fractures. It has already been established that instability in trochanteric fractures results from comminution of the adjacent fracture surfaces particularly in the region of the calcar, and that when there is a classical four fragment injury there is very poor apposition of the two major fragments if a convential reduction and pinning is carried out. This has led to a number of modifications of surgical technique of which medial displacement of the femoral shaft is the most popular.

Fixation with medial displacement. The technique with medial displacement is illustrated diagrammatically in Figures 29.150 to 29.153. The thin lateral trochanteric portion of the distal fragment is divided to produce a subtrochanteric osteotomy (Fig 29.150). Sometimes this part of the femur is so fragmented that osteotomy is unnecessary, or is achieved merely by driving in the nail of the fixation device. However, the osteotomy allows the guide wire to be inserted directly into the exposed fracture surface of the proximal fragment (Fig 29.151). The distal shaft can then be displaced medially and the spike in the lower margin of the femoral neck impinged into it (Fig 29.152). A suitable angled pin and plate to maintain the displacement and the valgus position of the femoral neck is inserted in the usual way (Figs 29.153 to 29.155).

Condylo-cephalic nailing. To avoid the use of a pin and plate with its attendant problems of stability, Kuntscher in 1966 introduced a technique of intramedullary nailing of intertrochanteric fractures using a long curved Kuntscher nail introduced through the medial femoral condyle.[156, 157] This rather cumbersome method has been overtaken by the multiple nail technique of Enders. The principle of both methods is the same, that is, to thread an intramedullary nail, or nails, (under an image intensifier), from the lower end of the femur along its whole length until the fracture at the intertrochanteric region is crossed and the proximal fragment firmly impinged. This method seems to have little to commend it, except the low blood-loss at operation and possibly that the patients can weight-bear earlier. It is more suited to undisplaced fractures which are in any case easily fixed with a pin and plate; and is apparently difficult in displaced fractures,[158] for which one would have hoped it would prove useful. Technically, good fixation is not easy to achieve and a fairly large number of problems associated with the insertion of the nails have been listed. In one survey of 98 unstable fractures treated by the Ender, 46 per cent required re-operation.[158a] Even in stable fractures a re-operation rate of 20 per cent has been reported.[158b] Perhaps

the technique is best summed up in the words of Poigenfurst and Schnabl: 'This operative procedure may appear simple but the impression is misleading. It must be carried out with great care and requires some technical skill. Incorrect nailing will not produce stability, the pain will persist and many problems ensue'.[159]

The use of acrylic cement as adjunct to internal fixation.[160] For some years already bone cement has been used successfully to fill large defects resulting from secondary deposits in bone. The same technique can be used in old people who are severely debilitated and suffering from marked osteoporosis. All the cancellous bone around the fracture site right up to the junction with the femoral head is removed and used later as an extra-periosteal graft. The pin and plate to be used is given a trial fit before the bone cavity is filled with acrylic cement. The nail plate is then reinserted while the cement is malleable and screwed on to the femur after it has set hard. This method should be confined to the management of fractures complicated by severe osteoporosis. Because of the risks of infection and the possibility of delayed union it is not indicated in young patients whose fractures can be effectively treated by more orthodox methods of fixation.[160]

Post-operative care. The management of these cases is exactly the same as that already recommended for transcervical fractures. It is unusual for the fracture not to be soundly united in three months, and union may occur in an even shorter time. But in order to reduce the residual varus deformity which may result from early weight-bearing the patient should be persuaded to walk partially weight-bearing and to use crutches until the fracture is united. Surgeons must constantly remember that these appliances are not guaranteed to withstand the forces of weight-bearing, and that they may be held responsible for any breakage if weight-bearing is allowed before the fracture is united (see Chapter 16).

Conservative treatment. *Treatment by traction.* Skin traction tapes or Steinmann pin tibial traction should be applied to the injured limb and Hamilton Russell traction used to reduce and immobilise the fracture. An encircling bandage over wool pads on the lower thigh attached to a suspended weight over a beam can be added to prevent lateral rotation of the limb. An overhead handle by which the patient can lift herself for bedpans, or move from one position to another, is most important. With good nursing, there is little doubt the results can be excellent and it has been claimed by Murray that the functional results of such conservative treatment are better than after operation, and that the mortality is lower.[161] This view is also held by Horn and Wang who reported a mortality of only just over 5 per cent in 170 patients treated conservatively.[162] However, the results in other series are less encouraging, and Horowitz quotes a 35 per cent mortality from conservative treatment compared with 17 per cent after operation.[163]

It must be emphasised also that although trochanteric fractures of the femur can be treated successfully, even in the most elderly patients, by conservative methods, it is essential to have the cooperation of the patient in moving about in the bed and generally taking a share in the nursing problem. When the patient is senile or very frail, or where skilful nursing facilities are not available to employ conservative treatment for a pertrochanteric fracture, it may result in disaster, and in these circumstances (which are commonly the case) internal fixation should be used. It must also be appreciated that to treat this fracture by traction means bed rest for at least 10 weeks, and if acute beds are at a premium it may be completely impracticable to use them in this way.

Trochanteric fractures with interposition of soft tissues. Very occasionally a trochanteric fracture can not be reduced by manipulation because there is an interposed band of fibrous tissue tightly stretched over the surface of the proximal fragment.*

* H. L. Greene, in a personal communication, reported such an inter-trochanteric fracture in which manipulative reduction was impossible. He wrote: 'There was found a very dense fibrous longitudinal band tightly stretched over the end of the proximal fragment ... It was incised transversely and then the fragments could be accurately apposed'.

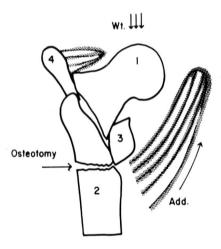

Fig 29.150

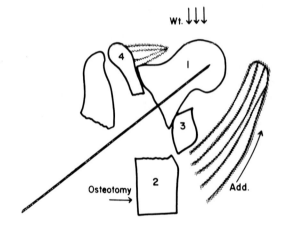

Fig 29.151

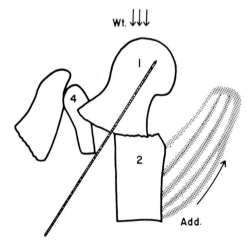

Fig 29.152

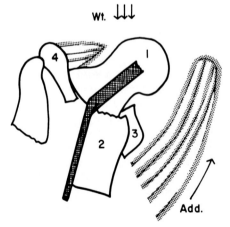

Fig 29.153

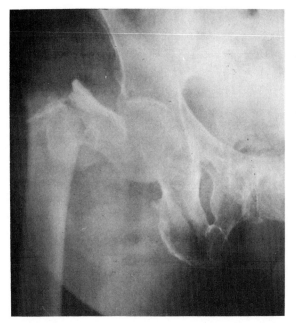

Fig 29.154

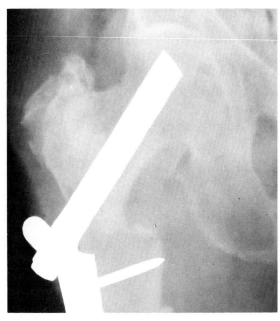

Fig 29.155

Figs 29.150 to 29.155 Steps in medial displacement fixation for trochanteric fractures. Figure 29.150 outlines the principle of osteotomy of the lateral trochanteric fragment of the femoral shaft. This allows the open end of the proximal fragment to be displayed and a guide wire inserted (Fig 29.151). The femoral shaft is then displaced below the inferior angle of the femoral neck which is made to engage the medullary cavity of the shaft (Fig 29.152). The proximal and distal fragments are then joined together by a suitably angled pin and plate (Fig 29.153). Figures 29.154 and 29.155 show the pre-operative and post-operative X-rays of an unstable trochanteric fracture treated by this technique. (Reproduced by the kind permission of the Editor of the *Journal of Bone and Joint Surgery* and Drs Dimon and Hughston from their paper in the *Journal of Bone and Joint Surgery* (1967)

In such cases there is no alternative: open reduction is essential. Failure to do this accounts for the rare instances of non-union of a trochanteric fracture as seen in Figure 29.156. If manipulative reduction by turning the limb into various positions of rotation and applying slight abduction is proved by radiographs to have failed to secure reasonable apposition of the fragments, this possibility of interposition of soft tissues must be considered. It is interesting to note that in the fracture shown in Figure 29.156 the greater trochanter along with the external rotators remains attached to the proximal fragment which is externally rotated. If there had been no soft tissue obstruction the fracture should have reduced accurately on externally rotating the lower limb.

In elderly patients interposition of soft tissues can almost be ignored. It is only in young athletic men whose fractures are sustained from severe violence, driving the upper shaft of the femur forcibly through muscle planes, that the problem of non-union need ever be thought about. Even in this rare group of injuries in young men, fractures with interposition of soft parts causing non-union are nearly always at the subtrochanteric level, or sometimes at the lowest part of the femoral neck itself. In patients in their eighth, ninth or tenth decades of life who sustain trochanteric fractures, the preference for operative treatment depends not upon the position or stability of the fracture, but upon the sure knowledge that very many of these patients will not survive the long period of immobilisation required for conservative treatment.

UNUNITED FRACTURES OF THE NECK OF THE FEMUR

The essential object of any operation for non-union of a fracture of the neck of the femur, other than a Girdlestone excision of the head and neck of femur, is to correct the telescopic instability produced by the fracture and to restore again direct transmission of weight from the femur to the acetabulum, pelvis and

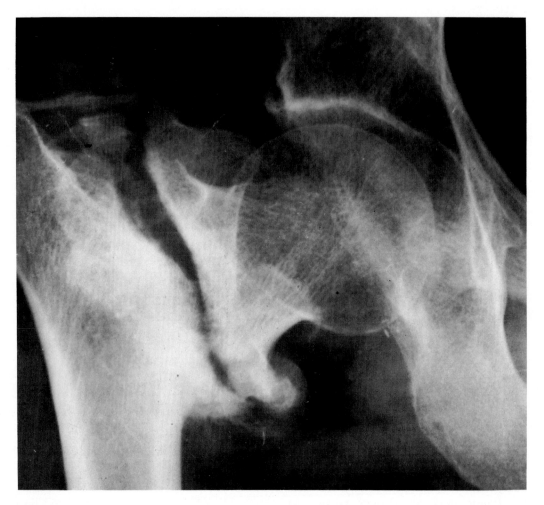

Fig 29.156 Intertrochanteric fracture of the femur, ununited because there was interposition of soft parts between the fractured surfaces. These fractures at the intertrochanteric or pertrochanteric level almost invariably unite whatever the treatment may be; but in rare cases, and this is one, soft tissue interposition demands open operative reduction. Note that the upper fragment is externally rotated.

spine. In the past before the advent of prosthetic replacement of the femoral head, a number of classical operations were devised, the indications depending on the degree of absorption and disappearance of the femoral neck and the vitality of the femoral head. However, there is only one which has survived the course of time and that is the original McMurray osteotomy.[164]

1. When there is minimal absorption of the femoral neck and no evidence of avascular necrosis of the head of the femur the ununited fracture should be treated either by a subtrochanteric abduction osteotomy to produce a more valgus femoral neck and

impact the fragments, or by internal fixation with a nail and fibular graft. These operations are only suitable for cases of delayed union.

2. When there is absorption of the femoral neck and a likelihood that the head of the femur is dead the fracture can sometimes be stimulated into union by carrying out a McMurray's bifurcation osteotomy, and even if the fracture does not unite the displacement of the osteotomy will usually regain stability and relieve pain. However, more usually nowadays frank non-union is treated by either hemi-arthroplasty, using an Austin Moore or Thompson prosthesis, or the insertion of a total hip replacement.

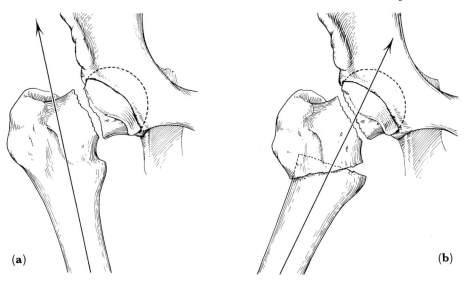

(a)   **(b)**

Fig 29.157 In the abduction osteotomy for delayed union of transcervical fractures the lower fragment must be sufficiently abducted to convert the shearing stress of weight bearing (a) to an impaction force (b) which passes directly from the shaft of the femur, through the fracture, to the femoral head.

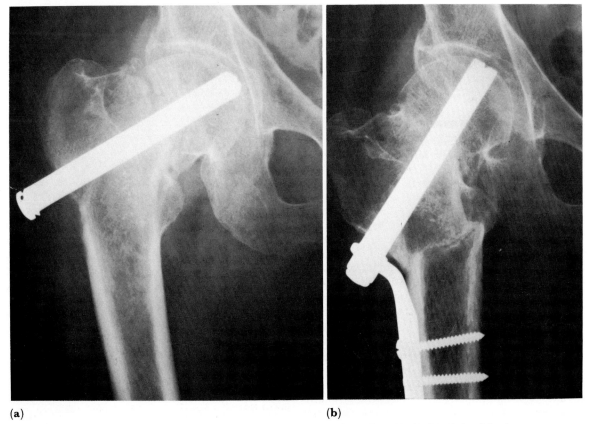

(a)   **(b)**

Fig 29.158 This femoral neck fracture showed no sign of union five months after nailing (Fig 29.158(a)). An abduction subtrochanteric osteotomy was carried out to remove the shearing strain at the fracture site and allow some impaction. A pin and plate was used for fixation and the patient kept ambulant on crutches. Figure 29.158(b) shows union of the fracture three months later.

Abduction osteotomy to produce valgus impaction. The purpose of an abduction osteotomy is to turn the shaft from the adducted to the abducted position, so that the shearing stress of weight-bearing and muscle retraction becomes an impaction force. The operation is therefore applicable to a fracture with delayed union in which final consolidation is prevented by the stresses of adduction deformity, but not to a fracture with established non-union, or to one in which most of the femoral neck has disappeared. The degree of correction must be such that the long axis of the femur will pass directly through the fracture and the head of the femur (Fig 29.157). The angle can be accurately calculated from radiographs and before the bone is divided parallel wires are inserted above and below the level of osteotomy so that the correction can be checked by measuring the angle between the wires. A pin and plate is used to fix the osteotomy, and where the fracture has been nailed in the usual way the same track can be used and the osteotomy performed immediately below the nail. A wedge of bone based laterally is removed, the angle of the wedge being precisely calculated to correct the varus deformity of the femoral neck. The osteotomy is closed by abducting the femoral shaft and fixed by attaching a plate to the nail already positioned in the femoral neck. Dickson reported good results when this operation is performed for delayed union.[164] (Fig 29.158).

Nailing and grafting the fracture. A graft alone is not strong enough to be relied upon for fixation of the fracture. King,[115] many years ago, showed that there is ample space within the neck of the femur for both a graft and a nail. Two guide wires are introduced, one into the upper and one into the lower part of the neck. A three-flanged nail is driven over the lower wire, and the other is used to guide cannulated drills which prepare a track for the fibular graft, the surface of which is freshened and drilled before it is introduced (Fig 29.159). This combined operation can be useful in patients below the age of 65 years. It should not be attempted, however, if there has been evidence that the blood supply of the femoral head is impaired.

McMurray's bifurcation osteotomy. The bifurcation osteotomy with inward displacement of the femoral shaft has the advantage that it is applicable to any type of ununited fracture of the femoral neck.[165] It can be employed equally in the treatment of non-union of intracapsular fractures, or trochanter fractures, and in the latter it is to be preferred to any

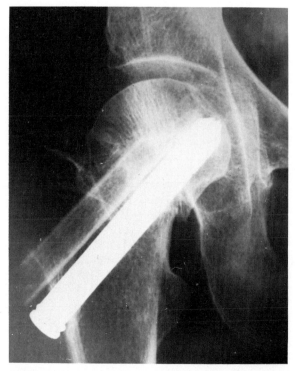

Fig 29.159 Delayed and non-union of the femoral neck can sometimes be healed by using nail fixation supplemented by a fibular graft.

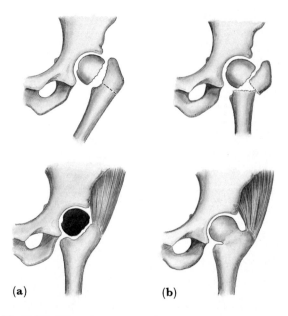

(a)   (b)

Fig 29.160 Bifurcation osteotomy for any type of ununited femoral neck fracture. If the head of the femur is dead an excellent arthroplasty is produced (a), and if it is alive the fracture unites (b).

attempt to bone graft the fracture. Through a lateral approach the trochanteric area of bone is exposed and the muscles overlying the anterior surface retracted to visualise the lower margin of the femoral neck. McMurray advised that the femoral head should be seen in order that after osteotomy the displaced shaft can come to lie under it. He emphasised that the success of the procedure depended upon siting the osteotomy correctly. If it was too high the shaft could not be displaced: if it was too low the weight was not borne through the shaft of the femur. The osteotomy is carried out with an osteotome immediately above the level of the lesser trochanter, and using the blade of the osteotome as a lever the shaft of the femur is displaced inwards so that it lies under the femoral head. If union of the fracture is merely delayed and the blood supply of the head is normal, the operation has the same effect as a simple abduction osteotomy and the fracture unites. On the other hand, if non-union is established and the femoral head has lost its blood supply, the osteotomy still succeeds because it has produced an excellent arthroplasty (Fig 29.160). If the conditions for prosthetic replacement are unsuitable, or if the patient is young, it is the operation of choice in any fracture with considerable absorption of the femoral

neck, paticularly when the blood supply of the head of the femur is in doubt. It has, unfortunately, the disadvantage of necessitating immobilisation in a plaster double hip spica, for internal fixation devices cannot be satisfactorily used and, indeed, may interfere with the correct positioning and repair of the fracture. For the first three weeks the hip is kept abducted and a little flexed to stabilise the femoral shaft under the femoral head. At the end of that time the limb is brought back to neutral, but the plaster maintained for a further eight weeks. It is therefore an operation for the young and intermediate age groups and it is not usually applicable in the treatment of the elderly.

The sources of failure of attempted bifurcation osteotomy were described clearly by McMurray.[165] For success the level of osteotomy must be immediately below the lower margin of the head of the femur so that the shaft can be placed beneath the head; the osteotomy must be slightly oblique in an inward and upward direction, and the outer angle of the shaft should be broken up and freshened in order that it shall certainly unite with the trochanteric fragment; and the limb should be immobilised in plaster with the femur in its inwardly displaced position until the osteotomy is united (Figs 29.161 and 29.162).

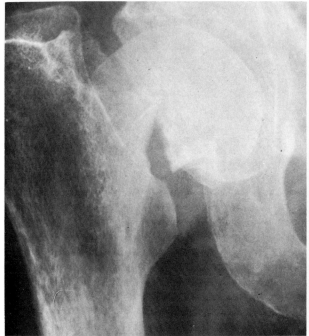
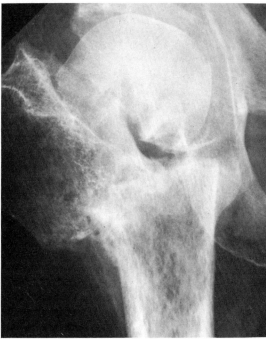

Fig 29.161   **Fig 29.162**

Figs 29.161 and 29.162 Ununited fracture neck of femur before and after bifurcation osteotomy. It is obvious from the first radiograph that the femoral head is relatively dense and therefore avacular. No type of nailing or grafting operation is justifiable.

Prosthetic replacement of the femoral head.
The classical reconstruction operations have been rendered almost completely obsolete by the introduction of prosthetic replacement of the femoral head. This procedure is certainly the operation of choice in the elderly patient with an ununited fracture or a painful avascular necrosis. The early Judet type of prosthesis has, of course, been completely superseded by the modern stem prosthesis of Austin Moore or Thompson, and on the whole these appliances give very satisfactory results. Provided the acetabulum has not been deformed by secondary arthritic change it is unnecessary to replace the whole joint with a total hip prosthesis. The operative procedure is therefore identical with that described in the management of the acute fracture.

REFERENCES

1. Hamilton Bailey 1940 Physical signs in clinical surgery, 7th edn. Wright, Bristol, p 252
2. Betto O 1926 Isolated fracture greater trochanter. Chirurgia degli Organi di Movimento 22: 58
3. Key J A 1926 Epiphyseal coxa vara or displacement of the capital epiphysis of the femur in adolescence. Journal of Bone and Joint Surgery 8: 53
4. Burrows H J 1957 Slipped upper femoral epiphysis. Characteristics of a hundred cases. Journal of Bone and Joint Surgery 39–B: 641
5. Perkins G 1932 Treatment of adolescent coxa vara. British Medical Journal, i: 55
6. Griffiths M J 1976 Slipping of the capital femoral epiphysis. Annals of the Royal College of Surgeons of England 58: 34
7. Mayer L 1937 The importance of early diagnosis in the treatment of slipping femoral epiphysis. Journal of Bone and Joint Surgery 19: 1046
8. Farrow R 1953 Displacement of the upper femoral epiphysis in a man of 26 years suffering from Simmond's disease following head injury. Journal of Bone and Joint Surgery 35–B: 432
9. Heatley F W, Greenwood R H, Boase D L 1976 Slipping of the upper femoral epiphysis in patients with intracranial tumours causing hypopituitarism and chiasmal compression. Journal of Bone and Joint Surgery 58–B: 169
10. Price N L, Davie T B 1937 Renal rickets. British Journal of Surgery 24: 548
11. Harris W R 1950 The endocrine basis for slipping of the upper femoral epiphysis. An experimental study. Journal of Bone and Joint Surgery 32–B: 5
12. Mickelson M R, Ponseti I V, Cooper R R, Maynard J A 1977 The ultrastructure of the growth plate in slipped capital femoral epiphysis. Journal of Bone and Joint Surgery 59–A: 1076
13. Rennie W, Mitchell N 1974 Slipped femoral capital epiphysis occurring during growth hormone therapy. Report on a case. Journal of Bone and Joint Surgery 56–B: 703
14. Milch H 1937 Epiphysiolysis or epiphyseal coxa anteverta. Journal of Bone and Joint Surgery 19: 97
15. Schlesinger A 1905 Zur Aetiologie und pathologischen Anatomie der Coxa Vara. Archiv fur Klinische Chirurgie Von Lagenbeck 75: 629
16. Clark K C 1956 Positioning in radiography, 7th edn. Heinemann, London, p 111
16a Billing L 1954 Roentgen examination of the proximal femur end in children and adolescents. Acta Radiologica Supp 110
17. Capener N 1956 Modern trends in orthopaedics (4) (2nd series) Edited by Sir Harry Platt. Butterworth, London
18. Jacobs P 1962 A note on the diagnosis of early adolescent coxa vara (slipped epiphysis). British Journal of Radiology 35: 619
19. Durbin F C 1960 Treatment of slipped upper femoral epiphysis. Journal of Bone and Joint Surgery 42–B: 289
20. Bloomberg T J, Nuttall J, Stoker D J 1978 Radiology in early slipped femoral capital epiphysis. Clinical Radiology 29: 657
21. Dunn D M 1964 The treatment of adolescent slipping of the upper femoral epiphysis. Journal of Bone and Joint Surgery 46–B: 621
22. Dunn D M, Angel J C 1978 Replacement of the femoral head by open operation in severe adolescent slipping of the upper femoral epiphysis. Journal of Bone and Joint Surgery 60–B: 394
23. Casey B H, Hamilton H W, Bobenchko W P 1972 Reduction of acutely slipped upper femoral epiphysis. Journal of Bone and Joint Surgery 54–B: 607
24. Aadalen R J, Weiner D S, Hoyt W, Herndon C H 1974 Acute slipped capital femoral epiphysis. Journal of Bone and Joint Surgery 56–A: 1473
25. Fahey J J, O'Brien E T 1965 Acute slipped capital epiphysis. Journal of Bone and Joint Surgery 47–A: 1105
26. Wardle E N 1933 Slipped epiphysis of the head of the femur. British Journal of Surgery 21: 313
27. Boyd H B 1950 Discussion of paper by C. L. Compere: Correction of deformity and prevention of a septic necrosis in late cases of slipped femoral epiphyses. Journal of Bone and Joint Surgery 32–A: 362
28. Southwick W O 1967 Osteotomy through the lesser trochanter for slipped capital femoral epiphysis. Journal of Bone and Joint Surgery 49–A: 807
29. O'Brien E T, Fahey J J 1977 Remodelling of the femoral neck after in situ pinning for slipped femoral epiphysis. Journal of Bone and Joint Surgery 59–A: 62
30. Klein A, Joplin R J, Reidy J A 1943 Treatment in cases of slipped capital femoral epiphysis at the Massachusetts General Hospital. Archives of Surgery 46: 681
31. Compere C L 1950 Correction of deformity and prevention of a septic necrosis in late cases of slipped femoral epiphysis. Journal of Bone and Joint Surgery 32–A: 351
32. Newman P H 1960 The surgical treatment of slipping of the upper femoral epiphysis. Journal of Bone and Joint Surgery 42–B: 280
33. Ireland J, Newman P H 1978 Triplane osteotomy for severely slipped upper femoral epiphysis. Journal of Bone and Joint Surgery 60–B: 390
34. Watson-Jones R 1926 Spontaneous dislocation of the hip joint. British Journal of Surgery 14: 36
35. Funsten R V, Kinser P, Frankel C J 1938 Dashboard

dislocations of the hip. A report of 20 cases of traumatic dislocation. Journal of Bone and Joint Surgery 20: 124

36. Campbell W C 1936 Posterior dislocation of the hip joint with fracture of the acetabulum. Journal of Bone and Joint Surgery 18: 842

37. Smith E J, Buxton St J D 1933 Traumatic anterior dislocation of the hip. Proceedings of the Royal Society of Medicine 27: 579

38. Macfarlane J A 1936 Anterior dislocation of the hip. British Journal of Surgery 23: 607

39. Amihood S 1975 Anterior dislocation of the hip. Injury 7: 107

40. Wulff H B 1936 Ein Fall doppelseitiger traumatischer Hüftgelenkverrenkung. Acta Chirurgica Scandinavica, 77: 626

41. Marquard W 1936 Die doppelseitige traumatische Hüftluxation. (Bilateral traumatic dislocation of hips. Review of 52 reported cases.) Archiv für Orthopädische und Unfall-chirurgie 37: 189

42. Goetz A G 1934 Traumatic dislocation of the hip (head of femur) into the scrotum. Journal of Bone and Joint Surgery 16: 718

43. Henderson R S 1951 Traumatic anterior dislocation of the hip. Journal of Bone and Joint Surgery 33–B: 602

44. Stewart M J, McCarroll H R 1970 Fracture-dislocation of the hip: a follow-up and comparative study. Journal of Bone and Joint Surgery 52–B: 773

45. Epstein H C 1974 Posterior fracture-dislocations of the hip. Long-term follow-up. Journal of Bone and Joint Surgery 56–A: 1103

46. Gartland J J 1967 Traumatic dislocation of the hip in children. Journal of Bone and Joint Surgery 49–A: 1017

47. Schlonsky J, Miller P R 1973 Traumatic hip dislocations in children. Journal of Bone and Joint Surgery 55–A: 1057

48. MacFarlane I J A 1976 Survey of traumatic dislocation of the hip in children. Journal of Bone and Joint Surgery 58–B: 267

49. Urist M R 1948 Fracture-dislocation of the hip joint. Journal of Bone and Joint Surgery 30–A: 699

50. Wilson J N 1960 The management of fracture dislocation of the hip. Proceedings of the Royal Society of Medicine 53: 39

51. Pringle J H 1943 Traumatic dislocation at the hip joint. An experimental study in a cadaver. Glasgow Medical Journal 139: 25

52. Epstein H C 1973 Traumatic dislocation of the hip. Clinical Orthopaedics and Related Research 92: 115

53. Amihood S 1975 Anterior dislocation of the hip. Injury 7: 107

54. Stimson L A 1908 A Treatise on Fractures and Dislocations, p 743. New York: Lea & Febiger

55. Henry A K, Bayumi M 1934 Fracture of the femur with luxation of the ipsi-lateral hip. British Journal of Surgery 22: 204

56. Chakraborti S, Miller I M 1975 Dislocation of the hip associated with fracture of the femoral head, Injury 7: 134

57. Brav E A 1962 Traumatic dislocation of the hip. Army experience and results over a twelve-year period. Journal of Bone and Joint Surgery 44–A: 1115

58. Fina C P, Kelly P J 1970 Dislocation of the hip with fractures of the proximal femur. Journal of Trauma 10: 17

59. Riggs T F, Slocum R C 1951 Fracture-dislocation of the hip. Report of an unusual case. Journal of Bone and Joint Surgery 33–A: 779

60. Ratcliff A H C 1968 Traumatic separation of the upper femoral epiphysis in young children. Journal of Bone and Joint Surgery 50–B: 757

61. Cooper, Sir Astley 1823 A treatise on dislocation and on fractures of the joints, 2nd edn. Longman, Hurst, Rees, Orme & Browne, London, p 62

62. Dehne E, Immermann E W 1951 Dislocation of the hip combined with fracture of the shaft of the femur on the same side. Journal of Bone and Joint Surgery 33–A: 731

63. Helal B, Skevis X 1967 Unrecognised dislocation of the hip in fractures of the femoral shaft. Journal of Bone and Joint Surgery 49–B: 293

64. Wadsworth T G 1961 Traumatic dislocation of the hip with fracture of the shaft of the ipsi-lateral femur. Journal of Bone and Joint Surgery 43–B: 47

65. Lyddon D W, Hartmann J T 1971 Traumatic dislocation of the hip with ipsi-lateral femoral fracture. Journal of Bone and Joint Surgery 53–A: 1012

66. Bohler L 1957 The treatment of fractures, 5th English edn. Grune & Stratton, New York, vol 2, p 1119

67. Stewart M J, Milford L W 1954 Fracture-dislocation of the hip—an end-result study. Journal of Bone and Joint Surgery 36–A: 315

68. Glass A, Powell H O W 1961 Traumatic dislocation of the hip in children. An analysis of 47 cases. Journal of Bone and Joint Surgery 43–B: 29

69. Thompson V P, Epstein H C 1951 Traumatic dislocation of the hip. A survey of 204 cases covering a period of 21 years. Journal of Bone and Joint Surgery 33–A: 746

70. Nicoll E A 1953 The management of dislocation of the hip associated with fractures of the acetabulum. Journal of Bone and Joint Surgery 35–B: 147

71. Nicoll E A 1952 Traumatic dislocation of the hip—review of 144 cases. Journal of Bone and Joint Surgery 34–B: 503

72. Piggott J 1961 Traumatic dislocation of the hip in childhood. Journal of Bone and Joint Surgery 43–B: 38

73. Pennsylvania Orthopaedic Society 1968 Traumatic dislocation of the hip joint in children. Final report by the Scientific Research Committee. Journal of Bone and Joint Surgery 50–A: 79

74. Haliburton R A, Brockenshire F A, Barber J R 1961 Avascular necrosis of the femoral capital epiphysis after traumatic dislocation of the hip in children. Journal of Bone and Joint Surgery 43–B: 43

74a. Armstrong J R 1948 Traumatic dislocation of the hip joint: review of 101 dislocations. Journal of Bone and Joint Surgery 30–B, 430

75. Repo R U, Finlay J B 1977 Survival of articular cartilage after controlled impact. Journal of Bone and Joint Surgery 59–A: 1068

76. Heinzelmann P R, Nelson C R 1976 Recurrent traumatic dislocation of the hip. Report of a case. Journal of Bone and Joint Surgery 58–A: 895

76a. Hollingdale J P, Aichroth P M 1981 Recurrent post-traumatic dislocation of the hip in children. Journal of the Royal Society of Medicine 74: 545

77. Sullivan C R, Bickel W H, Lipscomb P R 1955 Recurrent dislocation of the hip. Journal of Bone and Joint Surgery 37–A: 1266

78. Leibenberg F, Dommisse G F 1969 Recurrent post-traumatic dislocation of the hip. Journal of Bone and Joint Surgery 51–B: 632

79. Scott J E, Thomas F B 1974 Delayed presentation of post-traumatic posterior dislocation of the hip with acetabular rim fracture. Injury 5: 325

80. Huckstep R L 1971 Neglected traumatic dislocation of the hip. Journal of Bone and Joint Surgery 53–B: 355

81. Gupta R C, Schravat B P 1977 Reduction of neglected traumatic dislocation of the hip by heavy traction. Journal of Bone and Joint Surgery 59–A: 249

82. Paterson I 1957 The torn acetabular labrum. Journal of Bone and Joint Surgery 39–B: 306

83. Dameron T B, Raleigh M D 1959 Bucket-handle tear of acetabular labrum accompanying posterior dislocation of the hip. Journal of Bone and Joint Surgery 41–A: 131

84. Judet R, Judet J, Letournel E 1964 Fractures of the acetabulum; classification and surgical approaches for open reduction. Journal of Bone and Joint Surgery 46–A: 1615

85. Eichenholtz S N, Stark R M 1964 Central acetabular fractures. A review of 35 cases. Journal of Bone and Joint Surgery 46–A: 695

86. Knight R A, Smith H 1958 Central fractures of the acetabulum. Journal of Bone and Joint Surgery 40–A: 1

87. Lansinger O 1977 Fractures of the acetabulum. A clinical, radiological and experimental study. Acta Orthopaedica Scandinavica, supp. 165

88. Pearson J R, Hargadon E J 1962 Fractures of the pelvis involving the floor of the acetabulum. Journal of Bone and Joint Surgery 44–B: 550

89. Meggitt B F, Wilson J N 1972 The battered buttock syndrome—fat fractures. A report on a group of traumatic lipomata. British Journal of Surgery 59: 165

90. Tipton W W, D'Ambrosia R D, Ryle G P 1975 Non-operative management of central fracture-dislocation of the hip. Journal of Bone and Joint Surgery 57–A: 888

91. Rowe C R, Lowell J D 1961 Prognosis of fractures of the acetabulum. Journal of Bone and Joint Surgery 43–A: 30

92. Austin R T 1971 Hip function after central fracture-dislocation. A long-term review. Injury 3: 114

93. Bohler L 1957 The treatment of fractures, 5th English edn. Grune & Stratton, New York, vol 2, p 1138

94. Devas M 1978 Fractures in the elderly. Journal of Bone and Joint Surgery 60–B: 135

95. Wyman J B 1953 Symposium on problems of fractures in the aged—anaesthesia. Proceedings of the Royal Society of Medicine 46: 106

96. Nystrom G 1938 Die Behandlung der frischen medialen Schenkelhalsfrakturen. Ergebnisse der Chirurgie und Orthopadie 31: 667

97. Per Linton G 1944 On the different types of intracapsular fracture of the femoral neck. Acta Chirurgica Scandinavica. Supplement 86: 90

98. Per Linton G 1949 Types of displacement in fractures of the femoral neck. Journal of Bone and Joint Surgery 31–B: 184

99. Garden R S 1961 Low-angle fixation in fractures of the femoral neck. Journal of Bone and Joint Surgery 43–A: 647

100. Garden R S 1961 The structure and function of the proximal end of the femur. Journal of Bone and Joint Surgery 43–B: 576

101. Pauwels F 1935 Der Schenkenhalsbruch: ein mechanisches problem. Enke, Stuttgart

102. Nicoll E A 1963 The unsolved fracture (Editorial). Journal of Bone and Joint Surgery 45–B: 239

103. Nicolaysen J 1897 Lidt om Diagnosem og Behandlingen av Fr. Colli Femoris. Nordiskt Medicinskt Arkiv 8: 1

104. Lambotte A 1913 Chirurgie operatoire des fractures. Masson, Paris

105. Groves E W Hey 1916 On modern methods of treating fractures. Wright, Bristol

106. Smith-Petersen M N, Cave E F, Vangorder G W 1931 Intracapsular fractures of the neck of the femur. Archives of Surgery 23: 715

107. Johansson S 1932 On the operative treatment of medial fractures of the neck of the femur. Acta Orthopaedica Scandinavica 3: 362

108. Cubbins W R, Callahan J J, Scuderi C S 1939 Fractures of the neck of the femur. Open operation and pathological observations. A new incision and a new director for the use of a simplified flange. Surgery, Gynecology and Obstetrics 68: 87

109. Plummer W W 1938 Comments on internal fixation in fresh fractures of the neck of the femur. Journal of Bone and Joint Surgery 20: 100

110. Selig S 1939 Objections to the use of Kirschner wire for fixation of femoral neck fractures. Journal of Bone and Joint Surgery 21: 182

111. Moore A T 1937 Fracture of the hip joint. Treatment by extra-articular fixation with adjustable nails. Surgery, Gynecology and Obstetrics 64: 420

112. Putti V 1938 Treatment fracture neck of femur. Chirurgia degli Organi di Movimento 23: 399

113. Henderson M S 1938 Internal fixation for recent fractures of the neck of the femur. Annals of Surgery 107: 132

114. Godoy Moreira F E 1940 A special stud-bolt screw for fixation of fractures of the neck of the femur. Journal of Bone and Joint Surgery 22: 683

115. King T 1939 Closed operation for intracapsular fracture of the neck of the femur. British Journal of Surgery 26: 721

116. Charnley J, Blockey N J, Purser D W 1957 The treatment of displaced fractures of the neck of the femur by compression. Journal of Bone and Joint Surgery 39–B: 45

117. Brown J T, Abrami G 1964 Transcervical femoral fracture. A review of 195 patients treated by sliding nail-plate fixation. Journal of Bone and Joint Surgery 46–B: 648

118. Garden J 1964 Fractures of the neck of the femur. Journal of Bone and Joint Surgery 46–B: 355

119. Smyth E H, Ellis J, Manifold M C, Dewey P R 1964 Triangle pinning for fracture of the femoral neck. A new method based upon the internal architecture. Journal of Bone and Joint Surgery 46–B: 664

120. Garden R S 1964 Stability and union in subcapital fractures of the femur. Journal of Bone and Joint Surgery 46–B: 630

121. Barnes R, Brown T, Garden R S, Nicoll E A 1976 Subcapital fractures of the femur. A prospective review. Journal of Bone and Joint Surgery 58–B: 2

122. Bracey D J 1977 A comparison of internal fixation and prosthetic replacement in the treatment of displaced subcapital fractures. Injury 9: 1

123. Garden R S 1977 Selective surgery in medial fractures of the femoral neck: a review. Injury 9: 5

124. D'Arcy J C, Devas M 1976 Treatment of fractures of the femoral neck by replacement with the Thompson prosthesis. Journal of Bone and Joint Surgery 58–B: 279

125. Boyd H B, Salvatore J E 1964 Acute fracture of the femoral neck: internal fixation or prosthesis? Journal of Bone and Joint Surgery 46–A: 1066

126. Lunt H R W 1971 The role of prosthetic replacement of the head of the femur as primary treatment for subcapital fractures. Injury 3: 107

127. Arnold W D, Lyden J P, Minkoff J 1974 Treatment of intracapsular fractures of the femoral neck with special

reference to percutaneous Knowles pinning. Journal of Bone and Joint Surgery 56–A: 254

128. Durbin F C 1959 Avascular necrosis complicating undisplaced fractures of the neck of the femur in children. Journal of Bone and Joint Surgery 41–B: 759

129. McDougall A 1961 Fracture of the neck of the femur in childhood. Journal of Bone and Joint Surgery 43–B: 16

130. Leadbetter G W 1933 A treatment for fracture of the neck of the femur. Journal of Bone and Joint Surgery 15: 931

131. Flynn M 1974 A new method of reduction of fractures of the neck of the femur based on anatomical studies of the hip joint. Injury 5: 309

132. MacConaill M A 1953 Closely packed position of joints and its practical bearing. Journal of Bone and Joint Surgery 35–B: 486

133. Compton E A 1977 Accuracy of reduction of femoral subcapital fractures. Injury 9: 71

134. Smith F B 1959 Effects of rotatory and valgus malpositions on blood supply to the femoral head. Journal of Bone and Joint Surgery 41–A: 800

135. Sylvester B S, Boston D, Grant C, Galasko C S B 1977 Peak flow measurement as a guide to prognosis in patients undergoing hip surgery. Journal of Bone and Joint Surgery 59–B: 500

136. Brittain H A 1942 The low nail. British Medical Journal i: 463

137. Kuntscher G 1953 Die vollanatomatische Schenkelhals-nagelung. Zeitschrift für Orthopädie und ihre Grenzgebiete 84: 17

138. Fielding W J, Wilson H J, Zickel R F 1964 A continuing end-result study of displaced intracapsular fractures of the neck of the femur. Journal of Bone and Joint Surgery 44–A: 965

139. Fielding W J, Wilson S A, Ratzan S 1974 A continuing end-result study of displaced intracapsular fractures of the neck of the femur treated with Pugh nail. Journal of Bone and Joint Surgery 56–A: 1464

140. Jarry L 1964 Transarticular nailing for fractures of the femoral neck. A preliminary report. Journal of Bone and Joint Surgery 46–B: 674

141. Trueta J, Harrison M H M 1953 The normal vascular anatomy of the femoral head in adult man. Journal of Bone and Joint Surgery 35–B: 442

142. Catto M 1965 The histological appearance of late segmental collapse of the femoral head after transcervical fracture. Journal of Bone and Joint Surgery 47–B: 777

143. Strange F G St C 1969 Pinning under local anaesthesia for subcapital fractures of the femoral neck. Injury 1: 100

144. Bolton H 1961 Treatment of displaced subcapital fractures of the femoral neck in the aged by immediate replacement arthroplasty. Journal of Bone and Joint Surgery 43–B: 606

144a. Søreide O, Alho A, and Rietti D 1980 Internal fixation versus endoprosthesis in the treatment of femoral neck fractures in the elderly. Acta Ortho Scand 51: 827

145. Dandy D J 1971 Fat embolism following prosthetic replacement of the femoral head. Injury 3: 85

146. Sevitt S 1972 Fat embolism in patients with fractured hips. British Medical Journal ii: 257

147. Anderson L D, Hawsa W R, Waring T L 1964 Femoral head prostheses. A review of 356 operations and their results. Journal of Bone and Joint Surgery 46–A: 1049

148. Wrighton J D, Woodward J E 1971 Prosthetic replacement for subcapital fractures of the femur: a comparative study. Injury 2: 287

149. Knight W E 1978 Preliminary report on the Bateman universal proximal femur prosthesis. Journal of Bone and Joint Surgery 60–B: 293

150. Devas M B 1979 Personal communication

151. Evans E M 1951 Trochanteric fractures. Journal of Bone and Joint Surgery 33–B: 192

152. Dimon J H, Hughston J C 1967 Unstable intertrochanteric fractures of the hip. Journal of Bone and Joint Surgery 49–A: 440

153. May J M B, Chacha P B 1968 Displacements of trochanteric fractures and their influence on reduction. Journal of Bone and Joint Surgery 50–B: 318

154. Evans E M 1949 The treatment of trochanteric fractures of the femur. Journal of Bone and Joint Surgery 31–B: 190

155. Clawson D K 1957 Intertrochanteric fracture of the hip. American Journal of Surgery 93: 580

156. Kuntscher G 1970 A new method of treatment of pertrochanteric fractures. Proceedings of the Royal Society of Medicine 63: 1120

157. Collado F, Vila J, Beltran J E 1973 Condylo-cephalic nail fixation for trochanteric fractures of the femur. Journal of Bone and Joint Surgery 55–B: 774

158. Wynn Jones C, Morris J, Hirschowitz D, Hart G M, Shea J, Arden G P 1977 A comparison of the treatment of trochanteric fractures of the femur by internal fixation with a nail plate and the Ender technique. Injury 9: 36

158a. Jensen J S, Sonne-Holm S 1980 Critical analysis of Ender nailing in the treatment of trochanteric fractures. Acta Orth Scand 51: 817

158b. Jensen J S, Tøndevold E, Sonne-Holm S 1980 Stable trochanteric fractures. A comparative analysis of four methods of internal fixation. Acta Orth Scand 51: 81

159. Poigenfürst J, Schnabl P 1977 Multiple intramedullary nailing of pertrochanteric fractures with elastic nails: operative procedure and results. Injury 9: 102

160. Harrington K D 1975 The use of methylmethacrylate as an adjunct in the internal fixation of unstable comminuted intertrochanteric fractures in osteoporotic patients. Journal of Bone and Joint Surgery 57–A: 744

161. Murray R C, Frew J F M 1949 Trochanteric fracture of the femur—a plea for conservative treatment. Journal of Bone and Joint Surgery 31–B: 204

162. Horn J S, Wang Y C 1964 The mechanism, traumatic anatomy and non-operative treatment of intertrochanteric fracture of the femur. British Journal of Surgery 51: 574

163. Horowitz B G 1966 Retrospective analysis of hip fractures. Surgery, Gynecology and Obstetrics 123: 565

164. Dickson J A 1953 The unsolved fracture. Journal of Bone and Joint Surgery 35–A: 805

165. McMurray T P 1936 Ununited fractures of the neck of the femur. Journal of Bone and Joint Surgery 18: 319

30

Injuries of the Thigh

'If it should be discovered that I have added one atom to the principle it will give me much more satisfaction than if I should succeed in burdening practice by ingenious means'.   Hugh Owen Thomas, 1886

'Our aim should be to help Nature's normal healing processes rather than to hinder them'.   F G St Clair Strange, 1963

The principles taught by Hugh Owen Thomas are certainly not to be forgotten. The Thomas knee splint is still an essential feature for the conservative management of most fractures of the shaft of the femur in many centres and compares favourably with every other method of treatment. Most fractures of the femoral shaft can be dealt with successfully by this technique of immobilisation. At the same time it should be recognised that in some fractures, particularly in the middle and upper thirds of the shaft of the femur, internal fixation of a long intramedullary nail offers notable advantages.

The femur is richly supplied with blood, and the repair of uncomplicated fractures of this bone is usually rapid, particularly in young people amongst whom the fracture is more common. Non-union is relatively infrequent provided that there has been no serious infection, no major loss of bone substance, no unrecognised soft tissue interposition and no distraction of the fracture surfaces by the use of excessive traction. On the other hand it should be recognised that final consolidation is sometimes slow, and that the distribution of muscle forces is such that angulation may arise. The powerful abductor muscles are all inserted in the region of the greater trochanter, whereas the equally powerful adductor muscles are inserted into the medial aspect of the lower femoral shaft and the medial femoral condyle, so that there is always a tendency for the proximal fragment to be abducted and for the distal fragment to be adducted. Such lateral angulation may develop even in later stages of treatment, after a fracture of the femoral shaft has been suitably immobilised for 12 or 15 weeks, and it is in fractures which are slow in uniting

that the continued protection of an intramedullary nail finds its greatest benefit.

Thus, in considering the management of fractures of the shaft of the femur we must review:

1. Conservative treatment by skin or skeletal traction, usually with a Thomas splint.
2. The use of cast bracing in the later stages of immobilisation.
3. Operative treatment by the internal fixation with an intramedullary nail, a heavy-duty plate, or a blade plate.

We must also review the results of treatment in fractures at four levels:

1. Fractures in the mid shaft.
2. Subtrochanteric fractures.
3. Supracondylar and condylar fractures.
4. Injuries to the lower femoral epiphysis.

Finally we will discuss the complications of these fractures and in particular the management of the stiff knee. But first the clinical and radiological appearances of the fracture must be considered.

Clinical features in femoral shaft fractures.
In contradistinction to fractures of the neck of the femur which typically occur in the elderly, fractures of the shaft of the femur are injuries of the young and are usually the result of severe trauma. Road traffic accidents, and in particular motor cycle accidents, are the most common cause and it is not unusual for the femoral fracture to be only part of a complex multiple injury. To break the normal femoral shaft of a healthy young adult requires considerable force and

it is therefore not surprising that many of these fractures are widely displaced, and even if the femur is the only bone to be broken the degree of initial shock can be profound. Gross swelling of the thigh is present within a very short time of the injury and it has been estimated that over a litre of blood can be lost from bleeding fracture surfaces.[1] This blood loss must be taken into consideration when planning the patient's treatment; and operative procedures, particularly if there are other severe injuries, should not be carried out until blood replacement is readily available. Spasm of the large muscles which surround the femur commonly result in considerable overlap of the bone ends with obvious shortening of the leg, and any unprotected movement of the limb will lead to increase in the spasm and further deformity. Sometimes the angulatory and rotatory deformities can be grotesque, indicating again the severe forces involved in this fracture. Uncontrolled movement at the fracture site can also be responsible for increasing the degree of shock, partly as the result of repeated pain stimuli and partly by increasing the bleeding around the fracture. Therefore an important first aid measure, even at the roadside, is to immobilise the limb and if possible apply some traction (see Chapter 7); and it is equally important that this temporary traction, preferably in a Thomas splint, should be maintained on admission to hospital while preliminary investigations and X-rays are being carried out. When compared with the tibia open fractures of the femoral shaft are relatively infrequent, but when they do occur the wounds and soft tissue complications can be extensive, particularly if the fracture has been caused by a gunshot wound. In general, however, complications associated with this fracture are rare and this is probably a reflection of the considerable degree of protection afforded to the main vessels and nerves by the large mass of muscle around the femur. These complications are discussed at the end of the chapter.

Radiological appearance. The basic fracture pattern of a femoral shaft injury associated with the severe trauma of a road traffic accident is usually transverse, indicating direct trauma. But this appearance may have many variations which at their worst may take the form of gross destruction of continuity of a whole section of the femoral shaft (Fig 30.1). Pure spiral fractures resulting from indirect violence are less common and tend to occur in an older age group. Because of the pull of the abductors on the upper fragment most femoral shaft fractures tend to angulate laterally. A persistently adducted upper

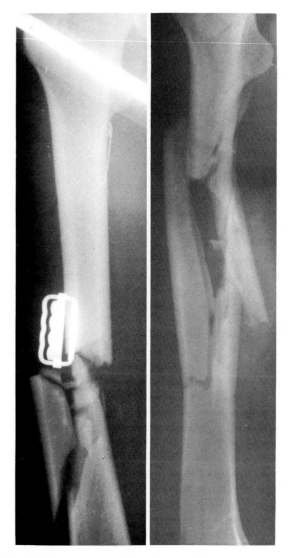

Fig 30.1 Two grossly comminuted fractures of the middle third of the femoral shaft both resulting from a motor-cycle injury. To produce this amount of damage the femur must be exposed to direct injury involving enormous forces. Is it any wonder that patients sustaining such fractures are in a state of severe shock?

fragment (despite manipulation) in a transverse fracture should always be examined carefully to exclude an unseen dislocation of the hip;[2] or sometimes a fracture of the neck of the femur (see p. 1022). Usually femoral shaft fractures can be lined up with an acceptable position by manipulation and this can be maintained satisfactorily by traction. A gap between the bone ends, seen in both the anteroposterior and lateral views, should lead the surgeon to suspect either distraction from excessive pull on the lower fragment, or what is more common, interposition of soft tissues between the bone ends. Both of these conditions need urgent correction if delayed union of the fracture is to be avoided.

CONSERVATIVE TREATMENT OF FRACTURES OF THE SHAFT OF THE FEMUR

Technique of immobilisation of the limb by traction in a Thomas splint.

Most fractures of the femoral shaft can be treated satisfactorily in a Thomas knee splint with skin-traction or skeletal-traction. It must be emphasised at once that, as with every other fracture, displacement should first be reduced by manipulation, the splint being expected only to hold the reduction that has been achieved. Many failures in the treatment of fractures of the femoral shaft have arisen from endeavours to secure gradual reduction by long-continued traction without ever giving an anaesthetic and deliberately manipulating the fragments into apposition. Surgeons who, in the treatment of other fractures, would never have doubted the need for manipulative correction of displacement with maintenance of correction thereafter by suitable splintage, have expected miracles from a Thomas splint, supposing that it would reduce the fracture as well as immobilise it. The displacement should be reduced by manipulation within a few hours of injury. No more is to be expected of the splint, whether used with skin-traction or skeletal-traction, than to maintain the replacement so achieved. Reduction of the fracture should be completed before the surgeon leaves the bedside, with the fractured surfaces in reasonable apposition and with alignment controlled by local wool padding or sometimes plaster slabs, as well as by the main support of the Thomas splint with light traction.

There are many methods of supporting a fractured thigh in a Thomas splint but they differ only in detail. It must be said quite clearly and definitely that, after manipulative reduction, the simplest and safest of all methods is fixed traction with adhesive skin-tapes tied to the lower end of a Thomas splint, with the end of the splint tied to the raised end of the bed in order to relieve pressure in the groin from the ring (see Fig 30.2). The method has been used extensively in underdeveloped countries for the treatment of femoral shaft fractures of all ages. If the simple technique is followed with proper attention to detail, nearly all fractures of the shaft of the femur can be treated successfully—without serious shortening, without

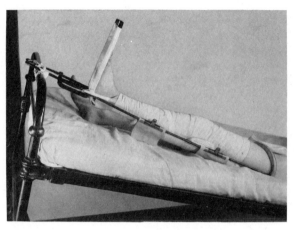

Fig 30.2 Fixed traction from adhesive skin-tapes in a Thomas splint. The end of the splint is fastened to the raised foot of the bed to reduce the pressure of the ring of the splint on the ischium. This is the simplest of all methods of treating fractures of the shaft of the femur and it is safe and satisfactory, and is particularly useful in treating childrens' fractures. It is less well tolerated in teenage and adult life where some form of balanced traction is usually necessary. (See Fig 30.4.)

deformity, without stiffness of the knee joint, and without any serious threat of non-union. It is an admirable method of treatment which for long years has stood the test of time. It is certainly the treatment of choice for fracture of the femoral shaft in children up until teenage. In adolescents and adults it is usually necessary to add weights to the end of the splint in order to avoid ring sores (Fig 30.4). Displacement must of course be reduced by manipulation and the corrected position can be maintained for about 12 weeks if this is necessary in order to obtain solid union. However, with the advent of the cast brace the time of immobilisation in the Thomas splint has been reduced by half (see later). Even with the longer periods in the splint there need be no fear of permanent stiffness of the knee joint. Such stiffness does not arise just from immobilisation. The causes of stiffness of the knee in fractures of the shaft of the femur will be discussed later, but meanwhile let it be clear that in young and middle-aged patients, fixation of the knee joint for two, three or even four months in the treatment of a simple fracture of the femoral shaft, provided there is no joint injury, rarely does any harm to the knee.

Thomas splint. A Thomas splint consists of a ring $\frac{3}{8}$ inch (10 mm) iron, padded with boiler felt and covered with basil-leather or plastic. The ring is set at such an angle to two side bars so that it fits round the upper thigh, with the posterior, more curved part of the ring under the tuberosity of the ischium and the flatter part just below and parallel to the inguinal ligament (Fig 30.3). The outer bar is joined to the middle of the ring, the medial bar slightly in front of the middle, and they converge at the lower ends where they are continuous at a level 3 or 4 inches (7.6 or 10.2 cm) below the foot, a notch on the crossbar serving for the attachment of extension cords. The limb rests upon strips of canvas, calico or domett bandage which are slung between the side bars of the splint.

Pearson knee-flexion attachment. There are occasions when it is wise to begin movement of the knee joint before union of the fracture is sound enough for the splint to be discarded or even for a cast brace to be used. Such early mobilisation may be necessary when there has been an associated intra-articular injury and is facilitated by the use of a Pearson knee-flexion attachment—a U-shaped metal frame hinged at its upper end to short clamps, fitting over the side bars of the Thomas splint just above the level of the knee.

This attachment can only be used effectively in combination with skeletal-traction using a tibial pin (Fig 30.5). The thigh is supported in the main part of the splint by broad strips of canvas stretched between its bars, the leg and foot are supported in a Pearson knee-flexion attachment on similar canvas strips. The Pearson attachment may be fixed at any desired angle with the main splint, or, with a movable junction, it may become part of a balanced system of weights and pulleys so that active flexion exercises of the joint can be practised by the patient.

Slinging the splint and special fracture beds. Whether skin-traction or skeletal-traction is used, suspension of the splint from an overhead beam increases the comfort of the patient, allows him to move more freely in bed, and facilitates the nursing problems. Many types of fracture bed are available, the essential feature of them all being a rigid overhead beam supported by two uprights, one clamped to the foot of the bed and the other to the head of it. Provision is made for the attachment of pulleys at any desired point on the beam or on the uprights.

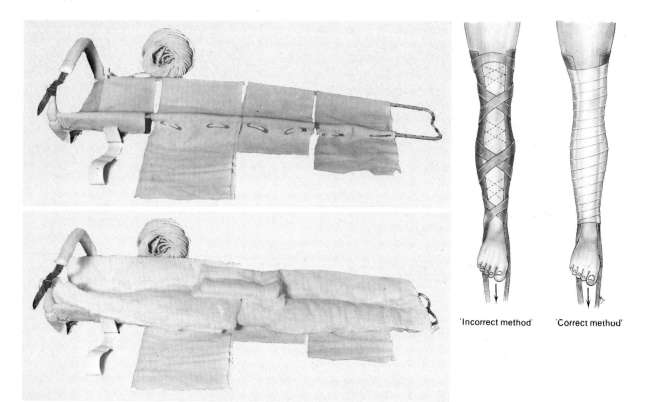

'Incorrect method'   'Correct method'

Fig 30.3 A modern Thomas bed knee splint with a detachable half-ring. Supporting slings and gamgee padding are shown. The inset shows the correct and incorrect method of applying skin-traction if this is to be used. If spiral adhesive strapping is applied pressure sores are produced.

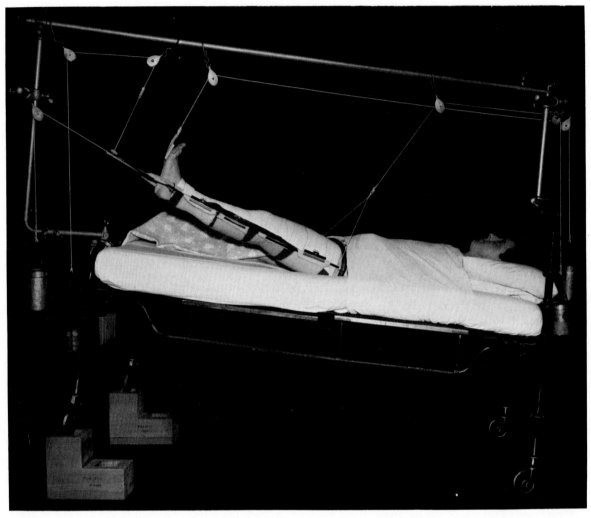

Fig 30.4 Combined fixed and backward suspended splint. Fracture of the shaft of the femur treated in a Thomas splint with fixed skin-traction combined with weights over the end of the bed to relieve ring pressure. The splint is suspended by pulleys and weights in order to facilitate movement of the patient in bed. The foot of the bed is elevated to give counter-traction. Note that an extra weight has been used in this case to support the foot.

Application of traction. Two methods of traction are available:

1. Skin-traction by adhesive strapping.
2. Skeletal-traction from a Steinmann pin, Denham pin or Kirschner wire in the upper part of the tibia.

Each has its advantages and limitations—sometimes one is better and sometimes the other. In general, children can be treated by skin-traction, whereas adults who require heavier traction are usually better treated with a skeletal pin. However,

surgeons should be ready to use either skin-traction or skeletal-traction according to the needs of the case.

Skin-traction with adhesive strapping. When no more than light traction of about 10 lb (4.5 kg) is required strapping affords a sufficient hold and is entirely satisfactory if the skin is healthy. When the skin is atrophic and inelastic, as it may be in elderly patients, even light traction may cause discomfort or give rise to ulceration of the skin, and in these patients skeletal-traction from a tibial pin is better—but adhesive strapping is usually good enough so long as it is used properly. Three inch (7.6 cm) wide, non-extensile

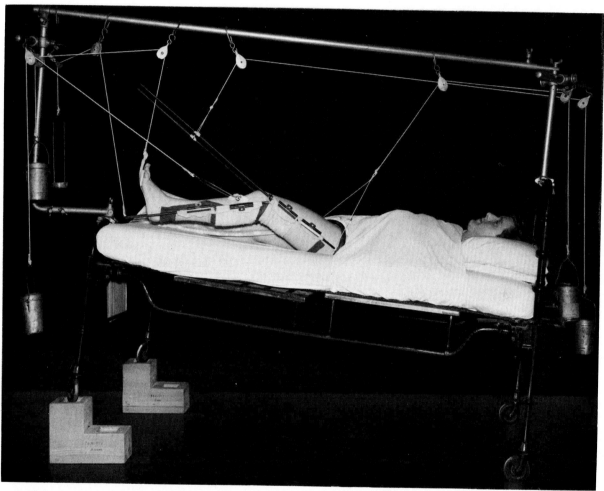

Fig 30.5 Balanced traction—suspended splint. Fracture of the shaft of the femur treated by balanced traction from a skeletal pin in the upper end of the tibia, the Thomas splint with Pearson flexed-knee attachment being suspended by pulleys and weights, thus permitting mobilisation of the knee joint while the traction on the fractured femur is still maintained.

adhesive traction tapes are applied, one on each side of the limb from just above the ankle to the mid-thigh. The outer strip should be centred slightly behind the mid-line of the limb, the inner strip slightly in front, so that when the tapes are fixed to the crossbar at the lower end of the splint the tendency for the limb to roll into external rotation is controlled. The strapping must not be allowed to adhere to the skin over the malleoli, which should be protected with a thin layer of felt. The traction strapping must never be bound to the limb by spiral turns of adhesive strapping because this always causes pressure sores (Fig 30.3). Day after day, as the strapping is pulled, it must tend to slide down the limb, and over a period of six or eight weeks it may slide as much as 2 inches

(5.1 cm). The encircling bandages must be constantly watched to make sure that they are not cutting into the front of the ankle, over the tendo-Achillis, or the crest of the tibia, or in the region of the knee joint. It is particularly important to protect the neck of the fibula from pressure; a tight strand of bandage can be sufficient to produce a paralysis of the external popliteal nerve. The longitudinal strips of traction strapping should be bound in position only with soft encircling bandage which does not adhere to it. After some weeks it may be necessary to replace the adhesive strapping and apply new traction tapes; but there should really be no difficulty in avoiding pressure sores.

Other methods of skin-traction. Where the skin condition is unsatisfactory for the use of adhesive strapping and where conditions such as osteoporosis or infection prevent the use of skeletal-traction, it is sometimes possible to obtain sufficient traction by using tapes incorporated in an Unna's paste bandage applied to the lower leg. Where only light traction is required 'Ventfoam' rubber strips applied directly to the skin and held there by soft bandaging may be satisfactory.

Skeletal-traction. When the skin is injured or ulcerated, when it is atrophic and inelastic, or on the few occasions when a very heavy pull is needed, skeletal-traction should be used. A Steinmann pin, or one of its threaded variants, is driven through the tibia in the region of the tubercle and a U-shaped stirrup applied from which a cord is attached to a suspended weight. On theoretical grounds it might seem more logical to insert such a pin through the lower end of the femur, but pins driven into the bone at this level have been found to increase the tendency to adhesion formation within the suprapatellar pouch and to aggravate stiffness of the knee. Wherever a pin may be inserted there is always some danger of low-grade infection of the track of the pin, and this is more serious if it is in the supracondylar region than if it is in the upper end of the tibia.

When inserting the pin there must be every precaution of aseptic surgery including meticulous cleaning of the skin, preparation with antiseptics, and non-touch technique by the surgeon, who is fully masked, gowned and gloved. A short stab incision is made at the level of the tibial tubercle 1 inch (2.5 cm) behind the lateral side of the crest. A Steinmann pin, mounted rigidly in its holder, is thrust through the bone at right angles to the long axis of the limb in the coronal plane, and sterile gauze dressings are applied over the ends of the pin and bandaged lightly with a 3 inch (7.6 cm) crepe bandage. A U-shaped stirrup is then slipped over the projecting ends of the pin with a suitable length of cord attached, a weight of about 10 lb (4.5 kg) being suspended from the cord. It is better to use stout Steinmann pins rather than thin Kirschner wires; and of course the more rigidly the pin or wire is fixed in the bone, the less danger there is of infection of the track. In an attempt to prevent side-to-side movement some surgeons prefer a pin which is threaded in the part which engages one tibial cortex (Denham pin (see Fig 14.31, p. 303)). This requires more care in the insertion than the simple Steinmann pin in order to make sure that the threads engage in cortical bone, and is often easier to introduce using a hand drill. If a smooth surface Steinmann's pin is used side-to-side movement can be prevented by putting metal collars on either exposed

ends of the pin and protecting them from pressing on the skin by felt washers (see Fig 14.30, p. 302).

Reduction of the fracture and application of the splint. A general anaesthetic with relaxant is preferable. However, local anaesthesia can be used if necessary because usually the fragments are not impacted, and it is easy to inject about 20 ml of 1 per cent lignocaine (plain) into the fracture-haematoma. Throughout the time that the surgeon is applying skin-traction or inserting a skeletal-traction pin, an assistant should hold the foot, pulling strongly and steadily upon the limb so that it can be moved and raised without injury to the soft tissues from sharp fragments of bone. When overriding of the fragments has been corrected by traction and the fragments have been replaced in apposition by direct pressure of the surgeon's hands, the ring of the splint is guided over the limb, which is supported on strips of bandage slung between the side bars of the splint, the normal anterior curve of the femur being maintained by a pad of wool behind the popliteal space and the back of the femoral condyles. The slings should be tight enough to keep two-thirds of the thigh in front of the side bars of the splint and only one-third behind, and the slings should be padded with a length of cotton wool or Gamgee dressing. The knee joint should be in a position of slight flexion; it should never be allowed to hyperextend, not only because this may cause backward bowing of the fragments at the site of fracture but also because it tends to stretch the posterior ligaments of the knee joint, perhaps even causing genu recurvatum and certainly increasing the tendency to stiffness of the joint. (The correct amount of knee bend and anterior bowing of the thigh can sometimes be more easily achieved by bending the Thomas splint into about 15 degrees of flexion at the level of the knee). When reduction has been achieved and the limb is secure in traction in the Thomas splint, suitable local splintage can be applied to correct any lateral angulation, using gutter splints, plaster slabs or pressure pads bandaged to the opposite side bar of the splint.

Methods of traction. A distinction should be made between fixed traction and balanced or sliding traction. In children where fixed traction alone can be used adhesive straps are attached firmly to the end of the Thomas splint with as much tension as is needed. They are checked, and if necessary tightened, at least once a day. In adults the counter-thrust of the splint in the region of the ischium must be reduced by fixing the lower end of the splint to the foot of the bed which is raised (Fig 30.2), or better still by attaching a weight to the end of the splint (combined fixed and balanced traction) (Fig 30.4). In balanced traction the cord attached to the strapping or skeletal pin is passed directly over a pulley at the foot of the bed to a weight of about 10 lb (4.5 kg) suspended from it and the foot of the bed elevated to give counter-traction. The choice between fixed traction with weights on the end of the splint and balanced traction is largely a matter of preference (Figs 30.4 and 30.5). Satisfactory results can be achieved by each of these methods. By suspending the splint with weights both techniques allow the patient to raise himself in bed and to move with freedom without disturbing the position of the fractured bone, but balanced traction offers the advantage of allowing earlier mobilisation of the knee joint. The arrangements of cords, pulleys and weights necessary for suspension shown in Figures 30.4 and 30.5 are commonly used, but there are alternatives which are satisfactory (see Chapter 14).

Other methods of suspension traction. The methods of fixed or balanced traction from skin-tapes or skeletal pins already described are adequate for most fractures of the femoral shaft, but other systems of traction may sometimes be preferred (Figs 30.6 to 30.12).

Fisk traction.[3] This method of treating fractures of the femoral shaft does not differ basically from the technique of skeletal tibial traction in a balanced Thomas splint with a Pearson flexed-knee attachment as illustrated in Figure 30.5, but the splintage is more simplified and makes it possible for a still greater range of knee movement at an even earlier stage of treatment. Fisk rightly decided that if there was to be a Pearson knee-flexion attachment to a Thomas splint, the lower half of the bars of the Thomas splint no longer served any useful purpose—and so he cut them off. From the sawn ends, just above the level of the knee, he attached suspension cords passing over a

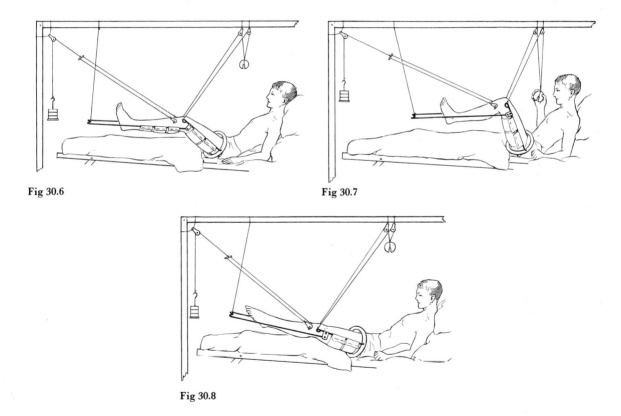

Fig 30.6

Fig 30.7

Fig 30.8

Fig 30.6 to 30.8 Fisk traction for fractures of the shaft of the femur. In this method a Thomas splint is used with a Pearson flexed-knee attachment and skeletal-traction from a tibial pin. The lower part of the bars of the Thomas splint, being no longer needed are sawn off. The idea of Fisk was that in this way the knee joint could be mobilised from the beginning. There is considerable doubt as to whether it is a good idea immediately after the fracture. When the shaft of the femur is fractured the limb should be rested for a few weeks—and this means that the knee joint should be rested. It is a useful technique, however, in the later stages of treatment.

pulley to a 4 lb (1.8 kg) weight near the head of the bed which the patient could seize and pull, thus adding his own active flexion exercises of the hip and knee joints even to the right angle, while still depending on the continuous traction of about 10 lb (4.5 kg) from a skeletal pin in the upper end of the tibia (Figs 30.6 to 30.8). Whether it is right to encourage such vigorous movement over so wide a range at so early a stage of treatment is still open to doubt. In most young and adult patients (provided there is no intra-articular injury) it does not matter in the least that the knee joint is immobilised for several months; a full range of movement will always be regained— it just takes a little longer. But there are more elderly patients whose arthritic knee joints may suffer from a long period of immobilisation, or others whose knees have been injured at the time that the femur was fractured and in whom earlier movement may be advisable. This compromise of firm fixation of the limb in a sawn-off Thomas splint with Pearson attachment and early active mobilisation of the knee is certainly to be preferred to the abandon of those who advocate Hamilton Russell or Perkins traction, or tibial skeletal-traction on a Bohler-Braun frame, where every principle of immobilisation is discarded and traction alone is relied upon to maintain length and alignment.

Hamilton-Russell traction.[4] In this method, not advised for the routine treatment of femoral shaft fractures, no splint is used. A system of cords, pulleys and weights as shown in Figure 30.9 permits the limb to be supported in a comfortable position with continuous traction in the line of the femur. By flexing the knee and supporting the limb on pillows it is claimed that both angulation and rotatory deformity are controlled. By reason of the mechanical advantage afforded by two pulleys at the foot, the longitudinal pull is theoretically twice as great as the upward pull,

and the resultant traction is in an axis of 30 degrees to the horizontal, roughly in the line of the femur. Russell traction is certainly comfortable for the patient, and it facilitates the exercise of a wide range of movement at the hip and knee joints; but it is not recommended as a routine treatment for fractures of the shaft of the femur because it makes no real provision at all for protection of the bone fragments against backward sagging or lateral angulation and requires very careful attention to prevent those deformities occurring. However, this method of treatment sometimes has a place in the management of femoral fractures in patients with multiple injuries, and is also a useful method of traction in the later stages of treatment.

Perkins traction.[5, 6] This method of treatment popularised by the St Thomas school gives even less support for the fracture than Russell traction and depends entirely upon skeletal-traction over pillows to control deformity. This can be modified to give more support by applying a sling under the fracture (Fig 30.10). Immediate knee bending is carried out using a split bed, even to the extent of allowing angulation at the fracture site, and it is difficult to believe that such a regime will not lead to mal-union in a number of cases. With up to 30 lb (13.5 kg) of traction recommended it is not surprising that consolidation cannot be expected before six months have elapsed.[5] These disadvantages would seem to outweigh the rather doubtful advantage of immediate knee movement. However, the method can be recommended for its simplicity with little or no

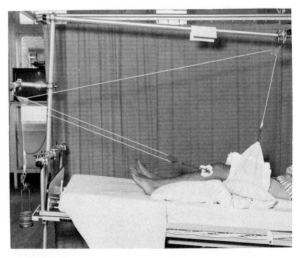

Fig 30.10 Modified Perkins traction. Skeletal-traction is applied to the femoral fracture by a pin through the tibia. No splint is used but the fracture site is supported by a sling.

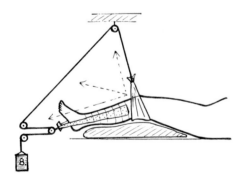

Fig 30.9 Hamilton Russell traction. This technique has often succeeded, but it is not recommended for fractures of the femur.

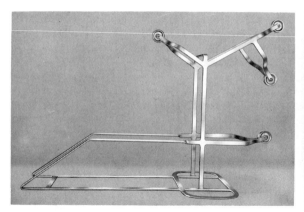

Fig 30.11 Bohler-Braun splint with four pulleys for fractures of the shaft of the femur.

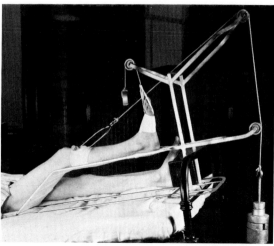

Fig 30.12 Braun splint with tibial traction. This is not recommended for fractures of the femur.

maintenance, and is useful in centres where Thomas splints are scarce and good nursing supervision is at a premium.

Skeletal-traction in a Bohler-Braun splint. Under the influence of Bohler of Austria many surgeons in European countries have treated fractures of the femur by tibial skeletal-traction with the limb resting on a Braun splint (Figs 30.11 and 30.12). This method of treatment offers no control of alignment of the fragments except by the degree of traction. Very commonly the weight needed to maintain proper alignment causes distraction, whereas if the weight is reduced sufficiently to keep the fragments in contact it is not enough to prevent angulation. But the worst defect of this type of splint when used to treat femoral shaft fractures is that the heavy frame is virtually part of the bed and cannot move with the patient during nursing procedures, with a result that constant angulation must occur at the fracture site every time the patient is lifted on to a bedpan. The distraction and movement so produced can be one of the causes of delayed union or non-union of fractures of the femoral shaft. The only merit to be claimed for such treatment of fractures of the shaft of the femur is that it is easy and often succeeds. But it is certainly not comfortable and may be responsible for some cases of delayed union. Ideal though the splint may be for the treatment of certain cases of fractures of the tibia it is not recommended for the routine treatment of femoral shaft fractures.

Bryant traction for fractures of the femur in infants.[7] The problem of treating fractures of the shaft of the femur in newborn babies and young infants is of course quite different and much more simple. At this young age the growth of bone is so vigorous that fractures of the shaft of the femur always unite, and the power of bone-modelling is such that even right-angled deformity soon grows straight. All that is needed is to support both lower limbs by skin-traction to an overhead beam for a few weeks, with the knees straight and the hips flexed to a right angle (Fig 30.13). Although this is a perfectly safe method of treatment in young infants it has been shown that after the age of $2\frac{1}{2}$ to 3 years there is an increasing danger of vascular complications—often occurring in the normal limb.[8] The blood pressure is insufficient to maintain an adequate peripheral circulation when the limbs of the larger child are elevated to a right angle. This, combined with the effect of hyperextension of the knee on the popliteal vessels, may result in severe peripheral ischaemia. Modification of the method for use in older children, with the limbs less elevated and the knees flexed, has been suggested,[9] and there are reports of the traction being used in children up to 6 years of age,[10] but it is probably wiser to use more orthodox splintage in children over the age of $2\frac{1}{2}$ years.

Day-by-day management of fractures of the femur in traction in a Thomas splint. Close supervision is essential, and no matter whether skin-traction or skeletal-traction is used, a constant watch must be maintained day-by-day, and in the early stages, even hour-by-hour. When skin-traction is used, care must be taken to see that pressure sores are not developing behind the heel, over the malleoli, or

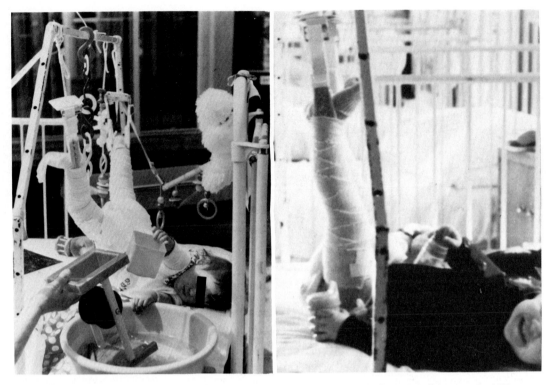

Fig 30.13 Bryant's traction. This is an efficient and simple method of immobilisation of the femoral shaft fractures in children up to the age of 2½ to 3 years. Despite the contortions performed by some children in this traction (left) the femoral fractures treated by this method unite without residual deformity.

in the region of the knee. When tibial skeletal-traction is used, there must be care to see that the pin is not sliding or rotating in its track and that infection of the pin track is not developing. The canvas slings upon which the limb is resting should be tightened regularly. Adjustment of padding is often required in order to maintain perfect alignment of the fragments. The position of the pulleys and the amount of weight must be constantly under review so that the splint remains in its correct position with the limb properly balanced. The ring of the splint should not cause excessive pressure in the groin, and it should not slide too far down the thigh. There is usually need to adjust the pulleys every day.

Control of alignment. The position of the fragments should be checked radiographically, at first every few days and then every few weeks. Forward or backward angulation should be corrected by reducing or increasing the tightness of the slings and supporting padding; and lateral angulation is to be controlled by correcting the position of the side splints or plaster slabs, by the alteration of pressure pads on the side bars of the Thomas splint, or by adjustment of bandages round the thigh and over the inner or outer stems of the splint. The effects of rotatory deformity must not be forgotten, particularly in fractures of the upper third of the bone. It is natural to put the leg up in the Thomas splint in neutral rotation with the patella pointing directly forwards. But sometimes the upper fragment is externally rotated and abducted and if the lower fragment is in neutral rotation the lateral angulation at the fracture site will be increased. It will be corrected by fully externally rotating the Thomas splint (Figs 30.14 to 30.16).

Danger of excessive traction. Within the first few hours of injury, when the fracture is being reduced, heavy traction may sometimes be needed to correct overriding and secure apposition of the fragments; but after reduction has been achieved the weight should be reduced to about 10 lb (4.5 kg), or sometimes in heavily built men with powerful muscles to 15 lb (6.8 kg)—thus just balancing the tendency to muscle

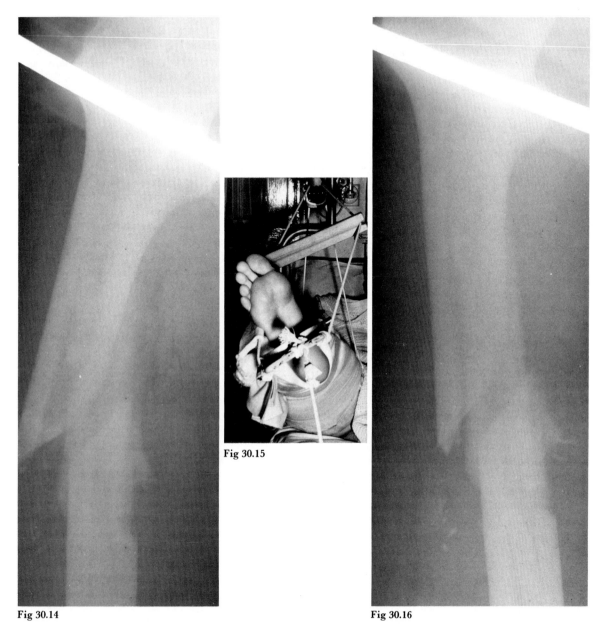

Fig 30.15

Fig 30.14

Fig 30.16

Figs 30.14 to 30.16 In femoral fractures abduction and external rotation of the upper fragment can produce marked lateral angulation (Fig 30.14). This will not be corrected by abducting the limb alone. The splint and lower leg require to be externally rotated in the abducted position in order to correct the angulation (Fig 30.15 and 30.16).

retraction. If heavy traction is maintained for a long time there is danger of distraction of the fragments with serious delay in the rate of union.

Muscle exercises. Throughout the period of immobilisation the patient must practise toe and foot exercises. For five minutes every hour of the day the

foot should be dorsi-flexed, everted, inverted and circumducted. Clawing of the toes should be prevented by regular flexion exercises. After three or four days the patient is encouraged to start gentle quadriceps drill. Between five and seven weeks, provided union of the fracture is beginning to be firm, active movements of the knee joint may be encouraged, these relatively early movements being safer when the fracture is high in the shaft but more dangerous when the fracture is low. The application of a cast brace, a change to Russell traction, or the use of a Pearson knee piece may be valuable in encouraging knee movement at this stage.

Estimating union of the fracture. Immobilisation of the fracture in some form or another is usually necessary for at least 12 weeks, after which time clinical and radiographic tests of the degree of union are made. The clinical criteria of union are firmness at the fracture site and freedom from pain when angulatory strains are applied. It is to be emphasised that these clinical tests are often misleading, and before unprotected weight-bearing can be regarded as safe there should also be radiographic evidence of union. Charnley has observed that a rapid return of knee movement always indicates that sound bony union is progressing, and conversely, slow return of knee movement is suggestive of delayed union.[11] It will of course be recognised that young callus, not yet fully ossified, does not always show on X-ray films. If there is uncertainty about the soundness of union it is better to defer unprotected weight-bearing until the evidence is more sure, meanwhile continuing active non-weight-bearing exercises in bed and perhaps allowing the patient to be up and around with crutches, but without taking full weight on the injured limb. If the patient is already up in a cast brace this should not be discarded before he is able to take weight through the brace on the affected leg for 10 seconds.[12]

Delayed union. If at the twelfth or fourteenth week the evidence of union is still unsure—perhaps by reason of earlier distraction, imperfect immobilisation or infection—a decision must be made whether to continue immobilisation either in a Thomas splint, or in a cast brace, even to the sixteenth or twentieth weeks, or whether to advise a bone graft. Certainly the fracture may unite if the support is maintained, but it will take a very long time. Slow union is not in itself an indication for operative intervention. Many years ago in a survey of 142 fractures of the shaft of the femur treated conservatively[13] Watson-Jones and Coltart found no single case of non-union. There had been delaying factors in many of them—interrupted immobilisation, excessive traction, distraction, infection and so on—but they all united in the end, though many needed to be immobilised for much longer than the usual period of 12 weeks, and a few as long as 24 weeks or even more. However, it is this very long period of immobilisation which may force the hand of the surgeon towards a bone grafting procedure,

particularly in cases where there is a wide fracture gap—probably due to interposition of soft tissues.

The use of a walking caliper splint. A patient with a very comminuted fracture of the femoral shaft, such as is illustrated in Figure 30.1, may be clinically united after 12 weeks on a Thomas splint, but unsafe to allow to weight-bear without support. A walking caliper can be useful in the management of such a case and preferable to a cast brace because it can be removed at night and for bathing. However, there is a difference of opinion among surgeons as to whether the so-called 'weight-relieving caliper' does prevent weight from being transmitted through the site of fracture and whether it offers real protection from angulatory or rotatory stresses. Late bowing or even refracture of unsoundly united fractures has occurred when walking in a caliper splint has been permitted. If union is sound, a caliper splint is clearly unnecessary and the patient can rapidly progress from crutch walking to full weight-bearing. However, if union is not sound, a caliper splint is often safer than crutch walking because it gives some protection if the patient should slip or fall, particularly if there is limited knee movement. A caliper splint need not hinder mobilisation of the knee joint since exercises can be continued in recumbency free of the splint.

Cast bracing for femoral shaft fractures. There is little doubt that the cast brace applied correctly and used intelligently, can shorten considerably the period of hospitalisation required for conservative treatment of femoral shaft fractures. The first brace used for fracture care was described as long ago as 1855 by H H Smith.[14] He designed a prosthetic device with a waist-band, ischial support and thigh laces which could be used for ununited fractures of the femur. Much to his surprise all the fractures so treated united within a few months. The modern version is the cast brace which has been popularised by Vert Mooney and his colleagues in Los Angeles.[15] It uses the principle of the bucket top thigh piece used in artificial limbs, to give support to the fracture without loss of alignment. The steps in its application are illustrated in Figures 30.17 to 30.20. Careful attention to detail is important if this method is to be successful. The plaster must be tightly fitting and this is achieved by lining the whole length of the limb with either an elastic stocking or double thickness 'Tubigrip'. Over the knee a length of stockinet is drawn to allow the edges of the plaster above the hinge to be tidied up later. The cast is put on in two sections, the thigh portion being moulded into the quadrilateral shape of an artificial limb socket either by using a predetermined plastic socket and moulding the plaster of Paris around it,[16] or by moulding the plaster as it sets, using pieces of board clamped on side to side and antero-posteriorly to prevent the mould becoming too loose.[17] The front of the knee (centre of patella) must be marked as a reference point to help in locating the hinge axis (Fig 30.18). The axis of the knee joint is sometimes surprisingly difficult to find but it is roughly two-thirds posterior from the front of the mid-point of the patella. By using an adjustable transverse bar temporarily screwed into the hinges on either side it is possible to locate the hinges fairly accurately at the site of the expected axis. The knee hinges should be clamped into place using Jubilee clips (Fig 30.19) and the range of movement tested. The plaster can then be completed (Fig 30.20) and the patient allowed to weight-bear on it in 48 hours. Some surgeons favour the idea of a waist-band made of thick tape which is attached to the thigh portion of the cast and taken around the waist just above the iliac crest. It is said that this helps to control any tendency for the fracture to angulate laterally.

The timing of application. There is some variation amongst surgeons as to exactly when they apply a cast brace; but there is general agreement that the method is not suitable for treatment in the very early stages when the fracture is still painful and freely mobile, although recent reports suggest that by using traction on the cast brace whenever the patient is recumbent it is possible to apply a modified appliance within a few days of the fracture.[18] This method, however, requires an adjustable thigh piece which must be tightened as swelling subsides and needs intelligent cooperation on the part of the patient if complications are to be avoided. Significant shortening of more than 2 cm has been reported when comminuted fractures are braced before two weeks[18a], but it has been suggested that by three weeks the reactionary swelling of the thigh has subsided and that it is safe to apply a cast brace, and provided it is put on under traction and a hip hinge is used to keep the leg abducted 20°, pressure generated under the upper part of the cast should prevent further shortening.[18b] Fractures treated thus when they are still unstable have certainly been shown to unite, but only in the most expert hands, and sometimes at the expense of a persisting varus deformity at the fracture site. On the whole earlier application is not recommended. Mostly, the cast is applied at five to six weeks after the accident when the bones feel both stable and firm, and when there is *no pain on stressing the fracture,* or on active straight leg raising.[10]

Removal. The average length of time in a cast brace is five to six weeks; the time of removal depending partly upon the X-ray appearance, but mainly on the clinical findings, particularly the ability to take full body weight through the plaster without discomfort.

TREATMENT OF FRACTURES OF THE UPPER AND MIDDLE THIRD OF THE FEMORAL SHAFT BY INTRA-MEDULLARY NAILING

'To nail or not to nail'. There are a number of orthopaedic surgeons who are so obsessed with the idea of quick restoration of knee movement after fracture of the femoral shaft that they advise intramedullary nailing for fractures which would heal perfectly satisfactorily with conservative treatment. Figures for the speed of recovery with regard to ambulation, knee movement and time spent in hospital are quoted in support of this regime.[19, 20, 21] Undoubtedly these figures are impressive when compared with the classical conservative regime of immobilisation on a Thomas splint for three months; but the advent of the cast brace has drastically shortened the period of hospitalisation and therefore lessens the attraction of operative treatment. Also, the advantages of operation must be weighed against the fact that uncomplicated fractures of the femur treated conservatively are not associated with permanent knee stiffness and that intramedullary nailing is not without its complications. In one series alone there was a 14 per cent error in operative technique,[22] emphasising that this is an operation which requires skill and considerable attention to detail. Infection after nailing can have disastrous consequences, and bent and broken nails associated with delayed union are by no means unknown. Thus the advantages must be weighed against the disadvantages, and the operation must not be advised routinely, particularly if theatre asepsis is in doubt, or the necessary surgical skill is not available. Above all, the surgeon must never be influenced in his decision by demands from the patient to have a quick 'cure' of his fracture (see Figs 30.21 and 30.22).

History. This method of treatment was first introduced in 1916 by Hey Groves,[23, 24] who used three types of steel nail. He tried solid nails, nails cruciform in section, and hollow steel tubes with perforations which he drove from the trochanter across the fracture site. He also introduced the method of retrograde nailing—exposing the fracture, driving a nail into the medulla of the proximal fragment and then, after correcting displacement of the fracture, hammering the nail back into the distal fragment; which is the technique used by most surgeons today when carrying out open nailing. For some years this method of internal fixation lay in abeyance, but it was revived and developed in the circumstances of war by Kuntscher,[25] who was faced with the emergencies of rapid evacuation of patients from bombed hospitals and the difficulties of nursing. He used intramedullary nails of trefoil section for nearly all femoral fractures and achieved great success—although it should be admitted that his admirable enthusiasm led him to use the technique very widely, possibly too widely. One of the advantages of the trefoil shape has been emphasised by Bohler—that is its ability to be compressed a little during insertion, thereby improving the intramedullary fixation. None of the solid nails has this property and should be regarded more as intramedullary bolts.[26] Although many variants of the nail have been devised the basic clover leaf type still remains the most popular, and the methods of introduction almost unchanged since the original descriptions by Hey Groves almost 70 years ago.

Indications. Although it has already been emphasised that the routine treatment of fractures of the femoral shaft should preferably be by traction in a Thomas splint followed by cast bracing, it must be recalled that there is sometimes difficulty in the management of fractures of this bone by the conservative method. The strong abductor muscles of the hip which are attached to the trochanteric region on the lateral side, and the strong adductor muscles which are inserted into the lower shaft of the femur on the medial side, account for a powerful deforming influence which always tends to angulate the fragments. There may be difficulty in controlling this deformity by conservative treatment, and in fractures with slow union, even though perfect alignment may have been maintained for 12 or 14 weeks, the imbalance of muscle power often causes late deformity with outward bowing. For this reason there is much to be said for treating displaced fractures of the upper and middle parts of the shaft of the femur by intramedullary nailing, the nail remaining in the bone and thus protecting it from angulation until the fracture is solidly united. Figures 30.23 to 30.28 show examples of suitably chosen cases.

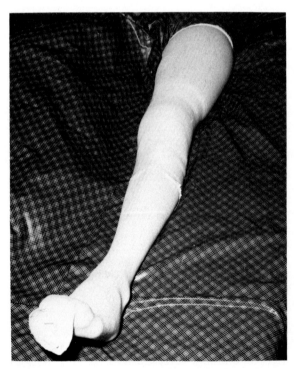

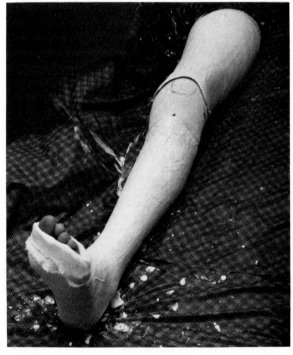

Fig 30.17

Fig 30.18

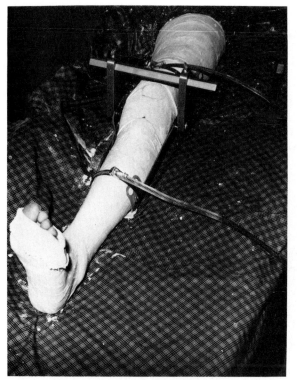

Fig 30.19

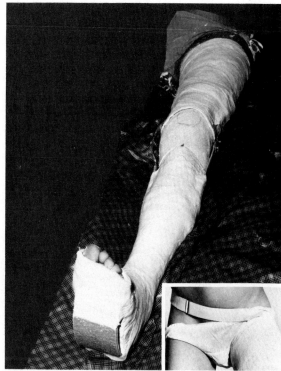

Fig 30.20

Figs 30.17 to 30.20 The application of a cast brace for femoral shaft fracture. The limb is covered with a double thickness of 'tubigrip' which must extend from the toes to the inguinal ligament (Fig 30.17). The patient is asked to pull this up to the iliac crest during the application of the cast. The knee is covered with an extra layer of stockinette which is later turned back to protect the plaster edges around the knee. The thigh piece is applied first and moulded very firmly with a quadrilateral socket. A plastic former may be used for this but a satisfactory moulding can be obtained by hand moulding. The below knee section extends to the patella tendon insertion which should be marked on the stockinette (Fig 30.18). Figure 30.19 shows the method of lining up the hinges using a cross-piece anchoring the hinges and Jubilee clips to hold them while the knee movement is tested. It is important to mark in the position of the patella and the estimated position of the knee axis (2/3 back from mid-patella). The final appearance of the cast brace is shown in Figure 30.20. Note that no pelvic strap has been used in this case (but see inset).

There are also fractures which cannot be reduced and in which, despite repeated manipulation, a wide gap remains between the fracture surfaces. These are certain indications of soft tissue interposition between the bone ends and such fractures require early open reduction.

It must also be remembered that in some circumstances it may be impossible to maintain even a simple fracture in a reasonable position by conservative methods—for example, severe head injury with marked muscle spasm; traumatic paraplegia requiring constant turning of the patient to avoid sores; multiple injuries necessitating neutralisation of the femoral fracture; sometimes in femoral shaft fractures complicated by a major vascular injury requiring arterial surgery. Such cases demand the use of internal fixation, and the Kuntscher nail often provides the most satisfactory method. In fractures with a large segmental third fragment the treatment of choice is open reduction and Kuntscher nailing, sometimes with additional wiring of fragments (see Figs 16.11 to 16.14 and 30.77 and 30.78). Fractures of the mid-shaft of the femur with patellar fractures on the same side should also be treated by nailing.

Fractures of the lower third of femur. It will have been noted that all preceding indications for intramedullary nailing specify fractures in the upper and middle shaft of the bone. Lower third fractures are unsuitable for this type of fixation unless special techniques are used. These fractures should be fixed with a heavy duty plate, or a knee blade plate.

Technique—open or closed nailing? Kuntscher and many of his surgical colleagues in Europe have

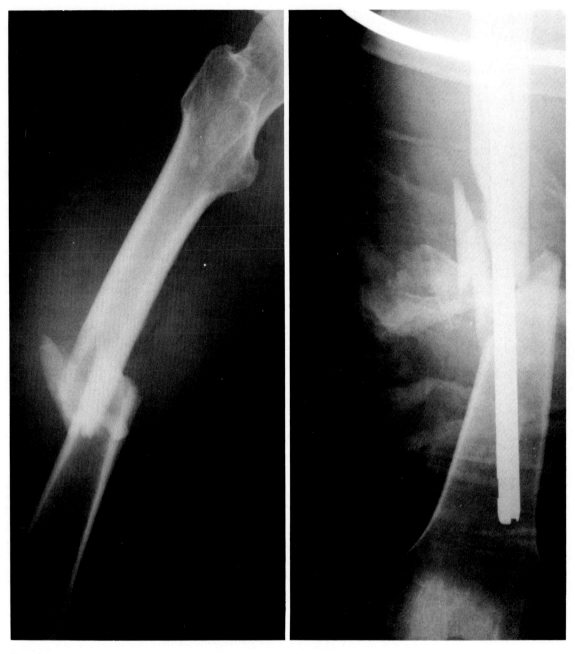

Fig. 30.21   Fig 30.22

Figs 30.21 and 30.22 This patient was knocked over by a car and sustained a closed transverse fracture of the shaft of his right femur (Fig 30.21). He ran a one man business as a riding instructor and persuaded his surgeon to perform a Kuntscher nailing in order to reduce his period of incapacity. The nailing was difficult and produced further comminution; the fixation was inadequate and the fracture became infected (Fig 30.22). This necessitated many operations and a further two years of treatment before the fracture finally healed.

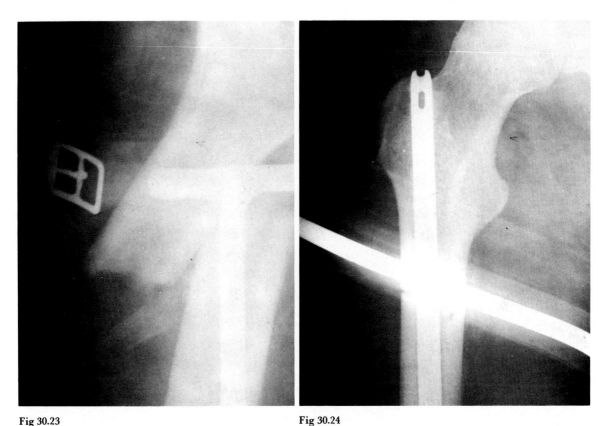

Fig 30.23   **Fig 30.24**

Figs 30.23 and 30.24 A displaced transverse fracture through the upper third of the femur is an ideal case for an intramedullary nail.

always advocated the technique of closed intramedullary nailing under X-ray control, the fracture itself never being exposed thereby greatly reducing the risk of infection.[27] All papers advising this technique emphasise the low infection rate compared with the open operation.[19, 21, 28]

The introduction of the image intensifier and the special traction tables which go with it have greatly increased the scope of the closed operation and it is doubtful if this method of nailing should be attempted in the absence of these facilities. Ability to reduce the fracture is all important and this may require some patience and considerable expertise. Kuntscher advised a few days on a distraction apparatus to bring the limb out to the correct length before embarking on a closed operation. The technique is not easy for the occasional operator, and if it is to be used at all it is probably wiser to nail all femoral shaft fractures routinely. This again brings up the question of the choice between conservative and operative methods of fracture treatment and the surgeon should choose

the method best suited to his local circumstances. For those who choose to treat most of the fractures conservatively and only require to nail an occasional irreducible fracture the open method of retrograde nailing is the operation of choice despite the higher risk of infection. Whereas those surgeons working in units where long stay beds are expensive and at a premium, and who have the necessary equipment, operating conditions and expertise will, of necessity, be forced into routine of operative management and should make themselves expert in the closed method. Whichever method is used, whether conservative or operative the end result will be the same and this should not influence the choice of treatment in the uncomplicated fracture.

Closed nailing. The patient must be set up on the traction table on his side with the affected leg uppermost (Fig 30.29). Traction can be applied to the leg and if necessary side-to-side correction obtained by wooden rings applied around the fracture

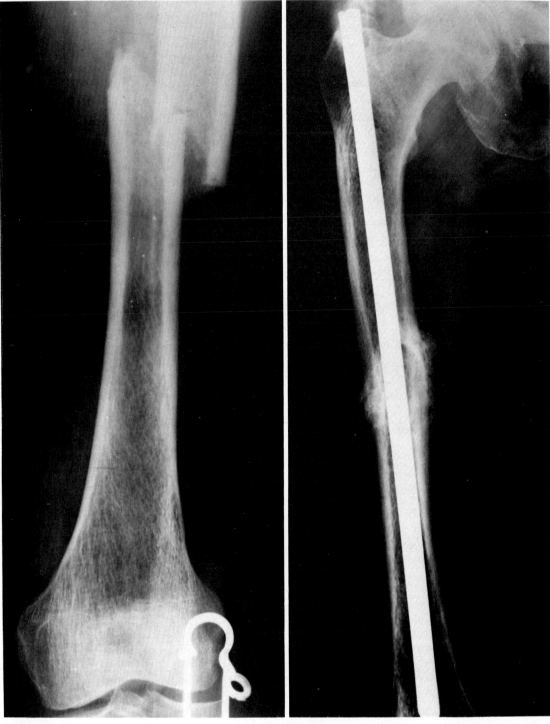

Fig 30.25   **Fig 30.26**

Figs 30.25 and 30.26 Oblique fracture of the upper middle third of the shaft of the femur treated by open exposure of the fracture and intramedullary nailing.

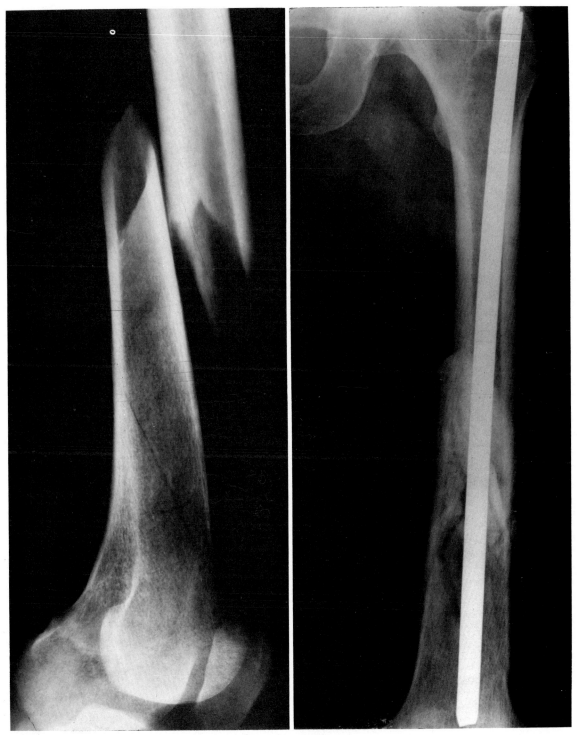

Fig 30.27   **Fig 30.28**

Figs 30.27 and 30.28 Spiral fracture of the lower middle third of the shaft of the femur treated by operative exposure of the fracture with intramedullary nailing. This fracture is nearing the lower limit for this type of fixation.

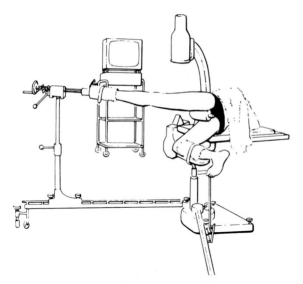

Fig 30.29 Closed nailing of femoral shaft fractures. The patient is placed on the operating table with the fractured leg uppermost. With a T-piece perineal post traction can be applied to the fracture with the hip flexed to expose the trochanteric region for operation. In this way the C arm of the image intensifier has access for X-rays in two planes at right angles. (Reproduced by kind permission of the Editor of the *Journal of Bone and Joint Surgery* and from the authors A. G. Rothwell and C. B. Fitzpatrick from their paper in the *Journal of Bone and Joint Surgery* (1978) 60-B, 504 (Ref 21).)

site.[26] The fracture must be capable of reduction by manipulation, and an almost perfect reduction is essential.[21] With the aid of an image intensifier a guide-wire is driven from the trochanter through the medulla of the proximal fragment into the distal fragment, the intramedullary cavity reamed using a cannulated mechanical reamer, and a nail threaded down the guide-wire. If it is intended to ream the medulla to receive a large diameter Kuntscher nail, motorised reamers with detachable heads increasing in $\frac{1}{2}$ mm sizes must be available, used with a guide-wire which has a bulbous end to allow easy removal of a broken or detached reamer. This technique has its complications. In the first place even with an image intensifier, there is danger to the hands of the surgeon and his assistants from X-ray exposure; and in the second place there is danger to the patient, because where reduction has been difficult nails have sometimes been driven through the cortex of the bone, or have failed to engage the medulla of the distal fragment, and have damaged the femoral artery. These disasters from blind intramedullary nailing although mainly the result of faulty operative technique, lack of the correct instrumentation and poor selection of patients do offset some of the objections to open operation as far as infection is concerned. Much nonsense has been written about the ease of the closed nailing technique, indicating to the unwary that it is applicable to virtually any fracture. This is just not true! Blind nailing is not an easy operation and should only be carried out in a fully equipped theatre by dexterous surgeons fully conversant with the technique; and then only on carefully selected cases.

Open nailing. Many surgeons in Britain prefer the technique of open exposure of the fracture, so that the fragments can be seen as they are replaced with accuracy and the nail can be seen as it passes from the proximal to the distal fragment, without the worry of obtaining an accurate manipulative reduction and the obscurity of X-ray screening which can sometimes be misleading.

Even when the fractured fragments are exposed and intramedullary nailing is performed under direct visual control, there are still possibilities of serious trouble.[22, 29, 30] It is obvious that if too slender a nail is introduced the fixation with be imperfect; but it is sometimes better to err on the side of safety than to take the still greater risk of driving in a nail that is too wide for the medulla of the femur—for that may even be disastrous. When this has been attempted the femur has sometimes been shattered. Still more often, when too wide a nail was hammered in, it became so tight that it could neither be driven further nor extracted. There is one record of surgical heroism throughout a four-hour operation in which a nail has been driven through the site of fracture of a femur into the proximal fragment and, having seized, was with very great difficulty removed. Then a guide-wire that was driven up from the site of the fracture to the trochanter, together with a nail that was driven over it from the trochanter into the femur, where both became inextricably fixed—and the surgeon was then faced with the horrible situation of a length of guide-wire protruding from the wound of the thigh, and more than half a nail protruding through the incision over the hip, neither being capable of removal. Even worse situations have been reported where surgeons have been rash enough to use another intramedullary nail in an attempt to disimpact one which is jammed, ending with both nails interlocked within the medulla. A longitudinal saw-cut along the whole length of the bone segment involved may release the nails, but sometimes the projecting ends must be removed with a hacksaw and the operation abandoned. There can be no doubt about the merit of this operative procedure, but at the same time there is also no doubt that unless the technique is followed with attention to every detail there are many sources of grave complications.

Operative technique of open nailing. The fracture should be exposed through a postero-lateral incision (see Chapter 15). The first step is to clear the bone surfaces and, if the fracture is more than a few weeks old, to remove the young callus and open the medulla of the fragments. A series of long-handled drills, or preferably motorised reamers corresponding to the diameter of the nails are then passed, first proximally, and then distally, to ream the medullary cavity to the exact diameter of the nail chosen to be used. Motorised reamer heads increase in diameter by steps of 0.5 mm and it is important to have the full range of heads if the medullary cavity is to be increased to take a large diameter nail. Motorised reamers must not be used without a guide-wire and the end of the wire must be bulbous, so that if a reamer bit becomes detached or stuck it can be extracted by pulling on the guide. The smallest reamer is introduced into the proximal fragment. If it passes too easily the next size is introduced and so on until the medulla is reamed to take the selected nail with a comfortable push fit. Now the diameter of nail is known, all that is needed is to estimate the exact length. From the site of fracture a guide-wire is passed down the medulla of the distal fragment and resistance is felt when it approaches the articular surface of the knee; by measurement of the length of wire outside the bone the exact length from the site of fracture is known. The guide-wire is then passed up the medulla of the proximal fragment until resistance is felt against the trochanter, so that once again there can be an exact measurement of the length. Thus is known the required length of nail—but we must add that the length finally chosen should be about 1 inch (2.5 cm) less than the measurements shown by the exploration of the guide-wire because it is far better that the point of the nail should lie about 1 inch (2.5 cm) short of the femoral articular surfaces than that it should be so long as to penetrate the joint surface. The diameter of the nail to be used will vary with the size of the medullary cavity, the function expected of the limb, and the personal views of the surgeon. In a young athletic adult a simple transverse fracture in the upper third of the bone may have an intramedullary cavity at the fracture as small as 6–7 mm,[31]* although

more usually a 9 to 10 mm nail can be passed through the narrow isthmus at this level without reaming. Whenever possible in the adult a nail of not less than 11 mm in diameter should be used. If unsupported weight-bearing is to be permitted, or there is a particularly large medullary cavity, nails up to 18 mm in diameter have been advised.[32] However most patients with a fracture in the mid-shaft are well stabilised by an 11 mm nail[21] and can safely be allowed to partially weight-bear with crutches. This size of nail is usually easy to pass and carries with it few of the technical hazards sometimes associated with the use of a very large nail.

The guide-wire driven from the fractured surface into the proximal fragment is then pushed still further, and short incision is made over the point of its emergence from the trochanter. A flanged nail, already known to be correct in both width and length, is driven from the trochanter over the guide-wire until the point is seen to appear at the site of fracture. The guide-wire is removed. An alternative method of inserting the nail is to introduce it retrograde from the fractured site, hammering it through the trochanter until it appears in the buttock where it can be exposed through a short incision. If the nail is used in this way it is important for it to have extractor holes at either end—just in case it becomes impacted in the first stage.* The fragments are then held in correct apposition and alignment while the nail is driven into the distal fragment. Great care must be taken to see that alignment is maintained with complete accuracy throughout this last step, because otherwise the point of the nail can easily be driven through the cortex of the distal fragment, especially when the bone is porotic or the femoral shaft is unusually bowed, such as in Paget's disease.

With the precaution of using a preliminary drill or reamer by which to determine the width of the medullary canal, there should no longer be disasters from the seizing of nails in a narrow femoral medullary canal. At the same time it is always wise to have a sterilised hacksaw on the table so that if by chance the nail does become locked it can be cut off.

After-treatment. Many surgeons rely entirely on the intramedullary fixation of a nail and allow patients to move freely in bed and to resume weight-bearing activity within a few days of operation. This can only succeed if very large diameter nails are inserted, with

* This problem may be further compounded by an abnormal amount of natural bowing of the femoral shaft. This should be carefully assessed before operation, for no amount of reaming with the usual flexible instruments will straighten out the medullary canal to take a large, close fitting nail. In these circumstances a narrow diameter nail is the only solution.

* The nail should advance steadily with each blow of the hammer and it is wise to stop immediately if there is no sign of progression.[31, 33] Kuntscher has observed that an increase in pitch as the hammer is applied to the nail can be an indication that the nail is impacting.[27]

all their attendant dangers. If a small nail (11 mm and below) is used the internal fixation must be protected by resting on a Thomas splint for about four weeks, and follow this up by crutch walking (partially weight-bearing) for three months.

Sometimes a cast brace or walking caliper can be used when the patient starts to weight-bear; for example, in a comminuted fracture of the middle third of the bone. The nail should never need to be removed until after the fracture is radiographically united, and its protection from late angulation in cases of delayed union is of course invaluable. There may be discomfort in the trochanteric region at the site of the head of the nail when the patient lies in bed on one side, but this is seldom important. Sometimes, however, the nail migrates proximally and comes to project in the gluteal region, or occasionally a large bursa may form over it. If this occurs before union the nail should be re-impacted, but if the union is solid the nail should be removed. In one interesting case a distinguished scientist complained of discomfort in the region of his nailed femur whenever he took a glass of sherry, or any other form of alcohol. This effect disappeared immediately once the nail was removed. This symptom, recorded by a shrewd observer, is of interest in relation to the deep pain that is known to be caused by alcohol in patients with lymphadenomatous glands, but it seems to be exceptional and in the ordinary way it is quite safe to leave an intramedullary nail in position indefinitely, although it is usual to remove it as soon as the fracture is soundly consolidated; most surgeons would advise removal at one year.

Complications. These have already been discussed in Chapter 16. The problem of infection after Kuntscher nailing is discussed in Chapter 17.

Operative treatment of lower third fractures of the femoral shaft. Because the medullary cavity of the femur widens out in its lower third, orthodox Kuntscher nailing gives inefficient fixation of a fracture at the junction of the middle and lower thirds of the femoral shaft (Fig 30.30). If conservative treatment cannot be used for this fracture it should be stabilised with a heavy-duty plate of the A.O. pattern, contoured to the lower third of the femur, and screwed to its lateral aspect. Retrograde intramedullary nailing using two heavy Rush nails passing upwards in a curve from the femoral condyles gives tolerably good fixation, but the nails are difficult to insert (see Fig 30.52). Good results in the lower third fracture have been reported from the use of the Enders long flexible intramedullary nails which have been used in the same way, introduced through the femoral condyles

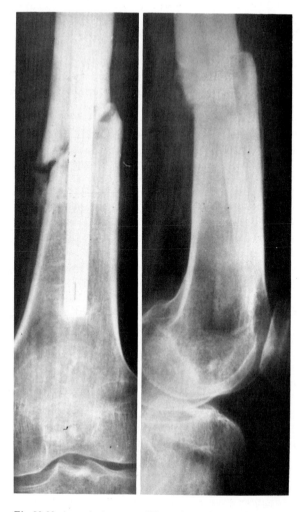

Fig 30.30 An orthodox type of Kuntscher nail is unsuitable for the fixation of fractures at the junction of the middle and lower third of the femur. Figure 30.30 shows the inadequate hold the nail has on the lower fragment and how easily movement can occur.

and passed up the femur to cross in an 'Eiffel Tower' formation.[34] It is, however, been pointed out that this method is unsuitable for lower third fractures which extend distally into the supracondylar area, because the nails may become loose or cause additional fracture.[34a] Satisfactory fixation from the Hansen-Street nail has also been reported in lower thigh fractures.[35] This appliance consists of a diamond nail split in its lower third to give two diverging prongs. These are claimed to give improved fixation by spreading out in the wide medulla of the lower end of the femur. Whichever method of fixation is used assisted knee movement in recumbency should be started early even while the patient is still resting in a Thomas splint. This is important in order to avoid adhesions forming in the quadriceps at the site of incision—a frequent cause of knee stiffness after open reduction of a fracture at this level.

Kuntscher nail variants. There are now many varieties of intramedullary nail, and many variations of the original surgical technique have been devised. A number of these modifications have been made, sometimes at the expense of operative safety, in order to improve the fixation (particularly rotation), and to allow early weight-bearing. The original Kuntscher nail design depends upon its irregular cross-section and its open compressible slot for establishing firm intramedullary contact, thereby minimising rotatory instability. Solid nails with an angular cross-section, such as the Schneider four-flange nail,[36] have been designed to further stabilise rotation; and more recently a fluted nail with eight cutting flanges to engage the endosteal cortex has been devised.[37] Huckstep[38] has designed a solid nail, now made out of titanium, perforated with screw holes at intervals of 1.5 cms. This is inserted by the open method and by using a special jig it is possible to locate the position of the holes in the nail and insert cross screws. Not only is rotation controlled by this technique, but also compression can be applied to the fracture (see Fig 30.31). Halloran[39] has also used a

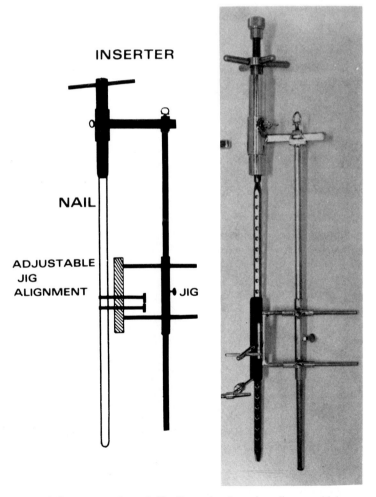

INSERTER

NAIL

ADJUSTABLE
JIG
ALIGNMENT   JIG

Fig 30.31 Huckstep's intramedullary compression nail. The illustration shows the nail set up with its compression apparatus and jig for locating the screw holes in the nail. Screws are inserted into the lower fragment and across the nail by using the drill jig which has been previously located by a pin inserted into a screw hole at the fracture site. The fracture is then compressed and screws applied to the upper fragment to maintain this compression.

solid nail with a figure-of-eight cross-section perforated by slots at regular intervals for the insertion of cross screws, or the addition of one or even double plates. It is difficult to believe that such a combination of two plates and an intramedullary nail would not have a deleterious effect upon the blood supply to the bone. A simple variation of the open nailing technique to control rotation, which can be used with the standard type of Kuntscher nail, is to insert four screws (two above and two below the fracture) through the outer cortex of sufficient length to engage the open trough of the nail which must, of course, be inserted facing laterally (Fig 30.32).* It is claimed that torque investigations show that this simple additional fixation greatly increases the torsional strength of the fracture.[40] Also, the nail can still be extracted without the need to expose the femoral shaft—a distinct advantage over the perforated nails of Halloran or Huckstep.

* I am indebted to Mr Paul Moynagh for permission to publish Figure 30.32B showing the application of the side plate to prevent rotation after Kuntscher nailing. The technique does not lock the nail, which can be extracted later without interfering with the plate. (J.N.W.)

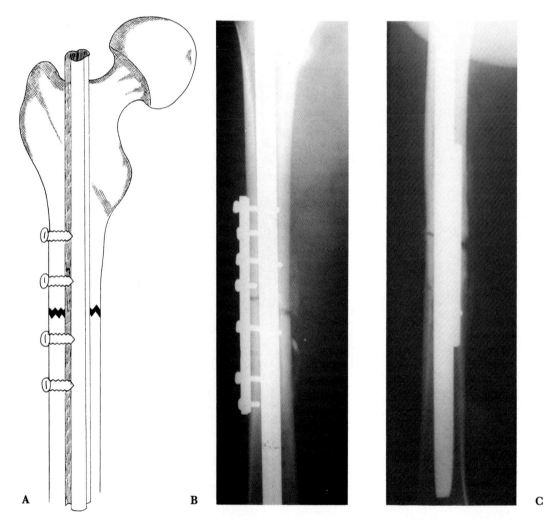

A   **B**   **C**

Fig 30.32 This diagrammatic drawing illustrates how screws can be used in combination with a Kuntscher nail to improve its rotational stability (Fig 30.32A). Two screws are inserted above the fracture and two below and made to engage the open slot of the nail, which must be introduced with its open side facing laterally. A. O. cortical screws of the correct length are the right size at their tip to lock against the open flange of the nail and prevent rotation at the fracture site. It is sometimes necessary to use a plate, placing the screws either against the nail, or to one side of it (Fig 30.32B)(Operation by Mr. Paul Moynagh).

Although all of these variations may have a place in the management of certain complicated fractures, they add nothing to the speed of recovery in a simple fracture and do not allow earlier weight-bearing. Indeed it is salutary to be reminded that the average sized nail of 13 mm diameter has a bending strength three times less than that of the intact femur.[37] Thus, unless very large diameter nails are used, full weight-bearing on the fractured limb should not be permitted until bone union is shown to be well advanced. Therefore, there is much to be said for retaining the nail form first advised by Kuntscher, certainly for the treatment of uncomplicated fractures. Oversize nails and fluted nails may lead to jamming, and the other devices all complicate what is a relatively simple procedure. Their use should be limited to the problem fracture where very rigid fixation is essential. The clover leaf nail, inserted by the standard closed or open technique, is still the most satisfactory form of internal fixation for the properly selected femoral shaft fracture.

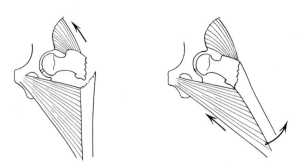

Fig 30.33 Stable subtrochanteric or intertrochanteric fracture. The proximal fragment of a subtrochanteric fracture is fully abducted by the gluteal muscles, and the shaft of the femur must be similarly abducted. If the fracture is oblique from the outer side inwards and downwards, reduction is stable.

SUBTROCHANTERIC FRACTURES OF THE FEMUR

Fractures of the upper shaft of the femur near the level of the trochanter show a typical displacement: The upper fragment is flexed due to spasm of the iliopsoas and abducted. The strong gluteal muscles which are the abductors of the hip, are attached to the proximal fragment in the region of the greater trochanter, whereas the adductor muscles are inserted below the level of the fracture, so that the proximal fragment is sometimes abducted even as much as 45 degrees. The first principle of conservative treatment of these fractures is to immobilise the limb in a similar position of at least 45 degrees of abduction. Often the fracture is oblique, with the obliquity from above downwards and medially, but sometimes the obliquity is in the opposite direction from above downwards and laterally (Figs 30.33 and 30.34). The first type of oblique fracture is stable when the limb is abducted, and it is enough to immobilise the limb in wide abduction. The second type is not stable unless there is continuous traction (Figs 30.35 and 30.36), because the shaft of the femur tends to be pulled upwards, and there is therefore a danger of non-union (Fig 30.37). But sometimes the fracture is transverse and this is particularly common in pathological fractures from secondary tumour deposit. The displacement is similar to that of the oblique fracture, but because of the transverse element it is difficult to reduce or hold

reduced, and the majority of these fractures require internal fixation.

Conservative management—Treatment in traction. This is only applicable to oblique fractures and fractures in children. No matter what the plane of obliquity may be, subtrochanteric fractures can often be treated successfully in Hamilton Russell traction with skin- or skeletal-traction, and with the limb in abduction and flexion so that the pull of the gluteal and iliopsoas muscles is neutralised. It is fortunate that the fracture lies so close to a ball-and-socket-joint that perfect accuracy of alignment is not essential and minor degrees of angulation cause little or no functional disability.

Immobilisation in a plaster spica. In children subtrochanteric fractures of the stable type, oblique from above downwards and medially, can be treated quite safely in a plaster spica with the lower limb in

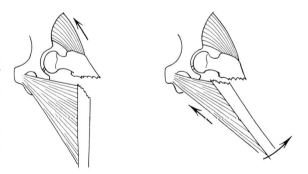

Fig 30.34 Unstable subtrochanteric fracture. If the fracture is oblique in the opposite direction and runs from the outer side *upwards* and inwards, reduction is unstable. Retraction of the adductors causes complete loss of apposition and there is danger of non-union. Continuous traction or internal fixation is essential.

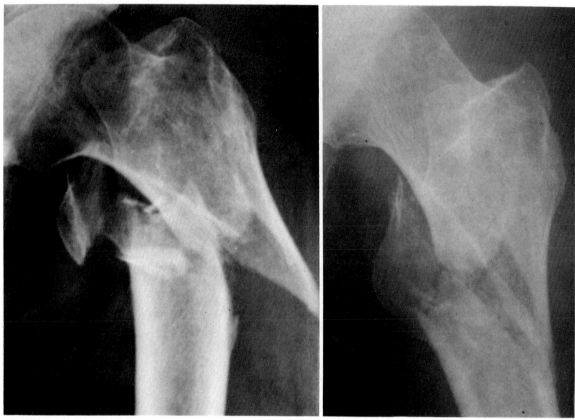

Fig 30.35   Fig 30.36

Figs 30.35 and 30.36 Subtrochanteric fracture of femur before reduction and after immobilisation in abduction with continuous traction. The obliquity of the fracture is such that it is an unstable injury. Continuous traction is needed.

abduction and some flexion. It is wise to use a double spica including both hip joints in order to control movements of the pelvis. It must be emphasised, however, that this treatment should not be used for fractures oblique in the opposite direction, because the upper end of the shaft of the femur may then displace under the capsule of the hip joint and the surfaces of the fragment are often sealed by overlying muscles so that there may be failure of union. Also, it may be impossible even in a child to reduce the fracture to an acceptable position, and open reduction and fixation with a Rush nail must be undertaken (Figs 30.38 and 30.39).

Operative treatment of subtrochanteric fractures. Although some oblique fractures will reduce into good alignment with traction in abduction and can be treated conservatively; others may remain widely displaced, particularly if there is a large

butterfly fragment, and these may require open reduction and internal fixation. Also, the transverse type of subtrochanteric fracture in adults can rarely be reduced satisfactorily by traction and more often than not requires open reduction. In addition, it must be remembered that this fracture is fairly common in the elderly who tolerate badly long periods of traction; and that, also, it is not an infrequent site for a pathological fracture, occurring in a debilitated cancer patient and demanding internal fixation as the only hope of stabilising the bone.

There are three methods at our disposal for the internal fixation of these difficult fractures. These are: (1) simple intramedullary nailing; (2) pin and plate fixation; and (3) combined intramedullary nail and femoral neck pin (the so-called 'signal arm' fixation).

Simple intramedullary nailing (Figs 30.40 and 30.41). This is carried out by the usual technique for open nailing. It is a very suitable fixation for the

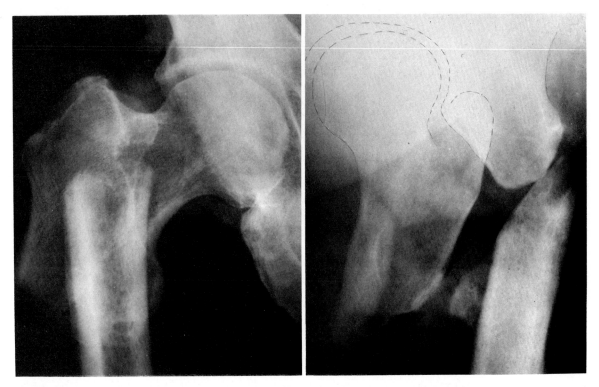

Fig 30.37 Unstable type of subtrochanteric fracture of the femur treated without sufficient traction and fixation, so that there was non-union from inadequate apposition and muscle interposition. There should have been traction by Hamilton Russell in abduction, or alternatively internal fixation with an intramedullary nail.

uncomplicated transverse fracture and is a relatively easy operation even when the fragments are widely displaced, provided it is combined with open reduction. The medullary canal, which is equally narrow in both proximal and distal fragments, must be reamed to give a good push fit of the nail against cortical bone on both sides of the fracture. Because the fracture is so proximal, and because the intramedullary nail will fit equally well into both fragments, it is unnecessary to use a long nail and it can terminate at the junction of the mid and lower thirds of the femur. Stability may be so firm that splintage can be discarded and patient allowed up partially weight-bearing with crutches very soon after the operation. However, if there is any doubt about the rigidity of the fixation it is wise to maintain the limb in Hamilton Russell traction and defer crutch walking for at least a few weeks.

Pin and plate fixation (Figs 30.42 to 30.45). This is suitable for the high oblique subtrochanteric or intertrochanteric fracture. There is a wide variety of appliances which can be used. The easiest to insert is

the two piece pin and plate, but the strain on the connecting bolt can be very high and the appliance may fail, particularly if early walking is allowed (Fig 30.45). A fixed angle pin and plate is favoured by some, but it has the disadvantage of being a little more difficult to introduce. Both forms of fixation require a plate with not less than seven holes, and in the long spiral fracture a 12 hole plate is advisable (see Figs 29.148 and 29.149). But so great are the forces involved that even with this degree of plate fixation disasters can occur and the plate break or cut out of the bone (Figs 30.44 and 30.45).

'Signal arm' fixation. The failure of the pin and plate to hold the unstable subtrochanteric fracture, and the desire to produce a form of stabilisation which would allow direct weight-bearing, has lead to the development of the 'signal arm' device. Basically, this appliance consists of an intramedullary nail fixing the fracture, with an interlocking cervical pin to give extra fixation in the upper fragment. There are two varieties (Figs 30.46 and 30.47): in one type (the Kuntscher-Y nail[41]) the cervical nail is inserted first

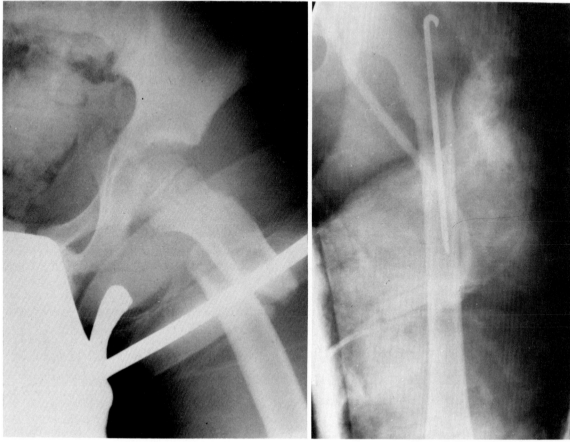

Fig 30.38   **Fig 30.39**

Figs 30.38 and 30.39 This 4-year-old child sustained a subtrochanteric fracture of the left femur when he was knocked over by a car. Traction in abduction failed to reduce the fracture (Fig 30.38). It was a simple operation to restore the alignment by open reduction and the insertion of a Rush nail (Fig 30.39). The fracture united in good position after six weeks immobilisation in a double hip spica.

and then a straight Kuntscher nail is driven through a hole in the base of the cervical component (Fig 30.46; in the other (Zickel nail[42]) the intramedullary part is put in first, and a triflange cervical nail passed through it (Fig 30.47). Both methods require a full exposure of the fracture and the area at the tip of the great trochanter. The medullary cavity of both fragments must be reamed to the size of the intramedullary component. Of the two devices the Zickel nail is slightly easier to introduce and will be described in more detail; although it must be made clear that there can be difficulties with both methods, and in comminuted fractures it is sometimes necessary to supplement the fixation with circlage wires or Partridge bands (see Chapter 16).

Zickel nail technique. The operation is carried out on the ordinary theatre table with the patient turned slightly to the opposite side with a sandbag under the buttock. A curved postero-lateral incision gives good access to the tip of the greater trochanter. The fracture is exposed and a test reduction is carried out. The medullary cavity of the distal fragment is reamed out as far as the cortex and the appropriate Zickel nail tried for a comfortable push fit. The upper fragment is then prepared. The tip of the trochanter is osteotomised to allow access for the larger reamers, for this fragment must be reamed out to 17 mm in order to accommodate the large upper end of the nail. The fracture is again reduced and firmly stabilised with bone clamps. The Zickel nail is then

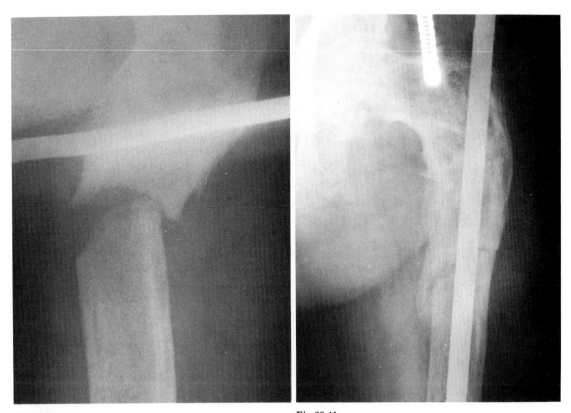

Fig 30.40   **Fig 30.41**

Figs 30.40 and 30.41 This subtrochanteric fracture occurred in an elderly pedestrian and resulted from being struck by a car. It could not be reduced satisfactorily by traction. Simple Kuntscher nailing (Fig 30.41) not only stabilised the injury but allowed the patient to be ambulant very shortly after the accident. Her fracture was united within three months.

assembled with the tunnel locator gauge secured to the top by the driver. With the hip adducted the nail is then driven across the fracture, allowing about 15 degrees of anteversion in relation to the top of the operating table. With the nail in place the femoral neck fixation must be inserted. A guide-wire is passed through the tunnel locator. This allows the guide-wire and triflange nail to find the hole in the intramedullary nail and then pass up the femoral neck. Once the right length of nail has been introduced it can be locked into position by a set screw.

The commonest cause of comminution of one or other fragment is inefficient reaming. In one series of 84 patients there were four with shattered trochanters requiring wire repair. This complication should not occur if the proper reaming tools are readily available.

SUPRACONDYLAR AND CONDYLAR FRACTURES OF THE FEMUR

Few injuries present more difficult problems than those sometimes associated with supracondylar and condylar fractures of the femur. The small supracondylar fragment is nearly always displaced backwards and to one or other side, and may be held flexed by the unopposed action of the gastrocnemius (Fig 30.48). If this tilting is not corrected and the fracture unites with backward angulation, a serious disability arises from genu recurvatum. Another and even more urgent hazard may arise from the vulnerable position of the popliteal artery, which is sometimes damaged at the time of injury, or may at a later stage be compressed by the sharp margin of the lower fragment of the femur. Also, Figure 30.48 shows in diagrammatic form the close association of the suprapatellar structures to the fracture site, which may lead to extra-articular adhesions and gross limitation of knee-flexion—yet another hazard of the supracondylar injury. If the fracture communicates with the joint as a T-shaped injury, or if one or other condyle is fractured separately, the problem of management becomes even more difficult; for in addition to the limited movement of the knee from extra-articular adhesions there will be stiffness from the intra-articular injury, compounded by possible irregularity of the joint surfaces from displaced condylar fragments.

Supracondylar fracture. Efficient control of the distal fragment in this fracture has exercised the ingenuity of generations of surgeons. Although it may be possible to improve the position by manual manipulation and traction, there is always difficulty in maintaining the reduction, and the long period of

immobilisation previously advised to allow the fracture to unite when treated conservatively led to further problems with knee stiffness. It was originally taught that if the fracture was immobilised with traction in a Thomas splint the muscle spasm would subside and tilting of the lower fragment would be corrected—but unfortunately this is not true. Bohler advocated the use of a Braun frame with the angle of the splint behind the fracture and not behind the knee joint—but again the results were often disappointing. The fracture must be first reduced and traction only used to maintain that reduction. The difficulties with reduction and the increased risk of knee stiffness has led many surgeons to abandon conservative treatment completely in favour of operative reduction and internal fixation. This point of view is understandable but should be discouraged. Internal fixation of these fractures is not an easy exercise and there are hazards associated with the method.[43] In addition, the intelligent use of conserv-

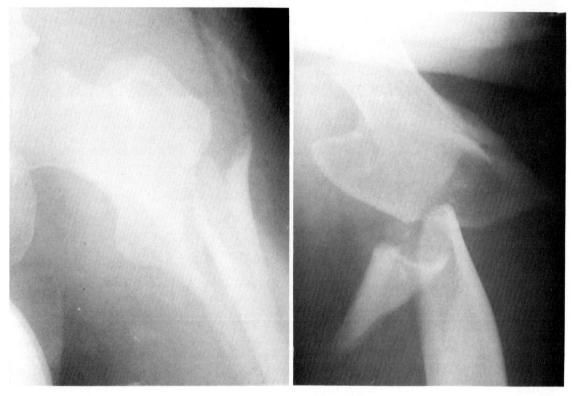

Fig 30.42

Figs 30.42 and 30.43 This patient who was struck by a car on the motorway sustained a severely comminuted spiral subtrochanteric fracture of the right femur (Fig 30.42). At the same time he had compound fractures of both tibiae. The subtrochanteric fracture was neutralised by the insertion of a pin and plate (Fig 30.43) and was united by three months. This method of fixation was very successful in this case because, by virtue of his other injuries, he remained at rest in bed for several months, and the fracture was not exposed to any weight-bearing stress until it was soundly united.

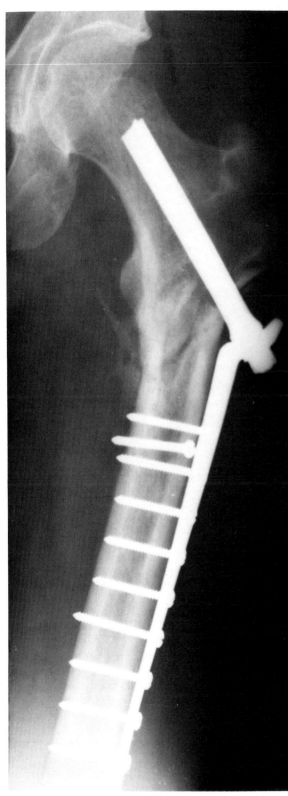

ative treatment, avoiding the long periods of complete immobilisation used in the past and employing a cast brace early on in treatment, can produce results at least equivalent to those obtained by operation. Both methods must be considered.

Conservative treatment. There are, of course, many supracondylar fractures of the femur which can be easily reduced into an acceptable position and controlled quite adequately on a straight, or slightly bent, Thomas splint with fixed traction. There is little advantage in using a Braun frame, and a distinct disadvantage in that it immobilises the knee in more flexion than is necessary and may produce a tiresome extension lag which persists long after the fracture has united. Very gentle knee movement and quadriceps exercises should be encouraged early, the patient being told to attempt to bend the knee a little within the limits of the bandages and traction a few days after the fracture. Charnley[44] has pointed out that as these fractures are usually in cancellous bone they become firm very rapidly provided they are allowed to impact, and he recommends 'controlled collapse' of the fracture using only skin-traction to the end of the Thomas splint and no weights. Although knee movement should be started early there must be time allowed for the fracture to become reasonably firm before the physiotherapist is permitted to give periods of assisted knee mobilisation with the traction detached. The time to make this change will depend upon the surgeon's assessment of the fracture stability and the patient's confidence in making small knee movements while still on the splint, but it is unlikely to be possible before three weeks and may be several weeks longer. It is important for the patient to rest on the splint between treatments and for the physiotherapist to concentrate as much on maintaining full extension as in restoring flexion. By four to five weeks there should be sufficient union to allow the application of a hinged cast brace in which the patient can weight-bear, first with elbow crutches and then unaided. This should be worn until there is radiological evidence of bony consolidation and the patient is able to take full weight on the cast brace without discomfort for 10 seconds.[12] For many years Perkins[45] and the Thomas's school have advocated immediate knee movement using skeletal-traction through the upper tibia with only the support of a pillow behind the knee and calf. Although excellent results are reported from the use of this method it has the danger of producing a troublesome extension lag at the knee and has only its simplicity to commend it over the Thomas splint method.

Operative treatment. Sometimes displacement of the

Fig 30.43

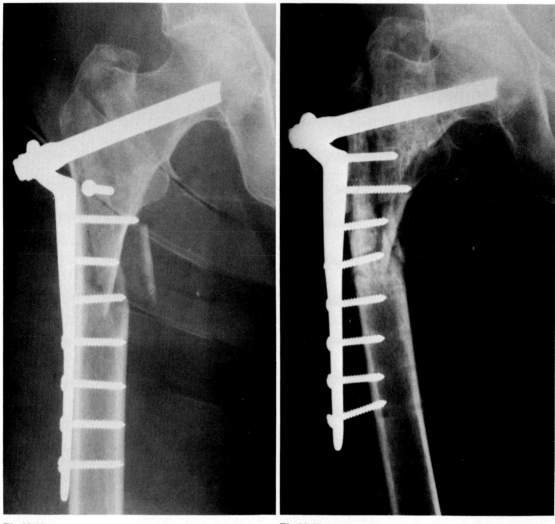

Fig 30.44   **Fig 30.45**

Figs 30.44 and 30.45 The subtrochanteric fracture shown in Figure 30.44 seemed to be adequately fixed, and as the patient was of very light build she was allowed to take a steadying weight with crutches. The fixation disintegrated under the strain (Fig 30.45).

small distal fragment of the femur by unopposed pull of the gastrocnemius is so pronounced that the simple technique of closed reduction and traction in a Thomas splint does not reduce the fracture into an acceptable position. These are the really difficult fractures to treat conservatively, and although some success has been claimed from combining longitudinal skeletal-traction to the tibia with vertical pin traction to the supracondylar fragment (diagrammatically represented in Figure 30.49), this method has all the

hazards of inserting traction pins through the supracondylar region, and in addition requires fixation in plaster. It is probably better in these cases which cannot be controlled by simple traction in a Thomas splint to undertake operative reduction with internal fixation. There is also a place for elective surgery in supracondylar fractures of the elderly who may deteriorate because of the enforced recumbency associated with treatment on traction, and who would find it difficult to tolerate the inconvenience of a cast

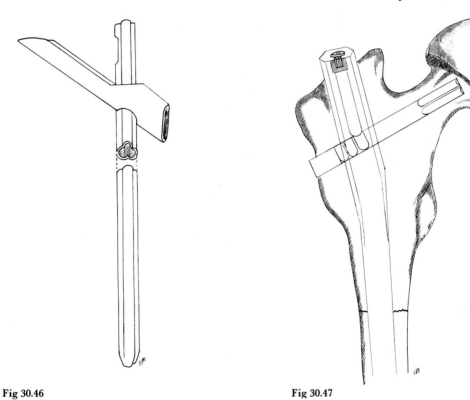

Fig 30.46   Fig 30.47

Figs 30.46 and 30.47 Illustration of the 'signal arm' method of fixation of subtrochanteric fractures. Figure 30.46 illustrates the Kuntscher-Y nail method, where an ordinary K nail is passed through a hole in a large semi-cylindrical cervical nail. The Zickel nail is shown in Figure 30.47. This is a solid cobalt-chrome-molybdenum nail with an enlarged upper end through which is passed a triflange cervical nail which is introduced by using a special jig attached to the top of the nail.

brace. But it must be remembered also that in these patients the fracture will have occurred through osteoporotic bone, and under these circumstances even the most rigid of internal fixation may have to be supplemented by some form of external splintage.[43] It is sometimes possible to strengthen the hold of the bone screws by using a Gallanaugh high density polyethylene plate on the contralateral cortex and engaging the tips of the screws into this plate (see Chapter 16). Brown and D'Arcy[46] have modified a blade plate for these cases, to provide a transverse compression across the condyles by applying a bolt and a compression washer to the end of the transverse blade (see Fig 30.54). As a general rule internal fixation can be achieved by two methods:* either by inserting two retrograde Rush nails through each

* Some writers[47,48] have advocated an extensive exposure of the front of the knee in order to carry out a meticulous repair of the fracture, using multiple screws in addition to a nail plate. No doubt this method may restore perfect anatomy, but fortunately it is not necessary because equally good results can be obtained by the simpler methods already outlined.

femoral condyle (Figs 30.50 to 30.52), or by using a right angle blade (Fig 30.53). The former method is difficult to carry out—the right point of insertion into the condyle and the correct bend in the nail being very critical, and on the whole it is not an operation to be recommended except occasionally in compound fractures. It is unlikely to succeed where there is osteoporosis and is therefore unsuitable for the elderly. Blade-plate fixation is easy to apply and has the added advantage that the effects of compression can be added to the fixation and the technique can be modified to cope with osteoporotic bone (see Fig 30.54 and Chapter 16). Usually active and passive knee exercises can be started immediately and the patient soon allowed to walk with crutches, partially weight bearing, as soon as the stitches have been removed. Unprotected weight-bearing should not be allowed until there is radiological evidence of bone union.

Condylar fractures of the femur. One or both condyles of the femur may be fractured, the line of injury, of course, extending into the knee joint so that

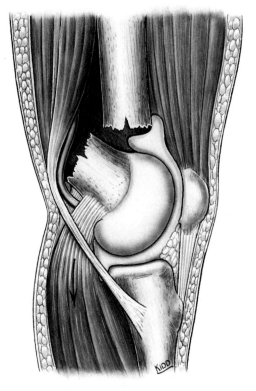

Fig 30.48 The distal fragment of a supracondylar fracture of the femur may be held in the flexed position by the unopposed action of the gastrocnemius muscle. The vulnerable position of the popliteal vessels is clearly shown, as well as the close association of the suprapatellar pouch and extensor mechanism with the fracture site.

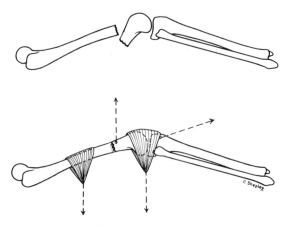

Fig 30.49 The two pin method of reducing a supracondylar facture. Tibial traction is applied to the knee joint slightly flexed. From a pin in the supracondylar fragment, close to the fracture, vertical traction is then applied against the counter-pull of a canvas sling over the front of the knee.

there is a haemarthrosis. If both condyles are separated by a T or Y fracture it is often possible to reduce the displacement by applying traction, with compression of the fragments between the surgeon's hands. For example, an elderly man sustained a fracture of both condyles with considerable displacement. Almost perfect reduction was secured by simple traction and manual compression, the limb then being supported in a Thomas splint with simple skin-traction. An excellent functional result was regained with a good range of movement (Figs 30.56 and 30.57). Provided a good reduction can be obtained by this method, and provided there is no contra-indication to pursuing a conservative regime, nothing will be gained by embarking on operative treatment, except to shorten the period as an in-patient. By following the conservative measures already outlined for the treatment of supracondylar fractures, it should be possible to obtain the same return of function

without submitting the patient to the hazards of open reduction and internal fixation. However, a good result from conservative treatment of these fractures is dependant upon the maintenance of a good reduction. In particular, residual flexion deformity at the fracture site will result in a disabling loss of extension at the knee which can only be corrected by supracondylar osteotomy. The physiotherapist responsible for supervising the early assisted exercises must concentrate as much on maintaining full extension of the knee as in regaining flexion (Fig 30.58).

Operative treatment. It is in single condylar fractures that open reduction and internal fixation are commonly used. One condyle may be fractured as a result of valgus or varus strain, the separated condyle being displaced upwards with resulting genu valgum if the fracture is of the lateral condyle, or genu varum if it involves the medial condyle. Sometimes it is still easy to correct the displacement by traction and direct manipulative compression as in bicondylar fractures. Sometimes, however, there is a rotatory displacement which is difficult to correct. Certainly if manipulative procedures fail to secure perfect replacement there should be no hesitation in exposing the lower end of the femur, replacing the condyle with accuracy and fixing it in position with screws (Fig 30.60) or transcondylar bolt (see Fig 16.18). Cancellous screws should be used in preference to the simple type of bone screw illustrated in Figure 30.60. It is necessary to expose the joint surfaces in order to be sure that

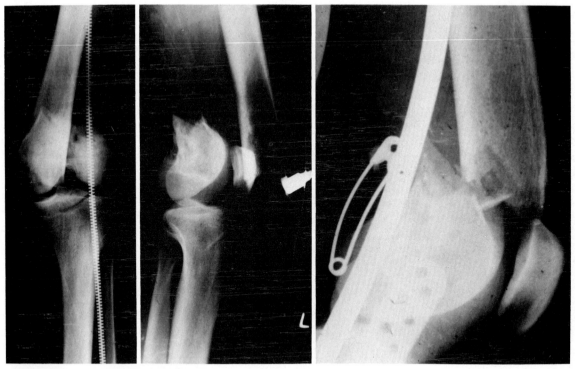

Fig 30.50

Fig 30.51

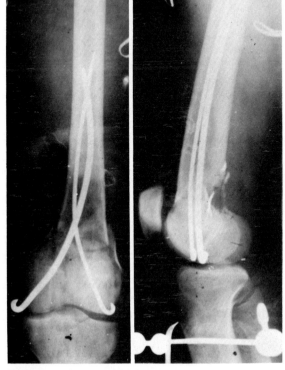

Fig 30.52

Figs 30.50 to 30.52 A compound supracondylar fracture of the femur which could not be reduced satisfactorily by conservative methods (Figs 30.50 and 30.51). Fig 30.52 shows the improvement in position after the insertion of retrograde Rush nails.

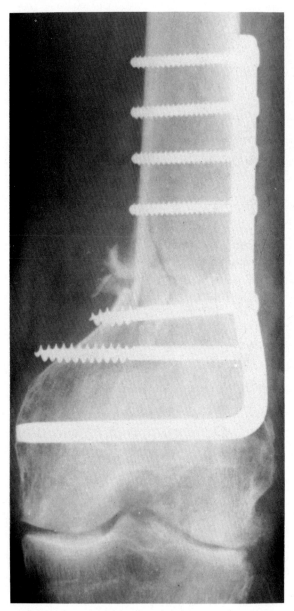

Fig 30.53 A supracondylar fracture of the femur can be fixed very securely with a blade-plate.

exact reposition has been gained and an extensive para-patellar approach gives the most satisfactory access to the fracture, allowing a clear view of the intra-articular reduction. Following operation the limb should be immobilised in a Thomas splint with fixed traction for three weeks to allow the reaction within the knee to subside, quadriceps exercises being encouraged throughout this period. Active and assisted flexion of the knee in recumbency is started in three weeks, the patient being allowed up wearing a weight-relieving caliper at six weeks (or non-weight-bearing on crutches). There should be no direct weight-bearing for three months.

In one unusual case shown in Figures 30.59 and 30.60 the lateral condyle was fractured by direct violence and the patella, being rotated through 90 degrees, was driven edgewise into the femur with its lateral margin forced into the articular surface and splitting off the condyle just as if a blunt chisel had been hammered in. The patella itself was damaged so seriously that it had to be excised. The condylar fragment of the femur, and the other comminuted fragments, were replaced accurately and fixed with screws. The quadriceps tendon was repaired and excellent function was regained.

DISPLACEMENT OF THE LOWER FEMORAL EPIPHYSIS

Epiphyseal separation of the lower end of the femur is classically described as an injury with gross displacement produced by a violent hyper-extension strain, the epiphyseal fragment being tilted forward in front of the femoral shaft and often rotated to one or other side. This severe type of displacement is a rare injury nowadays, and many orthopaedic surgeons in the Western World may see only two or three cases in their professional lifetime. But this was not so in the far off days of horse drawn transport, when the injury could easily be sustained by a child who swung himself up onto a moving vehicle and caught his leg in the spokes of a wheel.[49, 50] The gross hyper-extension and torsional strain submitted to the knee by such an injury—not uncommon a century ago—explains its relatively high incidence and vascular complication rate compared with the injury seen today. At the end of the last century Hutchinson was able to collect 58 children with this injury, half of them having compound fractures and with an amputation rate of 35 per cent:[49] whereas in two recent papers,[50, 51] which together report the results in a total of 54 patients, there were no amputations and only one vascular problem, which was unrelated to the epiphyseal injury.[50]

Typical displacement of the classical injury is shown in Figure 30.61. This injury is much more easy to treat than supracondylar fractures of the femur in adults. All that is needed is to apply traction, and then flex the joint to just beyond the right angle, pressure being applied over the front of the knee so as to push the epiphysis back. The shape of the separated

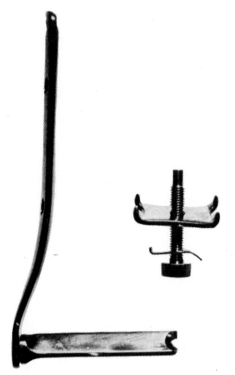

Fig 30.54

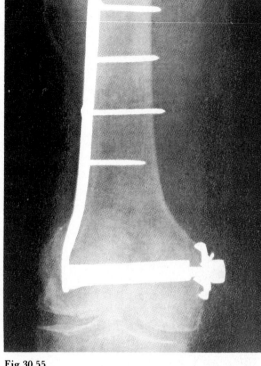

Fig 30.55

Figs 30.54 and 30.55 Brown and D'Arcy's modification of a blade plate for use in osteoporotic supracondylar fractures. The blade part of the device consists of a triflange nail coarsely threaded at either end (Fig 30.54). By using a compression washer on the other side to the main plate it is possible to obtain a very rigid fixation in the condyles of an osteoporotic femur (Fig 30.55). (Reproduced by the kind permission of the Editor of the *Journal of Bone and Joint Surgery* and Mr Austin Brown and Mr J. C. D'Arcy from their paper in the *Journal of Bone and Joint Surgery* (1971) 53-B, 420).

surfaces is such that they fit accurately together, and if the knee joint is immobilised in the flexed position reduction is stable. The limb can be supported for the first three weeks by a plaster slab over the front of the thigh and leg (Fig 30.62). An alternative method of treatment is to use fixed traction on a bent Thomas splint for three weeks with a pad supporting the upper fragment and the knee flexed through about 30 degrees. This is followed by a period in plaster in the same position for a further five weeks.

In many ways this injury is comparable to supracondylar fractures of the humerus in children. The displacement is to be reduced by flexing the joint after traction has been applied—but only after traction has been applied. The flexed position must not be forced because there is such swelling around the joint that fixation in too much flexion may compress the popliteal vessels and endanger the circulation of the limb.

There is particular danger of vascular complication in displacements of the lower femoral epiphysis, exactly as there is in similar injuries of the lower end of the humerus, because the popliteal vessels are stretched over the back of the lower margin of the diaphysis. Injury to the artery may cause vasospasm with ischaemic contracture of the leg and foot. There may even be such a degree of vascular injury as to cause thrombosis of the popliteal vessels with gangrene of the foot. Care must obviously be taken to apply traction before flexing the joint and not to flex the joint too much. If the right-angled position is used, an anterior plaster slab held in place with a crepe bandage should be applied so lightly as to exert no pressure in the popliteal space. After three weeks flexion may be reduced to about 30 degrees and the plaster maintained in this position for up to eight weeks. Movements of the knee joint are then regained by the patient's own active exercise. Recovery should

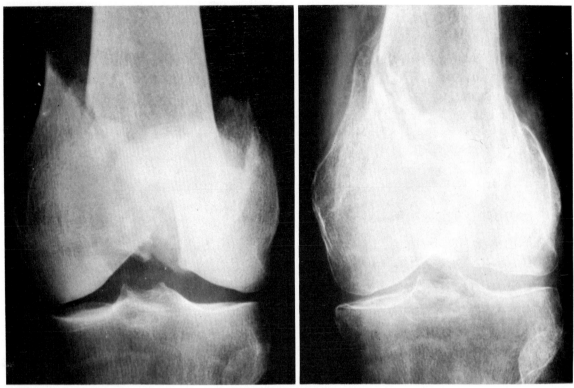

Fig 30.56   **Fig 30.57**

Figs 30.56 and 30.57 Fracture of both condyles of the femur reduced manually and immobilised in a Thomas splint with skin-traction. The final position after union of the fracture is shown in Figure 30.57.

be complete within about six months. It is important to reduce these epiphyseal injuries accurately and as soon as possible, and to check that the reduction is maintained by repeated X-ray examination. A delay of a few days can make manipulative correction impossible and necessitate a difficult open reduction, which increases the possibility of damage to the epiphysis and a late growth deformity.

Other displacements of the lower femoral epiphysis. The classical displacement has been described where the epiphysis is tilted and displaced forwards. But this is rare and more commonly the displacement is incomplete and often in other directions. There may be lateral or medial displacement and occasionally, as shown in Figure 30.64 the lower femoral epiphysis may be displaced backwards. If the injuries are classified by the Salter-Harris method the majority fall into Type II (separation of the whole epiphysis with a metaphyseal injury). The pure epiphyseal injury (Type 1), representing the classical anterior displacement, is very rare in all the recent series of cases.[50, 51] There are a few hemi-epiphyseal injuries (Types III and IV) and the very occasional crush injury (Type V). In one series a quarter of the cases were undisplaced and required no treatment other than immobilisation for a period of six to eight weeks.[51] All cases need protection from full weight-bearing for three months. Displaced fractures require meticulous reposition and there is little doubt that optimum results are directly related to the accuracy of the reduction.[51] In Type III and IV injuries (displacement of hemi-epiphysis) open reduction with screw or Kirschner wire fixation should be carried out so that an accurate and stable position can be achieved.[51a]

Arrest of growth after displacement of the lower femoral epiphysis. It is generally taught that traumatic separation and displacement of any epiphysis seldom interrupts growth because the line

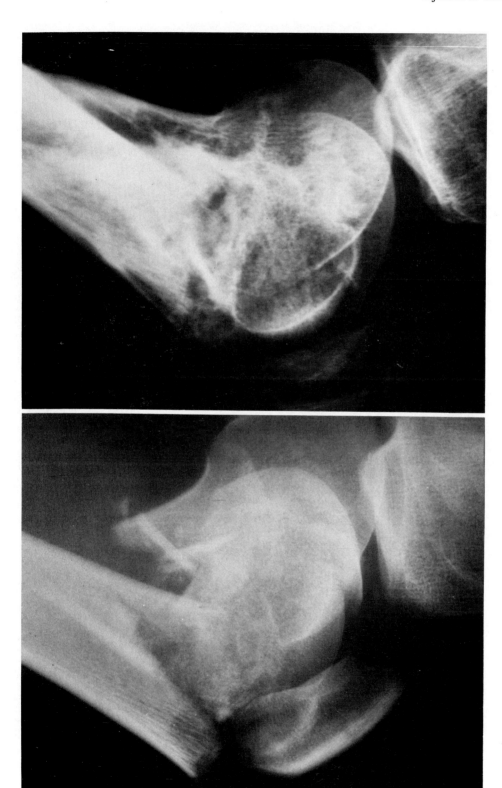

Fig 30.58 This man's condylar fracture was put up in traction with the knee flexed and allowed to unite with a flexion deformity at the fracture site of 20 to 30 degrees. This caused a permanent loss of extension at the knee of the same amount, which can only be corrected by a supracondylar osteotomy. This deformity should never have occurred if the physiotherapist treating the patient while still in traction had concentrated as much on extension exercises as she did on flexion.

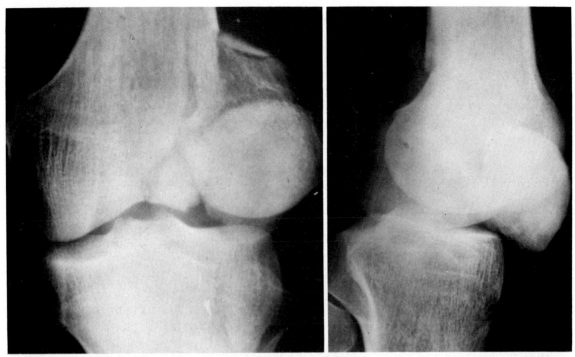

Fig 30.59

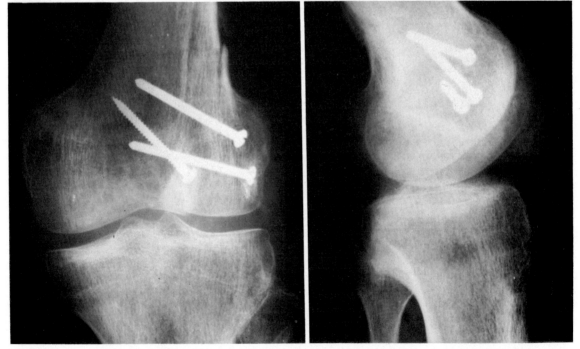

Fig 30.60

Figs 30.59 and 30.60 As the result of direct violence the patella was rotated through 90 degrees and its lateral margin was driven into the femur, splitting off the condyle. The patella itself was so damaged that excision was needed. The condylar fragments were fitted together and fixed by stainless steel screws. (Operation by Sir Henry Osmond-Clarke).

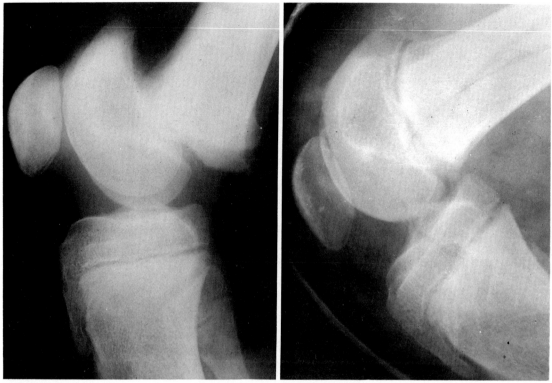

Fig 30.61 A classical anterior displacement of the lower femoral epiphysis.

Fig 30.62 After reduction of displacement.

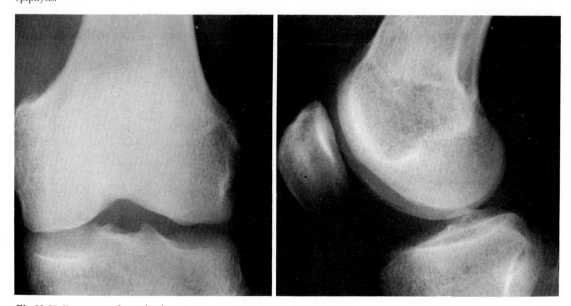

Fig 30.63 Four years after reduction.

Figs 30.61 to 30.63

Classical anterior displacement of the lower femoral epiphysis (Fig 30.61). The displacement was completely reduced by traction and flexion (Fig 30.62). Four years later it is evident that there has been no interference with epiphyseal growth; recovery was complete (Fig 30.63).

of injury is in the metaphysis (Fig 30.63), and that it is usually a segmental injury or crushing injury of the epiphyseal line that causes arrested growth (Salter-Harris Types III, IV and V). But Figure 30.65 shows that deformity can sometimes arise from interference with growth in separations of the lower femoral epiphysis when there is no clear evidence of crushing of the epiphysis, or segmental damage. Stephen and

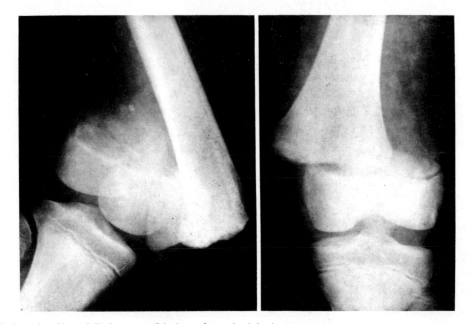

Fig 30.64 Backward and lateral displacement of the lower femoral epiphysis.

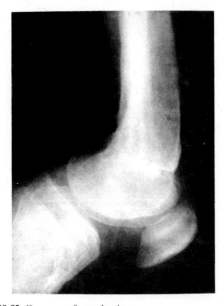

Fig 30.65 One year after reduction.

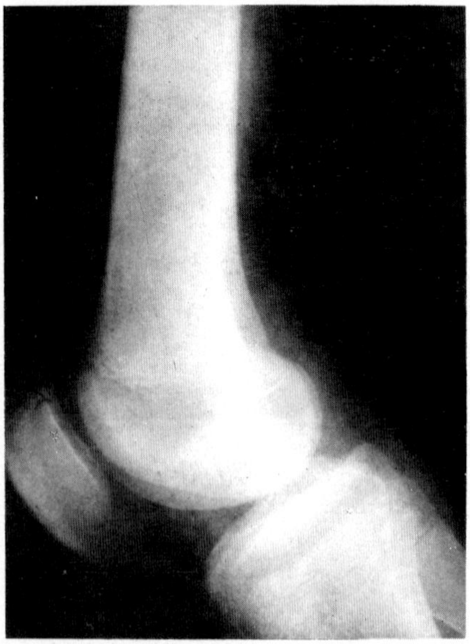

Fig 30.66 Normal knee for comparison.

Figs 30.64 to 30.66

The injury occurred from a motor accident. Backward displacement is unusual (Fig 30.64). In displacing backwards the posterior part of the epiphyseal line was evidently crushed; it fused prematurely and caused slight flexion deformity (Fig 30.65). Compare the injured knee joint with the normal knee (Fig 30.66).

Louis observed that 'the distal femoral epiphysis is prone to growth disturbances not seen with roentgenographically equivalent injuries at other sites'.[50] The prognosis therefore on the Salter-Harris classification is unreliable, and subsequent disorder of epiphyseal growth seems to depend more upon the degree of initial displacement and the accuracy of reduction than on the type of injury sustained; and it has certainly been shown that as far as limb length discrepancy is concerned this is greater with fractures displaced more than one half the diameter of the bone.[51] However, it is fortunate that these injuries usually occur at an age when the growth potential of the lower femoral epiphysis is almost exhausted, with a result that large discrepancies of limb length are rare and progressive valgus or varus deformities confined to the younger children. If premature fusion is to occur it will probably be seen within about 12 months of the injury. In these circumstances in the younger child it will be necessary to take steps to retard the growth of the epiphysis on the normal side, and consider leg lengthening procedures at a later date. Where a progressive varus or valgus deformity results from fusion of one side of the epiphysis, repeated corrective supracondylar osteotomies may be required, depending upon the age of the child. With respect to this unusual complication Langenskiold has reported an exciting new approach to the problem and has obtained promising results from excision of the bar of bone fusing the epiphyseal line and replacing it with a graft of fat.[52]

STIFFNESS OF THE KNEE JOINT IN FRACTURES OF THE SHAFT OF THE FEMUR

'*A soldier who has had a fracture of the femur is unlikely to return to duty, not because of mal-union of the fracture, but because of disability resulting from stiffness of the knee joint*'.
(*Young, 1942*)[53]

With modern advances in conservative and operative treatment of femoral shaft fractures the above quotation should no longer ring true, but it helps to emphasise that the penalty of stiffness applies more severely to the knee than to any other joint of the lower limb. Sound fusion of the hip, the ankle and the tarsal joints, provided they are in good position, causes little or no disability. But when a knee is stiff the limp can scarcely be concealed, and everyone falls over the outstretched leg in buses, trains and theatres: stairs can be climbed only one at a time, and as a result the patient has difficulty entering public

transport; driving a car is not easy; and taking part in any competitive sport impossible.

It is wise, therefore, that in the treatment of fractures of the shaft of the femur surgeons should direct their attention to preventing stiffness of the knee. However, at the same time it is foolish to suggest that these fractures differ from all others in that vigorous movement must be practised from the beginning. These are panic measures. *Provided the joint is undamaged* it is no more harmful to immobilise a knee for three or four months in treating fractures of the shaft of the femur than to immobilise an ankle in fractures of the tibia, a wrist in fractures of the radius, an elbow in fractures of the humerus or, indeed, to immobilise any joint in the treatment of any fracture. If, however, there has been an intra-articular injury, particularly a fracture of the patella, conservative treatment may have to be abandoned in favour of early internal fixation in order to stabilise the fracture and allow early knee movement.

The first essential to prevent permanent knee stiffness is to secure rapid union or rigid stabilisation of the fracture. As a corollary of this Charnley has pointed out that union of the fracture can be assumed when knee movement starts to improve.[11] Any attempt, therefore, to move and exercise joints which interferes with immobility of the fractured bone defeats its own object. The aim of treatment must be to secure prompt union of the fracture, because it is only when union is slow or delayed that serious problems of stiffness arise. In the conservative treatment of fractures of the femur uncomplicated by knee injury the sure method of preventing permanent stiffness of the knee is to maintain uninterrupted immobilisation until there is at least early union of the fracture, and then to regain movement by active exercise without forcible stretching or manipulation.

Three types of stiffness of the knee after fracture of the shaft of the femur. We have considered stiffness from the immobilisation of uncomplicated fractures, but there are three different causes of stiffness of the knee in fractures of the femur:

1. Stiffness from adhesion formation in and around the joint.
2. Stiffness from fixation of the patella to the femoral condyles.
3. Stiffness from anchorage of the quadriceps muscle to the femur at the site of fracture.

Stiffness from simple adhesion formation around the knee. This has already been recognised as an inevitable consequence of the necessary immobilisation of fractures of the femoral shaft; but there need be no concern because a full range of movement will nearly always be regained by active exercise provided only that passive stretching, repeated manipulation and other such forcible methods are avoided. The tendency to stiffness will have been minimised:

1. By ensuring that throughout the period of immobilisation the joint is in a slightly flexed position, short of full extension, and never in hyperextension.

2. By maintaining functional activity with active exercises of the toes, foot and ankle, and repeated static contraction of the quadriceps muscle.

3. By arranging that a physiotherapist prevents fixation of the patella to the femoral condyles with daily passive lateral movements from one side to the other.

4. By the intelligent use of a cast brace when the fracture feels clinically firm (usually six weeks or so after the injury). Whether the fracture has been treated by fixed traction, balanced traction, intramedullary nail fixation, or even immobilisation in a plaster spica, the time comes when there is clinical union of the fracture but not yet sound consolidation. More vigorous exercises should then be encouraged and the increased freedom in a cast brace with knee hinges is the obvious answer to the problem. It allows the fracture still to be protected while weight-bearing, and yet gives the patient the opportunity to move the knee naturally while walking. At this stage of the treatment it is the duty of the surgeon and the physiotherapist to encourage the patient—to stimulate, urge, cajole and inspire—but not to force. With this regime very few knee joints stiff from simple adhesion formation need be manipulated under anaesthetic and this should never be done in the early stage before the fracture is fully consolidated.

Stiffness of the knee joint from fixation of the patella. Fixation of the patella to the front of the femoral condyles is an important cause of stiffness. In young and healthy patients this should usually be prevented by a physiotherapist who not only supervises static quadriceps contraction but also maintains lateral movement of the patella by gentle passive movement repeated every day. Sometimes, however, when the shaft of the femur is fractured there is also injury to the knee with traumatic synovitis, damage to the articular surfaces, or even a stellate fracture of the patella. If the patella is thus fixed to the femur, forcible manipulation of the joint under an anaesthetic is still more disastrous—the quadriceps tendon, or the patellar ligament, will be avulsed, or the bone itself may be fractured. It is important to recognise patellofemoral ankylosis before attempting mobilisation of

a stiff knee by forcible manipulation. Not uncommonly the limitation of movement is due to dense adhesions between the superior pole of the patella, suprapatellar pouch and front of the femur. These give the false impression of patello-femoral ankylosis. An arthrogram of the knee can be valuable in making the diagnosis: 10 ml of 35 per cent diodone are injected under the patella and the patient laid prone with the body tilted steeply head downwards. In the normal knee the suprapatellar pouch fills with dye (Fig 30.67), whereas in a knee with suprapatellar adhesions the dye is held up at the upper border of the patella (Figs 30.68 and 30.69). This is a useful investigation to carry out before performing a quadricepsplasty in order to determine whether it is necessary to divide adhesions in the suprapatellar pouch. A gentle examination of the knee under anaesthetic regains a few degrees of movement and may help the physiotherapist in her work of mobilisation, but any forcible manipulation can do no good and runs the risk of rupture of the patella or its ligament.

Fixation of the quadriceps muscle to the shaft of the femur near the site of fracture. At the moment that a fracture of the femur is sustained, the fragments of the shaft of the bone may tear into the deep surface of the quadriceps and cause fixation of muscle to bone. When there is an open or compound fracture, perhaps with infection, the muscle becomes still more firmly anchored. This is probably the most serious of all cases of stiffness of the knee joint in fractures of the shaft of the femur, especially if endeavours are made to gain mobility by forcible manipulation under anaesthesia, which must almost inevitably fracture the patella or avulse the patella ligaments (Fig 30.70). Every effort should first be made to restore movement by active exercise continued hour by hour and day by day over many months.

Restoration of knee flexion by quadricepsplasty. If conservative measures fail (and one should wait not less than six months and probably about a year before deciding this) and there is still serious incapacity from stiffness, the only hope of restoring flexion is to free the scarred quadriceps tendon from its point of anchorage to the femur. The most successful way to do this is by the quadricepsplasty devised by Campbell Thompson.[54] The principle of this operation depends upon the fact that the rectus femoris component of the quadriceps is rarely involved in the adherent scarring. This part of the muscle can be isolated and left as the main extensor of the knee while the other components are

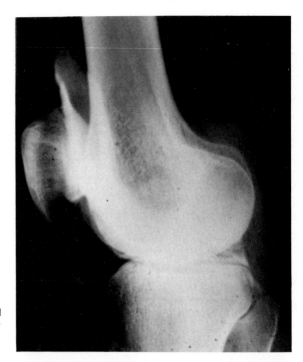

Fig 30.67 A prone-lying arthrogram of a stiff knee after femoral shaft fracture, demonstrating a normal suprapatellar pouch. The limitation of movement in this case was due to quadriceps scarring.

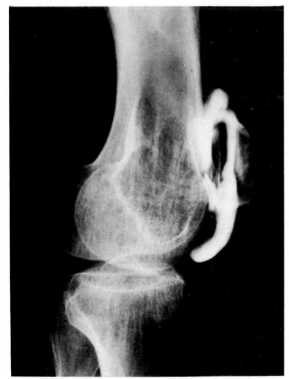

Fig 30.68

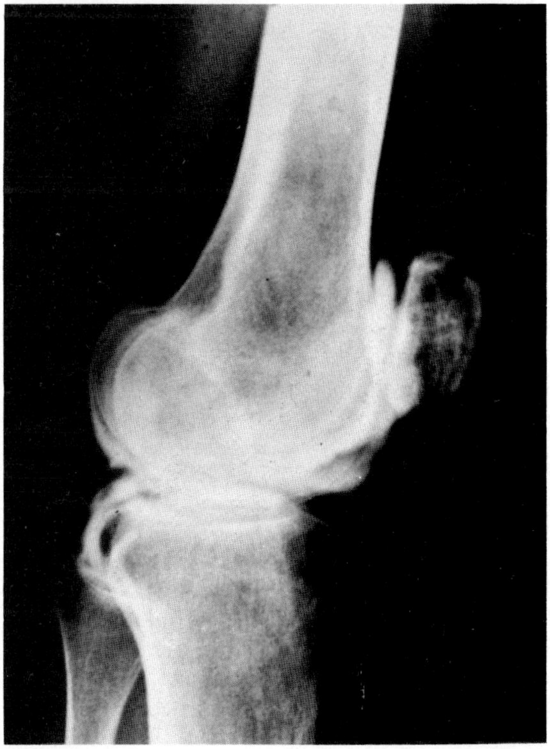

Fig 30.69

Figs 30.68 and 30.69 Arthrograms of stiff knees due to quadriceps scarring plus suprapatellar adhesions. The adhesions were divided at the time of quadricepsplasty and almost full range of flexion was restored.

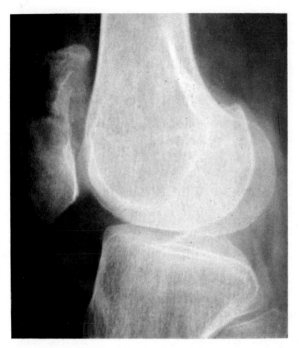

Fig 30.70 Fracture of the patella from forcible manipulation under anaesthesia of a knee joint stiff from anchorage of the quadriceps muscle to the femur.

detached from their insertion and allowed to displace proximally. In the original operation of quadriceps-splasty devised by Bennett[55] the rectus femoris was lengthened, but if this has to be done it always results in a permanent extensor lag. Fortunately it is usually unnecessary. In one series of 30 cases only three required lengthening of the rectus femoris and on each occasion this was done there was a permanent extensor lag.[56] Judet has described a method of muscle slide[57] which avoids lengthening the rectus, but this involves an extensive release of the whole of the vastus lateralis muscle origin and has little to commend it over the Thompson operation.

The Campbell Thompson technique. No tourniquet should be used for this operation, partly because it interferes with quadriceps movement, and partly because careful haemostasis is essential for success. Through an anterior mid-line incision extending from the mid-third of the thigh to the lower pole of the patella, the vastus lateralis and medialis are detached from the patella and retracted to expose the vastus intermedius component of the quadriceps muscle. The intermedius is frequently replaced by dense scar tissue which must be excised. At this stage in may be possible to flex the knee, but if there is still

a complete block to flexion the ilio-tibial band should be inspected and divided if it is taut. If the arthrogram has shown there to be obliteration of the suprapatellar pouch the knee joint must be opened and the dense adhesions of the upper pole of the patella divided. Only as a very last resort should the rectus femoris tendon be lengthened, for if this is done the restoration of flexion is necessarily slowed down to allow repair of the tendon, and an extensor lag is inevitable. Once the knee can be flexed to beyond the right angle, the vastus medialis and lateralis can be reattached to the sides of the rectus while the joint is held flexed. The skin must be carefully repaired with close sutures and a suction drain inserted.

Attention to detail in the after-care is as important as the operation itself. The limb should be set up in a Thomas splint using skin-traction and a Pearson knee piece, with the knee flexed about 30 degrees (Fig 30.71). Twice a day for at least two weeks the knee must be moved through the whole range obtained at operation (Fig 30.72); it is quite useless moving it a small amount hoping that the range will gradually improve—adhesions will reform and all will be lost. The treatment is painful and requires a devoted physiotherapist and an enthusiastic patient. Heavy sedation in the early stage is necessary. A manipulation under anaesthetic should be carried out after three weeks if the post-operative range has not been maintained, and the skin sutures must be retained until then. After the manipulation the patient is allowed up, usually walking at first with crutches, and sometimes using a back splint if the active extension lag is very marked. From this stage on the progress is slow and the patient must be encouraged to work hard on active exercises over the next few months. It usually takes at least six months for the joint to reach the final stage of recovery, and the same length of time for the patient to overcome extensor lag. The same result can be achieved by using alternating plasters in flexion and extension, changing the position every few days for two weeks.[58] If this technique is used great care must be taken in applying the cast in order to avoid wound breakdown.

If there was gross limitation of movement pre-operatively it is unusual for the patient to regain more than about 100 degree range of flexion, and there may be permanent extensor lag of 5 to 10 degrees. The considerable gain in function resulting from the restoration of movement far outweighs the minor disability from the loss of the last few degrees of active extension. This is a rewarding procedure but the careful attention to detail, both in operation and after-care, must be stressed.

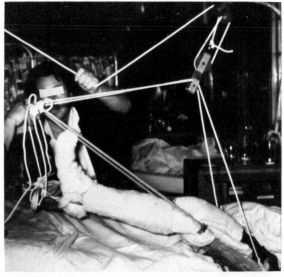

Fig 30.71

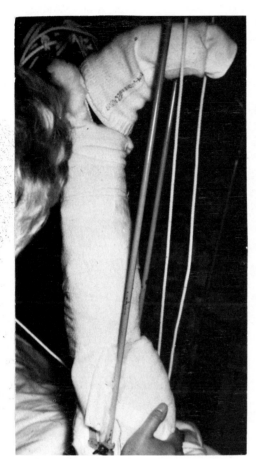

Fig 30.72

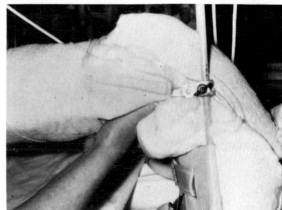

Figs 30.71 and 30.72 The Thomas splint and Pearson knee piece used in the treatment following quadricepsplasty. In the resting position the knee should be flexed through about 30 degrees, with below knee skin-traction attached to the end of the knee piece (Fig 30.71). This component must be carefully positioned to allow the physiotherapist to use the splint as a lever when exercising the knee (Fig 30.72).

The problem of fixed flexion deformity. So far we have only considered the restoration of flexion of the knee following post-fracture stiffness. A greater disability can result from fixed flexion deformity, even though the patient has regained some active flexion, enabling him to sit and ascend stairs normally. Fixed flexion of only 10 or 20 degrees causes real shortening of the limb and a very obvious limp. It is usually the result of adhesions around a fracture of the patella which has been immobilised partly flexed, but can also be caused by malunion of a supracondylar or T-shaped condylar fracture (see Fig 30.58). These fractures should never be immobilised for long periods in flexion and the physiotherapist must concentrate as much on extension as she does on flexion; otherwise the fracture will unite with the lower fragment already flexed and a fixed flexion deformity is inevitable. Only supracondylar osteotomy can correct this deformity.

COMPLICATIONS IN FRACTURES OF THE SHAFT OF THE FEMUR

It has already been said that the femoral shaft fractures may be only one part of a serious multiple injury and that to some extent the form of treatment of the fracture may be dictated by other priorities. In addition, however, there can be local complications at, or immediately adjacent to, the fracture which can radically alter the management of the injury. These are now briefly discussed in this last section.

Fractured shaft femur with ipsi-lateral dislocation of the hip. The diagnosis and management of this combined injury has already been fully described in Chapter 29 but is included again to emphasise how frequently the injury of the hip is missed at the initial examination. The fracture of the femoral shaft obscures, of course, the typical deformity of a hip dislocation; however, if on examination of the post-reduction X-rays of the shaft fracture the upper fragment is adducted, and particularly if it is also a transverse fracture, suspicions should be immediately aroused that there is an accompanying hip injury and appropriate X-rays taken.

Associated fracture of the neck of the femur. Very little has been written in the literature about this complication,[59, 60] but what little is available indicates that, like ipsilateral dislocation of the hip,

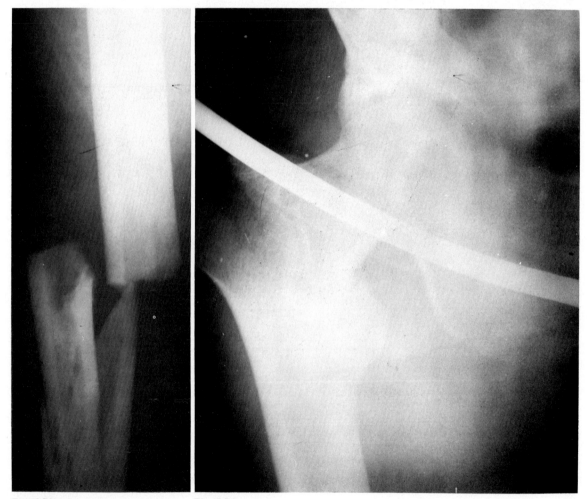

Fig 30.73   Fig 30.74

Figs 30.73 and 30.74 This patient's fractured shaft of femur was reduced and immobilised on a Thomas splint. The upper fragment was adducted and the fracture was basically transverse (Fig 30.73). A film of the hip on the same side showed an adducted pertrochanteric fracture (Fig 30.74).

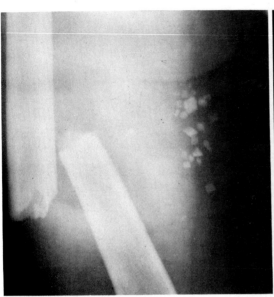
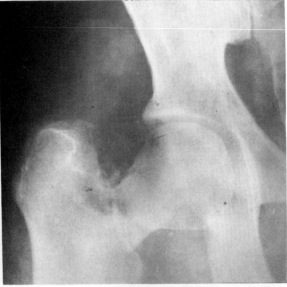

Fig 30.75

Figs 30.75 and 30.76 This 20-year-old patient sustained
multiple fractures of the lower limbs including a fracture of the
femoral shaft and basal transcervical fracture on the same side
(Fig 30.75). There was also a fracture of the mid third of the tibia
on this side. Note the marked comminution of the transcervical
fracture. Despite early stabilisation of the shaft fracture with a
plate followed by skeletal-traction and then a plaster spica, there
was no evidence of bone union at the femoral neck fracture. A
McMurray displacement osteotomy was carried out at six
months (Fig 30.76).

this second injury often goes untreated because it has
not been recognised early. It is all too easy to be so
involved with treatment of the shaft fracture that the
upper part of the X-ray is not studied properly; and
in a number of the cases reported the fracture was
missed despite the fact that it could be seen in the
initial X-rays.[59] Here again, persistent adduction
deformity of the upper fragment of the femoral shaft
should demand an X-ray of the hip (Figs 30.73 and
30.74). Treatment should first aim at stabilising the
shaft fracture with either an intramedullary nail or
a plate, so that the neck fracture can be more easily
controlled. A pertrochanteric fracture will almost
certainly unite satisfactorily by conservative treatment in traction, but basal fractures of the neck and
true transcervical fractures are more difficult. If left
on traction alone they will commonly go on to non-
union (Figs 30.75 and 30.76). Good results have been
reported in these cases from combining intramedullary nailing of the fractured shaft with multiple pin-
fixation of the femoral neck fracture.[60] Conrad
reported 11 cases treated by nail plate for the hip

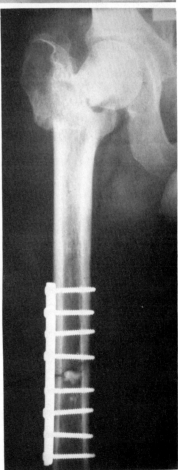

Fig 30.76

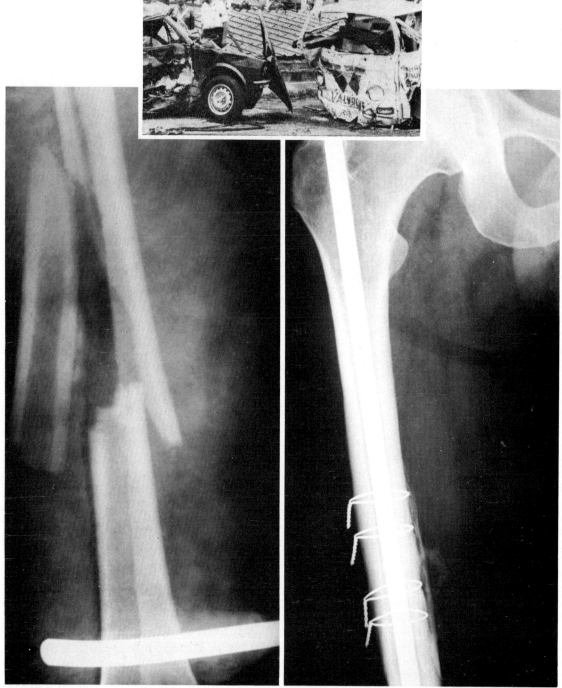

Fig 30.77   Fig 30.78

Figs 30.77 and 30.78 The segmental fracture of the femur illustrated in Figure 30.77 was one of many injuries sustained by the driver of a car involved in a high velocity collision with another vehicle (inset). Internal injuries prevented early fixation of the fracture, but even after three weeks it was possible to stabilise the comminuted middle fragment with circumferential wires, and immobilise all the fractures with a 10 mm diameter nail which easily traversed the reconstituted middle fragment (Fig 30.78).

fracture and compression plate for the femoral shaft fracture carried out in a single operation.[61] There was only one case of delayed union. It is also possible that the articulated femoral neck and intramedullary nails recommended in the treatment of difficult pertrochanteric fractures may have a place in the management of this double fracture.[41]

Fracture of the patella with fracture of the femoral shaft on the same side. This combination of fractures requires early stabilisation of the femur in order to allow knee movement to be started within a few weeks of injury. Very often in these cases the limb fractures are only part of a more serious multiple injury and the patient is unfit for a major reconstructive programme. In these circumstances the patella should be excised first, followed a week later by intramedullary nailing (or plate fixation if the fracture is unsuitable for a nail). Mobilisation of the knee can be started two to three weeks from the time of patella excision. There is little doubt that with definitive treatment and early mobilisation a satisfactory return of knee movement can be expected.[62]

Segmental fractures of the femoral shaft. The incidence of segmental fractures, sometimes with large comminuted central fragments (Fig 30.77), is on the increase, and this is the direct result of the mounting injury rate from road traffic accidents; particularly, high velocity collisions which are now so commonplace (Fig 30.77 inset). Surprisingly, this fracture is rarely compound and should always be treated by intramedullary nailing unless there is a very serious contra-indication to operation. Where the middle segment is intact there is little difficulty in threading a Kuntscher nail down the femur to stabilise the fracture. In these circumstances no attempt should be made to obtain very rigid fixation; instead, a nail should be used of such a diameter that it will slide easily through the middle fragment. *Reaming of this fragment is contra-indicated.* Fixation becomes more difficult when the fragment is split into two parts; but it is still possible provided there are two major pieces which can be wired together (Fig 30.78). In the author's opinion it is important to reconstitute the middle fragment with circumferential wires before proceeding to nail the fracture. Attempts to wire fragments after nailing can be very unrewarding. Following such a procedure it is essential to support the limb for some weeks in a Thomas splint before allowing the patient to weight-bear in a cast brace.

Fracture with major loss of diaphysis. Two cases of extensive loss of the femoral shaft have been recorded in high velocity collisions involving motorcyclists.[63, 64] In both injuries the lower fracture was through the supracondylar region and there was an associated fracture of the patella. It is suggested[63] that in this injury the femoral shaft above the condyles is forced out through the compound wound, stripping the periosteum in the process, and finally breaks off proximally (Fig 30.79). In both the recorded cases the fragments were recovered from the scene of the accident, sterilised and replaced successfully using intramedullary fixation some time later when the initial wound was healed. The early appearance of periosteal callus and the rapidity of bone repair suggests that a periosteal tube remains bridging the gap in this injury; and at least one case has been reported of repair by traction alone.[65] Certainly in children the powers of bony reconstruction after extensive bone loss are quite remarkable (Figs 30.80 and 30.81). Where there is loss of a segment in the middle third of the bone and the fragment is not available for re-insertion, Kuntscher nailing with a spacer bone graft will be necessary. Two blocks of iliac bone of a suitable length should be packed around a stabilising nail and maintained in place with cerclage wiring. An ingenious method of blind nailing combined with a cancellous graft injected

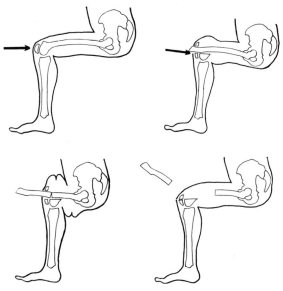

Fig 30.79 Diagrams illustrating the probable sequence of events leading to extrusion of the lower femoral shaft. (Reproduced by kind permission of the *Journal of Bone and Joint Surgery* and of J. R. Kirkup from his paper (1965) Traumatic femoral bone loss. *Journal of Bone and Joint Surgery*, 47-B, 106).

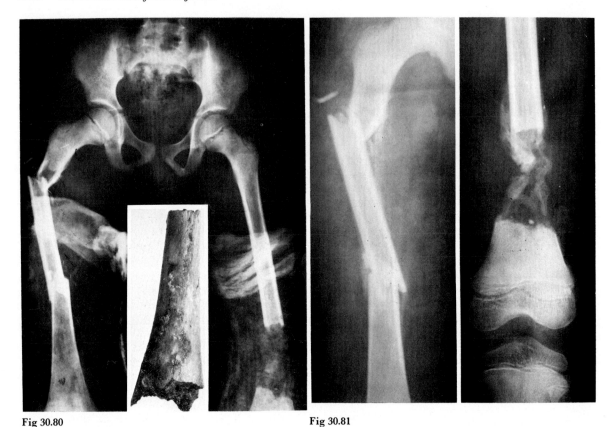

Fig 30.80

Fig 30.81

Figs 30.80 and 30.81 A 6-year-old West African child was knocked over by a car and sustained bilateral fractures of the femoral shafts with extensive diaphyseal loss on the left side (Fig 30.80). Three weeks later there was already evidence of bone bridging the gap (Fig 30.81).

down the nail track has been described, with a successful reconstitution of the femoral shaft in two out of three cases.[65a] Whatever method of reconstruction is adopted it is important to remember that the femoral vessels can become interposed between the bone fragments and that a pre-operative arteriogram may be necessary.[65a]

Ipsilateral fracture of the femur and tibia. When fractures of the femur and tibia occur simultaneously in the same limb there is a high risk of complications and often poor end results. There is fairly general agreement that the results are better if at least one fracture is treated by internal fixation,[66, 67, 68] and that conservative treatment of both fractures is associated with a higher complication rate, a high incidence of secondary operations, and a significantly longer healing time. However, it has been observed by Fraser and his colleagues that the

incidence of bone infection when both fractures are fixed at the same time is three times as high than when only one bone is stabilised.[66] This is, of course, to be expected because of the longer operating time, and sometimes the less satisfactory operative conditions. These authors suggest that whenever possible the femur should be fixed rigidly with a Kuntscher nail and the tibia stabilised by an external fixateur. Unfortunately it is not uncommon for both fractures to be unsuitable for Kuntscher nailing (Fig 30.82) and in these circumstances conservative treatment in a Thomas splint using a below-knee cast with a Steinmann's pin in the upper and lower tibial fragments is the treatment of choice (Fig 30.83). If the fractures are suitable for internal fixation the femur should be stabilised in preference to the tibia (which can be treated by the two pin method), in order to allow early mobilisation of the knee. If the fractures are segmental both bones may require

Figs 30.82 and 30.83 Although fractures of the ipsilateral tibial and femoral shafts are best treated by neutralisation of one fracture (preferably the femur), on some occasions both fractures are quite unsuitable for internal fixation (Fig 30.82). In these circumstances the fractures can be treated conservatively on a Thomas splint by using a pin through the upper tibia and another just above the ankle incorporating them in a below knee plaster. The upper pin can be used for applying femoral shaft traction in the usual way (Fig 30.83).

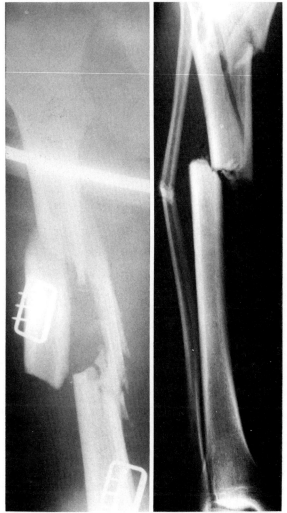

Fig 30.82.

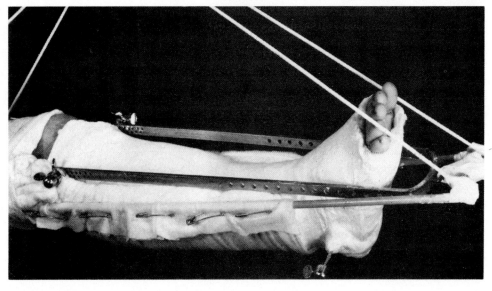

Fig 30.83

intramedullary nailing (Figs 30.84 and 30.85). These operations, however, can be carried out as separate procedures, and preferably not as an emergency. The initial treatment should be conservative, and the Thomas splint and two pin plaster technique is probably the best form of temporary immobilisation.

Nerve injury. Sciatic or femoral nerve damage is rarely associated with fractures of the shaft of the femur, except in compound fractures due to missile injuries. Drop foot weakness and sensory loss below the knee are more commonly due to local pressure on the peroneal nerve, either from inadequate padding

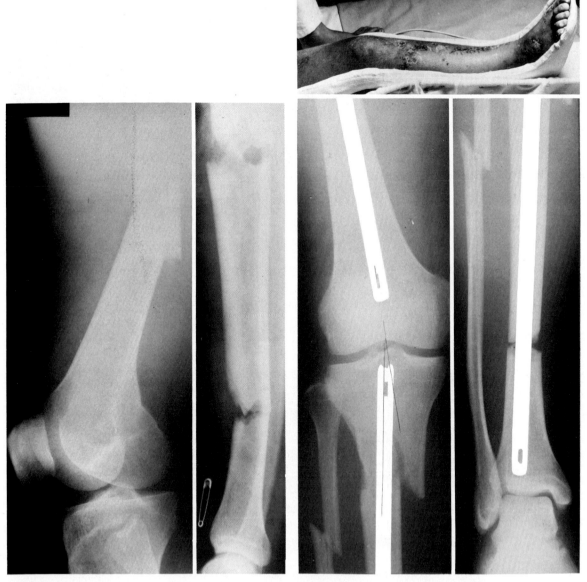

Fig 30.84   Fig 30.85

Figs 30.84 and 30.85 Ipsilateral segmental fractures of the femur and tibia demand Kuntscher nailing at both fracture sites. These operations are usually carried out as separate procedures but the fractures illustrated in Figures 30.84 sustained by a racing motor-cyclist, were very successfully nailed at one operation (Fig 30.85). The tibial fracture was grossly compound and yet the wound healed perfectly (inset) (Operation by Mr T. R. Beatson of the Isle of Man).

of a Thomas splint or pressure from an encircling bandage used to fix skin extensions.

Vascular complications. Arterial injuries are infrequent complications of femoral fractures, but when they do occur they are usually more common in injuries of the lower third of the bone or the supracondylar region, because at this site the femoral artery is relatively fixed, either in Hunter's canal, or in the popliteal space. It is now generally agreed that reconstructive arterial surgery in the limbs must be carried out early if this treatment is to have any chance of success.[69] Femoral artery injuries associated with fractures of the shaft of the femur are no exception, and an aggressive attitude towards re-establishing the arterial blood supply should be taken as soon as the patient has recovered from his initial shock.[70] Stabilisation of the fracture by an intramedullary nail or a plate although it protects the arterial repair and is sometimes desirable, is by no means essential, and the general condition and the local situation at the fracture site often dictates that a conservative regime is followed. Indeed, in one report it is stated that during the application of a plate 'inadvertently the arterial repair was thereby disrupted'.[71] This type of incident and high infection rate has resulted in a swing away from internal fixation[72, 73] for fractures complicated by damage to the main vessels. However, it is possible that the use of external fixation may be valuable in the management of these cases.[73] The techniques of arterial repair has already been fully described in Chapter 11.

Delayed union. Although non-union of fractures of the femoral shaft is uncommon, delayed union occurs not infrequently, and particularly when the initial displacement of the fracture has been severe. Prompt recognition of soft tissue interposition between the bone fragments followed by internal fixation can forestall a long period of unsuccessful conservative treatment; but remember—there must be no unpro-

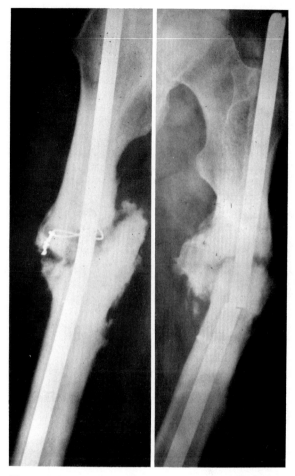

Fig 30.86 Bent and broken Kuntscher nails in fractures of the femur are often the penalty of unprotected weight-bearing. They pose a major problem in the subsequent treatment of the fracture.

tected weight-bearing until there is sound bony consolidation at the fracture site. Bent and broken Kuntscher nails can present a major problem of management (Fig 30.86). For the treatment of delayed union and non-union see Chapter 18.

REFERENCES

1. Clarke R 1959 Resuscitation and transfusion in severe injuries. In: Clarke R, Badger F G, Sevitt S (eds) Modern trends in accident surgery and medicine. Butterworth, London, ch 5, p 63
2. Helal B, Skevis X 1967 Unrecognised dislocation of the hip in fractures of the femoral shaft. Journal of Bone and Joint Surgery 49-B: 293
3. Fisk G R 1944 The fractured femoral shaft—new approach to the problem. Lancet i: 659
4. Russell R H 1924 Fracture of the femur: a clinical study. British Journal of Surgery 11: 491
5. Perkins G 1958 Fractures and dislocations. Athlone Press, London, ch 28, p 268
6. Usdin J 1967 Treatment of fractures of the femur by Perkins' traction. Journal of Bone and Joint Surgery 49-B: 200
7. Bryant T 1879 A manual for the practice of surgery, 3rd edn. Churchill, London, vol II, p 22
8. Nicholson J T, Foster R M, Heath R D 1955 Bryant's

traction. A provocative cause of circulatory disturbance. Journal of American Medical Association 157: 415

9. Ferry A M, Edgar M S 1966 Modified Bryant's traction. Journal of Bone and Joint Surgery 48-A: 533

10. Pearson C A 1977 Early protected weight-bearing in African patients with fracture of the femur. Injury 9: 89

11. Charnley J 1961 The closed treatment of common fractures, 3rd edn. Livingstone, Edinburgh, ch 13, p 190

12. Meggit B F 1978 Personal communication.

13. Watson-Jones R, Coltart W D 1943 Slow union of fractures with a study of 804 fractures of the shafts of the tibia and femur. British Journal of Surgery 30: 260

14. Smith H H 1855 On the treatment of ununited fracture by means of artificial limbs which combine the principle of pressure and motion at the seat of fracture, and lead to the formation of an ensheathing callus. American Journal of Medical Science 29: 102

15. Mooney V, Nickel V L, Harvey J P, Snelson R 1970 Cast-brace treatment for fractures of the distal part of the femur. Journal of Bone and Joint Surgery 52-A: 1563

16. Wardlaw D 1977 The cast-brace treatment of femoral shaft fractures. Journal of Bone and Joint Surgery. 59-B: 411

17. Adair I V 1976 The use of plaster casts in treatment of fracture of the femoral shaft. Injury 7: 194

18. Lesin B E, Mooney V, Ashley M E 1977 Cast-bracing for fractures of the femur. A preliminary report of a modified device. Journal of Bone and Joint Surgery 59-A: 917

18a. Hardy A E, White P, Williams J 1979 The treatment of femoral fractures by cast-brace and early walking. Journal of Bone and Joint Surgery 61-B: 151

18b. Hardy A E 1979 Pressure recordings in patients with femoral fractures in cast-braces and suggestions for treatment. Journal of Bone and Joint Surgery 61-A: 365

19. Rokkanen P, Slatis P, Vanka E 1969 Closed or open intramedullary nailing of femoral shaft fractures. A comparison with conservatively treated cases. Journal of Bone and Joint Surgery 51-B: 313

20. Nichols P J R 1963 Rehabilitation after fractures of the shaft of the femur. Journal of Bone and Joint Surgery 45-B: 96

21. Rothwell A G, Fitzpatrick C B 1978 Closed Kuntscher nailing of femoral shaft fractures. A series of 100 consecutive patients. Journal of Bone and Joint Surgery 60-B: 504

22. Denker H 1965 Technical problems of medullary nailing. A study of 435 nailed shaft fractures of the femur. Acta Chirurgica Scandinavica 130: 185

23. Hey Groves E W 1916 On modern methods of treating fractures. Wright, Bristol

24. Hey Groves E W 1918 Ununited fractures, gunshot injuries and bone grafting. British Journal of Surgery 6: 203

25. Le Vay A D 1950 Intramedullary nailing in the Kuntscher Clinic. Journal of Bone and Joint Surgery 32-B: 698

26. Bohler J 1968 Closed intramedullary nailing of the femur. Clinical Orthopaedics and Related Research 60: 51

27. Kuntscher G 1965 Intramedullary surgical technique and its place in orthopaedic surgery. Journal of Bone and Joint Surgery 47-A: 809

28. Denker H 1965 Shaft fractures of the femur. A comparative study of the results of various methods of treatment in 1003 cases. Acta Chirurgica Scandinavica 130: 173

29. Watson-Jones R et al 1950 Medullary nailing of fractures after fifty years with a review of the difficulties and complications of the operation. Journal of Bone and Joint Surgery 32-B: 694

30. Wickstrom J, Corban M S, Vise G T 1968 Complications following intramedullary fixation of 324 fractured femurs. Clinical Orthopaedics 60: 103

31. Broad C P, Percy A J C 1977 The jammed Kuntscher nail: a method of releasing the nail and report of a case. Injury 9: 135

32. Clawson D K, Smith R F, Hansen S T 1971 Closed intramedullary nailing of the femur. Journal of Bone and Joint Surgery 53-A: 681

33. Nimberg G A, Rosenfeld H 1970 Method of removing an incarcerated Kuntscher nail. Clinical Orthopaedics and Related Research 71: 205

34. Firica A, Troianescu O, Petre M 1978 Osteosynthesis of fractures of the femur with flexible metallic intramedullary nails. Italian Journal of Orthopaedics and Traumatology IV: 23

34a. Pankovich A M, Goldflies M L, Pearson R L 1979 Closed Ender nailing of femoral-shaft fractures. Journal of Bone and Joint Surgery 61-A: 222

35. Street D M, Vesley D G 1959 The split diamond nail. Journal of Bone and Joint Surgery 41-A: 1361

36. Schneider H W 1968 Use of the 4-flanged self-cutting intramedullary nail for fixation of femoral fractures. Clinical Orthopaedics and Related Research 60: 29

37. Allen W C, Heiple K G, Burstein A H 1978 A fluted femoral intramedullary rod. Biomechanical analysis and preliminary clinical results. Journal of Bone and Joint Surgery 60-A: 506

38. Huckstep R L, Hubbard M J S, Kongstad S, Hansen H, Patel A P 1972 Rigid intramedullary fixation of femoral shaft fractures with compression. Journal of Bone and Joint Surgery 54-B: 384

39. Halloran W X 1976 The slotted intramedullary rod. Orthopaedic Review V: 1

40. Jenkins D H R, Lewis M H, Downes E M 1978 Simple supplementary support in Kuntscher medullary nailing of the femur. Injury 9: 286

41. Cuthbert H, Howat T W 1975 The Kuntscher-Y nail in the treatment of intertrochanteric and subtrochanteric fractures of the femur. Journal of Bone and Joint Surgery 57-B: 113

42. Zickel R E 1976 An intramedullary fixation device for proximal part of the femur. Nine years experience. Journal of Bone and Joint Surgery 58-A: 866

43. Neer C S, Grantham S A, Shelton M L 1967 Supracondylar fracture of the adult femur. A study of one hundred and ten cases. Journal of Bone and Joint Surgery 49-A: 591

44. Charnley J 1961 The closed treatment of common fractures, 3rd edn. Livingstone, Edinburgh, ch 14, p 197

45. Perkins G 1958 Fractures and dislocations. University of London, Athlone Press, London, ch 29, p 287

46. Brown A, D'Arcy J C 1971 Internal fixation for supracondylar fractures of the femur in the elderly patient. Journal of Bone and J Surgery 53-B: 420

47. Olerud S 1972 Operative treatment of supracondylar-condylar fractures of the femur. Technique and results in fifteen cases. Journal of Bone and Joint Surgery 54-A: 1015

48. Muller M E, Allgower M, Willenegger H 1965 Techniques of internal fixation of fractures. Springer-Verlag, New York

49. Hutchinson J 1894 Lectures on injuries to the epiphyses and their results. British Medical Journal 1: 669

50. Stephens D C, Louis D S 1974 Traumatic separation of the distal femoral epiphyseal cartilage plate. Journal of Bone and Joint Surgery 56-A: 1383

51. Lombardo S J, Harvey J P 1977 Fractures of the distal femoral epiphysis. Factors influencing prognosis: a review of thirty-four cases. Journal of Bone and Joint Surgery 59-A: 742

51a. Salter R B, Czitrom A A, Willis R B 1979 Fractures involving the distal femoral epiphyseal plate. Journal of Bone and Joint Surgery 61-B: 248

52. Langenskiold A 1975 An operation for partial closure of an epiphyseal plate in children, and its experimental basis. Journal of Bone and Joint Surgery 57-B: 325

53. Young R H 1942 The prophylaxis and treatment of the stiff knee following fracture of the femur. Proceedings of the Royal Society of Medicine 35: 716

54. Thompson T C 1944 Quadricepsplasty to improve knee function. Journal of Bone and Joint Surgery 26: 366

55. Bennett G E 1922 Lengthening of the quadriceps tendon. Journal of Bone and Joint Surgery 4: 279

56. Nicoll E A 1963 Quadricepsplasty. Journal of Bone and Joint Surgery 45-B: 483

57. Judet R 1973 Mobilisation of the stiff knee joint. Journal of Bone and Joint Surgery 55-B: 441

58. Hesketh K T 1963 Experiences with the Thompson quadricepsplasty. Journal of Bone and Joint Surgery 45-B: 491

59. Kinborough E E 1961 Concomitant unilateral hip and femoral shaft fractures—a too frequently unrecognised syndrome. Report of five cases. Journal of Bone and Joint Surgery 43-A: 443

60. Delaney W M, Street D M 1953 Fracture of the femoral shaft with fracture of neck of same femur. Treatment with medullary nail for shaft and Knowles pins for neck. Journal of International College of Surgeons 19: 303

61. Conrad J J 1973 Fractures of the hip with simultaneous fracture of the shaft of femur on same side. Journal of Bone and Joint Surgery 55-A: 1320

62. Fitzgerald J A W 1970 The management of fractures of ipsilateral patella and femur. Injury 1: 287

63. Kirkup J R 1965 Traumatic femoral bone loss. Journal of Bone and Joint Surgery 47-B: 106

64. Abell C F 1966 Extrusion of femoral shaft fragment by trauma and successful replacement. Journal of Bone and Joint Surgery 48-A: 537

65. Strange F G St. Clair 1963 Union of fractures. Lancet i: 305

65a. Chapman M W 1980 Closed intramedullary bone-grafting and nailing of segmental defects of the femur. A report of three cases. Journal of Bone and Joint Surgery 62-A: 1004

66. Fraser R D, Hunter G A, Waddell J P 1978 Ipsi-lateral fracture of the femur and tibia. Journal of Bone & Joint Surgery 60B: 510

67. Karlstrom G, Olerud S 1977 Ipsilateral fracture of the femur and tibia. Journal of Bone and Joint Surgery 59A: 240

68. Ratcliff A H C 1968 Fractures of the shaft of the femur and tibia in the same limb. Proceedings of the Royal Society of Medicine 61: 906

69. Hardy E G, Tibbs D J 1960 Acute ischaemia in limb injuries. British Medical Journal i: 1001

70. Kirkup J R 1963 Major arterial injury complicating fracture of the femoral shaft. Journal of Bone and Joint Surgery 45-B: 337

71. Isaacson J, Louis D S, Costenbader J M 1975 Arterial injury associated with closed femoral-shaft fracture. Report of 5 cases. Journal of Bone and Joint Surgery 57-A: 1147

72. McNamara J J, Brief D K, Stremple J F, Wright J K 1973 Management of fractures with associated arterial injury in combat casualties. Journal of Trauma 13: 17

73. Rich N M, Metz C W, Hutton J E, Baugh J H, Hughes C W 1971 Internal versus external fixation of fractures with concomitant vascular injuries in Vietnam. Journal of Trauma 11: 463

31

Injuries of the Knee

E. L. Trickey

Redevelop the quadriceps: exercise for five minutes hourly throughout the day. This instruction is of the utmost importance in the treatment of every knee-joint injury. Manipulations and operations may be performed, and the joint may be immobilised, but no matter what other treatment may be needed, active non-weight-bearing exercises must be practised. Simple strains, traumatic synovitis, rupture of ligaments, tearing of semilunar cartilages, fractures into the joint—almost every injury of the knee should be treated from the first day by regular qaudriceps drill. Injuries such as open wounds of the joint or traumatic haemarthrosis which may be complicated by infection or continued haemorrhage are the only exceptions, and even in these cases quadriceps exercise should be practised after two or three weeks.

Wasting of the quadriceps muscle is itself a source of disability. The knee joint is imperfectly protected from the twists and strains of weight-bearing. Repeated stretching of ligaments and nipping of synovial fringes cause recurrent effusion, and the swelling may persist for many months. If such muscle wasting is accompanied by rupture of ligaments or a tendency to arthritis, the disability is still more serious. It is seldom relieved by the operative construction of new ligaments, because if the muscle-guard is lost the ligaments stretch as soon as weight-bearing is resumed. It is not relieved by the use of a knee cage, because the protection of such an appliance is inadequate and still more wasting of muscles is encouraged. But if the quadriceps can be fully redeveloped, relaxation of ligaments and early osteoarthritis cause little or no incapacity. The joint is protected; it is no longer strained whenever weight-bearing is attempted; and the symptoms subside.

Muscle wasting occurs as a direct consequence of injury of the knee joint. An almost total reflex inhibition of the quadriceps may be observed, and the muscle is completely flaccid—it might well be paralysed, for no flicker of active contraction seems possible. Wasting is unusually rapid, and the volume of the muscle disappears far more rapidly than it can subsequently be regained. Treatment is therefore urgent. The inhibition must be overcome as soon as possible by the patient's own exercise. This can be practised without weight-bearing, without movement of the joint and without aggravation of the injury. Massage and faradism are relatively useless because the treatment is purely passive: it does not restore voluntary control, it encourages the patient in his apathy, and it is possible only for limited periods. Moreover, it is not enough to advise the patient vaguely to practise exercise. Specific instruction is essential. Quadriceps contraction must be demonstrated. The muscle shoud be made as tight as possible and the contraction sustained. The limb is raised against gravity with the knee straight, and after a few days it is raised against the resistance of a flat-iron or a brick suspended over the ankle (Fig 31.1). The exercise should be repeated every hour for not less than five minutes. Boredom may be relieved by practice to the beat of music. Such treatment prevents wasting of the thigh even when the limb is completely immobilised in splints or plaster. Even if the muscle

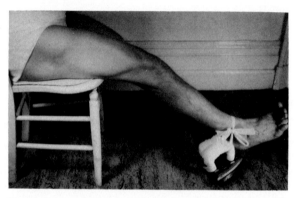

Fig 31.1 Active quadriceps exercise is of the greatest importance in all injuries of the knee joint.

is already wasted, it is possible, by quadriceps drill and by the non-weight-bearing exercises of cycling and swimming, to regain normal volume and tone of the muscle within six or eight weeks.

The injuries to be considered in this chapter include:

Internal derangements of the knee joint
  Traumatic synovitis and haemarthrosis.
  Injury of the medial, lateral and cruciate ligaments.
  Dislocation of the knee.
  Injury of the semilunar cartilages.
  Loose bodies in the knee.
Injuries of the extensor mechanism of the knee
  Avulsion of the quadriceps.
  Fracture of the patella.
  Avulsion of the ligamentum patellae.
  Injuries of the tibial tubercle and 'Schlatter's disease'.
  Dislocation of the patella.
Fractures of the tibial tuberosities

TRAUMATIC SYNOVITIS AND HAEMARTHROSIS OF THE KNEE JOINT

Traumatic synovitis. A strain or twist of the knee may cause synovial effusion with filling of the joint hollows, distension of the suprapatellar pouch, and 'floating' of the patella, which can be made to tap against the femoral condyles. The joint should be bound firmly with crêpe bandage and, if there is a marked effusion, immobilised on a back splint in the position of almost full extension. Exercise of the quadriceps muscle should begin at once and be continued hourly throughout the day. Weight-bearing is resumed in a few days and the back splint is discarded after 10 days. Recovery should be complete within two or three weeks.

Recurrent synovitis. If the muscles are allowed to waste recurrent synovitis may develop, particularly in middle-aged patients whose joints show a tendency to degenerative arthritis. Weight-bearing activity should be reduced until normal muscle control has been regained by regular quadriceps drill. Injury to one of the semilunar cartilages with recurrent displacement of a pedunculated fragment must be excluded.

Traumatic haemarthrosis. A severe blow or twist may tear the blood vessels of the synovial membrane and cause haemarthrosis. Haemorrhage into the joint also accompanies every fracture of the tibial spine and of the patella, and it may complicate tears of the peripheral part of a semilunar cartilage and operations for removal of the cartilage. The joint fills rapidly and is swollen within an hour, whereas in simple synovitis the swelling reaches its maximum only after six or eight hours. The joint contents feel firmer and less fluid than in synovitis, pain is greater and there is a febrile reaction. The temperature rises to 100°F or more (37.5°C) and the joint feels hot. The blood should be aspirated, the joint firmly bound with crêpe bandage and immobilised on a back splint. Quadriceps drill is begun after 10 or 14 days when the danger of recurrent haemorrhage is over. A spontaneous haemarthrosis in osteoarthritis has been described,[1] characteristically producing rapid swelling of the joint. Prompt aspiration greatly diminishes the disability from this condition. An acute traumatic haemarthrosis in a football injury may be due to an isolated tear of the anterior cruciate ligament. If such pathology is suspected action should be taken as indicated in the section dealing with cruciate ligament injuries (page 1040).

INJURIES OF THE LIGAMENTS OF THE KNEE JOINT

Whenever there is doubt about the extent of injury to knee-joint ligaments it is essential to complete the examination under general anaesthesia.

Medial ligament. The medial ligament is a broad, strong structure extending from the medial femoral condyle downwards and slightly forwards to a point on the tibial condyle distal to the mid-point of the medial semilunar cartilage. At this point it is firmly attached to the capsule and so to the tibial condyle and semilunar cartilage. It continues down the shaft of the tibia for a further 2 inches (5.1 cm) blending with the periosteum. At its upper portion the ligament blends in with the posterior joint capsule which covers the medial femoral condyle.

This ligament can be torn anywhere throughout its length, but injuries are common at the femoral or tibial attachments. A minor injury will involve the ligament in isolation, but more complete ruptures always include a tear of the postero-medial capsule.

The ligament complex is tight in extension and with external rotation of the tibia. It is torn by an abduction strain and by forced external rotation of the tibia. The diagnosis is made from the history together with swelling, ecchymosis and tenderness localised to the site of injury and by pain when the joint is forced into valgus. The joint can be made to open up on the medial side with valgus strain, but only when examined in some 20 degrees or more of flexion. The terminal degrees of extension movement are sometimes restricted, and during the first 14 days before limitation of movement has disappeared, it may be difficult to differentiate a simple sprain from a combined ligament and cartilage injury. If the injury is simply a sprain no more than a few fibres are torn and stability of the joint is normal.

The treatment of the injury depends on the degree of damage, and as degree of damage is determined by the amount of abnormal movement it may be necessary to examine the joint under anaesthesia to determine this correctly. A torn medial ligament will produce an opening of this side of the joint on valgus strain in flexion and an abnormal degree of external rotation movement of the tibia on the femur.

A minor strain needs little more than a crêpe bandage and possibly a stick or crutches for a while. It is important that further stress should be avoided by forbidding sport for two to three months.

A definite ligament tear requires treatment urgently to prevent permanent instability. An isolated tear of the medial ligament will heal if the joint is immobilised in plaster. It has been traditional to immobilise such an injury with the knee in extension. However, operative and dissection studies show that the divided ends of the ligament are separated in this position; this is particularly evident if the posterior capsule is involved. Torn ends are approximated by flexion of the joint. The optimum position for immobilisation in plaster in flexion of 45 degrees, which should be maintained for eight weeks.

There is a place for surgical repair of the damaged ligament. It should be undertaken in all cases in which the abnormal movement is gross as it is likely that one cruciate ligament at least is also torn. It should also be undertaken if there is suggestion that the ligament is displaced downwards or upwards by the palpation of a swelling which could be the rolled-up ligament near the joint level. Surgery should be undertaken within a few days of injury and not later than 10 days. An exposure on the medial side of the joint must be large enough to allow thorough inspection of the whole length of the ligament, the posterior capsular extension and the medial cartilage. It is desirable that the damaged structures are sutured into the bone rather than that soft tissue is sutured to soft tissue.

Late operative reconstruction of medial ligament of the knee. If a completely torn or avulsed medial ligament of the knee has not been protected by complete immobilisation at the time of injury a valgus and external rotatory instability of the joint persists. The disability can be reduced by a determined effort to regain normal muscle control. Operative treatment

must not be considered in late cases until exercises have been practised regularly for two or three months; often it will be found that operation is no longer necessary. If instability does persist stability can be improved either by constructing a new ligament from semitendinosus tendon[2] or by a medial capsular repair[3] supplemented by the pes anserinus transplant described by Slocum.[4] This transplant is effected by turning upwards the attachment of sartorius, gracilis and semitendinosus as a combined tendon from the shaft of the tibial to the medial tibial condyles, so that the action of these muscles is to actively control external rotation of the tibia, rather than to flex the knee joint. The joint is immobilised in plaster for eight weeks whichever procedure is undertaken, quadriceps exercises being continued throughout this time.

These procedures can be expected to improve knee-joint stability if instability is caused by medial ligament damage. They will not help if the instability is caused by a torn anterior cruciate ligament. It is a fact that the two types of instability are not sufficiently differentiated by clinicians.

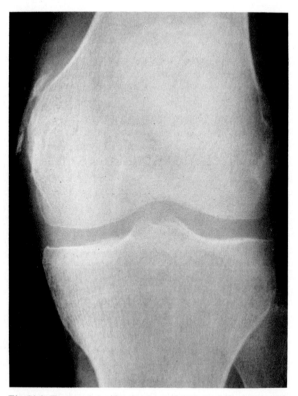

Fig 31.2 Traumatic ossification in a subperiosteal haematoma of an avulsed medial ligament of the knee—the so-called Pellegrini-Stieda disease.

Pellegrini-Stieda disease. When the medial ligament of the knee is avulsed from the femur, the periosteum at the site of its attachment is elevated and the subperiosteal haematoma undergoes ossification. Spicules, spurs or plaques of bone are formed (Fig 31.2). This bone formation has been described as Pellegrini-Stieda disease, but it does not differ from the ossification occurring at the periosteal attachment of any ligament or tendon that is avulsed from bone. It is not a disease of obscure origin, but a simple example of traumatic subperiosteal ossification. The condition is due to a partial tear of the ligament and is never associated with valgus instability. It does not, therefore, require any repair. The injury can be diagnosed before the appearance of calcification by the constant finding of gross limitation of flexion with pain over the femoral attachment of the ligament on forcing further movement, or palpating the part. Restoration of movement is always complete, but the range may take many weeks to return to normal. Manipulative treatment will only hinder progress, and physiotherapy should be confined to quadriceps strengthening exercises, with immobilisation in the acute stage.

The distinction should be clearly noted between this very common condition of subperiosteal ossification after avulsion of the ligament from the femur, and the rare condition of calcification within the ligament, which is comparable to calcification of the supraspinatus tendon of the shoulder.[5]

Lateral side of the knee joint. Stability of the lateral side of the knee joint is produced by the lateral ligament, the fascia lata and the popliteus and biceps femoris muscles. The lateral ligament is a small structure, taut when the joint is extended and floppy in flexion. The fascia lata is strong and broad. It is firmly attached to the tibial condyle and glides over the femoral condyle and lateral ligament in flexion and extension movements of the joint. It is attached by fascia to the strong tendon of the biceps femoris muscle, and to the lateral intermuscular septum of the thigh.

The lateral structures are damaged less commonly than the medial side. Damage is caused by a varus strain. A blow, however, may be transmitted from one knee to the other. A person who is struck on the outer side of the right knee by the bumper of a car can sustain ruptures of the medial ligament of the right knee and the lateral of the left knee (Fig 31.3).

It is incorrect to consider the lateral ligament in isolation. If damage occurs it is to the lateral structures as a whole. The injury may be a sprain or a complete rupture as demonstrated by marked opening up of the outer side of the joint on varus strain (Figs 31.4 and 31.5). A complete rupture is a rupture of all structures on the outer side. Marked widening of the joint does not occur without additional damage to one or both cruciate ligaments. The rupture of the lateral structures may be associated with an avulsion of the styloid process of the fibula (Fig 31.6), pulled off by the biceps tendon, or of bony fragments from the edge of the lateral tibial condyle, pulled off by the fascia lata (Fig 31.7). The bony injuries do not alter the diagnosis or treatment. Sprains require no more than regular muscle exercises with the avoidance of sport. Ruptures require open repair followed by plaster immobilisation in 30 degrees of flexion for eight weeks (Fig 31.8).

Old, untreated cases with persistant laxity cause less disability than do untreated ruptures of the medial ligament unless associated with genu varum. In such cases a high tibial osteotomy with correction of the varus is a more successful method of correcting instability than attempts at late repair of the soft tissue damage.

Rupture of the lateral structures with paralysis of external popliteal nerve. It is not surprising that this soft tissue injury is associated sometimes with damage to the external popliteal nerve. The nerve is vulnerable to any varus strain of the knee joint in the position of extension. There are two types of damage to the nerve. The nerve may be swollen and bruised at the level of the knee joint with or without loss of function. In such cases an expectant attitude should be adopted if there is paralysis. Alternatively the nerve may be completely torn. This injury occurs about 9 inches (23 cm) proximal to the joint and the distal end of the nerve lies rolled up in a ball at the level of the joint line. In such cases no effort should be made to repair the nerve damage as the intraneural damage is extensive. Active dorsiflexion of the foot should be restored as soon as convenient by anterior transplantation of the tibialis posterior tendon to the dorsum of the foot.

INJURIES OF THE CRUCIATE LIGAMENTS

Surgical anatomy. The *anterior cruciate ligament* is attached to the anterior part of the intercondylar area of the tibia and passes upwards and backwards to be attached to the intercondylar surface of the lateral femoral condyle. This ligament is taut in full flexion and with internal rotation of the tibia. It can

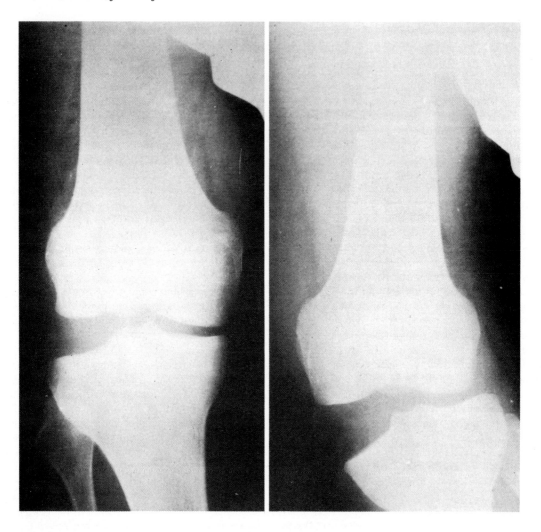

Fig 31.3 A young man was struck by a car on the lateral side of the knee. He ruptured the medial ligament of the left knee and the lateral structures of the right knee. The cruciate ligaments were torn in each knee.

be damaged by two quite separate mechanisms. It can be ruptured in isolation by forced full flexion with internal rotation of tibia. Such an injury can occur in gymnasts, basketball or soccer players or in a child who falls with the knee flexed while riding a bicycle. Alternatively it can be damaged in association with a ruptured medial ligament when the force that has ruptured the medial ligament continues and the anterior cruciate is stretched over the lateral femoral condyle, causing some fibres to be pulled apart or the whole ligament to rupture.

The classical teaching is that a ruptured anterior cruciate ligament produces an anterior draw sign of excessive mobility of the tibia on the femur at 90 degrees of knee flexion. Yet we have all seen cases of rupture of this ligament with very little abnormal movement in this position.

Abnormal movement in an anterior direction is always detectable, however, when the examination is undertaken in 10 degrees of flexion and may be abolished with a sudden jerk when the joint is flexed to 30 degrees. Only recently have clinicians come to appreciate this point. An examination carried out in 10 degrees of flexion is called *Lachman's sign* (Fig 31.9). An examination of anatomical specimens reveals that when the anterior cruciate ligament is divided in

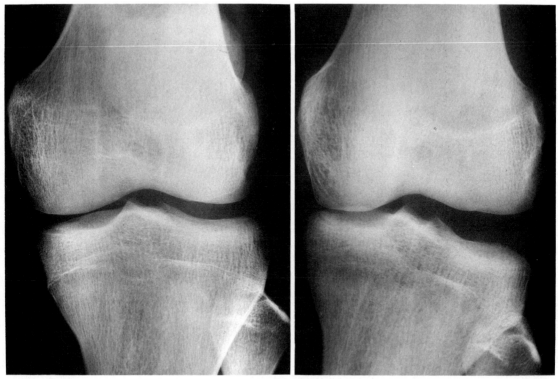

Fig 31.4

Fig 31.5

Fig 31.4 and 31.5 Avulsion of the lateral ligament. There will be no radiographic evidence of injury unless films are taken while the knee is adducted (Fig 31.5).

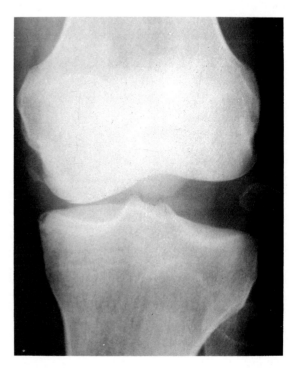

Fig 31.6 Avulsion of the lateral ligament of the knee with a fragment from the styloid process of the fibula.

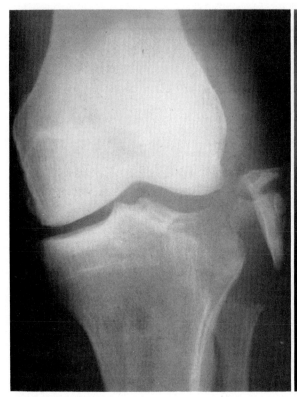

Fig 31.7 The lateral structures of the knee joint have been torn. The styloid process of the fibula is avulsed by the biceps femoris; the tibial plateau by the fascia lata.

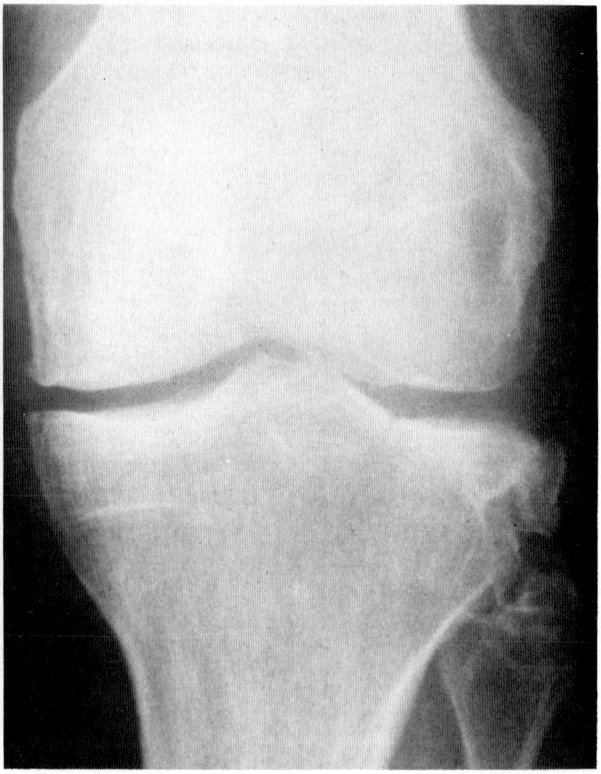

Fig 31.8 The same case as illustrated in Figure 31.7 after the avulsed fragments have been replaced by open repair.

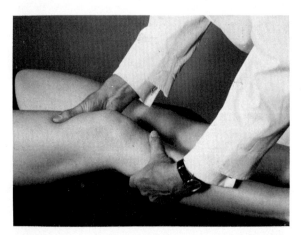

Fig 31.9 Testing for rupture of the anterior cruciate ligament. If abnormal forward mobility of the tibia is possible in 10° of knee flexion, the ligament is ruptured.

isolation the abnormal mobility is always rotatory. The lateral tibial condyle can be subluxed forwards. The tibia come forwards internally rotating. The extent of this rotatory movement is dependant on the integrity of the postero-lateral joint capsule. A divided medial ligament will allow a forward subluxation of the medial tibial condyle with tibia externally rotating. If the tibia can be displaced forwards without significant rotation, then there must be a combination of damage to medial and anterior cruciate ligaments. This is the pathology of true anterior draw sign at 90 degrees of flexion.

Therefore, when examining for a torn anterior cruciate ligament tear, first we will look for abnormal anterior subluxation of the lateral tibial condyle in 10 degrees of flexion. Then we undertake the jerk test.[6] With the knee in extension and internal rotation, the lateral tibial condyle is pushed forwards with palm of one hand. The joint is flexed. If the anterior cruciate ligament is torn the lateral tibial condyle will sublux forwards at 10 degrees of flexion. Further flexion is produced while the internal rotation is maintained and at 30 degrees of flexion the lateral tibial condyle will relocate with a characteristic jerk (Fig 31.10).

Lachman's sign is always positive and can be elicited in a conscious patient even when the joint is painful, because it involves so little joint movement.

The jerk test is not always positive and is dependant on the laxity of the postero-lateral joint capsule. Commonly it is painful and therefore sedation or anaesthesia may be required for the examination. However, the experienced examiner usually can elicit it without difficulty.

The *posterior cruciate ligament* is attached to the intercondylar surface of the tibia behind the inter-condylar eminences. It passes upwards and forwards to be attached to the front of the intercondylar surface of the medial femoral condyle. As with the anterior cruciate ligament this ligament can be damaged in isolation or as part of a combined injury. In isolation it is caused by blow on the front of a flexed knee, a mechanism common in motor-cycle injuries. It may be combined with damage to medial or lateral

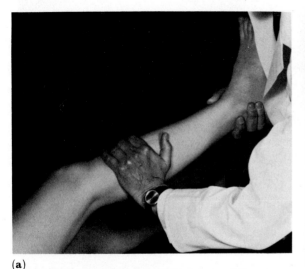

(a)

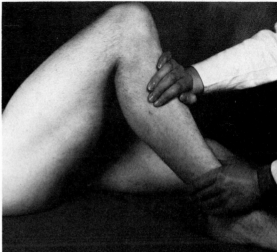

Fig 31.11 Testing for rupture of the posterior cruciate ligament. Excessive backward mobility of the tibia shows that the ligament is torn.

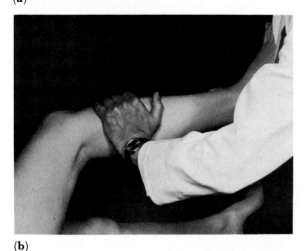

(b)

Fig 31.10 The jerk test. (a) In 5° of flexion the lateral tibial condyle is pressed forward to produce anterior subluxation. (b) As the knee is flexed, the lateral tibial condyle relocates with a jerk.

structures, and in such instances the posterior cruciate ligament damage may not be noticed, though the signs are there if one only looks for them. In combined injuries the posterior cruciate ligament damage is very important and its repair is just as important as that of the collateral ligament. The clinical sign of a ruptured posterior cruciate ligament is an abnormal posterior mobility of the tibia on the femur, detected when the knee is examined at flexion (Fig 31.11).

Fractures of the intercondylar area of the tibia. Formerly these injuries were named fractures of the tibial spine. This is incorrect naming. The fractures are fragments of bone avulsed by the cruciate ligaments. The so-called tibial spine consists of two intercondylar eminences, one on either side of the intercondylar space. The ligaments are attached to the space and not to the eminences (Figs 31.12 and 31.13).

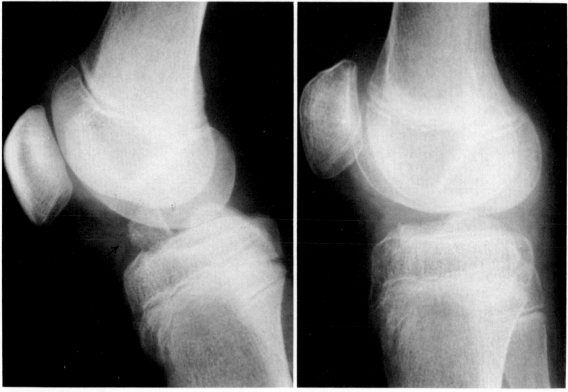

Fig 31.12   **Fig 31.13**

Figs 31.12 and 31.13 Avulsion of the anterior intercondylar area of the tibia by the anterior cruciate ligament (Fig 31.11). Minor displacements can be reduced by extending the knee under general anaesthesia. If operative replacement is necessary the reduction is usually stable on simple extension of the knee and internal fixation is unnecessary (Fig 31.12).

Anterior intercondylar fractures are caused by avulsion of the anterior cruciate ligament. The majority of these occur between the ages of 10 and 20 years and are common after a fall while riding a bicycle.[7] Undisplaced fractures should be immobilised in a plaster cylinder for six weeks. The bony fragment may be lifted up and may be rotated 90 degrees. Minor displacements will be replaced simply by fully extending the knee joint under anaesthesia. The mechanism of reduction is that the fragment is wide enough for the femoral condyles to push it back into its bed. If reduction is incomplete, and this is likely with grossly rotated fragments, open reduction is indicated. Usually the large fragment can be slipped under the anterior horn of the semilunar cartilages and remains stable in reduction without fixation, as long as the knee is kept extended. Smaller fragments, which may be avulsed in adults, will need some form of fixation, such as with a screw.

Posterior intercondylar fractures are fragments avulsed by the posterior cruciate ligament. These injuries occur at an older age than the anterior fractures. Undisplaced avulsions can be treated conservatively but displaced ones should be replaced by open operation and will need fixation with a single screw.[8]

Treatment of ruptures of the cruciate ligaments. Isolated ligament injuries commonly are missed, unless there is an intercondylar fracture, because the history of the mechanism of injury is not taken in detail and because physical signs of abnormal movement cannot be elicited in a painful knee without anaesthesia. It is essential that such an examination is undertaken, after aspiration of an effusion if it is large and under anaesthesia if necessary, in any case in which there is doubt about the diagnosis. If a torn anterior cruciate ligament is suspected as an isolated lesion an arthroscopy should be undertaken to assess the possibility of a primary repair. Cruciate ligament injuries associated with ruptures of medial or lateral structures often are unnoticed because the damage to the other structures is more obvious. It is not possible to produce gross abnormal mobility from ruptured medial or lateral ligaments without some cruciate ligament damage.

Minor damage of cruciate ligaments need not be repaired. When the ligament fibres are pulled apart in the middle so that each end looks like the bristles of a toothbrush repair is always unsatisfactory and healing does not take place between the two ends. As far as the cruciate ligament injury is concerned the joint is immobilised for pain, although often a more treatable ligament injury will determine management. When the anterior or posterior ligament is torn

out from bone at either end, repair is more easily accomplished and the ligament should be fixed to bone and not to soft tissues as this is unreliable (Figs 31.14 and 31.15). When the collateral ligament is torn an exposure is made large enough to repair both injuries and in such a case the knee opens up to allow the cruciate ligament to be repaired first. The surgical exposure of the posterior cruciate ligament from the back of the knee is not difficult and is described in Chapter 15.

Primary surgical repair of ruptured cruciate ligaments should be undertaken soon after injury and not later than 10 days. Whichever method of management is considered necessary it is most important to continue exercising the quadriceps muscles. This aspect of treatment becomes particularly important when mobilisation commences. There

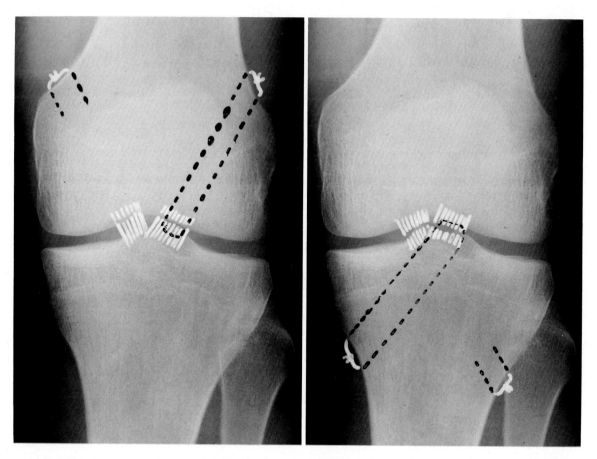

Fig 31.14 In this antero-posterior X-ray of the knee the direction of the stay sutures for the repair of a cruciate ligament avulsed from the femoral attachment has been drawn in.

Fig 31.15 Shows the same type of suture as in Figure 31.14 taken through the tibial condyle when the ligaments are avulsed from their lower attachments. Where the rupture is in the middle either method can be used.

can be marked incapacity from cruciate ligament injuries which have not been repaired and the knee may be unstable. The incapacity from instability is diminished by keeping up muscle tone and sometimes by changing sporting activities to something less strenuous. No attempt should be made to undertake late surgery for knee ligament damage until any semilunar cartilage damage has been treated.

In rotatory instability due to an old rupture of the anterior cruciate ligament MacIntosh has devised an operation which prevents medial rotation of the lateral tibial condyle. A long strip of fascia lata, attached to the tibia and 1 inch (2.5 cm) wide, is sutured to the lateral femoral condyle under the lateral ligament and to the lateral intermuscular septum, with the knee flexed and in full external rotation. The knee is immobilised in plaster for six weeks. The foot must be included so that the position of external rotation of the tibia is maintained. This operation is described in detail with illustrations elsewhere.[9]

Recurrent dislocation of the superior tibio-fibular joint.[10] This rare condition occurs in adolescent girls, usually before the age of 18. There may be a vague history of trauma, but quite often the symptoms start without reason, and unless the possibility of the diagnosis is brought to mind the condition may be mistaken for a derangement of the meniscus and an unnecessary exploration of the knee may be carried out.

The fibular head usually displaces forwards producing a prominence on the lateral side of the knee; this hypermobility of the fibula can be demonstrated clinically and radiologically and the movement may be accompanied by pain. Treatment is unnecessary— the girls should be advised to wear a supporting bandage around the knee when playing games and reassured that the instability will disappear by the time adult life is reached.

DISLOCATION OF THE KNEE JOINT

Complete rupture of the medial, lateral or cruciate ligaments of the knee must be associated with momentary dislocation. Less frequently, direct violence applied to the head of the tibia, or indirect twisting or hyperextension strain, causes more severe injury, and the tibia is dislocated backwards, forwards or laterally and does not slip back into position spontaneously. Five types of dislocation are described according to the direction in which the tibia is displaced: anterior, posterior, lateral, medial and

rotatory;[11] of these the anterior displacement predominates. Not only are the ligaments ruptured but the capsule is extensively torn, the semilunar cartilages may be displaced, and chip fractures of the tibial spine, tibial tuberosities or femoral condyles may occur. As a rule, reduction is accomplished quite easily by traction and direct pressure over the displaced bones.

The treatment of this condition is the same as the treatment of each ligament torn in isolation. Whenever possible the torn ligaments are repaired. It is not possible to predict the ease of repair without exploration and a seemingly impossible situation may be easy to solve. It must be emphasised that attention be paid to the cruciate ligaments first while the knee is widely open before the collateral ligament is repaired. The repair of the collateral ligament must be as thorough as the extent of damage will allow.

Occasionally it will be considered advisable to treat the injury conservatively for such reasons as the poor general condition of the patient, gross local skin damage or inadequate facilities for extensive surgery. In such cases the joint is immobilised in plaster for six to eight weeks. Sometimes an excellent function result is obtained but always there is abnormal laxity somewhere. This can be treated according to merit at a later date (Fig 31.16 and 31.17).

Dislocation with interposition of capsule. Sometimes the dislocation cannot be reduced by manipulation because the femoral condyle is driven through a short tear in the capsule and gripped like a button in a button-hole. A flap of capsular tissue is interposed between the articular surfaces. It has been suggested by the findings at operation that this injury is produced by an abduction-medial rotation strain of the tibia on the femur. A rather similar lesion, with inclusion in the joint of the styloid process of fibula and a temporary lateral popliteal palsy, has been described in a case of medial dislocation.[12] This can be compared to the lateral dislocation of the elbow joint with capsular interposition on the inner side and an ulnar nerve palsy.

The postero-lateral dislocation of the knee joint shown in Figures 31.18 to 31.20 sustained by a Czech pilot during the Second World War illustrates the clinical findings when there is interposition of the capsule. Repeated manipulation failed to reduce the dislocation. The backward displacement was easily corrected, but no matter what pressure was applied the joint space remained wide on the inner side, and on attempting to force reduction there was dimpling of skin over the medial joint line from the pull of

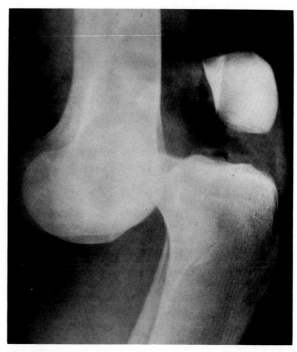

Figs 31.16 and 31.17 A forward dislocation of the knee joint
was associated with rupture of skin and deep tissues over the
femoral condyles in the popliteal space. The wound was excised,
the dislocation reduced, the joint immobilised and the muscles
redeveloped. An excellent recovery of joint function was
obtained. (Mr J. R. Armstrong's case.)

Fig 31.16

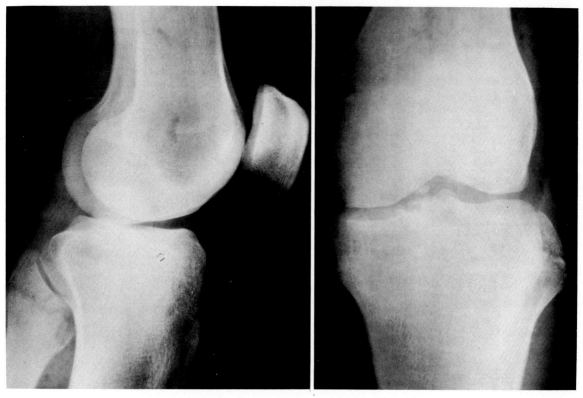

Fig 31.17

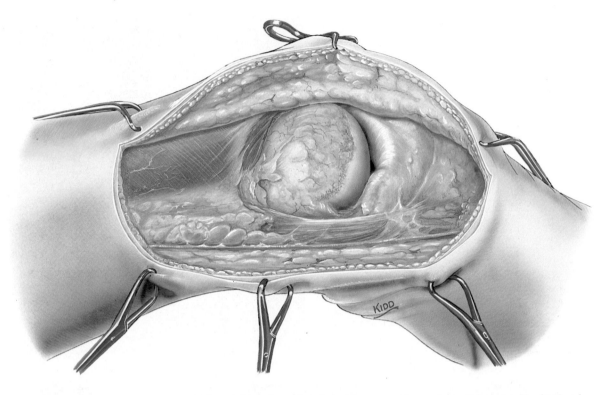

Fig 31.18 Dislocation of the knee joint with interposition of capsule and quadriceps expansion on the medial side (see Figs 31.19 and 31.20).

underlying tissues imprisoned in the joint. Operative reduction was necessarily delayed for over two months because the initial violence drove the medial femoral condyle so hard against overlying skin that an area lost its blood supply and an ulcer developed— a trophic sore from pressure by bone on the deep surface of the skin. At operation the medial femoral condyle and its articular surface were visible as soon as skin and fascia were divided, the medial ligament, capsule and quadriceps expansion being tucked into the joint. Six months later, after immobilisation of the joint in plaster with early quadriceps exercise, free movement to the right angle has been regained, with excellent stability of the joint, and a determined pilot of magnificent spirit went back to operational duties.

The open reduction in this case was of necessity delayed because of the poor skin condition; but in most cases it should be possible to proceed with operation as soon as possible after the injury—the sooner the articulation is restored to normal the better will be the result.

Nerve complications. Lateral popliteal palsy is likely to occur in medial dislocations of the knee joint. The prognosis depends upon the degree of stretching and the length of nerve trunk subjected to traction. In over 50 per cent of recorded cases there has been permanent paralysis.[13] The management of this complication has already been discussed (p. 1035).

Vascular complications. Dislocations of the knee joint are sometimes complicated by injury to the popliteal artery. The vessel is fixed by fibrous arches at the upper and lower limits of the popliteal space and cannot accommodate itself readily to the displaced position of the bones. The complication occurs more frequently in anterior dislocation of the tibia. In one series of 22 dislocations there were five with vascular complications, all of which were anterior displacements.[11] The incidence of almost 25 per cent gives a fair indication of the frequency of the problem. The evidence of vascular injury is obvious at once if the artery is completely torn; but when simple contusion or stretching causes later thrombosis there may only be delayed evidence of such injury on the third or fourth day. In either case the only hope for saving the

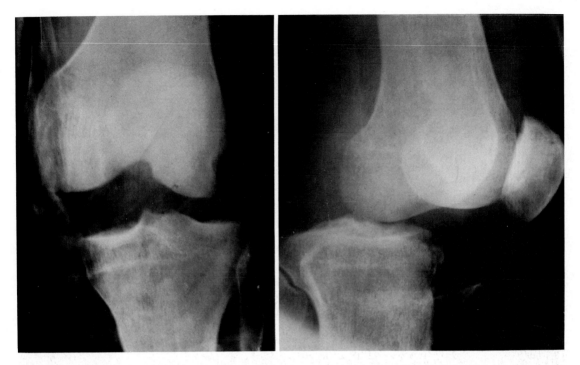

Fig 31.19 Postero-lateral dislocation of the knee joint. Manipulative reduction proved impossible. Widening of the joint space on the inner side is shown in this radiograph, and the clinical sign of dimpling of the skin over the inner side during manipulation confirmed the diagnosis of capsular interposition (see Fig 31.18).

limb is by exploration of the artery at the earliest possible opportunity after vascular impairment has been diagnosed. A delay of more than a few hours may result in an amputation, whereas early restoration of blood flow by direct suture, vein graft or insertion of Dacron prosthesis can give a successful outcome (see Chapter 11).

INJURIES OF THE SEMILUNAR CARTILAGES

Place one finger over the joint line of the knee in front of the medial ligament where the curved margin of the medial femoral condyle approaches the tibial tuberosity. Now externally rotate the foot and leg. It is easy to feel the medial semilunar cartilage disappearing from the surface, leaving a sulcus between the bones as it is sucked towards the middle of the joint. The cartilage is approaching the weight-bearing areas. When the tibia is also strongly abducted, the meniscus must lie actually between the weight-bearing areas. If the movement is sufficiently forcible, and at the same time weight is driven through the joint, the cartilage is split longitudinally.

The mechanism of injuries of the semilunar cartilage. This is the mechanism of all injuries to the medial meniscus of the knee joint. Whereas rupture of the medial ligament arises from abduction strain of the extended knee, tearing of the semilunar cartilage occurs from weight-bearing stress of the flexed knee.[14, 15] The joint must be flexed because otherwise the tibia is not free to rotate; body-weight must be carried through the joint at the moment of strain to give the grinding, splitting force; the tibia must be rotated laterally on the femur (or if the tibia is fixed, the femur rotated medially on the tibia) and at the same time abducted, to displace the medial cartilage between the weight-bearing surfaces. The degree of mobility of the meniscus accompanying rotation of the tibia varies in normal individuals and upon this depends its susceptibility to injury. It is therefore possible to forecast which individual is most likely to sustain a torn cartilage by estimating the laxity of the joint and the range of mobility of the meniscus. The footballer who tears a cartilage in one knee will usually be found to have excessive mobility of the cartilages of the opposite knee which as yet are uninjured. Moreover, it is not unusual to find a professional footballer who

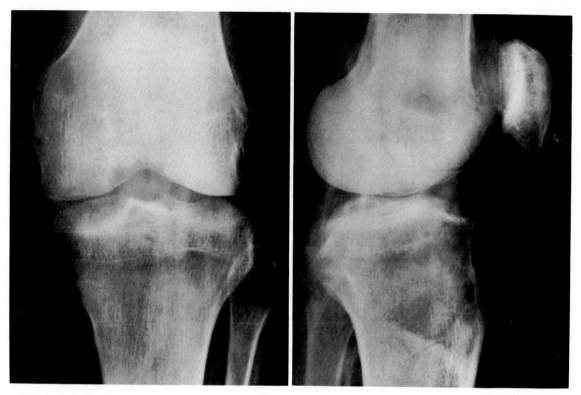

Fig 31.20 Same case as in Figures 31.18 and 31.19 after operative reduction. The patient eventually returned to full duty as a fighter pilot in the Second World War.

ruptures two or even three of his semilunar cartilages during a short career, whereas fellow-players exposed to similar stresses escape without one such rupture.

Redisplacements and secondary tears of cartilage. The first injury which actually splits the meniscus of the knee must necessarily be a weight-bearing stress. The footballer has all his weight on one foot which is fixed to the ground; in turning sharply towards the opposite side, so that the femur is internally rotated, he falls with the knee flexed and abducted. Subsequent displacements may of course occur with or without weight-bearing. Any lateral rotation strain of the tibia on the femur slides the meniscus towards the middle of the joint and may displace the loose fragment into the intercondylar region. If subsequent redisplacements do occur during weight-bearing, the same grinding force is applied once more and a secondary injury may be sustained. When a meniscus has been displaced many times, double bucket-handle tears, triple or even quadruple bucket-handle tears, combined bucket-handle and posterior horn tears, or secondary tears of the free margin of central or

peripheral fragments are very often found (Figs 31.21–31.28). Moreover, the lateral meniscus may be torn, especially when the first injury was associated with rupture of the posterior cruciate ligament leaving the joint unstable so that at the time of redisplacements either cartilage may be displaced between the weight-bearing areas.

Occupational hazards. Injuries of the semilunar cartilages occur most frequently in professional and amateur footballers, carpet layers and miners. The occupational hazard of the carpet layer arises mainly from the instrument shaped like a toasting fork, with sharp prongs, which he uses to tighten a fitted carpet. The workman kneels on the left knee, and with his right foot fixed on the ground and the knee flexed to the right angle, the inner surface of the knee is used as a 'punch' to strike the instrument. The medial meniscus is torn and displaced. Miners who work in low seams in a crouching position with the knee joints flexed often tear the back of the cartilage, for the more flexed the knee joint is at the moment of injury, and the farther back on the head of the tibia the

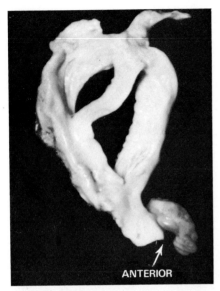

Fig 31.21 Double bucket-handle tear.

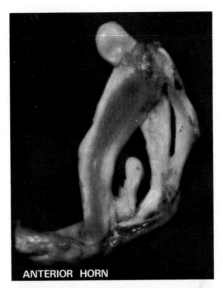

Fig 31.22 Triple bucket-handle tear.

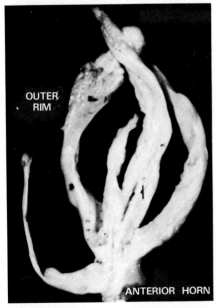

Fig 31.23 Quadruple bucket-handle and early fifth tear.

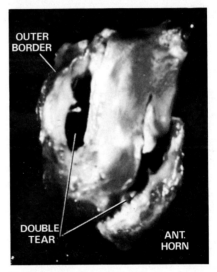

Fig 31.24 Double bucket-handle tear of congenital discoid cartilage.

Figs 31.21 to 31.24 Multiple cartilage injuries.

weight is borne, the farther back is the lesion of the cartilage.

Injuries of the lateral meniscus. The lateral cartilage tends to displace towards the middle of the joint by the opposite strain—internal rotation and adduction of the tibia on the femur. This twist is less frequent than the opposite one, and the mobility of the lateral meniscus from the periphery to the central part of the joint is more restricted than that of the medial meniscus. The frequency of injuries of the lateral

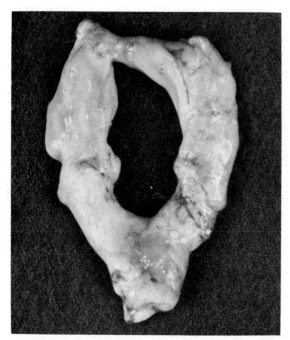 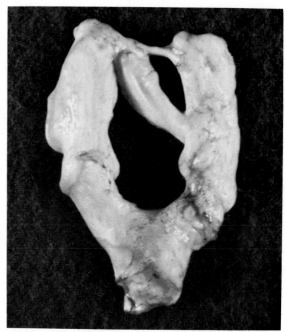

Fig 31.25   **Fig 31.26**

Figs 31.25 and 31.26 Concealed second bucket-handle tear. When the cartilage is first exposed it appears that the lesion is a simple bucket-handle tear (Fig 31.25). Only after the whole cartilage including the peripheral fragment is excised does the second bucket-handle split appear (Fig 31.26).

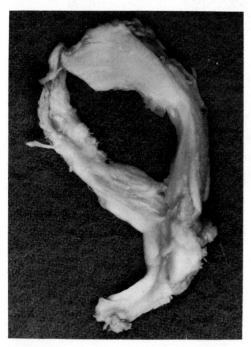 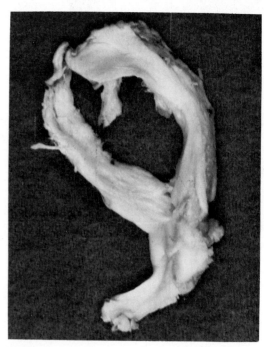

Fig 31.27   **Fig 31.28**

Figs 31.27 and 31.28 Concealed second tear in the posterior horn. Bucket-handle tear with secondary horn tear of the peripheral fragment (Fig 31.28).

meniscus is therefore six or eight times less than that of the medial meniscus.

Types of cartilage tear. The injury may consist of a longitudinal split separating a central 'bucket-handle' fragment which is displaced across the joint into the intercondylar space. On the other hand, the split may lie in the peripheral capsular attachment so that the whole meniscus is displaced. Again there may be a localised tear of the posterior part of the peripheral attachment which loosens the posterior horn, or a localised split of the central free margin of the cartilage separating a small pedunculated fragment. These injuries may be divided into two clinical groups: (1) bucket-handle tears and peripheral attachment tears, in which a large fragment or the whole cartilage is displaced centrally and the joint is therefore locked and (2) posterior horn tears and tears of the central free margin, in which a small pedunculated fragment is displaced and the joint does not lock.

Clinical features of a bucket-handle tear of the medial cartilage. The classical history of a torn medial cartilage is elicited when the lesion is of the bucket-handle type. The patient sustains an abduction-lateral rotation strain of the tibia on the femur. Immediate severe pain over the medial side of the joint is often accompanied by a tearing sensation. The joint locks in the semiflexed position, and extension movement is limited not only by pain but by an elastic resistance. Within a few hours the joint swells. After several days the range of movement increases, but the terminal degrees of extension remain limited, and even if the joint looks straight to the surgeon it does not feel straight to the patient. A history of sudden unlocking is sometimes but not always given. Within three or four weeks the pain disappears, the swelling subsides and the joint seems to be normal. Some weeks or months later, repeated stress of the same type causes recurrent locking pain and effusion. On this occasion the disability is of shorter duration. Every time the cartilage is displaced, reactionary swelling and pain become less marked. Finally the patient may suffer locking and unlocking of the knee almost without interference with his normal routine. With such a history with tenderness over the joint line in front of the medial ligament, and radiographic evidence excluding loose body formation, the diagnosis of a bucket-handle tear of the medial semilunar cartilage is seldom beyond doubt. If the last few degrees of extension movement are limited by an elastic block it is clear that the loose fragment, or even the whole cartilage, is still displaced across the joint and is lying in the intercondylar region.

Clinical features of posterior horn tear of the medial cartilage. When the lesion of the cartilage is not a longitudinal split, with displacement of a fragment so large that it locks the joint, but a localised tear which separates a small pedunculated fragment or loosens the posterior horn, the classical history is not elicited. The injury again arises from abduction-lateral rotation strain of the flexed joint, and pain is usually on the medial side, but there is no locking and unlocking, no localising tenderness and sometimes no effusion. The patient reports that the joint feels unstable. It feels as if the joint is about to lock but it never actually does so. It tends to give way, especially when going down stairs, and this sensation of insecurity may recur many times a day. There may be a sensation of something slipping, but localisation is so difficult that the patient usually puts his hands on each side of the joint and says 'it is in the middle'. The history is characteristically vague, and with the exception of one important sign clinical examination may not help to establish the diagnosis. The sign was described by McMurray.[16] and is of the greatest value. Without it, the diagnosis may be overlooked in a group of cartilage injuries which are no less common than bucket-handle tears—or alternatively the surgeon is driven to an 'exploration of the knee' which often fails to disclose the lesion because it lies so far back that it cannot be seen until the cartilage has actually been removed.

Test for posterior horn cartilage lesions. The surgeon stands on the side of the injured knee, places the fingers of one hand over the joint line and with the other hand firmly grasps the foot. The knee is flexed fully so that the heel is almost touching the buttock. The tibia is then rotated inwards and outwards on the femur, and is moved sideways from the adducted to the abducted position and back again. If the tear is at the posterior limit of the cartilage the loose fragment can be felt slipping between the femoral condyle and tibial tuberosity, and the resulting click is localised to the postero-medial compartment of the joint. If this manoeuvre fails to disclose a typical click, the leg should be rotated and abducted at the knee whole the joint is slowly extended. An easily palpable and often audible click may then be produced as the pedunculated fragment slips between the femoral condyle and tibial tuberosity. The more extended the knee at the moment that the click is produced, the farther forward in the cartilage is the tear. Care must be taken to differentiate this click from the posterior-horn cartilage click which is normal in the relatively lax joints of children, and which sometimes can be elicited in adults even in the uninjured knee. The thin quality of this click, the fact that it is not audible, that it is unaccompanied by any jerking movement between the femur and tibia, and that it does not reproduce the pain which had been experienced every time that the knee gave way, all indicate that it arises from laxity of the cartilage within normal limits, and not from a loose fragment or tearing of the posterior horn from its peripheral attachments.

Clinical features of torn lateral cartilage. Bucket-handle tears and detachment of pedunculated fragments from the posterior horn or from the central free margin of the lateral cartilage occur less commonly than in the medial cartilage, but the frequency is nevertheless greater than is generally recognised. This lesion is the result of an adduction-medial rotation strain of the tibia on the femur, and pain is usually localised to the lateral side of the joint. Tenderness is absent from the medial side but may be elicited on the lateral side over the anterior horn of the cartilage, the middle of the lateral ligament, or the posterior horn of the cartilage, according to the site of injury. Bucket-handle tears with displacement of the fragment always account for limitation of the terminal degree of extension and sometimes cause typical locking. Posterior horn lesions are recognised by the cartilage click elicited when the fully flexed tibia is adducted, medially rotated and gradually extended. Anterior horn lesions often cause very clicking, audible at a distance, occurring as the joint is actively extended and usually in the position of about twenty degrees short of full extension. The loud click or 'clunk' is also the characteristic feature of congenital discoid cartilages, which represent the persistence of the discoid form of cartilage seen in the knee joints of certain apes and reproduced in the early stages of development of the human fetus by a plate of mesodermal tissue.[17]

Arthrography and arthroscopy. Arthrography is undertaken as an out-patient procedure using local anaesthesia.

This examination should be undertaken by someone specialising in the technique and the success is dependant on experience. The success rate should be very high in the diagnosis of meniscal lesions, which are its main indication. In particular, the posterior horn of the medial meniscus is clearly demonstrated. It will demonstrate lesions of the articular cartilage of the femoral condyles. It is not helpful for patellar cartilage wear and the true state of the anterior cruciate ligament is not shown.

Arthroscopy is undertaken under general anaesthesia, therefore admission to hospital for one day at least is necessary. The arthroscopy is introduced by a stab incision just lateral to the patellar tendon. A good view is obtained of the patella, the femoral condyles, both menisci and the anterior cruciate ligament. The most difficult area to visualise is the postero-medial corner. This is the weakness of the method as this is the site of commencement of nearly all medial meniscal tears, and the commonest for false negative findings.

If an ancillary method of examination is considered necessary in a particular instance arthrography as an out-patient should be undertaken first, if the facilities exist. As a result of the findings the next step, if any, can be discussed with the patient.

Treatment of torn semilunar cartilage. *Treatment of first injury.* The peripheral attachment of a cartilage to the capsule of the joint is well supplied with blood vessels, and tears in this region can unite. Tears of the avascular cartilage itself seldom unite and recurrent displacement of the loose fragment is then inevitable. It is wise after a first injury to immobilise the knee with a pressure bandage or in a plaster cylinder for three to four weeks in the hope that the lesion may be in the peripheral attachment. Operative treatment is advised only when recurrent locking proves that this is not so.

A torn cartilage should of course be removed as soon as the diagnosis is certain; but it should be emphasised that the diagnosis must be certain. At first many injured knee joints seem to show signs of a torn cartilage, whereas in fact the injury is no more than a traumatic synovitis.

No harm comes from allowing time for the reaction to settle and for the diagnosis to become more certain, and some unnecessary operations will be avoided. After a severe wrench of the joint with acute synovitis there is often limitation of extension which may be misinterpreted as a block to movement from displacement of the cartilage, and yet this sign disappears after two or three weeks of simple rest.

The patient who fears that loss of the function of the semilunar cartilage will cause weakness of the joint may be reassured not only by the experience of surgeons, but also by that of experimental pathologists. Firstly, by keeping a damaged semilunar cartilage, articular cartilage is worn away, and secondly, a growth of fibrous tissue from the deep layers of the capsule produces a new cartilage which replaces the old one and resembles it in contour and position, although not in size, mobility or vulnerability to further injury. A regenerated cartilage is distinguished easily from a normal cartilage by its tri-radiate shape and white colour. Very occasionally a regenerated cartilage is fractured once more, with the separation of a pedunculated or bucket-handle fragment, and the surgeon who operates for recurrent disability after an earlier operation and finds a split cartilage must not jump to the conclusion that a previous surgeon had failed completely in his task of removing the cartilage.[18, 19, 20.]

Treatment of recurrent cartilage displacement. If the cartilage has been displaced on more than one occasion, no doubt remains as to the necessity for operative treatment. The disability cannot be cured by immobilisation or by manipulation, and any attempt to prevent displacement by the fitting of a knee cage or other surgical appliance is uncertain and unsatisfactory. If the cartilage is not removed the recurrent trauma of repeated displacement leads ultimately to osteoarthritis of the joint.

Treatment of torn cartilage in an osteoarthritic knee. It is sometimes said that operative treatment is not indicated for recurrent cartilage displacement if osteoarthritic changes are present in the joint. This view is entirely unjustified. Every time the cartilage is displaced the joint is traumatised and the arthritis is aggravated.

Treatment of torn cartilage with ruptured ligaments. It has also been suggested that excision of the cartilage is not advisable when the cruciate ligaments are ruptured. This view is equally unjustified. Far from refusing to excise the torn cartilage it is the duty of the surgeon to make certain that both cartilages are not torn.

Manipulative treatment. Although it is possible to reduce a locked knee by manipulation claims to cure cartilage instability are unjustified. The disabilities permanently relieved by manipulation have not been from torn cartilages: they may have been from adhesions in the region of the cartilage, from recurrent synovitis with hypotonicity of the quadriceps, or from early arthritis of the knee joint with loss of muscle control. Adhesions can be cured by manipulative treatment, and injured knee joints are always improved by simple redevelopment of the quadriceps, but there is little more than this to the work of osteopaths and other manipulators in their treatment of this joint.

Technique of excision of medial semilunar cartilage. A pneumatic tourniquet is applied and the leg is hung over the end of the table with the knee flexed. The medial cartilage is removed through an oblique incision two inches (5.0 cm) in length over the anteromedial compartment of the joint. If the incision begins near the patella and passes downwards and inwards, a small branch of the saphenous nerve may be divided, causing anaesthesia of the skin over the tibial tubercle, and sometimes persistent tenderness of the scar from nerve bulb formation. An incision that begins over the margin of the femoral condyle and passes downwards and outwards avoids injury to the nerve and gives equal access to the joint. The capsule and synovial membrane are divided in the same line.

An accurate idea of the type of meniscal damage will have been formed before the joint is opened from either the history or physical signs or from the ancillary investigations of arthrography or arthroscopy. Because of this the exact technique necessary will vary on account of the type of pathology. A basic principle is that torn portions of a meniscus are removed and normal portions are left alone. Here a strong word of warning is necessary because it may not be absolutely certain that the hidden posterior horn of the medial meniscus is normal. If reasonable doubt exists then the posterior horn must be removed together with any more obvious torn segments.

The joint has been opened and now it is inspected with medial and lateral retractors. A blunt hook is passed round the anterior horn of the meniscus and is pulled forward hard. This may improve the view of the posterior horn. A particular inspection is made of the postero-medial corner of the meniscus to look for a split running parallel with the peripheral attachment.

A simple tag tear is removed. A bucket handle fragment is removed without disturbing the rim whether or not the central fragment is displaced or remains in situ.

If it is considered right to remove the whole meniscus the anterior horn is freed first by sharp dissection, grasped by a cartilage clamp and pulled forwards. The peripheral attachment is freed by sharp dissection bit by bit, pulling the meniscus forward all the time. When it comes to the time to free the posterior horn, it is wise to use a tenotomy knife, a single piece scapel or a Smillie knife. A disposable blade scapel should not be used in case the blade breaks off at the back of the joint. It is essential that the knife used is sharp. It is safer.[21]

It must always be remembered that, as well as the main popliteal vessels, the geniculate arteries lie just behind the menisci and that a tenotome, pointed knife or a sharp, narrow chisel driven carelessly into the back of the knee joint may perforate these arteries and cause an aneurism.[22, 23]

Excision of the posterior horn of the medial cartilage. If by an error of technique the back of the cartilage is not completely removed through the anterior exposure (and it should be emphasised that this is always possible) a second incision should at once be made behind and parallel to the medial ligament, the capsule and synovial membrane being divided in the same line (Fig. 31.29). A retractor is held over the margin of the ligament, and the posterior capsule of the joint is retracted. The back of the cartilage with its posterior horn is thus removed without very great difficulty.

Excision of lateral cartilage. The technique of operation is the same as for the excision of the medial cartilage, but if a second incision is made for removal of the posterior horn, care must be taken not to damage the popliteus tendon, which lies in contact with the cartilage.

Post-operative treatment after excision of the cartilage. After operation, the knee should be protected by means of a plaster-slab bound to the limb with a crêpe bandage. The degree of joint reaction depends upon the number of times the cartilage has previously been displaced. If an operation is performed after a first or second displacement, considerable effusion

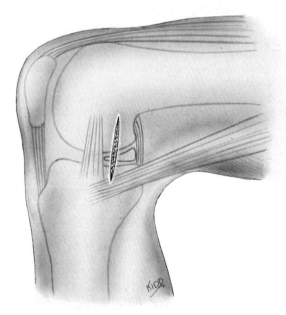

Fig 31.29 If through an error of technique the posterior horn is left in the back of the joint it is essential to remove it through a second incision over the posterior compartment.

must be expected and six or eight weeks may elapse before recovery is complete. If the cartilage has been displaced many times, the reaction is slight and recovery is often complete within four weeks. Rapid recovery is possible only if the tone of the thigh muscles is maintained. The patient should be taught quadriceps drill before operation. The day after operation, attempts should be made to overcome the reflex inhibition of the muscle. Part of the weight is taken by the surgeon while the patient tries to elevate the limb with the knee straight. With suitable encouragement and persuasion the patient takes more and more of the weight, until quite suddenly the knack of contracting the muscle is regained. Non-weight-bearing quadriceps contraction is then continued for five minutes hourly throughout the day. Flexion movements are begun after about 14 days, and weight-bearing is permitted.

Cysts of the semilunar cartilage arise from mucoid degeneration of the cartilage substance, possibly as a result of contusion of the cartilage from a direct blow, or indirectly by vertical compression between the femur and tibia.[15, 24, 25] The cystic area involves the peripheral part of the middle third of the lateral cartilage and very occasionally of the medial cartilage. It is multilocular and gives rise to a swelling beneath the lateral ligament so tense that it is sometimes mistaken for a bony exostosis. The size of the cystic mass may be anything up to two inches (5.0 cm) in diameter. The diagnosis is easily made by precise localisation of the swelling, which can be seen and felt. It is the only tense swelling that is situated exactly in the middle of the lateral surface of the knee at the level of the joint line. The patient complains of persistent aching pain but not of locking, giving way or recurrent swelling. The whole of the cyst and the cartilage from which it is developing should be removed.

Arthroscopic removal of a torn semilunar cartilage. Since 1970 earnest attempts have been made to undertake intra-articular surgery of the knee joint with the aid of an arthroscope. This has reached the stage that it is possible to deal effectively with nearly all meniscal tears, remove loose bodies, divide constricting bands as well as inspecting the joint and undertaking synovial biopsy.

The arthroscope is used to control the surgical procedure either by direct vision or through a television monitor attached to the arthroscope. The surgery is undertaken by the introduction of appropriate instruments such as scissors, knives or grasping forceps through a separate stab incision.

The technique has reached the stage that this method of meniscal surgery is the preferred one in the hands of those experienced in its use. It is possible to be more conservative by the removal of torn fragments only. Detention in hospital need be no more than a day or two and return to full function is rapid. This management fulfils the best principles of surgery.

This method is new and must be learnt carefully. There is no better guide than the book by Dandy[26] on this subject.

Calcification and ossification of semilunar cartilage. Aching pain in the knee joint sometimes occurs from calcification of one or both semilunar cartilages, a pathological process which possibly follows compression injury. It should be remembered that this may be only a manifestation of the generalised calcification of cartilage seen in chondro-calcinosis or pseudo-gout.

LOOSE BODIES IN THE KNEE JOINT

Loose bodies in the knee joint may arise from four sources: (1) osteochondritis dissecans, in which a fragment of articular cartilage and underlying bone is separated from the femoral condyle and less commonly from other parts of the articular surfaces; (2) osteoarthritis of the knee with detachment or fracture of marginal osteophytes from the patella, femoral condyles or tibial tuberosities; (3) chondrification of the synovial membrane with the formation of a large number of loose bodies (osteochondromatosis); (4) injuries producing osteochondral fracture. The symptoms of recurrent locking, effusion and pain in the joint may be identical with those of displacement of a torn semilunar cartilage, and radiographic examination is necessary before operation is performed for suspected cartilage injury (Fig 31.30 (a)). Prolonged and careful examination of the joint will often result in a momentary palpating of the loose body before it shoots away into one of the recesses of the synovial lining: it is not without reason that these fragments have been labelled 'joint mice'. An isolated loose body should be removed through a short incision over it. Multiple bodies from synovial chondrification may require synovectomy.

Osteochondral fractures of the femoral condyles. Fractures of the articular surface of the femoral condyle, with the production of a loose body

within the knee, can be produced in two ways:[27] by direct injury, such as a fall into the point of the knee or a kick on the front of the joint, when either condyle can be fractured (exogenous type); or by indirect injury, either as a result of a twist injury or from displacement of the patella,[28] when usually the lateral condyle is affected (endogenous type). These injuries are commonly missed in the initial radiograph (Fig. 31.30b and c). The fracture nearly always occurs in the adolescent and should be suspected where there is a history of a direct blow on a flexed knee or a violent twist on a flexed knee. Pain is severe, particularly if weight-bearing is attempted, and there is usually a frank haemarthrosis or a bloodstained effusion which may contain globules of fat. The fragment separates through the subchondral bone and should be visible in X-ray, but tangential and tunnel views may be necessary to show it. The treatment is operative: small fragments should be excised; in fresh cases it may be possible to relocate large fragments in their bed and fix them with Smillie pins, but if some time has elapsed since the injury even the large fragments should be excised.

RUPTURE OF THE EXTENSOR APPARATUS OF THE KNEE JOINT

The extensor apparatus of the knee joint consists of the rectus femoris and the vasti muscles, together called the quadriceps muscles. This group is inserted into the upper tibia by a strong central band which contains the patella, and medial and lateral expansions which cover the femoral condyles.

Isolated tearing of the individual muscle bellies of the apparatus does not cause great trouble. The injury heals by fibrous tissue and the other muscles can compensate for the damage. However, extensive adhesions of the muscle bellies to the underlying femur or extensive fibrosis along the length of one muscle can cause a disabling loss of flexion of the knee joint.

The rupturing of the extensor apparatus that matters, is the rupture of any part of the fibrous structure lying across the front of the knee joint. This structure contains the patella, which is a sesamoid bone in the central thick portion. The patella provides a smooth glide to movement by virtue of the conformity of its shape to that of the femoral condyle. This bony structure covered by articular cartilage, protects the tendon of the extensor apparatus from unwanted friction and provides some mechanical advantage to the movement of extension.

Ruptures of this attachment part of the extensor

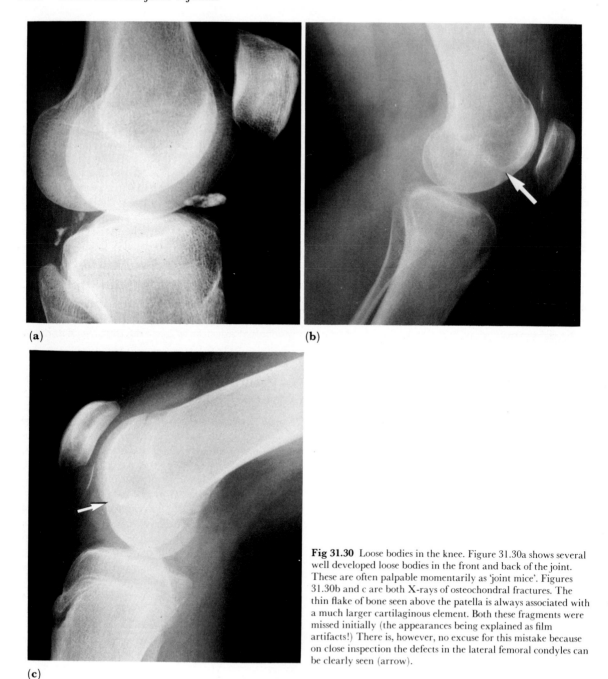

(a)

(b)

(c)

Fig 31.30 Loose bodies in the knee. Figure 31.30a shows several well developed loose bodies in the front and back of the joint. These are often palpable momentarily as 'joint mice'. Figures 31.30b and c are both X-rays of osteochondral fractures. The thin flake of bone seen above the patella is always associated with a much larger cartilaginous element. Both these fragments were missed initially (the appearances being explained as film artifacts!) There is, however, no excuse for this mistake because on close inspection the defects in the lateral femoral condyles can be clearly seen (arrow).

apparatus may or may not include a fracture of the patella. There are two types of injury: (1) a direct blow in which the patella may be fractured without displacement or with great comminution but in each case without damage to the medial and lateral expansions; and (2) by indirect violence of forced flexion of the knee against resistance in which there is a disruption with separation across the front of the joint of a variable degree, with or without a separation across the patella. In the first group the power of extension is not lost and surgery is rarely necessary. In the second group surgical repair must be undertaken immediately.

Commonly it is stated that the patella is an unnecessary structure and that it can be sacrificed without fear of disability. There is no doubt that in widely separated and comminuted fractures, it's removal may be correct treatment. Particularly is this so in the older age of patients. However, in the young and middle aged persons, the patella should be conserved if it can be reconstituted to give a smooth articulating surface with the femur. There are very few patients who can get up easily from the full crouch position after removal of the patella. The power of extension from the position of full flexion is diminished.

Rupture of the quadriceps tendon at four levels will be considered—1. Upper margin of the patella; 2. Across the patella; 3. Lower margin of patella; 4. Avulsion of tibial tubercle.

QUADRICEPS RUPTURE AT THE UPPER MARGIN OF PATELLA

This is commonly known as an avulsion of the rectus femoris. It occurs in elderly patients. It is diagnosed by the palpation of a gap in the extensor apparatus just above the patella; two fingers can be placed in the gap. Usually the lateral expansions are intact.

Unfortunately this injury is missed commonly through inadequate clinical examination and because the radiograph is not abnormal.

The fresh injury should be repaired by suturing tendon to the bone of the patella with immobilisation in a plaster cylinder for four weeks.

In late cases attending after two months, repair and immobilisation is not possible because of retraction of the proximal end. Usually in time, the person learns to walk by locking the knee just as in a case of poliomyelitis with quadriceps palsy.

RUPTURE OF THE QUADRICEPS TENDON WITH FRACTURES OF THE PATELLA

When the patella is fractured, the quadriceps muscle retracts with the proximal fragment of the bone. The distal fragment is usually tilted, with its fractured surface forwards, the surface being covered by aponeurotic fibres of the tendon which fall in towards the joint. The rupture of the tendon extends laterally on each side of the patella. The joint is filled with blood and clot. Without operative treatment the

muscle and proximal fragment of bone remain retracted, the gap fills with scar tissue, and repair takes place with lengthening of the tendon and permanent limitation of active extension movement. Operative suture is advisable as soon after injury as the condition of the skin will permit.

Suture of tendon and of patella. Although excision is the treatment of choice for fracture of the patella with separation, there is a place for open reduction and internal fixation when the fracture is in a young adult providing that the articular surface can be reconstituted. The most effective method of maintaining reduction is by using a tension suture of wire through quadriceps muscle and patella tendon. It is crossed anterior to the patella (Fig 31.31). The repair of the quadriceps expansion on either side of the patella must be carried out at the same time and the limb immobilised afterwards in a plaster cylinder for two to three weeks. Non-weight-bearing mobilisation of the knee is started after this time, but the patient should not be allowed to walk without a protective back splint for six weeks.

Indications for excision of the fractured patella. The best treatment for osteoarthritis confined to the patello-femoral compartment of the knee joint is excision of the patella. A comminuted fracture of the patella in a middle-aged or elderly patient usually causes osteoarthritis of this part of the joint. It is still better therefore to excise the patella at the time of the fracture and thus avoid the complication (Fig 31.32). The quadriceps tendon can be sutured so much more firmly after excision of the bone that prolonged splinting is unnecessary. Active movement and flexion exercises may begin within three or four weeks. With carefully directed treatment normal movement is soon regained (Figs 31.33–31.37). The operation avoids the necessity for prolonged after-treatment, reduces the incapacity period from about 12 months to about four months, minimises the danger of permanent stiffness of the joint and avoids the late complication of osteoarthritis of the knee.

Indications for excision of one fragment of the fractured patella. If a fracture of the patella lies near the upper or lower poles, there need be no hesitation in excising the smaller fragment. Excision of one small fragment has all the advantages and none of the disadvantages of total excision of the bone.

Excision of the patella with suture of quadriceps tendon. Though a vertical or tranverse incision the fracture and the tear in the tendon are exposed, and blood clot is evacuated from the joint. The fragments of the

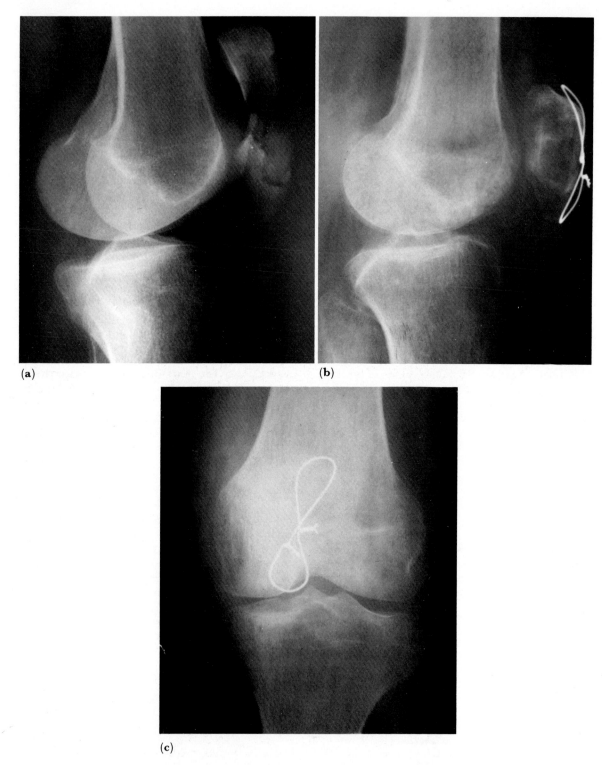

(a)

(b)

(c)

Fig 31.31 This comminuted fracture of the patella in a young man was held reduced very satisfactorily by using the technique of crossed tension wiring.

patella are shelled out by dissection close to the bone. It is then very easy to suture the tendon with strong catgut mattress sutures or with fascia. The upper and lower flaps should be overlapped and bunched together in the gap from which the bone was excised. If this is done the final contour of the knee is surprisingly normal despite loss of the bone—at any rate in the extended position. Some flattening of the contour is usually evident when the joint is flexed to the right angle. The joint is bound firmly over several layers of wool and at first the limb is supported in plaster. Active flexion and extension exercises should begin after two or three weeks using a plaster back splint to immobilise the knee when walking. Weight-bearing free of protection should not be allowed for six weeks. Recovery is usually complete within three or four months.

Un-united fracture of the patella. An un-united fracture of the patella of many weeks' or months' duration should usually be treated by excision of the bone fragment and repair of the quadriceps tendon with as much correction of muscle retraction as possible. Some surgeons have used strips of fascia lata, but the simpler method of catgut suture is usually better.

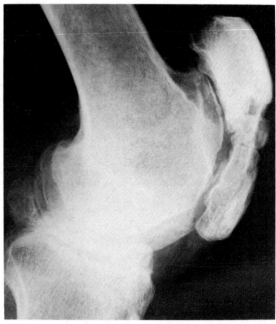

Fig 31.32 Grossly mal-united fracture of the patella with secondary arthritis of the patello-femoral compartment. It was treated by excision of the patella and suture of the quadriceps tendon. The result was satisfactory, but not as good as it would have been after early excision.

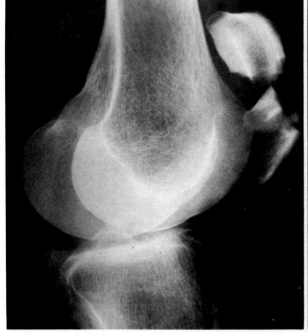

Fig 31.33

Fig 31.33 Comminuted fracture of the patella in a patient aged 68.

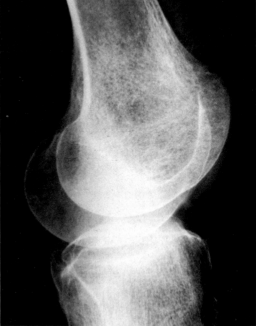

Fig 31.34

Fig 31.34 Radiograph after excision of the patella and suture of the quadriceps tendon.

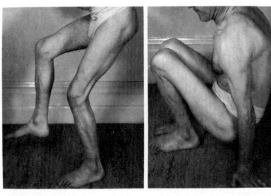

Fig 31.35   **Fig 31.36**

Figs 31.35 and 31.36 Power of the knee and range of movement two months after comminuted fracture of the patella treated by excision of bone and suture of tendon. (Same case in Figs 31.33 and 31.34.)

AVULSION OF THE LIGAMENTUM PATELLAE FROM THE PATELLA

Avulsion of the ligamentum patellae from the patella is again a rupture of the quadriceps tendon, and the tear involves not only those fibres which are attached to the patella itself, but the whole of the lateral quadriceps expansion. Active extension movement is therefore lost, and the patella is displaced upwards by retraction of the quadriceps muscle. If the rupture is not repaired by early operative suture the haematoma below the lower pole of the patella undergoes ossification and the new bone either fuses to the patella or becomes scattered—myositis ossificans traumatica—this depending upon whether or not the knee joint is immobilised. If the tendon is sutured within a few days of injury, no more than a few spicules of bone are formed. Small fragments of bone which remain attached to the distal part of the tendon may be excised in order to facilitate suture. It may be possible to stitch the tendon so securely that early active movements are safe, but since the injury occurs in young patients who show little susceptibility to stiffening of the joint, the knee should usually be immobilised in almost full extension for six or eight weeks.

FRACTURE AND EPIPHYSEAL INJURIES OF THE TIBIAL TUBERCLE

The ligamentum patellae, which is inserted into the tibial tubercle, is no more than the central part of the tendon of insertion of the quadriceps muscle. The tubercle is the apex of a triangular area of insertion spreading laterally over the tibial tuberosities. This apical region takes the first strain of an extensor injury, but with so wide an area of insertion, complete avulsion of the tendon is exceptional.

Fracture of the tibial tubercle. In the adult, where the tubercle is firmly fused to the tibia by a broad base, avulsion injuries are rare. When a very stiff knee joint is forcibly manipulated under anaesthesia, the tubercle may occasionally be cracked and slightly separated, but it will usually be found that the greater part of the quadriceps insertion to the tuberosities is still intact. The power of active extension is not reduced and it is unnecessary to immobilise the knee. Active flexion exercises may be practised at once and the value of the manipulation need not be lost. Passive stretching movements must of course be avoided.

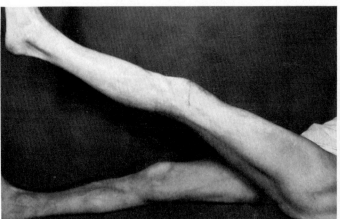
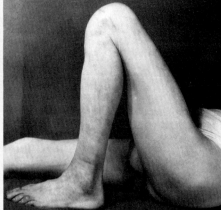

Fig 31.37 Movement of the knee joint six months after excision of a fractured patella.

Complete avulsion of the epiphysis of the tibial tubercle. More violent injury may cause avulsion of the tendon of insertion of the quadriceps together with one or more fragments from epiphyses of the tibial tubercle and head of the tibia. The typical injury is that sustained by the boy of 14 whose radiographs are shown in Figures 31.41 and 31.42. He was attempting the high jump at school sports and landed with his body-weight slightly behind his feet so that he fell backwards into the sitting position. The knee joint was forcibly flexed against the resistance of the strongly contracting quadriceps muscle and the tendon of insertion was avulsed.

The injury is most common before the age of 18, when the epiphyses of the tubercle and head of the tibia fuse to the shaft of the bone. Three types of injury may be differentiated. (1) A small fragment representing part of the tibial tubercle may be avulsed and retracted upwards (Fig 31.38). This part of the tubercle sometimes develops as a separate centre of ossification which fuses to the ossific centre of the upper tibial epiphysis at the age of 16. Before that age the cartilage between the two centres is a weak junction, susceptible to separation. The small fragment cannot be replaced accurately by manipulation, and operative treatment is necessary. It may be held in its normal position by suture of the overlying soft tissues, or by passing a suture through drill holes in the bone. Screws or pins are usually unnecessary. The limb is immobilised in plaster for 8 or 10 weeks, and movements are then regained by active exercises. (2)

When there is no separate centre of ossification for the tubercle, or if there has been such a centre when it is fused to that of the upper tibial epiphysis, the quadriceps tendon is more securely fixed to a broad area of bone. Instead of a small fragment being avulsed the whole lip formed by the front of the upper tibial epiphysis is hinged upwards being completely fractured at its base (Fig 31.39). The fragment can usually be replaced by manipulation, and operative reduction is unnecessary. (3) Sometimes the injury is of such severity that even this broad lip of bone is fractured at its base, the line of fracture passing upwards and backwards into the joint surface (Fig 31.40). The large piece of bone which is displaced can sometimes be reduced accurately by manipulation, but if manipulative reduction fails or if the fragment is comminuted as is the case shown in Figures 31.41 and 31.42 operative suture may be indicated.

Osgood's or Schlatter's sprain. The fact that the tibial tubercle takes the first strain of extension movement but is supported laterally by the insertion of the tendon into the tibial tuberosities explains the condition described as Osgood's or Schlatter's 'disease'.[29, 30] The tubercle is developed as an epiphysis, either by extension of the upper epiphysis of the tibia or from a separate centre of ossification, and it does not fuse firmly to the tibia until the age of 18. Before that age the epiphysial line is a weak point in the extensor mechanism of the knee. A sudden flexion movement of the joint against the resistance of the

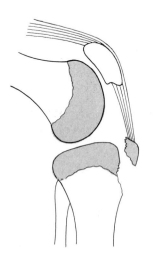

Fig 31.38

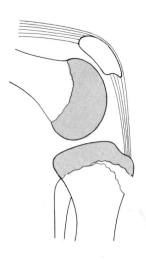

Fig 31.39

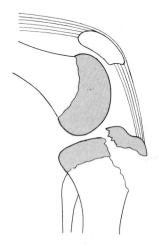

Fig 31.40

Figs 31.38 to 31.40 Three types of avulsion fracture of the upper tibial epiphysis.

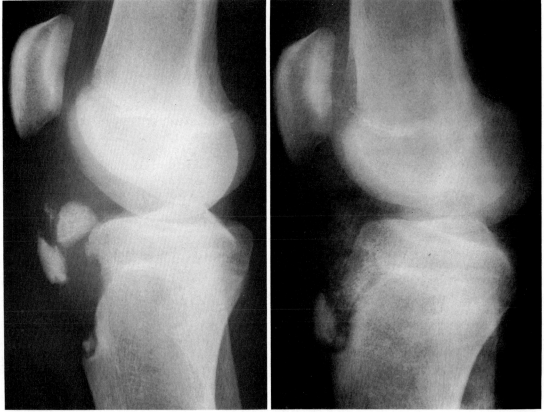

Fig 31.41   Fig 31.42

Figs 31.41 and 31.42 Avulsion of the tibial tubercle epiphysis before and after operative reduction.

quadriceps muscle tends to avulse the epiphysis from the tibia. Actual avulsion is prevented by the lateral insertions of the tendon to the tibial tuberosities, but the epiphysial line of the tubercle is strained. The patient complains of tenderness, which is localised accurately to the tubercle. The pain is increased by active extension against resistance. If the joint is not protected by immobilisation repeated strains cause increased separation of the epiphysis and bony thickening develops. These are the characteristic features of Schlatter's 'disease'. It is not a disease. It is a simple traumatic condition comparable to the separation of other epiphyses.

It may sometimes be necessary to support the knee in plaster in the position of full extension for about two months. Protection should be continued until relief of pain and tenderness proves that the epiphysis has become reattached to the tibia.

This epiphysial separation does not necessarily undergo spontaneous fusion at the age of 18 when it should normally join with the tibia; it may fail to fuse. A patient aged 40 years complained of pain, tenderness and bony thickening in the region of the tibial tubercles of both knee joints, and of inability to kneel. The symptoms had been present since adolescence. Radiographs showed evidence of an old, untreated, bilateral Schlatter's sprain (Figs 31.43 and 31.44). Failure to immobilise the joints at the time of the original injury allowed repeated separation and elevation of the epiphyses throughout the period of active growth, with deposition of successive layers of bone. Despite this bone formation, continued strain prevented fusion of the epiphysial lines, and the epiphyses remained as separate ossicles, joined to the tibia only by fibrous tissue which was susceptible to strain. The symptoms were relieved by excision of the fragments of bone and immobilisation of the joint in extension for two months. Sometimes a local

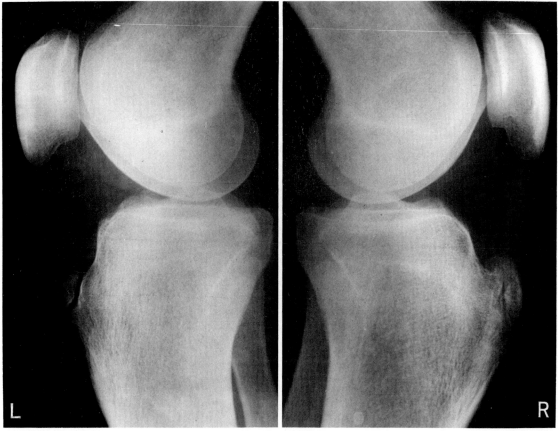

Fig 31.43   **Fig 31.44**

Figs 31.43 and 31.44 Bilateral Schlatter's sprain, the result of strain of the epiphyses during adolescence, causing recurrent symptoms in the adult because the epiphyses never united by bone.

injection of 25 mg of hydrocortisone will relieve symptoms.

COMMINUTED FRACTURE OF THE PATELLA FROM DIRECT VIOLENCE

The fractures of the patella described earlier in this chapter are incidental to a primary rupture of the quadriceps tendon. The patella may also be injured by a direct blow, crushing the bone against the femoral condyles, so that a comminuted stellate fracture is produced. Since the quadriceps tendon is not ruptured there may still be a full range of active extension movement, and operative treatment is often unnecessary. If displacement of the fragments is minimal and the articular surface is smooth, there is need only to protect the joint for two or three weeks by a posterior plaster slab, and immediate weight-

bearing may be permitted. Flexion movements are allowed after a few weeks. However, in the specimen shown in Figure 31.45 it is obvious that damage to the articular cartilage may be of such severity that a perfect joint surface cannot be possibly be restored. All comminuted fractures of the patella with more than minimal displacement and in which the joint surface is seriously damaged are best treat by excision of the bone. Since the quadriceps tendon is intact the operation is easy, and early active movements may be practised with safety.

Excision for old mal-united fracture of patella. A window-cleaner sustained a comminuted fracture of the patella which united with marked irregularity of the articular surface. Physiotherapy continued for many months failed to relieve the pain or to increase the range of flexion movement beyond 80 degrees, and the patient was totally incapacitated. At two years

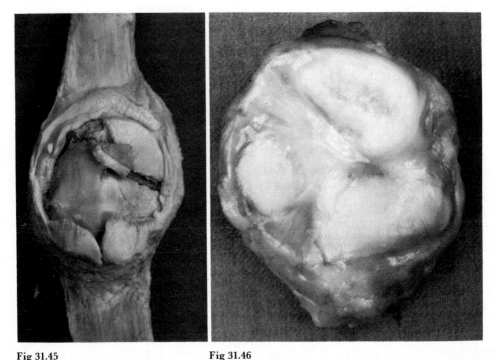

Fig 31.45   **Fig 31.46**

Fig 31.45 Comminuted fracture of patella. The quadriceps expansion has not been ruptured, but the articular surface is severely damaged. Excision is advisable in such cases.

Fig 31.46 Patella excised from the knee joint of a window cleaner who sustained a comminuted stellate fracture. Mal-union, causing irregularity of the articular surfaces, gave rise to persistent pain and limitation of movement.

the patella was excised, the joint fully flexed and the tendon repaired (Fig 31.46). After three months of active exercise the range of movement of the joint was normal, pain was relieved, and the man went back to work.

Marginal fracture of the patella. A direct blow may chip a large fragment of bone from one of the angles of the patella.[31] The bone is not crushed, the fragment is not displaced, and the articular surface is smooth. Operation is unnecessary and immobilisation is not indicated. The fracture is to be distinguished from congenital bipartite patella, in which a supernumerary bone develops at the upper outer angle from a second centre of ossification.[32] This anomaly may be bilateral and seldom causes disability.

Chip fracture of articular surfaces. Contusion of the patella against the femoral condyle may bruise the articular cartilage and cause a localised area of osteochondritis dissecans. A number of cases have been described of detachment of a fragment from the inferior medial angle of the articular surface of the

patella by impact of the bone against the lateral femoral condyle, the loose fragment in each case being removed from the lateral pouch of the knee.[21, 33] In many injured knee joints where there has been forcible impact of the patella against the femoral condyles, it will be found at operation that apart from detached fragments of bone there are quite large detached fragments of articular cartilage with are not disclosed in radiographs. Very often chip fractures involving the articular surface of the bone were sustained during momentary lateral dislocation of the patella, and of course they occur still more frequently in recurrent lateral dislocations where frequent displacement of the patella over the lateral femoral condyle gives rise to so many more opportunities for fracture. The skyline X-ray projection of the patella can be valuable in diagnosing these injuries.

LATERAL DISLOCATION OF THE PATELLA

The mobility of the patella varies in normal individuals. If the capsule of the joint is lax and the lateral femoral condyle is poorly developed so that the patellar groove is shallow, the patella may be so mobile that relatively slight pressure is sufficient to displace it over the margin of the femoral condyle. An injury sustained while the muscles of the thigh are relaxed may completely dislocate the bone.[34] The tibia is forcibly abducted and laterally rotated, or the patella is struck on its medial side by a glancing blow. The capsule is stretched or torn; sometimes there is a flake fracture of the medial border of the patella which can only be seen in the X-ray skyline view (Figs 31.47 to 31.49); the patella rotates through 90 degrees, and its articular surface lies in contact with the outer side of the lateral femoral condyle. The dislocation is often reduced spontaneously as the joint is extended, or it is replaced by the manipulation of onlookers. When the surgeon examines the knee the only clinical signs remaining may be those of traumatic synovitis and tenderness over the patellar margin at the attachment of the vastus medialis. It may be difficult, therefore, to differentiate dislocation of the patella from displacement of a semilunar cartilage. The history must be elicited carefully, the site of greatest tenderness determined, and the degree of lateral mobility of the patella estimated. The joint should be immobilised on a back splint or in plaster

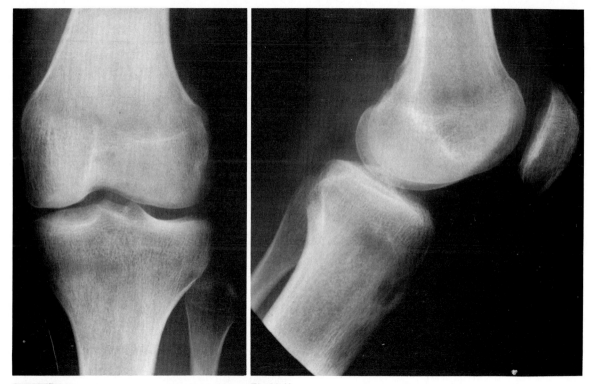

Fig 31.47   **Fig 31.48**

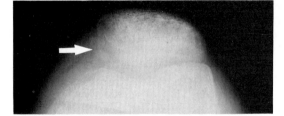

Fig 31.49

Figs 31.47 to 31.49 Traumatic dislocation of patella. The standard antero-posterior and lateral X-ray after reduction of traumatic dislocation of the patella (Figs 31.47 and 31.48). No obvious bony injury can be seen. The skyline view (Fig 31.49) shows the characteristic medial flake fracture which occurs in an acute traumatic dislocation.

for two months, wasting of the quadriceps being prevented by regular active exercise.

The forceful lateral dislocation of the patella may cause a shearing osteochondral fracture of either the posterior surface of the patella or of the prominent anterior ridge on the lateral femoral condyle. The fragment may be large. It consists mainly of articular cartilage. In a lateral radiograph it appears as a thin line of bone which can be missed Fig 31.30b and c. When such a fracture is recognised the fragment must be removed as soon as convenient.

Recurrent dislocation of the patella. The relation between the axes of the quadriceps muscle and the ligamentum patellae predisposes to outward displacement of the patella. The muscle passes downwards and inwards, but the ligament lies vertically, and the patella is situated at the angle between the two (Fig 31.50). When the muscle contracts it tends to form a straight line between its origin and insertion so that the angle is obliterated and the patella is displaced outwards. This tendency is normally corrected by the lowermost fibres of the vastus internus, which lie in an almost horizontal axis. The vastus internus contracts simultaneously with the other muscles of the quadriceps group so that it pulls the patella inwards at the moment that it

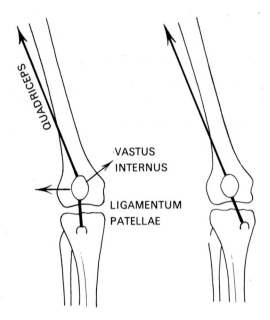

Fig 31.50 The relative axes of the quadriceps and patella ligament encourage lateral displacement of the patella, normally prevented by the vastus medialis. Transplantation of the tibial tubercle corrects the tendency.

would otherwise displace over the lateral femoral condyle. Very occasionally there may be a lateral rotation deformity of the tibia which predisposes to the dislocation, but a far more important predisposing factor (in almost 50 per cent of cases) is generalised joint laxity.[35, 36]

Operative treatment. Many operative procedures have been devised in the attempt to cure recurrent dislocation of the patella; this large number in itself is an indication that no one operation is wholly satisfactory. Of all the procedures, probably that described by Hauser[37] has, because of its success, deservedly become the most popular. Basically, the operation consists of detaching the attachment of the ligamentum patellae from the tibia along with its underlying portion of bone and implanting it in a new bed one diameter medially where it can be impacted or fixed with a screw. At the same time the lateral retinaculum of the quadriceps is divided from alongside the ligament to well above the patella in order to allow the patellar tendon to swing medially; plication of the capsule on the medial side although not essential, also helps to maintain stability. The limb should be immobilised in a plaster cylinder for six weeks; weight-bearing is allowed and quadriceps exercises practised throughout the time.

There is one serious disadvantage of this operation: if carried out before the age of 14 there is a grave risk of damage to the anterior part of the tibial epiphysis with resulting genu recurvatum.[38] If possible, operation should be delayed until after this age. The best results can be expected between teenage and 30 years of age, when the restoration of normal patello-femoral contact can be expected to improve any secondary cartilage change.

In patients younger than 14 years in which surgery is necessary, it should be restricted to a soft tissue procedure with extensive vertical division of the lateral retinaculum and plication of the medial side.

Congenital recurrent dislocation of the patella. In the congenital type of recurrent displacement of the patella there is no history of injury or of acute dislocation followed by recurrent dislocation. For as long as the patient could remember, the patella had displaced over the lateral condyle every time the joint was flexed Fig 31.51. Examination usually demonstrates a thick band of tendon of the quadriceps attached to the superior lateral corner of the patella.

The treatment consists of a vertical division of the lateral expansion and in particular complete division of the aforesaid band attached to the upper lateral

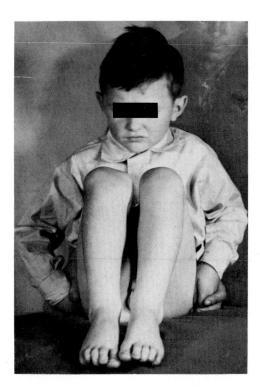

Fig 31.51 Congenital recurrent lateral dislocation of the right patella in a child.

the ligaments of the joint and then causes depression, splitting or comminution of the tuberosity by the impact of the femoral condyle against it: occasionally the fracture is associated with a subluxation of the whole of the tibia on the femur. Treatment of the soft tissue injury is often no less important than treatment of the fracture.

The fate of the joint depends on a number of factors, namely the restoration of a satisfactory joint surface, maintainance of the reduction of deformity until bone union, early joint movement without weight bearing and the strength of the muscles.

The two essentials of treatment are therefore: (1) to correct the displacement and depression of the tuberosity, restoring the smoothest possible joint surface; (2) to prevent wasting of the quadriceps muscle by active non-weight-bearing exercise begun immediately and continued throughout the period of immobilisation. No matter what the type of fracture and no matter whether it is reduced by manipulation or by operation, the secret of success is the tone of the muscles of the thigh. Quadriceps drill should begin the day after injury and be repeated for five minutes hourly throughout the day. It must continue until the patient is weight-bearing free of splintage. Within three months of injury the muscles should be as strong as those of the normal limb. They should be so powerful that any permanent support for them becomes unnecessary.

corner. But this is not enough. The medial retinaculum must be plicated also.

On no account should the patella be removed.

FRACTURE OF THE TUBEROSITIES OF THE TIBIA

Although either condyle of the tibia may be fractured, by far the most common injury is to the lateral side. A blow on this side of the extended knee forces the joint into the abducted position, tears the medial ligament, and may sometimes stretch the cruciate ligaments. A more severe injury such as the impact of a motor vehicle or the dropping of a heavy weight on the outer side of the limb causes still greater valgus deformity and, in addition to rupture of the medial and cruciate ligaments, the lateral tuberosity of the tibia may be fractured. A strain in the opposite direction may result in a similar fracture of the medial condyle, but this is a rare injury. Sometimes the fracture occurs without rupture of the ligaments, but usually a severe valgus or varus strain first tears

Types of fracture of the tibial tuberosities.
Many groups of fracture of the tuberosities have been described. However, these can be simplified into the following groups based on the types of treatment necessary

1. Cleavage condylar fracture
2. Depressed condylar fracture
3. Comminuted fracture of one or both condyles.

Cleavage condylar fracture.
This can be of two types. In the first type the whole of one condyle is depressed and the fracture line involves the knee joint surface in the intercondylar area (Fig. 31.52 and Fig. 31.54, 31.55). The weight bearing articular cartilage is not damaged. There is little compression of the cancellous bone and the deformity is of angulation. This fracture can be treated conservatively with manipulative correction of the deformity and immobilisation in plaster. It is important avoid weight bearing until the fracture is united. Otherwise the deformity will recur. If the initial deformity cannot be reduced, it must be

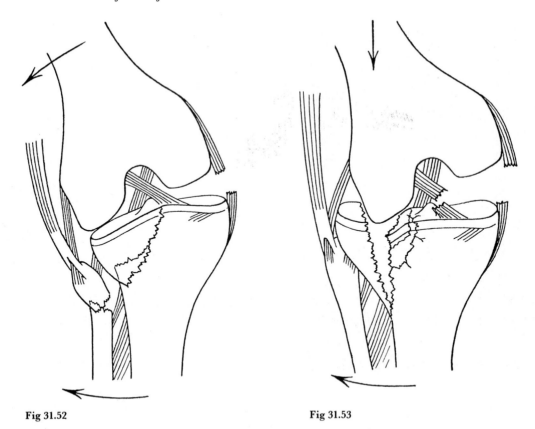

Fig 31.52   Fig 31.53

Figs 31.52 and 31.53 Mechanism of injury in the two types of fracture of the lateral tuberosity of the tibia. In the first type the tuberosity is depressed by the surface of the lateral femoral condyle (Fig 31.52). In the second type the tuberosity is split by the margin of the femoral condyle, and a marginal fragment is displaced (Fig 31.53). In both there may be ligamentous damage to the medial ligament and sometimes to the cruciate ligaments.

achieved by open reduction and internal fixation. Usually the bone is of good texture and screw fixation will suffice.

In the second type, the fracture line is vertical and commences across the articular surface of the tibial condyle. Usually there is a gap across the fracture. The fragment is not always depressed. The fracture separation must be closed. Sometimes this can be undertaken by manipulation (Fig. 31.56 and 31.57) followed by plaster immobilisation. Manipulation may be unsuccessful, in which case the fracture should be fixed and usually screw fixation is adequate (Fig. 31.61 and 31.62).

Depressed condylar fracture. (Fig. 31.53). In this fracture the femoral condyle has been driven into the middle of the articular surface of the tibial condyle which is comminuted and depressed. A small

portion of the articular surface may be rotated 70°. The cancellous bone deep to it is severely compressed so that if this fragment is elevated a significant hole remains beneath it. Lateral to the depressed central fragment the remainder of the condyle is split off laterally. With this widening of the tibial plateau something must happen to the peripheral attachment of the meniscus. Usually it is detached at its periphery and it remains near the more central depressed portion. It may be lodged in the fracture gap.

It is in the treatment of this and the third group of fractures that quite considerable differences of opinion exist. It is not possible to restore the joint surface correctly by conservative means. Yet conservative treatment can produce a good functional knee joint, despite some initial unevenness of the joint surface.

There are three possible methods of treatment:—plaster immobilisation, skeletal traction with imme-

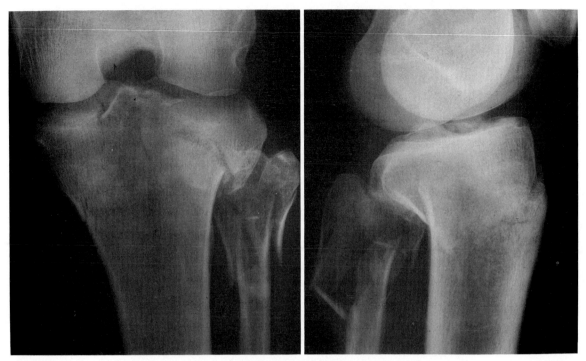

Fig 31.54

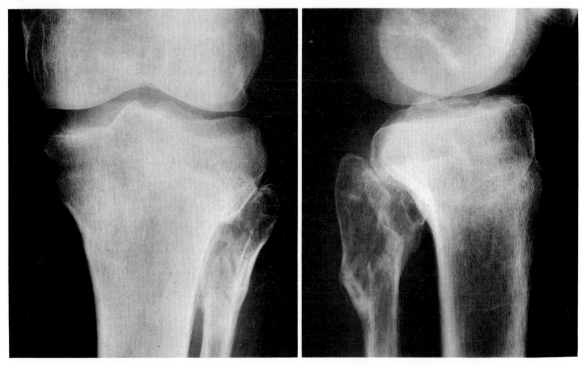

Fig 31.55

Figs 31.54 and 31.55 Fracture of the lateral tuberosity of the tibia without comminution or separation of a marginal fragment, before and after manipulative reduction.

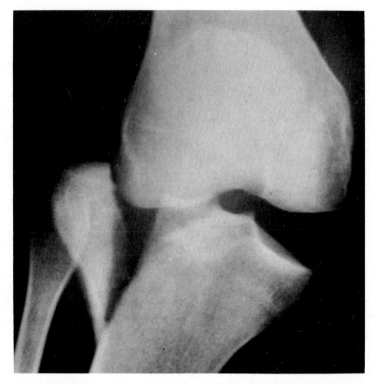

Fig 31.56 Fracture of the lateral tuberosity of the tibia. The medial and anterior cruciate ligaments are torn. It is obvious how the tibial tuberosity has been split and crushed by the impact of the margin of the femoral condyle.

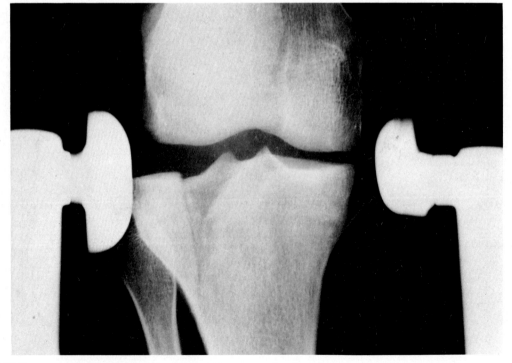

Fig 31.57 Same case as Figure 31.56 during reduction with a compression clamp.

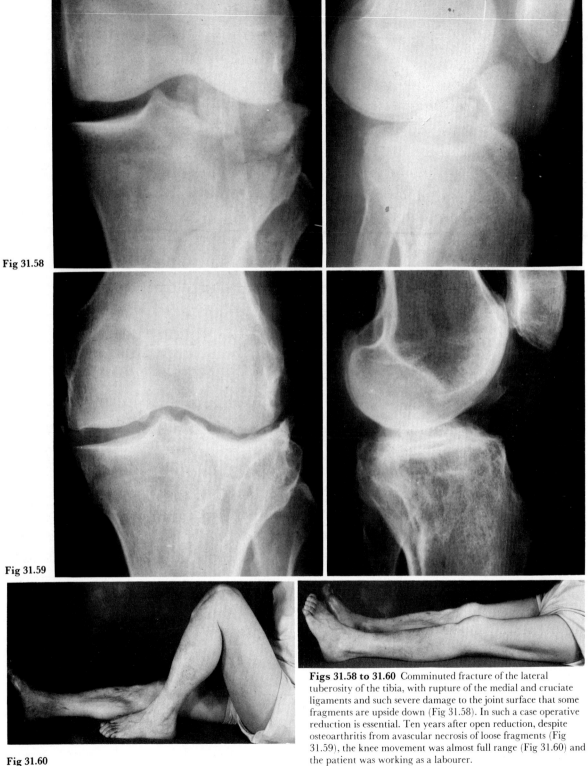

Fig 31.58

Fig 31.59

Fig 31.60

Figs 31.58 to 31.60 Comminuted fracture of the lateral tuberosity of the tibia, with rupture of the medial and cruciate ligaments and such severe damage to the joint surface that some fragments are upside down (Fig 31.58). In such a case operative reduction is essential. Ten years after open reduction, despite osteoarthritis from avascular necrosis of loose fragments (Fig 31.59), the knee movement was almost full range (Fig 31.60) and the patient was working as a labourer.

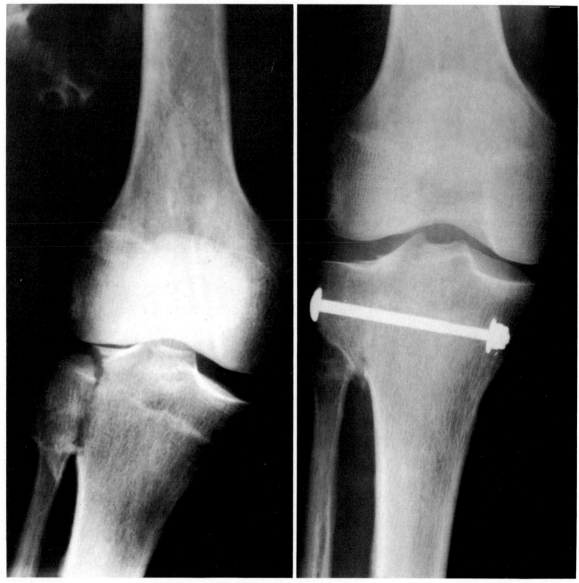

Fig 31.61   Fig 31.62

Figs 31.61 and 31.62 This depressed fracture of the lateral tibial tuberosity (Fig 31.61) could not be reduced satisfactorily by conservative means. The position obtained by open reduction and fixation with a compression bolt is shown in Figure 31.62.

diate knee joint movement and open reduction with internal fixation and bone grafting.

The decision as to the appropriate method depends on a number of factors, age and motivation of the patient, strength of the bone, associated fractures, condition of the skin and the demands that will be placed on this one joint. A considerable proportion of these fractures occur in middle aged or elderly women with poor skin and demineralised bones. Surgical treatment is additional trauma to skin and joint.

Plaster immobilisation. This is preceded by an attempt at manipulation under anaesthesia to improve the joint surface as much as possible and to correct angular deformity. This can be an out-patient procedure. Weight bearing is not permitted before about six weeks and the plaster is removed at ten to twelve weeks. Thereafter physiotherapy is required for at least three months to regain movement. The treatment is prolonged but by one year a surprising number of patients have a useful knee with near right angle knee flexion.

Skeletal traction. This method has been advocated by Apley.[39] A strong traction pin is used through the tibial shaft. This must be located at least 15 cm below the joint to avoid the traumatic haematoma, and must be placed exactly parallel to the plane of knee movement. While traction is maintained knee movements are started immediately and continued for four weeks. Traction corrects some of the joint displacement and the early movement ensures that the opposing joint surfaces develop a corresponding shape. This is a comfortable method of treatment but does involve impatient treatment for four to six weeks. Thereafter non weight mobilisation is continued until fracture consolidation.

Open reduction. This sounds very attractive. Yet it has big problems. The skin incision must be carefully placed and carefully repaired. It must allow inspection of the joint and of the whole lateral condyle. In most cases the incision should start as a vertical lateral, parapatellar approach and then extend distally with a curve to finish near the neck of the fibula. The approach to the fracture should be from under the meniscus and not from above it, and the meniscus must be retained and sutured back into its bed at all costs. Rarely is it torn except at its vascular periphery. After elevation of the depressed central fragment there is a gap which must be filled with bone graft from ilium or elsewhere, otherwise the depression will recur. The depression must be slightly overcorrected. The fracture complex must be fixed rigidly so that external support is unnecessary and early knee movement can be commenced. For such fixation screws and bolts alone are insufficient. A buttressing plate is essential.[40]

For the right fracture internal fixation properly undertaken can produce complete restitution of the joint surface with excellent movement, and in the hands of the experienced surgeon is the method of choice. However, if the fracture and joint are assaulted by incomplete reduction, incomplete bone fixation, absence of bone graft buttressing and removal of the meniscus the final result is inevitably a stiff and painful knee which is worse than such a fracture treated by any other means.

After adequate internal fixation knee flexion is commenced early and progress is dependant to some extent on the healing of the skin. Weight bearing is not permitted before twelve weeks.

Comminuted fractures of one or both condyles. These fractures are associated with severe trauma. In many of them it is still possible for the experienced surgeon to openly reduce and use internal fixation. In some it is necessary to expose both condyles and to use two buttressing plates. However, for the ordinary orthopaedic surgeon it is safer to treat these injuries by skeletal traction and early movement. The exception is where bone fragments are displaced with the joint cavity (Figs 31.58 to 31.60).

REFERENCES

1. Wilson J N 1959 Spontaneous haemarthrosis in osteo-arthritis of knee. British Medical Journal i: 1937
2. Bosworth D M 1952 Transplantation of the semitendinosus for repair of laceration of medial collateral ligament of the knee. Journal of Bone and Joint Surgery 34—A: 196
3. O'Donoghue D H 1973 Reconstruction for medial instability of the knee. Journal of Bone and Joint Surgery 55-A: 941
4. Slocum D B, & Larson R L 1968 Pes anserinus transplantation. Journal of Bone and Joint Surgery 50-A: 226
5. Lamb D W 1952 Deposition of calcium salts in the medial ligament of the knee. Journal of Bone and Joint Surgery 34-B: 233
6. Galway R D, Beaupre A, MacIntosh D L 1972 Pivot Shift: a clinical sign of symptomatic anterior cruciate insufficiency. Journal of Bone and Joint Surgery 54-B: 763
7. Meyers M H, McKeever F M 1959 Fracture of the intercondylar eminence of the tibia. Journal of Bone and Joint Surgery 41-A: 209
8. Trickey E L 1968 Rupture of the posterior cruciate ligament of the knee. Journal of Bone and Joint Surgery 50-B: 334
9. Trickey E L 1979 Repair of knee ligament injuries. In Robb C, Smith R (eds) Orthopaedics II. Butterworths, London p 768
10. Owen R 1968 Recurrent dislocation of the superior tibio-fibular joint. Journal of Bone and Joint Surgery 50-B: 342
11. Kennedy J C 1963 Complete dislocation of the knee joint. Journal of Bone and Joint Surgery 45-A: 889
12. Watson-Jones R (1931) Styloid process of the fibula in knee joint with peroneal palsy. Journal of Bone and Joint Surgery 13: 258
13. Highet W B, Holmes W 1943 Traction injuries to the lateral popliteal nerve and traction injuries to peripheral nerves after suture. British Journal of Surgery 30: 212
14. Bristow W R 1928 Cysts of the semilunar cartilages of the knee. In: Robert Jones Birthday Volume. Oxford Medical Publications, Oxford, p 269

15. Bristow W R 1935 Internal derangement of the knee joint. Journal of Bone and Joint Surgery 17: 605

16. McMurray T P 1928 The diagnosis of internal derangements of the knee. In: Robert Jones Birthday Volume. Oxford Medical Publications, Oxford, p301

17. Fairbank H A R 1937 Internal derangement of the knee in children and adolescents. Proceedings of the Royal Society of Medicine 30: 427

18. Gibson A 1931 Regeneration of internal semilunar cartilage after operation. British Journal of Surgery 19: 302

19. Bruce J, Walmsley R 1937 Replacement of semilunar cartilages of the knee after operative excision. British Journal of Surgery 25: 17

20. Goldenberg R R 1935 Refracture of regenerated internal semilunar cartilage. Journal of Bone and Joint Surgery 17: 1054

21. Smillie I S 1978 Injuries of the knee joint, 5th edn. Churchill, Livingstone, Edinburgh

22. Ross W T 1951 Injury to the popliteal artery during meniscectomy. Journal of Bone and Joint Surgery 33-B: 571

23. Patrick J 1963 Aneurysm of the popliteal vessels after meniscectomy. Journal of Bone and Joint Surgery 45-B: 570

24. Taylor H 1935 Cysts of the fibro-cartilages of the knee joint. Journal of Bone and Joint Surgery 17: 588

25. Ollerenshaw R 1921 Development of cysts in connection with the external semilunar cartilage of the knee joint. British Journal of Surgery 8: 409

26. Dandy D J 1981 Arthroscopic surgery of the knee. Churchill Livingstone, Edinburgh

27. Kennedy J C, Grainger R W, McGraw R W 1966 Osteochondral fractures of the femoral condyles. Journal of Bone and Joint Surgery 48-B: 436

28. Rosenberg N J 1964 Osteochondral fractures of the lateral femoral condyle. Journal of Bone and Joint Surgery 46-A: 1013

29. Osgood R B 1903 Lesions of the tibial tubercle occurring during adolescence. Boston Medical and Surgical Journal 148: 114

30. Schlatter C 1903 Verletzungen des Schnabels—förmigen Fortsatz des oberen Tibia-Epiphyse. Beitrage Zur Klinischen Chirurgie 38: 874

31. Botto Micca A, Teramo M 1938 Vertical fractures of patella. Polichinico (Sezione Chirurgica) 45: 53

32. George R 1934 Bilateral bipartite patellae. British Journal of Surgery 22: 555

33. Meekison D M 1937 A hitherto undescribed fracture of patella. British Journal of Surgery 25: 64

34. Kleinberg S 1932 Traumatic lateral dislocation of patella. Annals of Surgery 95: 635

35. Heywood A W B 1961 Recurrent dislocation of patella. A study of its pathology and treatment in 106 knees. Journal of Bone and Joint Surgery 43-B: 508

36. Carter C, Sweetnam R 1960 Recurrent dislocation of the patella and of the shoulder. Their association with familial joint laxity. Journal of Bone and Joint Surgery 42-B: 721

37. Hauser E. D. W 1938 Total tendon transplant for slipping patella; a new operation for recurrent dislocation of the patella. Surgery, Gynecology and Obstetrics 66: 199

38. Harrison M H M 1960 Results of a realignment operation for recurrent dislocation of the patella. Clinical Orthopaedics 18: 96

39. Apley A G (1956) Fractures of the lateral tibial condyle treated by skeletal traction and early mobilisation. Journal of Bone and Joint Surgery 32-B: 699

40. Ackroyd C E 1979 Fractures of the tibial condyles. In: Robb C, Smith R (eds) Operative surgery. Orthopaedics I, Butterworths, London, p 154

32

Injuries of the leg

'We have still a long way to go before the best method of treating a fracture of the shaft of the tibia can be stated with finality'.
Sir John Charnley.[1]

Why are there so may differing opinions on the management of fractures of the lower leg and why does the above quotation still ring true over 20 years after it was first written? Fractures of the shaft of the tibia are among the most common long bone injuries presenting for treatment; and certainly, because of the subcutaneous location of the tibia it provides the widest experience in the management of an open fracture and all the complications associated therewith than any other injury to a long bone. Why then the problem? Why should the writer, along with Charnley, 'find the chapter on fractures of the tibia the most difficult to revise'? It is because, of all bone injuries, the management of the fractured tibia requires the widest experience, the greatest wisdom and the nicest of clinical judgement in order to choose the most appropriate treatment for a particular pattern of injury. Fracture treatment in general has a tendency to produce enthusiasts for one method or another who are sometimes easily influenced by the glib tongue or well written word. Beware of the master craftsmen who have no difficulties, for their words can be responsible for much suffering if believed implicitly by surgeons less blessed with their surgical expertise. However skilful, such men often lack the most important asset in fracture treatment—that of common sense. The surgeon who internally fixes every ski fracture of the tibia may become a superb carpenter, but he lacks the wisdom and judgement of a physician; for otherwise he would quickly learn that most fractures of this type will unite more rapidly, more solidly, and with less risk if they are treated by conservative means. What is more disturbing is that enthusiasm for one form of treatment for one particular fracture may lead the unwary to apply the same methods to every fracture. Surely there can be fewer surgical disasters greater

than the conversion of a previously closed uncomplicated fracture of the tibia into one which is compound, infected and ununited. Those who would religiously follow the advice of the surgeons who advocate rigid internal fixation of almost every tibial fracture should bear in mind that the *majority of amputations* which follow several years of disability can be traced to the injudicious use of these techniques.

However, the difficulties that may arise in the treatment of fractures of the shafts of the leg bones should not be underrated. They include: (1) a high incidence of open and infected fractures because the tibia lies superficially just beneath the skin; (2) a tendency to redisplacement of the fragments when swelling subsides, particularly in oblique and spiral fractures; (3) cosmetic and sometimes functional disability if the alignment or rotational position of the fragment is imperfect because the knee and ankle joints normally move in the same parallel axis; (4) conspicuous disfigurement if apposition of the fragments is imperfect because the tibia lies subcutaneously; (5) slow union as a result of severity of the fracture, poor blood supply to one fragment, and sometimes distraction of the bone fragments; (6) the occasional limitation of joint movement in the knee, ankle and foot, usually caused by associated joint, soft tissue, or vascular injury.

It is these difficulties that have given rise to so much controversy between surgeons as to the best method of managing tibial fractures. There are those who earnestly hold the view that the majority of these injuries, whether open or closed fractures, should be treated by open reduction and internal fixation; and in papers supporting this method of treatment the figures of fractures healed without major complications are very convincing.[2, 3] However, at the other end of the scale, Nicoll, after a detailed study of 705 fractures, concludes that as yet no case has been made for internal fixation as the method of choice in the treatment of fractures of the tibial shaft.[4] In Nicoll's view there is only one good reason for the use of internal fixation and that is that a satisfactory result is unlikely from conservative treatment and is more likely to be attained by operative intervention.[5] Van der Linden and Larsson in a randomised trial of a 100 displaced fractures treated either conservatively, or by A.O. plating, found that complications in the A.O. group were more numerous, the stay in hospital longer, and delayed union more frequent. The A.O. cases gained only in the average speed of union and the more rapid return to work, and in compound fractures even this gain was eliminated.[5a] Other workers have found the complication rate so high, particularly infection, that they have advised that the method should be abandoned.[5b] Where therefore, is the truth? As it is so often the case in the management of fractures the answer is a compromise between the two extreme points of view. 'Virtue is situated at an equal distance between two vices' (Aristotle).[5a] Choice of treatment should be dictated by the local circumstances, the type of fracture and the facilities available. What may be an ideal and safe treatment in a first-class and fully staffed traumatic unit in Europe, could be disastrous if employed in an underdeveloped country with very limited surgical resources. In America Preston Wade has issued a salutory warning to those who would follow in the footsteps of the Swiss surgeons who have done so much to popularise the operative treatment of tibial fractures. He makes the comment: 'They are master surgeons who have spent years in developing their technique ... This then is their problem. The beginners can no more hope quickly to emulate the work of these surgeons than a week-end skier can successfully duplicate the efforts of an Olympic champion'.[6] While in Great Britain Ellis has summed up the problem as follows: 'However attractive the possibilities of operative treatment may seem, operation still entails the conversion of a closed fracture into an open one, and the consequent risk must be weighed against the theoretical advantages. Though the risk may be small *when the operation is undertaken by an expert,* few would deny that the picture is very different when considered as a whole.[7]

There is certainly no convincing case for the abandonment of a conservative regime merely on the excuse of the inconvenience of plaster fixation, or the unproven disability of stiff joints. Nor have the protagonists of internal fixation proved their case of a decreased incidence of non-union as a result of operative treatment. Every fracture of the tibial shaft must be assessed individually, and it can be dangerous to establish fixed routines of treatment. Surgeons should remember that most of these injuries can be treated safely by closed methods, and before embarking upon operative treatment the surgeon must ask himself three questions: Is open reduction and internal fixation essential? Is the condition of the skin over the fracture site satisfactory for operation? And finally, are the facilities and surgical skills necessary for the operative treatment of fractures readily available?

SOFT TISSUE INJURIES OF THE CALF

Before going on to discuss in detail the management of tibial shaft fractures it is important to spend a little time outlining the diagnosis and treatment of two common injuries, often misdiagnosed, often confused one with the other, and often inadequately or badly treated: these are (1) ruptures of the calf; and (2) ruptures of the tendo-Achillis. Both injuries occur in patients of roughly the same age group; with always a characteristic history of sudden muscle strain, and with physical signs if properly elicited, which can leave little doubt as to the correct diagnosis. And yet still the significance of the findings are commonly misunderstood and the diagnosis either missed altogether, or, in the case of tendo-Achillis rupture, made so late that treatment can have little hope of success.

Rupture of the calf (*Tennis leg*[8]). The injury occurs usually in adults of early middle age who are still actively involved in competitive sport. It is rare in young adults and less common in the later stages of life, with the possible exception of the keen, elderly sportsman. The strain which produces the rupture may seem so insignificant to the victim that he denies any injury; or on some occasions, accuses his opponent of striking him on the calf with a ball or racquet. The cause is always due to a sudden calf contraction in response to effort, such as leaping for a high ball at tennis, turning for a run at cricket, or, not infrequently, from trying to make a spectacular 'get away' in the parent's race. The result is dramatic and devastating. There is immediate and excruciating pain in the mid-third of the calf and if the patient is able to walk at all he can only hobble along taking weight on his toes with his foot in equinus. The rupture is invariably in the gastrocnemius, and swelling and bruising of the calf becomes apparent within an hour or so of the injury. It is of the utmost importance to distinguish this injury from that of the

Achilles tendon rupture. Both injuries may present with a very similar history, but whereas failure to recognise a simple calf rupture will cause only temporary impairment of function, neglect to treat a complete tear of the Achilles tendon will leave serious permanent disability.

Although ruptures of the calf muscles have a high immediate morbidity, the acute effects rarely last more than a week or two and these can be substantially reduced by adequate treatment. The lack of any permanent disability led some writers to suggest that the rupture was confined to the plantaris muscle. However, this diagnosis is not supported by operative findings. Bristow is reported to have explored sixteen calf ruptures and found that the plantaris muscle was intact in all of them.[9] Also, a plantaris rupture should not produce pain on dorsiflexion of the ankle to the extent invariably seen in calf injury.[8]

Treatment. In the acute stage the limb should be rested in elevation and the calf supported in a crepe or elastic bandage applied from the toes to the knee. Daily application of ultra-sound therapy is helpful in dispersing a tense haematoma. Cyriax has suggested that up to 50 cc of 0.5 per cent lignocaine should be injected into the tender area and dorsiflexion exercises of the ankle encouraged.[8] As soon as possible the patient should be encouraged to walk on his toes, using elbow crutches and gradually forcing his heel to the ground. The use of 1 inch (2.5 cm) sorbo heel elevators is a very helpful support in the first two weeks, but it must be remembered that the heels of both feet must be elevated otherwise the irregular gait will increase the strain on the ruptured calf. Further participation in sport should be prohibited until the patient is able to run on tiptoe without pain.

Rupture of the tendo Achillis. The same injury which can produce a calf rupture can also be responsible for a rupture of the Achilles tendon. The usual cause is athletic activity in a patient who is in early middle age and out of training. The mean age in the major series ranges from 34 to 44 years,[10] although partial ruptures have been reported in much younger athletes who are at the peak of their training; and there is some evidence to suggest that a complete rupture may be preceded by a series of minor intratendinous ruptures resulting in a degenerative change in the tendon.[11]

Provided there is an adequate examination there should be no difficulty in making the diagnosis. A gap in the tendon can always be felt at the site of the rupture and this is usually situated about 1½ inches (3.5 cm) from the distal insertion into the heel. Loss of tendon continuity can be demonstrated by squeezing the calf with the patient lying face downwards (Thompson's test).[11a] In the normal calf the foot will plantar-flex on compression of the muscle, whereas no movement occurs when the Achilles tendon is divided. Because of the inability to maintain a tiptoe position the patient adopts a flat-footed, plodding type of gait, and completely loses the active plantar-flexion against body weight so necessary for taking part in competitive physical exercise. In lateral radiographs of the ankle the shadow formed by the tendo Achillis can be clearly seen to be distorted, and the radio-translucent triangle formed between its anterior surface and the toe flexor muscles (Kager's triangle) is partially obliterated in every case.[12]

Treatment. Although most surgeons favour operative repair as the treatment of choice for this condition there are some who advocate conservative management,[13,14] treating the rupture in an equinus plaster for eight weeks, followed by another four weeks using a 1 inch (2.5 cm) heel elevator and partially weight-bearing with the aid of crutches. Those who recommend conservative treatment rightly point out that operative repair is not without its complications, particularly with regard to wound healing and infection. However, several comparison series of surgical and conservative treatment[15,16] have shown that re-rupture of the tendon is not uncommon after treatment by equinus plasters, a complication almost unknown after surgery, and this alone makes operative repair the safest form of treatment. Even where there is some doubt whether the rupture is complete exploration is advisable, for in at least one series of cases all the so-called partial ruptures were found to be complete when they were explored.[17] The repair can be carried out through a postero-lateral or postero-medial incision. If the postero-lateral approach is used care must be taken to avoid damage to the sural nerve which lies lateral to the tendon accompanied by its vein. The ruptured tendon will be found to be very frayed and the insertion of efficient sutures can be difficult. It is important to obtain a good hold on both sides of the rupture by using a standard 'zigzag' tendon suture technique. The foot must be put into full equinus during the suturing in order to bring the two ends into good apposition, and in delayed cases it may be necessary to mobilise the upper section to achieve this. After a careful repair using number 1 thread or thick Dexon the skin is closed and a heavily padded below-knee plaster applied with the foot in full equinus. It is important to relax the skin incision as much as possible by plantar flexing the foot. A tense operative scar combined with plaster pressure over the heel cord is the cause of many of the wound complications. The plaster should be changed at three weeks, the equinus reduced, and a walking cast applied. This is maintained for a further three to five weeks. Heel elevators should be used for at least a month after coming out of plaster.

Late repair. Regretfully there are still too many cases where the diagnosis has been missed for many months. Although the results of surgery are less than good in a fresh case it is still a rewarding exercise to carry out a repair even as late as 12 months after rupture. It will certainly be necessary to expose the gastrocnemius and soleus more proximally in order to bring down the proximal fragment of the tendon. Sometimes an intact plantaris tendon can be used as a living graft to augment the sutures. A V-Y tendinous flap raised from the musculo-cutaneous surface of the mid-calf may be required if there is a wide defect which cannot be closed by the equinus position[18] (see Fig 32.1). A longer period of immobilisation in plaster is required after this repair—six to eight weeks in an above-knee plaster with the knee flexed 30 degrees and the foot plantar-flexed 20 degrees, followed by a further four to six weeks in a below-knee walking plaster.

FRACTURE OF THE SHAFTS OF THE LEG BONES WITHOUT DISPLACEMENT

The treatment of undisplaced fractures of the tibia and fibula should always be conservative. There is no justification to interfere surgically with a fracture which is stable and in good alignment merely to relieve the patient of the inconvenience of a plaster cast and the surgeon of its routine management.

Isolated fractures of the shaft of the fibula. These may be sustained from direct violence; they cause little functional incapacity. The shaft of this

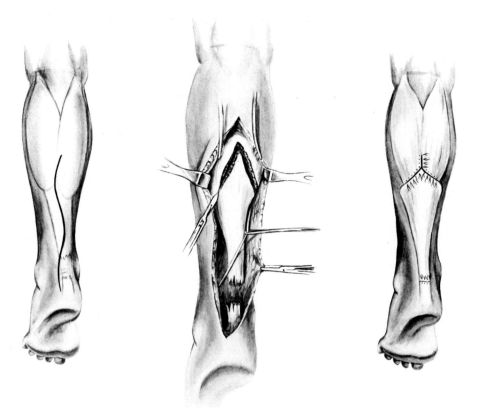

Fig 32.1 V-Y tendinous flap for repair of an old rupture of the Achilles tendon. (A) shows the lazy S posterior midline incision used to expose the tendon rupture and musculo-tendinous junction. (B) An inverted V flap of musculo-tendinous tissue is fashioned and advanced to close the tendon defect. (C) Final closure of the fascia using a Y repair and anastomosis of the tendon rupture. Reproduced by kind permission of the Editor of the *Journal of Bone and Joint Surgery* and Drs Abraham and Pankovitch from their paper in the *Journal of Bone and Joint Surgery* (1965) 57-A, 253.

bone serves only for the attachment of muscles and ligaments, and it bears no weight, so that immobilisation of the fracture is only necessary for the relief of pain and the patient may often be allowed to walk with only the protection of a crepe bandage or adhesive strapping. Sometimes a below-knee walking plaster is required to relieve pain in the first four weeks. Some precaution is needed to be sure that the fracture is in fact an isolated injury, because the shaft of the tibia may be fractured at a very different level. Fractures of the neck and upper shaft of the fibula are sometimes associated with ruptures of the medial and cruciate ligaments of the knee joint; fractures of the lower shaft of the fibula are almost invariably part of fracture-dislocation of the ankle joint; and spiral fractures of the upper third of the shaft of the fibula may be associated with dislocations of the ankle joint (see Maisonneuve's fracture, Chapter 33).

Greenstick and subperiosteal crack fractures of the shaft of the tibia. These are often sustained by children, and a similar type of fracture may be seen in adults, particularly as a result of a direct kick from a football injury (Fig 32.2). There is no overriding or loss of apposition of the fragments but only angulation, which is easily corrected by gentle moulding. This can often be done in the adult without an anaesthetic, although in a child it is often easier and kinder to give one. When working single-handed it is sometimes convenient to hang the limb over the end of a table with the knee flexed to the right angle and the leg in the line of gravity while applying a padded plaster from the toes to the tibial tubercle (Fig 32.2 inset), but it is usually as easy to do this with the leg horizontal. When the plaster is hard it is extended to the groin with the knee in a position slightly short of full extension. If post-reduction radiographs show the alignment is not perfect the angulation should be corrected by wedging the plaster (see Chapter 14). After 8 or 10 weeks the degree of union may be tested clinically; if it is not sound, immobilisation should be continued for a further period either is a full length above-knee plaster, or in a Sarmiento patellar tendon bearing cast (see later).

Valgus deformity following fracture of the proximal metaphysis of the tibia in children. Sometimes in greenstick fractures of the tibia just distal to the upper epiphysis where an initial valgus deformity has been corrected, further deformity may recur after removal of the plaster cast. This is thought to be due to the loss of restrictive tension on the growing epiphysis by the medial periosteum which has been divided by the

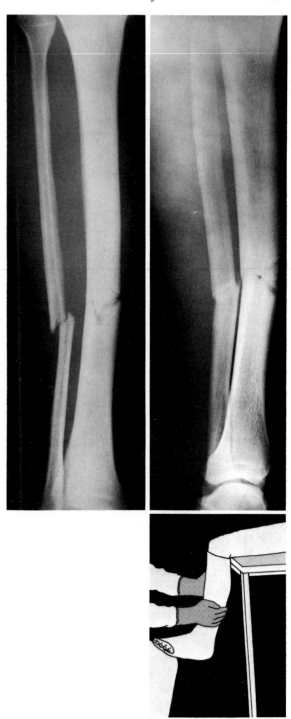

Fig 32.2 Fractures of the shaft of the tibia resulting from football injuries are often minimally displaced transverse fractures due to a direct injury from a kick. They should be treated conservatively in a long-leg plaster. When working single-handed it is sometimes convenient to apply the below-knee part of the plaster with the leg hanging over the end of a table (inset).

original fracture, and on rare occasions a periosteal flap can be trapped within the fracture line. In these circumstances unless anatomical reduction can be achieved by manipulation surgical exploration must be considered.[18a]

FRACTURES OF THE SHAFTS OF THE LEG BONES WITH DISPLACEMENT

Where a tibial fracture is transverse and can be reduced to a stable position, or where a long oblique fracture feels stable, such as is seen in some ski-ing injuries, closed reduction and immobilisation in a long-leg cast will give excellent results. It is when faced with the problem of unstable reduction, the irreducible fracture, and the open fracture with extensive soft tissue involvement that the surgeon must turn to other methods of treatment.

It is always difficult and sometimes impossible to reduce and immobilise fractures of the shafts of the leg bones when there is overriding and complete loss of apposition of the fragment of a horizontal fracture, or sliding of the fragments of an oblique or spiral fracture. Simple manual reduction may be unsuccessful. Moreover, if the fracture line is oblique and swelling is severe, redisplacement often occurs despite the application of a well-fitting plaster. Some form of stabilising traction can be essential, especially in the treatment of serious open fractures—the only alternative being immediate internal fixation.

Treatment by manipulative reduction and plaster fixation

It is often possible to reduce a displaced fracture of the shaft of the tibia by simple manipulation, and to maintain the reduction by applying a plaster cast while the limb hangs vertically over the end of a table, or having an assistant apply counter-traction in the horizontal position. Good relaxation under general or spinal anaesthesia is essential. The use of local anaesthetic has no place in the treatment of tibial shaft fractures. If the fracture is grossly unstable the insertion of a traction pin, either through the lower fragment of the tibia or through the os calcis, greatly facilitates the application of the cast and can be used afterwards to maintain stability by continuous traction (Fig 32.3). Controversy still exists as to the merit of a tibial pin and an os calcis pin. The fact that both are used widely indicates that both have their uses. The dangers of os calcis traction have been grossly overrated in the past, and the incidence of infection at this site is no worse than when a pin is used in the tibia provided it is incorporated in plaster.

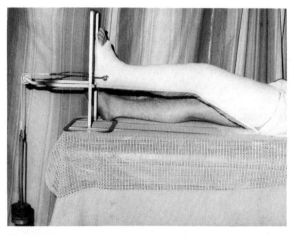

Fig 32.3 Continuous traction of a tibial fracture in an above-knee plaster on a Braun frame. Although the method has a slight danger of distraction, it is useful in the management of an unstable fracture, particularly in compound injuries.

Low-grade serous infections as a result of os calcis pins are residues of the past when tibias were treated by traction on Braun frames without plaster support. Also, on the credit side, the os calcis pin is much easier to incorporate into plaster while traction is being applied, and has the added advantage that by pulling directly on the calf there is a corrective effect on any anterior angulation.[19]

Reduction of the fracture. The technique is the same whether the injury is a closed fracture, an open fracture after excision of the wound or an infected fracture after drainage of the wound. If skeletal-traction is to be used a stirrup is fitted to the traction pin, the thigh is supported on a sorbo-covered rest, and the limb is lengthened by manual traction on the stirrup. Traction is increased until the limb is taut and the operator feels the crepitus of fragments in apposition. This indicates that overriding has been corrected. If the axis of the pin is correct there should be no rotational displacement, and the toe and patella point in the same direction. The fragments are then locked against each other by the firm lateral pressure of the operator's two hands. This is an essential step without which accurate reduction cannot be expected. Strong lateral pressure is needed. Radiographs in at least two planes are then taken, and if the reduction is satisfactory a plaster is applied.

Application of plaster. The limb is completely covered with plaster wool. If skeletal-traction is being used a plaster slab is guided through the stirrup and applied over the layer of wool from the toes to the upper calf. Special care should be taken to insure that there is adequate padding over the malleoli, the back of the heel and the neck of the fibula. The padding helps to accommodate swelling and if, after a few hours, impairment of circulation of the toes indicates that the plaster is too tight it can easily be cut longitudinally over the front of the foot and leg and through the wool bandage without injury to the skin. The plaster is then completed, and while it is setting strong lateral pressure is again maintained with the palms of the operator's hands. As soon as the plaster is hard, traction is released and the knee is straightened to a position of 10 degrees short of full extension. The plaster is then extended to the upper thigh and moulded round the knee in order to prevent rotational displacement. The knee should never be completely straight because the tibia and femur can then rotate together, and even the above-knee plaster extended to the upper thigh will not prevent rotation strain at the fracture.

Continuous traction after reduction. Although this method sometimes results in distraction of the fracture with the possibility of delayed union, it must be accepted that skeletal-traction to the lower fragment is a valuable way of preventing loss of reduction in cases of compound fractures, or where there is gross comminution interfering with internal fixation. If this technique is to be used it is essential to put only a steadying weight on the leg, for example, about 5 lb (2.3 kg). The traction should be maintained for about four weeks, after which time the long-leg plaster should be changed and the pin either removed or incorporated in the plaster.

The two-pin method of fixation of the tibia. This technique has already been described in Chapter 7 (Fig 7.19). It is extremely valuable in the treatment of infected open fractures which may require extensive local treatment to the skin over the fracture site, and also in combined injuries of the tibia and femur, where the fixation from the two-pin technique allows the tibia to be immobilised in a below-knee cast. It has been suggested that two pins in the upper fragment prevent pivotting of the bone and control anterior angulation at the fracture site.[20] However, a pin above and a pin below the fracture is usually all that is required.

Replaster after two or three weeks. After the swelling of a simple fracture of the tibia has subsided a new plaster is nearly always needed. This should be almost completely unpadded except for the bony prominences—perhaps with one or two layers of stockinet beneath it—extending to the groin with the knee slightly flexed.

Wedging the plaster. If the alignment is not accurate

it should be corrected after the plaster has set by wedging. The technique of such wedging of the plaster is described in Chapter 14 (Fig 14.12). It is of special value in fractures of the tibia because the slightest trace of medial or lateral angulation can cause serious incapacity, and whereas a surgeon may hesitate to remove a plaster and apply a new one with the object of correcting a few degrees of angulation, fearing that some other displacement may arise, he need not hesitate to use the wedging method with its accurate control and safety (Figs 32.4-32.7). It is important, however, not to wedge a wet plaster for it may buckle and produce a plaster sore. Inadequate padding under the angle of the wedge may also be responsible for skin breakdown (Fig 32.7).

Preventing rigid clawing of the toes. Rigid transverse flat foot with rigid clawing of the toes sometimes complicates leg fractures and may cause persistent disability long after the fracture has united. In applying plaster to the forefoot there is a tendency to pull up the first and fifth metatarsal heads by the turns of bandage and to hyperextend the metatarso-phalangeal joints of the toes so that the transverse arch is convex towards the sole. Even before the fracture was sustained, many patients have had mobile transverse flat foot with clawing of the toes— symptomless because it was mobile and correctable. After long immobilisation in the faulty position, with neglect of active exercises, mobile clawing becomes rigid clawing; the toes cannot be flexed to the ground. With every step body-weight is carried through the metatarsal heads and there is crippling pain and a sensation as of walking on small stones. Two precautions are needed to prevent this complication: (1) the plaster over the forefoot should be so moulded that the metatarsal heads lie in their normal, slightly arched position so that the metatarso-phalangeal joints can be flexed; (2) the toes must be prevented from clawing over the end of the plaster by extending it to their tips, either as a platform on the plantar surface, or preferably as a complete cast (see Chapter 14).

It is important always to keep in mind that toe clawing, particularly when it is severe or accompanied by calf contracture, may be a manifestation of vascular impairment. In a study of 343 tibial fractures no less than one-third of the patients with persistent limitation of ankle and foot movement showed signs of ischaemic contracture.[21]

Duration of immobilisation. After 10 or 12 weeks, if radiographic examination shows continuity of bone trabeculae between the fragments, the plaster is removed to allow clinical tests of union. Union is

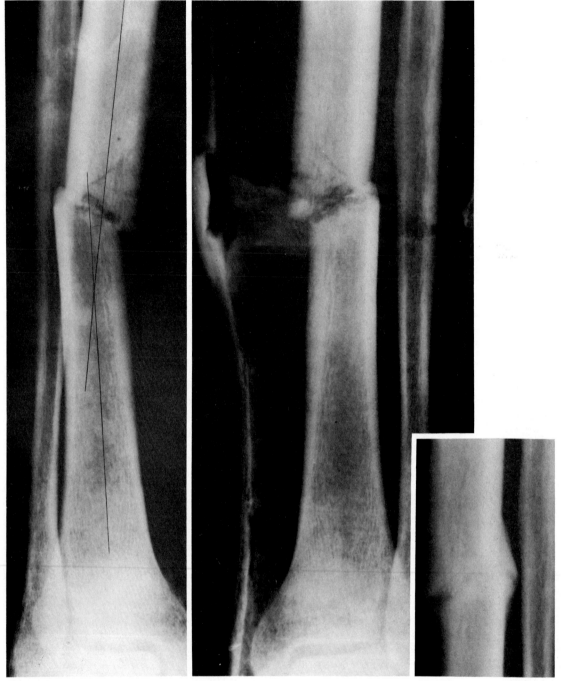

Fig 32.4   **Fig 32.5**   **Fig 32.6**

Figs 32.4 to 32.6 The fallacy of an intact fibula preventing alignment or apposition of the fragments of a fractured tibia. A displaced fracture of the shaft of the tibia was manipulated and put in plaster. Radiographs then showed that there was lateral angulation (Fig 32.4). It was suggested that this could not be corrected without operation because the fibula was intact; it was proposed that the fibula should be divided by osteotomy; but this of course is nonsense. The alignment was easily corrected by simple wedging of the plaster (Fig 32.5), and the fracture united in perfect position (Fig 32.6 inset). Far too much stress has been placed on the supposed problem of the intact fibula, not only in such a matter as this but also in the treatment of fractures of the shaft of the tibia with delayed union or established non-union. There is no need at all to divide the fibula by osteotomy in any of these cases. In recent fractures a simple bone-grafting procedure succeeds without there being any need at all to osteotomise the fibula.

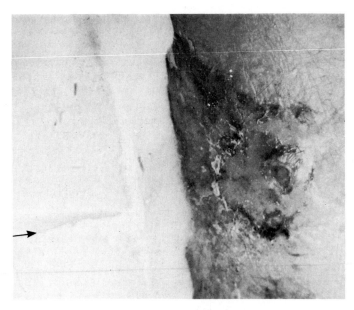

Fig 32.7 This sore produced directly under the wedged plaster used to correct angulation was due to inadequate padding. Do not wedge an unpadded plaster, or one which has not yet dried out completely.

sound when tenderness has disappeared, when no pain is elicited by straining the fracture, and when there is no longer elasticity or springing of the fragments. If union is not firm either a complete plaster should again be applied from the toes to the upper thigh, or a Sarmiento type weight-bearing plaster applied (see later).

Weight-bearing in plaster. Weight-bearing should not be permitted until the fracture is stable and only allows a rock of movement on clinical testing. Also, when union is clinically sound, but there is not yet sufficient radiographic evidence of consolidation for the plaster to be discarded, a short period in a walking-plaster may stimulate solid bony union. The plaster should still extend from the toes to the upper thigh, again with the knee slightly flexed or be of the Sarmiento type. A sorbo-rubber pad may be fixed to the heel with strapping, and a boot is fitted so that the patient dresses normally; or if preferred, a walking rocker can be used (see Figs 14.13 and 14.15). The plaster is not discarded until there is clinical and radiographic evidence of firm union of the fracture.

In recent years a number of papers have been published advocating immediate weight-bearing for tibial shaft fractures treated in a straight long-leg cast without internal fixation.[22,23] It is maintained that the straight position of the knee facilitates a proper gait and prevents stiffness of the ligaments. It is also claimed that scanogram studies show that weight-bearing does not cause shortening.[24] It is very doubtful if either of these arguments are valid, and the position is not recommended. Both closed and open fractures have been treated in this way, most of the patients being service personnel, and many of them combat victims. At first sight the results from this method are impressive: 'average time to discard plaster—19 weeks'; 'average shortening only 9 mm'; 'swelling rarely a problem'; 'all fractures united'. However, it must be remembered that these fractures were being treated in fit young soldiers who could be expected to unite their bones rapidly, particularly if they were not allowed to develop disuse osteoporosis by long periods off their feet. If the technique is used the surgeon must be prepared to change the plaster frequently ('average of six casts per patient') and be constantly on the lookout for angulation or rotatory deformity which may require wedging or change of cast. Perhaps it has a place in war-time conditions, when rapid evacuation to base is the order of the day. It has very little place in civilian practice, where the more orthodox approach already outlined can usually be guaranteed to give satisfactory results.

The use of the Sarmiento below-knee plaster.
A conventional below-knee plaster has little place in the treatment of fractures of the tibial shaft. Neither

rotational strain or angulation of the fracture is controlled by this type of plaster, and the strain delays consolidation and can even cause resorption of the newly formed callus, thus giving rise to non-union. However, there is now convincing evidence that these disadvantages can be overcome by using a carefully moulded patellar-bearing below-knee plaster which has now come to be known as the Sarmiento plaster.[25, 26] Experimental work using transducers located on the inner walls of carefully moulded patellar-bearing braces has revealed that most of the pressure is taken over the gastro-soleus mass rather than over the bony prominences of the upper end of the tibia.[27] It has also been shown that over 80 per cent of the weight is still taken through the leg and that with an unstable fracture increase in the shortening occurs under weight-bearing load. However, in the experimental model this displacement was seen to return to the preload state on release of pressure, and it has been postulated that there is a hydraulic environment provided by the soft tissues of the calf which is responsible for returning the fracture to its initial position of displacement. Although enthusiasts for the method advocate it as 'the treatment of choice for fractures of the tibial shaft'[28] it is admitted that the use of a weight-bearing plaster of this type even after a week or two in a long-leg cast, can result in angulation and marked shortening.[26] However, undoubtedly this method of splintage has a place in the later stages of conservative treatment when the fracture is more stable and requires the stimulus of direct weight-bearing, and it can be particularly useful in the management of fractures of the femur and tibia in the same limb.

The essential points in the moulding technique of this plaster are shown in Figs 32.8 and 32.9. It is recommended that the cast is applied over a thin layer of stockinet in three stages.[29] With the patient sitting on the edge of a table the knee is allowed to flex to 90 degrees (see Fig 32.2 inset). The ankle and foot are first immobilised and when this part of the cast is set the plaster is extended up the leg to the tibial tubercle. The bandages must be applied very smoothly but firmly, and without wrinkles. Firm moulding is required over the anterior tibial surface, the lateral peroneal mass and the posterior aspect in order to achieve a triangular shape which will prevent rotation of the fragments. Before the second part of the plaster is completely set the patellar tendon bearing component is added by extending the plaster up to the proximal pole of the patella while the knee is extended about 45 degrees. This part of the plaster extends backwards to cover the lower

femoral condyle and then falls away to just below the knee joint level (Fig 32.9). Firm moulding marks must be made on either side of the patellar tendon and over the tibial flares. Attention to detail is essential for success in this technique and it is well to remember that 'the method requires understanding and some skill'.[28]

Short above-knee plasters and calipers. Other methods can be used, however, at this stage to allow some knee movement. A short above-knee cast with the knee flexed about 15 degrees prevents rotation at the fracture site and allows a small amount of knee movement. It is lighter and more acceptable to the patient than a full-length plaster. Another method is to use a full length weight-relieving caliper with a cylindrical shin-guard from the knee to the ankle, made out of moulded leather or plastic. If a caliper is used it is important to have fixed sockets in the heel to prevent angulating strain at the fracture site provoked by ankle movement. Knee hinges are an optional luxury. They are not essential unless the instrument is to be worn for a very long period. A caliper is particularly valuable if there has been a fracture of the tibia and femur in the same limb. If a conventional long-leg plaster is used in this combined

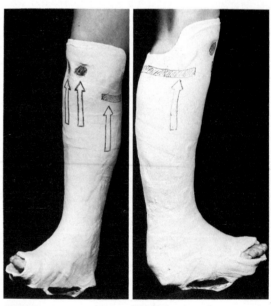

Fig 32.8   **Fig 32.9**

Figs 32.8 and 32.9 The Sarmiento below-knee plaster. This is a patellar tendon bearing fixation which is applied with maximum moulding on either side of the patellar tendon (Fig 32.8) and around the upper tibial flare on the medial and lateral sides (Figs 32.8 and 32.9).

injury the weight of the cast immobilising the tibia may result in undue strain at the femoral fracture with resulting delayed union (Figs 32.10 and 32.11).

Danger of distraction. It has been said in the past that distraction on the tibia may cause delay in union of fractures of the shaft and the average delay in one reported series of 804 lower limb shaft fractures was

in the region of four weeks.[30] Even when excessive pull and distraction were avoided only 22 per cent of tibial fractures treated with traction united soundly in 12 weeks or less, whereas 45 per cent of fractures treated without traction were united at that time. Nicoll, in a survey of 705 cases, came to the conclusion that the case against traction was not proved.[4] He

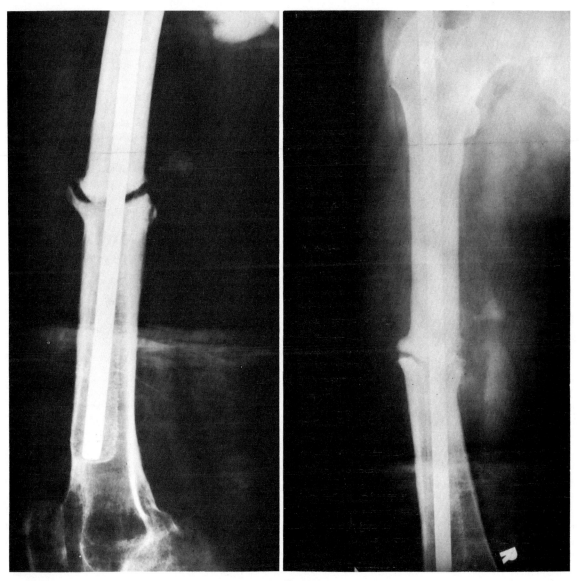

Fig 32.10

Fig 32.11

Figs 32.10 and 32.11 X-rays of a fractured lower half of the right femur in a state of delayed union. The injury was complicated by a seriously comminuted fracture of the tibial shaft on the same side. The weight of the long-leg cast used to hold the tibial fracture is clearly causing increased strain at the femoral fracture site. Note that the above-knee part of the plaster has been left short to allow some knee movement. It has only succeeded in *immobilising* the knee and *mobilising* the femoral fracture!

rightly pointed out that severity of the fracture was of importance in promoting the state of delayed union and that most cases treated by traction were of the severe type. Ellis, after a study of 576 fractures, holds the same view.[31] However, if traction is unduly heavy, and the fragments are allowed to distract, there is no doubt that delay can occur. Even if separation of the fragments amounts to only ¼ inch (6 mm), and even if it is corrected within a week or two, few distracted fractures of the tibia unite in less than four months and many unite only after 6 or 12 months. In the series previously mentioned[30] 63 per cent of distracted fractures took up to a year to unite. It is therefore clear that although light skeletal-traction may sometimes be needed during the first few weeks in unstable open fractures of the shaft of the tibia, it should be avoided if possible in simple closed fractures. If the fracture is so unstable that manipulative reduction with immobilisation in plaster does not suffice to prevent redisplacement, the two-pin method may control the instability, or it may be better to resort to operative reduction and internal fixation. However, it must be remembered that some fractures are so comminuted that internal fixation is not practicable and may be responsible for actually delaying union,[32] it is in these cases that traction, two-pin fixation, or external skeletal fixation is indicated.

Refracture of tibial shaft fractures. The treatment of refracture rarely presents any more of a problem than did the original fracture and is usually conservative. The complication occurs mainly in young adults who are still involved in contact sports. The incidence has been reported as between 3 and 4 per cent.[33, 34] In the series reported the refractures were rather more common in conservatively treated fractures, although it has been pointed out by several workers that refractures may occur after internal fixation through screw hole defects unless time is allowed for these to fill in.[33, 35] It is important to advise those taking up contact sports again that there is a possibility of refracture if they return to the sport too soon. It has been suggested that tomograms should be taken before allowing full sporting activities, and if there is still a defect in the cortex strenuous sports should be forbidden until later films confirm that the defect is filled in.[33] Others have ruled that union should only be considered complete when the medullary cavity is reconstituted. Clearly the decision to allow unrestricted exercise must depend largely upon the X-ray appearance, but in practice it is usually wise to err on the side of safety and forbid any

severe contact sports for at least one year after the accident.

Summary of conservative management. Study of the preceding section leaves little doubt that conservative measures form the basis of the safest method of treatment of tibial shaft fractures. Their management is summarised below.

1. Stable undisplaced fractures require only the application of a long-leg cast until the fracture is healed, and weight-bearing can be allowed within a few weeks of the injury. If preferred a Sarmiento type of plaster may be used at four to six weeks.
2. Displaced fractures should be reduced under general anaesthetic and if stable treated in a long cast. Weight-bearing should be deferred for four to six weeks. A Sarmiento cast may be used at about eight weeks.
3. Displaced, unstable fractures, if unsuitable for internal fixation, can be treated by a long-leg plaster with skeletal traction through the os calcis for three to four weeks, followed by a long-leg non-weight-bearing plaster for a further four to six weeks. It may be possible to use a Sarmiento cast after this time, depending upon the stability of the fracture.
4. Grossly comminuted fractures may require additional stabilisation, either using the two-pin plaster technique, or an external skeletal fixateur[35a] (Hoffmann apparatus, see Chapter 17, Figure 17.8).
5. Tibial shaft fractures complicated by an ipsilateral fracture of the femur can be treated in a below-knee cast incorporating an os calcis pin and the upper tibial pin used for femoral traction.

TREATMENT BY OPERATIVE REDUCTION AND INTERNAL FIXATION

'I make this appeal—keep the closed fractures closed'. J. R. Moore[36]

The surgeon who proposes to avoid the delays of continuous traction and distraction by operating on a fracture of the shaft of the tibia must remember that infection of the wound causes even more serious delay. Distraction and infection are both harmful in delaying union; but whereas the penalty of distraction is limited to slow union, the penalty of infection may also include chronic osteomyelitis with persistent discharge from sinuses and established non-union. There is no justification for the treatment of closed fractures of the shaft of the tibia by operative reduction and internal fixation except in the hands of surgeons who can rely on first-intention healing of the wound with complete certainty. It is not enough that most wounds heal without infection; every wound must heal without infection, for despite constant advances in chemotherapy there are still many infections which cannot be controlled. There can be few greater disasters than to convert a closed fracture into an open infected fracture with its sequestration and non-union. In this respect it is well to be reminded of the words of Sir John Charnley— 'I feel it true to say that amputations after one or two years disability are always traced to injudicious plating of the tibia'.[37] Let no surgeon consider using operative reduction with internal fixation unless he is fully competent in the operative technique, unless proper operative facilities are available to insure perfect sterility, and unless the skin condition over the fracture is satisfactory.

It is clear, therefore, that open reduction and internal fixation should be reserved for the treatment of grossly unstable or irreducible fractures. Rate of union will not necessarily be increased by operative measures—in fact there is evidence to suggest that the rate is better in conservatively treated fractures.[38] Urist, in a very complete study of matched united and ununited tibial fractures, observed that in extensively comminuted fractures open reduction and internal fixation 'always prolonged healing and never encouraged it',[32] While Sarmiento discussing the roles of conservative and operative treatment makes the comment—'Fractures of the appendicular skeleton treated by means of internal fixation, heal not because of surgery but in spite of it'.[39]

Timing of the operation. It has been shown that the complications from immediate internal fixation are high—approximately one in three cases being affected. The rate of union and the incidence of complications showed marked improvement when operation was delayed for one to three weeks.[40]

Screw fixation of oblique and spiral fractures.
Although supporters of the present vogue for rigid internal fixation have rather poured scorn on the screw method of fixation alone there is still a place in unstable oblique and spiral fractures without comminution for internal fixation by two or more screws transfixing the fragments. (Fig 32.12) Through a 4 or

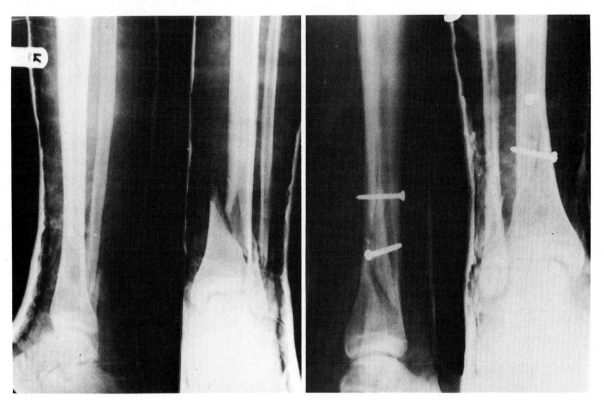

Fig 32.12 Spiral fractures in the lower third of the tibia can be stabilised satisfactorily by the insertion of one or two screws across the fracture site.

5 inch (10.2 or 12.7 cm) incision the fracture is reduced with minimal disturbance of the periosteum and the bone ends are held secure in a suitable bone clamp. The axis in which the screws will lie must be selected carefully so that an equal thickness of bone will be engaged in each fragment. The hole proximal to the head of the screw should be overdrilled to the thickness of its pitch, while the hole in the other fragment for the tip of the screw should be tapped. This allows the fragments to be compressed together as the screw is tightened in the bone (see Chapter 16, Figure 16.6). One screw may suffice but usually two, and sometimes three, are necessary. To avoid subcutaneous projection the screw heads are counter-sunk into the bone and the length of drill holes must be measured accurately. A great deal of nonsense is written about the angle at which these screws should be inserted. The plain fact of the matter is that the direction is usually dictated by the fracture anatomy and varies to some extent with every injury. Screws of the correct length are driven home, the stability of

reduction is tested, the periosteum is closed, the skin sutured and a padded plaster applied. The plaster is changed after two or three weeks. Full weight-bearing in plaster should not be permitted until about eight weeks and the plaster maintained 10 to 12 weeks. It will be appreciated, therefore, that the screwing of the fracture is merely an incident in the conservative management of the case. The method is best suited to an uncomminuted spiral fracture of the lower quarter of the tibia. It should be remembered that for most comminuted spiral fractures screw fixation alone will not give sufficient stability and in these circumstances the surgeon must be prepared to use a plate.

Percutanous cerclage wiring of spiral fractures.[41, 42] Percutaneous cerclage wiring, first introduced by Goetze in 1933,[41] has been widely used in the treatment of spiral ski fractures by orthopaedic surgeons in Austria. Undoubtedly the method works (see Figs 32.13 and 32.14) and this gives the lie to the previously strongly held view that cerclage wires

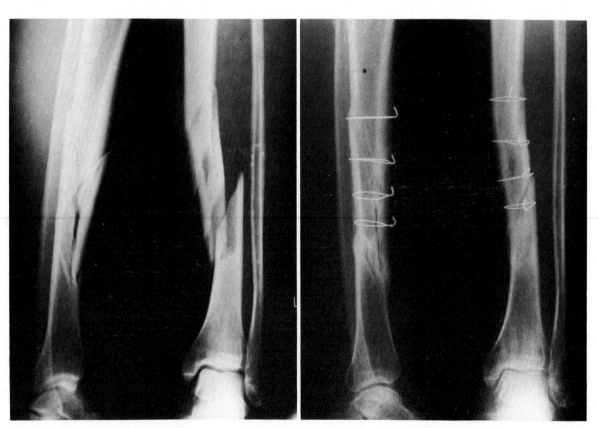

Fig 32.13 This air-line pilot sustained a spiral comminuted fracture of the tibia from a fall ski-ing. Satisfactory reduction was obtained by traction and the position stabilised by percutaneous wiring.

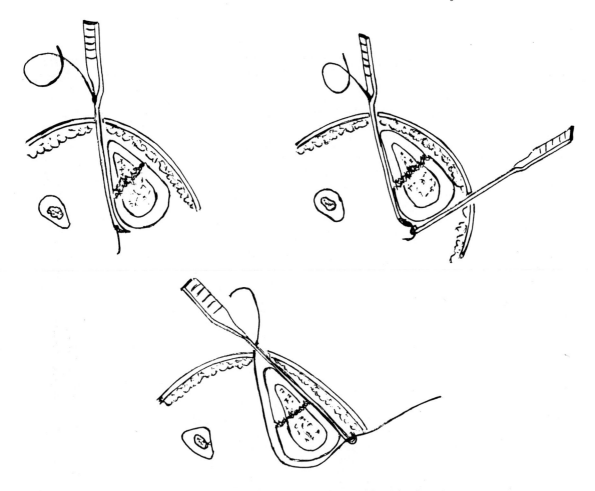

Fig 32.14 Diagrammatic illustrations of the technique of percutaneous cerclage wiring (after Goetze).

always cause absorption of bone and are responsible for refracture.[43] This technique, however gives a relatively inefficient form of fixation, particularly if there is wide displacement with marked instability. Its success in the treatment of ski fractures is probably dependant on the fact that, although often comminuted, these fractures are usually inherently stable and many would have united in good alignment without operation. If the fracture is widely displaced percutaneous wiring has the danger of picking tendons, and even vessels, and is considered unsuitable unless the displacement can be accurately reduced by traction beforehand. On the whole, the method is not recommended for the management of tibial fractures.

Plating fractures of the tibial shaft. In transverse fractures it is rarely possible to use screws—the fixation is relatively inefficient and the selection of the correct axis for the screws more difficult than in the uncomplicated spiral fracture. Also, comminuted spiral fractures cannot be safely stabilised by screws alone, although screwing of individual fragments may be a valuable additional fixation. Even if the comminuted element is still undisplaced screw fixation alone should be used with caution, and every spiral fracture must be carefully studied to exclude undisplaced comminution (Fig 32.15). For these reasons, irreducible transverse as well as comminuted fractures should be treated by means of a plate, or sometimes an intramedullary nail. Whenever possible at least a six-hole plate should be used. There are many varieties of plates and techniques advocated. Those who wish to dispense with external splintage make a great fetish of 'rigid fixation' as opposed to

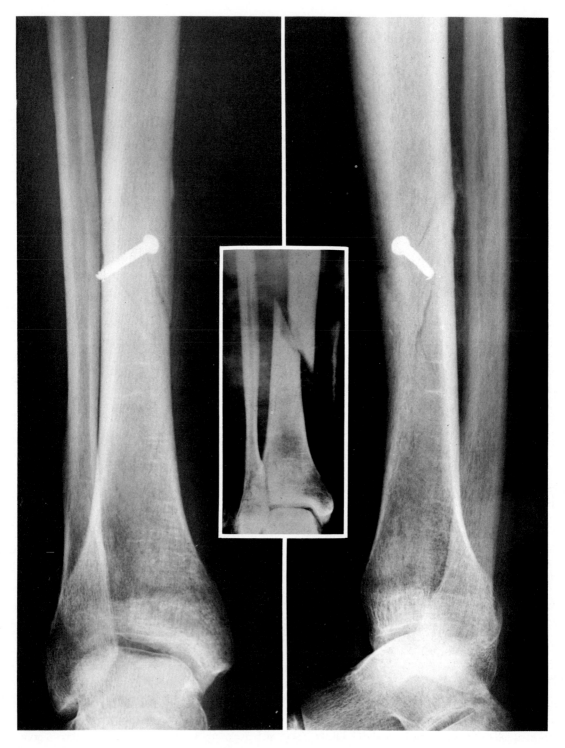

Fig 32.15 Oblique fracture of shaft of tibia treated by open reduction and transfixion with a screw. Inset shows an apparent spiral fracture without comminution, but the reduction X-rays show that there is a comminuted element. This type of fracture is fixed more safely with a plate. Respective films should be examined critically to exclude comminution.

'bone suture'. Hicks[44] has devised a plate with lugs which carry the holes for the screws and allow them to be inserted obliquely (see Chapter 16). It is claimed that this gives more rigid fixation, but this plate can be difficult to apply to a tibia and has little to commend it over the more standard varieties. Muller[45] has introduced the element of compression into the plating of fractures (see Chapter 16). Much mystique surrounds this technique which simply depends on the proper use of precision instruments. It is now generally accepted that compression cannot have any influence upon the rate of union—it merely improves the fixation, and in this respect it is useful if plaster fixation cannot be used. It has the grave disadvantage that very large plates with many screws are necessary, and the lack of callus formation makes it very difficult to know when the fracture has united.

Provided a reasonably stout plate is used the particular variety does not matter very much. Some authorities have insisted that it should be always applied on the muscular surface, but very many plates have been applied to the subcutaneous surface and have served their purpose well. No rules should be laid down about this—the plate is applied on whichever surface seems most appropriate in the circumstances prevailing at the time; the technique has been described in Chapter 16.

The use of plaster after plating depends to some extent upon the local conditions. Provided that solid fixation has been obtained there is no contraindication to allowing the limb free of plaster for the first three weeks while the patient is in bed and can carry out exercises for the knee, ankle and foot. Following this a long-leg cast is applied and the patient allowed to walk with crutches–his subsequent management following the conservative regime already outlined.

Removal of tibial plates. Subcutaneous plates should always be removed after the fracture is soundly united. If the patient is a young adult who wishes to return to contact sports he should be advised against this until the plate has been removed. After plate removal a period of about three months should be allowed for obliteration of screw holes before taking part in strenuous sport again. If the patient is unfortunate enough to have had his fracture fixed with two plates (a procedure for which there is very little indication) it is important to remove these singly at an interval of two months or more. Simultaneous removal creates a hazard of refracture.[45a]

Fixation of tibial fractures by an intramedullary nail. Intramedullary nail fixation, which is so successful in fractures of the shaft of the femur, fractures of the upper shaft of the ulna, and fractures of the shaft of the humerus where insertion of a straight nail is so easy, has also been advocated in fractures of the shaft of the tibia where the insertion of a curved nail through the upper tibial plateau down the shaft of the bone is far from easy; and it is not yet clear that there is real merit in the attempt to secure fixation of simple fractures of the shaft of the tibia by intramedullary nailing. It has a place in the stabilisation of some compound fractures, but it must be remembered that the method gives poor fixation when the fracture is close to the upper or lower end of the bone.[46]

There is, however, one fracture where the use of an intramedullary nail can be invaluable—this is the double fracture of the tibial shaft with a large middle fragment (Figs 32.16 to 32.18). In these cases it may be possible to carry out the nailing by the closed method, but if difficulties are encountered it only requires a small incision over the fracture site to align the bones.

The technique of intramedullary nailing of the tibia has been fully described by Alms and others[46,47] and is usually carried out under X-ray control by the closed nailing technique, although some papers have suggested that the open method gives better results.[48] As a preliminary to nailing a Kirschner wire is inserted through the os calcis and 5 lb (2.3 kg) of traction is applied to the fracture. This is maintained until the time of operation, which can be delayed for several days according to convenience. The normal leg is measured from anterior margin of ankle joint to anterior margin of knee joint, and a nail $\frac{1}{2}$ inch (1.3 cm) shorter than this is selected. The procedure is carried out with the knee flexed to at least a right angle. If a suitable fracture table and image intensifier is not available (Fig 32.19) the operation is made easier by using the special support shown in Figures 32.20 and 32.21, although some surgeons use only a prop which holds the knee acutely flexed (Fig 32.22). If possible traction is maintained during operation, and whichever support is used to hold the knee flexed it must be well padded to avoid pressure on the popliteal vessels and nerves. It is advised that the operation should be carried out without a tourniquet in order to allow the intramedullary canal to fill with blood between insertion of each instrument. The knee must be flexed to a right angle or more* to allow

* It is important to remember that nailing by this technique may be impossible in some late cases where the knee is not fully mobile—for example, in combined fractures of the femur and tibia in the same limb.

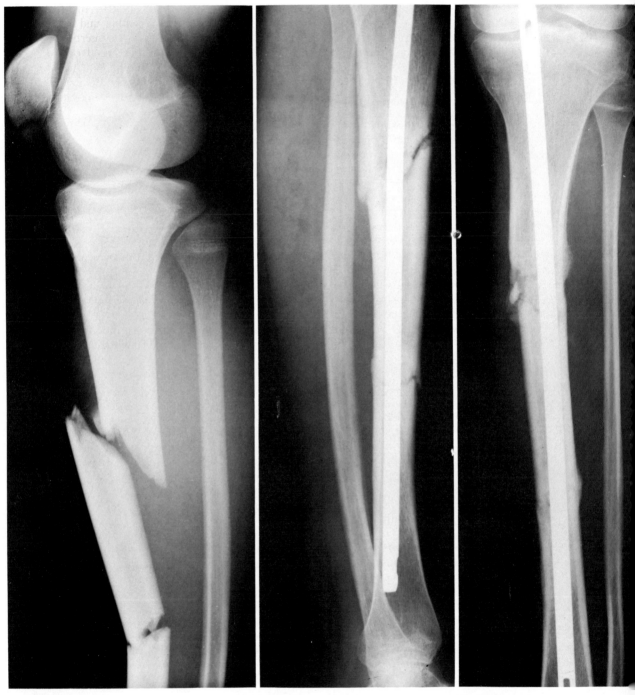

Fig 32.16   Fig 32.17   Fig 32.18

Figs 32.16 to 32.18 Double fracture of the shaft of the tibia for which the treatment of choice is.intramedullary nailing. Figures 32.17 and 32.18 show the fracture three months after Kuntscher nailing.

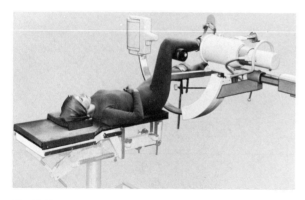

Fig 32.19 The leg position for tibial Kuntscher nailing using a Maquet table and an image intensifier unit. (Reproduced by kind permission of Downs Surgical Limited).

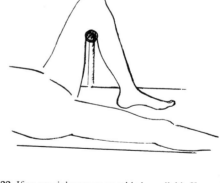

Fig 32.22 If no special support or table is available Kuntscher nailing of the tibia can be performed with the knee flexed over a prop attached to the operating table. (After Merle d'Aubigne).

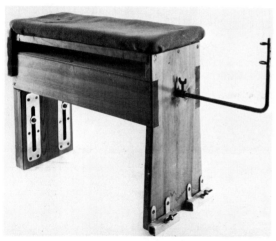

Fig 32.20

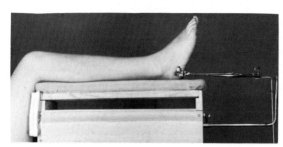

Fig 32.21

Figs 32.20 and 32.21 The adjustable support recommended for Kuntscher nailing of the tibia by Alms.[46] Note the rod for securing traction and the slot for X-ray plates. The appliance is heavily padded to prevent neurological complications. Figure 32.21 illustrates the position of the leg with traction applied.

insertion of the nail, and it may be necessary to adjust the height of the support to achieve this position. A medial incision is made just to the side of the patellar ligament, and the space occupied by the retro-patellar pad of fat and the infra-patellar bursa is developed; the knee joint should not be opened. A point on the tibial plateau just behind the patellar tendon and near the anterior margin (Fig 32.23) is selected for nail entry; a pointed punch starts the hole, and this is followed by a guide-wire which is passed across the fracture site into the lower fragment to the calculated length required and checked by X-ray. The flexible reamers (Fig 32.24), essential for the operation, are passed over the guide-wire and enlarge the medulla to the requisite size (an 11 mm diameter nail is the usual size for an adult). Extensive reaming to allow the introduction of oversize nails is not recommended. Undoubtedly it produces more rigid fixation, but it does so at the expense of considerable thinning of the endosteal cortex, and this, combined with the very rigid fixation, may be responsible for delay in natural bone healing. Also, there are some who feel that the infection rate is higher in reamed cases.[46-48a] Some difficulty may be encountered when passing the guide-wire because of the point passing out through the back of the fracture site and, as a result of this, it is important not to use guides with pointed ends. If the fracture cannot be reduced sufficiently well to pass the guide it is better not to waste time and immediately proceed to open reduction.[48a] The nail to be used must be carefully angled at its upper end to accommodate the bend from the point of insertion to the middle of the medullary cavity; usually 10 to 20 degrees of angulation at a point quarter of the length from the upper end is sufficient, and this can

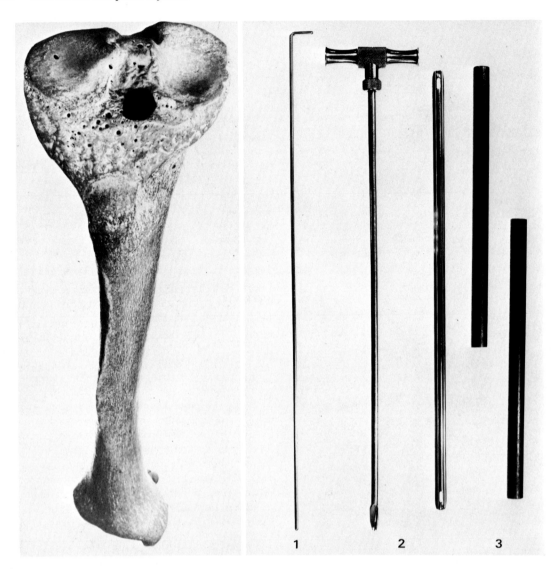

Fig 32.23 Photograph of the tibial plateau with the site of entry of the Kuntscher nail in black (after Alms).

Fig 32.24 Instruments required for Kuntscher nailing of the tibia: 1. Blunt-ended guide-wires. 2. Flexible reamers. 3. Kuntscher nail and pipes used for bending it.

be made by bending the nail over a wedge using the lengths of piping as levers (Fig 32.24). It is vital to the technique that the nail should be bent with the open channel on the convex side; in this way the nail cannot slip off the guide-wire and find a false passage through the fracture site. The nail is driven along the guide wire until the upper end is just below the cortex of the tibial plateau. It is important to impact fully the nail for a projection even as small as a half an inch

(1 cm) can interfere with full extension of the knee (Fig 32.25). During the insertion pressure should be kept on the foot to prevent distraction of the fracture surfaces. Check X-rays should be taken, the knee wound sutured and the os calcis pin removed. If the immobilisation is completely rigid no plaster is necessary, but the patient should be kept non-weight-bearing. A long-leg cast should be used if there is any doubt about the rigidity of the fracture.

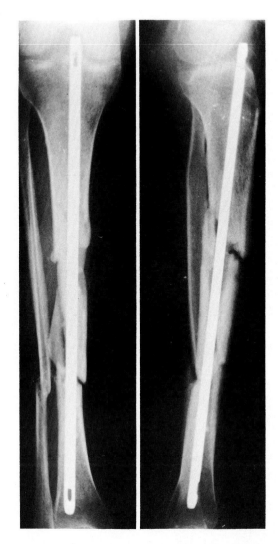

Fig 32.25 This severely compound and comminuted fracture of the tibia was adequately immobilised by a Kuntscher nail which was just too long to allow it to be fully impacted at the upper end. This resulted in 5 to 10 degrees of limitation of knee extension. Tibial Kuntscher nails must be accurately measured to give adequate hold at the lower end but still allow the upper end to be impacted.

The use of Rush nails. In some cases where there are multiple fragments, it may be impossible to thread a Kuntscher nail through the bone without producing further fragmentation of the small tibial segments. In these circumstances it is wise to use the intramedullary fixation merely to string the pieces of bone into alignment again, and a much narrower Rush type of nail may be passed down the medulla, usually under the direct vision of an open reduction. If circumstances permit, more than one Rush nail can be used to improve fracture stability. This must be followed by external fixation as would be used for a fracture being treated conservatively (Figs 32.26 to 32.30). Indeed Charnley regards Rush nail fixation as a most satisfactory adjunct to the conservative management of tibial fractures.[49] It has none of the disadvantages of rigid internal fixation, only assisting in maintaining a satisfactory alignment, and does not interfere with the natural method of healing by periosteal callus.

Rush nails can sometimes be used to advantage in compound fractures which are complicated by severe soft tissue damage. To avoid opening the knee the nail can be introduced through the medial malleolus (Fig 32.31).

COMPLICATIONS OF FRACTURES OF THE SHAFT OF THE TIBIA

Fracture of the tibial shaft is one of the most common bony injuries to occur, and because of the situation of the bone it is the most common of the compound fractures: the displacement of the fragments and the severity of the soft accompanying tissue injury may be extensive. It is therefore not surprising that complications are frequent. They can be listed as follows:

1. Slow union and non-union.
2. Vascular problems.
3. Nerve injury.
4. Severe skin and soft tissue loss.
5. Loss of bone substance.

Slow union and non-union. The average time of union varies from 10 to 15 weeks in an adult fracture of the tibial shaft—the speed of healing decreasing rapidly with the increase in initial severity of the fracture.[31] It has been suggested previously that a fracture through the lower third of the tibia is more liable to go on to delayed union because the lower fragment becomes relatively avascular. Nicoll, however, in his large series of 705 cases,[4] has shown that the number of cases of delayed union is almost exactly the same for upper, middle and lower third fractures. However, anyone who has performed a number of grafting operations for delayed union must have been impressed by the avascular appearance at the fracture site, and Nicoll's work shows that this is common to all fracture sites. He has also shown that, contrary to common belief, an intact fibula associated with a

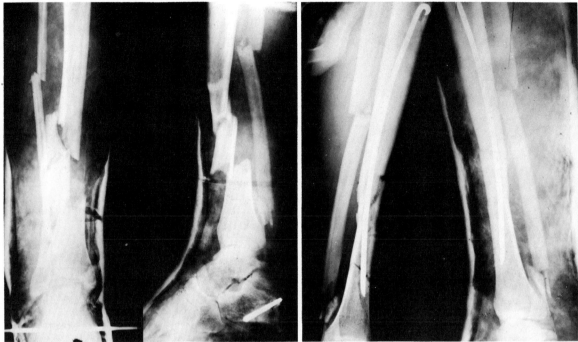

Fig 32.26   Fig 32.27

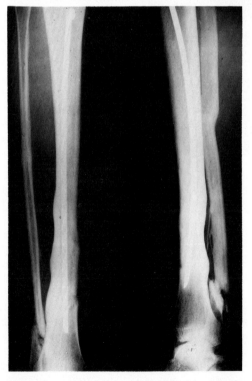

Fig 32.28

Figs 32.26 to 32.28 Figure 32.26 is an X-ray of a multiple fracture of the shaft of the tibia after attempted manipulation and immobilisation in plaster with os calcis traction. Figure 32.27 shows the position of the open reduction and the insertion of a Rush nail, and Figure 32.28 is an X-ray taken six months after operation.

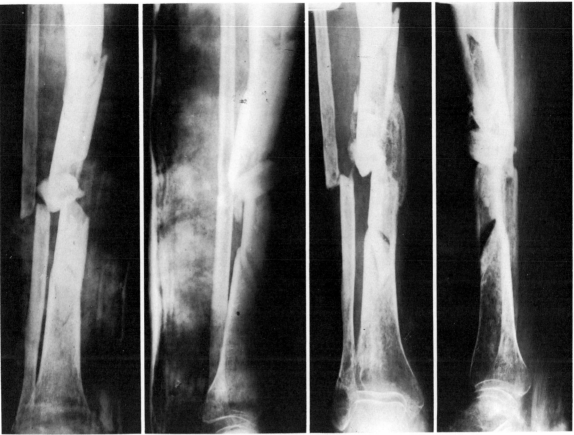

Fig 32.29   **Fig 32.30**

Figs 32.29 and 32.30 Compare the management of this multiple fracture of the tibia with that of the case shown in Figures 32.26 to 32.28. Figure 32.29 shows the degree of union six months after conservative treatment and cancellous strip grafting.

fractured tibial shaft causes no increase in the incidence of delayed union (Figs 32.4 to 32.6).

Other workers have formed the opinion that in open fractures an intact fibula gives a better prognosis for union.[50] However, this view has been challenged more recently,[50a] where a clinical study of over 100 tibial fractures with an intact fibula (backed by experimental work) has revealed 26 per cent delayed union and 26 per cent varus malunion in patients over the age of 20. Delayed union was rare when the fracture occurred in adolescents. Thus there are two directly opposing views on the importance of the intact fibula. The difference of opinion probably lies in the failure to recognise the significance of the varus deformity. If this can be corrected as suggested in the legend to Figures 32.4 to 32.6 no problem should

arise. If this cannot be achieved by manipulation surgery must be considered.

Although it is true that prolonged and uninterrupted immobilisation of these fractures will eventually result in union, it is not justifiable to withold bone grafting for longer than about six months. Charnley considers that the introduction and wider use of the Phemister bone graft is one of the greatest advances in the management of the fractured tibial shaft,[49] and he advocates grafting as early as three months after injury. Certainly the results of the cancellous strip graft applied by the Phemister technique are so good and the operation is so simple that it should be considered as soon as the diagnosis of delayed union is made (see Chapter 18). Union of the fracture can be almost guaranteed within three

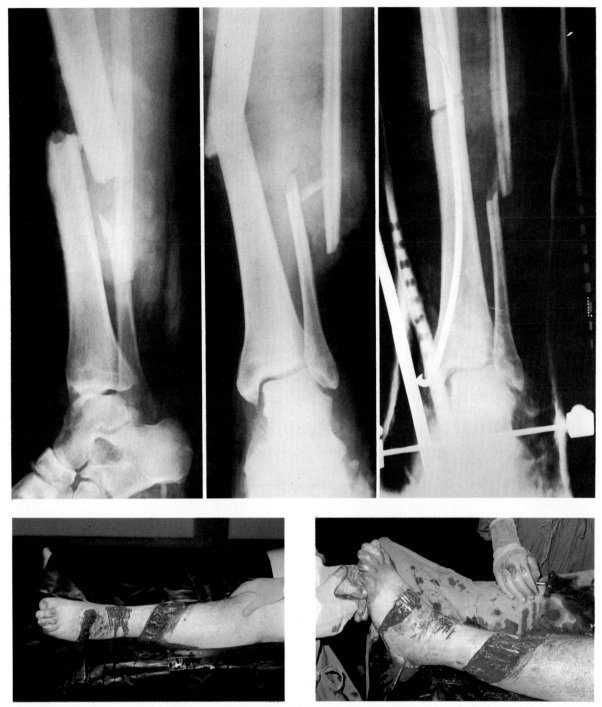

Fig 32.31 This patient sustained a severe compound fracture of the left tibia with a large soft tissue wound. The injury was complicated by a fracture of the shaft of the femur and a compound fracture of the tarsus, both in the same limb. It was not possible to close the wounds over the tibia or over the foot and extensive skin grafting was necessary as a secondary procedure. This was greatly facilitated by neutralisation of the tibial fracture with a Rush nail inserted at the time of the initial debridement. Very stable fixation was obtained by inserting a large diameter nail by the retrograde method through the medial malleolus, thereby avoiding opening up the tissues around the knee.

months of grafting and early operation may prevent many months of delay and frustration. As a conservative measure in cases where it is inconvenient to operate, or where bone grafting must be delayed indefinitely, a full-length weight-relieving caliper with a shin guard and *fixed* ankle stops is a very welcome change to continuous plaster and allows mobilisation exercises of the knee and ankle. A well moulded Sarmiento brace may serve almost the same purpose,[25] but this has the disadvantage that, even though the knee and ankle can be exercised freely, the cast itself cannot be completely removed.

The use of electrical stimulation with further prolonged immobilisation is much in vogue at present but is not yet proven (see Chapter 18).

Vascular complications. The management of the frankly ischaemic leg has been fully discussed in Chapter 11 and is easily recognised; but it has been pointed out that lesser degrees of ischaemic change may be very much more common than was previously supposed;[51] and in one series of cases no less than one-third of the patients with persistent ankle and foot stiffness showed signs of ischaemic change.[21] Unexplained cavus, with clawing of the toes and inversion of the foot is almost certainly due to vascular impairment,[52] and has been attributed to compression within the deep posterior compartment of the calf. It should be suspected in the acute phase when there is pain and tenseness in the distal and medial side of the calf. Pain on passive extension and diminished active flexion of the toes, associated with plantar hypoaesthesia, are characteristic of the compartment syndrome. Early diagnosis is essential if permanent disability is to be avoided; for those cases where decompression has been delayed for more than 12 hours can be expected to have some ischaemic contracture.[53] The anterior compartment is, of course, also affected and manometric readings have shown compartmental pressures in over 50 per cent of displaced fractures of the upper third of the tibia resulting from high energy trauma.[53a]

Nerve complications. These are neither frequent nor serious.[54] Except in compound injuries nerves are unlikely to be divided, and in the rare case when a nerve is involved it is usually the posterior tibial nerve which is affected, being stretched over fracture surfaces in the upper third of the tibia where it lies close to the bone.[55] An unusual case has been reported associated with an ankle injury where tarsal tunnel symptoms occurred and were completely relieved by decompression.[54] However, before leaving the subject it is only right to remind the reader of the vulnerability of the external popliteal nerve—sometimes damaged by a fracture of the fibular neck, but more often as the result of pressure from a badly padded plaster or splint. *Never forget* that if a drop-foot develops while a patient is under treatment for a tibial fracture *it is mandatory* to inspect the area around the neck of the fibula.

Severe soft tissue injury. Compound wounds and severe crushing injuries to the soft tissues are relatively frequent complications of tibial fractures and responsible for much of the residual joint stiffness. The presence of a wound with extensive skin loss may dictate the treatment of the bony injury, and on occasions it may be necessary to 'neutralise' the fracture by some means in order to free the limb for the treatment of the soft tissues; for example, where extensive skin-grafting is necessary or frequent dressings are needed. Under these circumstances, plating of a compound fracture is quite justifiable and is preferable to the use of an intramedullary nail (see Chapter 7), although a Rush nail, which can be slipped down the medulla with minimal disturbance of the bone, can be very useful. External skeletal fixation with the Hoffman apparatus is also a valuable method. Contrary to general belief the introduction of metal itself cannot *cause* infection and is unlikely to contribute to it provided wounds are submitted to the treatment of any compound fracture, that is, no tight closure and delayed primary suture as required.

Fractures with loss of bone substance. Because of its subcutaneous position the fractured tibia is more likely to suffer the loss of a bone fragment through a compound wound than other fractures, and there are instances of pieces of bone being recovered from the scene of the accident, brought to the theatre and reinserted after sterilisation. Usually, however, the bone gap must be temporarily accepted. If this is small—less than 1 inch (2.5 cm)—it may be possible to reshape the bone ends, bring them together and fix them with a plate. But often the gap is too big to close in this simple way, and in these circumstances the preliminary treatment must be directed towards skin closure and maintenance of limb length by use of continuous traction, two-pin fixation, Hoffman apparatus or even a 'spacer' plate (Figs 32.32 to 32.34). When the wound is soundly healed the gap can be filled with a block of iliac bone, using supplementary internal fixation with a bone plate.[56] This technique is quite different from the Phemister method of inlay grafting without disturbance of the pseudarthrosis;

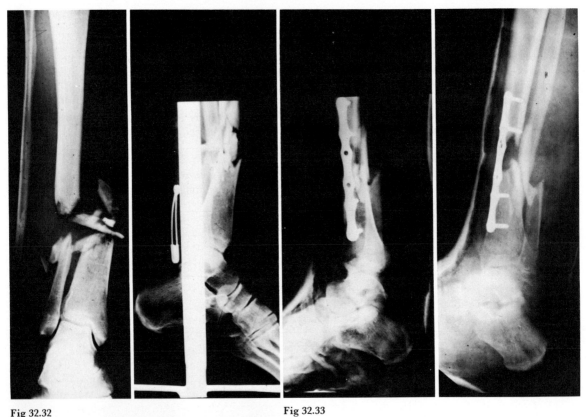

Fig 32.32

Fig 32.33

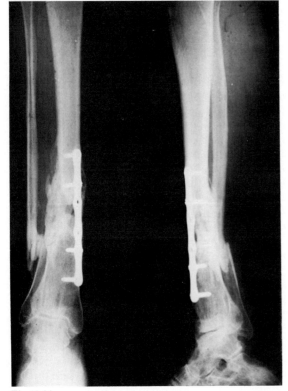

Fig 32.34

Figs 32.32 to 32.34 Figure 32.32 shows the X-ray of the tibia of a pillion passenger injured in a motor-cycle combination accident. The injury was compound and there was a severe loss of bone substance. Figure 32.33 shows the 'spacer' plate used in the primary treatment to maintain length and stability. This defect was repaired with a cancellous graft five months later, and Figure 32.34 shows the united fracture 10 months after grafting with the original plate still in situ. (Initial treatment by the late Mr D. W. Purser).

for where a bone block is to be used, it is important to cut back any avascular tissue until a bed of bleeding bone is produced for the graft. The gap is carefully measured and a prepared cancellous bone block is inserted. This procedure has been successfully carried out in the face of infection, and although some of the graft may sequestrate, enough remains to restore continuity and heal the defect. Mowlem[57] used cancellous strips alone in the same way to restore bone defects, emphasising that they could survive in the face of infection; his technique is probably a safer method when operating upon infected, or potentially infected, fractures. Illustrative cases of the method of repairing defects are shown in Figures 32.32 to 32.38.

Fractures with interposition of soft tissues. It is unusual for this complication to be a problem in the treatment of fractures of the tibial shaft. However, in fractures of the upper quarter of the bone it is possible for reduction to be impeded by interposition of the pes anserinus. This should be suspected it a fracture at this site cannot be reduced by manipulation or traction (Figs 32.39 and 32.40).

COMPOUND FRACTURES OF THE TIBIA SUMMARY OF MANAGEMENT

Although the management of compound fractures in general has already been discussed in Chapters 7 and

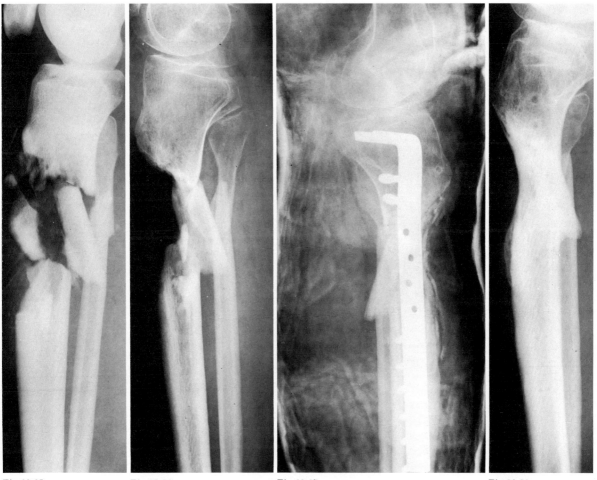

Fig 32.35   Fig 32.36   Fig 32.37   Fig 32.38

Figs 32.35 to 32.38 Figure 32.35 shows the initial X-ray of a motorcyclist who sustained a compound fracture of the upper tibia with severe skin loss and loss of bone. Figure 32.36 shows the defect remaining in the bone after skin cover restored by a cross-leg flap. The repair with a blade plate and cancellous graft is shown in Figure 32.37. Figure 32.38—repair 18 months later. (Treated by Mr E. L. Trickey.)

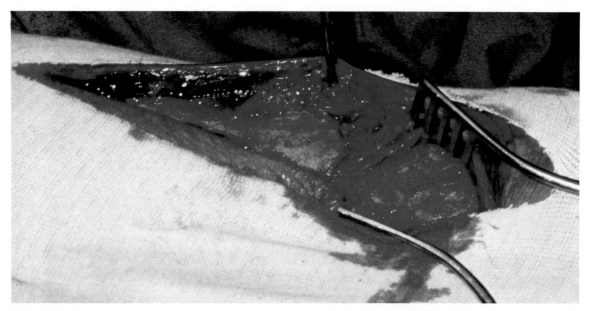

Fig 32.39(a)

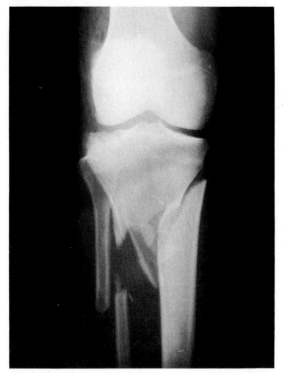

Fig 32.39(b)

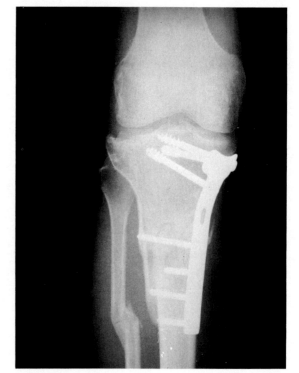

Fig 32.40

Figs 32.39 and 32.40 Soft tissue interposition in tibial fractures is rarely a problem. However in fractures of the upper quarter of the bone the pes anserinus can sometimes prevent reduction (Fig 32.39). Open reduction and internal fixation is essential in these rare cases (Fig 32.40).

16 it is appropriate that this chapter should end with a summary of the management of the most common of them all—the compound fracture of the tibial shaft. The fracture patterns and complications of this injury are so varied that dogma has little place in the treatment—each injury presenting its own problems. Therefore, only the general principles of management can be useful, and these are summarised below.

1. Classification. Difficulties in grading these injuries has lead to problems in assessing the results of treatment.[58] Most of the classifications are very similar, dividing the fractures into minor, moderate or severe according to the degree of soft tissue involvement, the extent of displacement and the amount of comminution.[4, 21, 59, 60] It is clear that the prognosis is more dependant upon the severity of the lesion than on any method of treatment employed: even though the choice of treatment may well be dictated by the severity of the original injury.

2. Management of the soft tissue wound. All wounds must have an adequate debridement. Small lacerations resulting from a compound fracture from within, and wounds through healthy skin which can be easily closed without tension and where there is no involvement of the deep tissues can be safely closed at the primary operation. Extensive wounds with devitalised skin and muscle destruction must *never* be closed initially. Closure will be possible later, either by delayed primary suture or by split skin grafting. But it is well to remember that 'the proper management of an open fracture is to convert it to a closed fracture at the earliest moment consistent with safety'.[50]

Management of the fracture. *A stable fracture* with minimal skin involvement should be treated as a closed injury in plaster. *Instability without a major soft tissue complication* may be managed by the two-pin method of fixation in plaster, or by continuous os calcis traction. *Unstable two fragment fractures* in the presence of extensive skin damage can be neutralised by rigid fixation with a plate, a Rush nail or by use of the extra-skeletal fixateur; both methods giving access to the wound for skin grafting procedures while still maintaining reduction of the fracture. *Segmental fractures* may often be controlled in reasonable alignment by the use of a Rush intramedullary nail, which is easy to insert and preferable to the more hazardous procedure of formal Kuntscher nailing.

4. Use of antibiotics. A broad spectrum antibiotic should be given with the premedication for the initial operation and continued until the immediate problems of wound healing have been overcome. Local antibiotic (1 g of chloramphenicol is useful in this respect) is also valuable, but in no way must this detract from the value of wide debridement of devitalised tissue.

5. Place of primary amputation. In hopelessly damaged legs the question of amputation should be considered early. Patients are more likely to accept it as an initial procedure than they will many months later when it is put to them as a final solution. Early amputation in these serious cases should not be regarded as an admission of defeat[50]—it may save the patient many months, or even years of unnecessary suffering.

REFERENCES

1. Charnley J 1961 The closed treatment of common fractures, 3rd edn. Livingstone, Edinburgh, ch 15, p 105
2. Burwell H N 1971 Plate fixation of tibial shaft fractures. A survey of 181 injuries. Journal of Bone and Joint Surgery 53-B: 258
3. Lucas K, Todd C 1973 Closed adult tibial shaft fractures. Journal of Bone and Joint Surgery 55-B: 878
4. Nicoll E A 1964 Fractures of the tibial shaft. A survey of 705 cases. Journal of Bone and Joint Surgery 46-B: 373
5. Nicoll E A 1974 Closed and open management of tibial fractures. Clinical Orthopaedics and Related Research 105: 144
5a. Van der Linden W, Larsson K 1979 Plate fixation versus conservative treatment of tibial fractures. A randomized trial. Journal of Bone and Joint Surgery 61-A: 873
5b. Bauer G, Hulth A 1973 Kompressionsosteosyntes enligt AO vid underbenets diafysfrakturer bor overges. (The AO-method for compression osteosynthesis when treating tibial shaft fractures ought to be rejected.) Lakartidningen 70: 4752
6. Wade P A 1970 A.S.I.F. Compression has a problem. (Editorial) Journal of Trauma 10: 513
7. Ellis J 1964 Treatment of fractures of the tibial shaft. (Editorial) Journal of Bone and Joint Surgery 46-B: 371
8. Cyriax J 1978 Textbook of orthopaedic medicine, vol 1: Diagnosis of soft tissue lesions. Balliere Tindall, London p 662
9. Groce E J, Carpenter G K 1944 Rupture of the plantaris muscle. Journal of Bone and Joint Surgery 26: 818
10. Barfred T 1973 Achilles tendon rupture. Acta Orthopaedica Scandinavica, suppl 152
11. Ljungqvist R 1968 Subcutaneous partial rupture of the Achilles tendon. Acta Orthopaedica Scandinavica suppl 113
11a. Thompson T G, Doherty J H 1962 Spontaneous rupture of tendon Achilles: a new clinical diagnostic test. Journal of Trauma 2: 126

12. Arner O, Lindolm A, Lindvall N 1959 Roentgen changes in subcutaneous rupture of the Achilles tendon. Acta Chirurgica Scandinavica 116: 496

13. Lee R B, Smith L 1968 Rupture of the Achilles tendon. Non-surgical treatment. Clinical Orthopaedics and Related Research 60: 115

14. Gillies H, Chalmers J 1970 The management of fresh ruptures of the tendo Achillis. Journal of Bone and Joint Surgery 52-A: 337

15. Davey K 1956 Comparison of operative and conservative treatment of acute rupture of the tendo calcaneus. Journal of Bone and Joint Surgery, 58-B: 384

16. Inglis A E, Scott W N, Sculco T P, Patterson A H 1976 Ruptures of the tendo Achillis. An objective assessment of surgical and non-surgical treatment. Journal of Bone and Joint Surgery 58-A: 990

17. Hooker C H 1963 Rupture of the tendo-calcaneus. Journal of Bone and Joint Surgery 45-B: 360

18. Abraham E, Pankovich A M 1975 Neglected rupture of the Achilles tendon. Treatment by V-Y tendinous flap. Journal of Bone and Joint Surgery 57-A: 253

18a. Rooker G D, Salter R B 1980 Prevention of valgus deformity following fracture of the proximal metaphysis of the tibia in children. Jounal of Bone and Joint Surgery 62-B: 527

19. Charnley J 1961 The closed treatment of common fractures, 3rd edn. Livingstone, Edinburgh ch 15, p 242

20. Anderson L D, Hutchins W C, Wright P E, Disney J M 1974 Fractures of the tibia and fibula treated by casts and transfixing pins. Clinical Orthopaedics and Related Research 105: 179

21. Ellis H 1958 Disabilities after tibial shaft fractures. With special reference to Volkmann's ischaemic contracture. Journal of Bone and Joint Surgery 40-B: 190

22. Dehne E et al 1961 Non-operative treatment of the fractured tibia by immediate weight-bearing. Journal of Trauma 1: 514

23. Brown P W, Urban J G 1969 Early weight-bearing of open fractures of the tibia. An end result study of sixty-three cases. Journal of Bone and Joint Surgery 51-A: 59

24. Brown P W 1974 The early weight-bearing treatment of tibial shaft fractures. Clinical Orthopaedics and Related Research 105: 167

25. Sarmiento A 1970 A functional below-the-knee brace for tibial fractures. Journal of Bone and Joint Surgery 52-A: 295

26. Sarmiento A 1974 Functional bracing of tibial fractures. Clinical Orthopaedics and Related Research 105: 202

27. Sarmiento A, Latta L, Zilioli A, Sinclair W 1974 The role of soft tissues in the stabilisation of tibial fractures. Clinical Orthopaedics and Related Research 105: 116

28. Mollan R A B, Bradley B 1978 Fractures of the tibial shaft treated in a patellar-tendon-bearing cast. *Injury* 10: 124

29. Sarmiento A 1967 A functional below-the-knee cast for tibial fractures. Journal of Bone and Joint Surgery 49-A: 855

30. Watson-Jones R, Coltart W D 1943 Critical review. Slow union of fractures with a study of 804 fractures of the shafts of the tibia and femur. British Journal of Surgery 30: 260

31. Ellis H 1958 The speed of healing after fracture of the tibial shaft. Journal of Bone and Joint Surgery 40-B: 42

32. Urist M R, Mazet R, McLean F C 1954 Pathogenesis and treatment of delayed union and non-union. Journal of Bone and Joint Surgery 36-A: 931

33. Chrisman O D, Snook G A 1968 The problem of refracture of the tibia. Clinical Orthopaedics 60: 217

34. Pinder I M 1973 Refracture of the shaft of the adult tibia. Journal of Bone and Joint Surgery 55-B: 878

35. Frankel V H, Burnstein A H 1968 Biomechanics of refracture of bone. Clinical Orthopaedics 60: 221

35a. Lawyer R B, Lubbers L M 1980 Use of the Hoffmann apparatus in the treatment of unstable tibial fractures. Journal of Bone and Joint Surgery 62-A: 1264

36. Moore J R 1960 The closed fracture of the long bones. Journal of Bone and Joint Surgery 42-A: 869

37. Charnley J 1961 The closed treatment of common fractures, 3rd edn. Livingstone, Edinburgh ch 15, p 206

38. Hoagland F T, States J D 1967 Factors influencing the rate of healing in tibial shaft fractures. Surgery, Gynecology and Obstetrics 124: 71

39. Sarmiento A 1974 Editorial comment. Fractures of the tibia. Clinical Orthopaedics and Related Research 105: 2

40. Smith J E M 1974 Results of early and delayed internal fixation for tibial shaft fractures. A review of 470 cases. Journal of Bone and Joint Surgery 56-B: 469

41. Goetz O 1933 Subcutane Drahtnaht bei Tibiaschrägfrakturen. Archiv für Klinische Chirurgie 177: 445

42. Buhler J 1974 Percutaneous cerclage of tibial fractures. Clinical Orthopaedics and Related Research 105: 276

43. Watson-Jones R 1955 Fractures and Joint Injuries, 4th edn. Livingstone, Edinburgh ch X, p 201

44. Hicks J H 1964 Rigid fixation as a treatment for non-union. Proceedings of the Royal Society of Medicine 57: 358

45. Muller M E 1963 Internal fixation for fresh fractures and for non-union. Proceedings of the Royal Society of Medicine 56: 455

45a. Jergeson F 1974 Double plating of tibial fractures. Clinical Orthopaedics and Related Research 105: 240

46. Merle d'Aubigné R, Maurer P, Zucman J, Masse Y 1974 Blind intramedullary nailing for tibial fractures. Clinical Orthopaedics and Related Research 105: 267

47. Alms M 1962 Medullary nailing for fracture of the shaft of the tibia. Journal of Bone and Joint Surgery 44-B: 328

48. Hamza K M, Dunkerley G E, Murray C M M 1971 Fractures of the tibia. A report on fifty patients treated by intramedullary nailing. Journal of Bone and Joint Surgery 53-B: 696

48a. Bintcliffe I W L, Vickers R H 1980 Tibial nailing: an open or shut case? Journal of Bone and Joint Surgery 62-B: 525

49. Charnley J 1961 The closed treatment of common fractures, 3rd edn. Livingstone, Edinburgh ch 15, p 208

50. Rosenthal R E, Macphail J A, Oritz J E 1977 Non union in open tibial fractures. Analysis for failure of treatment. Journal of Bone and Joint Surgery 59-A: 244

50a. Teitz C C, Carter D R, Frankel V H 1980 Problems associated with tibial fractures and intact fibulae. Journal of Bone and Joint Surgery 62-A: 770

51. Önnerfalt R 1978 Fracture of the tibial shaft treated by primary operation and early weight-bearing. Acta Orthopaedica Scandinavica, supp 171

52. Karlström G, Lönnerholm T, Olerud S 1975 Cavus deformity of the foot after fracture of the tibial shaft. Journal of Bone and Joint Surgery 57-A: 893

53. Matsen F A, Clawson D K 1975 The deep posterior compartmental syndrome of the leg. Journal of Bone and Joint Surgery 57-A: 34

53a. Halpern A A, Nagel D A 1980 Anterior compartment pressures in patients with tibial fractures. Journal of Trauma 20: 786

54. Seddon Sir Herbert 1975 Surgical disorders of the peripheral nerves, 2nd edn. Churchill Livingstone, Edinburgh, ch 5, p 88
55. Bateman H E 1962 Trauma to nerves in limbs. Sanders, Philadelphia, ch 14, p 397
56. Nicol E A 1956 The treatment of gaps in long bones by cancellous insert grafts. Journal of Bone and Joint Surgery 38-B: 70
57. Mowlem R 1944 Cancellous chip grafts for the restoration of bone defects. Proceedings of the Royal Society of Medicine 38: 171
58. Austin R T 1977 Fractures of the tibial shaft: is medical audit possible? Injury 9: 93
59. Karlström G, Olerud S 1975 Percutaneous pin fixation of open tibial fractures. Journal of Bone and Joint Surgery 57-A: 915
60. Clancey G J, Hansen S T 1978 Open fractures of the tibia. A review of one hundred and two cases. Journal of Bone and Joint Surgery 60-A: 118

33

Injuries of the Ankle

C. L. Colton

Although ankle injuries are so common and the name of Percival Pott is so closely associated with them, it is surprising how little has been written in the English language on this subject. The French, on the other hand, have written extensively, beginning with Baron Dupuytren's description in 1819[1] of the fracture that eponymously bears his name. According to Bonnin[2] the period 1815 to 1872 was dominated first by Dupuytren and then by Maisonneuve;[3,4] it was not until 1922 that we see the beginning of a proper understanding of the mechanism and classification of ankle fractures in the paper by Ashhurst and Bromer.[5] In accusing Pott of 'describing a fracture which did not exist' and Dupuytren of 'commending him for his acute observation and fidelity to nature' they highlighted the confusion which had existed about the anatomy and mechanism of these fractures. In 1950 Lauge-Hansen[6] proposed a classification of ankle injuries which is now almost universally accepted and which, in a simplified form, will be used in this chapter. Its particular value is that it brings together ligamentous and bony injuries.

To understand the treatment of any fracture or joint injury it is of paramount importance to understand the mechanism by which it was produced. How else can we know the best method to reduce the deformity? How else can we recognise or predict the degree of instability which may require surgical intervention, or the small indications of mal-position which, if left uncorrected, may lead to the eventual destruction of the joint?

This dictum has never been more important than in the treatment of ankle injuries. For their proper understanding we must have a thorough knowledge of the sequences of bony and ligamentous failures which produce the common patterns of ankle injury. It must be realised that most of these injuries are mixed bony and ligamentous and that while in some the treatment of the fracture or fractures may

dominate the scene, the appreciation and management of the ligamentous element is all important.

CLASSIFICATION OF ANKLE INJURIES

Based upon cadaveric experiments and the careful study of a series of ankle injuries from both clinical and radiological points of view, Lauge-Hansen[6] devised what has been termed the 'genetic classification'. It is based upon the concept that each of the various patterns of fracture-dislocation of the ankle is the end product of a sequence of bony and ligamentous failures which results from a deforming force, and that for any given deforming force the failure sequence usually occurs in the same order to produce the complete injury pattern which is pathognomonic of that deforming force. Should that force cease to act at any point in the sequence a partial failure pattern will result. With minor modification of terminology a simplified 'genetic' classification is used here. Throughout this chapter the description of the deforming force will refer to the direction in which movements of the talus occur within the ankle mortice.

There are six groups of ankle injuries:

1. Abduction injuries.
2. Adduction injuries.
3. External rotation injuries with diastasis of the inferior tibio-fibular joint: pronation-external rotation injuries.
4. External rotation injuries without diastasis of the inferior tibio-fibular joint: supination-external rotation injuries.
5. Vertical compression injuries.
6. Uncommon unclassifiable injury patterns.

INJURY MECHANISMS

Abduction injury. Here the talus is forcibly

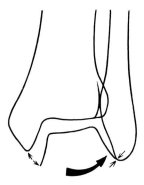

Fig 33.1 *Abduction injury.* The talus exerts a compressive force on the lateral malleolus and a distraction force on the medial ankle structures.

abducted in the ankle mortice producing a traction force on the medial ankle structures and a compression force laterally (Fig 33.1). The medial traction force may cause either a complete tear of the deltoid ligament or, more commonly, a 'pull-off' fracture of the medial malleolus.

The lateral compression force produces a lower fibular fracture at, and angling slightly upward from, the level of the ankle joint, always with comminution of the lateral fibular cortex of a greater or lesser degree (Fig 33.2).

In most cases the medial injury just precedes the lateral injury and partial failure is represented by an isolated traction fracture of the medial malleolus. As there is no rotational element to the abnormal talar movement the abduction fracture of the medial malleolus is horizontal on the lateral view (compare with Figure 30.15 due to a rotational injury). Isolated rupture of the deltoid ligament is hardly ever seen—some deny it ever occurs.[7] If the abduction force continues to act it will then produce a fracture of the fibula at the level of the junction of the lower shaft and the lateral malleolus, with characteristic comminution of the lateral cortex. With severe abduction violence the comminution can be considerable (Fig 33.2).

Abduction of the talus in the ankle mortice does not produce separation of the inferior tibio-fibular joint. The combined strength of the three ligaments of this joint—the anterior and posterior tibio-fibular ligaments together with the interosseous ligament—coming under tension simultaneously is greater than the resistance of the bone of the lateral malleolus to the abduction force. Separation, or diastasis, of the inferior tibio-fibular joint can only occur when the fibula is rotated so that the three ligaments are stressed one after another and yield in sequence; this will be considered again in more detail in the section on external rotation injuries. Very rarely, abduction of

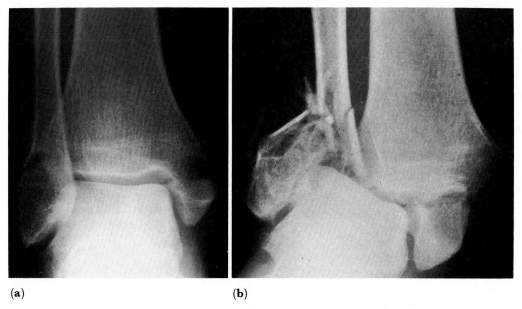

(a)   **(b)**

Fig 33.2 (a). In this abduction injury a traction fracture of the medial malleolus can be seen with a minimum of displacement: the 'push-off' fracture of the lateral malleolus is characterised by comminution of the lateral fibular cortex, in this case not gross. (b). A more severe abduction injury with considerable comminution of the lateral malleolus.

the talus, especially if associated with an element of vertical compression, can cause *en bloc* avulsion of the whole incisura fibularis,[8] as in Figure 33.3.

Adduction injury. In this group of ankle injuries the talus is forcibly adducted in the mortice so that a compressive force is exerted on the medial ankle structures and a traction force applied to the lateral structures (Fig 33.4). There is no rotational movement of the talus about a vertical axis as in external rotation injuries.

Traction failure of the lateral structures precedes the medial injury in the majority of instances. It may result in partial or complete disruption of the components of the lateral ligament of the ankle, or may cause a traction failure of the lateral malleolus. The lateral ligament injury may be a partial one with a tear of the anterior talofibular

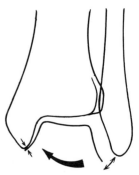

Fig 33.4 *Adduction injury.* Here the talus exerts a compressive force on the medial malleolus and a distraction force on the lateral ligament of the ankle and the fibular malleolus.

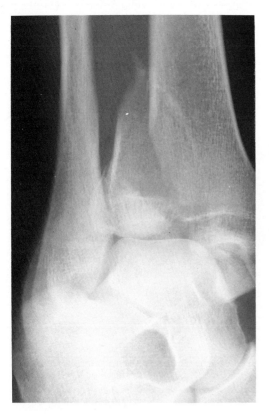

Fig 33.3 Abduction of the talus in the ankle mortice may occasionally, especially in combination with a vertical compression force, cause avulsion of the whole incisura fibularis followed by a fibular shaft fracture. In this case a fracture of the fibula occurred in the proximal half of the fibular shaft.

fasciculus only: this is caused by forcible inversion of the plantar-flexed foot,[9] in which position this anterior band of the lateral ligament is under tension. If the adduction force then stops, this will be the only injury, and, in fact, isolated injury of the anterior talo-fibular ligament is the common 'sprained ankle'.[10]

If forcible inversion is exerted on a foot which is at right angles to the tibia all three fasciculi of the lateral ligament of the ankle—the anterior and posterior talofibular ligaments and the calcaneo-fibular ligament—are stressed simultaneously and a complete lateral ligament tear may be produced. On the other hand, the combined resistance to traction of the three ligamentous bands may exceed the bony strength of the lateral malleolus causing it to fracture. Such a fracture may be represented by an avulsion fragment from the tip of the lateral malleolus at the insertion of the calcaneo-fibular ligament (Fig 33.5), or the whole lateral malleolus may be avulsed at the level of the ankle joint (Fig 33.6). This latter fracture is characteristically transverse with a 'clean' break in the outer fibular cortex (in contrast to the lateral cortical comminution which characterises the abduction fracture of the fibula, as in Figure 33.2).

Should the deforming force continue to act it will produce a compression injury of the medial malleolus. This consists of a near vertical fracture starting in the angle between the medial malleolus and the horizontal tibial articular surface, and frequently associated with depression of the articular surface in this angle where the adducting talus has compressed the subchondral bone (Fig 33.7).

Rarely the medial compression injury occurs without lateral structural failure (Fig 33.8).

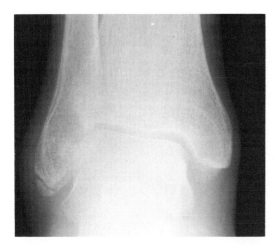

Fig 33.5 This radiograph shows the not uncommon avulsion flake fracture from the tip of the lateral malleolus. Here adduction of the talus in the mortice has caused traction on the lateral ligament and the middle fasciculus of the ligament (the calcaneo-fibular band) has pulled off its proximal bony insertion. This may be part of a total rupture of the lateral ligament, and if the history is one of considerable violence and there is gross soft tissue swelling stress radiographs under anaesthesia should be performed to exclude or confirm total ligament rupture.

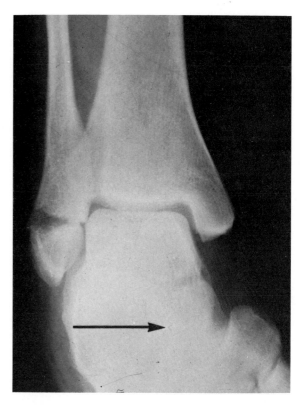

Fig 33.6 In this adduction injury the traction force on the lateral ankle structures has caused a 'pull-off' fracture of the lateral malleolus. (Note the clean break of the lateral fibular cortex in contrast to the comminution caused by abduction forces, as in Figure 33.2) This is a stress radiograph showing the opening up of the fracture on displacement of the hind-foot in the direction of the arrow.

External rotation injuries with diastasis of the inferior tibio-fibular joint (pronation-external rotation injury). The complete failure pattern in this group is the fracture-dislocation of the ankle described by Dupuytren.[1] There is a medial injury (either a traction fracture of the malleolus or a rupture of the deltoid ligament), diastasis of the inferior tibio-fibular joint and an indirect fracture of the fibular shaft between the upper level of the syndesmosis and the fibular neck (Fig 33.9). Monk[11] has pointed out that partial diastasis of the inferior tibio-fibular joint with a low spiral fibular fracture may occur as a variant of this injury complex (Fig 33.12).

Only a detailed analysis of the mechanisms of the various failure patterns within this group can lead to a complete understanding of the full extent of bony and ligamentous damage. Lauge-Hansen,[6] in his cadaveric experiments, found that by pronating the foot and forcibly externally rotating it at the ankle joint he could produce this type of injury. With the foot pronated the deltoid ligament is under tension, and as the talus starts to rotate externally in the ankle mortice it is the taut medial structures which fail first. The talus is then free of its medial tether and swings forwards out of the inner side of the mortice about a lateral axis (Fig 33.10). This imparts a torsion force

to the fibula which first tears the anterior tibio-fibular ligament (or avulses its attachment to the anterior lip of the incisura fibularis—the Tillaux[12] fracture) followed by rupture of the interosseous ligament of the inferior tibio-fibular joint (Fig 33.11).

At this point, where the only intact ligament of the syndesmosis is the posterior tibio-fibular ligament, one of two things may happen as the deforming force continues. If the force continues to rotate the fibula it will relax the posterior tibio-fibular ligament and a spiral fracture of the fibula will occur just above the syndesmosis (Fig 33.12): this is partial diastasis of the inferior tibio-fibular joint.[7,11] The spiral fibular fracture may be as high as the neck of the fibula (Fig 33.13) as in the injury described by, and associated with the name of, Maisonneuve.[3] It is of interest that Maisonneuve produced this injury complex experimentally in 1840 but the first account of it as a clinical entity is by Huguier some eight years later.[13]

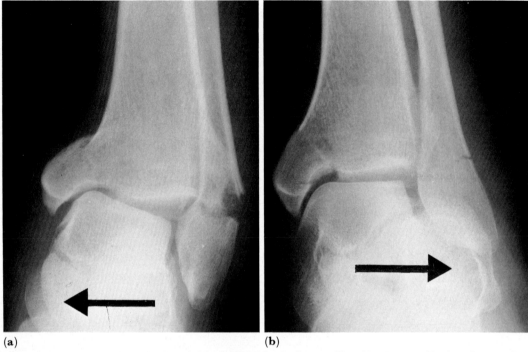

(a)   **(b)**

Fig 33.7 Radiographs showing the mechanism of a bimalleolar adduction fracture. The adduction stress film shows how traction on the lateral structures opens out to 'pull-off' fracture of the lateral malleolus and causes displacement of the medial malleolar fracture. Abduction stress reduces the fractures and on this film the separate compression fracture of the subchondral bone at the angle between the medial malleolus and the horizontal tibial articular surface can be seen; this is characteristic of the adduction compression fractures of the medial malleolus.

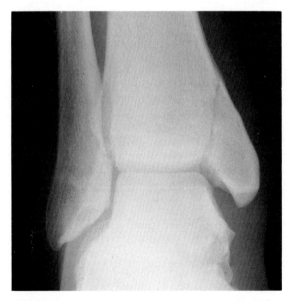

Fig 33.8 Very occasionally an adduction injury causes an isolated 'push-off' failure of the medial malleolus with its typically vertical fracture plane, frequently undisplaced.

If, however, from the point where only the posterior tibio-fibular ligament is intact, the tibia is pushed medially off the top of the rotating talus under the influence of body weight and forward thrust, as in a running injury, the posterior tibio-fibular ligament is ruptured (or its tibial attachment avulsed as a thin shell of bone, as in Figure 33.14) as the fibula is carried violently away from the tibia suffering an oblique bending fracture of its shaft (Fig 33.9).

As in all ankle injuries the deforming force may cease to act at any point in the sequence and so a number of possibilities exist for incomplete failure patterns.

Firstly, an isolated rotational traction fracture of the medial malleolus may be seen. Because the medial side of the talus is rotating anteriorly in this type of injury the malleolus is pulled off forwards and in consequence the fracture line characteristically slopes backwards and downwards (Fig 33.15). Such a sloping fracture may be difficult to see on routine radiographs and a 45 degree internal rotation oblique projection is a valuable additional film in cases of doubt[14] (Fig 33.16).

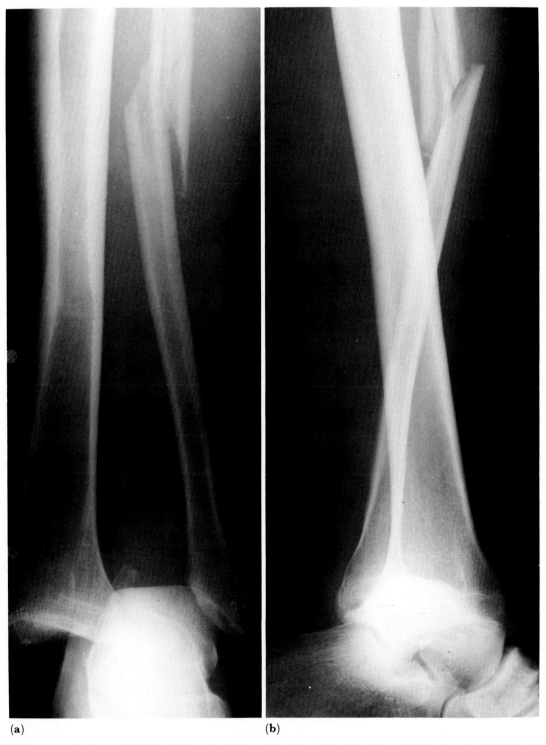

(a)   (b)

Fig 33.9 An example of a severely displaced Dupuytren fracture-dislocation of the ankle. The medial structures have failed (in this instance by rupture of the deltoid ligament), there is complete separation—or diastasis—of the inferior tibio-fibular syndesmosis and an indirect, bending fracture of the fibular shaft has occurred.

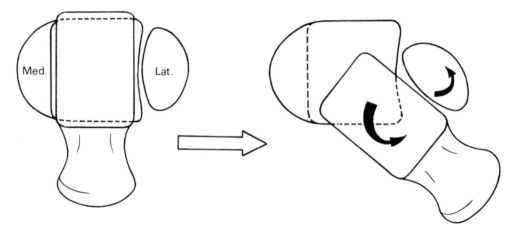

Fig 33.10 Diagram showing how in the pronation-external rotation injury, where the medial ankle structures fail first, the talus is free to rotate forwards out of the mortice and in so doing it imparts a torsional force to the fibula.

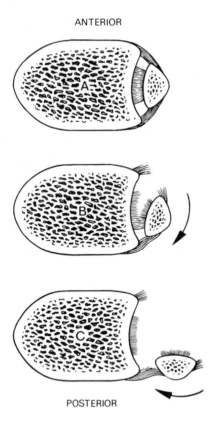

Fig 33.11 In the pronation-external rotation injury the talus twists the fibula, opening up the inferior tibio-fibular syndesmosis by rupturing first the anterior tibio-fibular ligament and then the interosseous ligament.

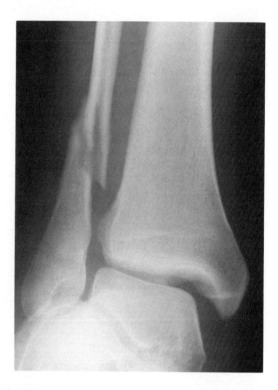

Fig 33.12 An example of partial diastasis of the inferior tibio-fibular joint. The posterior tibio-fibular ligament is intact and this stress X-ray shows how separation of the fibula from the tibia is limited and how the fibula is rotated by unrolling on the intact posterior ligament. Note that on this antero-posterior projection the profile of the distal fibular fragment is that normally seen on a lateral film, i.e. it is rotated through almost 90 degrees.

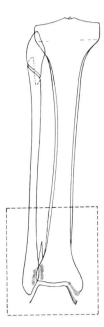

Fig 33.13 Diagram of the *Maissonneuve* injury. This is a partial diastasis of the inferior tibio-fibular joint where the spiral fracture is at the fibular neck. It can easily be missed if only standard ankle X-rays (dotted line) are taken and the initial displacement has reduced itself. Clinical examination of the fibula will always reveal high fracture tenderness and give an important clue to the presence of this injury complex. *Always palpate the whole length of the fibula* when examining any injured ankle.

Secondly, the medial injury may occur in conjunction with a rupture of the anterior tibio-fibular ligament. This latter would not be apparent radiologically unless, instead of a simple ligament rupture, the tubercle of Tillaux[12] is avulsed. Such a fragment can be quite large and may require open replacement and fixation.

Thirdly, it is possible for the first event in the failure sequence to be a deltoid ligament disruption and the second event a tear of the anterior tibio-fibular ligament, giving no radiological abnormality. Careful clinical examination (the necessity for which in the management of ankle injuries can never be over-stressed) will reveal, however, marked tenderness and swelling over the deltoid ligament immediately distal to the medial malleolus, and localised pain on pressure over the front of the inferior tibio-fibular joint. Such a combination should alert the surgeon to suspect a deltoid rupture which should be investigated further by stress radiography.

Lastly, it is not uncommon for this latter combi-

nation of ligamentous injuries to precede further torsion of the fibula and a spiral fracture at its neck—the Maissonneuve injury. In this event a routine radiograph of the ankle region alone may show no bony abnormality, or just slight widening of the medial talo-malleolar interval (Fig 33.13). Such a situation has frequently resulted in the failure to diagnose what is an unstable injury of the ankle. For this reason the examination of any injured ankle must include the palpation of the whole length of the fibula to elicit the tenderness of a high fibular fracture.

External rotation injury without inferior tibio-fibular joint diastasis (supination-external rotation injury). This injury pattern, although very different from that in the Dupuytren fracture-dislocation group, is also caused by the talus externally rotating in the ankle mortice.

This group is characterised by an oblique fracture of the fibula passing downward and forward to the level of the ankle joint, not infrequently a fracture of the posterior lip of the tibial plafond (the so-called posterior malleolus) and a medial traction failure, either a malleolar fracture or a deltoid ligament disruption (Fig 33.17).

How is it that the body of the talus externally rotating in the mortice can produce this injury pattern which is so different from that of the previous group? This injury can be produced consistently in the cadaver by forcibly externally rotating a supinated foot.[6] The probable explanation is that as the foot is in a supinated position at the moment when the talus starts to rotate, the medial structures are not in a state of tension (as they are in the pronation-external rotation injury) and therefore they do not fail first. In consequence, the talus is not free to rotate forwards out of the mortice on the medial side and so it starts to rotate backwards, pivoting on the medial structures. This causes it to push the lateral malleolus posteriorly, rupturing the anterior tibio-fibular ligament and producing the low oblique fibular fracture which is typical of this injury sequence (Fig 33.18). If at this stage the deforming force arrests, the only injury is the undisplaced fibular fracture—the commonest fracture around the ankle (Fig 33.19). The apparent paradox of this relatively simple injury is that whereas it is caused by the talus externally rotating in the mortice, the patient almost invariably describes an inversion twist of the foot. This is explicable, however, by a knowledge of the mechanics of subtalar joint function. The average axis about which movement takes place at the subtalar joint is angled 42 degrees above the horizontal and 16

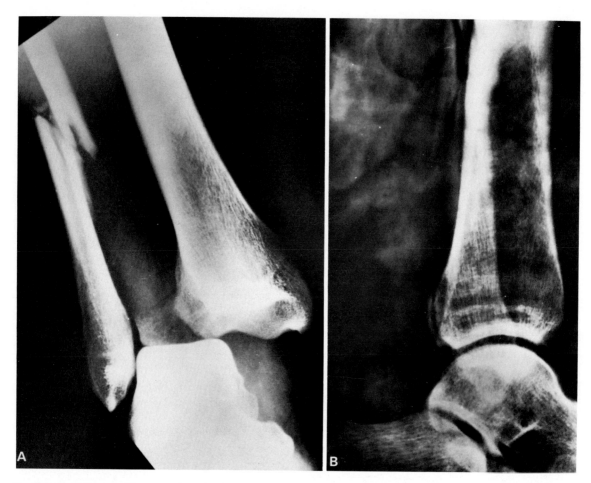

Fig 33.14 Complete pronation-external rotation fracture-dislocation (Dupuytren fracture). Note the bony fragment between tibia and fibula in the anteroposterior view. After reduction (Lateral X-ray) this is seen to be a thin shell of bone avulsed from the back of the tibia by the posterior tibio-fibular ligament.

degrees medial to the sagittal plane as depicted in Figure 33.20[15] so that the subtalar joint acts as a torque convertor (Fig 33.21), rotating the talus externally as the os calcis inverts.[16] Thus, with the foot fixed to the ground by body weight and then violently inverted, as in slipping off a kerbstone on to the lateral border of the foot, the talus is equally violently externally rotated in the tibio-fibular mortice, causing the failure pattern described above.

If after oblique fibular fracture, the deforming force does not cease, the talus will rotate further backwards right out of the mortice frequently pushing off the restraining posterior 'malleolus' as a large fragment at the moment of dislocation.[17] At the same time, the medial structures fail producing a complete,

tri-malleolar fracture-dislocation of the supination-external rotation type. In this injury, the distal fibular fragment and the posterior malleolar fragment displace together and simultaneously, remaining firmly bound to each other by the posterior tibio-fibular ligament, and moving as a single unit (Fig 33.22). Reduction of the fibula will sometimes relocate the posterior 'third' fragment.[18]

DIAGNOSIS AND TREATMENT

ABDUCTION INJURIES

Diagnosis. In general, the patient's account of the direction in which the foot was twisted is unreliable.

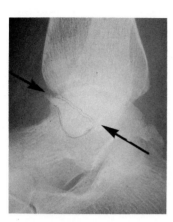

Fig 33.15 X-ray of an isolated fracture of the medial malleolus caused by a pronation-external rotation force. The medial malleolus has been pulled off forwards and so the fracture plane runs obliquely downwards and backwards (as arrowed). This contrasts with the horizontal fracture plane of the abduction fracture of the medial malleolus (see Fig 33.24).

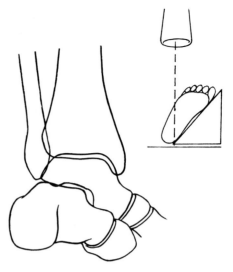

Fig 33.16 The antero-posterior oblique projection which will often clearly reveal a doubtful fracture of the medial malleolus. (Reproduced by kind permission of the *Proceedings of the Royal Society of Medicine* and Mr N. Cobb, from his article (1965) Oblique radiography in the diagnosis of ankle injuries. *Proceedings of the Royal Society of Medicine*, 58, 334.)

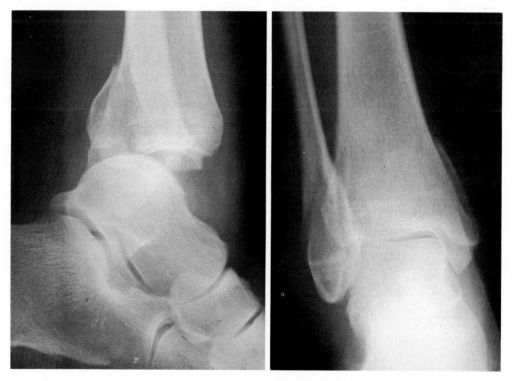

Fig 33.17 X-ray films of a supination-external rotation fracture-dislocation of the ankle. There is an oblique fracture of the lower fibula, a posterior tibial fracture and a medial disruption (in this case a deltoid ligament rupture). Note that the talus dislocates backwards out of the ankle mortice.

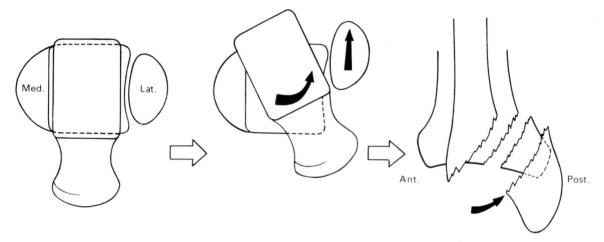

Fig 33.18 Diagram to show how in the supination-external rotation injury the talus rotates backwards out of the mortice, pivoting about a medial axis and pushing the fibula backwards. This causes the low oblique fibular fracture which characterises this injury and may also push of the posterior lip off the tibial articular surface.

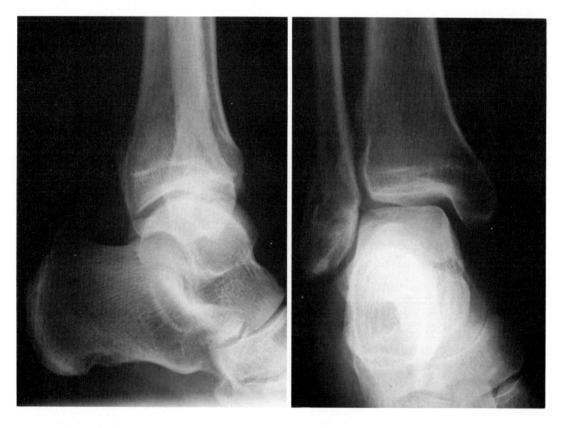

Fig 33.19 An isolated, undisplaced, oblique fracture of the distal fibula. This is the commonest ankle fracture and represents a supination-external injury arrested immediately after the first event of the sequence.

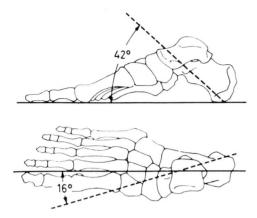

Fig 33.20 Movement occurs at the subtalar joint about an axis 42 degrees above the horizontal and 16 degrees medial to the sagittal plane. (Reproduced by kind permission of Butterworth and of Mr G. K. Rose, from his article (1962) Ankle injuries. In *Modern Trends in Orthopaedics*, **3**. Fracture Treatment, ed. Clark, J. M. P. London: Butterworth.)

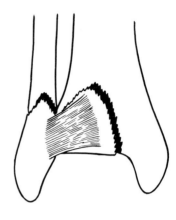

Fig 33.22 Diagram to show how, in the supination-external rotation injury, the distal fibular and the posterior tibial fragments are bound together as a single unit by the posterior tibio-fibular ligament.

Ankle injuries happen too quickly to be accurately observed—least of all by the patient: if accidents happened slowly they would be avoidable!

In the case of the full abduction failure pattern as in Figure 33.2b the foot is usually seen to be lying in a position of valgus deformity with swelling both medially and laterally. The medial tenderness may be directly over the medial malleolus where this is

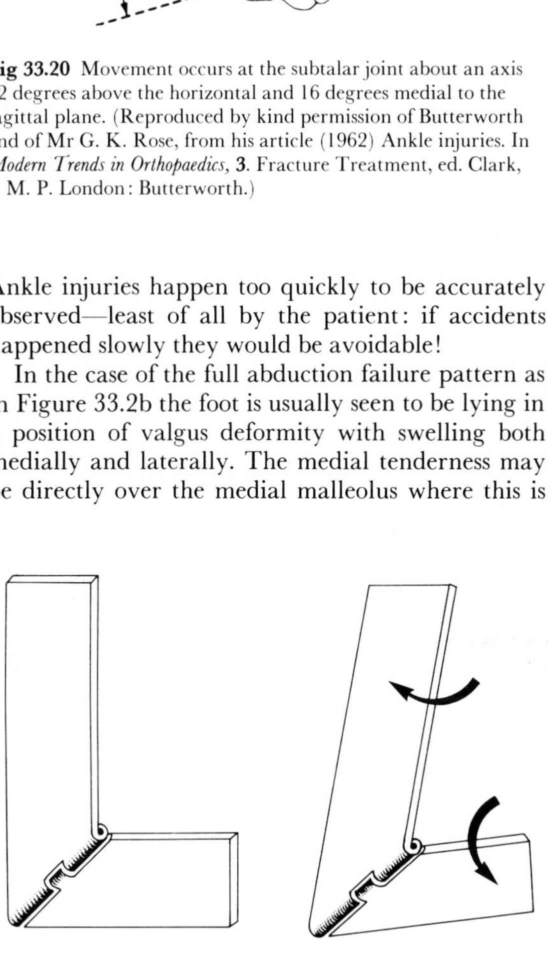

Fig 33.21 Because of the axis of movement at the subtalar joint it acts as a torque-convertor. The simplest example of this is the angled hinge as shown above: as one arm of the hinge is rotated so it rotates the other arm. Thus inversion of the foot at the subtalar joint externally rotates the talus in the ankle mortice. (Reproduced by kind permission of Butterworth and of Mr G. K. Rose, from his article (1962) Ankle injuries. In *Modern Trends in Orthopaedics*, **3**. Fracture Treatment, ed. Clark, J. M. P. London: Butterworth.)

fractured or just distal to the medial malleolus in the rarer event of a deltoid ligament rupture. The lateral swelling is considerable with bony tenderness over the base of the lateral malleolus.

Radiographs reveal the typical fibular fracture with varying degrees of comminution of the lateral cortex, and separation of a medial malleolar fracture (Fig 33.2).

Partial abduction failure causing a solitary traction fracture of the medial malleolus (Fig 33.23) may be easily missed if it is undisplaced, and should be suspected if there is swelling and localised tenderness over the medial malleolus. In cases of doubt the use of an oblique radiograph (see Fig 33.16) or a stress film is essential.

Treatment. An isolated abduction fracture of the medial malleolus which is undisplaced will unite if immobilised in a well-moulded below-knee plaster cast. There is rarely sufficient swelling to necessitate a change of plaster due to loosening, and a total of six weeks' immobilisation is all that is required. During the last two weeks weight-bearing in the cast is permitted.

A short period of physiotherapy after removal of the plaster cast will rapidly restore a good range of ankle and tarsal movement.

A separated traction fracture of the medial malleolus without fibular injury can sometimes be manipulated into a position of perfect apposition of the fracture surfaces and can then be treated as an

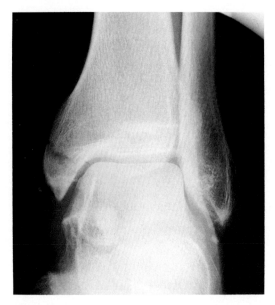

Fig 33.23 An isolated abduction fracture of the medial malleolus. Note that the fracture plane runs horizontally from before backwards (in contrast to the oblique medial malleolar fracture caused by a pronation external rotation injury, as in Figure 33.15).

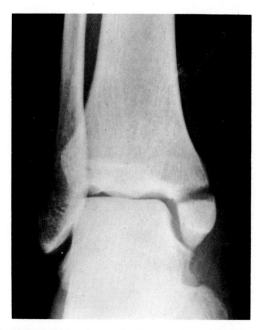

Fig 33.24 A displaced abduction fracture of the medial malleolus with soft tissue interposition. Such a fracture should be internally fixed with a lag screw or traction-absorption wiring.

undisplaced fracture. There is, however, a greater possibility of redisplacement and weekly radiological checks are essential during the first month. Redisplacement demands internal fixation.

Where the original manipulation fails to achieve anatomical reduction, as is frequently the case, it must be assumed that there is soft tissue interposition between the fragments. A flap, attached to the distal fragment and consisting of superficial fibres of the deltoid ligament, may tuck itself into the fracture gap. Such a fracture (Fig 33.24) must be explored and, after excision of the interposed flap, the malleolus is reduced and fixed with a screw, the distal fragment being over-drilled (or a cancellous lag screw used) to produce interfragmentary compression.

An alternative method of fixation, especially useful for smaller fragments, is the traction-absorption technique of wiring described by Weber and Vasey,[19] as illustrated in Figure 33.25. The reduced fragments are fixed using two parallel Kirschner wires at right angles to the fracture plane. A horizontal through-and-through drill hole is then made in the tibia about $1\frac{1}{4}$ inches (3 cm) proximal to the fracture and a length of 20 S.W.G. stainless steel wire is passed through the hole. The ends of the wire are crossed over, one end is passed deep to the projecting portions of the two

Kirschner wires and the two ends of the wire loop tightened and twisted. This gives rigid fixation which amply resists the pull of the deltoid ligament on the malleolar fragment.

After fixation of the medial malleolus, provided that there is minimal comminution of the fibula, the fracture will be unlikely to redisplace and the protection of a well-fitting below-knee plaster cast moulded into slight inversion for about eight weeks will be sufficient to ensure union. The severely

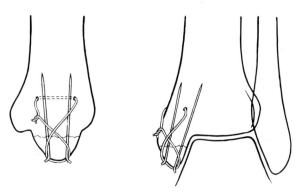

Fig 33.25 Diagram to show the technique of traction-absorption fixation of the medial malleolus. (After Weber and Vasey, 1963.)

comminuted abduction fracture of the fibula is difficult to manage by internal fixation, but fortunately it often falls into an acceptable position when the medial side of the joint is stabilised. If this does not occur fixation with a well-contoured plate is justifiable (Fig 33.26).

ADDUCTION INJURIES

Sprained ankle

This is a common injury caused by an inversion twist of the plantar flexed foot producing a tear of the anterior talo-fibular ligament (see page 1106).

Diagnosis. There is characteristic swelling over the lateral aspect of the ankle joint, maximally in front of and distal to the lateral malleolus. Generalised mild tenderness can be elicited over the whole bruised area, but in the line of the anterior talo-fibular ligament the tenderness is very marked. In this injury the middle band of the lateral ligament—the calcaneo-fibular ligament—is intact, and stressing this ligament by inverting the heel with the foot at a right

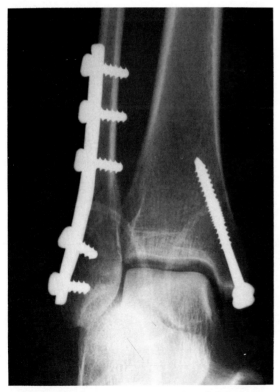

Fig 33.26 This figure shows how a comminuted abduction fracture can be managed by a well-contoured fibular plate.

angle produces little pain. If, however, the foot is then plantar-flexed at the ankle and the heel inversion test repeated, severe pain is felt just in front of the lateral malleolus. This test is pathognomonic of isolated anterior talo-fibular ligament injury. Usually the only abnormality seen in the X-ray is a lateral soft tissue shadow, although in complete tears of the anterior talo-fibular ligament minor degrees of talar tilt on inversion stress radiographs have been reported.[9] It is, however, important in the management of all injuries of the lateral ankle ligament to perform inversion stress films whenever there is a suspicion of a major tear in order to exclude a complete lateral ligament rupture. The place of arthrography in the accurate diagnosis of ligamentous injuries of the ankle remains the subject of much debate. Broström[20] (1964) advocates surgical exploration of the lateral ligament complex in all patients with an abnormal arthrogram with a view to surgical repair—he found arthrographic abnormality in 75 per cent of patients presenting with 'sprained ankle' Staples[21] (1965), however, stresses the good results of non-surgical treatment and Spiegel and Staples[22] report a large number of false negative results following arthrography. Careful clinical examination remains the mainstay of diagnosis.

Treatment. Isolated injuries of the anterior talo-fibular ligament may be treated by bandaging to control inversion. Despite its disadvantages of minor irritation and discomfort on removal, elastic adhesive strapping is widely used with excellent relief of symptoms permitting early walking. It is essential first to apply an 'eversion stirrup'—this is a strip of non-elastic adhesive strapping (as used for skin traction) applied to the inner aspect then the plantar surface of the heel and the outer aspect of the lower leg whilst the foot is held everted. Over this is applied a spiral of adhesive elastic bandaging from the base of the toes to the upper third of the calf, the foot being held at a right angle and great care being taken to avoid creasing the bandage (Fig 33.27). After two weeks this dressing may be removed and a firm crêpe bandage worn until all symptoms have settled.

In cases of skin allergy or in hot climates a crêpe bandage should be applied as an alternative, firm turns passing from within outwards around the inner margin of the foot, under the sole and across the front of the ankle to the inner side of the leg in such a manner that inversion is controlled. Lettin,[10] in his excellent review of the management of sprained ankle, advocated local infiltration of the tender area with 1,500 units of hyaluronidase dissolved in 5 ml of

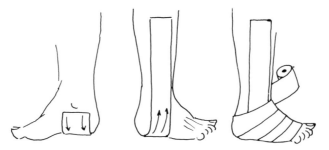

Fig 33.27 Diagram showing the technique of applying an eversion stirrup of non-elastic adhesive strapping beneath a spiral of elastic adhesive bandage. This technique affords rapid pain relief in the management of minor ankle sprains.

normal saline. The ankle should then be bound with crêpe bandage and early active movements with full weight-bearing encouraged. This regime resulted in more rapid relief of pain and an earlier return to full function than the Elastoplast strapping technique. The long-term results of the two methods were, however, indistinguishable.

Adhesion formation. The formation of adhesions in and around a sprained ankle ligament is minimised by preventing swelling and oedema with the use of a supporting bandage, elevation of the limb and early active exercise. If adhesions still develop, the patient may complain of continued pain on the lateral side of the joint with weakness and 'giving way'. It is sometimes helpful to raise the outer side of the heel of the shoe by $\frac{1}{8}$ inch (3 mm), or to 'float out' the heel $\frac{3}{8}$ inch (1 cm) so as to broaden its outer side.[23] Occasionally it may be necessary to infiltrate the area of persistent tenderness with a few millilitres of a mixture of 25 mg of hydrocortisone acetate and 1,500 units of hyaluronidase made up in 5 ml of 1 per cent lignocaine. This should be followed by a course of active exercises under the supervision of a physiotherapist, including a programme of 'wobble-board' exercises (see Fig. 33.32).

Complete avulsion of the lateral ligament
A complete tear of the anterior and middle fasciculi of the lateral ligament should be suspected in every violent inversion injury of the ankle joint. Severe swelling and ecchymosis should alert the surgeon to the possibility of such an injury and the clinical sign of abnormal mobility of the talus on inversion movement of the foot may be present.

Clinical diagnosis. In a normal foot the lateral surface of the body of the talus can be felt just in front of the lateral malleolus, and it remains in close contact with the malleolus even when the foot is inverted at the subtalar joint. On the other hand, if the lateral ligament is torn, inversion movement occurs at the ankle joint as well as at the subtalar joint and it is sometimes possible to feel the talus tilt and move away from the malleolus as a well-defined sulcus appears between the two bones, deep enough to admit the tip of the examiner's finger (Fig 33.28). To perform this test it is necessary to infiltrate the haematoma with local anaesthetic. Minor degrees of tilting of the talus from tear of the lateral ligament cannot always be appreciated clinically and radio-

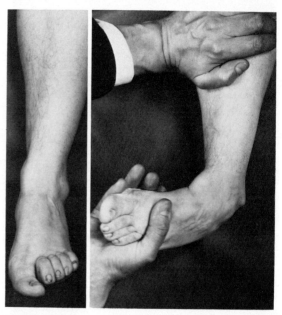

Fig 33.28 Complete avulsion of the lateral ligament of the ankle joint with momentary dislocation. The joint may seem to be normal unless it is examined with the foot in full inversion; then there is clinical evidence of the talus separating from the malleolus. This should, of course, be confirmed by taking radiographs of the inverted foot (Figs 33.29 and 30).

graphic examination of the ankle with the foot stressed into inversion is essential.

Radiographic diagnosis. Under regional or general anaesthesia antero-posterior radiographs are taken of the ankle joint with the heel forcibly held in the fully inverted position. If the injury has been a simple sprain the talus remains stable in the mortice (Fig 33.29). If the lateral ligament tear is complete, well-marked talar tilt is evident (Fig 33.30). The disruption of the middle fasciculus may be represented by avulsion of its attachment to the tip of the lateral malleolus (Fig 33.5).

If total lateral ligament rupture is not correctly treated, recurrent dislocation of the ankle may develop with still greater tilting of the talus (Fig 33.31). This radiographic investigation is misleading unless the heel is fully inverted, and this should be carried out by the surgeon himself under general anaesthesia or at least infiltration of the haematoma with local anaesthetic. It has been shown that 30 per cent of normal ankles will tilt 5 degrees or more and that 20 per cent have unequal tilts.[24] It is, therefore,

essential to take similar views of both ankles. Compared with the uninjured side, an increase in talar tilt of 5 to 15 degrees denotes a complete tear of the anterior talo-fibular ligament, 15 to 30 degrees denotes disruption of both the anterior and middle fasciculi of the lateral ligament, whereas a difference of more than 30 degrees of tilt can only occur with total rupture of all three components of the lateral ligament.[25] Arthrography of the ankle joint may help to confirm the diagnosis of lateral ligament disruption with exravasation of dye laterally into the subcutaneous tissues and occasionally into the peroneal tendon sheaths.[20]

Treatment. Complete immobilisation in plaster is essential. A lightly padded below-knee plaster cast is applied with the foot at right angles to the leg, the heel being in the neutral position or slightly everted. It may be necessary to renew the cast after two weeks if loosening occurs as the swelling settles. The patient may weight-bear in the cast, which must be retained for six to eight weeks. Attention has been drawn to the value of re-education of the proprioceptive

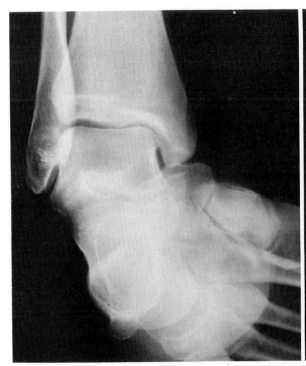

Fig 33.29 After simple sprain of the anterior talo-fibular ligament the talus remains stable within the ankle mortice.

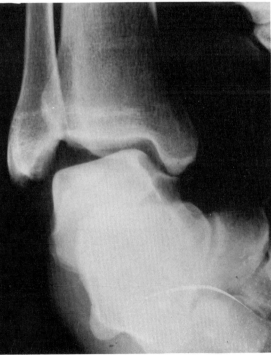

Fig 33.30 After complete tear of the lateral ligament stress radiography under general anaesthesia will reveal a major degree of talar tilt.

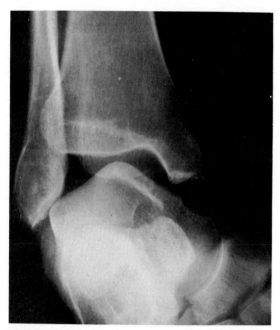

Fig 33.31 If total lateral ligament rupture is not correctly treated recurrent dislocation of the ankle will occur with still greater tilting of the talus.

function of the healed ligamentous structures after removal of the plaster cast,[26] and 'wobble-board' exercises have proved of value in increasing the sense of ankle stability where there has been major ligamentous damage (Fig 33.32).

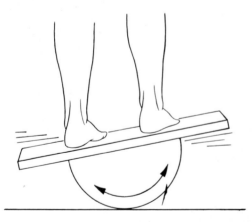

Fig 33.32 Wobble-board exercises are of value in re-education of the proprioceptive function of the muscles controlling the foot and ankle after major ligamentous injury. The boards are of two types: one with a hemicylindrical under-surface permitting rocking in a single plane and a second type with a hemispherical undersurface which rocks in any direction. The patient graduates from the former to the latter as treatment progresses.

If this regime is followed repair will be complete and normal stability of the ankle will be regained. Hughes[27] has drawn attention to the common incidence of articular damage, finding a lesion at the supero-medial margin of the talus in 50 per cent of cases explored for surgical repair of the ligament. This may occasionally form a loose body which can necessitate arthrotomy later, but there seems little support for immediate surgical repair. Certainly it was felt by Freeman[26] that routine surgical repair of tears of the lateral ligament of the ankle produces results inferior to those following the conservative regime, although surgical repair in the young athletic subject has its advocates.[20, 22, 28]

Recurrent subluxation of the ankle joint

When an avulsed lateral ligament has been mis-diagnosed as a simple sprain and incorrectly managed, recurrent subluxation* of the talus often follows. The patient complains of a sensation of insecurity, weakness and giving way of the joint. It is impossible to walk in narrow-heeled shoes or on a heel which is worn down on the outer side. On uneven surfaces a sudden inversion twist may throw the patient to the ground and he learns to walk cautiously watching for irregularities. Games and recreations become impossible.

Diagnosis. Routine clinical and radiographic examinations show no abnormality, and the nature of the disability can pass unrecognised. Patients with this disability have been treated for years with many forms of physiotherapy based upon a wide range of diagnoses from 'weak ankle' (a descriptive but unhelpful term) to neurosis.

If the heel is forcibly inverted it may sometimes become obvious that the talus tilts inwards and forwards leaving a well-defined sulcus in front of the lateral malleolus, but the diagnosis must be confirmed (or refuted) by inversion stress radiographs. While holding the foot for such films the surgeon must use protective gloves which are cumbersome. A Thomas

---

*Traumatic dislocation or subluxation? Some surgeons insist that this injury should be described as recurrent subluxation since the talus and tibia do not totally lose contact, whereas dislocation refers to a situation where there is no remaining contact between the two articular surfaces. This distinction has special significance in congenital dysplasias of joints, notably the hip, but injuries of joints cause so wide a spectrum of displacement from momentary total separation spontaneously reduced, to persistent or recurrent displacement of various degrees. Is it not better to think only of traumatic dislocation whilst recognising that there is an imperceptible merging of every degree of displacement—momentary, temporary, persistent or recurrent?

wrench applied to the heel (Fig 33.33) not only gives excellent leverage but also allow the hands to be kept well away from the X-ray beam, without obscuring the view of the ankle joint (Fig 33.34). The occasional association between osteochondritis dissecans on the supero-medial ridge of the talar articular surface and excessive talar tilt due to lax lateral ligaments has been reported[29] (Fig 33.35).

Non-operative treatment. The displacement can sometimes be controlled by the use of a laterally

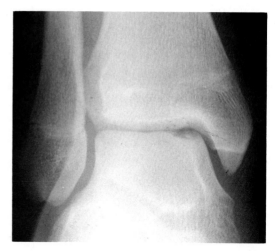

Fig 33.35 X-ray showing osteochondritis dissecans of the talus in a young man with marked laxity of his lateral ligament and recurrent dislocation.

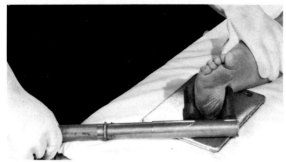

Fig 33.33

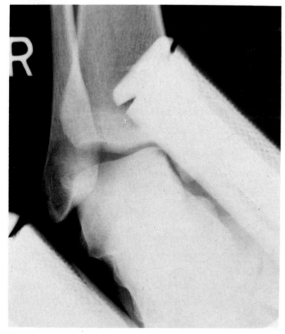

Fig 33.34

Figs 33.33 and 33.34 A Thomas wrench is very useful for inverting the heel during stress radiography of the ankle joint. It affords good purchase and keeps the surgeon's hands (albeit in protective gloves) away from the X-ray beam. Figure 30.34 shows how the wrench does not obscure the ankle joint on the X-ray film.

raised and flared heel combined with a programme of 'wobble-board' exercises for education and development of the peroneal muscles and their reflex protective action. A below-knee inside iron with an outside T-strap will prevent recurrent dislocation, but it is cumbersome and whenever possible operative reconstruction is preferable.

Operative reconstruction of the lateral ligament. The classical Watson-Jones operation is a complex and difficult tenodesis of peroneus brevis aimed at reconstructing both anterior and middle fasciculi of the lateral ligament. Evans[30] and Pennal[31] pointed out that in order to produce lateral ankle instability experimentally it is necessary to divide both anterior talo-fibular *and* calcaneo-fibular ligaments. Evans therefore described the simpler procedure where the peroneus brevis tendon is detached from its muscle belly and threaded from in front backwards through an oblique hole drilled upwards and backwards in the lateral malleoleus (Fig 33.36). The wound is closed and the foot is immobilised in plaster for eight weeks. Weight-bearing is permitted after the change of plaster at the second or third week. This procedure is simple and reliable and has superseded the Watson–Jones operation.

Adduction fracture of the lateral malleolus
It may be that the traction injury on the lateral side of the ankle when the talus is adducted in the mortice is not a ligamentous tear but a 'pull-off' fracture of the whole lateral malleolus. This fracture occurs at

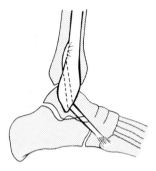

Fig 33.36 Evan's tenodesis for lateral ankle instability. The peroneus brevis tendon is detached at its musculo-tendinous junction and mobilised down to its insertion into the fifth metatarsal. A tunnel is drilled upwards and backwards from the tip of the lateral malleolus, the tendon is then passed up this tunnel and secured to the back of the fibula as tightly as possible. The peroneus brevis belly is sutured to the peroneus longus muscle.

the level of the ankle joint and is typically horizontal with a 'clean' break of the lateral fibular cortex. The malleolar fragment bears the attachments of all three components of the lateral ligament and so causes lateral instability equivalent to total disruption of the lateral ligament (Fig 33.6).

Diagnosis. The patient may occasionally be able to give a precise account of adduction violence, but will

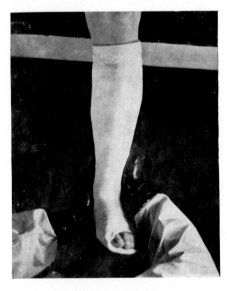

Fig 33.37 Reduction of an adduction fracture of the ankle. While the plaster is setting the foot must be pushed outwards. The displacement will not be over-reduced even with strong pressure.

always have pain and gross swelling over the outer aspect of the ankle. Bony tenderness is present at the base of the lateral malleolus and a fracture gap may be felt to open up if gentle attempts are made to invert the heel. The radiological features of this fracture have been described above and are shown in Figure 33.6. The films should be carefully inspected to exclude a compression fracture of the medial malleolus (Fig 33.7).

Treatment. Conservative management of adduction fracture of the lateral malleolus usually gives excellent functional results. A lightly padded below-knee cast is applied and the heel is moulded into slight eversion: the palm (not the fingers) of one hand—the left hand for the left foot and vice versa—exerts gentle pressure over the inner aspect of the heel whilst the other hand applies counter-pressure over the lower fibular shaft proximal to the fracture (Fig 33.37). As the medial structures are intact the talus cannot be displaced laterally and so over-reduction cannot occur.

The leg should be rested in elevation as much as possible during the first week or 10 days, after which walking non-weight-bearing is permitted provided a check X-ray shows that the reduction has been maintained. A walking heel may be applied after four weeks and the plaster removed at eight weeks. At this stage radiological union will generally be observed and mobilisation exercises started. Troublesome swelling after removal of the cast can be relieved by wearing an elastic support and by exercise in elevation.

In the event of failure to secure or hold anatomical reduction of the fracture, internal fixation becomes essential. The fracture is exposed through a longitudinal incision skirting the posterior border of the fibula. Open reduction of the fresh fracture is rarely difficult but perfect reduction must be obtained and internal fixation by intramedullary screwing requires great care. The screw should be inserted at the very tip of the lateral malleolus and angled as vertically as possible. The malleolar fragment is over-drilled to produce a lag effect and the screw should be long enough to engage the medial cortex of the fibula well above the fracture (Fig 33.38). Because the lateral malleolus is set at an angle of 10 to 15 degrees valgus in relation to the fibular shaft it is impossible to fix it with a long, straight intramedullary screw or rod without tilting the malleolus into varus. As an alternative the traction-absorption wiring technique may be used (see page 1116).

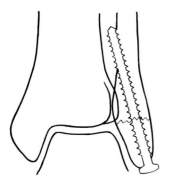

Fig 33.38 Diagram to show how an intramedullary screw is inserted to control an adduction fracture of the lateral malleolus. Because of the normal valgus set of the lateral malleolus on the fibular shaft a straight screw must engage the medial fibular cortex proximally.

Post-operative care after rigid internal fixation of ankle injuries. If rigid fixation of the isolated adduction fractures of the lateral malleolus has been possible active exercises of the foot and ankle can be permitted immediately after operation. Such daily exercise performed with the leg in elevation rapidly restores a full range of movement and reduces swelling and bruising. Because of the rigidity of the fixation the patient rarely experiences pain during physiotherapy once early wound swelling has subsided after two or three days. Such a regime should be followed only when completely rigid fixation of all components of an ankle injury has been secured: if there is any doubt plaster must be used. Because of the tendency to hold the foot relaxed in plantar-flexion between periods of exercise and the consequent danger of ankle stiffness in a position of equinus, the foot is supported during these intervals in a strong right-angled plaster back slab which can be removed for frequent exercises. Use of the plaster back slab may be abandoned when the patient can actively and comfortably dorsiflex the foot above the right angle. Immediate joint mobilisation where rigid fixation has been achieved aids nutrition and healing of the articular cartilage. After two weeks when there is usually a full range of ankle and tarsal movements a protective below-knee plaster cast can be applied permitting the patient to leave hospital walking non-weight-bearing with crutches. A walking heel is applied at four weeks, and when the plaster is finally removed after eight weeks there will be little residual stiffness and a full range of movements will be regained within a few days.[32, 33] Such a programme, however, demands extreme accuracy of surgical technique and constant supervision by both surgeon and physiotherapist during the early post-operative period.

Bimalleolar adduction fracture
It has already been shown (page 1106) that continued adduction of the talus in the ankle mortice will cause traction failure of lateral structures to be followed by a compression fracture of the medial malleolus. The supero-medial ridge of the talar articular surface percusses the angle between the tibial plafond and the medial malleolus—the 'medial corner'—splitting off the medial malleolus along a near-vertical fracture plane (Fig 33.7). Frequently, there is crushing of a plate of the subchondral bone at this site, which may be so severe as to form a depression into which the talus cannot be prevented from subluxating (Fig 33.39).

Very occasionally the medial compression injury occurs before traction on the lateral structures can cause their disruption, and the vertical 'push-off' fracture of the medial malleolus is seen as an isolated injury (Fig 33.8).

Treatment. Bimalleolar adduction fractures, when widely displaced, are very unstable injuries and it is rarely possible to achieve and maintain anatomical reduction by conservative methods. For this reason internal fixation is the treatment of choice. The lateral malleolus should be internally fixed by the method already described and the medial malleolar fragment secured with one or two almost horizontal screws. Where there is marked depression of a large segment of the 'medial corner', this should be disimpacted, reduced and the resultant defect filled with cancellous bone chips. This must be done before fixation of the medial malleolar fragment. These fractures require a long period of plaster immobilisation—10 weeks at least—with no weight-bearing for the first six weeks. If the surgeon is satisfied that his fixation is truly rigid the patient may be allowed to exercise the foot and ankle in recumbency for the first two weeks after operation (as outlined above).

EXTERNAL ROTATION INJURIES WITH INFERIOR TIBIO-FIBULAR JOINT DIASTASIS (PRONATION-EXTERNAL ROTATION FRACTURE)

These injuries are the consequence of an external rotation force being applied to the pronated foot. In the section on ankle fracture mechanisms we have

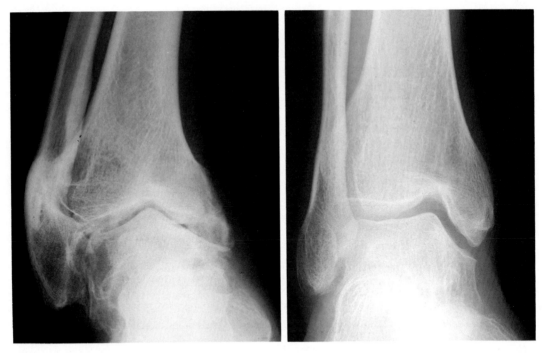

Fig 33.39 Two examples of mal-union following bimalleolar adduction fractures each demonstrating the crushed 'medial corner' in the ankle between the horizontal tibial articular surface and the medial malleolus.

seen that in this injury the medial structures fail first, permitting the talus to rotate externally and forwards out of the mortice, twisting the fibula and sequentially tearing the anterior tibio-fibular ligament and the interosseous ligament. From this point the force on the fibula may continue as a torsional one causing a spiral fibular shaft fracture and leaving the posterior tibio-fibular ligament intact (Fig 33.40A), or the force on the fibula may be exerted in a lateral direction tearing the posterior tibio-fibular ligament and causing an oblique, often comminuted bending fracture of the fibula (Fig 33.40B). If the spiral fibular fracture is in the upper quarter of the bone, the injury corresponds to that described by Maisonneuve (Fig 33.13), whereas complete diastasis of the syndesmosis produces the classical Dupuytren fracture-dislocation.

Isolated fracture of the medial malleolus

This is the first event in the sequence described above, a traction fracture of the medial malleolus as it is pulled forward by the rotating talus. If the injuring force now stops, the remainder of the failure sequence is frustrated, leaving an isolated fracture of the medial malleolus which, because of the forward direction of the 'pull-off' force, is angled as shown in Figure 33.15.

Diagnosis. These fractures are rarely grossly displaced and may be accompanied by only a little swelling in the immediate vicinity of the bony injury. Radiologically, they can be easily missed as the fracture plane is parallel to the X-ray beam only in the lateral projection. In cases of doubt the 45-degree internal rotation view of Cobb should be used (Fig 33.16).

Treatment. A number of these fractures can be treated in a below-knee plaster for six to eight weeks, but because of the possibility of soft tissue interposition[34, 35] and the danger of non-union many surgeons prefer to internally fix medial malleolar fractures, either by a screw or by the traction absorption wiring technique (Fig 33.25).

Partial diastasis of the inferior tibio-fibular joint

Diagnosis. In this injury there is medial pain and swelling together with tenderness over the fibular fracture above the syndesmosis. There is rarely sufficient displacement to produce clinical deformity as the lateral excursion of the talus is limited by the

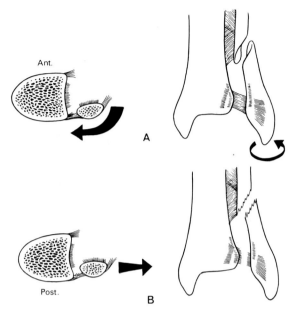

Fig 33.40 A. Shows how external torsion of the fibula in a pronation-external rotation injury leaves the posterior tibio-fibular ligament intact and causes a spiral fibular shaft fracture—partial diastasis of the inferior tibio-fibular joint. B. If, after external torsion of the fibula has ruptured the anterior and interosseous tibio-fibular ligaments, the force pushes the fibula laterally, the posterior tibio-fibular ligament is torn and the fibular shaft fractures by bending—complete diastasis of the inferior tibio-fibular joint.

intact posterior tibio-fibular ligament (Fig 33.12). The Maisonneuve variety of the injury, if in combination with deltoid ligament disruption rather than a medial fracture, is easily missed on routine ankle radiographs because the talus may spring back into a normal relationship with the tibia, either after injury or when the foot is positioned by the radiographer. Palpation of the whole fibula is an integral part of the clinical examination of the injured ankle and unexplained medial swelling demands a full length radiograph of the fibula. External rotation stress films under general anaesthesia will resolve any question of suspected ankle instability.

Treatment. This injury is usually easily reduced provided a ruptured deltoid ligament is not interposed between the talus and the medial malleolus. The leg must be immobilised in an above-knee plaster cast moulded so that the foot is slightly inverted and firmly internally rotated. As the foot is internally rotated the fibula 'winds itself up' on the intact posterior ligament which serves to locate it well in its

groove in the tibia—the incisura fibularis. Care must be taken to ensure that a medial malleolar fracture is perfectly closed and if this is in doubt it is wiser to internally fix the whole fracture complex.

Where fixation is necessary it is sound practice to fix the medial malleolar fragment first, followed by fixation of the diastasis. Occasionally difficulty can be experienced in getting the fibula to lie neatly in the incisura and this may be due to a small unnoticed avulsion fracture of the anterior tibial tubercle (a Tillaux fragment) being trapped between the two bones.[36] In order to locate perfectly the fibula in the incisura, attention must be paid to the anatomical reduction and fixation of the fibular fracture:[37, 38] then the diastasis is secured by an oblique screw across the syndesmosis inserted through the lateral fibular cortex opposite the level of the ankle joint. If this is angled upwards 20 degrees it will traverse approximately the centre of the inferior tibio-fibular joint,[39] tending to tilt the fibular neither into valgus nor varus (Fig 33.41). The insertion of a screw across the inferior tibio-fibular syndesmosis is deprecated by some authorities on the grounds that it causes synostosis. This does not occur if certain basic rules are followed: (1) The screw should only be inserted after perfect reduction and fixation of the fibular fracture; (2) the foot should be held in dorsiflexion when the screw is inserted so that the widest portion of the talar body is engaged in the ankle thus avoiding 'pinching' the mortice; (3) the screw should not compress the inferior tibiofibular joint—a lag screw should be tightened and then 'backed off' 90° ($\frac{1}{4}$ turn). Any fibulo-tibial screw must be removed about 10 weeks later when healing is complete and before weight is transmitted through the ankle.

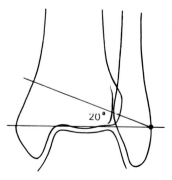

Fig 33.41 A fibulo-tibial screw, fixing a diastasis of the inferior tibio-fibular joint, should be inserted at the level of the ankle joint and angled upwards approximately 20 degrees. (After Danis, 1949.)

Complete diastasis of the inferior tibio-fibular joint—the Dupuytren fracture-dislocation

Clinical examination of this injury leaves little doubt that a major dislocation of the ankle joint has occurred and radiographs will confirm the features of the injury complex (Fig 33.42).

Treatment. The treatment of choice is open reduction and internal fixation[7, 32, 37, 40-43] As in the partial diastasis group, any medial malleolar fracture is stabilised first. Where the medial injury is a deltoid ligament rupture, it should be explored through a small, submalleolar incision to exclude entrapment and the ligament lightly sutured to keep its fibres out of the joint. Occasionally it is necessary to excise some of the deep fibres if exploration has been delayed and the ligament has already started to organise inside the joint.[44]

The fibular fracture is then explored and fixed after reduction, using a small plate or oblique screws across the fracture. If this precaution is neglected, the

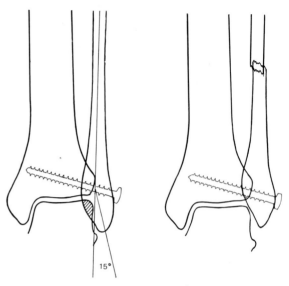

Fig 33.43 In a Dupuytren fracture-dislocation the fibular fracture must be accurately reduced and fixed; if this precaution is neglected the fibula may shorten and widen the mortice by virtue of the fact that the lateral malleolus is set at an angle of about 15 degrees in relation to the fibular shaft.

fibula can shorten and widen the mortice by virtue of the fact that the lateral malleolus is set at an angle of about 15 degrees of valgus in relation to the shaft (Fig 33.43). Also, failure to fix this fracture can leave the fibula free to tilt into varus or valgus and lead to fibular non-union with inferior tibio-fibular joint instability (Fig 33.44).[37, 38]

Following fibular fixation the syndesmosis is stabilised with an angled screw as already described. Where all components of the fracture-dislocation have been rigidly fixed a programme of immediate post-operative mobilisation followed by a plaster cast can be undertaken (see page 1123), but if the medial injury is a deltoid ligament disruption plaster immobilisation must be used immediately after operation. In either event the plaster is removed 8 to 10 weeks after injury. Gentle weight-bearing is permitted during the last two weeks in plaster. As already mentioned weight-bearing out of plaster must not be permitted until the fibulo-tibial screw has been removed (p. 1125).

EXTERNAL ROTATION INJURY WITHOUT DIASTASIS OF THE INFERIOR TIBIO-FIBULAR JOINT (SUPINATION-EXTERNAL ROTATION FRACTURES)

This group of injuries is caused by external rotation of the supinated foot. As already described (pages

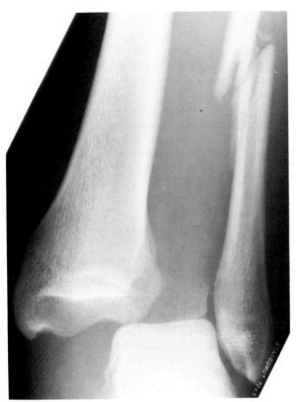

Fig 33.42 An example of a Dupuytren fracture-dislocation of the ankle. The medial structures have failed, the inferior tibio-fibular syndesmosis completely ruptured and the fibular shaft fractured by abduction.

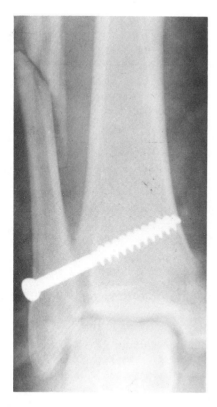

Fig 33.44 In this case of Dupuytren fracture-dislocation the fibular fracture was not fixed and the syndesmosis was screwed with the fibula in varus. The fibular fracture failed to unite, the screw later broke (see Fig 33.50) and the talus redisplaced laterally.

1111 and 1112) the talus twists backwards out of the ankle mortice, pushing the fibula posteriorly, first tearing the anterior tibio-fibular ligament, and then producing an oblique fibular fracture which runs downwards and forwards to the level of the ankle joint (Fig 33.19). Cessation of the deforming force at the moment of the fibular fracture results in an isolated, undisplaced oblique fracture of the lower fibula—probably the commonest ankle fracture.

Oblique fracture of the lower fibula

This has been referred to as the 'mixed oblique' fibular fracture.[5] It has been shown that in the absence of displacement and of injury on the medial side this fracture is quite stable, and in fact a number of patients present with the fragments totally undisplaced after having walked—abeit somewhat painfully—for a week or two. On rare occasions the first stage of the injury is seen alone, i.e. damage to the anterior tibio-fibular ligament, the diagnosis being made clinically by finding acute local tenderness. The bony equivalent of this is the isolated fracture of the anterior tibial tubercle—the Tillaux fracture (Fig 33.45).

Diagnosis and treatment. There is often a history of inversion violence, such as tripping down a kerb, the talus being caused to flick into external rotation because of the torque convertor effect of the subtalar joint (pages 1111 and 1112). Pain is felt mainly laterally where there is moderate swelling and bony

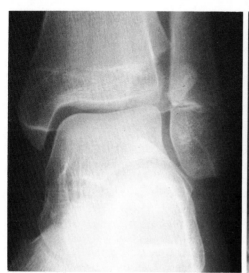
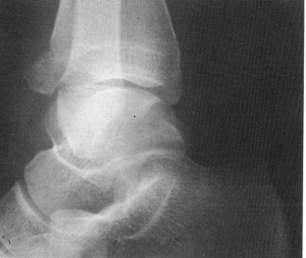

Fig 33.45 Avulsion of the inferior tibio-fibular ligament with a fragment of bone from the tibia (Tillaux fracture). Operative replacement of the displaced bone fragment is needed as the fragment usually bears a significant area of articular cartilage. Fixation with a small cancellous lag screw is ideal.

tenderness over the fibula just above the level of the ankle joint. There should be no tenderness over the medial structures; if this is present stress radiographs must be taken with an external rotation force applied to exclude talar instability, for this will demand reduction and immobilisation for six weeks in a plaster cast. In the absence of medial injury, the fibular fracture remains undisplaced; it is inherently stable and will unite in excellent position even without any immobilisation.[45] However, it is painful to walk on, and four weeks in a below-knee walking casts renders the patient comfortable and will often permit early return to work. Rarely is ankle stiffness troublesome after this line of management, but a light elastic support to control any swelling should be worn for a few weeks after removal of the cast, and a short programme of mobilisation exercises ordered if necessary.

Fracture-dislocation without inferior tibio-fibular joint diastasis

If the injuring force continues after causing an oblique fibular fracture, the talus then impinges against the posterior lip of the tibial articular surface and may fracture it. In fact, the fibular fracture and the so-called 'posterior malleolar' fragment comprise a single unit being united by the posterior tibio-fibular ligament (Fig 33.22). The medial structures then fail as the talus dislocates backwards.

Diagnosis. There is always a history of considerable violence to the ankle—a heavy person falling off a step-ladder, a high speed stumble during a fast game, a road traffic accident—and it is usually clinically obvious that the ankle joint is greatly deformed and swollen. Prominence of the heel with shortening of the forefoot denote a posterior dislocation. Good quality radiographs are essential to appreciate all components of the complex bony failure.

Treatment. The only acceptable result of treatment of fracture-dislocations of the ankle is union in an anatomical position, and nothing short of perfect reduction should satisfy the surgeon. Even a displacement of the talus as small as 2 mm can result in such incongruity of the joint surfaces as to produce point loading of the articular cartilage sufficient to result in early degenerative arthritis: in nearly all published studies of the treatment of ankle fractures it has been shown that the functional result is proportional to the quality of the final reduction of the displacement.[32, 37, 46–50].

The gross instability of this fracture-dislocation of the ankle makes it extremely difficult to achieve these high standards by conservative methods and in most instances open reduction and internal fixation is the treatment of choice. Nevertheless, there is a place for conservative treatment in the elderly and infirm, in the presence of unhealthy skin or poor vascularity, or where the necessary surgical facilities are not available. In managing this injury it is wise to bear in mind that it has been produced by violent talar rotation and so an above-knee plaster cast with the knee flexed 5 to 10 degrees is necessary to control rotatory strain. Reduction of the displacement is achieved not only by correcting the posterior displacement but also by internally rotating the foot on the leg. It is impossible to over-reduce the displacement by manual pressure because the malleolar fragments lock against each other. With the limb hanging over the end of the table a plaster is applied from toes to just below the knee with the foot at right angles and neutral to inversion and eversion. It is wise to apply a padded plaster at the first reduction and to be prepared to change it in a week or so when the swelling has reduced. Provided the wool padding is applied smoothly and firmly and the plaster is wound over it to give an even compressive effect, padding should increase rather than decrease the stability of the reduction.[51] While the plaster is setting the surgeon should use both hands, one over the medial side of the shaft of the tibia and the other cupping the back of the heel pushing it forwards and inwards (Fig 33.46). It is futile to try to reduce the displacement by inverting the foot as this externally rotates the talus.

In the presence of a large posterior lip fragment, the foot must never be dorsiflexed by plantar pressure during reduction as this will cause displacement (Fig 33.47). Rather, the heel is pulled downwards and forwards as an essential part of the manipulation.[51]

The reduction must be checked radiographically each week for the first three weeks as redisplacement may occur, and most authorities regard loss of an initial good reduction, or the failure of an experienced surgeon to secure anatomical reposition in the first place, as an indication to proceed to open reduction and internal fixation.[33, 37, 52-57]

Open reduction should start with reduction of the fibular fracture which is exposed by incision along its posterior border and, after cleaning of the fracture surfaces, the ankle is manipulated as already described. Difficulty in reduction may be due to a number of problems: a ruptured deltoid ligament may be turned into the ankle joint (a small medial incision will permit this to be hooked out and sutured); the tibialis posterior tendon is occasionally

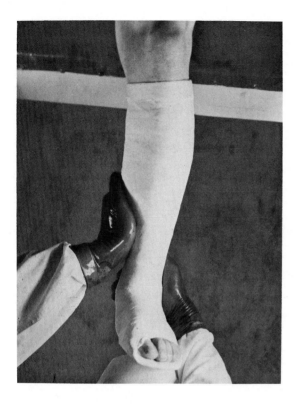

Fig 33.46 The first stage of this plaster is applied as a lightly padded below-knee cast. While the plaster is setting, posterior dislocation is prevented by the surgeon cupping the back of the heel in one hand, gently pulling forwards and inwards; at the same time the other hand applies firm counter-pressure over the medial side of the tibial shaft. The surgeon's knee maintains the foot dorsiflexed to a right angle.

trapped in the ankle joint;[58] there may be failure of the posterior fragment to reduce, or an unreduced 'Tillaux' fragment may be present.[36] After reduction, the position of the talus is checked by X-ray, and the fibula is fixed. The best method is to insert two screws across the fracture from in front backwards, over-drilling the anterior fragment to produce interfragmentary compression. A screw is then passed obliquely from the distal fibular fragment, across the inferior tibio-fibular joint, and into the tibia. Alternatively a small, contoured plate may be applied to protect the interfragmentary fixation. Any posterior fragment of significant size (and that includes nearly all those associated with this particular fracture-dislocation) should be fixed with one or two screws—two being preferable as there is a tendency for a large fragment to rotate as well as to displace proximally. After fixation of the fibula it is rare that the large posterior tibial fragment is sufficiently stabilised by the intact posterior tibio-fibular ligament as to need no fixation. When necessary the posterior tibial fracture may be explored through the incision along the post border of the fibula and this may be adequate to permit fixation of a postero-lateral fragment. However, screw fixation of a large fragment will usually require a postero-medial incision deepened between the lateral edge of the lower fibres of the belly of flexor hallucis longus and the peroneal tendons; or alternatively a large fragment may be held in position temporarily by Kirschner wires and then fixed by two lag screws inserted from in front: this manoeuvre, however, requires a sizeable fragment and considerable technical skill (Fig 33.48).

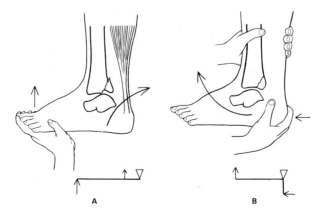

Fig 33.47 A. Shows the disastrous effect of struggling to secure a plantigrade foot, especially if the tendo Achillis is tight, by forcing the forefoot upwards. This pushes the talus out of the ankle joint posteriorly by the system of levers illustrated. B. Shows how the plantigrade position should be obtained by lifting the heel forwards—dorsiflexing the forefoot through the medium of the system of levers illustrated. This method enhances the security of the reduction. (Reproduced by kind permission of Professor Sir John Charnley, from his book (1957) *The Closed Treatment of Common Fractures*, 2nd edn. Edinburgh: Livingstone.)

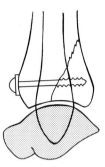

Fig 33.48 Diagram showing the technique of fixing, after reduction, a large posterior tibial fragment by the use of one or two cancellous lag screws inserted through a small anterior incision. In all but the young adult, the anterior tibial cortex is thin and the use of a washer on each screw is advisable.

If there is a medial malleolar fracture this should then be fixed either by a screw or by a traction-absorption suture (Fig 33.25). When the surgeon is satisfied that rigid fixation of all three elements of the bony injury has been secured mobilisation of the ankle and foot in the immediate post-operative period, as described in the section on adduction fractures, can be permitted (see page 1123). If a medial injury is a deltoid rupture, immediate plaster immobilisation after operation is necessary to allow the ligament to heal. In either event a non-walking below-knee cast is used until six weeks after operation, followed by a weight-bearing cast for a further two to four weeks.

Where an oblique screw across the inferior tibio-fibular joint has been used this must be removed at 8 to 10 weeks after injury, before weight is transmitted through the ankle joint unprotected by plaster. Lambert[59] has demonstrated that the fibula bears about one-sixth of the body weight and both rotational and gliding movements normally occur at the inferior tibio-fibular joint during walking;[60] therefore, if the screw is left across the joint it will either loosen in the fibula (Fig 33.49)—not necessarily an untoward event—or, more seriously, it may break (Fig 33.50).

VERTICAL COMPRESSION INJURIES OF THE ANKLE

The ankle joint is designed to bear weight and supports up to three times body weight during the push-off phase of normal gait. Hirsch and Lewis[61]

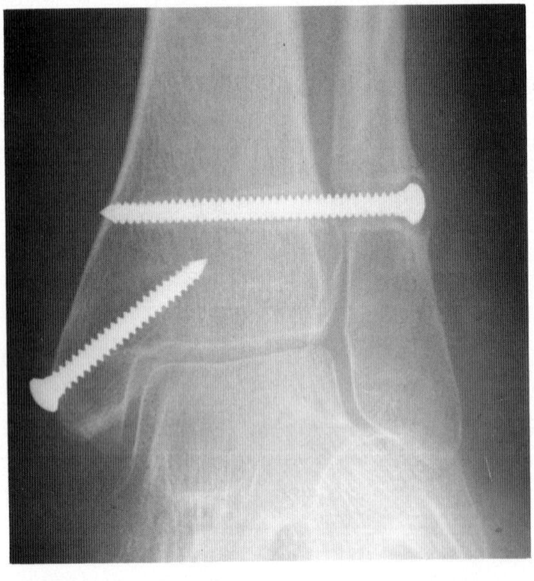

Fig 33.49 A fibulo-tibial screw has been left *in situ* (albeit improperly placed) after resumption of weight-bearing. Because of the normal movement of the fibula in relation to the tibia it can be seen that the screw has become loose in the fibula.

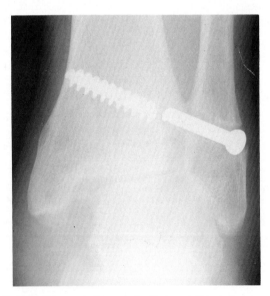

Fig 33.50 Movement between the fibula and tibia during walking has caused fatigue fracture of a fibulo-tibial screw which should have been removed prior to permitting the patient to weight-bear. In fact the fibular fracture in this Dupuytren fracture-dislocation had not been reduced and fixed, had proceeded to non-union in varus mal-position, and the talus has in consequence shifted laterally—a disaster which should have been avoided!

demonstrated experimentally the ankle joint's remarkable resistance to compressive forces, but nevertheless high velocity percussion of the dome of the talus on to the lower tibial articular surface may cause its failure. The talus splits the lower tibia into a number of fragments of varying size and impacts them into the cancellous bone of the supramalleolar region. As the deformation occurs the fibular shaft usually fractures.

Rüedi and Allgöwer[62] divided these injuries into two main types: anterior compression fractures caused by axial impaction of the dorsiflexed talus, the commonest variety (Fig 33.51), and posterior compression fractures caused by a fall on to the plantar-flexed foot (Fig 30.52). A third, combined group is also described.

Diagnosis. A history of considerable violence is available and the ankle region is grossly swollen with widening of the bony diameter in the malleolar area. Many cases are the result of falls from a height as well as road traffic accidents. Radiography will reveal the degree of comminution of the lower tibia.

Treatment. These injuries cause severe disruption of the tibial articular surface which is highly likely to lead to secondary degenerative arthritis, and where possible surgical reconstruction of the joint should be undertaken by an experienced surgeon. It has to be remembered, however, that these injuries are always associated with considerable swelling and therefore the skin condition must be very carefully assessed before embarking upon any operative procedure.

If the degree of comminution is excessive, especially in the combined type of compression fracture, the outlook for ankle joint function is grave and arthrodesis is the likely outcome. However, there are occasionally surprisingly good results following union

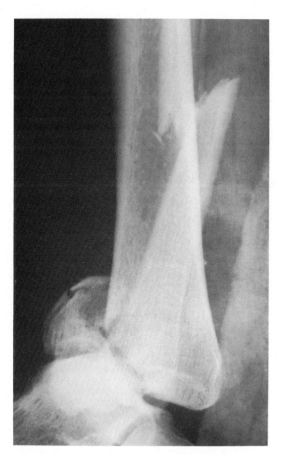

Fig 33.51 An anterior crush injury of the lower tibia caused by a fall from a height with the foot in a dorsiflexed position.

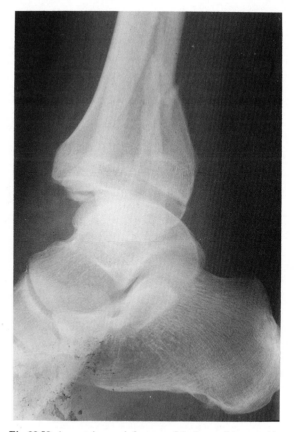

Fig 33.52 A posterior crush fracture of the lower tibia caused by a violent compressive force acting upwards on the plantar-flexed foot.

in an apparently poor position, and for this reason an expectant line of management is worthwhile where primary reconstruction is not possible.

Conservative treatment consists of os calcis pin traction on a Braun frame with gentle active movements of the foot and ankle for three to four weeks followed by a non-weight-bearing plaster cast for a further nine weeks.[63] Unprotected weight-bearing is not permitted until 12 to 20 weeks after injury according to the radiographic evidence of union.

Operative treatment. The first step is to reduce and fix the fibular fracture out to length. This frequently locates a major lateral tibial fragment which has retained its attachments to the fibula. The tibial fragments are then exposed through a curved antero-medial incision (Fig 33.53), disimpacted and patiently fitted together on to the dome of the talus to reconstruct the joint surface, followed by fixation with interfragmentary screws and a medial buttress

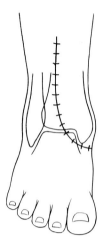

Fig 33.53 Curved antero-medial incision used to expose the distal tibia for reconstruction of compression fractures of the anterior and combined types.

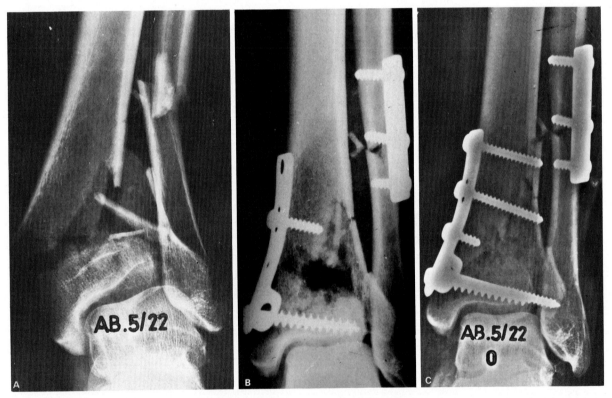

Fig 33.54 Severe compression fracture of the ankle and supramalleolar region of the tibia. A fissure fracture runs into the ankle joint and frequently the joint surface is deformed. The first step in its reduction is to fix the fibula out to length. B. With the fibula plated the major distal tibial fragments relocate themselves approximately. A lower tibia plate (in most cases a T-plate is used) then holds these fragments in position after perfection of their reduction. Note the gap thus created. This is the result of crushing of tibial cancellous bone at the time of injury. C. The final stage is the filling of the supramalleolar gap with cancellous bone chips from the iliac crest or greater trochanteric region. (Reproduced by kind permission of *Injury* and Dr Rüedi and Professor Allgöwer, from their article (1969) Fractures of the lower end of the tibia into the ankle joint. *Injury*, 1, 92.)

plate (Fig 33.54). Where cancellous bone was crushed by impaction of the tibial fragments a gap will now exist, and an essential part of the operation is to fill this gap with cancellous bone chips from the iliac crest (Fig 33.54). Early post-operative movements in elevation are then practised for two to three weeks, after which a light, protective, non-weight-bearing, below-knee plaster cast is worn until eight weeks after operation. When the cast is removed non-weight-bearing mobilisation of the foot and ankle under the care of an experienced physiotherapist is necessary. These injuries are often associated with considerable swelling after removal of the plaster, and an elastic supporting bandage should be used. Overenthusiastic mobilisation at this stage will only aggravate the swelling and must be resisted lest it hinder the return of movement. Weight is not transmitted through the ankle until at least 12 weeks have elapsed since operation. *It cannot be over-emphasised that such surgery is difficult and should only be carried out by an experienced surgeon,* but with patience and skill it can yield most

rewarding results from an otherwise hopeless injury of the ankle joint.

Primary arthrodesis of these injuries has been advocated,[64, 65] but this is a very difficult procedure and is better undertaken at a later stage after a full programme of either conservative or surgical care.

INJURIES OF THE EPIPHYSES AT THE ANKLE

The types and degrees of displacement of epiphyseal injuries of the lower ends of the tibia and fibula are broadly comparable with the fracture dislocations of adults, and the principles of treatment are similar. Displacement is often accurately reduced by manipulation, the fragments frequently lock into position and over-reduction is nearly impossible. However, the form of treatment and certainly the final result will depend upon the type of epiphyseal injury which has occurred. Salter and Harris[66] have classified epiphyseal injuries in general into five types according to the pattern of failure (Fig 33.55). Injuries of the

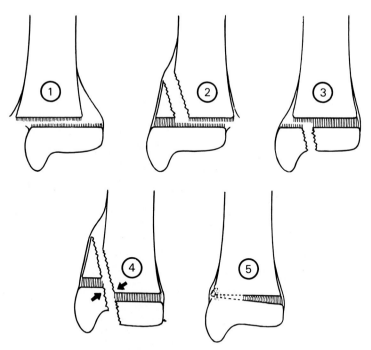

Fig 33.55 The five types of epiphyseal injury. Type 1 is a pure shear injury of the growth plate. Type 2 is the commonest epiphyseal injury. A shear injury of a portion of the growth plate occurs in association with the fracture of a metaphyseal fragment united to the epiphysis by an area of undamaged growth plate. Type 3 injury is where a fracture of the epiphysis occurs at right angles to the articular surface and then an epiphyseal fragment displaces by shearing its associated growth plate. Type 4 injury consists of a single fracture plane running from the articular surface through the epiphysis, the growth plate and the metaphysis. If it remains displaced the bone of the epiphysis may unite with that of the metaphyseal region—as arrowed—causing an area of premature growth plate fusion and a resultant deformity. Type 5 injury is a crushing injury of the growth plate where the bone of the epiphysis is impacted into the metaphysis—this is always followed by premature fusion of the damaged area of the growth plate. (After Salter and Harris, 1963.)

distal tibial and fibular epiphyses are conveniently grouped using this classification but subdivided according to the direction of the deforming force.

Type 1 injuries. In this type of injury the epiphysis is displaced on the metaphysis following a shearing injury of the growth plate (Fig 33.55). There is no bony injury to either the ossific nucleus or the metaphysis. The epiphyseal shear takes place between the hypertrophic layer of the growth plate and the zone of provisional ossification,[67] and provided that there is no interference with the blood supply to the epiphysis, growth will continue from the layers of the growth plate which remain with the epiphysis. At the ankle the epiphyses have wide soft tissue attachments so that their vascularity would not be imperilled by this type of injury and in theory growth should not be affected.

Type 1 injury rarely occurs in its pure form at the ankle, although rotational displacement of the lower tibial epiphysis, without associated fracture, has been described.[68, 69, 70] The reported cases were reduced with ease and were followed by normal healing and growth.

A variety of the type 1 injury form is the 'lamellar injury of Werenskiold[71] where an epiphyseal shear injury occurs but in a small area a thin lamella of metaphyseal bone separates with the growth plate. In the virtually undisplaced epiphyseal injury the presence of this lamella may be the sole clue to the true nature of the damage. A lamellar injury of the fibular growth plate may be seen in association with other types of displacement of the tibial epiphyses (see 'railing' fracture, page 1135).

Type 2 injury. This is probably the most common type of epiphyseal injury. Here, the epiphysis shifts on the metaphysis as in the type 1 injury but it carries with it a triangular metaphyseal fragment which remains attached to the epiphysis by a portion of uninjured growth plate (Fig 33.55). The soft tissue attachments of the epiphysis are always preserved and subsequent growth is normal. At the ankle this is caused either by external rotation or by abduction strain.

External rotation injury causes separation of a posterior tibial metaphyseal fragment. The injury may be virtually undisplaced and without concomitant fibular injury (Fig 33.56). These injuries heal rapidly and require only three to four weeks in a well-moulded below-knee plaster cast. Subsequent growth is normal.

Displaced type 2 injuries occurring by external

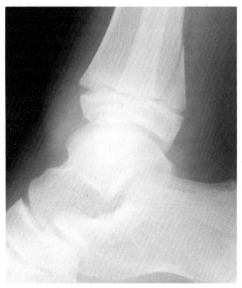

Fig 33.56 X-ray showing an undisplaced type 2 external rotation injury of the tibial epiphysis associated with posterior metaphyseal fragment and an intact fibula.

rotation are accompanied by a spiral greenstick fracture of the lower fibular shaft (Fig 33.57). They must be reduced by internal rotation of the foot, at the same time pulling the heel forward, followed by

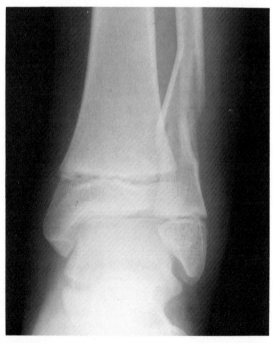

Fig 33.57 X-rays showing a displaced type 2 external rotation injury with a spiral greenstick fracture of the fibula.

immobilisation in an above-knee plaster cast. After two weeks there will be no further tendency to rotational redisplacement and the above-knee portion of the cast can be removed. The remaining plaster may be taken off six weeks after injury.

The severely displaced type of this injury is often rapidly followed by tibial epiphyseal fusion, but this rarely produces deformity as these injuries occur mostly in the period immediately before natural fusion. The significance, however, of the likelihood of this injury being followed by early growth plate closure is that residual displacement may be permanent in the absence of subsequent growth with its potential for remodelling. Carothers and Crenshaw[72] have observed that valgus displacement of more than 12 degrees does not correct spontaneously after this kind of injury.

An abduction injury of the foot may produce a type 2 displacement of the distal tibial epiphysis with a lateral metaphyseal fragment and a bending fracture of the lower fibular shaft (Fig 33.58). Reposition by manipulation under anaesthesia is usually easily accomplished and, as with all type 2 injuries, over-reduction is impossible. Careful moulding of a lightly padded, below-knee plaster cast is essential to maintain the reduction, and a check radiograph must be taken at the end of the first week. The cast may be removed after six weeks, and subsequent growth is likely to be normal.

Type 3 injuries. The type 3 epiphysiolysis consists of a fracture of the epiphysis running from the articular surface into the growth plate, and a shear injury of that portion of the growth plate related to one or other of the epiphyseal fragments. There is no metaphyseal injury (Fig 33.55). At the ankle this can be produced by adduction or external rotation injury.

Adduction injury—'railing fracture'.[73] This fracture is caused by adduction of the talus in the mortice pushing off the medial malleolus as in Figure 33.59. With any degree of displacement a fibular injury occurs which is either a lamellar injury of Werenskiold or an avulsion fracture of the tip of the fibular epiphysis (Fig 33.60).

Reduction of the tibial malleolar fragment is occasionally difficult and sometimes fixation with a horizontal lag screw is permissible. If screw fixation is used the screw's course must be entirely intra-epiphyseal in order not to damage the growth plate (Fig 33.61), and it must be removed after two to three months. Usually, however, replacement of the fragment, if required, is achieved by manipulation using direct pressure over the malleolus followed by a below-knee cast for four to six weeks.

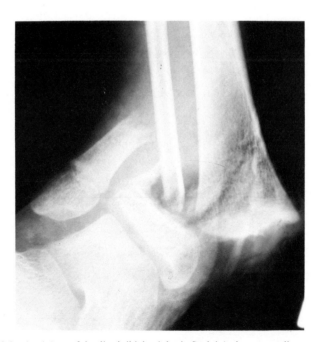

Fig 33.58 X-ray of a type 2 abduction injury of the distal tibial epiphysis. Such injuries are usually caused by extreme violence and are frequently compound. This patient's foot was caught beneath the rotating platform of a fairground carousel.

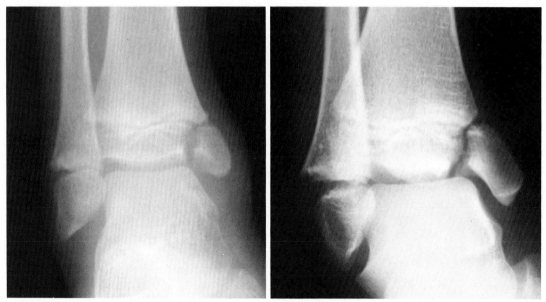

Fig 33.59   **Fig 33.60**

Figs 33.59 and 33.60 X-rays showing a type 3 adduction injury of the distal tibial epiphysis. There is sometimes a degree of crushing of the medial growth plate if the medial malleolar fragment is more markedly displaced (Fig 33.60) and growth disturbance may follow such damage. This was called the 'railing' fracture by McFarland, who recorded that it often followed a fall from railings with the foot firmly wedged between two of the upright posts.

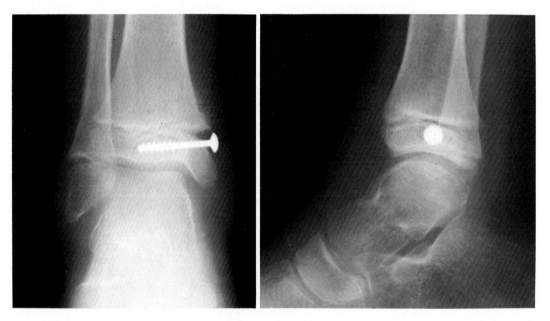

Fig 33.61 A displaced, unstable 'railing' fracture may be fixed with an intra-epiphyseal lag screw as shown here. Great care must be taken to ensure that the growth plate is not damaged, and the operation is always performed with radiological control.

It has been stated[73-75] that the railing fracture often causes premature fusion of the medial portion of the tibial growth plate leading to progressive varus deformity. Undoubtedly this occurs but it is not common; nevertheless, all children who have suffered this injury should be followed up radiologically until normal growth is observed. In the event of a bony bridge forming medially across the growth plate repeated 'open wedge' valgus osteotomy may be necessary to control deformity. Recent experimental work by Österman[76] has suggested that resection of the fused area of the growth plate and filling the resultant defect with a free fat graft may result in normal growth being re-established. The application of this principle by Langenskiold[77] to the problem of post-traumatic partial growth plate fusion in the human has been encouraging.

External rotation injury. The antero-lateral quadrant of the distal tibial epiphysis is the last portion of this epiphysis to remain unfused during the fifteenth year of skeletal age. At this age an external rotation strain of the anterior tibio-fibular ligament can avulse a 'block' of this unfused tibial epiphysis as a type 3 injury[78, 79] (Fig 33.62). This is equivalent to the Tillaux fracture in the adult. An undisplaced fragment rapidly heals after four weeks in a below-knee walking cast. A displaced fragment must be reduced and fixed as it not only represents an area of ligamentous instability, but an intra-articular defect. Fixation with a small screw may be practised without fear of growth disturbance as this portion of the tibial epiphysis would have fused naturally within a month or two.

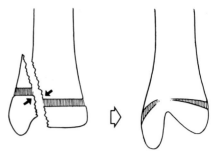

Fig 33.63 A displaced type 4 epiphyseal injury may result in bony union between the epiphysis and the metaphysis as indicated by the arrows. This causes a bony bridge across the growth plate and a 'fish-tail' deformity of the articular surface.

Type 4 injury. This type of epiphyseal injury comprises a longitudinally running fracture plane starting at the articular surface and passing up through the epiphysis, the growth plate and the metaphysis (Fig 33.55). With any degree of displacement, there is a danger of union between epiphysis and metaphysis as arrowed in Figure 33.63. This may result in an epiphysiodesis causing deformity of the articular surface.

This type of epiphyseal injury is rare at the ankle (Fig 33.64) and is caused by adduction of the talus in the mortice, analogous to the vertical adduction fracture of the medial malleolus in the adult (Fig 33.8).

As well as the possibility of growth disturbance resulting from union of the type 4 injury in a displaced position, a deformity of the tibial articular surface will result with no possibility for remodelling.

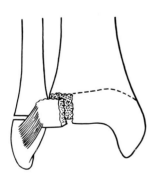

Fig 33.62 External rotation injury may cause the interior tibio-fibular ligament to avulse an antero-lateral fragment from the distal tibial epiphysis. This fragment is the last portion of the epiphysis to fuse with the metaphysis and so such an injury only occurs in the final six months of skeletal maturation. It is equivalent to the Tillaux fracture in the adult (see page 1107).

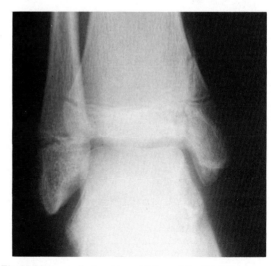

Fig 33.64 An undisplaced type 4 injury of the distal tibial epiphysis.

Such mal-union of the articular fracture must be avoided and open reduction with internal fixation of the metaphyseal fragment is the treatment of choice if significant displacement is present.

Type 5 injury. This is a crushing injury of the growth plate where the bone of the epiphysis is impacted into the metaphysis (Fig 33.55), and premature fusion is an inevitable result.[66] There is usually a greater or lesser portion of the growth plate which will continue to function and cause severe growth asymmetry; the earlier the age at which the injury occurs, the more serious the resultant deformity will be. The crushing nature of the injury often results in the extrusion of a small metaphyseal fragment adjacent to the growth plate, and this can be a most helpful diagnostic feature (Fig 33.65). At the ankle it is usually the medial tibial growth plate which is crushed, causing a progressive varus deformity[72] (Fig 33.66). The management of the resultant growth asymmetry should be along the lines suggested in the section on 'railing' fracture (page 1137).

Avascular necrosis in epiphyseal injury. Post-traumatic osteochondritis of the distal tibial epiphysis due to avascular necrosis is rare but has been described.[80, 81] One recorded case was followed eventually by reconstitution and normal development of the epiphysis, but another led to degenerative arthritis of the ankle, which eventually had to be arthrodesed.

Lateral ligament injuries in children
Major disruptions of the lateral ligament complex in children have hitherto been regarded as virtually unknown. Jani and Baumgartner[82, 83] however have drawn attention to the fact that they are less rare than previously thought. They stress the diagnostic significance of minute osteochondral flakes from the lateral aspect of the talus or oscalcis visible on good quality radiographs. In cases of suspicion of such injury, stress inversion radiographs should be taken and where excessive talar tilt is present they recommend exploration and suture of the ligament

MISCELLANEOUS ANKLE INJURIES

Isolated fracture of the posterior tibial lip. In the discussion of supination-external rotation injuries we have observed that as the talus rotates laterally and backwards out of the mortice the first three events in the failure sequence are:

1. Rupture of the anterior tibio-fibular ligament.
2. Oblique fibular fracture.
3. A push-off fracture of the posterior lip of the tibial plafond.

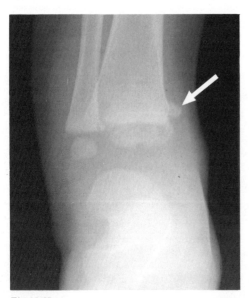

Fig 33.65

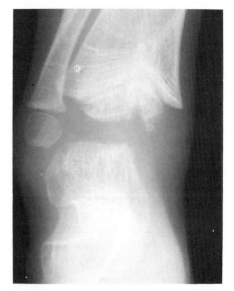

Fig 33.66

Figs 33.65 and 33.66 X-ray showing a crushing injury of the medial growth plate. Note the small extruded metaphyseal fragment (arrowed) which is a valuable clue to the true nature of the injury. This patient, a child of 2½ years of age, developed a severe deformity of the tibial articular surface, as depicted in Figure 33.66, an X-ray taken two years later.

Bröstrom and colleagues[84] postulated that isolated fracture of the posterior tibial 'tubercle' represented a situation where the third event of this normal sequence occurred immediately after the first and then the injuring force ceased before fibular fracture could occur. Arthrography of 18 cases of isolated posterior lip fracture revealed consistent rupture of the anterior tibio-fibular ligament—an observation which supports their hypothesis.

These injuries are not common; the fragments are usually undisplaced and heal rapidly in a below-knee plaster cast.

Dislocation of the ankle without associated fracture. This is a rare event but has nevertheless been recorded by a number of authorities[85-92] (Fig 33.67) and is due to forced plantar flexion of the foot.[87] There is usually dislocation of the inferior tibiofibular syndesmosis and the fibula may become trapped behind the tibia.[93-97] Many are open injuries with an extensive lateral wound, but provided that the blood supply to the foot is adequate after reduction and that infection is averted by careful wound débridement and closure, a guarded prognosis for reasonable ankle function may be given.

Recurrent sprain of the inferior tibio-fibular joint. A partial tear of the anterior tibio-fibular ligament represents a 'forme fruste' supination-external-rotation failure and has a reputation for becoming a chronic lesion. It may be differentiated from the more common anterior talo-fibular sprain by localisation of the tenderness over the front of the syndesmosis, and pain at this site if the foot is gently flicked into external rotation by the examiner.

Mullins and Sallis[98] believe that 70 per cent of recurrent ankle sprains are due to injury of the anterior tibio-fibular ligament and have recommended screw fixation of the inferior tibio-fibular joint for persistent disability. Usually one or more infiltrations of the tender ligament with hydrocortisone acetate 25 mg and 1 per cent lignocaine will cure the symptoms.

Le Fort-Wagstaffe fracture (Fig 33.68). In the late nineteenth century Le Fort (of maxillary fracture fame) and Wagstaffe of St. Thomas' Hospital independently described an avulsion fracture of the anterior cortex of the lateral malleolus.[99, 100] It is a rare pull-off injury of the fibular attachment of the anterior tibio-fibular ligament and is much loved for its scarcity value and eponym. Its recognition is a source of delight to the 'ankle devotee' but of doubtful value to the patient! Most instances are missed.

Recurrent dislocation of the peroneal tendons. Recurrent dislocation of the peroneal tendons

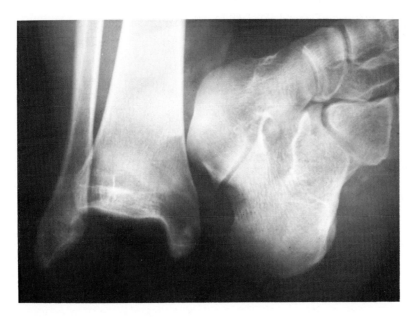

Fig 33.67 X-ray showing dislocation of the ankle without an associated fracture.

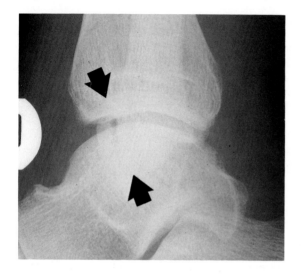

Fig 33.68 X-ray showing the rare Le Fort-Wagstaffe fracture. This is a supination-external rotation injury where, instead of a rupture of the anterior tibio-fibular ligament, the anterior surface of the lateral malleolus is avulsed.

from the groove behind the lateral malleolus is a rare cause of ankle instability. The depth of this groove, and the mobility of the tendons, vary considerably in normal individuals. If the groove is shallow and the annular fibres forming its roof are lax, both tendons may slip over the margin of the bone on to the subcutaneous surface of the malleolus. The displacement occurs when the foot is actively dorsiflexed and

it is reduced when the foot is plantar-flexed. Sharp jerking movement of the tendons from one position to the other causes pain, weakness and giving way of the joint.

Conservative treatment. At the time of the first displacement, treatment by strapping, encircling the limb immediately above the malleoli and keeping them in position for about six weeks, may prevent recurrence of displacement of the tendons. Raising the heel of the shoe by about $\frac{1}{4}$ inch (5 mm) may also help to prevent recurrence. If the symptoms persist, operative treatment is needed.

Operative treatment. The peroneal groove of the lateral malleolus which should hold the tendons of the peroneus brevis and peroneus longus in position may be deepened by a bone-flap operation. Sir Robert Kelly of Liverpool[101] devised a procedure by which a thick flap of the subcutaneous surface of the lateral malleolus was swung back through at least $\frac{1}{4}$ inch (5 mm) so as to form a more prominent lip to the peroneal groove. He held the displaced 'veneer of bone' in position by two screws. In another case he used more complicated carpentry to avoid the necessity for screw fixation. But the fact is that a thick osteoperiosteal flap cut from the surface of the lateral malleolus with an intact pedicle of periosteum and soft tissue, swung back and held in position by one or two sutures, is all that is needed (Figs 33.69 and 33.70).

Anterior ankle joint instability. *'Footballer's ankle'.*[102, 103] The anterior capsule of the ankle joint is

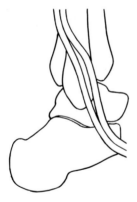

Fig 33.69 Recurrent dislocation of the peroneal tendons which slip to and fro over the lateral margin of the malleolus.

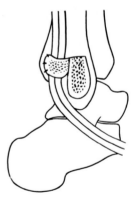

Fig 33.70 A thick bone flap is cut from the subcutaneous surface of the lateral malleolus with its periosteal and soft tissue attachments preserved so that there will be no interference with the blood supply. The veneer or sliver of bone is swung back so that it lies over the peroneal tendons and deepens the peroneal groove. It is held in position by a simple suture. The ankle is then protected in plaster for two months.

sometimes torn from its distal attachment to the neck of the talus, but there is seldom complete avulsion. The injury is often sustained by footballers, who, on kicking the ball, usually take its weight on the dorsum of the foot so that there may be separation of the capsular fibres from the neck of the talus with resulting traumatic subperiosteal ossification (see Fig 4.41). Very seldom is there complete separation of the anterior capsule from the talus with resulting recurrent forward dislocation of the joint. Sometimes the avulsion may be from the tibial attachment of the capsule, associated with a fracture of the anterior articular margin. Ossification during repair forms an anterior spur which may limit dorsiflexion (Fig 33.71). Removal of this spur will restore some movement, but it must be remembered that late traumatic arthritis can occur in these cases.

Recurrent forward dislocation of the ankle. Complete avulsion of the anterior capsule from the neck of the talus associated with momentary forward dislocation of the talus is unusual, but Watson-Jones described two cases in 1952[104] (Fig 33.72). Each time these patients stepped out the tibia slipped backwards on the body of the talus and then slid forwards again as weight was taken off. With the foot fixed firmly on the ground the tibia could be displaced backwards at will. There was such great disability that a reconstruction operation was devised, using the tendon of

peroneus longus as a tenodesis (Figs 33.73–33.75). The symptoms were relieved and weight-bearing radiographs showed that normal stability had been regained.

Landeros and colleagues[105] reported a number of cases where the talus could be seen radiographically to move anteriorly on the tibia if the dorsiflexed foot was pulled forwards. Plantar-flexion abolished this sign due to tightening of the anterior capsular structures. These patients gave a consistent history of a forced plantar-flexion sprain, anterior ankle pain with swelling, and reported improvement by wearing high-heeled shoes. Plication of the anterior capsule and repair of the usually torn anterior talofibular ligament were recommended.

MAL-UNION AT THE ANKLE

Most severely displaced ankle injuries involve the articular surfaces, and the irregularities produced by failure to anatomically reduce the bony fragments lead to degenerative arthritis of the joint. The ankle joint tolerates badly any incongruity of its surfaces for its articular cartilage is relatively thin and relies upon perfect adaption of its joint surfaces to avoid damage to this precious hyaline veneer.[106]

Post-traumatic degenerative arthritis is the usual sequel to mal-union at the ankle, although some

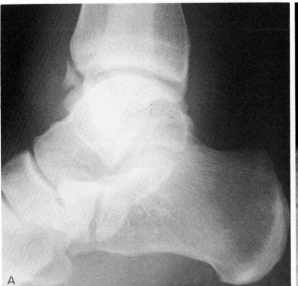 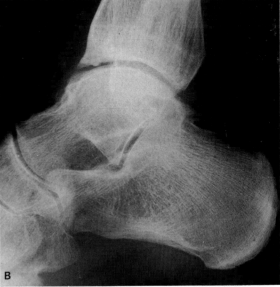

Fig 33.71 A. X-ray showing how a forced plantar-flexion injury may cause avulsion of the anterior lip of the tibia—'footballer's ankle'. B. Union of this injury causes an anterior spur which may limit dorsiflexion; on occasions this spur may have to be excised.

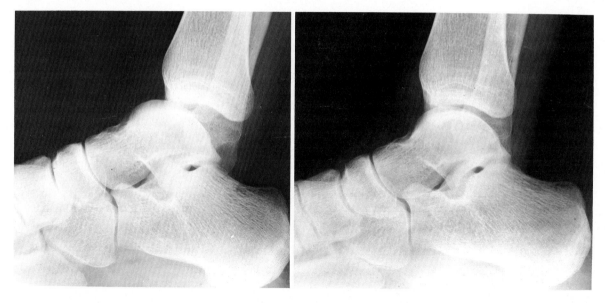

Fig 33.72 Radiographs of the first case recorded of recurrent forward dislocation of the ankle joint.[104] The patient displaced the foot forwards and backwards at the ankle whenever he put weight upon it. Radiographs show the displacement and occurred with every step (see also Figs 30.73 to 30.75).

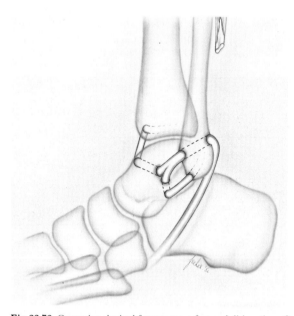

Fig 33.73 Operation devised for recurrent forward dislocation of the ankle joint. It is a simple modification of the tenodesis used for recurrent inward subluxation, but this time the tendon of peroneus longus was used. Half the tendon was passed back through the lateral malleolus in the ordinary way; the other half was passed through the neck of the talus to the medial side in order to provide an additional check to forward displacement of the tarsus.

surgeons will deny this on the grounds that they are not frequently presented with patients requiring arthrodesis after trauma: this is rather more a tribute to the stoicism of the patients and their readiness to accept some residual disability after a severe injury than to the resilience of the ankle joint in the face of insult. Not only will incongruity of the joint surfaces predispose to degenerative arthritis, but it must be remembered that trauma severe enough to cause fracture-dislocation of any degree can effectively cause direct damage to the articular cartilage of the ankle and lead to osteo-arthritis, which will develop within one or two years.[107]

Arthrodesis of ankle. Our constant aim must be the union of fractures at the ankle joint in *anatomical* position, but regrettably this is not always achieved and arthrodesis may be necessary. Fortunately the penalty of arthrodesis, with its restriction of movement, applies far less to the ankle than to most other joints because the subtalar and mid-tarsal joints contribute so great a range. In fact these joints alone provide such good plantar-flexion and dorsiflexion movement of the foot that after sound arthrodesis of the ankle joint it is often quite difficult to know that movement is restricted at all. The patient walks without a limp, runs, jumps and pursues most

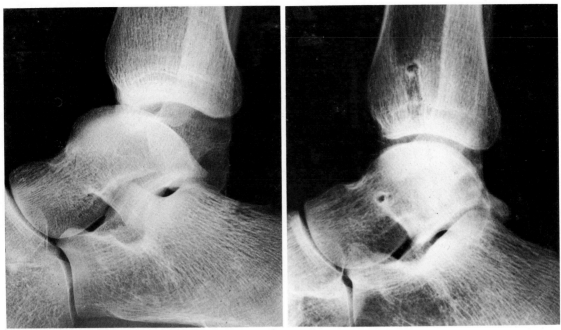

Fig 33.74

Fig 33.75

Figs 33.74 and 33.75 Radiographs of the ankle joint of a patient with recurrent forward dislocation, before and after tenodesis by the technique shown in Figure 33.73. Note the drill hole in the talus and the lower end of the tibia through which the two halves of the long peroneal tendon were united. The radiographs show that there is now perfect stability despite every passive movement or strain. (Case of the late Sir Reginald Watson-Jones recorded by Mr W. C. Robinson.)

recreations and occupations with a negligible disability. It is wrong, therefore, to explain an arthrodesis of the ankle to a patient as a stiffening procedure. Recognising the stiffness that is already present he imagines something worse and quite probably will refuse the operation. It should be described as an operation which will not alter the range of movement of the foot but will relieve the pain and allow him to walk and run without disability.

The position in which the ankle joint is fixed is of great importance. Tilting into valgus or varus must be corrected completely because otherwise the patient will walk on the inner or outer border of the foot where painful callosities will develop, and there will be constant strain of the tarsal joints. The foot must not be fixed in the inverted position. This is not a position of strength—it is a deformity which causes disability quite similar to that of the opposite deformity of fixed eversion. The ankle should be fixed in about 5 to 10 degrees of equinus, which is the usual position of standing in shoes. To arthrodese the foot exactly at right angles to the leg would be satisfactory if our lives were spent in bare feet, but since we stand and walk in shoes with heels, it is not satisfactory. Still worse is to arthrodese the ankle joint in a position of dorsiflexion above the right angle. This causes serious disability, because no matter how free may be the mobility developing at the mid-tarsal joints the patient is then unable to stand flat on the sole of his foot except with the knee joint flexed.

Arthrodesis of the ankle by screwing the fibula to the tibia and the talus. In this technique described by Crawford Adams[108] the joint is exposed from the lateral side and the lower 4 inches (10.2 cm) of fibula with its malleolus are removed. The articular cartilage and subchondral bone of the tibia and talus are then excised in such a way that any deformity of varus or valgus is corrected at the same time. A bed is prepared on the lateral aspects of the tibia and talus to which is screwed the freshened fibular fragment. Because of the application of a lateral graft there is a tendency for the ankle to be tilted into valgus as the graft is screwed home. Great care must be taken to ensure that the bones are firmly clamped together in the correct position before the fibula is fixed into place. The fixation secured in this way is so sound that after simple protection of the limb in plaster for about 12 weeks, firm fusion of the joint is assured (Figs 33.76 and 33.77).

Compression arthrodesis of the ankle. Early compression techniques[109, 110] were further developed by Charnley[111] and his technique has a very high fusion rate but is technically a little more difficult than the previous operation. Charnley has emphasised the importance of adhering to the operative details he describes, and although a number of surgeons have attempted various modifications these have often led to difficulties and it is wiser to follow carefully the original method.

The operation is carried out through a transverse incision extending to the tips of the malleoli and curving distally towards the foot in order to avoid a scar immediately over the site of tendon division. All structures over the front of the ankle (including vessels and nerve) are divided at joint level, stay sutures having been previously inserted on each side of the site of tendon section. This approach allows the joint surfaces to be resected transversely with a saw in a similar way to the method described by Charnley for knee fusion. During the resection it is important to protect the vessels at the back of the medial malleolus by passing a lever behind this part of the tibia, since the posterior tibial artery and vein are the only remaining major vessels of supply to the foot. The resected surfaces can then be clamped together using Steinmann pins through the talus and tibia (Fig 33.78). A common error is to place the talar pin too far back—it should pass through the front half of the body of the talus and the talus should be located well back on the cut tibial surface or the heel will be foreshortened (Fig 30.79). The compression clamps are tightened daily initially and retained for four weeks. The pins are then removed and the plaster changed to a well-fitting, below-knee walking cast which is worn until 12 weeks from operation.

Union after compression arthrodesis is rapid and certain (Fig 33.79) and, contrary to widespread belief, the swelling and stiffness of the toes which theoretically might be expected rarely occurs. There are, however, two disadvantages: firstly, if the

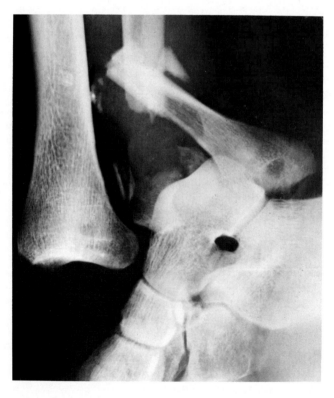

Fig 33.76 Severe fracture-dislocation of the ankle joint which was first reduced by manipulation and immobilised in plaster, but in which the injury to the joint surfaces was so grave that traumatic arthritis soon developed.

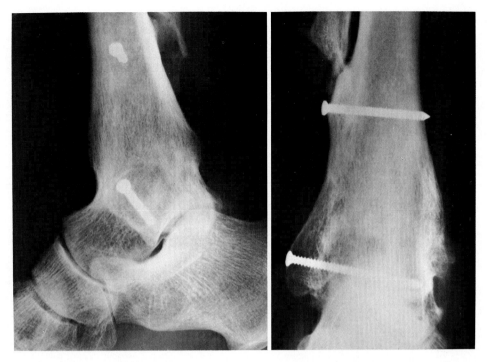

Fig 33.77 Two years later the ankle joint was arthrodesed by the method described in the text of denuding the ankle joint surfaces of cartilage and screwing the lower part of the fibula to the lateral side of the talus and tibia. This resulted in a patient able to walk without a limp and with apparently virtually normal foot movement. (Case of the late Sir Reginald Watson-Jones.)

transverse osteotomies are not made correctly there is little margin for refashioning them to adjust the position and very great care is required at this stage of the operation; secondly, if there is any suspicion of posterior tibial arterial insufficiency, possibly resulting from previous trauma, an alternative method of arthrodesis which does not divide the anterior tibial neurovascular bundle must be employed.

Posterior arthrodesis of the ankle joint (Fig 33.80 and 33.81). White described an excellent technique where, with the patient prone, a midline, straight skin incision is made over the Achilles tendon, which is then divided as for the standard tendon lengthening procedure in a long Z-fashion[112]. The posterior capsule of the ankle joint can then be widely exposed and divided. A slot is cut into the tibia and talus, extending well anteriorly into the ankle joint, the foot being carefully held in the desired degree of plantar flexion—usually 5 to 10 degrees. A full thickness, tailored, slightly oversized cortico-cancellous graft is then cut from the posterior iliac crest and

when this graft is impacted into the prepared slot the ankle is firmly held. The wound is closed after suture of the joint capsule and Achilles tendon and plaster cast immobilisation is continued for 12 to 16 weeks until radiological union.

The author has modified this technique by internally fixing the ankle joint using two cancellous lag screws on either side of the prepared slot, the screws passing obliquely downwards and forwards from the tibia, across the joint and into the talus. As rigidity of fixation is provided with the screws, a block of graft is no longer required and the slot can then be filled with cancellous iliac chip grafts providing more reliable and rapid incorporation. Protection with a simple below knee cast is then used for 12 to 16 weeks (Fig 33.81).

OPEN FRACTURE-DISLOCATIONS OF THE ANKLE JOINT

Dislocations and fracture-dislocations of the ankle joint are not infrequently compound because the

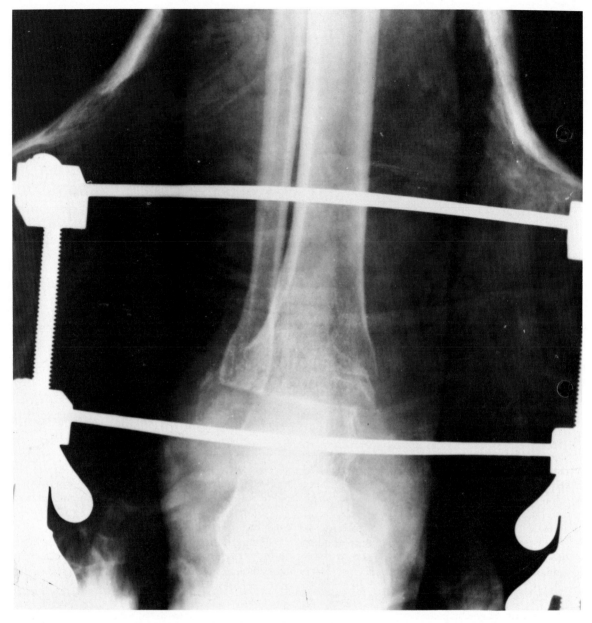

Fig 33.78 X-ray showing a Charnley compression arthrodesis of the ankle for degenerative arthritis following mal-union of an ankle fracture.

malleoli of the tibia and fibula are situated immediately beneath the skin. If there is severe deformity with gross displacement of the foot to one side the skin over the opposite side of the ankle may be split, and the flaps are button-holed round the lower end of

the leg bones leaving the articular surface of the joint exposed in the wound. The soft tissue injury may be very extensive, but nevertheless the injury is compound from within (Fig 33.82). The wound occurs because the tibia or fibula bursts outwards (Fig

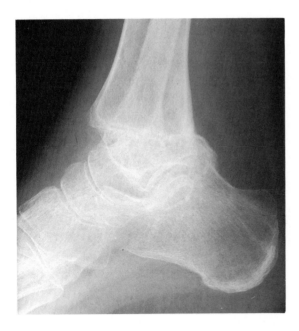

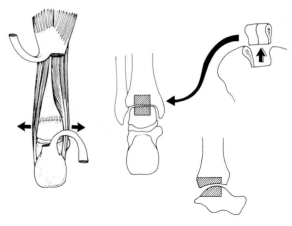

Fig 33.80 White posterior ankle fusion. The back of the ankle is exposed by dividing the Achilles tendon, a slot is cut across the ankle joint as shown and tailored cortico-cancellous iliac grafts punched into this cavity.

Fig 33.79 After 10 weeks fusion is certain. This X-ray, taken 12 weeks after a compression arthrodesis, shows how the talus should be set well back on the tibia to avoid the appearance of a shortened heel.

33.83), and rarely by reason of a direct crushing injury which devitalises tissues and drives foreign bodies into deep recesses. The prognosis is therefore excellent. By suitable operative treatment, first-intention healing is usually possible over most of the length of the wound.

The principles of the management of all open skeletal injuries apply. The wound should be thoroughly cleansed and a meticulous layer by layer excision of all devitalised tissues undertaken.

Any unstable fracture must be stabilised as this greatly aids soft tissue healing. The method of achieving such stability will depend on the experience of the surgeon and the facilities available, but if internal fixation is indicated and practicable, the fact that one is faced with an open injury is not a contraindication. Indeed, the greater the soft tissue wounding, the more imperative is it to stabilise the skeletal injury adequately.

There is no better account of the principles of the management of open fractures than that of Hampton (1955)[113] which should be compulsory reading for any surgeon dealing with injured patients.

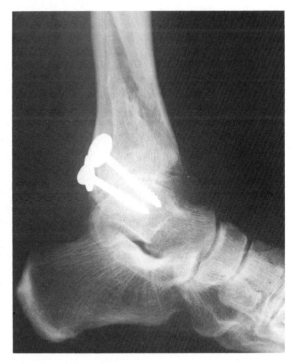

Fig 33.81 The author (CLC) has modified the White posterior fusion by internally fixing the ankle using two cancellous lag screws inserted after cutting the slot. The slot is then packed with cancellous bone chips (rather than blocks) to achieve earlier incorporation).

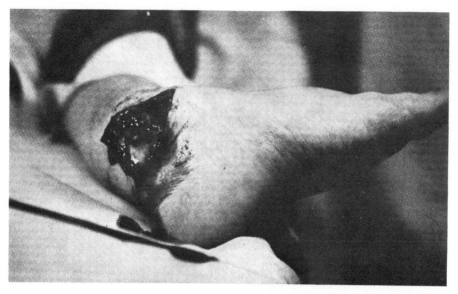

Fig 33.82 Compound fracture-dislocation of the ankle with open wounding from within out. This is the most common type of wound associated with ankle fractures and results in little devitalisation of tissue. The degree of contamination is variable.

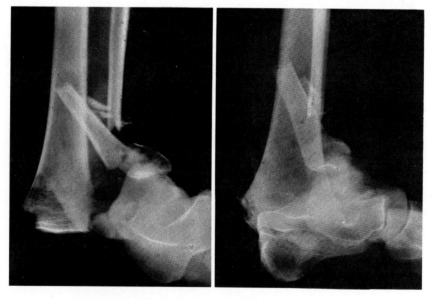

Fig 33.83 Same case as shown in Figure 33.82. The injury is a severe pronation-external rotation fracture-dislocation with an additional fracture of the lateral malleolus.

REFERENCES

1. Dupuytren G 1819 Mémoire sur la fracture de l'extrémité inférieure du péroné, les luxations et les accidents qui en sont la suite. Annuaire médico-chirurgical des Hôpitaux et Hospices Civils de Paris 1 : 1

2. Bonnin J G 1950 Injuries to the ankle. Heinemann Medical Books, London, p 3

3. Maisonneuve J G 1840 Recherches sur la fracture du péroné. Archives générales de médecine 1 : 165 and 433

4. Hughes S P F 1975 An historical review of fractures involving the ankle joint. Mayo Clinic Proceedings 50 : 611

5. Ashhurst A P C, Bromer R S 1922 Classifications and mechanism of fractures of the leg bones involving the ankle. Archives of Surgery 4 : 51

6. Lauge-Hansen N 1950 Fractures of the ankle. II Combined experimental-surgical and experimental-roentgenologic investigations. Archives of Surgery 60 : 957

7. Golterman A F L 1964 Diagnosis and treatment of tibio-fibular diastasis. Archivum Chirurgicum Neerlandicum 16 : 185

8. Kleiger B 1968 Ankle fractures due to lateral strains. Bulletin of the Hospital for Joint Diseases 29 : 138

9. Leonard M H 1954 Sprained ankle may be more serious injury than fracture. The American Surgeon 20 : 660

10. Lettin A W F 1963 Diagnosis and treatment of sprained ankle. British Medical Journal i : 1056

11. Monk C J E 1969 Injuries of the tibio-fibular ligaments. Journal of Bone and Joint Surgery 51-B : 330

12. Tillaux (reported by Gosselin) (1872). Rapports Recherches; cliniques et expérimentales sur les fractures malléolaires. Bulletin de l'Académie de Médecine, Series 2, 1 : 817

13. Huguier P C 1848 Mémoire sur les luxations du pied considérées en général et sur une nouvelle espèce de luxation par rotation du pied en dehors. Union Médicale de Paris 2 : 120

14. Cobb N 1965 Oblique radiography in the diagnosis of ankle injuries. Proceedings of the Royal Society of Medicine 58 : 334

15. Manter J T 1941 Movements of the subtalar and transverse tarsal joints. The Anatomical Record 80 : 397

16. Rose G K 1962 Ankle injuries. In : Clark J M P (ed) Modern trends in orthopaedics, 3. Fracture treatment, Butterworth, London, p 161

17. Phillips R S, Balmer G A, Monk C J E 1969 The external rotation fracture of the fibular malleolus. British Journal of Surgery 56 : 801

18. Iselin M, de Vellis H 1961 La primauté du péroné dans les fractures du cou-de-pied. Mémoire de l'Académie de Chirurgie 87 : 399

19. Weber B G, Vasey H 1963 Osteosynthese bei olekranonfraktur. Zeitschrift für Unfallmedizin und Berufskrankheiten 56 : 90

20. Broström L 1964 Sprained ankles. Acta Chirurgica Scandinavica 128 : 483

21. Staples O S 1965 Ligamentous injuries of the ankle. Clinical Orthopaedics and Related Research 42 : 21

22. Spiegel P K, Staples O S 1975 Arthrography of the ankle joint : problems in diagnosis of acute lateral ligament injuries. Radiology 114 : 587

23. Coltart W D 1951 Sprained ankle. British Medical Journal ii : 957

24. Rubin G, Witten M 1960 The talar-tilt angle and the fibular collateral ligaments. A method for the determination of talar tilt. Journal of Bone and Joint Surgery 42-A : 311

25. Dziob J M 1956 Ligamentous injuries about the ankle joint. American Journal of Surgery, 91 : 692

26. Freeman M A R 1965 Treatment of ruptures of the lateral ligament of the ankle. Journal of Bone and Joint Surgery 47-B : 661

27. Hughes J R 1955 The articular damage in complete ruptures of the lateral ligaments of the ankle. Journal of Bone and Joint Surgery 37-B : 723

28. Sherrod H H, Phillips J D 1961 The surgical care of severe sprains of the ankle. Southern Medical Journal 54 : 1379

29. Davis M W 1970 Bilateral talar osteochondritis dissecans with lax ankle ligaments. Journal of Bone and Joint Surgery 52-A : 168

30. Evans D L 1957 Recurrent instability of the ankle joint. Journal of Bone and Joint Surgery 39-B : 795

31. Pennal G F 1943 Subluxation of the ankle. Canadian Medical Association Journal 49 : 92

32. Burwell H N, Charnley A D 1965 The treatment of displaced fractures at the ankle by rigid internal fixation and early joint movement. Journal of Bone and Joint Surgery 47-B : 634

33. Hachez-Leblanc M 1950 Le vissage direct des fractures trimalléolaires basses par torsion, avec diastasis tibio-astragalien. Acta Orthopaedica Belgica 16 : 307

34. Meekison D M 1945 Some remarks on three common fractures. Journal of Bone and Joint Surgery 27 : 80

35. Sneppen O 1972 Malleolar pseudarthrosis. Munksgaard, Copenhagen

36. Duval P, Basset A 1923 Traitement des fractures bi-malléolaires. Bulletin et Mémoires de la Société de chirurgie de Paris 49 : 1415

37. Colton C L 1971 The treatment Dupuytren's fracture-dislocation of the ankle. Journal of Bone and Joint Surgery 53-B : 63

38. Denham R A 1964 Internal fixation for unstable ankle fractures. Journal of Bone and Joint Surgery 46-B : 206

39. Danis R 1949 Théorie et pratique de l'ostéosynthèse. Masson, Paris, p 142

40. Desenfans G 1959 Réflexions au sujet du traitement du diastasis tibio-péronier à la suite d'une dislocation importante ouverte du tarse. Acta Orthopaedica Belgica 25 : 279

41. Jergesen F 1959 Open reduction of fractures and dislocations of the ankle. American Journal of Surgery 98 : 136

42. Rienau G 1970 Manuel de traumatologie, 3rd edn. Masson, Paris

43. Vasli S 1957 Operative treatment of ankle fractures. Acta Chirurgica Scandinavica, Suppl. 226 : 40

44. Cargill A J 1974 Personal communication.

45. Lapidus P W, Guidotti F P 1968 Immediate mobilisation and swimming pool exercises in some fractures of foot and ankle bones. Clinical Orthopaedics 56 : 197

46. Braunstein P W, Wade P A 1959 Treatment of unstable fractures of the ankle. Annals of Surgery 149 : 217

47. Burgess E 1944 Fractures of the ankle. Journal of Bone and Joint Surgery 26 : 721

48. Cedell C.-A 1967 Supination-outward rotation injuries of the ankle. Acta Orthopaedica Scandinavica, Suppl. 110

49. Desenfans G, Evrard H 1952 Le traitement chirurgical des fractures du cou-de-pied. Acta Orthopaedica Belgica 18 : 303

50. Stören G 1964 Conservative treatment of ankle fractures. Acta Chirurgica Scandinavica 128: 45

51. Charnley J 1957 The closed treatment of common fractures, 2nd edn. Livingstone, Edinburgh, p 243

52. Devlies A 1959 Résultats éloignés du vissage direct dans les fractures malléolaires par torsion. Acta Orthopaedica Belgica 25: 131

53. Frankel C J, McCue F, Humphries D 1963 Injuries to the ankle. Southern Medical Journal 56: 402

54. Hodgkinson R 1967 Surgical management of fracture-dislocations of the ankle. Medical Journal of Australia 1: 1014

55. Lee H G, Horan T B 1943 Internal fixation in injuries of the ankle. Surgery, Gynecology and Obstetrics 76: 593

56. Lewis R W, Graham W C 1940 Secondary osteoarthritis following fractures of the ankle. American Journal of Surgery 49: 210

57. Martinez C, Rienau G, Gay R, Mansat C H 1970 Résultats du traitement sanglant des fractures malléolaires. Revue de Chirurgie Orthopédique 56: 665

58. Coonrad R W, Bugg E I 1954 Trapping of the posterior tibial tendon and interposition of soft tissue in severe fractures about the ankle joint. Journal of Bone and Joint Surgery 36-A: 744

59. Lambert K L 1971 The weight-bearing function of the fibula. Journal of Bone and Joint Surgery 53-A: 507

60. Close J R, Inman V T 1952 The action of the ankle joint. Prosthetic Devices Research Project, Institute of Engineering Research, University of California (Berkeley), Advisory Committee on Artificial Limbs, National Research Council, Series II: Issue 22

61. Hirsch C, Lewis J 1965 Experimental ankle joint fractures. Acta Orthopaedica Scandinavica 36: 408

62. Rüedi T P, Allgöwer M 1969 Fractures of the lower end of the tibia into the ankle joint. Injury 1: 92

63. Gay R, Evrard J 1963 Les fractures récentes du pilon tibial chez l'adulte. Revue de Chirurgie Orthopédique 49: 397

64. Müller M E 1964 Les fractures du pilon tibial. Revue de Chirurgie Orthopédique 50: 557

65. Weber B G 1965 Behandlung der Sprunggelenks—Stauchungsbrüche nach biomechanischen Gesichtspunkten. Hefte Unfallheilkunde 81: 176

66. Salter R B, Harris W R 1963 Injuries involving the epiphyseal plate. Journal of Bone and Joint Surgery 45-A: 587

67. Harris W R 1958 Epiphyseal injuries. In: Instructional course lectures of the American academy of orthopaedic surgeons. Edwards, Ann Arbor vol 15, p 206

68. Broock G J, Greer R B 1970 Traumatic rotational displacements of the distal tibial growth plate. Journal of Bone and Joint Surgery 52-A: 1666

69. Lovell E S 1968 An unusual rotatory injury of the ankle. Journal of Bone and Joint Surgery 50-A: 163

70. Nevelos A B, Colton C L 1977 Rotational displacement of the lower tibial epiphysis due to trauma. Journal of Bone and Joint Surgery 59-B: 331

71. Werenskiold B 1927 A contribution to the röntgen diagnosis of epiphyseal separations. Acta Radiologica 8: 419

72. Carothers C O, Crenshaw A H 1955 Clinical significance of a classification of epiphyseal injuries at the ankle. American Journal of Surgery 89: 879

73. McFarland B 1931 Traumatic arrest of epiphyseal growth at the lower end of the tibia. British Journal of Surgery 19: 78

74. Aitken A P 1936 The end results of the fractured distal tibial epiphysis. Journal of Bone and Joint Surgery 18: 685

75. Böhler L 1958 The treatment of fractures. Vol. III, p. 1857. London & New York: Grune & Stratton

76. Österman K 1972 Operative elimination of partial premature epiphyseal closure. Acta Orthopaedica Scandinavica Suppl., 147

77. Langenskiold A 1975 An operation for partial closure of an epiphyseal plate in children, and its experimental basis. Journal of Bone and Joint Surgery 57-B: 325

78. Kleiger B, Mankin H J 1964 Fracture of the lateral portion of the distal tibial epiphysis. Journal of Bone and Joint Surgery 46-A: 25

79. Mølster A, Søreide O, Solhaug J H, Raugstad T S 1977 Fractures of the lateral part of the distal tibial epiphysis (Tillaux or Kleiger fracture). Injury 8: 260

80. Robertson D E 1964 Post-traumatic osteochondritis of the lower tibial epiphysis. Journal of Bone and Joint Surgery 46-B: 212

81. Siffert R, Arkin A 1950 Post-traumatic aseptic necrosis of the distal tibial epiphysis. Journal of Bone and Joint Surgery 32-A: 691

82. Baumgartuer R, Jani L, Herzog B 1975 Verletzung des Ligamentum fibulo-talare im Kindesalter. Helvetica Chirurgica Acta 42: 443

83. Jani L, Baumgartner R, Mayer S 1976 Lesione del legamento peroneo-astragalico nei bambini. Bolletina dell' AO Italiano 14: 1

84. Bröstrom L, Liljedahl S O, Lindvahl N 1964 Isolated fracture of the posterior tibial tubercle. Acta Chirurgica Scandinavica 128: 51

85. D'Anca A F 1970 Lateral rotatory dislocation of the ankle without fracture. Journal of Bone and Joint Surgery 52-A: 1643

86. Fonda M P 1952 Dislocation of the tibio-fibular joint without fracture. An unusual ski injury. Journal of Bone and Joint Surgery 34-A: 662

87. Ikpeme J O 1970 Compound complete dislocation of the ankle joint without fracture or diastasis. Injury 1: 186

88. Olerud S 1971 Subluxation of the ankle without fracture of the fibula. Journal of Bone and Joint Surgery 53-A: 594

89. Poinot J, Doutre L P 1946 Un cas de luxation tibio-tarsienne totale, sans fracture. Bordeaux Chirurgical 3-4: 74

90. Scott J E 1974 Dislocation of the ankle without fracture. Injury 6: 63

91. Wilson M J, Michele A A, Jacobson E W 1939 Ankle dislocations without fracture. Journal of Bone and Joint Surgery 21: 198

92. Woods R S 1942 Irreducible dislocation of the ankle joint. British Journal of Surgery, 29: 359

93. Bosworth D M 1947 Fracture-dislocation of the ankle with fixed displacement of the fibula behind the tibia. Journal of Bone and Joint Surgery 29: 130

94. Fahey J J, Murphy J L 1965 Dislocations and fractures of the talus. Surgical Clinics of North America 45: 79

95. Fleming J L, Smith H O 1954 Fracture dislocation of the ankle with the fibula fixed behind the tibia. Journal of Bone and Joint Surgery 36-A: 556

96. Langer B 1967 Fracture-dislocation of the ankle with trapped fibula: report of two cases. Canadian Journal of Surgery 10: 308

97. Meyers M H 1965 Fracture about the ankle joint with fixed displacement of the proximal fragment of the fibula behind the tibia. Clinical Orthopaedics 42: 67

98. Mullins J F P, Sallis J G 1958 Recurrent sprain of the ankle joint with diastasis. Journal of Bone and Joint Surgery 40-B: 270

99. Le Fort 1866 Note sur une variété non-décrit de fracture verticale de la malléole externe, par arrachement. Bulletin Général de Thérapie, Paris 110: 93

100. Wagstaffe W W 1875 An unusual form of fracture of the fibula. St. Thomas's Hospital Reports 6: 43

101. Kelly R E 1920 An operation for the chronic dislocation of the peroneal tendons. British Journal of Surgery 7: 502

102. McMurray T P 1950 Footballer's ankle. Journal of Bone and Joint Surgery 32-B: 68

103. Morris L H 1943 Athlete's ankle. Journal of Bone and Joint Surgery 25: 220

104. Watson-Jones R 1952 Recurrent forward dislocation of the ankle. Journal of Bone and Joint Surgery 34-B: 519

105. Landeros O, Frost H M, Higgins C C 1968 Post-traumatic anterior ankle instability. Clinical Orthopaedics 56: 169

106. Simon W H, Friedenburg S, Richardson S 1973 Joint congruence. Journal of Bone and Joint Surgery 55-A: 1614

107. Cox F J, Laxson W W 1952 Fractures about the ankle joint. American Journal of Surgery 83: 674

108. Adams J C 1948 Arthrodesis of the ankle joint. Journal of Bone and Joint Surgery 30-B: 506

109. Anderson R 1945 Concentric arthrodesis of the ankle joint. Journal of Bone and Joint Surgery 27: 37

110. White J W 1945 In discussion on arthrodesis of the ankle. Journal of Bone and Joint Surgery 27: 58

111. Charnley J 1951 Compression arthrodesis of the ankle and shoulder. Journal of Bone and Joint Surgery 33-B: 180

112. White A A 1974 A precision posterior ankle fusion. Clinical Orthopaedics, and Related Research. 98: 239

113. Hampton O P, Jnr 1955 Basic principles in management of open fractures. Journal of American Medical Association 159: 417

34

Injuries of the Foot

Injuries of the foot are all too often a neglected part of traumatic surgery. Yet this is an area of the body where soft tissue, joint, or bone disorders can be responsible for long standing periods of morbidity, structural deformity, and occasionally severe functional disability. The foot has a complex structure and joint mechanism with a result that many of the fracture patterns and joint injuries are bizarre, difficult to interpret, and even more difficult to treat. It is because of this very complexity that some surgeons have come to regard many of the injuries as impossible to treat by the conventional methods of reduction and immobilisation and to insist upon an immediate restoration of function as the first priority, completely disregarding the first principles of fracture treatment which would be applied to any other bone or joint injury elsewhere in the body. Very often difficulty in analysing a type of fracture leads to every variety of it being lumped together and given a common form of treatment. Fractures of the calcaneum are a good example of this philosophy, for many difficult fracture patterns exist and yet frequently the same treatment is applied to all. Also, minor fractures and joint displacements, particularly in the mid-tarsal and tarso-metatarsal joints, are sometimes passed off as unimportant soft tissue injuries, treated by exercises alone with the early chance to reduce displacement being lost forever. The blame of this can often be traced to blind adherence to negative X-ray reports when the history and findings on clinical examination should have made the diagnosis clear. If a negative X-ray report belies the severity of the clinical appearance, then the X-ray must be studied again. Other views may be required, particularly when considering injuries of the hindfoot (Figs 34.1 and 34.2). It is only by the careful study of both clinical and radiological findings that the true significance of many foot injuries can be fully understood.

The injuries will be considered under three headings:

1. Soft tissue injuries.
2. Fractures and dislocations of the hindfoot (calcaneum and talus).
3. Fractures and dislocations of the forefoot (distal tarsus, metatarsus and toes).

SOFT TISSUE INJURIES

Because of the vulnerable position of the feet soft tissue injuries resulting from direct trauma, from twisting or wrenching injuries, or from crush fractures are commonplace and are often associated with extensive swelling, gross pain and marked limitation of function. The less severe injuries, provided there is no serious skin loss, bone involvement, or vascular complication respond satisfactorily to elevation and bandaging, either at home or preferably in hospital. At the other end of the scale severe crushing injuries may be accompanied by considerable skin damage, with underlying injury to tendons and muscles (Fig 34.3). These injuries can present a formidable problem of treatment, particularly if there is an associated bone or joint injury, and their management will be discussed later. Nevertheless, let it be said now that it is rarely wise to attempt primary skin closure in these injuries and that the bone and joint complications which may be present often produce difficulties of management which are considerable. However, the soft tissue lesions we will now consider are not of this dramatic nature. None the less, if their significance is not fully understood and the appropriate treatment given, long periods of disability can be the result.

Minor crush and twist injuries. Because of their very frequency and minor nature, and in the absence

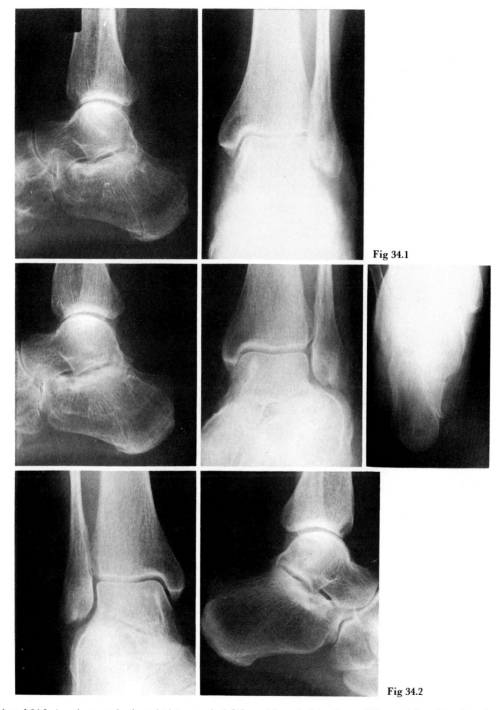

Fig 34.1

Fig 34.2

Figs 34.1 and 34.2 A patient sustained a twist injury to the left foot while on holiday. Several X-rays of the ankle taken after the injury were reported as normal (Fig 34.1). Comparison films of both ankles taken almost a year after injury showed a possible fracture of the thalamic part of the os calcis (Fig 34.2). This was confirmed by the heel view (inset). Although the patient had made an excellent recovery and had almost full function, she threatened to sue those who had failed to diagnose the fracture initially. Beware of the 'soft tissue' injury of the foot with persistent symptoms—careful re-examination of the X-ray films may reveal a previously unrecognised fracture.

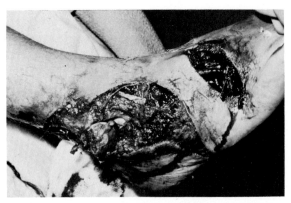

Fig 34.3 A severe soft tissue injury to the foot and ankle due to crushing under the wheel of a heavy earth moving vehicle. Primary skin closure cannot be carried out safely in this type of injury.

of X-ray changes, the treatment of these injuries is often neglected; and even though the local signs of trauma may be obvious the patient is told that 'as the X-ray is normal' no serious damage can have occurred. He or she is persuaded to keep the limb dependant and to continue to walk, and often despite vigorous protests encouraged to take weight on the injured foot; sometimes the victim is even shamed into removing the supporting bandages, which at least are controlling some of the soft tissue oedema. As has been said in an earlier chapter (see Chapter 4) oedema forms the glue which is later responsible for adhesion formation and sometimes permanent stiffness. Prevention of the detrimental effects of oedema is the very essence of the primary treatment of soft tissue injuries of the foot.

A careful clinical and radiological examination is mandatory to exclude bone injury or tarsal subluxation and provided there is no displacement which could require reduction, the limb should be elevated and supported by a firm wool and crepe bandage applied from the toes to the knee. Bed rest with elevation applied early for a few days is time well spent and may prevent many weeks of unnecessary swelling and pain. It should be followed by a graduated return to normal walking, maintaining the support of bandages until the postural oedema is reduced to a minimum. Surgeons should be particularly wary of the patient (usually a woman) whose foot remains persistently painful and swollen and who, after a relatively minor injury, develops a shiny, tender and atrophic skin. She may be developing the first signs of Sudek's atrophy (reflex sympathetic

dystrophy*). This has already been fully discussed in Chapter 4.

Spoke injuries from bicycle and moped accidents. An injury which is peculiar to this type of accident has been described by a number of authors.[2,3] It takes the form of a particularly unpleasant laceration of the heel. The victim is usually a child and is always the pillion passenger. As the result of a jolt or swerve the foot slips off the passenger's footrest (which in a number of the cases reported was found to be deficient) and the heel is caught up in the spokes of the back wheel. This can produce an avulsion flap of skin based caudally and medially which has a very uncertain blood supply. These injuries are commonly on the right side because on a motor-cycle the chain guard usually protects the left foot. When there is an avulsion injury the flap is often grossly contaminated and requires a wide and thorough debridement. *The skin should never be closed by primary suture.* Delayed primary suture a week or so after the injury may allow complete closure, or at least enable repair to be made by skin graft.

Foreign bodies in the foot. In Westernised societies where shoes are worn for most of the day foreign bodies in the foot are relatively uncommon and usually result from needles or wood splinters entering through the sole when walking around the house without shoes or slippers. However, there are a number of reports of larger foreign bodies presenting as deep infections without any clear history of previous trauma.[4,5] Some have even been mistaken for tumour. Such a case is illustrated in Figures 34.4 to 34.6. It should always be remembered that fairly large fragments of foreign material can be introduced into the tissues in any part of the body with minimal trauma and possibly no recollection of an injury. The foot, by virtue of its exposed position, is particularly vulnerable.

The post-traumatic sinus tarsi syndrome.[6,7] This condition has been reported as a cause of the persistent ache and tenderness which sometimes occurs over the outer side of the subtaloid joint after an ankle or foot sprain, and may be associated with hypertrophy of the lateral fat pad of the ankle. It has

* It is important to distinguish Sudek's atrophy (which is always post-traumatic) from transient painful osteoporosis of the lower extremities.[1] Although this presents as a painful osteoporosis with swelling it differs from Sudek's atrophy in that there is never any history of preceding trauma, no painful muscle spasm and the symptoms flit from place to place.

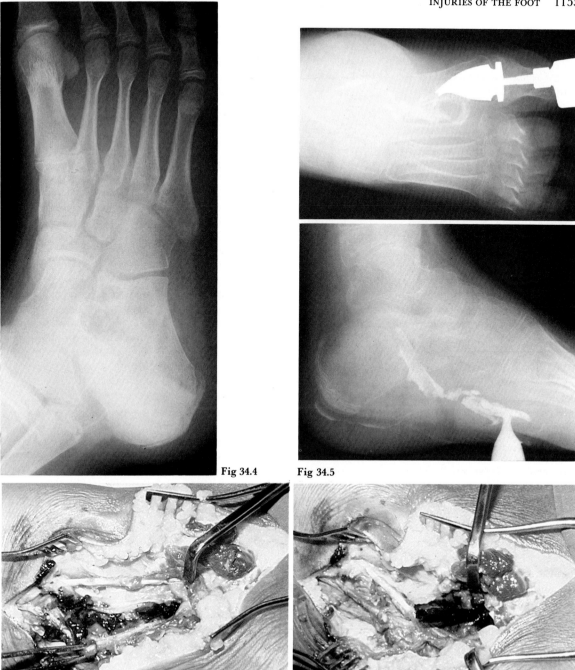

Fig 34.4   Fig 34.5

Fig 34.6

Figs 34.4 to 34.6 A boy of 12 presented with a tender swelling in the sole of his foot near to the neck of the third metatarsal. There was no history of injury. Any movement of the subtaloid joint was painful and X-rays showed an erosion of the sinus tarsi (Fig 34.4). Exploration of the swelling and the subtaloid joint showed only chronic granulations and did not relieve his symptoms. A sinogram some months later (Fig 34.5) suggested that the infection arose in a tendon sheath, but at further exploration (after a methylene blue injection) the sinus was found to lead down to a wooden splinter (seen dyed blue) lodged in the medial side of the subtaloid joint (Figure 34.6).

been attributed to synovial hyperplasia developing around the ligamentous tissue within the sinus tarsi secondary to a rupture of the calcaneo-fibular ligament.[7] Excision of the contents of the sinus tarsi with removal of the fat pad is claimed to relieve the symptoms.[6]

Plantar fascial strain.[8] The common ailment of a painful heel in the adult, although rarely associated with a history of injury, is nevertheless basically traumatic in origin and is closely related to other strains of fibrous tissue such as tennis elbow (see Chapter 22—the fibrilosis syndrome). Like all lesions of this nature it is characterised by a very localised area of tenderness. In the heel the tender spot is situated on the medial side of the calcaneum exactly corresponding to the attachment of the long plantar ligament. Pain is brought on by weight-bearing and is always at its worst when the patient first gets out of bed in the morning. X-rays may show that there is a plantar spur arising from the under surface of the calcaneum but this is not the cause of the condition and is often to be found also on the symptomless side. Provided the tenderness can be accurately localised the condition will usually respond to an injection of 2 ml of cortisone mixture.* This treatment should be augmented by phenylbutazone given in standard doses by mouth for 14 days. As this lesion is probably due to a minute tear of the fibrous attachments to the calcaneum it is important to protect the tender area for several months after the initial treatment by fitting the patient with high sorbo heel elevators. These must be at least 1 inch (2.5 cm) in height (the thin pieces of sorbo often sold for this purpose are quite useless) and they must be worn on both sides in order to give the patient an even gait. As a last resort in resistant cases a Steindler type of stripping of the plantar attachments to the heel can be carried out, and at the same time any bony prominence resulting from a plantar spur can be removed. However, it is never necessary to operate simply because of the presence of a spur.

Tendonitis around the foot. Any of the major tendons of the foot can become afflicted with a painful tendonitis or teno-vaginitis, but the tendo Achillis, the peroneal tendons and the tendon of tibialis posterior are by far the most common to be affected. Inflammation around the tendo Achillis is seen frequently in new army recruits wearing heavy boots

* Cortisone mixture consists of 25 mg of hydrocortisone acetate, 1500 units of hyalase with 1 per cent lignocaine made up at the time of injection.

for the first time. It produces disabling pain so long as boots continue to be worn and is accompanied by a creaking feeling whenever the tendon is put on stretch. The symptoms can be relieved immediately by a change to shoes and there is rarely any recurrence after a return to boots a week or so later. A chronic form of this condition is sometimes seen in long distance runners and may require local cortisone, or even stripping of the tendon to relieve the symptoms.

Peroneal tendonitis may occur as a late complication of fracture of the calcaneum and the clinical features and treatment will be considered later in this chapter. Tendonitis of the tibialis posterior tendon[9] is rarely associated with direct injury but is usually related to a gradually increasing strain in a valgus foot. Very occasionally it may present as the first sign of rheumatoid arthritis. The signs and symptoms are always the same, the patient complaining of pain over the inner side of the ankle which may sometimes be attributed to a minor injury, with obvious swelling and tenderness localised to the tendon as it passes around the medial malleolus. This condition quickly responds to a local injection of cortisone mixture (see footnote), followed by the fitting of a longitudinal arch support.

FRACTURES OF THE CALCANEUM

When a builder or window cleaner falls from a height and lands on his feet a vertical force is driven through the foot and ankle, and the talus is compressed between the tibia and calcaneum. Similarly when a soldier stands on a land-mine, or a sailor on deck suffers the effects of underwater explosion, there is vertical compression of the bones—this time from below up instead of from above down. The wedge-shaped inferior aspect of the talus is driven into the calcaneum in the angle between the anterior and posterior talo-calcaneal joints which has been described as the critical angle.[10] The calcaneum may be split, compressed and displaced; sometimes the talus itself is fractured; and if the vertical compression is applied in a slightly different direction it may cause fracture of the lower end of the tibia with forward displacement of the foot. Nor is the force necessarily expended on the foot or ankle alone. In 5 to 12 per cent associated fracture of the vertebral bodies has been reported,[11,12] and an important part of the examination of the patient with vertical compression injury of the foot is clinical and radiographic study of the lumbo-dorsal spine.

Minor fractures of the calcaneum are often overlooked because superficial examination may seem to show free mobility with no obvious deformity, the symptoms then being attributed to simple contusion or sprain. It should be enough to know that a patient has fallen from a height, sometimes only from a chair or table, and having landed flat on his foot complains of pain in the heel or mid-tarsal region. In the child, although a rare injury, the fracture is frequently misdiagnosed as a sprain.[13] Fortunately this is of little consequence because calcanean fractures give no residual disability in children. This is not the case however in adult fractures which are not infrequently missed, particularly those involving the anterior part of the bone.[14]

Classification

Many classifications of calcanean fractures have been suggested.[15-20] They are all broadly similar, emphasising the distinction between fractures of the calcaneum which do not involve the subtalar joint, and fractures into the joint with varying degrees of damage and displacement of joint surfaces. The fractures which do not affect the subtalar joint are in the minority and in 80 per cent of cases this joint is involved to a greater or lesser extent.[19] The classification presented below is based upon that proposed by Warrick and Bremner and many of the X-ray illustrations have been taken from their paper.[17]

Fractures of the calcaneum not involving the subtalar joint. (Figs 34.7 to 34.10).

1. Vertical fracture of the tuberosity (Fig 34.7).
2. Horizontal fracture of the tuberosity (Fig 34.8).
3. Fracture of the sustentaculum tali (Fig 34.9).
4. Fracture of the anterior end of the calcaneum (Fig 34.10).

Fractures of the calcaneum involving the subtalar joint (Figs 34.11 to 34.14).

5. Fractures adjacent to but not entering the subtalar joint (Fig 34.11).
6. Fracture site with displacement of the lateral part of the subtalar joint (Fig 34.12).
7. Fracture with central crushing of the whole subtalar joint (Fig 34.13).
8. Crush fracture of the subtalar joint and calcaneo-cuboid joint (Fig 34.14).

1. Vertical fracture of the tuberosity of the calcaneum (Fig 34.7). This fracture is caused by a shearing force sustained from a fall in the valgus position which often occurs as an isolated injury and causes relatively little disability. Imperfect reduction may give rise to local thickening and tenderness from projecting spurs. There may be tenderness under the heel in the region of the calcaneal tuberosity where the plantar fascia and muscles are attached, aggravated by the impact of weight-bearing.

2. Horizontal fractures of the tuberosity of the calcaneum (Fig 34.8). These are fractures involving the upper part of the tuberosity with upward tilting of a fragment and have been previously described as beak-fractures to distinguish them from pure avulsion fractures in which an oval-shaped piece of bone is pulled away by traction of the tendo Achillis. It is true that some of the horizontal fractures of the tuberosity are not avulsion fractures but are due to extension backwards into the tuberosity of a secondary horizontal fracture arising from a depressed subtalar joint. The lateral radiograph of Figure 34.12 shows just such an injury, which has been described by Aaron and Howat as a tongue fracture.[20] A few may be due to direct trauma, as suggested by Böhler.[21] But the vast majority of the fractures when explored will be found to be attached to the tendo Achillis and displaced upwards by it.[22,23] This may be caused by an abnormally high insertion of the tendon.[23]

3. Fracture of the sustentaculum tali (Fig 34.9). This fracture is produced by violence applied to the inner side of the foot while it is in an everted or valgus position. As an isolated injury it constitutes less than 1 per cent of all fractures of the calcaneum. The displacement is usually slight and the injury gives rise to little disability.

4. Fracture of the anterior end of the calcaneum (Fig 34.10). Isolated fractures of the anterior end of the calcaneum may be sustained as an avulsion injury from forcible inversion of the foot. The line of fracture extends obliquely into the calcaneo-cuboid joint so that a smaller triangular fragment is detached from the front of the bone. There is seldom displacement and the fracture unites quickly. This should be treated as a ligamentous injury with a short period of immobilisation in a walking plaster. Occasionally, however, the mechanism of injury may be different.[14] The forefoot is forcibly abducted on the hindfoot and a large fragment of the antero-superior articular margin is squeezed dorsally out of the calcaneo-cuboid joint, while at the same time the lower part of the articular surface is compressed backwards (Figs 34.15 and 34.16). This injury may be part of a fracture subluxation of the mid-tarsal joint.[24]

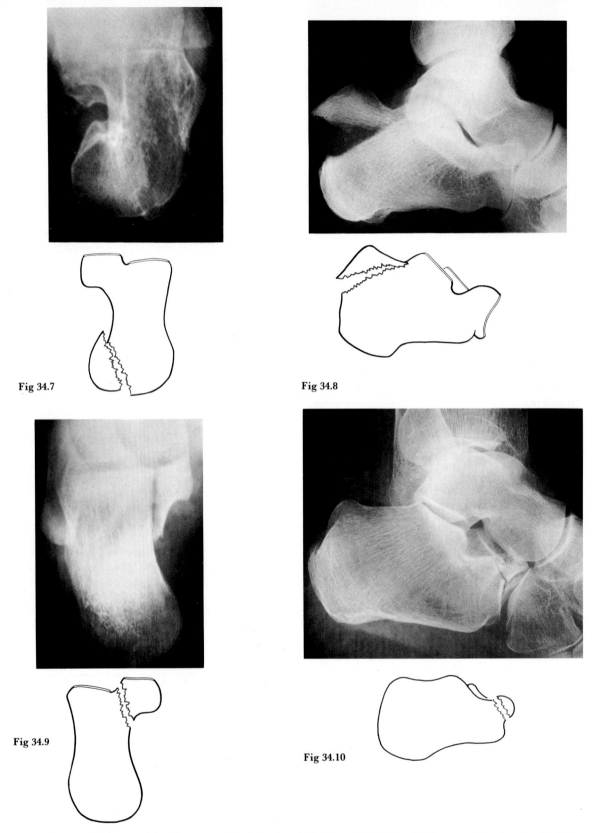

Figs 34.7 to 34.10 Fractures of the calcaneum not involving the subtalar joint. Fig 34.7: Vertical fracture of the tuberosity. Fig 34.8: Horizontal fracture of the tuberosity. Fig 34.9: Fracture of the sustentaculum tali. Fig 34.10: Fracture of the anterior end of the calcaneum.

5. Fractures of the body of the calcaneum without disturbing the subtalar joint (Fig 34.11). When there has been vertical compression with injury to the body of the calcaneum the basic line of fracture runs from the postero-medial to the antero-lateral aspect of the bone, separating a small postero-medial fragment, with the medial part of the subtalar joint and sustentaculum tali, from a large postero-lateral fragment, with most of the tuberosity of the bone and the lateral part of the subtalar joint. This fracture sometimes occurs without displacement of the subtalar surfaces because at its anterior limit it just escapes the joint and lies lateral to it (Fig 34.11).

6. Fractures with displacement of the lateral part of the bone and lateral half of the subtalar joint (Fig 34.12). The main line of fracture extending from the postero-medial to the antero-lateral aspect of the bone is usually associated with displacement of the lateral fragment carrying with it a large part of the subtalar joint surface. It is obvious that if such displacement cannot be corrected there will be serious disturbance of the subtalar joint with at least fibrous ankylosis and perhaps persistent and painful osteoarthritis. In addition to this primary fracture there is usually at least one secondary line of fracture, roughly parallel with the first, involving the lateral cortex of the bone. Between them the main mass of the tuberosity with the lateral part of the subtalar joint is crushed down, with the tilting described so graphically by Morestin[25] as 'like a see-saw, down in the front and up at the back'. The cancellous bone beneath it, in the middle of the calcaneum, is crushed. Nevertheless, there is no complete destruction of the whole subtalar surface, and it is in these fractures that manipulative or operative replacement may occasionally succeed in restoring joint alignment and improving the appearance of the foot. Also, some subtalar joint movement may be restored by operation.

7. Fractures with central crushing and displacement of the whole of the subtalar joint (Fig 34.13 and 34.14). There is sometimes even greater comminution and crushing of the subtalar joint—the fracture with the so-called centro-lateral compression—and often with comminution of the calcaneo-cuboid joint. Because there is depression of the whole of the subtalar segment the injury has been termed a 'thalamic' fracture by Soeur and Remy,[19] the thalamus of the calcaneus being the part which supports the posterior articular facet and extends forwards with the sinus tarsi.

Clinical features

Obvious swelling of the heel, acute local tenderness and gross loss of function of all tarsal joints are always present in any severely displaced fracture of the calcaneum. A valuable diagnostic sign, which can be seen even in the undisplaced fracture, is discolouration of the sole of the foot produced by blood tracking under plantar fascia. But it must be remembered that this may not appear for 24 hours or more (Figs 34.17 and 34.18).

The shape of the calcaneum is such that there is normally an angle between the axis of the tuberosity and the body of the bone which is known as the tuber-joint angle or the salient angle (see inset, Fig 34.19). This is the angle between a line projected back from the subtalar articular surfaces and the line of the upper margin of the tuberosity of the bone. In a normal calcaneum it measures about 40 degrees. If from a compression fracture the tuberosity is displaced upwards or the articular surface is displaced downwards, the angle may be reduced to 20 or 10 degrees. It may also be obliterated altogether, or it may even be represented by a negative angle. This angle should be estimated in determining the degree of upward displacement of the tuberosity, whether from fractures involving the joint or from fractures escaping the joint surfaces. Such upward displacement of the tuberosity, and therefore of the insertion of the tendo Achillis, causes difficulty in standing on tip-toe and impairment of the normal heel and toe movement of walking, which depends upon full power of the calf group of muscles. The upward displacement may amount to as much as 1 inch (2.5 cm). In its functional result this is just the same as if the tendo Achillis had been lengthened by 1 inch (2.5 cm). In consequence there is excessive passive dorsiflexion of the ankle joint as shown in Figure 34.19.

Broadening of the heel, which should be recognised from clinical examination and is seen by radiographs taken in the axial projection, may in itself cause disability, especially when it is associated with valgus displacement of the foot. Later there may be pain from impingement of the tarsal bones against the lateral malleolus,[26] but when this occurs the pain is in part due to compression of the peroneal tendons between the two bones while weight-bearing. A tenolysis during the later stages of recovery will often result in considerable relief of pain and general improvement in foot function.[27] Removal of the tip

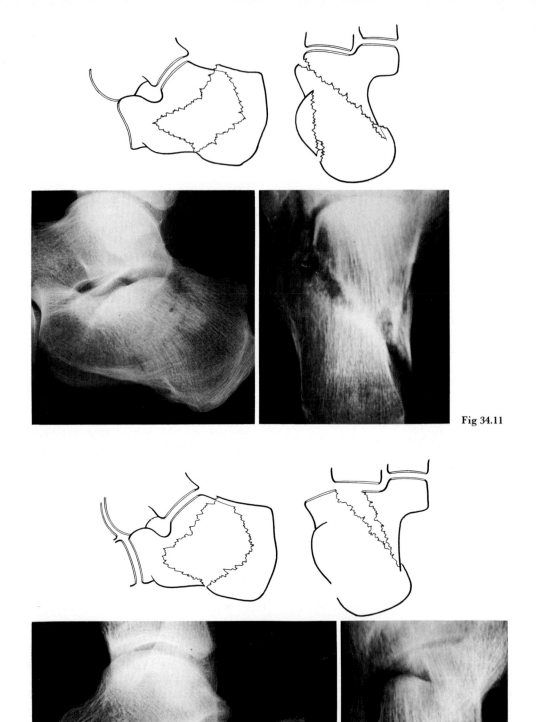

Fig 34.11

Fig 34.12

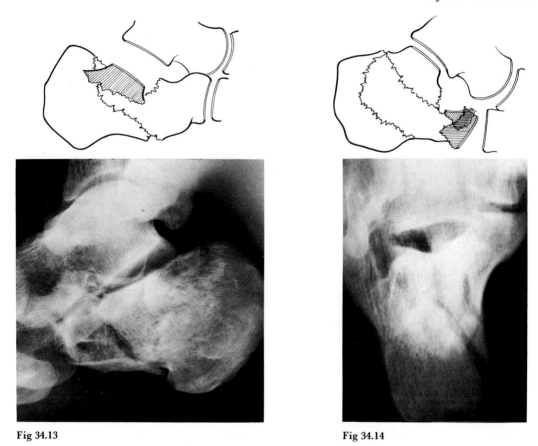

Fig 34.13   **Fig 34.14**

Figs 34.11 to 34.14 Fractures of the calcaneum involving the subtalar joint. Fig 34.11: Fracture of the calcaneum with displacement, adjacent to but not entering the subtalar joint. This is the basic line of fracture of the calcaneum from the postero-medial to the antero-lateral part but not involving the joint surface. Fig 34.12: Fracture of the calcaneum with displacement of the lateral part of the subtalar joint. The large postero-lateral fragment of the calcaneum is separated from the smaller antero-medial fragment. Figs 34.13 and 34.14: Fracture of the calcaneum with central crushing of the whole subtalar joint.

of the lateral malleolus[26] or the projecting part of the calcaneum[28] may be necessary.

X-ray examination

Care must be taken not to miss these fractures even after X-ray examination has been taken. The main lines of fracture are in the antero-posterior plane, and they are masked in lateral radiographs by overlying shadows of bone. There can be complete crushing of the lateral half of the subtalar joint while the intact medial half throws a normal shadow in lateral projections, thus suggesting that the joint is not seriously injured. It is essential that radiographic examination should include projections in the antero-posterior plane—the plantar-dorsal or axial plane.

Radiographs of the calcaneum in the plantar-dorsal or axial plane. The back of the foot is placed on the X-ray cassette, the ankle being dorsiflexed by means of a bandage held by the patient (Fig 34.20 (a)). The tube of the X-ray apparatus is tilted 45 degrees below the foot so that its axis is parallel with the posterior compartment of the subtalar joint. The body of the calcaneum with its lateral surface is then seen in profile, as well as the joint between the sustentaculum tali and the talus. At least one film should be taken, preferably with a Potter-Bucky diaphragm with such a degree of over-penetration that the tuber of the calcaneum scarcely appears at all, so that every detail of the subtalar joint and the region of the sustentaculum tali is outlined clearly despite the overlap of many bone shadows.

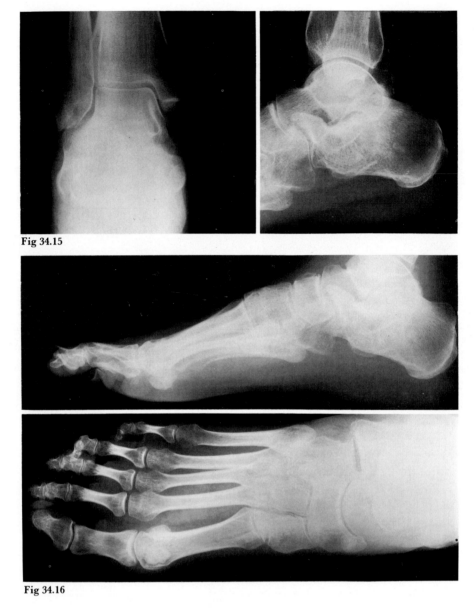

Fig 34.15

Fig 34.16

Figs 34.15 and 34.16 This patient sustained a relatively minor abduction strain of the right forefoot. X-rays taken of the ankle shortly after the accident were reported as normal (Fig 34.15). In the lateral view an irregularity can be seen in the anterior end of the calcaneum. Films of the foot taken some months later confirm the irregularity of the calcaneo-cuboid joint (Fig 34.16).

Anthonsen's oblique radiographic projection of the calcaneum. One other radiographic study is needed for the complete investigation of calcaneal fractures. This is the oblique projection described by Anthonsen,[29] which shows the subtalar joint with greater clarity than ordinary lateral projections. The foot is dorsi-flexed and placed on its lateral side on the cassette.* The central ray of the X-ray tube is directed to a

* The value of both this and the plantar-dorsal special X-ray projection will depend upon the patient being able to dorsiflex the foot into the required position. This is not always possible in the acute phase of the injury.[14]

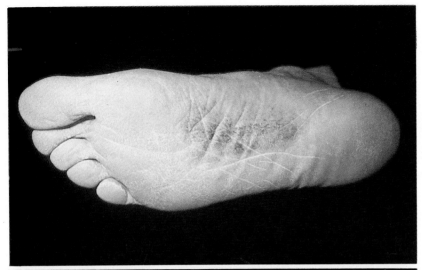

Fig 34.17

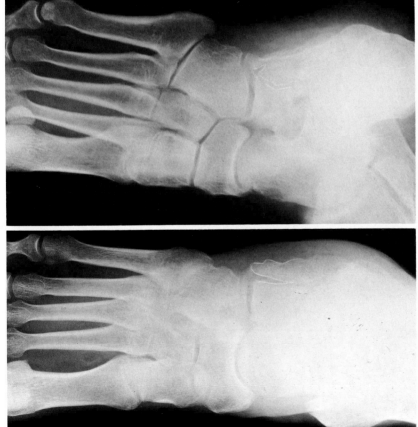

Fig 34.18

Figs 34.17 and 34.18 The bruising in the sole of the foot which is diagnostic of a fracture of the calcaneum and is found even in minor fractures. Figure 34.18 are X-rays of the same case illustrated in Figure 34.17, showing the minimal displacement of the bone fragments.

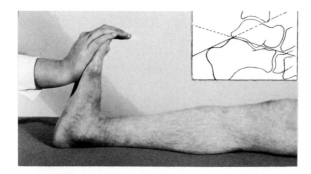

Fig 34.19 In all fractures through the body of the calcaneum the tuberosity is displaced upwards. This may amount to as much as 1 inch (2.5 cm) or even more, and if it is left uncorrected the functional effect is just the same as if the tendo Achillis had been lengthened by 1 inch (2.5 cm) or more. This is displayed clinically by the excessive passive dorsiflexion of the foot as shown in this patient. It explains the difficulty of standing on tip-toe or walking with a normal heel to toe spring. The normal tuber-joint angle, which is lost in compression fractures, is shown in the inset.

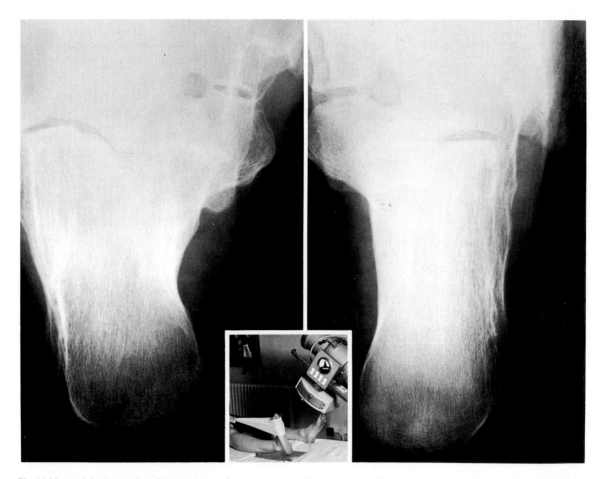

Fig 34.20a Axial (plantar-dorsal) projection used in radiography of the calcaneum. Deformity from an old fracture is shown on the left side. The inset shows the position of foot and X-ray tube for this view.

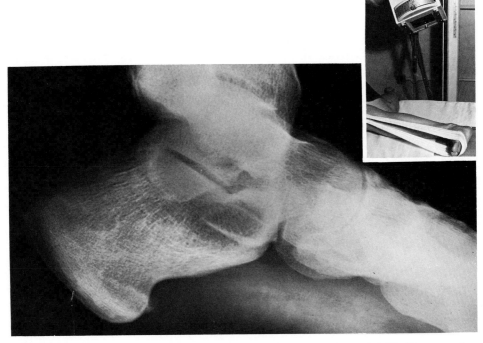

Fig 34.20b Anthonsen's oblique view of the calcaneum (see inset for positioning of the X-ray tube). The X-rays pass through the axis of the sulci calcanei and display the exact nature of many fractures, the displacement of which could not otherwise be understood.

point below the medial malleolus and is tilted 25 degrees towards the foot of the table (in a cranio-distal direction) and also 30 degrees towards the toes of the patient (since the foot is on its side this is in the dorsi-ventral direction). The rays of the tube strike the posterior part of the subtalar joint tangentially, passing in the axis of the sulcus calcanei and displaying the exact nature of many fractures, the displacement of which could not otherwise be understood. These radiographs disclose the outline of the calcaneum with its tuber behind, the recess of the upper surface receiving the wedge of the body of the talus between the posterior and anterior subtalar joint surfaces, and the anterior end articulating with the cuboid (Fig 34.20 (b)).

TREATMENT OF FRACTURES OF THE CALCANEUM

The treatment of fractures not involving the subtalar joint presents no special problem. For fractures which do involve the joint we must consider three plans of treatment:

1. Simple rest for a few weeks with the support of a bandage.
2. Attempted reduction with restoration of the subtalar joint surfaces by elevating the postero-lateral fragment.
3. Primary arthrodesis of the subtalar joint and probably also of the mid-tarsal joint.

Treatment of fractures not involving the subtalar joint. The treatment of fractures not involving the subtalar joint is relatively simple. When there is a *vertical fracture of the tuberosity* manipulation is seldom needed. After a short period of bed rest with elevation and bandaging to reduce swelling a walking plaster should be applied for about six weeks with a crepe bandage for some weeks thereafter. In occasional cases, when there is more severe displacement of the medial process of the tuberosity which might cause spur formation and resulting local tenderness, it should be corrected by compression between the surgeon's two hands before the plaster is applied. *In horizontal fractures of the tuberosity* (beak-fractures) the foot should be examined under anaesthesia to see if the upward tilting can be easily corrected by plantar-flexing the foot and applying direct pressure over the displaced fragment. If an accurate reduction can be achieved and the surgeon is confident that the attachment of the tendo Achillis is intact, the patient can be treated in a walking plaster with the ankle joint in a few degrees of plantar-flexion. The plaster may be removed after about six weeks, recurrent oedema being prevented by the support of a crepe bandage and active exercise. However, more often than not, these injuries are avulsion fractures of the tuberosity arising from the pull of a high attachment of the tendo Achillis, with a fragment torn from the back of the bone which is completely detached and displaced upwards; this should be replaced through a lateral incision over the heel and held in position by a cancellous bone screw. *Fractures of the sustentaculum tali* when isolated and not associated with other fractures of the calcaneum need only be immobilised in a walking plaster for about six weeks, unless by chance there is slight lateral displacement which should be corrected by manual pressure before the plaster is applied. In *isolated fractures of the anterior end of the bone* displacement is usually unimportant. The foot should be protected in a below-knee walking plaster for six weeks, after which time active exercise restores full movement and minimises gravitational oedema. Cases of non-union of the fragment have been reported.[30,31] A number of these have given sufficient disability to require excision of the fragment. Only when large fragments of the calcaneum are separated and tilted, with more severe damage to the calcaneo-cuboid joint, is immediate operative inter-vention needed. These latter injuries are usually produced by abduction of the forefoot on the hindfoot, squeezing a large antero-superior fragment of the calcaneum out of the joint and causing compression of the anterior end of the calcaneus. They are frequently missed in the acute stage (see Figs 34.15 and 34.16) but if recognised they should be treated by open reduction, using a cancellous graft to restore the compressed fragment to its correct position.[14] Cases recognised late may require calcaneo-cuboid fusion.

Treatment of fractures involving the subtalar joint. Fractures through the body of the calcaneum which do not disturb the alignment of the subtalar joint (see Fig 34.11) are no problem and can be treated conservatively on the lines indicated later. It is over the management of fractures which have split, or otherwise disorganized the joint that much controversy exists. For over 30 years argument has raged between those who sincerely believe that better

results can be obtained by operative reduction, and those who adamantly hold the view that the damage is so severe and the mechanism of the subtalar joint so complex that no operative procedure can be expected to improve function. The protagonists for either treatment can produce convincing evidence in support of the method they advocate, and true comparison series are difficult to obtain, sometimes resulting in misleading conclusions. However, one common factor does emerge from study of the papers on the subject, which is that those cases where the fracture is adequately reduced have subtalar move-ment restored,[10,20] and the long term follow up would seem to indicate that those with restoration of subtalar movement have a better chance of returning to heavy work.[20] There would seem, therefore, to be a case for considering operative treatment in the young patient engaged in heavy manual work, and to treat conservatively the elderly and those not engaged in a heavy occupation or strenuous sport. Those who choose operative reduction must constantly bear in mind that subtalar movement is only restored if the joint is properly reduced,[10] and that many of the bad results are due to inadequate surgery—'There is nothing wrong with the idea; it is the execution which is at fault'.[32]

Conservative treatment of bed rest and early mobilisation. No attempt is made to correct the displacement. The patient is put to bed and a firm crepe bandage is applied over a wool dressing which covers the whole of the foot from the toes to just above the ankle. The foot of the bed is elevated and the patient encouraged to carry out toe, foot and ankle exercises several times a day. The aim of this treatment is to prevent stiffness developing in joints which have not been damaged by the injury; the function of the subtalar joint can be regarded as totally lost, and no attempt is made to mobilise this part of the foot. The patient must be kept with his foot elevated until all the soft tissue swelling has subsided; this usually takes about three weeks. Direct weight-bearing on the heel is forbidden for three months, but the patient is encouraged to take steadying weight on the forefoot while using crutches. If the injury is bilateral the period of bed rest is increased to six weeks and then below-knee weight-bearing plasters applied for a further six weeks. It is important that after coming out of plaster the patient should wear a well-made longitudinal arch support with a sorbo-rubber heel elevator, and that he should continue to use this permanently. If the original injury caused such destruction of the subtalar and mid-tarsal joints as to cause fibrous ankylosis he will probably be able to return to sedentary work within about six months, with of course stiffness of the tarsal joints but without much pain. There may be lack of heel and toe spring because the tuber of the calcaneum is displaced upwards with relative lengthening of the tendo Achillis. There may also be thickening of the heel and valgus deformity which will distort the posterior part of the shoe. But even with these limitations the patient will often be capable of doing a full day at work provided this is not of a heavy nature. For patients over the age of 50 who are unlikely to engage in hazardous or strenuous occupations again, and for those with very comminuted fractures where the whole bone and subtalar joint is shattered completely, this form of conservative management is the treatment of choice.[10] There are, of course, many surgeons who believe it is the best routine treatment for all crush fractures of the calcaneum.[33–37] But to take this view is too fatalistic. We must move forward in our thinking and in time we will do better. We must know more surely which fractures to leave alone and which to treat by early operation. The segregation by age and comminution is perhaps a useful start in this direction.

Treatment by operative replacement. When the main line of fracture runs through the body of the calcaneum, with displacement of the lateral part of the subtalar surface, or with depression of the whole thalamic portion of the calcaneum, and where there is no complete crushing and destruction of the joint, and the patient is under 50, good results have been reported from operative replacement.[18,19] Maxfield

believes[38,39] that all fractures of the calcaneum with displacement or depression of the posterior articular facet should be treated by open reduction with the possible exception of some fractures with extreme comminution. The depressed subtalar joint surface and the upward displacement of the tuberosity which reduces the tuber joint angle should first be corrected by a skeletal pin driven through the back of the bone. The pin should not be longer than 6 cm, otherwise it will extend too far beyond the posterior subtalar joint. Part of a Steinmann's pin can be used for this purpose, but the Gissane spike and introducer is specially designed for this purpose and is preferable (Fig 34.21). The point of the spike should be aimed to lie under the subtalar fragment, with a result that when its introducer is depressed not only is the tuber angle restored, but also the subtalar joint surface is elevated (Figs 34.22 and 34.23). Then, through an incision over the side of the heel, just behind the peroneal tendons, the downwardly displaced lateral part of the bone with the lateral part of the subtalar joint surface is explored and if necessary further elevation carried out. This leaves a gap where the cancellous bone in the middle of the calcaneum has been crushed. This is filled with cancellus grafts taken from the ilium. It is wise to use a block of cancellous bone which will hold the fragment elevated. A graft cut in a diamond shape has been found very suitable for maintaining the reduction.[40] A plaster shoe is applied after operation, incorporating the spike used to correct the deformity. This allows mobilisation of the ankle, and to some extent the subtalar joint, without fear of

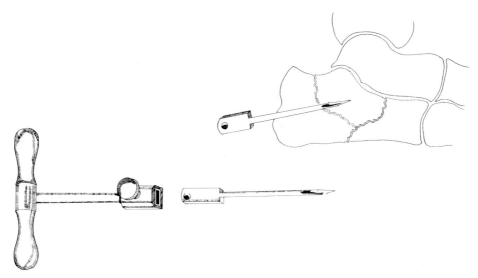

Fig 34.21 The Gissane spike and introducer for reduction of displayed fractures of the calcaneum. The inset shows the optimum position for the introduction of the spike to allow maximal correction of the tuber angle and subtalar fragment.

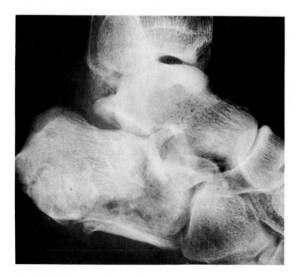

Fig 34.22 Fracture of the calcaneum with upward displacement of the tuberosity, loss of the tuber-joint angle, and depression of subtalar joint surface.

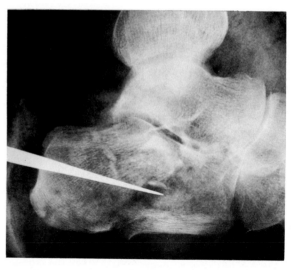

Fig 34.23 The upward displacement of the tuberosity of the calcaneum has been corrected by means of a skeletal pin driven through the back of the bone, and the depressed fragment of the calcaneum curtaining the posterior subtalar joint surface has been restored to its normal position. The calcanean pin shown in the X-ray is rather lower and more horizontal than is usual (see inset to Fig 34.21).

redisplacement of the bone fragments. The cast is changed to a below-knee plaster at about four to six weeks, the spike removed, and the patient kept non-weight-bearing for another four weeks. Good results have also been reported from reduction by the bone spike alone,[20] by elevation at open reduction without any bone graft using Kirschner wire fixation,[19] and by operating through a medial approach behind and below the neurovascular bundle with fixation of the medial cortex with a staple.[40a] Whichever of these techniques is used they all have one factor in common, and that is a simple elevation of the depressed articular fragment. Each method attempts to restore the posterior subtalar joint to reasonable alignment; no attempt is made to obtain anatomical perfection. Small fragment surgery with all its paraphernalia of multiple screw fixation has no place in the operative treatment of fracture of the calcaneum.

Treatment by primary arthrodesis. It has been suggested by some surgeons that when crushing of the whole subtalar joint is of such a degree that the best functional results to be expected is ankylosis, it is best to promote this by early operation. The operation may have to be deferred until two or three weeks after injury because of the condition of the skin. If this is so it is wise to correct serious deformity within the first few days by manipulation under anaesthesia—

particularly correcting the lateral spread and the valgus deformity of the heel by simple compression between the surgeon's two hands, the foot then being supported in a light plaster cast. As soon as the skin condition permits, the joint is exposed, fragments of cartilage are removed, the surfaces are thoroughly freshened and, if necessary, cancellous bone grafts cut free from the ilium are impacted. The lateral approach for stabilising operation on the paralytic foot is commonly used, especially since this allows fusion of the calcaneo-cuboid joint if it is required, although some surgeons prefer the posterior approach described by Gallie[41] and Lawson Dick.[42] But whichever approach is used these fusions should always be accompanied by reduction of the depressed subtalar fragment and restoration of the tuber angle.[39] A padded plaster is applied which should be replaced after two or three weeks by an unpadded cast, closely moulded on each side of the heel in such a way as to prevent recurrence of lateral thickening and to keep the heel in a strictly neutral plane with no valgus deformity—but it must be added, and with still greater emphasis, with no varus or inversion deformity, which is so much more disabling after subtalar arthrodesis.

In a recent study of the use of primary subtalar fusion more careful selection of cases has been suggested[42a]. If fractures with gross comminution are excluded, full function in over 80 per cent of cases was obtained by the Dick method of posterior fusion. In this method the subtaloid joint is exposed through an incision just lateral to the tendo Achillis, and without any attempt to reduce the fracture a trough is prepared across the subtaloid joint to take two cortico-cancellous grafts cut from the ilium. The authors advise early operation (i.e. within the first four weeks of injury) even though they found that operations carried out during this period had a higher complication rate from infection and delayed wound healing. This is a well thought out approach to the use of primary arthrodesis in fractures of the calcaneus, but it would seem wise to reduce the complication rate by delaying operation for at least three to four weeks to allow the soft tissues to recover from the initial trauma.

Those who favour a primary triple arthrodesis in severely damaged calcaneal fractures point out that in many cases not only the subastragaloid joint is involved, but also the calcaneo-cuboid joint. Careful study of the X-rays will often show this to be true (Figs 34.22 and 34.25); if this joint is damaged a triple arthrodesis would seem to be a better way of stabilising the damaged joint complex.

Treatment of fractures of the calcaneum by complete excision of the bone. It should be mentioned that Pridie suggested complete excision of severely comminuted fractures of the calcaneum.[43] One or two other surgeons have done the same operation.[44] It is astonishing that such excellent function can be regained after complete excision of this bone through a posterior split-heel incision, and it is possible that the procedure may have a very limited surgical application. The indications are few, but the operation probably has a place in the management of the severely displaced bursting injury associated with explosions and other major trauma. It is interesting to note that Pridie developed this technique because of the difficulties he encountered in carrying out a primary arthrodesis in this type of case. Perhaps this is a salutary warning to those who are about to embark upon early fusion.

LATE DISABILITY AFTER FRACTURES OF THE CALCANEUM

The late disabilities that may arise from this serious group of fractures are listed under the following headings:

1. Thickening of bone with undue prominence beneath the tuberosity and resulting pain under the heel from the impact of weight-bearing. Also, lateral thickening of the bone, which in itself is ugly and causes distortion in the shape of shoes and may cause pain from impingement against the lateral malleolus and secondary peroneal tendonitis.

2. Upward displacement of the tuberosity, which is the equivalent of lengthening the tendo Achillis and causes such loss of power as to make it difficult to stand on tip-toe or walk with a normal heel and toe spring.

3. Valgus deformity of the heel causing secondary strain on the other tarsal joints with traumatic flat foot.

4. Arthritis of the subtalar or mid-tarsal joints into which the fracture extends and where there is often grave damage of the articular surfaces.

Thickening of the calcaneum. Thickening of the heel results from vertical crushing and lateral spreading with separation of an antero-medial and a large postero-lateral fragment. The various types of fracture causing this thickening have already been outlined. The displacement can usually be corrected by manipulative treatment at the time of injury. In later stages when there is mal-union, it may sometimes be wise to remove the excess of bone from the lateral part of the body of the calcaneum. Sometimes the peroneal tendons are trapped between the calcaneus and the tip of the lateral malleolus. This produces an area of pain and acute tenderness directly over the peroneal tubercle and can often be relieved by a simple tenolysis,[27] or by removal of impinging bone.[26, 28] If there is thickening with pain under the heel from the impact of weight-bearing, the heel of the shoe should be hollowed out, the excavation being filled with sorbo-rubber.

Tarsal tunnel syndrome. The floor of the tarsal tunnel is formed by the medial wall of the calcaneus which is always damaged by fracture. It is not surprising therefore that cases of tarsal tunnel syndrome have been reported following calcanean fracture. In one review of 500 fractures it was found that 10 per cent developed symptoms.[44a] These took the form of pain and paraesthesia in the distribution of the posterior tibial nerve, frequently worse at night, or on walking or standing. The diagnosis can be confirmed by injection of local anaesthetic and by nerve conduction studies. Operative decompression may be required if local cortisone does not relieve the symptoms.

Upward displacement of the tuberosity with laxity of the tendo Achillis. Upward displacement of the tuberosity, which in its effect amounts to lengthening of the tendo Achillis with loss of power in the calf group of muscles, explains why it is often difficult to stand on tip-toe after this fracture and why it is difficult to walk with a normal spring. This can sometimes be corrected by manipulation in the early stages. But if, as is often the case, the deformity is left uncorrected, it is fortunate that by retraction of the calf muscles considerable compensation is often gained even when in earlier days there may have been marked excess of passive dorsiflexion and loss of power of active plantar-flexion. The patient gradually learns to stand on tip-toe so that the gait is much improved.

Valgus deformity of the heel. Valgus deformity of the heel, especially when a large postero-lateral fragment of the body of the calcaneum is displaced outwards, is associated not only with traumatic arthritis of the subtalar joint but often with secondary arthritis of the other tarsal joints. It can result in a painful flat foot deformity (Fig 34.24). It should always be remembered that a severely comminuted fracture of the calcaneum may extend forwards into the calcaneo-cuboid joint.[45] This explains why simple subtaloid arthrodesis is often unsuccessful in curing a late painful arthritis, and if operation is being considered it is usually wiser to complete the triple arthrodesis by fusing the mid-tarsal joint in addition to subtaloid arthrodesis (Fig 34.25).

Injury to the subtalar joint surface. Traumatic arthritis from direct injury to the subtalar and calcaneo-cuboid joints is the most serious disability in these injuries. The comminution of bone and destruction of articular surfaces may be so complete that fibrous ankylosis develops spontaneously. It is for this reason that success is often gained by treatment in which no attempt is made to reduce displacement. The simple support of an elastic bandage is relied upon. Because of the gross disorganisation of the subtaloid joint primary arthrodesis has been suggested. This is not an easy procedure to carry out as a primary operation, but the exponents of early operation make the point that reduction of heel deformity is an important factor in obtaining a satisfactory result,[46] this, of course, can only be achieved if the arthrodesis is performed shortly after the fracture.

SUMMARY OF THE TREATMENT OF FRACTURES OF THE CALCANEUM

From what has been said already it is obvious that there is still considerable divergence of opinion as to the best method of treating serious fractures of the calcaneum in which there is crushing of bone with involvement of the subtalar joint, and despite many comparative surveys of different treatments we are

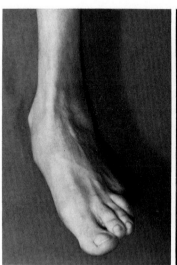

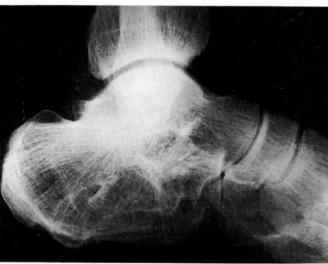

Fig 34.24 Valgus deformity of the foot after fracture of the calcaneum. This can result in a painful flat foot deformity and may require operative treatment.

Fig 34.25 Subtalar arthrodesis for fracture of calcaneum with complete destruction of the joint surfaces. Note that the calcaneo-cuboid joint has also been deformed by the fracture. This is a common cause of failure of subtalar arthrodesis after fracture of the calcaneus. It would have been wiser to carry out a triple arthrodesis in this case.

still none the wiser as to the best method. The correct choice of treatment depends upon the careful analysis of the fracture before treatment is instituted, followed by an equally careful consideration of the applicable therapeutic possibilities.[47] Meanwhile the principles of treatment to be accepted are listed below:

1. With certain exceptions *fractures not involving the subtalar joint* need only the support of a light plaster cast or a crepe bandage for a few weeks.

2. *Fractures in the same basic line of fracture but entering the subtalar joint* can be treated in *young patients* by operative reduction of the displaced fragment, using a spike to reduce the articular fracture and cancellous iliac grafts to fill the space of the compressed bone below. Early subtalar fusion by the posterior approach may also give good results in this category of patient.[42a]

3. *Similar fractures in middle-aged or elderly patients* should be treated by simple bed rest for a week or two with no more than simple endeavours to reduce the lateral thickening and valgus deformity by manipulation but without prolonged fixation in plaster.

4. *Severely comminuted fractures* with complete destruction of the joint surfaces in patients of all ages are best treated conservatively but may require early triple arthrodesis (preferably after the fracture has consolidated).

5. *There is no place for small fragment surgery and meticulous screw fixation in fractures of the calcaneum.*

FRACTURES, DISLOCATIONS AND FRACTURE-DISLOCATIONS OF THE TALUS

To understand the treatment of fractures of the neck of the talus and other fractures and fracture-dislocations of this bone, we must first study the mechanism of injury, because otherwise it is difficult to recognise the best methods of manipulative replacement. In earlier surgical contributions these injuries were described as simple and double luxations, or primary, secondary and tertiary luxations, depending upon whether there was involvement of one, two or three of the tarsal joints.[48] This was really no more than an academic exercise; it was also confusing and of little value in treatment. Others have preferred to classify the injuries according to whether they were fractures without dislocations, subluxations or complete dislocations.[49,50] Many injuries, however, are classified in accordance with their mechanism and the direction of displacement. For example, injuries of the ankle joint can be grouped into fractures due to abduction

or adduction, fractures associated with external rotation in pronation or supination, and fractures due to vertical compression. Similarly, fractures of the spine are classified as flexion, extension and rotatory injuries. So it is with fractures and fracture-dislocation of the talus which should also be grouped in accordance with the direction of violence into:

1. Inversion injuries.
2. Dorsiflexion injuries.
3. Adduction and abduction injuries.

Inversion injuries causing displacement of the talus (Figs 34.26 to 34.28). Forcible inversion of the foot may rupture the lateral ligament of the ankle and cause momentary dislocation—this has already been discussed. With similar stress, but with the foot more plantar-flexed at the time of injury, the interosseus ligaments of the subtalar joints may be torn—the tarsal bones being dislocated inwards while the talus remains undisplaced in the tibio-fibular mortise—*subtalar or talo-calcaneal navicular dislocation*. As this injury occurs around the combination of joints labelled by Shephard as the peri-talar joint[50] it has been described more accurately by Kenwright and Taylor as a peri-talar dislocation.[51] If all the ligaments, not only those of the subtalar joint but also those of the lateral side of the ankle joint, are torn simultaneously the talus is separated not only from the other tarsal bones but also from the tibio-fibular mortise so that there is total dislocation of the talus. This is a combined medial dislocation of the ankle joint with medial dislocation of the subtalar joint. The lateral ligament of the ankle joint and the interosseus ligament of the subtalar joint are both ruptured. At the moment of greatest inversion the talus is rotated 90 degrees about its vertical axis so that the head is directed medially; it is also rotated 90 degrees about its long axis so that its inferior surface is directed backwards. When violence ceases and the foot springs back to the neutral position, the dislocated talus remains in this rotated position and lies with the body in front of the lateral malleolus, the head on the medial side, the calcanean surface directed backwards and the tibial articular surface under the skin.

Dorsiflexion injuries (Figs 34.29 to 34.32). An entirely different injury causes fracture of the neck of the talus with dislocation of the body. The type of displacement is different, and the after-treatment is different. This injury is not to be classified with total dislocations of the talus. It arises from forced dorsiflexion of the foot. Violent dorsiflexion is an

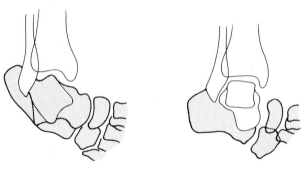

Fig 34.26 Dislocation of the ankle joint.

Fig 34.27 Dislocation of the subtalar joint—peri-talar dislocation.

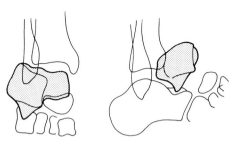

Fig 34.28

Figs 34.26 to 34.28 Total dislocation of the talus. Inversion strain ruptures the lateral ligament of the ankle joint (Fig 34.26), the interosseus ligament of the subtalar joint (Fig 34.27) or both the lateral ligament and the interosseus ligaments (Fig 34.28). Note that when the foot is inverted and plantar-flexed the talus is rotated (Fig 34.26), and that after total dislocation of the talus it remains locked in this position (Fig 34.28).

infrequent strain in civilian life, and fracture-dislocation of the neck of the talus are unusual injuries. Nearly all the reports in the literature are based on one or two causes. In war time it was a frequent complication of flying accidents, and in peace time it is occasionally seen in road traffic accidents after a head-on collision.

Graeme Anderson reported 18 such fractures sustained by members of the flying services in the First World War.[52] In the Second World War no less than 228 such injuries were treated, of which 70 per cent of the more serious injuries occurred as the result of flying accidents.[49] This represented an incidence of 1 per cent of all major fractures and dislocations, or 6 per cent of injuries of the foot and ankle.

It is therefore still reasonable to describe the injury as the 'aviator's fracture'.[51]* It is nearly always the result of a head-on crash, and is sustained by a pilot whose feet are on the rudder bar of a light aircraft, or the driver or passenger in a motor car trapped by the

* It is interesting to learn that a new type of fracture has arisen from helicopter crashes. In an attempt to right the aircraft the pilot applies heavy pressure to the tail rotor pedals. This has resulted in an explosive type of fracture of the lower end of the tibia.[53]

impact of a collision. The rudder bar or brake pedal lies under the instep or forefoot and, as it is driven backwards, the foot is forced into dorsiflexion. The neck of the talus is impacted against the anterior margin of the lower end of the tibia, which drives into the talus like a chisel and causes a vertical fracture of the neck of the talus. As a rule there is also damage to the anterior tibial margin. If violence continues, the line of injury extends from the neck of the talus to the ligaments of the posterior part of the subtalar joint and the whole foot subluxates forwards on the body of the talus—*fracture of the neck of the talus with subtalar disolocation.*† As the foot continues to

† It must be understood that only the posterior half of the subtalar joint is dislocated. There is usually no displacement between the head of the talus and the anterior facet of the calcaneum (but see page 1184). Described in full the injury is a fracture of the neck of the talus with dislocation of the posterior half of the subtalar joint, and the final degree of displacement is a fracture of the neck of the talus with dislocation of the posterior half of the subtalar joint with backward displacement of the body of the talus. For brevity it is described throughout the text as fracture of the neck of the talus with subtalar dislocation. The last degree of injury is described as fracture of the neck of the talus, subtalar dislocation with backward displacement of the body.

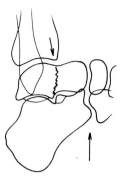

Fig 34.29 Fracture of the neck of the talus without displacement.

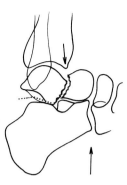

Fig 34.30 Fracture of the neck of the talus with subtalar dislocation.

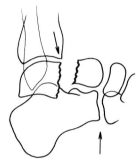

Fig 34.31

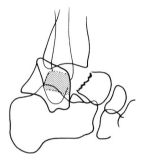

Fig 34.32

Figs 34.29 and 34.32 Fracture of the neck of the talus with subtalar dislocation and backward displacement of the body. Forcible dorsiflexion fractures the neck of the talus by impact against the anterior margin of the tibia (Fig 34.29). If violence continues the posterior half of the subtalar joint is dislocated (Fig 34.30). With still more displacement the tuber calcanei locks under the body of the talus (Fig 34.31), and when violence ceases, the foot is plantar-flexed once more and the body of the talus is displaced backwards (Fig 34.32).

dorsiflex and displacement increases, the tuber cal- canei comes to lie under the body of the talus. But it is obvious from examination of the disarticulated bones that it will be the medial surface of the tuber that lies under the talus (see Figs 34.44 to 34.47). The curved posterior facet of the calcaneum leads directly backwards to this surface. While it is in this position, the sustentaculum tali of the calcaneum locks in front of the medial tubercle of the body of the talus. Thus when violence ceases and the foot is once more plantar-flexed the locked body of the talus is displaced backwards out of the tibio-fibular mortise. It lies on the medial surface of the tuber calcanei with its fractured surface directed laterally, its trigonal tubercle medially, and its medial tubercle hooked behind the sustentaculum tali—*fracture of the neck of the talus with subtalar dislocation and posterior displacement of the body.*

DISLOCATION OF THE SUBTALAR JOINT—PERI-TALAR DISLOCATION (TALO-CALCANEO-NAVICULAR DISLOCATION)

The great majority of these injuries are a result of inversion plantar-flexion strain when the interosseus ligament is ruptured, the talus remaining within the tibio-fibular mortise while the foot is dislocated inwards at the subtalar and the talo-navicular joints.[54] This has been rightly described as a peri-talar dislocation. Very occasionally the injury is caused by a lateral strain, resulting in dislocation to the opposite side.[51] This is explained by the wedge shape of the body of the bone. The transverse diameter of the anterior part of the body is greater than that of the posterior part. When the normal foot is dorsiflexed to the right angle the wide anterior part of the talus is engaged in the tibio-fibular mortise, and the inferior tibio-fibular ligaments are stretched. Elastic recoil would tend to force the talus into the equinus position, but this is resisted by the tone of the anterior tibial muscles which keep the foot at the right angle. After dislocation of the subtalar joint this resistance is lost. The talus has no support from the foot bones, and no muscle is inserted into it so that it drops into the equinus position, with the narrow posterior part of the body engaged in the tibio-fibular mortise. This observation is significant in its bearing on fracture-dislocations of the neck of the talus. It is also important in the technique of manipulative reduction of subtalar dislocations. *The foot should be plantar-flexed and only then should it be everted and abducted.* When the dislocation is reduced it is usually stable. The limb is immobilised for six weeks in a walking-plaster with the foot in right-angled dorsiflexion and neutral to inversion-eversion. Recovery is rapid and complete. Occasionally there may be a fracture of the medial part of the head of the talus or of the lateral part of the navicular from the impact of those bones during dislocation, and if the separated fragments are so large that reduction is unstable the foot should be immobilised in full eversion for 10 weeks. Kirschner wire fixation of bony fragments can be a useful method of maintaining reduction.[55] Late arthritic change in the talo-navicular joint sometimes necessitates arthrodesis. Very rarely the dislocation may be irreducible by manipulation due to 'button-holing' of the capsule by the prominent head of talus and will require an open reduction.[51]

Subtalar dislocation with dislocation of the ankle joint. The case shown in Figures 34.33 to 34.35 illustrates the close relationship between dislocation of the subtalar joint and dislocation of the ankle joint. The subtalar dislocation shown in Figure 34.33 was manipulated and put in plaster. Post-reduction radiographs showed satisfactory reduction, but there was then evidence of dislocation of the ankle joint. A second manipulation was necessary (Figs 34.34 and 34.35).

Instability of the subtalar joint. Review of the literature suggests that 10 per cent of patients undergoing peroneal tenodesis for talar instability at the ankle also have subtalar instability.[56] This condition may be suspected clinically when there is excessive inversion of the hindfoot and can be confirmed by taking stress tomography views. The feet are strapped on to hinged boards which hold the feet fully inverted and antero-posterior tomograms

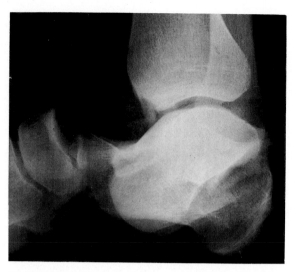

Fig 34.33 Peri-talar (subtalar) dislocation. When the talus is released from the resistance of the other foot bones it is pushed into equinus by elastic recoil of the inferior tion-fibular ligaments (see Figs 34.34 and 34.35).

taken at the level of the medial malleolus, and at 1 cm anterior and 1 cm posterior to it. The subtalar inversion angle averages 38 degrees in the normal and 57 degrees in the unstable joints.[56] This instability will not always be corrected by the Watson-Jones or Evans operation and Chrisman and Snook[57] have

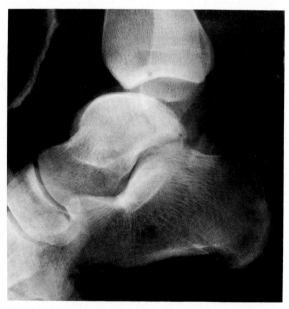

Fig 34.34 Same case as shown in Figure 34.33. After reduction of the subtalar dislocation there was obviously forward dislocation of the ankle joint.

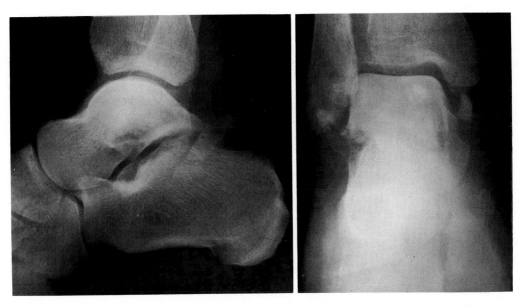

Fig 34.35 The final reduction of the case shown in Figures 34.33 and 34.34. This case illustrates the close relationship of dislocation of the ankle, subtalar dislocation and total dislocation of the talus.

devised a modification of the Elmslie procedure. Half of the peroneus brevis tendon is passed through the anterior talo-calcanean ligament, or a hole in the talus, through a hole in the fibular, through a hole or groove in the calcaneus, and finally secured to the base of the fifth metatarsal.* Late cases in which tenodesis has already failed may require a triple arthrodesis.

Dislocation of the calcaneum. This rare injury was first reported over 70 years ago as a complete dislocation at the subtalar and calcaneo-cuboid joints.[58] A recent report[59] describes the dislocation as a lateral displacement, but mentions another case where the bone, dislocated inferiorly, ended up with its long axis in the same plane as that of the tibia. If reduction cannot be achieved by manipulation open reduction through a lateral approach should be carried out. Kirschner wire fixation may be necessary to maintain the position, followed by plaster fixation for 10 weeks.

---

*This is a complicated procedure and positioning of the peroneus brevis tendon for the simpler Evans or Watson-Jones tenodesis should always be carried out first to see if it gives sufficient stability.

TOTAL DISLOCATION OF THE TALUS

The talus is liable to dislocation because it is the only bone in the leg without muscle attachments and because more than half of its surface is articular.[48] The mechanism of injury and the direction of displacement has already been discussed. Coltart described it in the following manner: 'The characteristic feature is that displacement is forwards and laterally so that the bone comes to rest under the skin in front of the ankle on the dorso-lateral-aspect of the foot'.[49] It is produced by violent inversion of the foot, which rotates the bone 90 degrees round its vertical axis so that the head is directed medially, and 90 degrees round its long axis so that the calcaneum surface is directed backwards (Fig 34.36 and inset). With such violence and such a degree of displacement it is not surprising that the skin is often torn over the dorso-lateral aspect of the foot. In four of the five cases here reported the dislocation was compound. Sometimes the talus has been extruded through the lateral wound and has been lost, or it has been thrown away with the sock and shoe. In other cases the foot springs back to the neutral position and the talus lies with the body in front of the lateral malleolus. Even if the skin is not torn, it is tightly stretched over the bone and in danger of sloughing from pressure on its

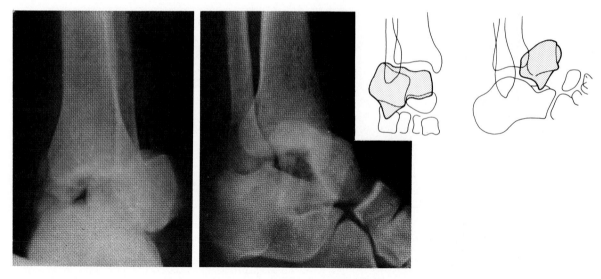

Fig 34.36 Total dislocation of the talus. The bone is rotated 90 degrees round its vertical axis and 90 degrees round its long axis. (The inset illustrates the displacement diagrammatically.)

deep surface with loss of its blood supply.* Treatment is therefore urgent whether the dislocation is open or closed.

Treatment. Two complications bedevil the treatment of total dislocation of the talus—infection and avascular necrosis; and the one potentiates the effect of the other. The blood supply of the talus depends mainly upon vessels entering the bone from the sinus tarsi.[60] These vessels must be destroyed in the fully displaced dislocation, producing at least some degree of avascular change. Many of the dislocations are compound, and even those which are closed often suffer skin breakdown after open reduction.† Infection, therefore, is common, and this combined with loss of blood supply, results in a massive sequestrum which can make talectomy inevitable. In one series of nine patients[61] late talectomy and tibiocalcanean fusion was required for infection in seven, leading the authors to the conclusion that talectomy and fusion

---

* As mentioned by Sir Astley Cooper in his most interesting 'Treatise on Dislocations and Fractures', published in London in 1822.

† An unusual case has been described of an apparently isolated anterior dislocation of the talus associated with anterior displacement of the fibula and an intact talofibular ligament. Stress views confirmed this, but also showed a complete rupture of the talonavicular and talocalcanean ligaments, indicating a total dislocation of the talus. No avascular necrosis occurred in this case, emphasising the importance of the blood supply received via the talofibular ligament.[60a]

should be considered as an initial treatment. This, however, is too fatalistic an attitude and in the acute case every effort should be made to avoid excising the talus. Excellent function is sometimes regained after reduction, and even if the bone loses its blood supply and undergoes avascular necrosis, revascularisation is possible and function may still be satisfactory. In the two cases of total dislocation reported by Kenwright and Taylor[51] there was no avascular necrosis, and in one of the patients who had been followed up for 11 years the symptoms were minimal and there was a normal ankle anatomy. Also, if degenerative arthritis supervenes, arthrodesis of the ankle joint or the subtalar joint—or, when necessary, arthrodesis of both joints—gives a result which is usually more satisfactory than that of excision of the talus and tibio-calcanean fusion. When the talus is missing, tibio-calcanean fusion, if necessary later, is far from easy. It is difficult to correct the inversion deformity which so often develops after excision of the talus, and shortening of the limb, which amounts to about 1 inch (2.5 cm), cannot be made good. Whenever possible, therefore, the talus should be reduced and not excised.

Open dislocations. The wound of the skin arises from a bursting force from within so that it is unlikely to be contaminated seriously. It should not be excised so thoroughly that all soft tissue attachments of the talus are destroyed. Moreover, it should not be enlarged with the object of aiding reduction. The blood supply of the bone is in peril and every soft tissue attachment must be preserved.

Manipulative reduction. The doubly rotated position of the talus, and the interlocking of the talus and calcaneum, may give rise to difficulty in reduction and open reduction is often required. The secret of success is to reproduce the deformed position of the foot which caused avulsion of the bone—that is to say, strong inversion and plantar-flexion. With an assistant holding the foot in this position the surgeon presses with both thumbs over the posterior part of the talus, pushing it inwards and backwards, and at the same time trying to correct the rotation round its long axis. If this fails a tibia traction apparatus may be used with a pin through the calcaneum by which to increase the tibio-calcanean gap, after which the same manipulation is repeated.

After-treatment. The limb is immobilised in plaster with the foot in right-angled dorsiflexion. Early weight-bearing should be strictly forbidden because the talus has been deprived of its blood supply and there is danger of crushing the avascular bone and articular cartilage. Even where there are no signs of avascular necrosis weight should not be allowed for the first three months. If radiographs show evidence of relative density, immobilisation in plaster or a Sarmiento type of removable brace should be continued for many months until revascularisation is almost complete. Early weight-bearing without protection accelerates the onset of degenerative arthritis of the ankle, subtalar and talo-navicular joints.

FRACTURE OF THE NECK OF THE TALUS

Forcible dorsiflexion of the talus against the anterior margin of the tibia causes a vertical fracture of the neck of the talus. It is possible for this fracture to occur without displacement, and the only treatment then needed is to immobilise the limb in plaster for 8 to 10 weeks. But the surgeon must beware. Fracture of the neck of the talus without displacement is unusual. There is very often a dislocation of the posterior half of the subtalar joint which is easily overlooked.[51] Examine the radiographs shown in Figure 34.37. There is a fracture of the neck of the talus. Is it a fracture without displacement? Look at Figure 34.38 and examine the outline traced from the radiograph. It is obvious that the line of injury extends through the neck of the talus into the posterior compartment of the subtalar joint which is dislocated. If the foot is immobilised in the right-angled position the dislocation remains unreduced. Only full plantar-

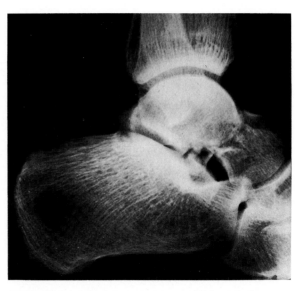

Fig 34.37 Fracture of the neck of the talus. Is there displacement of the fragments? See Figures 34.38 and 34.39.

flexion adjusts the position of the head of the talus and the calcaneum to the displaced equinus position of the body of the talus (Fig 34.39). See also Figures 34.40 to 34.42.

FRACTURE OF THE NECK OF THE TALUS WITH SUBTALAR DISLOCATION

'Fracture dislocations of the talus are one of the most challenging problems facing orthopaedic surgeons.'[61a]

Many feet have been permanently crippled by failure to recognise the displacement of fractures of the neck of the talus and the associated displacements of the posterior half of the subtaloid joint. Before reading on, look again at Figures 34.40 to 34.42 and study Figure 34.43. The clue to a displacement of a fracture of the neck of the talus with subtalar dislocation is in the shape of the body of the talus. It is wider in front than behind. In dorsiflexion the wide anterior part of the body is engaged in the tibio-fibular mortise and the inferior tibio-fibular ligaments are stretched. Tension of the ligaments would push the talus into equinus if it were not for the resistance of the other bones of the foot. This resistance may be released by subtalar dislocation (see p. 1174). It may also be released by fracture of the neck of the talus with dislocation of the posterior half of the subtalar joint. In this injury the body of the talus lies in the equinus position. If the foot is immobilised in right-angled

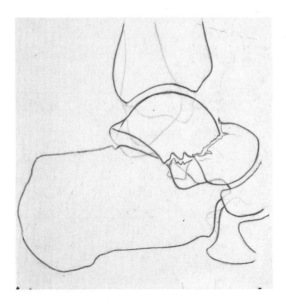

Fig 34.38 An accurate outline of the radiograph presented in Figure 34.37 shows that in addition to fracture of the neck of the talus there is dislocation of the posterior half of the subtalar joint.

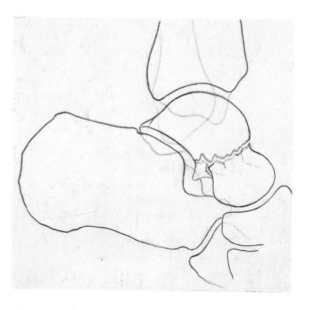

Fig 34.39 The fracture of the neck of the talus and the dislocation of the posterior half of the subtalar joint are reduced only when the foot is fully plantar-flexed.

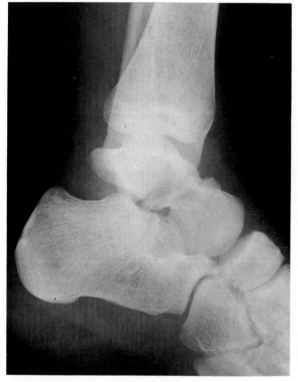

Fig 34.40 Fracture of the neck of the talus with subtalar dislocation.

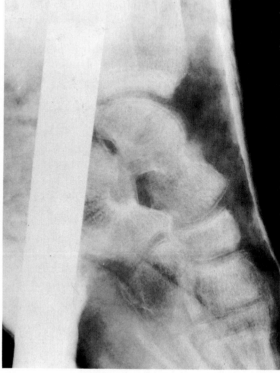

Fig 34.41 After manipulative reduction by full plantar-flexion and eversion of the foot.

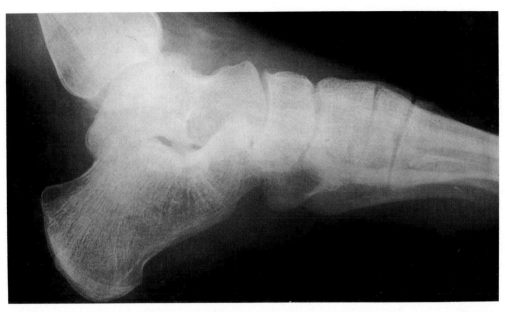

Fig 34.42 Same case as shown in Figures 34.30 and 34.41 six months after reduction and immobilisation. Movements of the ankle, mid-tarsal and subtalar joints are normal, and the patient has no disability. If the fracture-dislocation is completely reduced, there is no danger in immobilising the foot for eight weeks in full plantar-flexion and eversion.

dorsiflexion the head of the talus and the calcaneum do not occupy a similar position—the fracture is unreduced and the dislocation is unreduced.

Conservative treatment—manipulative reduction. *The equinus position.* The displacement is reduced only when the foot is immobilised in the position of full plantar-flexion. Figure 34.43 shows a typical fracture of the neck of the talus with subtalar subluxation. An accurate outline of the 'distal fragment'—that is to say, the head of the talus—the calcaneum and the other foot bones has been superimposed on the fracture through the neck of the talus, and it is clear that the tarsal bones are not in

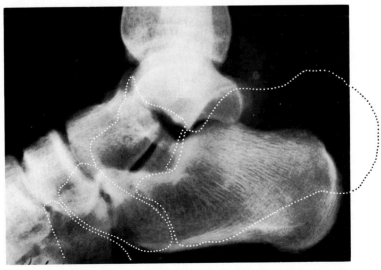

Fig 34.43 Typical fracture of the neck of the talus with dislocation of the posterior half of the subtalar joint. Only when the forefoot is fully plantar-flexed and displaced backwards are the tarsal bones in normal relationship (see outline). If the surgeon is not sure whether or not there is a subtalar dislocation, it is wise to take a tracing of the 'distal fragment' on tissue paper and adjust it in relation to the body of the talus.

normal relationship until the foot is pushed downwards and backwards into equinus.*

The everted position. As a rule the distal fragment represented by the head of the talus, the calcaneum and the other foot bones is inverted. It is therefore necessary not only to plantar-flex the foot but also to evert it. This position must be maintained in plaster for at least eight weeks until the fracture is united. Only then is the surgeon at liberty to apply a new plaster in less plantar-flexion; dorsiflexion at an earlier stage causes redisplacement of the fracture and of the dislocation.[49] Two or three weeks later, when the fracture is quite sound, a final plaster may be applied in right-angled dorsiflexion. There is no danger in immobilising fracture-dislocation of the neck of the talus in full equinus and full eversion. If the dislocation has been reduced and the fragments unite without displacement full movement will be regained. The only danger is the misapplication of a principle which is sound in other circumstances, namely, insistence on the right-angled position of the ankle in immobilisation. If this position is adopted the foot will be permanently crippled.

Operative reduction. Unfortunately it is not always possible to reduce the subtalar subluxation satisfactorily, and in one series of cases 10 out of 14 required open reduction.[51] By using either a Kirschner wire or screw fixation from the head of the talus into the body of the bone a stable position can be obtained and a plaster in the orthodox position used.[55,62,63]

Avascular necrosis. Fractures of the neck of the talus without displacement, where the ligament and blood supply are usually intact, rarely suffer from avascular necrosis, although it has been recorded.[63,64] Fractures with subtalar subluxation, however, where the interosseus ligaments may have been destroyed and the blood supply to the body of the bone reduced, have been estimated by some writers to have an incidence of avascular necrosis as high as 80 per cent.[65] The incidence is probably related to the degree of trauma and displacement, and in Kenwright and Taylor's series there was only a 36 per cent incidence in subluxation cases alone. An overall incidence of about 50 per cent is probably nearer the mark.[63] Treatment will be considered under fractures with subtalar dislocation and posterior displacement of the body, in which avascular necrosis occurs much more commonly.

* Traction distally and then posteriorly on a Steinmann's pin through the calcaneus greatly assists this manipulation.

FRACTURE OF THE NECK OF THE TALUS WITH SUBTALAR DISLOCATION AND POSTERIOR DISPLACEMENT OF THE BODY

The mechanism of injury and displacement was discussed on pages 1172 and 1173. There is a fracture of the neck of the talus with backward displacement of the body, which lies on the inner aspect of the tuber calcanei, rotated so that its fractured surface is directed laterally, and with its medial tubercle hooked behind the sustentaculum tali (Figs 34.44 to 34.47). The treatment is often complicated by:

1. The danger of sloughing of skin over the displaced body of the bone.
2. The difficulty of replacing the body of the talus in the tibiofibular mortise.
3. The frequent association of fractures of the medial malleolus with interposition of periosteal tissues.
4. The grave danger of avascular necrosis of the dislocated body. (Between 70 and 90 per cent.[63,64,65a])

There is also danger of compression of the posterior tibial neuro-vascular bundle by the displaced body of the talus, threatening gangrene of the forefoot and sometimes responsible for a paralysis of the medial plantar nerve. If operative replacement is needed, care must be taken to protect this bundle.

Urgency of reduction. When the body of the talus lies over the inner aspect of the tuber calcanei the skin is tightly stretched over it and there is danger of sloughing from pressure on the deep surface and loss of blood supply. If this occurs the bone forms a sequestrum in an infected wound. The only treatment then available is excision of the dislocated body, with the inevitable consequence of gross limitation of function in the foot and ankle. Reduction is urgent. The talus must be replaced at once, either by manipulation, skeletal-traction or by open reduction.

Closed reduction of dislocation. In most cases closed reduction is impossible and in three recent series the necessity for open reduction varied from 70 to 100 per cent.[51,63,64,65a] In attempting any manipulative reduction the mechanism of displacement should be remembered. The foot should be put back into the position of deformity which it occupied at the moment that the body of the talus and the tuber calcanei became interlocked—that is, full dorsiflexion with the heel pulled forward. This itself may replace the body of the talus in the tibio-fibular mortise. The

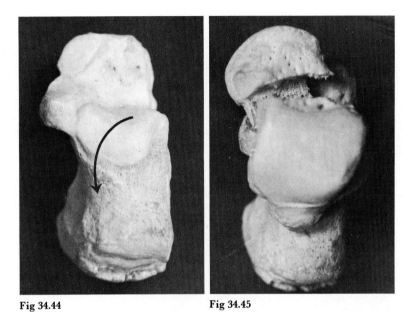

Fig 34.44   **Fig 34.45**

Figs 34.44 and 34.45 Superior aspect of calcaneum. The curved plane of the posterior facet leads directly to the medial surface of the tuber calcanei and guides the body of the talus to this position after fracture of the neck of the talus with subtalar dislocation.

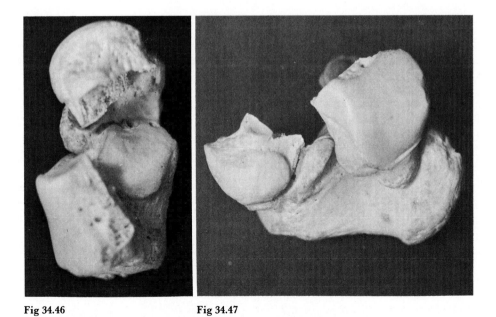

Fig 34.46   **Fig 34.47**

Figs 34.46 and 34.47 Position of the body of the talus in the third degree of displacement. The medial tubercle is locked behind the sustentaculum tali. With the disarticulated bones in his hand it is easy for the surgeon to teach himself the mechanism of displacement and the principle of reduction. Try it.

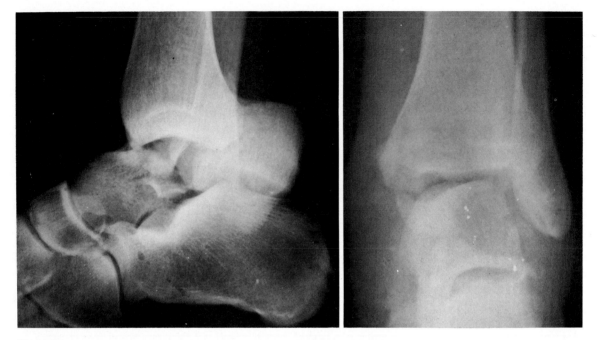

Fig 34.48

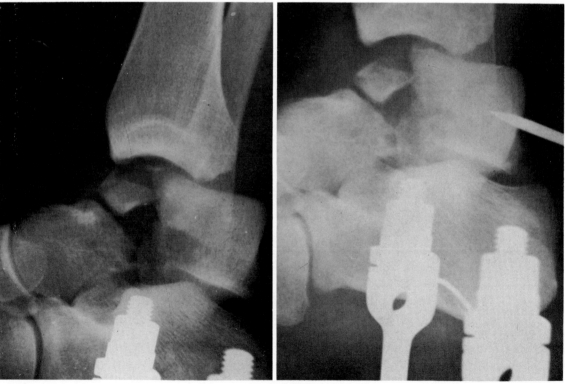

Fig 34.49   Fig 34.50

Figs 34.48 to 34.52 Fracture of the neck of the talus with subtalar dislocation and posterior displacement of the body during and after manipulative reduction by skeletal transfixion wire. Displacement is typical (Fig 34.48). The body of the talus lies on the inner aspect of the tuber calcanei, and it is rotated so that the fractured surface faces outwards. Simple manipulative reduction fails. It is reduced under radiographic control after transfixion of the bone by a Steinmann pin (Figs 34.49 to 34.51). The radiograph six weeks later confirms that reduction is still accurate but shows evidence of relative density and avascular necrosis of the body (Fig 34.52).

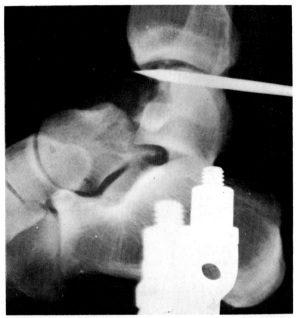

Fig 34.51

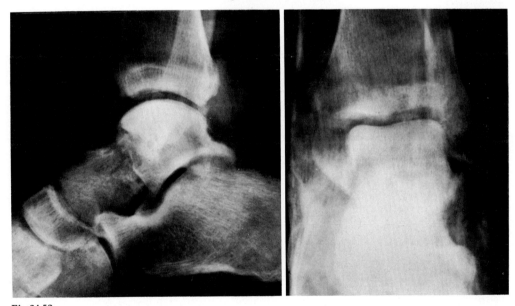

Fig 34.52

heel is then everted in order to unlock the sustentaculum tali. Finally, the foot is plantar-flexed to reduce the subtalar dislocation, while thumb pressure is maintained behind the ankle joint to prevent the body of the talus from redisplacing.

Closed reduction with skeletal-traction and manipulating pin. If this manipulation fails, traction may be used with a pin in the calcaneum so that the space between the tibia and calcaneum is increased. After everting the heel, thumb pressure is applied over the back of the body of the talus to push it forwards into the mortise. If there is still no success a second pin may be driven into the body of the talus by which to rotate it and guide it back to its socket (Figs 34.48 to 34.52).

Open reduction. The closed methods of reduction described above have a very limited chance of success, particularly if there has been a delay of 24 hours or so before definitive treatment is started. Preferably an incision should be made over the postero-medial aspect of the joint, but the condition of the skin may dictate a postero-lateral approach (Figs 34.53 and 34.54). The tendo Achillis can be split to give better access. Because the body of the talus has been displaced backwards the tuberosity and the insertion of the tendo Achillis are much closer than normal to the back of the ankle; and therefore the posterior capsule of the ankle and with it on the medial side, the neuro-vascular bundle, may present immediately under the skin incision. They must be carefully identified before opening the joint. Once the pathological anatomy has been displayed the reduction of the displaced body of the talus should be easy and the normal distance between the tibia and the tendo Achillis restored (Figs 34.55–34.57). Maintaining a stable position can be difficult and the addition of another Kirschner wire or Steinmann pin may be necessary (Fig 34.56).

Associated dislocation of the head of talus. Canale and Kelly have described a fourth type of fracture-dislocation of the talus, where not only is the body fragment completely displaced, but also the distal head of the talus is dislocated from the talo-navicular joint. In the three cases reported the results were poor or fair in all of them.[63]

Fracture of the medial malleolus. There is often an avulsion fracture of the medial malleolus, and when the body of the talus has been reduced there may be radiographic evidence that the malleolar fragment is not accurately replaced because a periosteal flap is interposed between it and the tibia (Fig 34.58). A short incision should be made to withdraw the flap and screw the fragment in position. In one case, after manipulative reduction, it was found that the medial malleolus was interposed between the head and body of the talus; it was obstructing accurate reduction of the fracture of the neck. The fragment was withdrawn and replaced in its normal position.

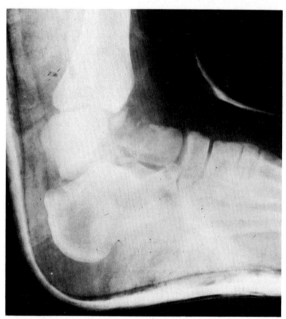

Fig 34.53

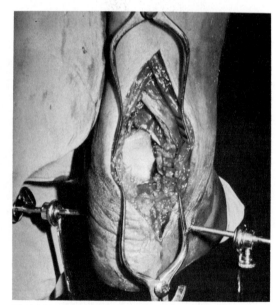

Fig 34.54

Figs 34.53 and 34.54 Figure 34.53 shows the lateral X-ray of a posteriorly displaced fracture of the body of the talus in the right ankle of the driver of a car involved in a head-on collision 10 days before. The ankle injury was complicated by a fracture of the lower third of the tibia. Closed manipulation and calcanean traction were unsuccessful. The poor condition of the skin demanded that the open reduction should be done through a posterior-lateral approach. Figure 34.54 shows the body of the talus pushed backwards and rotated through 90 degrees presenting its fibular trigonal surface posteriorly. The fracture surface of the neck of the talus lay against the fibula.

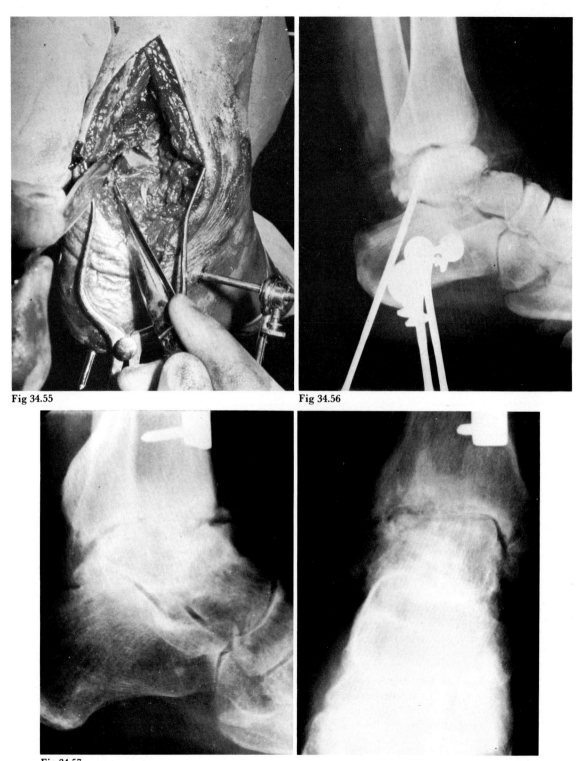

Fig 34.55

Fig 34.56

Fig 34.57

Figs 34.55 to 34.57 The same case as in Figures 34.53 and 34.54 showing the post-reduction operative appearance (Fig 34.55) and post-operative X-ray (Fig 34.56). Note how the normal relationship between the tuberosity of the calcaneum and the tibia has been restored. It was necessary to use a sagittal pin inserted through the tuberosity of the calcaneum to maintain reduction. The talo-tibial subluxation corrected itself later when the tibial shaft fracture became stable. Figure 34.57 shows the X-ray appearance two years later. The fracture has united but there is obvious avascular change in the body of the talus and degenerative changes in the ankle joint.

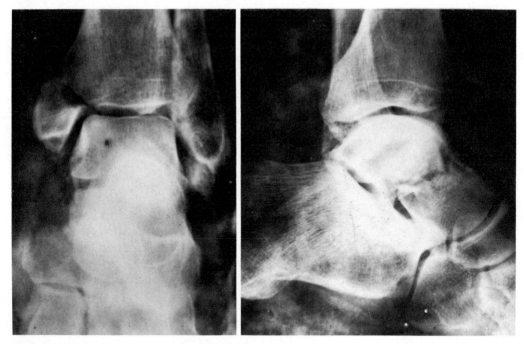

Fig 34.58 Fracture of the neck of the talus with subtalar dislocation and posterior displacement of the body after manipulative reduction, showing an associated fracture of the medial malleolus with interposition of a periosteal flap accounting for failure of accurate replacement.

Avascular necrosis of the body of the talus.
Figures for the incidence of this important complication are variable and the numbers in the series which have been reported have no statistical significance. But it seems clear that the incidence rises sharply according to the severity of the injury, and that an avascular necrosis rate of 75 to 80 per cent is not unrealistic for injuries with marked displacement of bone fragments. Certainly when the body of the talus is completely dislocated backwards all soft tissue attachments must be torn. It has been shown by injection studies that the main blood supply to the body of the talus enters the bone through the antero-inferior aspect of the neck from a complex of vessels originating from the tarsal sinus.[60] It would indeed be surprising if these vessels were not badly damaged in subtalar dislocation. If the bone is entirely deprived of its blood supply, avascular necrosis is inevitable. The diagnosis is established by the radiographic evidence of relative density. Care must be taken in accepting evidence of relative density of the talus, because in the lateral radiograph one part of the bone is overlapped by the shadows of both medial and lateral malleoli; the density of this area is always three times that of normal bone. The diagnosis of

avascular necrosis must be made on the evidence of relative density in the regions where there is no overlap of bone shadows. Weight-bearing in plaster should be deferred until the fracture of the neck of the talus is united.[65a] Immobilisation in a walking-plaster is then continued for several months longer. A removable patella bearing type of plastic gaiter with extensions into the heel of the shoe is useful at this stage (Sarmiento brace). Continued protection prevents crushing of the bone and minimises the danger of degenerative arthritis of the ankle joints. In some cases excellent function may be regained with a satisfactory range of painless movement (Figs 34.59 to 34.63), and certainly not all patients with avascular necrosis of the talus have severe disability or need surgery.[63]

Arthrodesis for degenerative arthritis. Degenerative arthritis may supervene in the ankle and subtalar joints after several months or years. If only one joint is involved it should be arthrodesed. Even when both joints are involved there should be no hesitation in performing a tibiocalcanean fusion. In a study of 75 fractures and dislocations of the talus, the most striking inference was that the results of excising the talus for degenerative change, or avascular necrosis were usually poor and the results of tibio-calcanean fusion were surprisingly good (Figs 34.64 to 34.67). Through an antero-lateral incision the lower shaft of the tibia, the ankle joint and the subtalar joint are exposed. Degenerated cartilage is removed from both joints, inversion deformity is corrected, and the foot is held in the optimal position, 10 degrees below the right angle. A trough is cut in the tibia and talus, with a socket in the calcaneum. A graft is removed from the opposite tibia, or slid down from the same tibia at a higher level. It is driven into the socket of the calcaneum and inlaid in the trough of the talus and tibia. Many years ago Blair described a similar fusion in which he utilised the intact head and neck of talus, driving his graft into this viable bone fragment without encroaching upon the subtalar joint.[61a,65b] If necessary, a screw may be used for fixation of the graft. Despite rigidity of the foot, the sound ankylosis and complete freedom from pain allows the patient to walk with little limp and resume all normal activities with the exception of strenuous contact games.

Arthrodesis after loss of the talus. It has already been said that the final results of excision of the talus are often unsatisfactory. Inversion deformity develops rapidly. The gait is halting and painful. A surgical boot with an inside iron and outside T-strap is sometimes needed. One patient whose talus was removed went back to heavy work as a miner, and for five years both the patient and the surgeon were satisfied. Two years later the patient was less satisfied; after three years he stopped work; and after four years he could scarcely walk. The joints were then arthrodesed. When the whole of the talus is missing, including the head, it is usually necessary to arthrodese the tibia, calcaneum and navicular. After freshening the opposing bone surfaces and driving a graft between the tibia and calcaneum, a second graft is inserted from the tibia to the navicular and the intervening spaces are filled with bone chips.

Comminuted fractures of the body of the talus. Even when the body of the talus is shattered into more than one piece the fragments should still be retained whenever possible. Despite the depression of the bone which will inevitably take place a stable ankle and plantigrade foot may be retained for some years, and the presence of talar bone substance within the ankle mortise greatly facilitates the tibio-calcanean fusion which will be required later (see Figures 34.68 and 34.69 and compare with figures 34.64 and 34.65). Excision of the talus should only be considered

for incorrectable deformity, gross contamination in compound fractures, and late sepsis.

Management of the late case of fracture-dislocation of the talus. When this injury is only seen for the first time many weeks or perhaps months after it has occurred, when it is still in the unreduced state, excision of the talus, despite its drawbacks, may be the only way to restore a plantigrade foot. Figures 34.70 and 34.71 show such a case in an 11-year-old boy with a six-week-old fracture-dislocation of the body of the talus. The excision of the talus gave an excellent correction of the deformity and function sufficiently good to allow the boy to take part in sport at school.

MINOR FRACTURES OF THE TALUS

Dome fracture. This rare injury has been described in detail by Nisbet[66] and later by Mukherjee and Young.[67] It is produced by a twist injury of the ankle, but it is not the same lesion as the fracture which has been described in association with a tear of the lateral ligament.[68] The site of the dome fracture is always on the lateral margin of the superior articular surface, resulting in the separation of a small fragment of bone, which is usually turned upside down (Fig 34.72). This fragment should be removed through a small antero-lateral incision.

Fractures of the lateral process. The lateral process of the talus is situated distal to its articular surface for the fibula and extends to the posterior inferior surface of the bone. A fracture through this process partially involves the subtalar joint and is therefore to be classified as an injury of that joint rather than of the ankle.[69] There has been some controversy over its mechanism, but experimental work and clinical studies have shown that the fracture can be reproduced by a compression force on the dome of the talus with the foot inverted and dorsiflexed.[69,70] As a result the fracture is sometimes present as a complication of an inversion strain of the ankle (Fig 34.73). The treatment should be by early operation, internally fixing large fragments with Kirschner wires, or excising small fragments.

Separation of the posterior tubercle of the talus. Separate ossicles are found not infrequently in association with the posterior margin of the talus and are usually attributed to a separate epiphysis which has not fused to the main mass—the so-called os trigonum. There is, however, good evidence to suggest

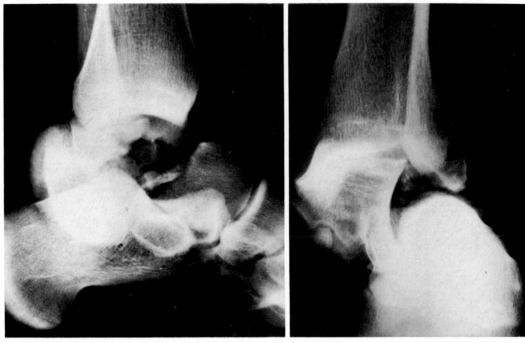

Fig 34.59

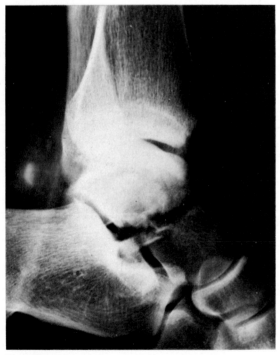

Fig 34.60

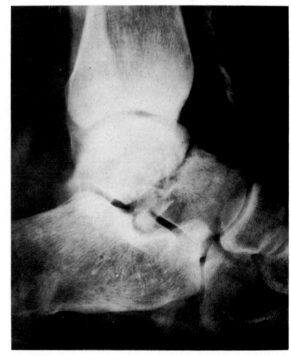

Fig 34.61

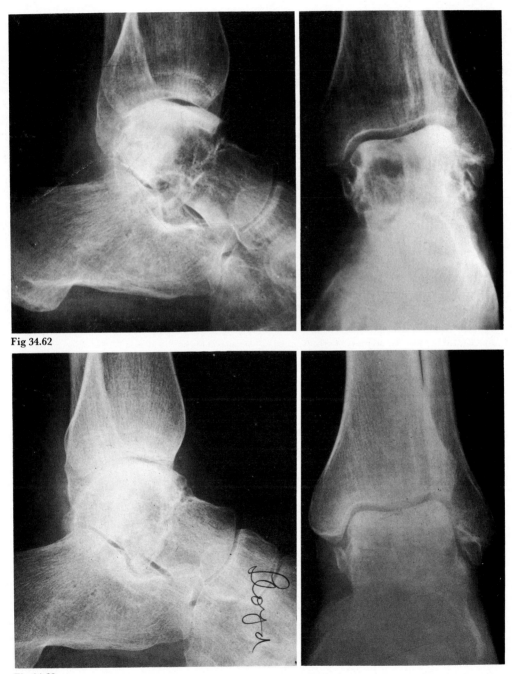

Fig 34.62

Fig 34.63

Figs 34.59 to 34.63 Fracture-dislocation of the talus with avascular necrosis of the body and revascularisation. Fig 34.59: Fracture of the neck of the talus with backward displacement of the body. Fig 34.60: Immediately after reduction. Fig 34.61: Six weeks after reduction. Fig 34.62: Six months after reduction. Fig 34.63: Twelve months after reduction. The radiograph six weeks after reduction shows relative density of the body of the talus, thus providing loss of blood supply. Immobilisation in plaster and protection from weight-bearing were continued for many months. Serial radiographs showed gradual revascularisation, proved by areas of decalcification beginning in the region of the fracture and gradually spreading backwards (Fig 34.62). The last area to revascularise was the subchondral region and articular surface of the ankle joint. Both ankle and subtalar joints suffered some degree of degenerative arthritis, shown in the narrowed joint space (Fig 34.63), but there was a satisfying range of painless movement and good function.

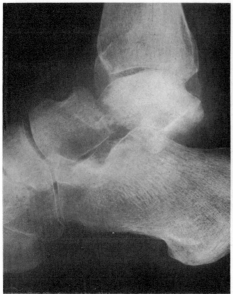

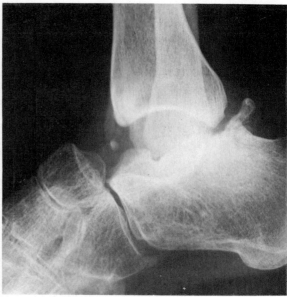

Fig 34.64 Old unreduced fracture of neck of talus with subtalar dislocation, complicated by avascular necrosis of the body of the talus, which is relatively dense.

Fig 34.65 Same case as shown in Figure 34.64. It was treated by excision of the body and head of talus. Function was good for two years, but it rapidly deteriorated after that until in five years' time the patient could scarcely walk. Tibio-calcean fusion was then performed.

that at least some of these fragments are detached as a result of repeated minor trauma. In full equinus the posterior rim of the talus impinges against the lower end of the tibia and acts as a 'natural bone block' to further plantar-flexion. This observation by Lambrinudi led to the development of his drop foot operation.[71] Repeated impingement of the tubercle against the tibia may eventually separate the tubercle from the body of the bone. This type of trauma is experienced repeatedly by footballers who kick the ball on the dorsum of the foot with the ankle in maximum equinus and may complain of pain in the back of the ankle when kicking.[72] The symptoms can be rapidly relieved by excision of the fragment. Some of the fragments can be of appreciable size and these are probably separate centres of ossification which have been strained by minor trauma.[73] Excision of the fragment is still the treatment of choice.

FRACTURES OF THE TARSAL NAVICULAR BONE

Three types of fracture of the navicular are to be distinguished:

1. Fracture of the tuberosity.
2. Fracture of the dorsal lip.
3. Transverse fracture with dislocation of the dorsal fragment.

Fracture of the tuberosity of the navicular. The tuberosity of the navicular may be avulsed by the tibialis posterior and may occur as an isolated fracture. This tendon has so many extensions to neighbouring bones that the separated fragment is seldom displaced widely and operative replacement is usually unnecessary. The foot should be immobilised in plaster for about four weeks and the functional

Figs 34.66 and 34.67 Tibio-calcaneal arthrodesis for avascular necrosis of the talus and degenerative arthritis of the ankle and subtalar joints (Fig 34.66). A graft cut from the upper shaft of the tibia has been inlaid in tibia and talus and impacted into a socket in the calcaneum. A simple screw was used to fix the graft at the upper end where it tended to spring. The radiograph four months after operation (Fig 34.67) shows sound fixation of both joints.

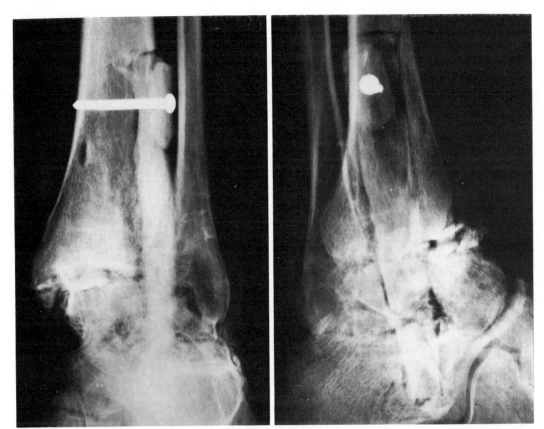

Fig 34.66

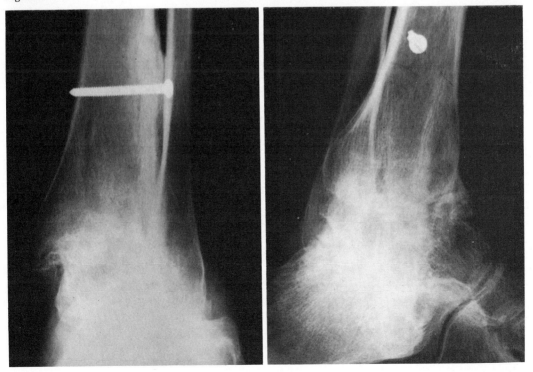

Fig 34.67

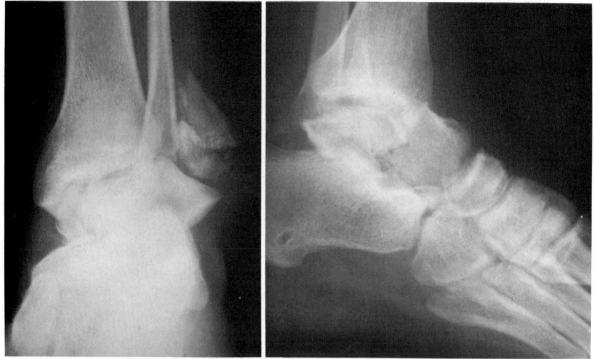

Fig 34.68

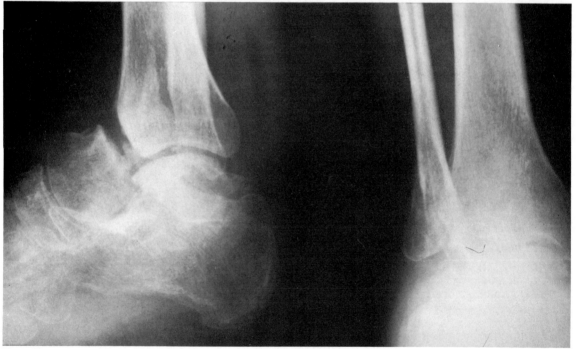

Fig 34.69

Figs 34.68 and 34.69 In this compound fracture of the ankle the neck of the talus was fractured, the body dislocated, and the displaced segment split into two parts (Fig 34.68). The fragments were replaced and despite considerable loss of height of the talus (Fig 34.69) a stable position of the ankle and foot was obtained greatly facilitating the tibio-calcanean fusion which was required later. (Compare with figures 34.64 and 34.65.)

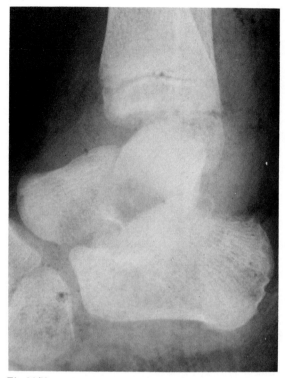

Fig 34.70

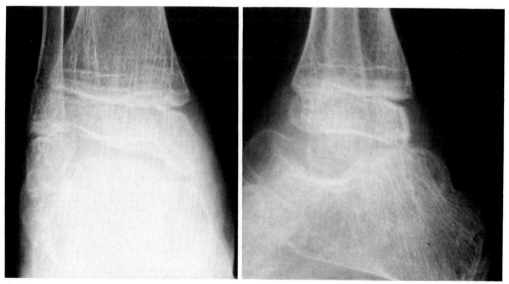

Fig 34.71

Figs 34.70 and 34.71 A case for excision of the talus. An 11-year-old boy sustained an injury to the right ankle, and X-rays taken at that time were not recognised as showing a fracture-dislocation of the body of the talus (Fig 34.70). Six weeks later the boy had a completely fixed ankle and foot with an inversion and equinus deformity. Complete excision of the talus gave a plantigrade foot with a useful range of movement at the tibio-calcanean joint. The boy was able to return to normal games activity at school (Fig 34.71).

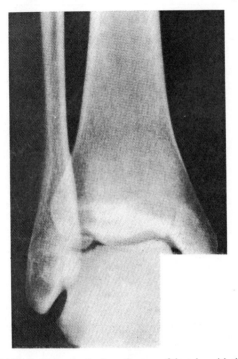

Fig 34.72 Radiograph of a dome fracture of the talus with the fragment lying upside down. (Reproduced by courtesy of the *Journal of Bone and Joint Surgery* and of Mr N. W. Nisbet from his paper (1954) Dome fracture of the talus. *Journal of Bone and Joint Surgery*, 36-B, 244).

result is nearly always good. It must be remembered, however, that this injury can be only a part of a more serious subluxation of the mid-tarsal joint and X-rays should be carefully scrutinised to exclude displacement of the forefoot.

Congenital os tibiale externum. Fracture of the tuberosity of the navicular is to be distinguished from the congenital anomaly of ossification in which the tuberosity develops from a second centre of ossification—known as the os tibiale externum. The line of separation is then quite smooth and regular and the congenital anomaly is usually bilateral. In both congenital and traumatic separations of the tuberosity, excision of the detached fragment may be needed if there is persistent pain.

Fracture of the dorsal lip of the navicular. A small flake of bone may be avulsed from the dorsal surface of the navicular. Immobilisation in plaster is required only for a short period. The results are usually excellent, but as they are avulsion injuries they may be part of mid-tarsal subluxation, particularly if associated with a calcaneo-cuboid injury.[24] Such an injury requires six weeks in plaster, followed by the use of a moulded longitudinal arch support.

Transverse fractures of the navicular. The body of the navicular is fractured transversely in a

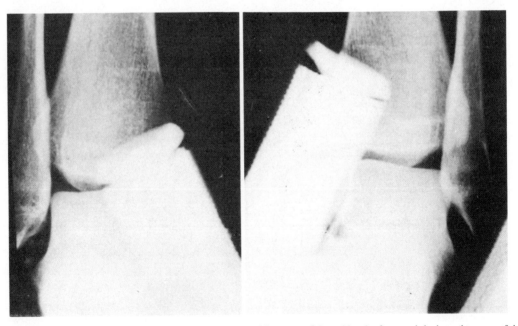

Fig 34.73 This patient, in addition to sustaining a tear of the lateral ligament of the ankle, also fractured the lateral process of the talus as a result of inversion strain at the ankle and subtalar joint.

horizontal plane so that the bone is divided into a large dorsal and a small plantar fragment. These injuries result from a longitudinal thrust along the metatarsal rays while the ankle is in equinus.[74] The large fragment is dislocated upwards from the talonavicular-cuneiform joints. It is often possible to replace the displaced bone by pressure over its dorsal surface while the foot is held in plantar-flexion, but redisplacement is liable to occur despite a closely moulded plaster. Redisplacement can be prevented by the counter-traction of a pin through the calcaneum and a Kirschner wire through the bases of the metatarsals, the pin and wire being left in position and incorporated in the plaster. Occasionally the navicular is impacted on the dorsal lip of the head of the talus ·and cannot be reduced except by open operation (Figs 34.74 to 34.76). It may be held reduced by transfixion with Kirschner wires. But whether the dislocated fragment is reduced by manipulation, skeletal transfixion or open operation, the sequel is usually the same. The fragmented bone often undergoes absorption and the small plantar fragment may disappear altogether. The keystone maintaining the longitudinal arch is lost and a traumatic flat-foot deformity is established. Arthritis develops in the talo-navicular and naviculo-cuneiform joints and good function is secured only when the joints become firmly ankylosed by dense fibrous tissue. The disability period is prolonged. If pain cannot be controlled by arch supports and shoe alterations there can be little doubt that the treatment of choice is an early arthrodesis of both joints. An incision is made over the bone, articular cartilage is denuded, the dislocated fragment is replaced, and a small graft cut from the tibia or ilium is inlaid in a trough cut from the head of the talus to the medial cuneiform. The foot is immobilised in plaster until union is sound, usually at least 10 weeks after operation.

Main and Jowett[74] have pointed out that if the ankle is in acute plantar-flexion the longitudinal

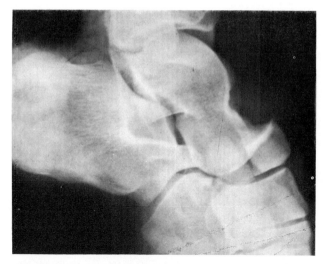

Fig 34.74

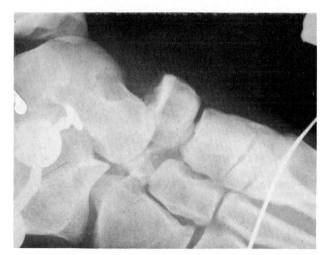

Fig 34.75

Figs 34.74 to 34.76 Transverse fracture of the navicular with dislocation of the large dorsal fragment. Attempted reduction by plantar-flexion and direct pressure over the fragment failed (Fig 34.74). An attempt was then made by skeletal-traction from a Steinmann pin in the calcaneum and Kirschner wire in the metatarsals (Fig 34.75); this also failed. The navicular was impaled on the dorsal lip of the head of the talus and it was reduced only by operative exposure (Fig 34.76). Transfixion with crossed Kirschner wires is a wise precaution to prevent redisplacement. Despite accurate reduction, degenerative arthritis of the damaged joints necessitated arthrodesis. (Treatment by the late Mr I. Lawson Dick).

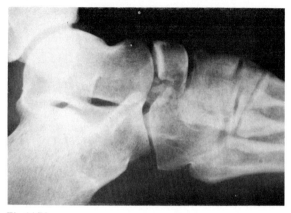

Fig 34.76

force may be expended towards the medial side of the navicular, resulting in a verticular fracture of the body—sometimes with extrusion of a medial fragment. The treatment for this injury is nearly always conservative. As the longitudinal arch is not disrupted the prognosis is less gloomy than in the case of the transverse fracture.

Avascular necrosis of the scaphoid. Avascular necrosis due to osteochondritis of the tarsal scaphoid (Kohler's disease) is a well known although fairly rare condition of childhood which always heals without any residual deformity. It is very unusual for avascular change to present in the adult bone. Wiley and Brown[75] described three cases of listhesis of the adult scaphoid resulting in approximation of the head of the talus to the cuneiforms. There was no suggestion that this was a sequel to childhood disease. Another example is illustrated in Figures 34.77 to 34.79. This patient complained of pain in the mid-tarsal region of the foot without any history of injury or childhood disease. It is possible that the adult manifestation of avascular necrosis may be the result of a stress fracture of the scaphoid (see Chapter 35, stress fractures). It should be treated by a period of rest in plaster. Triple arthrodesis of the foot may be required.[75]

FRACTURE-DISLOCATION OF THE MID-TARSAL JOINT

The mid-tarsal or talo-navicular calcaneo-cuboid joint is usually dislocated by abduction or adduction stresses to the foot. Sometimes only the talo-navicular joint is disrupted—the forefoot twisting medially around an axis of rotation which appears to be an intact interosseus talo-calcanean ligament (Figs 34.80 to 34.82). Main and Jowett have described this as the 'swivel dislocation'.[74] Manipulative reduction is seldom difficult, and if there is no associated fracture of the tarsal bones good function is restored quite quickly. Sometimes, however, the dislocations may be associated with fracture of the navicular or cuboid bones. A crushing injury, such as is produced when the wheel of a lorry is driven over the foot or when a heavy weight falls upon it, may comminute the tarsal bones and drive the navicular into the head of the talus, or the cuboid into the front of the calcaneum. Dewar and Evans[24] and other surgeons[22,23] have

pointed out how easily the subluxation of the foot can be missed in these cases if a fracture of the calcaneus is considered in isolation, and they have advised an aggressive attitude towards treatment. In these circumstances accurate reduction of the bone fragments may demand operative treatment and Kirschner wire fixation. But even when the mid-tarsal dislocation is replaced and the bone fragments reduced, there is often persistent disability from traumatic arthritis of the injured joints with widespread osteoporosis, adhesion formation, painful stiffness and other disuse changes. It is sometimes better to anticipate these disabilities after reduction of the dislocation by arthrodesing the calcaneo-cuboid or the mid-tarsal joint within two or three weeks, sometimes using free grafts of cancellous bone cut from the ilium to accelerate the surgical fusion. Of course, if the subtaloid joint is also involved a full triple arthrodesis should be carried out. In either case the foot should be immobilised in plaster after operation for about three months.

Mid-tarsal dislocation with paralysis of the plantar nerve. A dislocation of the mid-tarsal joint, shown in Figures 34.83 and 34.84, was associated with injury to the medial and lateral plantar nerves, causing anaesthesia of the plantar surfaces of the toes and paralysis of the lumbrical and interosseus muscles, with claw deformity of the toes just like 'main en griffe' from corresponding paralysis of the hand. Kenwright and Taylor describe a similar case with partial paralysis of the medial plantar nerve.[51] The phrase 'pied on griffe' gives an exact description of the disability. In tarsal and metatarsal injuries special attention should be paid to the possibility of associated injuries to the plantar nerves and the blood vessels of the foot, as well as the neurovascular bundle behind the medial malleolus.

FRACTURE-DISLOCATIONS OF THE TARSO-METATARSAL JOINT

Tarso-metatarsal dislocations were hallowed in history at Waterloo. In the campaigns of Napoleon and Wellington, Lisfranc developed his amputation at the tarso-metatarsal level for closed injuries of the foot. He knew the perils of gangrene from this injury long

---

Figs 34.77 to 34.79 This 63-year-old woman patient presented with a history of pain in the mid-tarsal joint of her right foot for several months. There was marked avascular change in the scaphoid with a possible linear defect (Fig 34.77). The symptoms were relieved by two months rest in a walking plaster but the changes in the bone were still apparent three years later (Fig 34.78). A defect seen in an earlier film taken elsewhere (Fig 34.79) suggests that this condition may have arisen as a result of a stress fracture (see Chapter 35—stress fractures).

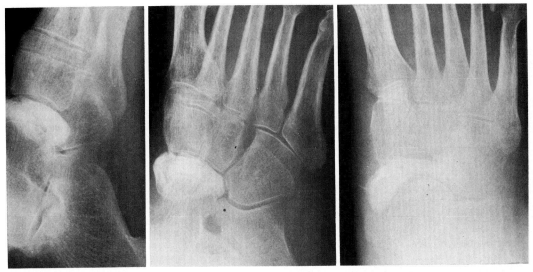

Fig 34.77

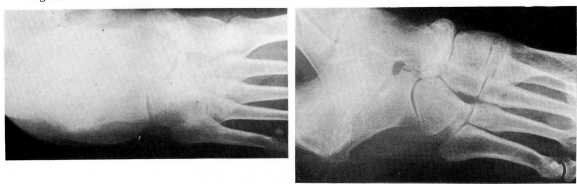

Fig 34.78

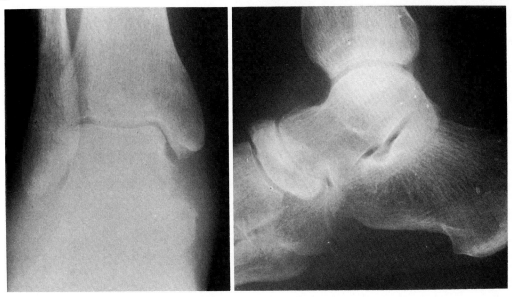

Fig 34.79

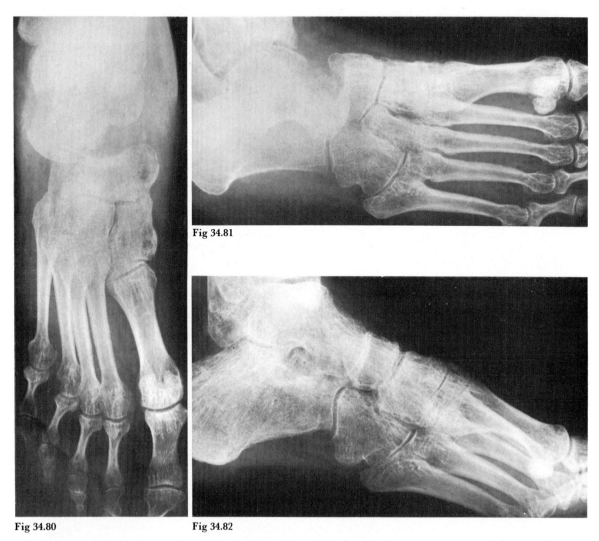

Fig 34.81

Fig 34.80   Fig 34.82

Figs 34.80 to 34.82 Medial swivel dislocation of the mid-tarsal joint. Figure 34.80 shows the antero-posterior view of the talo-navicular displacement in a medial swivel dislocation of the mid-tarsal joint. The calcaneum has swivelled beneath the talus on an axis formed by the talo-calcanean ligament. Figures 34.81 and 34.82 show that while the calcaneo-cuboid joint is undisplaced the talo-navicular joint is clearly subluxated and the forefoot is out of alignment with the hindfoot. (Reproduced by kind permission of the *Journal of Bone and Joint Surgery* and of Messrs B. J. Main and R. L. Jowett, from their paper (1975) Injuries of the mid-tarsal joint. *Journal of Bone and Joint Surgery*, 57-B, 89).

before we knew the pathogenesis of traumatic arterial spasm and ischaemia.[76,77] A number of investigations have attempted to elucidate the mechanism of this complex injury.[78,79,80] From clinical and experimental studies it would appear that there is no clear-cut series of strains responsible, but that the dislocation occurs as the result of a combination of forces, rotation with plantar-flexion being the most important. The dislocation may be due to direct injury, when the

metatarsals are displaced in any direction determined by the line of force; and indirect injury, when displacement follows certain set patterns. Basically, the indirect injury is first a dorsal dislocation of the metarsals which can be produced in a variety of ways.[81] Probably the most common cause is a car accident, where the forces applied to the braced and plantar-flexed foot are sufficient to displace the metatarsal heads dorsally. But the same injury can be

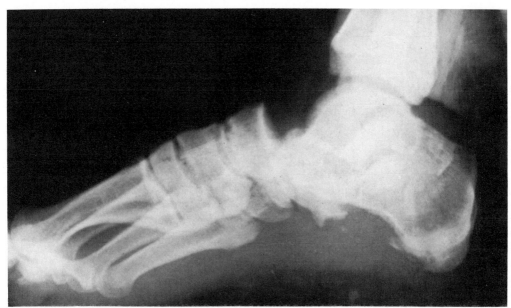

Fig 34.83

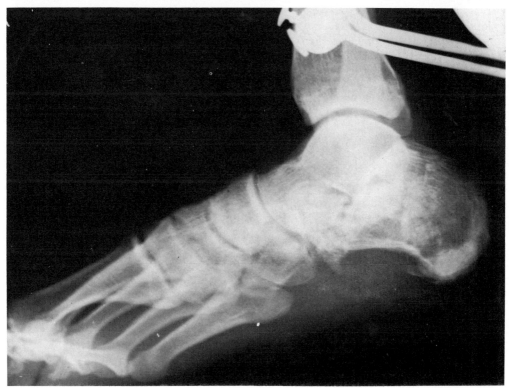

Fig 34.84

Figs 34.83 and 34.84 Fracture-dislocation of the mid-tarsal joint with injury of the plantar nerves causing 'pied en griffe'. This mid-tarsal dislocation was unusual in the association of a comminuted fracture of the calcaneum. There was also injury to the medial and lateral plantar nerves causing anaesthesia of the plantar surface of the toes with paralysis of the lumbrical and interosseus muscles, giving rise to clawing of the toes similar to that of 'main en griffe' deformity of the hand from paralysis of the ulnar nerve. In all tarsal, tarso-metatarsal and metatarsal injuries of the foot the possibility of injury to the plantar nerves and to the dorsalis pedis and posterior tibial vessels must be considered.

produced as a result of a fall from a horse, the foot trapped in the stirrup being forcibly bent at the tarso-metatarsal joint by the weight of the falling body. Displacement of the forefoot in the coronal plane to one or other side, or sometimes divarication of the first metarsal from the rest of the metatarsus, depend upon the subsequent forces which are applied. An essential factor in maintaining the stability of the whole joint is the shape of the second metatarso-cuneiform joint. The bone of the second metatarsal is dovetailed into the tarsus and a complete dislocation cannot take place until this joint is ruptured or fractured.[79] The dislocations have been classified as homolateral displacement (Fig 34.85) where the lateral four, or all five metatarsals, are displaced together, usually to the lateral side; or divergent displacements (Fig 34.86), when the first ray is displaced medially, sometimes along with the medial cuneiform bone, while the rest of the metatarsals move laterally.[81,82] These dislocations may sometimes be treated safely by manipulative reduction—the more promptly the better—with immobilisation in a padded plaster cast and elevation of the limb during the first few days, but the reduction can be very

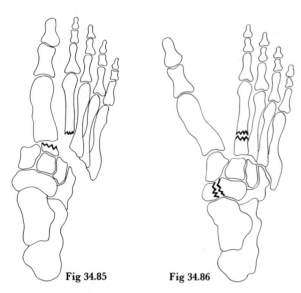

Fig 34.85   Fig 34.86

Figs 34.85 and 34.86 Drawings to show the two types of tarso-metatarsal dislocations. The homolateral variety is shown in figure 34.85 where the whole of the metatarsus displaces laterally. In the divergent type (Fig 34.86) the first metatarsal is displaced medially, sometimes taking with it the medial cuneiform and fracturing the tuberosity of the scaphoid, while the other metatarsals are dislocated to the lateral side. It is to be noted that neither of these dislocations can occur without a fracture of the base of the second metatarsal. (After Aitken and Poulson.)

unstable and it is usually necessary to maintain the position by the insertion of percutaneous Kirschner wires (Figs 34.87 and 34.88). Sometimes, however, particularly where the brunt of the deformity lies in the first metatarso-cuneiform joint, there may be obstruction, such as the tendon of tibialis anterior which can become trapped between the cuneiform bones.[83] In such a case there should be no hesitation in performing an open reduction. But as Gissane pointed out this is a dangerous type of fracture;[84] lateral rotation or pronation force, in dislocating the forefoot, may separate the bases of the first and second metatarsals and rupture the dorsalis pedis artery; it may also twist the main vessels behind the medial malleolus and cause arterial spasm and thrombosis of the main plantar vessels. The essential points of treatment are therefore:

1. To reduce the displacement promptly and completely, either by manipulation or by open operation. In either case the displaced bones should be stabilised with percutaneous Kirschner wires.
2. To maintain the reduction by means of a suitably padded plaster cast with high elevation of the limb.
3. To defer weight-bearing for at least two months.

The management of threatened ischaemia and gangrene has been discussed in Chapter 11.

FRACTURES OF THE METATARSALS

Avulsion fracture of the base of the fifth metatarsal bone (Jones fracture). The first report of this fracture was in 1902 when Sir Robert Jones described sustaining the injury himself when dancing.[85] Previous to this paper the condition had always been assumed to be due to a strain or rupture of the peroneus longus tendon. The peroneus brevis, however, is inserted into the tubercle at the base of the fifth metatarsal bone and severe inversion stresses applied to the foot may give rise to a crack fracture or to complete avulsion of the fragment of bone to which the tendon is inserted (Fig 34.89). This fracture must be distinguished from the normal epiphyseal line at the base of the tubercle which is present in children between the ages of 9 and 14, and also from the sesamoid bones which are sometimes present in association with both peroneal tendons. Usually there is no displacement and the only treatment required is simple strapping of the foot for a few weeks. Sometimes a walking plaster may be needed. Although a few rare cases of delayed or non-union have

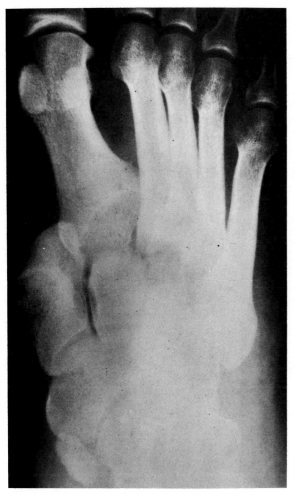 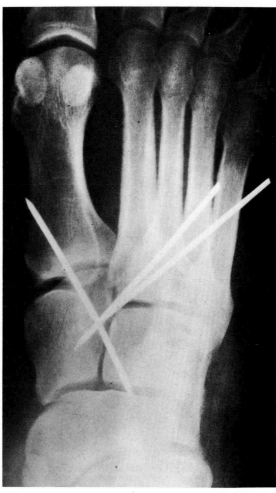

Fig 34.87   **Fig 34.88**

Figs 34.87 and 34.88 A homolateral dislocation of the tarso-metatarsal joint (Fig 34.87) has been stabilised by three percutaneous Kirschner wires (Fig 34.88). Even though it may be possible to reduce these dislocations by closed manipulation, they redisplace in plaster very readily unless fixed in this way.

been reported[86] they have given no functional disability.

However, a second type of basal fracture of the fifth metatarsal has been described where the fracture is in the shaft of the bone and just distal to the tuberosity flare.[86] These fractures may be slow to unite and some have even needed bone grafting. Such injuries should be treated with more respect than the avulsion of the tuberosity and require immobilisation in plaster for six weeks.

Fracture of the necks of the metatarsals.
Simple crack fractures of the necks of one or more

metatarsal bones occurring from simple weight-bearing stresses such as marching are considered with pathological fractures in Chapter 35. More complete fractures of the metatarsal necks arising from severe injury are still more serious because there is usually displacement of the metatarsal heads into the sole which if not reduced gives rise to serious disability (Fig 34.90). If the bones are allowed to unite in this position the undue prominence of the metatarsal heads in the tread causes pain every time an attempt is made to step forwards so that the patient may be completely crippled. It is usually possible to correct the displacement by simple manipulation with the

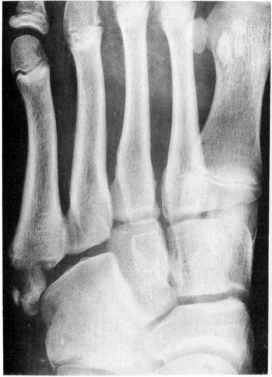

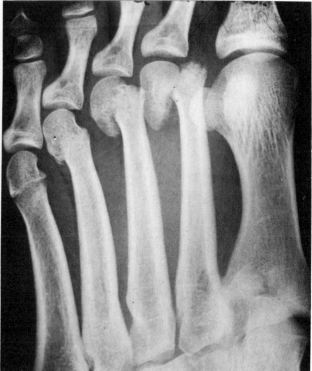

Fig 34.89 Avulsion of base of fifth metatarsal by peroneus brevis tendon (Jones fracture).

Fig 34.90 Fracture of necks of second to fifth metatarsals.

application of a plaster extending well beyond the metatarso-phalangeal joints to include the toes in their corrected position. There is never need for the traction that was formerly advised by means of loops of stainless-steel wire passed through the pulp of the toes and fixed to a spreader. Very occasionally when manipulative reduction fails it may be wise to correct the deformity by means of an open operation through two small dorsal incisions between the second and third and fourth and fifth toes.[87] The fractures can be easily stabilised with short Kirschner wires.

Fractures of the metatarsals with gangrene of the forefoot. The ischaemic changes already noted in tarsal and tarso-metatarsal injuries of the foot may also complicate fractures of the necks of the metatarsal bones. One such case is shown in Figures 34.91 and 34.92. It is true that in this case there had been long exposure on the side of a mountain, which in itself impaired the vascular supply.

Mal-united fracture of the necks of the metatarsal bones. When a fracture of the metatarsal bone has united with the head displaced into the sole and the patient complains of severe and persistent pain whenever weight is borne under the tread, with a sensation like that of 'walking on a stone', the disability should be relieved by excision of the metatarsal head through a dorsal incision.

FRACTURES OF THE TOES

Fractures of the proximal phalanges of the toes show the same displacement as the corresponding fracture of the phalanges of the fingers. The tension of the lumbrical and interosseus muscles causes angulation, and if this is not corrected the toe remains clawed and a bony lump develops on the plantar surface with persistent tenderness and pain. The symptoms may necessitate amputation, and if several toes are fractured the resulting disability is serious. With multiple toe fractures the displacement should be reduced by flexing the toes and immobilising them in a full length below-knee plaster extending to the tips of the toes and using a walking rocker to prevent any pressure on the distal end of the cast.

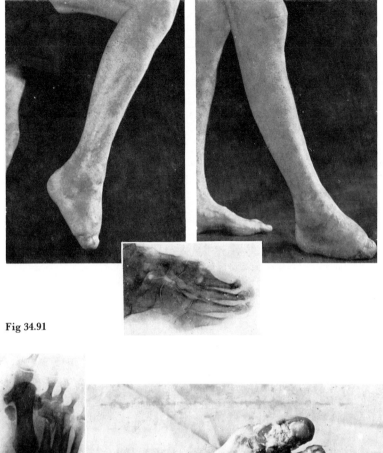

Fig 34.91

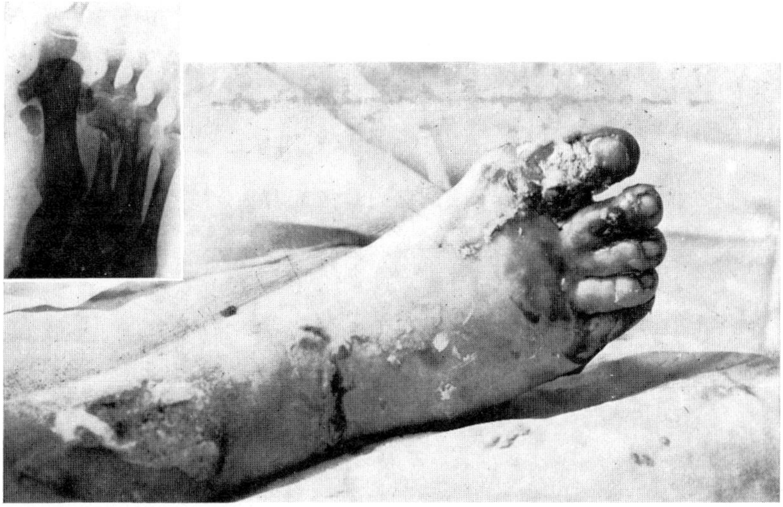

Fig 34.92

Figs 34.91 and 34.92 Fracture of the necks of the metatarsals with gangrene of the toes, to which an important contributory factor was long exposure on the side of a mountain. The important point of treatment to be recognised is that local amputation sufficed.

Comminuted fracture of phalanges of the great toe. The most frequent injury to the forefoot is a comminuted fracture of one or both phalanges of the great toe from the dropping of a heavy weight.

The fragments are seldom displaced and the protection of a collodion gauze dressing is adequate. Immediate weight-bearing is allowed in a boot with the toe-cap cut out and a metatarsal bar screwed on the sole at the level of the tread. A painful subungual haematoma should always be decompressed by drilling the nail.

Fracture of the sesamoid bones of the great toe. The dropping of a weight on the foot may crush the sesamoid bones of the great toe between the metatarsal head and the ground. The fracture is comminuted. One or both sesamoids may be involved, but the tibial (medial) sesamoid is more likely to fracture. The injury must be distinguished from congenital bipartite and tripartite sesamoids. In a true fracture the line is usually irregular whereas in bifurcation it is smooth.[88] Fracture of the bone involves the articular surface, and since the whole of the body-weight is transmitted through this joint with every step the resulting disability may be serious. It is sometimes necessary to excise the sesamoid. After operation a metatarsal bar may be fitted behind the tread of the sole in order to relieve weight-bearing.

The disability is sometimes prolonged and it is often necessary to continue suitable protection by metatarsal bars or sorbo-insoles for several months.

CHOPART'S FOREFOOT AMPUTATION

Severe crush injuries of the forefoot may require partial ablation. Up until recently the Chopart amputation through the midtarsal joint was considered inadvisable because of the frequent occurrence of an equino-varus deformity. However, this can be prevented at the time of amputation by transferring the tibialis anterior to the neck of the talus, and by suturing the extensor tendons into the sole of the foot.[89] It is also claimed that the same result can be achieved by carrying out a second stage subtalar fusion some months after amputation.[90] With such modifications Chopart's operation has been found to give superior results to the Symes amputation.[89]

REFERENCES

1. Langloh N D, Hunder G G, Riggs B L, Kelly P J 1973 Transient painful osteoporosis of the lower extremities. Journal of Bone and Joint Surgery 55–A: 1188
2. Viljanto J 1975 Bicycle and moped spoke injuries in children. An analysis of 103 consecutive cases. Annals Chirurgiae et Gynaecologiae Fenniae 64: 100
3. Ahmed M 1979 Motor cycle spoke injury. British Medical Journal 2: 401
4. Floman Y, Katz S 1975 Osseous lesion simulating a bone tumour due to unsuspected fragment of wood in the foot. Injury 6: 344
5. Rhydderch A I 1960 Chronic septic arthritis caused by foreign bodies. Two patients with infection of the ankle from wood splinters. Journal of Bone and Joint Surgery 42–B: 405
6. Brown J E 1960 Sinus tarsi syndrome. Clinical Orthopaedics and Related Research 18: 231
7. Meyer J M, Lagier R 1977 Post-traumatic sinus tarsi syndrome. An anatomical and radiological study. Acta Orthopaedica Scandinavica 48: 121
8. Furey J G 1975 Plantar fasciitis—the painful heel syndrome. Journal of Bone and Joint Surgery 57–A: 672
9. Williams R 1963 Chronic non-specific tendovaginitis of tibialis posterior. Journal of Bone and Joint Surgery 45–B: 542
10. Essex-Lopresti P 1952 The mechanism, reduction technique, and results in fractures of the os calcis. British Journal of Surgery 39: 395
11. Zayer M 1969 Fracture of the calcaneus. A review of 110 fractures. Acta Orthopaedica Scandinavica 40: 530
12. Nade S, Monahan P R W 1973 Fracture of the calcaneus—a study of the long-term prognosis. Injury 4: 201
13. Matteri R E, Frymoyer J N 1973 Fractures of the calcaneus in young children. Report of three cases. Journal of Bone and Joint Surgery: 55–A: 1091
14. Hunt D D 1970 Compression fracture of the anterior articular surface of the calcaneus. Journal of Bone and Joint Surgery 52–A: 1637
15. Böhler L 1958 The treatment of fractures, 5th English edn. Grune & Stratton, New York, Vol III, p 2046
16. Jaekle R F, Clark A G 1937 Fractures of the os calcis. Surgery, Gynecology and Obstetrics 64: 663
17. Warrick C K, Bremner A E 1953 Fractures of the calcaneum. Journal of Bone and Joint Surgery 35–B: 33
18. Palmer I 1948 The mechanism and treatment of fractures of the calcaneus. Journal of Bone and Joint Surgery 30–A: 2
19. Soeur R, Remy R 1975 Fractures of the calcaneus with displacement of the thalamic portion. Journal of Bone and Joint Surgery 57–B: 413
20. Aaron D A R, Howat T W 1976 Intra-articular fractures of the calcaneum. Injury 7: 205
21. Böhler L 1958 The treatment of fractures. 5th English edn. Grune & Stratton, New York, vol III, p 2047
22. Lowy M 1969 Avulsion fractures of the calcaneus. Journal of Bone and Joint Surgery 51–B: 494
23. Protheroe K 1969 Avulsion fractures of the calcaneus. Journal of Bone and Joint Surgery 51–B: 118
24. Dewar F P, Evans D F 1968 Occult fracture-subluxation of the mid-tarsal joint. Journal of Bone and Joint Surgery 50–B: 386
25. Morestin H 1902 Quoted by Schwartz M A 1929 in Bulletins et Memoires de la Societe Nationale de Chirurgie 55: 148
26. Isbister J F St C 1974 Calcaneo-fibular abutment following crush fractures of the calcaneus. Journal of Bone and Joint Surgery 56–B: 274
27. Farrow R C 1962 Peroneal release in calcaneal fractures. Journal of Bone and Joint Surgery 44–B: 961
28. Magnuson P B 1923 An operation for relief of disability in old fractures of os calcis. Journal of the American Medical Association 80: 1511
29. Anthonsen W 1943 An oblique projection for roentgen

examination of the talo calcanean joint particularly regarding intra-articular fracture of the calcaneus. Acta Radiologica 24: 306

30. Levine J, Kenin A, Spinner M 1959 Non-union of a fracture of the anterior superior process of the calcaneus. Case report. Journal of Bone and Joint Surgery 41–A: 178

31. Piatt A D 1956 Fracture of the promontory of the calcaneus. Radiology 67: 386

32. Trickey E L 1975 Treatment of fractures of the calcaneus. (Editorial.) Journal of Bone and Joint Surgery 57–B: 411

33. Roberts N W 1947 Symposium on fractures of the os calcis. (Annual Meeting of the British Orthopaedic Association, London, 1946.) Journal of Bone and Joint Surgery 29: 254

34. Roberts N W 1968 Fractures of the calcaneus. Journal of Bone and Joint Surgery 50–B: 884

35. Barnard L 1963 Non-operative treatment of fractures of the calcaneus. Journal of Bone and Joint Surgery 45–A: 865

36. Barnard L, Odegard J K 1970 Conservative approach in the treatment of fractures of the calcaneus. Journal of Bone and Joint Surgery 52–A: 1689

37. Evans J D 1966 Conservative management of os calcis fractures. Journal of the Royal College of Surgeons of Edinburgh 12: 40

38. Maxfield J E, McDermott F J 1955 Experiences with the Palmer open reduction of fractures of the calcaneus. Journal of Bone and Joint Surgery 37–A: 99

39. Maxfield J E 1963 Treatment of calcaneal fractures by open reduction. Journal of Bone and Joint Surgery 45–A: 868

40. Fisk G R 1978 Fracture of the os calcis treated by open reduction and iliac crest grafting. Hunterian Lecture given at The Royal College of Surgeons of England, 12th January 1978

40a. Urowitz E, Hall H 1980 The medial approach to fracture of the os calcis. Journal of Bone and Joint Surgery 62–B: 131

41. Gallie W E 1943 Subastragalar arthrodesis in fractures of the os calcis. Journal of Bone and Joint Surgery 25: 731

42. Dick I L 1953 Primary fusion of the posterior subtalar joint in the treatment of fractures of the calcaneum. Journal of Bone and Joint Surgery 35–B: 375

42a. Noble J, McQuillan W M 1979 Early posterior subtalar fusion in the treatment of fractures of the os calcis. Journal of Bone and Joint Surgery 61–B: 90

43. Pridie K H 1946 A new method of treatment for severe fracture of the os calcis. A preliminary report. Surgery, Gynecology and Obstetrics 82: 671

44. Cleminson K 1952 Excision of calcaneum for fracture. Journal of Bone and Joint Surgery 34–B: 158

44a. Garcia G, Garcia-Rubio M, Coneijero-Lopez V, Cachero Bernandiz D 1979 Tarsal tunnel syndrome: a report of fifty-six cases. Journal of Bone and Joint Surgery 61–B: 123

45. Thompson K R, Friesen C M 1959 Treatment of comminuted fractures of the calcaneus by primary triple arthrodesis. Journal of Bone and Joint Surgery 41–A: 1423

46. Hall M C, Pennal G F 1960 Primary subtalar arthrodesis in the treatment of severe fractures of the calcaneus. Journal of Bone and Joint Surgery 42–B: 336

47. Schottstaedt E R 1963 Symposium: treatment of fractures of the calcaneus. Introduction. Journal of Bone and Joint Surgery 45–A: 863

48. Bonnin J G 1940 Dislocations and fracture-dislocations of the talus. British Journal of Surgery 28: 88

49. Coltart W D 1952 Aviator's astragalus. Journal of Bone and Joint Surgery 34–B: 545

50. Shephard E 1951 Tarsal movements. Journal of Bone and Joint Surgery 33–B: 258

51. Kenwright J, Taylor R G 1970 Major injuries of the talus. Journal of Bone and Joint Surgery 52–B: 36

52. Anderson H 1919 Medical and surgical aspects of aviation. Henry Froude, London. Oxford University Press: Hodder and Stoughton

53. Dummit E S, Reid R L 1969 Unique tibial shaft fractures resulting from helicopter crashes. Clinical Orthopaedics and Related Research 66: 155

54. Shands A R Jr 1928 The incidence of subastragaloid dislocation of the foot with a report of one case of the inward type. Journal of Bone and Joint Surgery 10: 306

55. Taylor R G 1962 Immobilisation of unstable fracture-dislocations by the use of Kirschner wires. Proceedings of the Royal Society of Medicine 55: 499

56. Brantigan J W, Pedigana L R, Lippert E G 1977 Instability of the sub-taloid joint. Diagnosis by stress tomography in three cases. Journal of Bone and Joint Surgery 59–A: 321

57. Chrisman O D, Snook G A 1969 Reconstruction of lateral ligament tears of the ankle. Journal of Bone and Joint Surgery 51–A: 904

58. Ekehorn G 1904 Ein Fall von Isolierter Luxation des Calcaneus. Nordiskt Medicinskt Archiv Afd I (Kirurgi) Haft 4, N: r 15

59. Viswanath S S, Shephard E 1977 Dislocation of the calcaneum. Injury 9: 50

60. Halliburton R A, Sullivan C R, Kelly P J, Petersen L F A 1958 The extra-osseous and intra-osseous blood supply of the talus. Journal of Bone and Joint Surgery 40–A: 1115

60a. Segal D, Wasilewski S 1980 Total dislocation of the talus. Journal of Bone and Joint Surgery 62–A: 1370

61. Detenbeck L C, Kelly P J 1969 Total dislocation of the talus. Journal of Bone and Joint Surgery 51–A: 283

61a. Dennis M D, Tulles H S 1980 Blair tibio-talar arthrodesis for injuries of the talus. Journal of Bone and Joint Surgery 62–A: 103

62. McKeever F M 1963 Treatment of complications of fractures and dislocations of the talus. Clinical Orthopaedics and Related Research 30: 45

63. Canale S T, Kelly F B 1978 Fractures of the neck of the talus. Long term evaluation of 71 cases. Journal of Bone and Joint Surgery 60–A: 143

64. Lorentzen J E, Christensen S B, Krogsøe O, Sneppen O 1977 Fractures of the neck of the talus. Acta Orthopaedica Scandinavica, 48: 115

65. Dunn A R, Jacob B, Campbell R D 1966 Fractures of the talus. Journal of Trauma 6: 443

65a. Hawkins L G 1970 Fractures of the neck of the talus. Journal of Bone and Joint Surgery 52–A: 991

65b. Blair H C 1943 Comminuted fractures and fracture-dislocations of the body of the astragalus. American Journal of Surgery 59: 37

66. Nisbet N W 1954 Dome fracture of the talus. Journal of Bone and Joint Surgery 36–B: 244

67. Mukherjee S K, Young A B 1973 Dome fractures of the talus. A report of ten cases. Journal of Bone and Joint Surgery 55–B: 319

68. Hughes J R 1955 The articular damage in complete ruptures of the lateral ligaments of the ankle. Journal of Bone and Joint Surgery 37–B: 723

69. Mukerjee J K, Pringle R M, Baxter A D 1974 Fracture of the lateral process of the talus. A report of thirteen cases. Journal of Bone and Joint Surgery 56–B: 263

70. Hawkins L G 1965 Fracture of the lateral process of the talus. A review of thirteen cases. Journal of Bone and Joint Surgery 47–A: 1170

71. Lambrinudi C 1927 New operation on drop-foot. British Journal of Surgery 15: 193

72. McDougall A 1955 The os trigonum. Journal of Bone and Joint Surgery 37–B: 257

73. Weinstein S L, Bonfiglio M 1975 Unusual accessory (bipartite) talus simulating fracture. A case report. Journal of Bone and Joint Surgery 57–A: 1161

74. Main B J, Jowett R L 1975 Injuries of the mid-tarsal joint. Journal of Bone and Joint Surgery 57–B: 89

75. Wiley J J, Brown D 1974 Listhesis of the tarsal scaphoid. Journal of Bone and Joint Surgery 56–B: 586

76. Lisfranc J 1815 Nouvelle méthode opératoire pour l'amputation partielle du pieds dans son articulation tarsométatarsienne. Gabon, Paris.

77. Lisfranc J 1840 Fractures compliquées. Réflectiones sur l'époque la plus opportune pour application de l'appareil. Gazette des Hôpitaux Civils et Militaires, Deuxième Series 2: 205

78. Jeffreys T E 1963 Lisfranc's fracture-dislocation. A clinical and experimental study of tarso-metatarsal dislocations and fracture-dislocations. Journal of Bone and Joint Surgery 45–B: 546

79. Wiley J J 1971 The mechanism of tarso-metatarsal joint injuries. Journal of Bone and Joint Surgery 53–B: 474

80. Wilson D W 1972 Injuries of the tarso-metatarsal joints. Etiology, classification and results of treatment. Journal of Bone and Joint Surgery 54–B: 677

81. Aitken A P, Poulson D 1963 Dislocations of the tarso-metatarsal joint. Journal of Bone and Joint Surgery 45–A: 246

82. Trillat A, Lerat J L, Lerderc P, Schuster P 1976 Les fractures-luxations tarso-métatarsiennes. Classification. Traitement. A propos de 81 cas. Revue de Chirurgie Orthopedique 62: 685

83. Lowe J, Yosipovitch Z 1976 Tarsometatarsal dislocation: a mechanism blocking manipulative reduction. Journal of Bone and Joint Surgery 58–A: 1029

84. Gissane W 1951 A dangerous type of fracture of the foot. Journal of Bone and Joint Surgery 33–B: 535

85. Jones R 1902 Fracture of the base of the fifth metatarsal bone by indirect violence. Annals of Surgery 35: 697

86. Dameron T B 1975 Fractures and anatomical variations of the proximal portion of the fifth metatarsal. Journal of Bone and Joint Surgery 57–A: 788

87. Milch H, Milch R A 1959 Fracture surgery. A textbook of common fractures. Hoeber and Harper, New York, ch 23, p 456

88. Inman V T 1973 Du Vries' Surgery of the foot. Mosby, Saint Louis, ch 6, p 151

89. Christie J, Clowes C B, Lamb D W 1980 Amputations through the middle part of the foot. Journal of Bone and Joint Surgery 62–B: 473

90. Schnaid E, Otto Q S 1980 The place of Chopart amputations in trauma. Journal of Bone and Joint Surgery 62–B: 281

35

Pathological Fractures

Fracture surgery cannot be practised in total isolation from general orthopaedic surgery, and nowhere is this more clearly seen than in the treatment of pathological fractures. Such fractures may be the earliest manifestation of a genetic disturbance, hormonal imbalance or vitamin deficiency; they may be the first indication of a primary or secondary tumour of bone, or a deposit of lipoid granulomatosis, leukaemia or other disease of the marrow constituents. It must never be forgotten that changes in the structure of bone which at first may seem to be a localised abnormality may assume a quite different significance when other bones are examined radiologically and a general examination is completed. Until the rest of the skeleton has been fully examined, none but the most simple of pathological fractures should be regarded as due to localised disease alone. Also, it is important to appreciate the significance of localised bone pain. This can precede a complete break in the bone and often may be caused by an incomplete cortical fracture, as seen in the pseudo-fractures of osteomalacia or Paget's disease. Failure to record the presence of *localised bone pain* is too often the cause of delay in making a diagnosis and consequently, in some conditions, an unnecessary prolongation of functional disability.

Clearly it is not possible to list every condition which could be complicated by a pathological fracture, but surgeons who treat fractures must be alert to the many possible implications of bone injury and to the recognition of diseases of bone which have a particular predisposition to pathological fracture. Examples of the wide variety of conditions which can give rise to pathological fractures will be considered later under the following headings:

1. Developmental disorders of bone.
2. Nutritional and vitamin deficiencies.
3. Hormonal imbalance.
4. Atrophic conditions of bone.
5. Fractures through infected bone.
6. Cysts and fibrocartilaginous defects.
7. Paget's disease.
8. Primary and secondary tumours of bone.
9. Marrow cell disorders—granuloma of bone.
10. Parasitic disease causing pathological fracture.
11. Neurotrophic fractures.
12. Iatrogenic fractures.

Fatigue or stress fractures, although not strictly pathological fractures, are also included in the list because sometimes they can be the cause of mystifying bone pain and considerable functional disability. However, before describing this wide variety of conditions in more detail it is appropriate to first outline the measures which are available to the surgeon for the management of the fractures which may ensue from them.

GENERAL PRINCIPLES IN THE MANAGEMENT OF PATHOLOGICAL FRACTURES

When considering the local treatment of pathological fractures it is convenient to divide them into two main types. There are those resulting from disorders which cause a generalised weakness of the whole, or part of the skeleton, of which osteomalacia, rickets and osteoporosis are good examples; and there are those due to localised bone destruction or weakness such as is seen in secondary malignant disease, localised destructive primary tumours (both benign and malignant), and sometimes in bone infection. As a generalisation it may be said that the first group can be largely treated conservatively, while the second type often require operative treatment. Also, it must be emphasised that although it is the techniques of management of the second type with which this section is largely concerned it is equally important that the underlying disease should be fully understood and when available appropriate general treatment given.

Investigations. The cause of some pathological fractures, such as those due to simple cysts, is so obvious that very little investigation is called for. However, when the immediate diagnosis is in doubt, and particularly when there is a possibility of bone disease elsewhere, a general examination of the skeleton and investigations of other systems becomes mandatory.

The whole body isotope scan has largely replaced the extensive radiological survey which was advised in the past. If a suspicious area of uptake in bone is revealed in other parts of the skeleton this can be examined more fully by local X-ray studies. It must be remembered, however, that when dealing with a pathological fracture it is to other parts of the body to which attention should be drawn because the fracture itself will produce a 'hot spot' on the scan irrespective of whether it is due to abnormal bone disease.

Computerised axial tomography (CAT scan) is useful in displaying the local distribution of disease, particularly when it involves the soft tissues, and gives valuable information if local resection is contemplated. However, the facilities for this investigation are limited and the costs are high. It is by no means essential in every case.

Radiology. In addition to the routine antero-posterior and lateral views oblique projections can be helpful in making a diagnosis. Local tomography, and occasionally stereography, are also valuable; but arteriography, so popular for tumour investigation in past years, is rarely more than of academic interest. A routine chest X-ray should always be requested.

Blood and urine examination. As well as the routine tests for haemoglobin, white cell count and sedimentation rate, the patients should have a complete 'work up' with calcium, phosphorus, acid and alkaline phosphatase, serum proteins and blood urea (not forgetting a routine W.R.). In addition to the routine ward tests, the urine must be examined for casts and cellular debris.

Biopsy. If there is still doubt about the cause of the fracture a biopsy should be performed; and certainly the opportunity to obtain material should always be taken whenever internal fixation is necessary. Needle biopsies on the whole are not very satisfactory and should be confined to sites not readily accessible to surgery. A generous portion of bone should be removed and if a fracture has not yet occurred it is usually wise to protect the biopsy site with some form of internal fixation.

Conservative measures. Many pathological fractures, whether due to generalised bone disease or localised bone destruction, will unite if treated by orthodox conservative measures. This is particularly true of fractures resulting from treatable bone disease, and much nonsense has been written of the dangers of plaster fixation in such cases. The fact is that a pathological fracture, provided the diseased bone can be restored to normality by treatment, will unite perfectly satisfactorily in a plaster cast which, in the vast majority of instances, will cause no complication. The widely differing views on the treatment of fractures through areas of disuse osteoporosis is a good example of the confused thinking which surrounds the use of plaster in this context. And yet the answer is simple. The best treatment for osteoporosis is active use of the limb. The patient will only use the limb if it is pain free, and as in many cases operative fixation is impracticable, plaster becomes mandatory. Indeed, in some instances the use of operative measures using internal fixation may be positively harmful, particularly when there is a danger of reactivation of infection, and the majority of pathological fractures through infected bone (excluding those requiring sequestrectomy) should be treated conservatively.

The use of radiotherapy. Many pathological fractures occur through areas of bone which have been eroded by secondary neoplastic deposits sensitive to radiation. Although it is accepted that radiation has some destructive effect upon fracture healing it has been demonstrated experimentally that this effect is mainly upon the bridging callus, which is cartilage based and known to be very liable to radiation damage.

Observations on secondary deposits irradiated *before* a fracture has occurred have shown that under these conditions excellent recalcification can occur, indicating that osteogenesis (as opposed to chondrogenesis) is much less effected by the radiotherapy.[1] In fracture cases therefore the function of the cartilagenous bridging callus must be taken over by artificial means, and in the majority of pathological fractures this can only be done by using rigid internal fixation. Although there are some theoretical disadvantages to applying this fixation before radiation is given (for example, spread of tumour cells, ionisation around metal implants, and obstruction to the X-rays[2, 3]), the advantages of early fixation far outweigh the disadvantages, particularly with regard to the improvement of function and relief of pain, and whenever possible internal fixation should be carried out prior to radiotherapy. It may even be indicated as a prophylactic measure against a fracture occurring later during radiotherapy and can be conveniently carried out at the time of biopsy.

The use of bone grafts. Bone grafts are mainly used in the treatment of pathological fractures due to certain benign cystic lesions. They have a place in the treatment of unicameral bone cysts, in non-osteogenic fibroma of bone, and in giant cell tumour of bone and aneurysmal bone cyst. Usually autogenous cancellous bone is used to fill cavities and this is often augmented by homogenous grafts from the bone bank. Complete cadaveric allografts have been used where large segments of bone have been excised at the site of the pathological fracture, such as in giant cell tumour of the upper or lower end of the femur. But the results from these procedures are very unpredictable and they carry a very high morbidity rate. If such a wide excision of bone is required prosthetic replacement of the affected segment is to be preferred (see later).

Internal fixation of pathological fractures. Although internal fixation can, of course, be used in the treatment of pathological fractures from any cause, it is particularly applicable to the management of fractures due to secondary malignant disease. More and more surgeons have come to realise the improvement in the quality of life which results from this procedure, and no longer is it regarded as an unnecessary surgical insult to a patient who may have only a few months to live. In 1956 Devas and his colleagues laid down the following indications for internal fixation of pathological fractures from metastatic disease,[4] and these indications still hold good 25 years later. Internal fixation is indicated: (1) if the fracture is painful and immobilising; (2) when external fixation is not efficacious, or does not allow early ambulation; (3) when malignancy is such that widespread deposits can be expected; (4) when deposits are known to be elsewhere; and (5) when the primary tumour is hormone dependent. The type of fixation used depends to some extent on the site of the fracture but in the majority of cases intramedullary fixation is the method of choice. The theoretical disadvantage of spreading the tumour cells throughout the medulla is of little importance when treating metastatic disease.* Large nails should be used, if necessary their fixation should be augmented by

* It must be remembered however that this opinion does not apply to the treatment of pathological fractures resulting from certain primary tumours of bone. This is particularly relevant to the management of fractures through a chondrosarcoma, where the use of an intramedullary nail may completely jeopardise treatment later by excision and prosthetic replacement.

using acrylic cement to fill in large bone defects. Fractures in the trochanteric and subtrochanteric areas can be fixed more efficiently by using an articulating intramedullary nail and a femoral neck nail (Signal arm or Zickel nail—see Chapter 29).[5] Huckstep has reported good results in pathological fractures using a solid compression nail.[6,7] Whatever method is used the fixation should be as rigid as possible in order to relieve pain and to allow movement and positioning for the administration of radiotherapy.

Prophylactic nailing in metastatic bone disease. The following features in a metastatic deposit in long bones have been listed as having a high risk of fracture, and for which prophylactic nailing should be considered.[5] These are (1) pure lysis seen in X-ray; (2) the development of lesions previously not demonstrable in bone; (3) involvement of even small portions of the cortex; and (4) increasing pain. Fidler feels that it is mandatory to carry out prophylactic intramedullary nailing if more than half of the endosteal cortex is eroded;[8] while Beals et al recommend nailing for all femoral lesions which measure 2.5 cm or more in diameter and involve the femoral cortex.[9] There is one important technical point to remember in nailing the intact shaft of the femur. Unless the intramedullary nail is preset to compensate for the anterior bowing of the bone there is a danger of penetrating the anterior cortex with the lower end of the nail.[10]

The use of acrylic cement. There is a steadily increasing number of favourable reports on the use of methacrylate cement in conjunction with internal fixation for the treatment of pathological fractures from metastatic bone disease.[11,12,13] The presence of acrylic cement does not interfere with any subsequent radiation therapy, for the mass attentuation coefficient of bone and striated muscle is much the same as that for cement.[14] When using an intramedullary rod or a pin or plate for internal fixation, the appliances should be inserted first to check their position and then withdrawn beyond the defect to allow the cement to be inserted. Tumour tissue must be thoroughly curetted from the site of bone destruction and the space packed with the cement, and while this is still malleable the internal fixation is re-inserted[15] (Fig 35.1). Methyl-methacrylate has also been used successfully to fill large defects due to giant cell tumour, with or without pathological fracture, and there are now a significant number of cases reported in which there has been no recurrence for up to five years.[16]

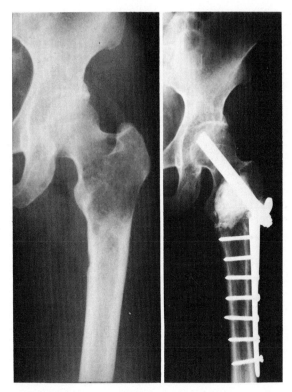

Fig 35.1 Use of acrylic cement with internal fixation in the treatment of pathological fractures. This patient sustained a pathological fracture after biopsy of a malignant round cell tumour of the upper end of the left femur. After insertion of a nail in the femoral neck the bone defect caused by the tumour was filled with acrylic cement and a plate applied in the usual way. Excellent fixation was obtained, and the tumour was later treated with radiotherapy and chemotherapy followed by major prosthetic replacement of the upper half of the femur.

Prosthetic replacement in the treatment of pathological fractures. Femoral head replacement for pathological fractures of the neck of the femur using a standard femoral prosthesis is now regarded as the treatment of choice when the fracture is due to metastatic disease. In one series of 163 patients operated on for pathological fracture or impending fracture, almost complete relief of pain was obtained in over half the cases, and there was significant improvement in the remainder. It was considered that—'if the anticipated life of the patient exceeds one month this constitutes an indication for the treatment of a pathological or impending fracture of the hip'.[16a]

However, in many cases the deposit extends well beyond the true femoral neck and may involve the upper third of the femur. Also, there are some primary bone tumours, such as chondrosarcoma and giant cell tumour which cause extensive destruction over a large segment of bone. These lesions are usually too extensive for internal fixation with metal and cement alone, but often they can be successfully treated (and amputation avoided) by a major bone replacement using a custom made prosthesis. This technique has a limited application, but is valuable when the alternative may be amputation. The femur and the humerus because of their thick covering of muscle particularly lend themselves to this form of treatment. It is unsuitable, however, in cases of pathological fracture due to infection and in conditions where there is spread of the disease into the soft tissues, such as occurs in fracture through hydatid disease, or in cases of fast growing lytic tumours of a high degree of malignancy.

Amputation. There are some cases of pathological fracture where the local diseased process cannot be controlled by treatment, and where there is no likely possibility of the fracture uniting. In these circumstances amputation of the limb is the kindest form of treatment. Pathological fracture of a long bone from extensive hydatid disease usually falls into this category, as does an ununited fracture through infected bone with extensive loss of bone substance and all pathological fractures occurring through highly malignant bone tumours, such as osteosarcoma and Ewing's tumour. Limited excisional surgery in these latter cases is fraught with the danger of local recurrence, a complication which usually results in a miserable terminal situation for the patient, by then often uncontrollable by radiotherapy, or even by amputation.

DEVELOPMENTAL DISORDERS OF BONE

There are many developmental disorders of bone, and for most of them the etiology is completely unknown. Although a large proportion are undoubtedly genetically controlled, there are a few which may have been caused by some insult to the embryonic cells during pregnancy, and the thalidomide disaster high-lighted the importance of this cause. There are others, such as the effect of rubella and of smoking during pregnancy; but we are only approaching the fringe of this fascinating study, and much more is to be learned before developmental disorders of bone growth can be controlled and prevented.

Congenital defects of bone tissue. Congenital disorders of the growth of bone tissue, as opposed to failures of epiphyseal development and modelling of individual bones, are typified in osteogenesis imperfecta and osteopetrosis. In *osteogenesis imperfecta* there is genetic damage to primitive mesenchymal cells so that although osteoblasts are differentiated in large numbers they are imperfect in their function, and the development of mature bone is retarded. In *osteopetrosis* genetic damage is seen in the impaired activity of osteoclasts, with failure of resorption of bone causing abnormal thickening and density. In some respects osteopetrosis is the counterpart of osteogenesis imperfecta; but in both conditions—whether the bones are stout or slender, sclerotic or porotic—the bone is immature, fragile and susceptible to fracture. Other condensing bone dystrophies, such as melorheostosis, osteopoikilosis, osteopathia striata, and Engelmann's disease are rarely, if ever, complicated by pathological fracture.

Disorders of cartilage growth. Congenital disorders of the epiphyseal cartilage, such as achondroplasia, and abnormal peripheral cartilage growth as is seen in diaphyseal aclasis (multiple exostoses) are never associated with bone weakness and do not present with fractures. On the other hand in dyschondroplasia (Ollier's disease) large masses of cartilage replace the metaphyseal bone and fail to ossify, with a result that pathological fractures are frequent occurrences.

Osteogenesis imperfecta presents such remarkable features that despite all the confusion of early surgical literature on bone diseases, clear descriptions can be traced back as far as the year 1700. The genetic aspect has been reviewed by Seedorff in 180 members of 55 Danish families.[17] The congenital form is nearly always sporadic and there is rarely more than one child affected. The late form shows a genetic determination with autosomal dominant inheritance.[18] The characteristic features and treatment of the bone fragility and deformity have been discussed fully in Chapter 19.

Osteopetrosis (marble bones, Albers-Schönberg's disease). This takes two forms: *osteopetrosis congenita* which has an autosomal recessive inheritance and is associated with severe loss of marrow activity and early death; and *osteopetrosis tarda*—probably of autosomal dominant inheritance and running a relatively benign course but usually with many pathological fractures. There is increase in the number and thickness of trabeculae with a disordered irregular architecture and complete failure of modelling resorption, so that continued periosteal apposition and surface thickening are accompanied by failure to develop a medullary cavity (Figs 35.2 to 35.5). Consequent reduction in the blood-forming marrow causes an anaemia which can sometimes be fatal. The abnormal growth of bone often continues uninterruptedly until the epiphyses fuse, and thereafter the dense and thickened skeleton remains unchanged; but there may be a curious periodicity, with intermission or even complete cessation of the developmental error, so that metaphyses show alternating bands of dense and normal bone. The vertebral bodies may show dense layers above and below, with a less dense layer between (the 'sandwich spine', Fig 35.6); in the pelvis there are curves of dense bone parallel to the iliac crests giving the appearance of 'miniature models lying within each bone',[19] the carpal and tarsal bones show circular distribution of dense bone surrounding a clear centre, or a dense centre surrounded by less opaque bone, or perhaps several concentric rings of dense and porous bone. Not only does encroachment of the sclerosed bone on the marrow cause anaemia, but constriction of the cranial foramina may give rise to optic atrophy, facial palsy, or other cranial nerve lesions. The bones are sometimes intensely hard, like marble, but in other cases they are more chalk-like in consistency and are susceptible to fracture. When fractures occur they are usually sharp and abrupt, in a strictly transverse axis corresponding to one of the planes of disordered epiphyseal growth. The patient shown in Figures 35.2 to 35.5 sustained symmetrical fractures of both femora (Fig 35.7). Another patient sustained 10 fractures in 20 years. Callus formation is sometimes slow but fractures always unite and consolidate soundly.

Dyschondroplasia (Ollier's disease, or multiple enchondromatosis) is characterised by such delayed and imperfect conversion of epiphyseal cartilage to bone that the metaphyses include a considerable proportion of unossified cartilage and are often expanded diffusely by enchondromata, but without exostoses as in diaphyseal aclasia. The growth disorder is seldom generalised—it may affect the epiphyses of a single bone, of several bones, of a single limb, of both lower limbs, or of both limbs on one side of the body. Moreover, it does not usually affect every part of an epiphysis equally. Sometimes there is normal growth on one side of an epiphysis with areas of unconverted cartilage and delayed ossification on

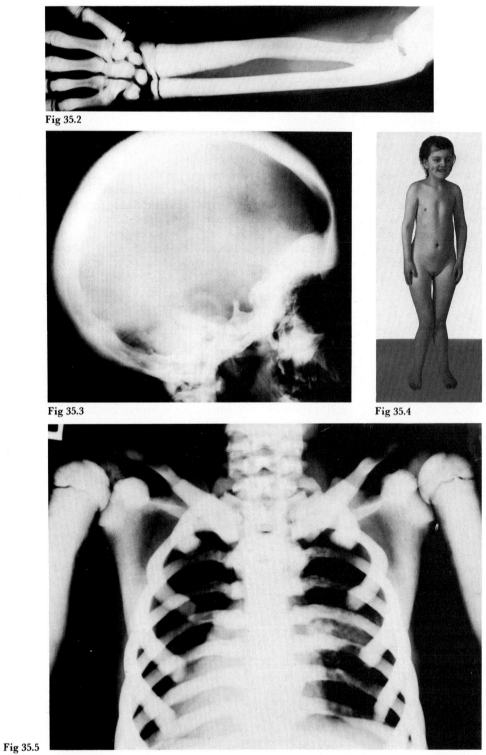

Fig 35.2

Fig 35.3

Fig 35.4

Fig 35.5

Figs 35.2 to 35.5 Osteopetrosis. There is abnormal density of all bones with club-like thickening of the metaphyses, encroachment on the medulla causing anaemia, and constriction of cranial foramina with paralysis of the facial and auditory nerves.

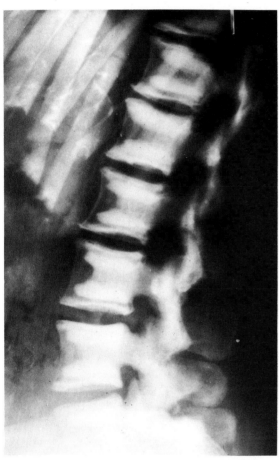

Fig 35.6 Osteopetrosis. Alternate bands of dense calcification and normal bone in vertebral bodies producing the 'sandwich spine'. (Reproduced by kind permission of the Radiological Museum, Royal National Orthopaedic Hospital, London.)

retarded and there is dwarfing or inequality of limb length (Fig 35.10), sometimes with spontaneous dislocation. If the radius alone is affected, the normally growing ulna dislocates at its lower end; and conversely if the ulna is more affected than the radius, and is proportionately shorter, the shaft of the radius curves and the upper end may dislocate. When there is still a considerable proportion of normal bone in the metaphysis, fractures are uncommon; but when a fracture is sustained union is often slow and delayed (Fig 35.11). If every part of an epiphysis is involved so that the metaphysis is expanded by a mass of pure hyaline cartilage, fractures are more frequent, despite the misleading appearance of density often observed from secondary calcification of the enchondroma (Fig 35.12).

The cause of dyschondroplasia is obscure. There seems to be no hereditary or familial influence, but several features—notably the curiously selective rather than generalised involvement of epiphyses, the normal blood chemistry, and the occasional association with congenital haemangioma (Maffucci's syndrome)—support the view that it is the result of a primary germ cell defect. The condition is compatible with a normal span of life. Sarcomatous changes have been reported but they are confined to cases of Maffucci's syndrome.[20] Infants and children with inherited rickets showing resistance to treatment with vitamin D may develop general skeletal deformity with dwarfing epiphyseal disturbance resembling some types of dyschondroplasia, and they respond to massive doses of vitamin D. But this is to say no more than that vitamin-resistant rickets has sometimes been mistaken for dyschondroplasia.

NUTRITIONAL AND VITAMIN DEFICIENCIES

Pioneer work on vitamins, first pursued in England by Mellanby and Bourne, has led to the virtual disappearance in many countries of scurvy and rickets. In Britain and American many years have passed since epiphyseal separation, subperiosteal haemorrhage and 'pseudo-paralysis' have been seen from scurvy; rickets, however, has reappeared in Britain in recent years among the immigrant Asian community. These nutritional deficiencies are still a cause of weakness, deformity and pathological fracture in parts of Africa, India and Asia. Moreover, minor deficiencies of vitamin C and the 'subscurvy state' may be of some importance in the healing of fractures and in various forms of vitamin-resistant rickets.

the other (Fig 35.8). In the knee joint, for example, genu valgum may develop from greater involvement of the lateral than the medial part of the epiphysis. Very often some columns of cartilage cells ossify normally, whereas adjacent columns remain unossified, thus accounting for the longitudinal striation of metaphyses seen in radiographs. The striae of reduced density, representing columns of unconverted cartilage, are based at one end on the epiphyseal plate and are lost at the other end in the shaft of the bone. In the ilium, unossified sectors of cartilage based on the epiphysis at the crest, alternating with areas of more normal bone, give the typical radiographic appearance of a fan which may be a diagnostic sign in doubtful cases (Fig 35.9). Even when there is limited involvement of an epiphysis, growth is usually

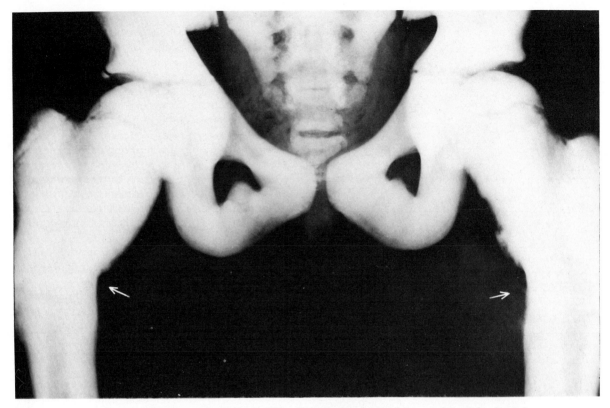

Fig 35.7 Osteopetrosis. Same case as that shown in Figures 35.2 to 35.5. There are united fractures of the shafts of both femora.

Vitamin C and scurvy. Deficiency of vitamin C, which is in highest concentration in citrus fruits and leafy vegetables, was formerly the dreaded peril of long sea voyages, sieges of war and polar explorations. Scurvy is characterised by extensive haemorrhage in muscles and subperiosteal planes, swelling and bleeding of the gums with loosening of teeth and failure of wounds to heal normally. In growing children there is osteoporosis, fibrosis of marrow, and epiphyseal separation or fracture. Vitamin C is needed for the growth and maintenance of collagen matrix and, if there is deficiency, the cells responsible for the elaboration of intercellular substance are not differentiated and may revert to fibroblasts. The calcifying zone of the epiphyses is widened. Preparatory calcificaton proceeds normally but osteoid is not laid down, or at best the osteoblasts produce a homogeneous matrix with little collagen content.

Fractures often occur at the costochondral junction of ribs or at the epiphyseo-diaphyseal junction of long bones. Periosteal spurs are laid down by the metaphysis (Pelkan's spurs).[21] There are haemorrhages because support of the capillary vessels is weakened by imperfect development of connective tissue around them. For the same reason, healing of wounds is delayed. Ascorbic acid is needed for the growth of collagen in repairing wounds of soft tissue, as well as for growth of osteoid in uniting fractures of bone.

The subscurvy state. There is a relationship between vitamin C and the adreno-cortical hormone controlling the growth of collagen. Apart from the direct influence on the healing of wounds of connective tissue, ascorbic acid is needed to support the potential of the adrenal cortex in defence against cold, fatigue and other stresses which initiate the adaption syndrome. If the intake of ascorbic acid is insufficient, the adrenal cortex becomes hypertrophied in its endeavour to meet the demand, and it soon loses all power of defence. The optimal daily intake of this vitamin may be estimated at 50 mg. Many individuals receive far less than this without usually showing ill effect, but they need much more when stresses are to be met. There is little doubt that deficiency of ascorbic acid or the 'subscurvy state' has often passed unrecognised

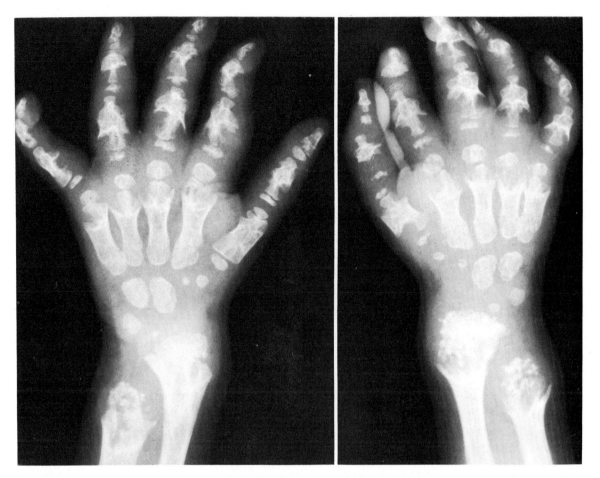

Fig 35.8 Dyschondroplasia. Typical changes in the hands in dyschondroplasia. At every epiphysis there is delayed conversion of cartilage to bone. Secondary calcification of the cartilage is seen in the radial and ulnar metaphyses.

as a cause of slow union of fractures, delayed healing of wounds and lessened resistance to shock. After severe injury, especially when coupled with exposure, fatigue or exhaustion, saturation should be achieved by giving 400 mg three times daily for three days, with a maintenance dose thereafter of not less than 50 to 100 mg daily.

Rickets. The vitamin D content of egg yolk and dairy products in an ordinary diet is low, but there is usually sufficient precursor, 7-dehydro-cholesterol, in the skin to be converted by ultraviolet irradiation to vitamin D. There is a striking seasonal variation in circulating levels of vitamin D metabolites.[22] Possibly the main cause of deficiency is insufficient exposure of the body to light. The function of this vitamin is the regulation of calcium and phosphorus metabolism, primarily by promoting absorption of calcium from the alimentary tract. Vitamin D plays a major role in calcium transport and thereby in the maintenance of normal plasma calcium. It has also been shown that active vitamin D metabolites promote phosphate reabsorption from the renal tubules.[23, 24]

The effects of deficiency of vitamin D may therefore be summarised as follows: absorption of calcium from the gut is reduced and hypocalcaemia develops early; calcium remaining in the alimentary tract may combine with phosphorus to form insoluble calcium-phosphate, and phosphorus absorption is also reduced; hypocalcaemia eventually stimulates parathyroid secretion and the glands hypertrophy, so that the level of blood-calcium may be restored to normal

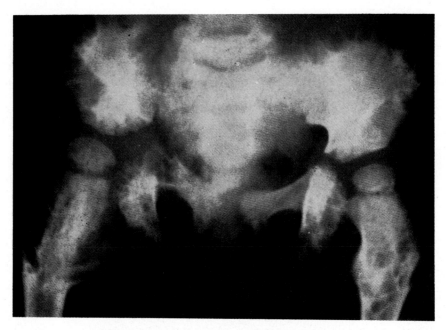

Fig 35.9 Dyschondroplasia. Typical fan-like ossification of the ilia in dyschondroplasia. (Reproduced by kind permission of the *Journal of Bone and Joint Surgery* and of Sir Thomas Fairbank, from his article (1948) Dyschondroplasia. *Journal of Bone and Joint Surgery*, 30–B, 689.)

despite continuing vitamin D deficiency; if the deficiency is very severe and long standing plasma-calcium may fall again. Calcium is not deposited in the bones and growth cartilage and it may even be withdrawn from them by parathyroid hyperactivity; phosphorus level is usually low; increasing osteoblastic activity producing uncalcified osteoid raises the level of serum-alkaline phosphatase. *The blood chemistry of rickets is therefore characterised by a low, or normal, serum-calcium, low blood-phosphorus, and raised alkaline phosphatase.*

In growing children the first consequence of vitamin D deficiency is failure of calcification at the epiphyses. The zone of proliferating cartilage cells becomes progressively deeper and osteoid remains uncalcified. Resistance of uncalcified bone to modelling resorption causes widening and broadening of epiphyses, with the characteristic 'rachitic metaphysis' of long bones (Fig 35.13) and 'rachitic rosary' of ribs. Similarly, in the shafts of long bones, appositional growth of osteoid remains uncalcified and unconverted to mature bone. The bones may be thick but they are weak and then become deformed. Incomplete crack fractures may develop on the convex side of the bent bones, and trivial injury may convert any of these cracks into a complete fracture

(Figs 35.14 and 35.15). The effect of giving adequate supplies of vitamin D (2000 units daily) is surprisingly prompt.

Primary hypophosphataemic (vitamin D-resistant) rickets. In some cases the rickets fail to respond to vitamin D in usual dosage. The blood chemistry is similar to ordinary rickets but serum-calcium is always normal and serum-phosphorus is always low; serum-alkaline phosphatase is raised; the serum-phosphorus remains low throughout life despite vitamin therapy sufficient to heal the rickets. Severe deformities develop in the untreated and there may be multiple pathological fractures (Figs 35.16 and 35.17). Vitamin resistance is believed to be congenital and the basic lesion is probably an excessive renal phosphorus leak.[25] Success has been reported from the administration of spectacularly high doses of the vitamin, long-term control being achieved with 0.5 to 2·0 mg daily.[26]

Malabsorption syndrome. In coeliac disease of children and adults (formerly classified as 'idiopathic steatorrhoea'), there is atrophy of the jejunal mucosa, causing incomplete digestion and absorption of fats, resulting from a special sensitivity to gluten in the diet. Both malabsorption of, and resistance to, vitamin D may result in defective calcium and phosphorus absorption as in true rickets. There is epiphyseal thickening,

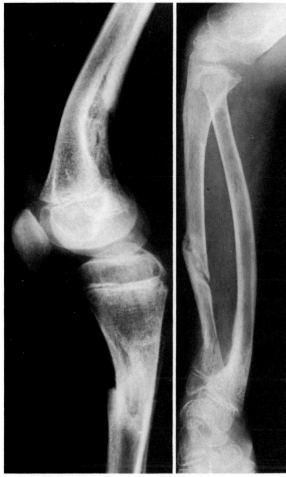

Fig 35.10   Fig 35.11

Figs 39.10 and 35.11 Dyschondroplasia. Boy aged 11 years
with dyschondroplasia causing arrested growth of the back of the
lower femoral epiphysis and the front of the upper tibial
epiphysis. A fracture of the ulna showed delayed union with
refracture from trivial injury; consolidation was unsound six
months later (Fig 35.11.)

general osteomalacia with deformity, and pathological fracture which unite slowly. Treatment consists of
putting the patients on to a strictly gluten-free diet
and combining this with high doses of vitamin D, up
to 5 mg daily for the first few weeks.[27]

Renal rickets. In some groups of renal diseases bone
changes occur exactly as in true rickets, with
secondary hyperparathyroidism. Occasionally the
defect does not become apparent until middle life
when it may present as osteomalacia. The disorder
may arise from congenital cystic disease or congenital

hydronephrosis causing total renal insufficiency,
glomerular as well as tubular; or from tubular defects
alone which appear to result from two mechanisms—
one in which the proximal tubules fail to reabsorb
phosphate, bicarbonate, glucose and amino-acids so
that there is low serum-phosphorus, acidosis, renal
glycosuria and amino-aciduria (*the Fanconi syndrome*),
and the other where acidosis is due to a failure of the
distal tubule to acidify the urine which further
depletes the serum of phosphorus. This latter disease
results in a relative hypercalcuria with renal calcinosis
or lithiasis. The prognosis depends on the nature of
the renal disease; the rickets may be cured by
treatment with large doses of sodium bicarbonate and
vitamin D,[28] and with potassium supplements as well
if necessary.

Osteomalacia in the adult is the counterpart of
rickets in the child; the causes are identical, blood
chemistry the same, and bone changes similar except
for the different X-ray appearances. There is bone
tenderness, kyphotic deformity with biconcave vertebral bodies, ballooned intervertebral discs, and
often spontaneous fracture of the rarefied long bones
(Figs 35.18 and 35.19). There may also be transverse
bands of uncalcified osteoid. These bands of malacic
bone have been described as pseudo-fractures, *umbau-
zoen*, or Looser's transformation zones. They are not
true fractures, and they disappear when the cause of
osteomalacia is removed.

Chalmers and others[29, 30] have drawn attention to
the incidence of osteomalacia in the elderly of this
country, mainly in women. A number of these cases
are undoubtedly due to malabsorption following
gastric surgery, but some must be attributed to dietary
insufficiency—an appalling admission to make in a
welfare state. The condition should be suspected in
patients complaining of weakness and continuous
bone pain with localised tenderness. It can be
confirmed by the finding of a raised serum-alkaline
phosphatase,* an X-ray showing pseudo-fractures,
and a positive biopsy. One or two days before a bone
biopsy the patient should be given an oral dose of
tetracycline, 2 g in an adult, in order to demarcate
the calcification front for histological study. It is also
a most important aid to obtain undecalcified sections.
If osteomalacia or even subclinical vitamin D deficiency is present during pregnancy, the great loss of
calcium from the lactating breast in the puerperium

* Fracture of the neck of the femur may be a complication of
osteomalacia. A raised serum-alkaline phosphatase *immediately* after
the fracture should alert the surgeon to the possibility of an
underlying osteomalacia.[31]

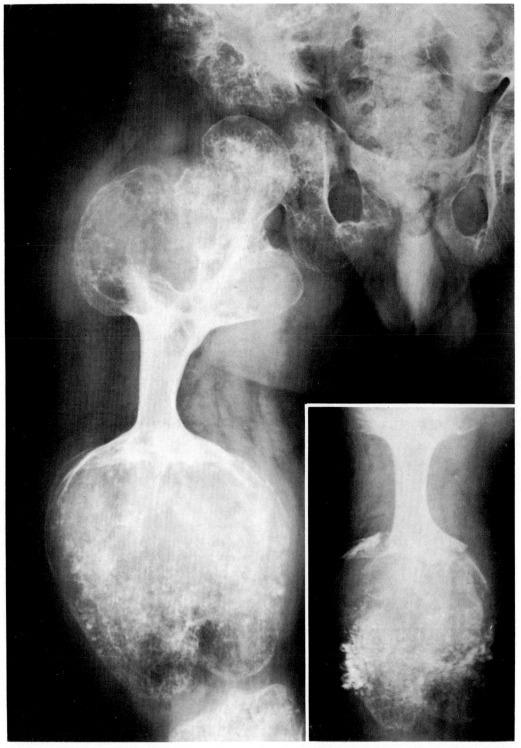

Fig 35.12 Dyschondroplasia. When all parts of the epiphyses are involved equally in arrested conversion of cartilage to bone, the metaphyses became widely expanded with masses of hyaline cartilage which are fragile despite secondary calcification. In this case there was a fracture at the junction of the metaphysis with the femoral shaft (see inset). It united soundly.

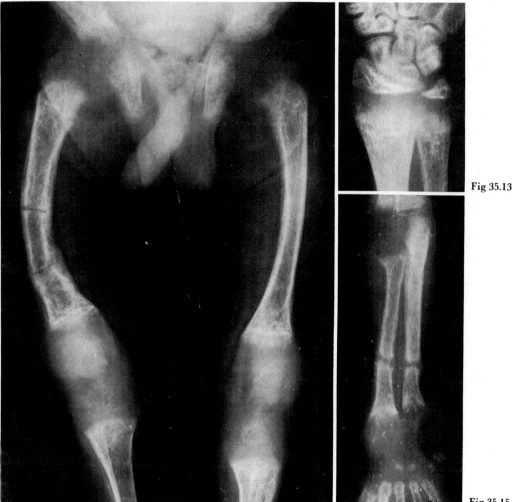

Fig 35.14

Fig 35.13

Fig 35.15

Fig 35.13 Typical rachitic metaphysis with epiphyseal widening and uncalcified osteoid.

Fig 35.14 and 35.15 Rickets. Indian child, aged 3 years, who has never walked. The epiphyses are wide and there is evidence of imperfectly calcified osteoid laid on the shafts of the femora. In one femur there is an ununited fracture of the lower shaft, and a recent fracture of the middle third. Fractures of the shafts of both forearm bones are uniting. (Reproduced by courtesy of Dr Mungo-Thompson, King Edward VIII Hospital, Durban.)

may cause severe tetany. Neonatal rickets may rarely occur in this situation.

A vitamin D-resistant osteomalacia can arise in well-fed, apparently healthy people, the condition corresponding in every respect to vitamin D-resistant rickets. It is usually a recrudescence of childhood hypophosphataemic rickets. Osteomalacia may also occur as a result of the malabsorption syndrome and from renal tubular insufficiency.

HORMONAL IMBALANCE CAUSING PATHOLOGICAL FRACTURE

We still only understand a little of the balance and interplay of the various hormones which control bone growth, and of the specific influence they have on different types of ossification—for example, pituitary growth hormone on periosteal ossification, and oestrogens on enchondral ossification. For the moment

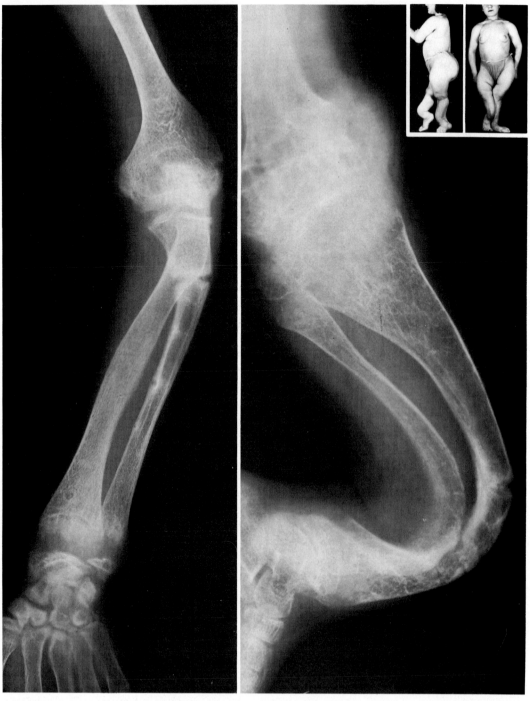

Fig 35.16   **Fig 35.17**

Figs 35.16 and 35.17 Vitamin D-resistant rickets. Radiograph of the patient shown in the inset who had evidence of rickets from infancy. Treatment by cod-liver oil and sunlight were of no avail. Severe deformities developed and pathological fractures of the tibiae, femora and forearm bones. Serum-calcium 11.5 mg; serum-inorganic-phosphate 3 mg; blood urea 35 mg; total fat in stool within normal limits. The patient had been unable to stand or walk before the age of 15 when these radiographs were taken. After treatment by a quarter-million units of calciferol daily the disease was arrested and the fractures united. The deformities were then corrected. (Presented at Staff Conference, Robert Jones and Agnes Hunt Orthopaedic Hospital; investigated at the Victoria Infirmary, Newcastle-on-Tyne.)

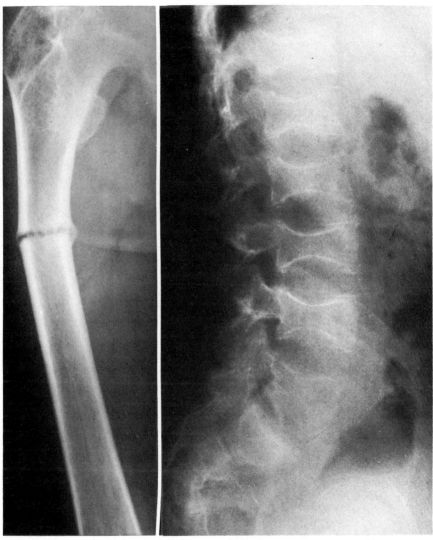

Fig 35.18   **Fig 35.19**

Figs 35.18 and 35.19 Osteomalacia causing fractures. This patient with proven osteomalacia sustained a pathological fracture of the shaft of the right femur through a typical Looser's zone (Fig 35.18). Lateral X-rays of the lumbar spine show the characteristic ballooning of the intervertebral discs seen in osteomalacia (Fig 35.19). (Illustrations reproduced by the kind permission of Dr. Trevor Stamp of the Metabolic Unit, Royal National Orthopaedic Hospital, Stanmore.)

we can do no more than outline the disorders that have proved relationship to recognised syndromes with pathological fracture.

Hyperparathyroidism. Increased parathyroid secretion from hyperplasia or neoplasia of the glands mobilises calcium from bone and raises the serum-calcium level. At first it was believed that the hormones acted only on bone promoting release of its

calcium; it is now recognised that the influence is less direct and that there is a specific action of parathyroid hormone (PTH) on the kidneys, causing both increased urinary excretion of phosphorus with consequent lowering of serum-phosphorus and increased absorption of calcium.[32] Raised serum-calcium is therefore associated with lowered serum-phosphorus. Hypercalcaemia causes hypercalcuria, and very often there are multiple renal calculi;

indeed, this complication is so frequent that the investigation of every patient with stones in the kidney should include study of the blood chemistry even if hyperparathyroidism is not suspected on other grounds.

The clinical manifestations of hyperparathyroidism are sometimes obvious because there is extensive cystic change in all bones, generalised rarefaction, osteoclastomatous cysts, peppery granulation of the skull, recurring spontaneous fractures, and renal colic with haematuria from calculi. Very often, however, the signs are much less obvious and some patients have suffered for many years before the diagnosis has been established. There may be no more than thickening of one or more bones with tenderness often diagnosed as 'fibrositis', and epulis or cyst of the jaw without changes elsewhere in the skeleton, generalised kyphosis with reduction of stature, or perhaps a fracture sustained from trivial injury. Sometimes there are no obvious bone changes; there may be muscle weakness mistaken for myasthenia gravis; polyuria and polydipsia wrongly diagnosed as diabetes insipidus; or stones in the kidney which are not recognised as part of a constitutional disease. Loosening of teeth without pocketing may be the first evidence and X-rays of the teeth which show a disappearance of the lamina dura (Figs 35.20 and 35.21). This appearance is said to be a specific sign of hyperparathyroidism,[33] so also are the X-ray changes in the hands (Fig 35.22) where there are characteristic subperiosteal erosions of the phalanges. The histological appearance of hyperparathyroidism can be mistaken for that of a giant cell tumour; but general rarefaction of bones, the multiplicity of the lesions

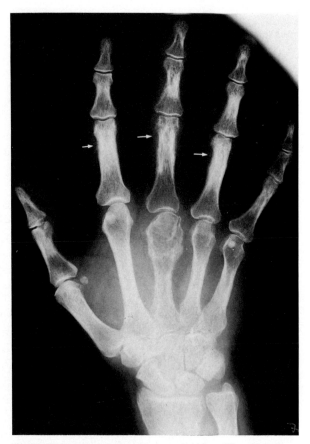

Fig 35.22 X-rays of the hand in hyperparathyroidism. Note the characteristic cortical erosions of the shafts of the phalanges and the cystic lesion in the head of the third metacarpal.

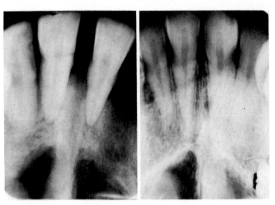

Fig 35.20   Fig 35.21

Figs 35.20 and 35.21 X-rays of the teeth in hyperparathyroidism show that the lamina-dura—the line of condensation around the roots—is missing (Fig 35.20). Compare this appearance with an X-ray of normal teeth (Fig 35.21).

and the absence of the typical radiographic appearance of giant cell tumour, should call for estimation of the blood-calcium and phosphorus and an X-ray of the hands (Figs 35.23 and 35.24).

Secondary hyperparathyroidism. Any condition that lowers the serum-calcium value stimulates increased secretion from the parathyroid glands. Thus secondary hyperparathyroidism occurs when there is rickets or osteomalacia causing failed absorption of calcium or any type of renal failure or insufficiency associated with phosphate retention.

Tertiary hyperparathyroidism.[34] It has been shown that a very small proportion of parathyroid tumours, confirmed by operation, have a long history of malabsorption syndrome or chronic renal failure. It is suggested that these cases first went through a phase of secondary hyperparathyroidism due to hypocalcaemia during which time an autonomous adenoma

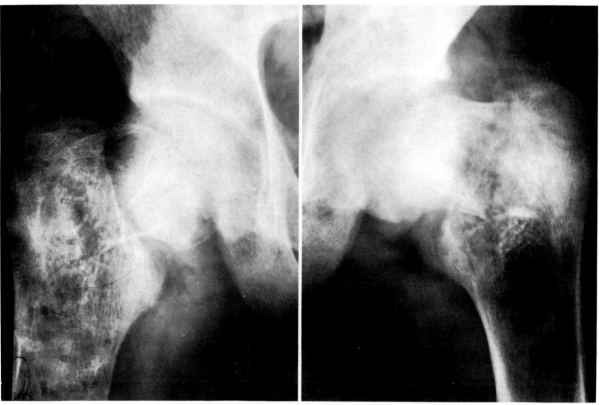

Fig 35.23   **Fig 35.24**

Figs 35.23 and 35.24 Hyperparathyroidism. A man, aged 26 years, turned quickly on a railway platform to greet his wife and collapsed. He was admitted to hospital with fractures of both femoral necks. There was obvious porosis of the bones, and study of the case showed that there was hyperparathyroidism from an adenoma.

was formed which eventually produced hypercalcae-mia. This complicated state of affairs has been termed tertiary hyperparathyroidism.

Calcitonin. The whole concept of plasma-calcium control has been altered greatly following the discovery of another hormone, calcitonin, which is able to reduce plasma Ca by direct action on bones.[35] Its significance in the treatment of metabolic bone disease is still to be worked out, but it is already proving useful in the treatment of Paget's disease, with relief of pain, reduction in the serum-alkaline phosphatase and diminution of hydroxyproline excretions.[36, 37]

Cushing's syndrome (pituitary-adrenal hyper-function). The syndrome may arise from a basophilic adenoma of the pituitary, or it may arise from a

tumour of the adrenal cortex itself. In either event there is increased secretion by the adreno-cortical hormones which promote the conversion of protein to sugar and are antagonistic to insulin. This catabolic action, causing breakdown of protein with release of glucose, discourages osteogenesis and apposition of new bone. There is osteoporosis with rarefaction of vertebral bodies which easily sustain crush fracture from trivial injury, kyphosis with reduced stature, persistent pain in the back from vertebral deformity, fractures of the ribs and clavicle and sometimes fractures of the long bones. Histological examination of bone shows osteoporosis with marked attenuation of trabeculae. On the other hand when fractures are sustained there is abundant formation of osteoid not only in surrounding callus but also within the bone fragments (Fig 35.25).

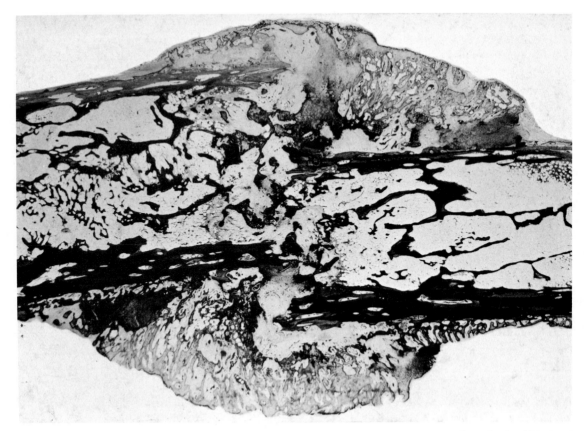

Fig 35.25 Cushing's syndrome. Section of fractured rib in Cushing's syndrome showing repair by surrounding callus in which there is much woven bone. There is osteoporosis, but the fracture simulated growth of osteoid within the bone fragments as well as in the abundant surrounding callus. (Dr Robb Smith's case; photomicrograph by Mr King, Bernhard Baron Laboratories, London Hospital, courtesy of Professor D. Russell; haematoxylin and eosin × 6.)

Pathological fractures from cortisone treatment. Since it is known that hormones of the adrenal cortex are catabolic, or at least anti-anabolic, and that in promoting breakdown of protein to glucose they suppress osteogenic activity—thus causing the osteoporosis of Cushing's syndrome—it is not surprising that cortisone treatment of rheumatoid arthritis and other diseases should predispose to pathological fracture. Experimental work with adreno-cortical hormones has shown that they retard all phases of healing of fractures.[38] Also, there is strong clinical evidence to support the view that long-term administration of cortisone is responsible for rapid deformation in joints affected with arthritis.[39]

Hypopituitarism (Fröhlich's syndrome). The syndrome of hypopituitarism described by Fröhlich in 1901 is a deficiency disease of the anterior pituitary.

In the first case he described there was a 'craniopharyngioma' with delayed sexual development and adiposity from spread of the tumour to the hypothalamus. These patients are dwarfed, or at least below average height, and defective secretion of testicular and adrenal adrogens causes retarded growth, slenderness of bones, weakness of muscles, and laxity of ligaments. Although these patients rarely present with pathological fractures they are particularly susceptible to separation and displacement of the upper femoral epiphysis, usually when they are excessively fat and much above normal weight. The classical Fröhlich syndrome from pituitary tumour is very rare indeed, but on the other hand hypogonadism with delayed sexual maturity and excessive adiposity without a detectable pituitary lesion occurs commonly and is sometimes complicated by slipped upper femoral epiphysis.

ATROPHIC CONDITIONS OF BONE

Disuse atrophy of bone was at one time attributed to decalcification or halisteresis. It was thought that demineralisation left the cellular structure of bone intact; but histological study has shown that the trabeculae themselves are destroyed. There is failure of normal osteoblastic apposition while normal osteoclastic resorption continues. The greater the functional inactivity, the more complete is the failure of bone apposition in keeping pace with osteoclastic resorption, and the more severe is the osteoporosis.

In every fracture, no matter how treated, there is at first osteoporosis. This can be minimised by prompt immobilisation of the fragments and continued active contraction of the muscles, but sometimes functional disuse is aggravated because muscle contraction is painful, or there may be other severe injuries which prevent an active exercise programme so that the osteoporosis is increased. Certain patients undoubtedly become more osteoporotic than others and those who develop Sudeck's atrophy after injury are good examples of this. The osteoporosis in these cases may continue long after union of the fracture, often associated with adhesion of muscles and stiffness of joints, and therefore with still greater difficulty in practising exercises. Thus a vicious circle of functional inactivity causing disuse change, and disuse changes inhibiting functional activity is set up, with the establishment of Sudeck's acute post-traumatic atrophy, already fully discussed in Chapter 4.

Disuse osteoporosis causing fracture. Osteoporosis induced by a fracture may be so severe as to cause secondary pathological fracture. This is an unusual complication but it may occur in patients who have been treated in recumbency for many months following severe trauma, or complicated fractures. Pathological fracture, however, is not uncommon in patients with disuse atrophy associated with a lower motor neurone disease which has caused excessive paralysis, such as poliomyelitis, muscular dystrophy or spina bifida. In the management of these patients care must always be taken to avoid fracture of long bones from careless handling of a limb, particularly after immobilisation for corrective procedures. The supracondylar region of the femur is particularly vulnerable.

Senile osteoporosis. In the same way that osteoporosis arises from functional inactivity because apposition of new bone fails to keep pace with normal osteoclastic resorption, it develops in old age because there is general retardation of cellular proliferation. Replacement of outlived osteocytes demands resorption of surrounding bone, and this goes on while osteoblastic apposition of new bone fails. Thus the bone trabeculae become progressively thinner, the fat content increases, and the cortex is thinned. This general osteoporosis predisposes to fractures of the neck of the femur, especially in elderly women, and more rarely, to fractures of the shafts of long bones. Fatigue fractures of the femoral neck have been shown to occur when relatively small loads are applied to ageing cadaveric femora,[40] and isolated trabecular fractures have been demonstrated in femoral heads of the elderly removed for fracture or for arthritic joint replacement.[41] However, the softening of bone and the predisposition to fracture are most pronounced in the spine. From time to time a vague discomfort and general aching may be accentuated by acute attacks of agonising pain, almost immobilising in its intensity, and it is then found that one or more vertebral bodies have been crushed. Pathological crush fractures are sustained from trivial incidents such as stooping to lift a weight, using a spade in the garden, or even stumbling on a carpet. Radiographic examination shows complete crushing of one vertebral body, often with evidence of former crushing of other vertebrae in the lumbar and dorsal regions (Fig 35.26). The serum-calcium and phosphorus values are normal and the alkaline phosphatase is only raised if there has been a recent fracture. Bone biopsy shows thinning of trabeculae, but with normal calcification.[42]

Treatment of fractures in senile osteoporosis. No constitutional treatment is known by which to stimulate bone formation in senile osteoporosis. It may be that the atrophy of old age represents underfunction of the steroid-producing glands—but we do not know. The intake of calcium and phosphorus should certainly be increased by giving calcium phosphate 3 g daily. A sufficient supply of vitamin D should be assured by giving from 5000 to 10 000 international units. If there is achlorhydria, dilute hydrochloric acid should be given with meals. Hormonal treatment is discussed below; but the management of senile osteoporosis is essentially symptomatic. This does not mean that there must be despair. It must be emphasised that the fracture will unite but may take a little longer than in a young person, and that function will be restored.

Acute fractures of the spine can be treated by rest in bed for about two weeks on a firm mattress with a soft pillow at the mid-dorsal level. After the first few

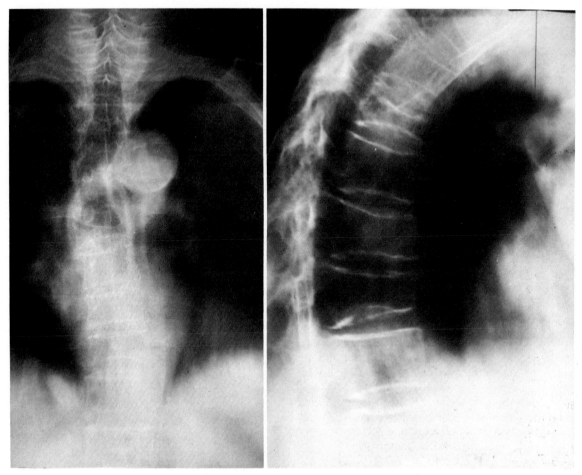

Fig 35.26 This 80-year-old patient developed severe pain in the back when lifting. She had sustained another osteoporotic crush fracture of her vertebral column. She had been quite unaware of any previous trouble although she did think she was 'growing smaller'.

days hyperextension exercises should be encouraged. Meanwhile a posterior spinal support should be ordered—a high lumbar corset for fractures in the lower part of the back, extending further proximally and using shoulder straps for fractures in the thoracic spine. A proper Thomas type of brace is too heavy to be tolerated by old people, and any support must be slender, with a comfortable abdominal corset and with well-padded shoulder straps; it should be moulded closely to the existing curves of the spine. Such a support may be needed indefinitely to relieve pain and prevent increasing deformity and also to protect the spine from further spontaneous fractures.

Menopausal osteoporosis. The greater frequency of senile osteoporosis in women than in men and the frequent onset of symptoms at about the age of 50 suggests that menopausal deficiency of gonadal hormones may be an important factor. The symptoms from menopausal osteoporosis can often be relieved considerably by the regular administration of sex hormones; the dose recommended is 0.5 mg of stilboestrol in the morning combined with a 5 mg linguette of testosterone at night.[43] There are many proprietary anabolic agents recommended for the treatment of osteoporosis but they are of doubtful value.

PATHOLOGICAL FRACTURES THROUGH INFECTED BONE

Very little has been written about the treatment of pathological fractures in bone affected by osteomyelitis: and yet this is not an uncommon complication of severe bone infection and may occur many months, or even years, after the acute infection has subsided (Figs 35.27 and 35.28). The treatment of the fracture should always be conservative, and the only surgery which may be necessary is that of surgical drainage and possible sequestrectomy. Any active infection must be controlled by appropriate antibiotic therapy given both parenterally and locally and augmented by surgical exploration when indicated. Removal of large sequestra should be deferred until an involcrum

is well established. When there are large gaps resulting from sequestration these can be filled by cancellous grafts, and it is interesting to remember that the first successful bone graft carried out by McEwen to repair a gap after osteomyelitis was achieved by using multiple bone chips. Despite the advice from some surgical sources that infected fractures are best treated by internal fixation this method should not be used in pathological fractures resulting from osteomyelitis, where the extent of the bone infection, unlike that of an infected compound

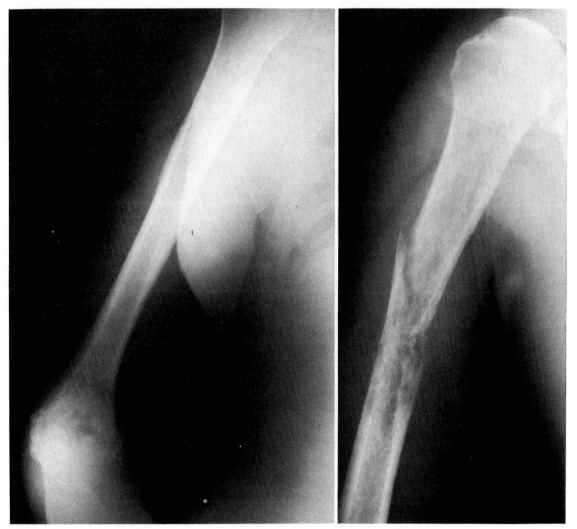

Fig 35.27 **Fig 35.28**

Figs 35.27 and 35.28 The patient whose upper arm X-rays are shown in Figure 35.27 presented with a large soft tissue abscess extending down to the humerus. There was no bony disease seen at that time. One month later when preparing to leave hospital his humerus fractured while lifting a suitcase (Fig 35.28). Acute osteomyelitis should be protected for several months after the acute infection has settled. This fracture united satisfactorily with conservative treatment.

fracture, cannot be assumed to be localised to the fracture site alone. Intramedullary nails in particular should never be used, for their use carries the grave hazard of spreading a localised infection along the whole length of the bone (Figs 35.29 and 35.30). If union of an infected pathological fracture is possible it will occur with a conservative regime. In some

cases the bone destruction is such that amputation may be the only solution. Such cases will not be improved by the enthusiastic use of even the most modern of internal fixation devices. At the most they can only defer the inevitable outcome, and in the process inflict upon the patient much unnecessary misery.

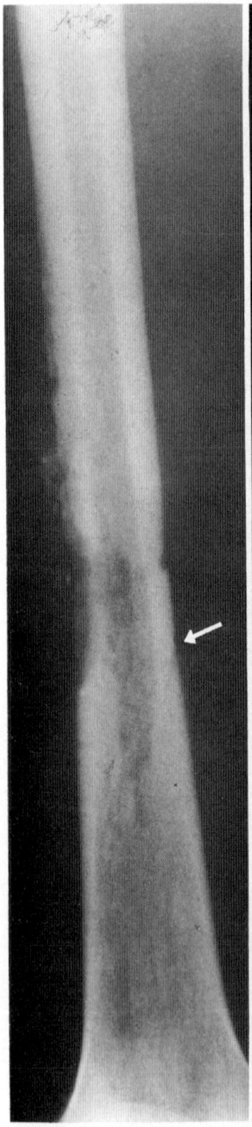

CYSTIC DISORDERS AND FIBROUS DYSPLASIA OF BONE

There are two localised cystic lesions and two fibrous lesions of bone which not uncommonly present as pathological fractures. These are: localised bone cyst and aneurysmal bone cyst; and non-osteogenic fibroma and fibrous dysplasia of bone. There are, of course, many other conditions which can present as apparent cysts, but these are often manifestations of tumour, such as giant cell tumour, or are due to a generalised bone disorder such as hyperparathyroidism. They are considered under separate sections.

Solitary cyst of bone (unicameral cyst). This is one of the commonest causes of pathological fracture in children and young adolescents (see Chapter 19). It presents in childhood and adolescence as a metaphyseal lesion with destruction of bone, slight expansion, and thinning of the cortex. There is no periosteal reaction or new bone formation such as occurs when there is infection. At first the cyst is juxta-epiphyseal but gradually moves down the shaft as the child grows, whereas other non-malignant cystic lesions tend to invade the epiphyseal area and are often eccentrically placed. Solitary bone cysts are more common in males, and are found most frequently in the upper ends of the humerus, femur and tibia.

The first evidence of a dystrophic cyst is often a fracture from trivial injury. If a fracture is sustained it always unites quickly and may even promote healing of the dystrophy, the cyst being obliterated by newly formed callus. There should certainly be no haste in considering surgical intervention (see Fig 19.23) and the fracture can be treated on conventional lines by immobilisation in splints or plaster. However, Stone has observed that spontaneous healing of the defect after fracture is less likely if the injury occurs before the age of puberty.[44] Only if the cyst fails to heal should it be explored and grafted in an attempt to prevent recurrent fracture. Part of the attenuated cortex should be removed; the brown or clear fluid within the cyst should be evacuated and the thin layer of tissue lining the wall curetted; the space should then be filled with cancellous chips of bone cut

Fig 35.29   Fig 35.30

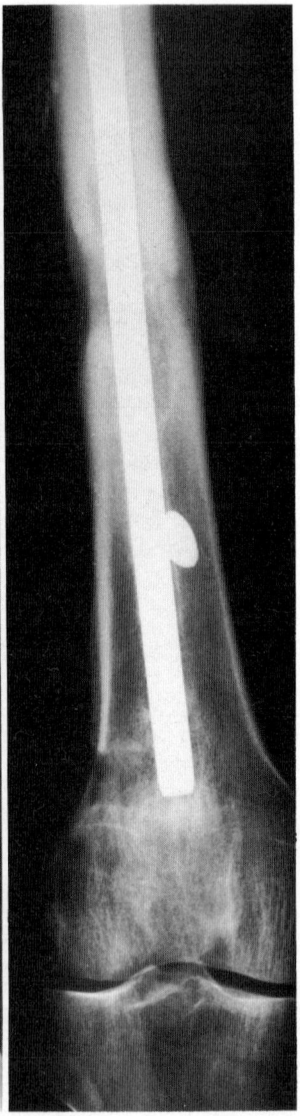

Figs 35.29 and 35.30 A patient with acute osteomyelitis of the femoral shaft sustained a crack fracture some weeks after the infection had subsided (Fig 35.29). Misguidedly this fracture was stabilised with a Kuntscher nail, resulting in a spread of infection the entire length of the bone. Fractures through zones of osteomyelitis should be treated conservatively.

from the ilium. Some cysts, particularly those requiring operation before puberty when the cyst is still active, can be more aggressive and may require a second graft. Agerholm and Goodfellow claim success in treating humeral cysts by subperiosteal block excision of the whole cyst and its cortex, followed by filling the remaining periosteal sleeve with bank bone. In the three cases reported there were no recurrences.[45]*

Aneurysmal bone cyst.[47] Although occurring also in the child or adolescent this lesion is entirely different from the unicameral cyst, and sometimes does not present until adult life. It derives its name not from its vascular nature but from its eccentric situation (Fig 35.31). It often involves the shaft of a long bone rather than the metaphyseal region, and is not uncommonly found in the vertebrae, affecting the body, the neural arch and the processes. Unlike the simple cyst the aneurysmal bone cyst is usually highly vascular and is semi-solid. Haemorrhage during curettage can, on occasions, be disturbing. In the cystic parts of the tumour the lining is clearly defined and can be peeled off the bone and, if examined in isolation, can be mistaken histologically for giant cell tumour. The situation, age of the patient and cystic nature of the lesion should, however, always make the diagnosis clear. Pathological fractures from trivial injury do occur but the presentation is often from pain or swelling. The fractures usually unite without difficulty. An aneurysmal bone cyst should be curetted and filled with bone chips, but it must be realised that because of the vascularity and more extensive nature of the lesion, the operation is a much bigger procedure than that of curetting a simple bone cyst. Fortunately, healing usually occurs, even after incomplete removal; it is also very radio-sensitive and any residual locules can often be dispersed by deep X-ray therapy. Very rarely the lesion remains locally aggressive despite all forms of treatment and may require wide excision or even amputation (Figs 35.32 and 35.33).

Non-osteogenic fibroma of bone. This localised fibrous lesion occurs towards the ends of long bones in children and adolescents. It is always eccentric and causes expansion and thinning of the cortex, often with pathological fracture (Fig 19.25). The clinical and radiographic appearances can sometimes be

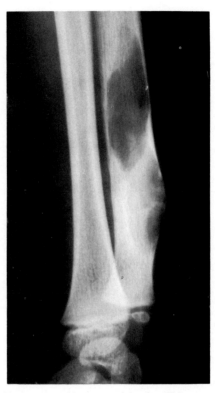

Fig 35.31 Aneurysmal bone cyst of the ulna. This eccentric cystic lesion of the ulna in a girl of nine is typical of aneurysmal bone cyst. Quite unlike a unicameral bone cyst it is localised and involves the shaft rather than the metaphyseal area of bone. It was successfully treated by local curettage and bone graft.

confused with those of a simple dystrophic cyst, but when exposed at operation the area is found to be filled with a solid mass of yellow or brown fibrous tissue and the whole lesion is relatively avascular. Giant cells are always found amongst the masses of fibrous tissue and this finding has occasionally resulted in the lesion being wrongly diagnosed as a giant cell tumour; also foam cells containing lipoid account for the view that the dystrophy represents a burnt out lipoid granuloma. More probably non-osteogenic fibroma of bone, or 'metaphyseal fibrous defect' as it is sometimes called, arises from developmental failure of metaphyseal ossification. Treatment is by curettage and bone graft.

Monostotic and polyostotic fibrous dysplasia. Fibrous dysplasia may occur more diffusely in a bone (monostotic dysplasia) or in several bones of one or more limbs (polyostotic dysplasia) with involvement not only of long bones but also of the pelvis, ribs and

---

* Remarkable results have been claimed from the injection of methyl prednisolone into bone cysts, with a 90 per cent favourable result in a series of 72 cases[46]. Unfortunately there is no indication of age groups or incidence of pathological fracture in this study.

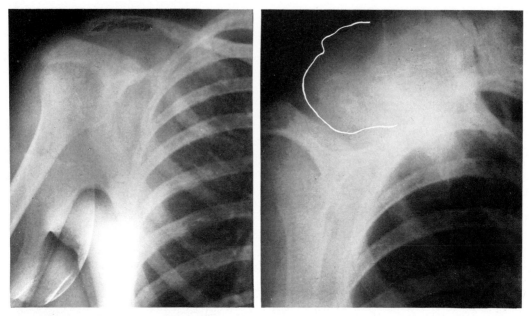

Fig 35.32   **Fig 35.33**

Figs 35.32 and 35.33 Aggressive aneurysmal bone cyst of clavicle. Figure 35.32 shows a small osteolytic lesion of the outer end of the right clavicle in a girl of 10. Biopsy showed this to be an aneurysmal bone cyst. It was treated by curettage and bone graft but within two months it had recurred in alarming proportions (Fig 35.33). It was eventually eradicated by complete excision of the outer three-quarters of the clavicle.

facio-maxillary bones. No bone is exempt.[48] There is often a curiously unilateral distribution. The association of predominantly unilateral fibrosis of bone with pigmentation of skin and precocious puberty is known as Albright's syndrome.[49] Fibrous dysplasia is believed by Jaffe to arise from a congenital developmental failure of ossification,[50] but the fact is that we do not know the etiology. It is possible that polyostotic fibrous dysplasia, and particularly Albright's syndrome, may have a hormonal basis, but we do not know what it is. The essential pathological change is replacement of large areas of bone by masses of dense fibrous tissue arranged in whorls, with small islands of fibre-bone produced by membrane ossification but with no tendency to multiplication of osteoclasts. Cyst formation is rare but may sometimes result from degenerative change within the fibrous defect (see Figure 35.35 inset).

Pathological fractures and severe deformity may occur in childhood but sometimes there is no evidence of abnormality until adult life, and even then it may be disclosed incidentally; there is, indeed, an almost infinite graduation in the severity of the dysplasia as it occurs in different patients. Figures 35.34 and 35.35 show an extreme example of monostotic fibrous

dysplasia in a young woman. The bony lesion had gradually enlarged over a period of five years and had been associated with several pathological fractures. Another patient with polyostotic disease suffered his first fracture at the age of 4, was bedridden for nearly 20 years, and sustained scores of fractures (Figs 35.36 to 35.38). The blood chemistry is always normal. There is diffuse thickening with loss of distinction between cortex and medulla so that the whole bone appears homogenous (so-called 'ground grass' appearance), but sometimes with areas of such complete translucency as to give the appearance of a simple bone cyst (Fig 35.34).

Even when the first evidence of dysplasia arises in childhood it may be relatively benign. Figures 35.39 to 35.41 are the X-rays of the right arm of a young boy with polyostotic fibrous dysplasia. At the age of 14 he sustained a fracture of the humerus from trivial injury, and radiographic examination showed that it was a pathological fracture through a previous area of fibrous replacement. Nevertheless the fracture united after simple conservative treatment and, moreover, the fibrous defect healed by new osteogenesis (Fig 35.42).

Where a bone is extensively weakened by the

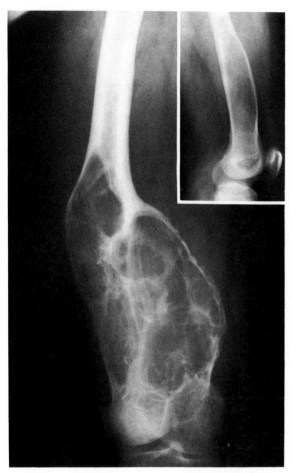

Fig 35.34

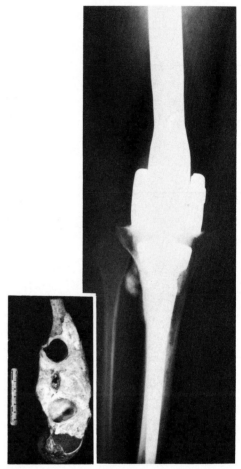

Fig 35.35

Figs 35.34 and 35.35 Monostotic fibrous dysplasia. This extensive bone defect involved most of the lower half of the right femur of a 20-year-old female patient. It was originally diagnosed as a simple bone cyst when it presented as a pathological crack fracture five years previously (Fig 35.34 inset). The lower half of the femur and the knee were successfully replaced by a prosthesis (Fig 35.35). Specimen removed at the prosthetic replacement operation showed that the lesion was basically solid, with areas of cystic degeneration (Fig 35.35 inset).

fibrous defect repeated fracture can be anticipated and a radical approach is usually necessary. The whole thickness of the affected bone may have to be excised, including the periosteum and subperiosteal layers, and replaced with cortical and cancellous grafts (Figs 35.43 and 35.44). Where the medullary cavity has been eroded as far as the subperiosteal layer (Fig 35.34) local curettage and even subperiosteal excision is doomed to failure. A wide extraperiosteal incision is required to eradicate the disease. If reconstruction cannot be achieved by grafts prosthetic replacement should be considered (Fig 35.35).

It must be reiterated that we are still unaware of the etiology of polyostotic fibrous dysplasia and still unable to cure it. Sometimes no more is needed than to prolong the period of immobilisation of a fracture, but in very severe cases surgical appliances or prophylactic internal fixation may be required to protect the limb from deformity (Figs 35.45 and 35.46). One last word of warning—cases of malignant transformation in both monostotic and polyostotic

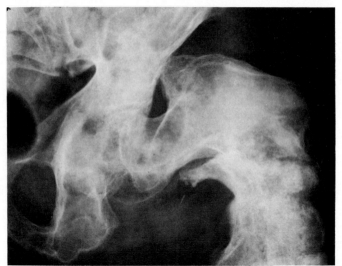

Fig 35.36

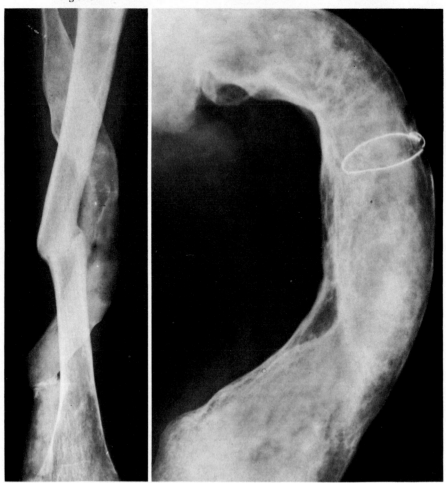

Fig 35.37   Fig 35.38

Figs 35.36 to 35.38 Polyostotic fibrous dysplasia with many pathological fractures and very severe deformities. This patient with polyostotic fibrous dysplasia sustained his first fracture at the age of four. Since then he has sustained scores of fractures—some treated rather stupidly with bits of wire. He was bedridden for nearly 20 years. After osteotomies the deformities were corrected enough for him to stand and walk, and all the osteotomies united quickly. But he still needed surgical appliances to prevent recurrent deformity.

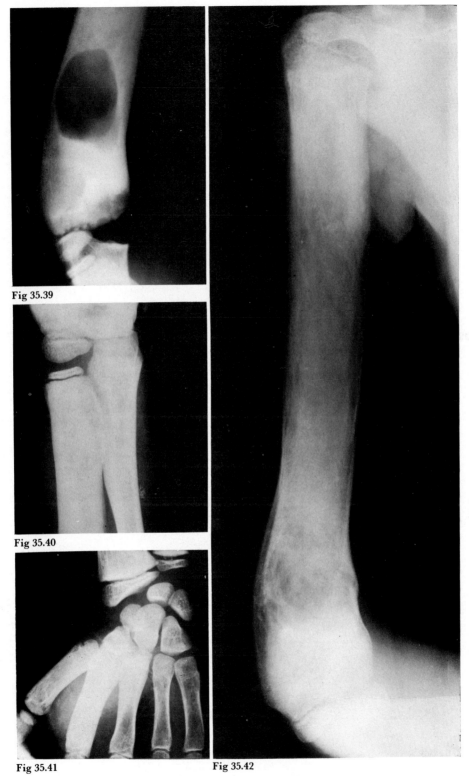

Fig 35.39

Fig 35.40

Fig 35.41   **Fig 35.42**

Figs 35.39 to 35.42 Polyostotic fibrous dysplasia (benign course). A young child showed areas of polyostotic fibrous dysplasia in the humerus, forearm bones and metacarpals of the right arm (Figs 35.39 to 35.41). At the age of 14 he sustained a pathological fracture through the lower end of the humerus. The fracture united with conservative treatment, moreover the fibrous defect ossified (Fig 35.42).

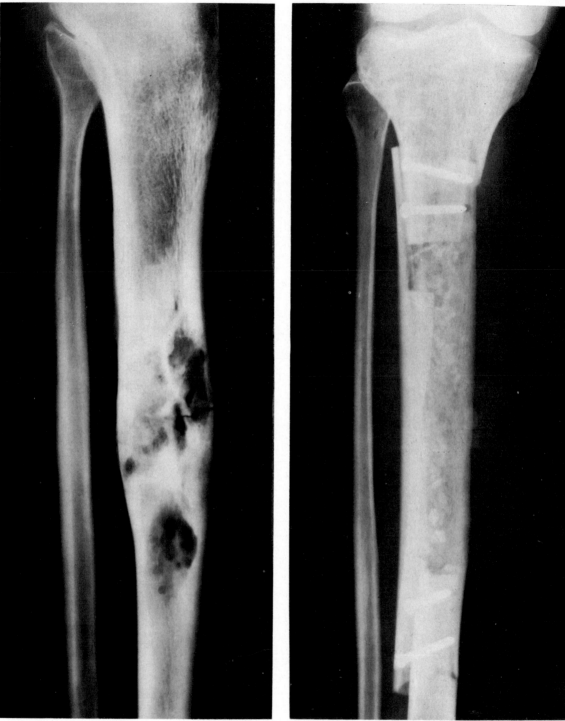

Fig 35.43

Fig 35.44

Figs 35.43 and 35.44 Monostotic fibrous dysplasia. A male aged 43 years sustained a fracture through a cystic area in the tibia. The cyst was curetted and bone grafts were implanted. It appeared that the lesion had healed, but two years later another spontaneous fracture was sustained (Fig 35.43). The blood chemistry was normal. The area of bone showing fibrous dysplasia was excised, the gap being filled with cancellous grafts cut from the ilium; stability was maintained by onlaid cadaveric grafts of whole-thickness bone (Fig 35.44). Histological examination confirmed the diagnosis.

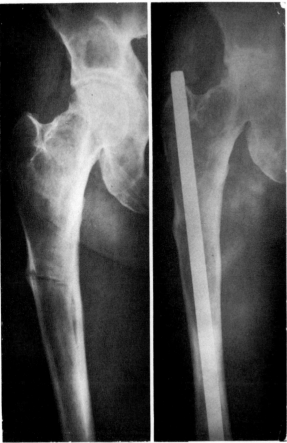

Fig 35.45   **Fig 35.46**

Figs 35.45 and 35.46 Protective intramedullary nailing for fibrous dysplasia. This patient with extensive fibrous dysplasia of the upper shaft of his right femur first developed pain from cortical stress fractures in his late thirties (Fig 35.45). Pain was relieved by intramedullary nailing of the femoral shaft (Fig 35.46).

fibrous dysplasia have been reported.[51] Many cases of fibrous dysplasia are symptomless unless a pathological fracture occurs. Beware of diagnosing simple fibrous dysplasia alone, without a fracture, if pain is the presenting symptom.

PAGET'S DISEASE OF BONE—OSTEITIS DEFORMANS[52]

This is another disorder of unknown etiology which is perhaps one of the commonest diseases of bone. Progression however, can be very slow indeed. Although bone changes may appear even before the age of 30, symptoms seldom arise before the sixth or

seventh decades. However, it is one of the common causes of pathological fracture (Fig 35.47) and in a small proportion of cases there is sarcomatous transformation (Figs 35.51 and 35.54).

The disease is often localised to one bone, the tibia being involved more often than other long bones. For 10 or 20 years the patient is unaware of abnormality; there may be clinical evidence of thickening of the shaft, reduced sharpness of the crest, or local heat from increased circulation, but there is little or no pain. As years go by the thickening becomes more obvious and there may be deep aching pain, sometimes with a tendency to forward and outward

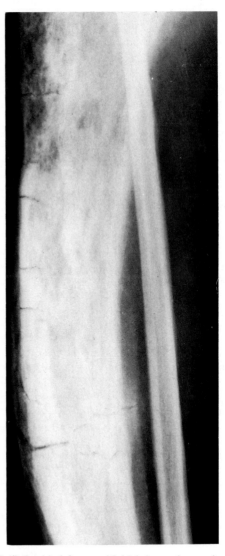

Fig 35.47 Osteitis deformans. Multiple incomplete cracks of the subcutaneous surface of the tibia in Paget's disease.

bowing of the shaft of the bone. If the disorder extends as far as the articular surface of the hip or knee joint secondary degenerative arthritis may develop.

Radiographic examination shows an irregular deposit of many trabeculae of new bone, first on the subperiosteal surface and then on the medullary surface, so that the distinction between cortex and medulla is lost (Figs 35.48 to 35.50). Collins[53] describes three stages in the appearance of the disease; the first process is always one of osteoclastic resorption of existing bone and can be seen on the advancing edge of every focus; the second one of osteoblastic regeneration of coarse-fibred bone in a highly vascular stroma; whereas the final burnt out stage produces the characteristic mosaic pattern of lamellar bone, formed by 'jerry built' blocks joined by irregular 'cement' lines. Unbridled formation of immature osteoid is reflected in the high level of serum-alkaline phosphatase. In relation to the area of bone involved, the phosphatase level is higher than in any other disease. Although the serum electrolytes are normal it has been shown by using radioactive calcium that there is an increased turnover of calcium in the affected bones, and many of these patients are in negative calcium balance. Administration of sodium fluoride has been used to restore the patients to positive calcium balance and it is claimed that this treatment reduces bone pain in the disease.[54] A good response in this respect is also claimed from the use of calcitonin[55] which inhibits osteoclast proliferation and activity. It is even more effective in reducing the serum-alkaline phosphatase and relieving pain when it is combined with mithramycin and diphosphonate therapy.[36] Salmon calcitonin in doses of 100 units daily has been shown to be effective in preventing pathological fractures in Paget's disease,[37] although it has been observed by some workers that fissure fractures may fail to unite while the patient is under treatment.[56] A variety of changes can occur in the skull as a feature of Paget's disease. As well as the uniform thickening with blurred contour from generalised apposition of osteoid, there may be wide areas of porosis of the calvarium with no change in adjacent bones (Fig 35.49).

To the surgeon who treats fractures the particular significance of Paget's disease is that replacement of mature lamellated bone by immature woven bone causes fragility despite thickening. Lack of normal resistance to weight-bearing is shown first in a tendency to bowing of the shafts, and then in multiple incomplete cracks through the thickened cortex, always on the convex side of the bowed bone and perpendicular to the surface (Figs 35.47 to 35.51).

Any of these cracks may be converted into complete fractures from trivial injury, and the complaint of acute pain in the area of a fissure may herald the onset of this complication.[56] In these circumstances it is tempting to forestall the fracture by prophylactic intramedullary nailing, but it must be remembered that even a small amount of bowing can make this a difficult undertaking, and the surgeon must be prepared to ream carefully and to use a relatively small nail. In the management of these fractures two important principles should be observed: First, there must be adequate and sustained immobilisation exactly as in the treatment of any other fracture—the

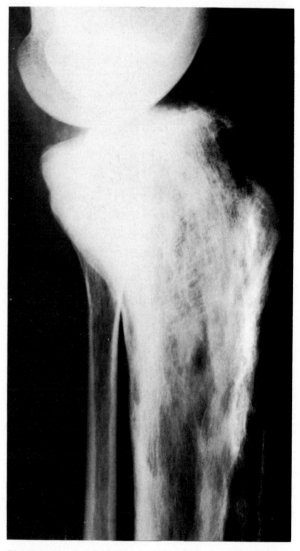

Fig 35.48 Osteitis deformans. Early stage showing deposition of osteoid on the surface of the original shaft of the tibia.

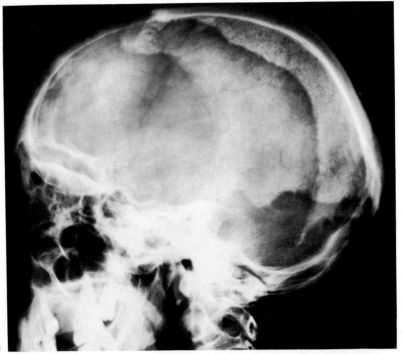

Fig 35.49

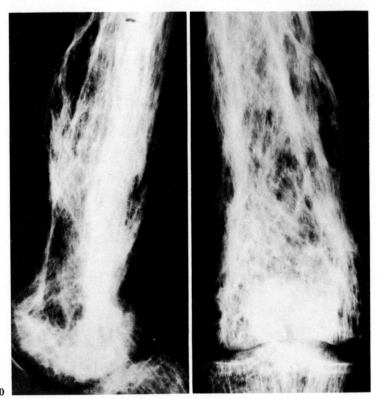

Fig 35.50

Figs 35.49 and 35.50 Osteitis deformans. Later stage showing unbridled new bone formation in the shaft of the femur, consisting largely of osteoid and woven bone which is fragile and susceptible to fracture. The skull shows porotic thickening of some bones of the calvarium from deposition of osteoid, while other adjacent bones are almost normal—a change quite typical of Paget's disease.

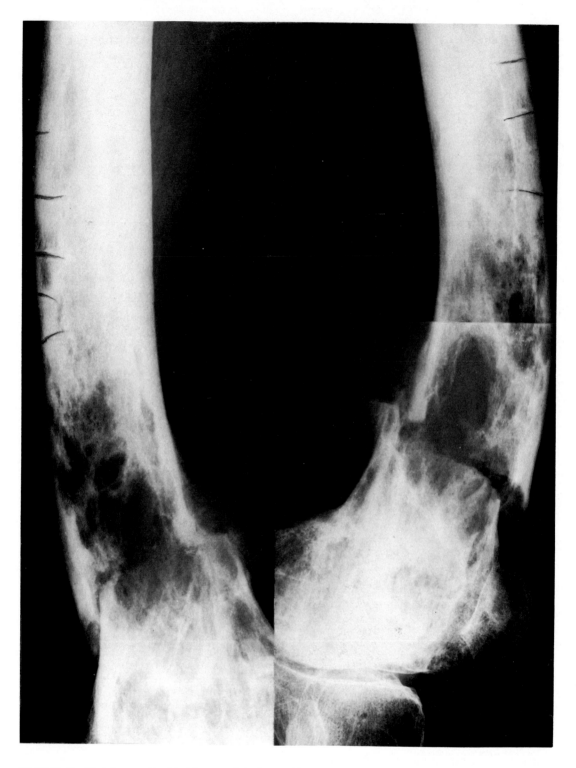

Fig 35.51 Osteitis deformans. Osteitis deformans of the femur with many incomplete cracks where the bone is bending, pathological fracture from trivial injury, and secondary sarcomatous transformation which necessitated amputation.

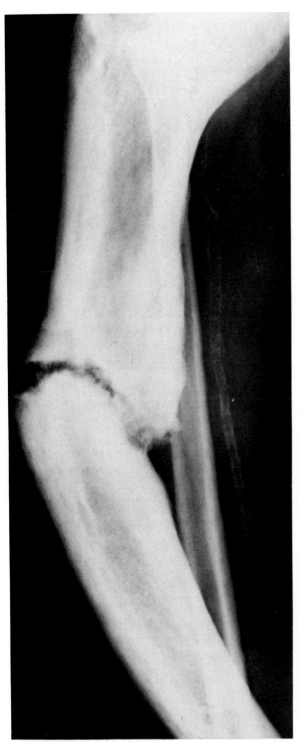

fragments will usually unite with abundant formation of osteoid or woven bone but, contrary to popular belief, repair is often slow and there is a significant element of non-union[56a] (Fig 35.52). Secondly, pre-existing deformity should usually be corrected at the site of fracture, because if bowing persists there will still be predisposition to further pathological fractures. Even when there has been no fracture it is sometimes wise to correct deformity by osteotomy, and advantage should certainly be taken of any fracture that is sustained. Fractures of the shaft of the tibia should be immobilised in plaster after alignment has been restored. Fractures of the femoral shaft can be treated successfully by traction in a Thomas splint, but they lend themselves to immobilisation by an intramedullary nail provided the bowing deformity is not too great. Care must be taken, however, to avoid jamming of the nail or splintering of the cortex; and because of the bowing of the bone, it is possible to drive the nail through the cortex and out of the medullary cavity (see above). Fractures of the femoral neck, which are very common in Paget's disease and occur in a strictly vertical plane unlike that of ordinary fractures in this situation (Fig 35.53), may be treated by intramedullary fixation of the usual

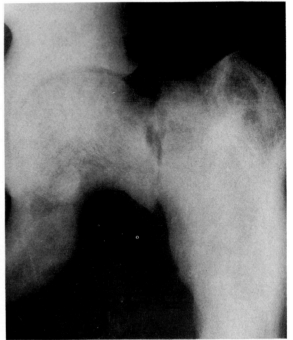

Fig 35.52 Osteitis deformans—Paget's disease. Un-united pathological fracture of the shaft of the tibia in Paget's disease. Despite abundant formation of osteoid in this disease fractures may fail to unite even though they are immobilised properly.

Fig 35.53 One of the commonest pathological fractures in osteitis deformans is a strictly vertical fracture through the femoral neck. Special care should be taken in fixing this fracture because the bone is liable to split.

type (see Chapter 29). Special care must be taken to avoid splitting the bone, and it is probably wise to use a screw device rather than a Smith-Petersen nail. In the very elderly, in widely displaced fractures, and where the fracture is complicated by Paget's arthritis of the hip, prosthetic replacement is the treatment of choice.

Paget's sarcoma. This complication has been given an incidence as high as 10 per cent by Jaffe[57] in cases of widespread Paget's disease. However, the overall incidence in the general Paget population is probably much lower and nearer to the order of 2 per cent. Price and Goldie have put it as low as 0.2 per cent.[58] The condition should be suspected when a patient with Paget's disease complains of increasing pain in one affected bone: a very high alkaline phosphatase value (for example, 200 Bodensky units) combined with a high sedimentation rate is usually found. The X-ray appearance typically shows marked osteolysis in a zone of Paget's disease (Fig 35.54) with a break through the cortex and often a pathological fracture. These sarcomata are always highly malignant with great variation in cellular structure. The prognosis is bad and the only hope of survival is immediate amputation.

PRIMARY AND SECONDARY TUMOURS OF BONE CAUSING PATHOLOGICAL FRACTURE

Pathological fractures are often caused by primary or secondary tumours of bone, particularly tumours of the osteolytic type which are responsible for the destruction of cortical bone without the production of reactive periosteal new bone. For example, multiple myeloma is a destructive neoplasm occurring in many sites without reparative bone formation, and fractures are sustained in more than 60 per cent of cases, whereas Ewing's sarcoma with its medullary destruction is characterised also by subperiosteal apposition of new bone in many 'onion-layers', and only 5 per cent of these tumours are complicated by fracture. Similarly, osteosarcoma with its considerable potential for new bone formation rarely presents with a pathological fracture. The incidence of fracture in various bone tumours was estimated by Geshickter and Copeland[59] as: multiple myeloma, 62 per cent; cysts and cystic tumours, 45 per cent; secondary carcinoma, 35 per cent; giant cell tumour, 14 per cent; osteosarcoma, 8 per cent; Ewing's tumour, less than 5 per cent.

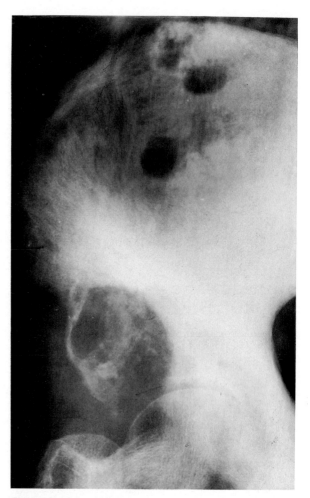

Fig 35.54 Paget's sarcoma of the pelvis. Note the destructive nature of the lesion which has broken into the soft tissues.

COMMON BENIGN TUMOURS PRESENTING WITH PATHOLOGICAL FRACTURES

Chondroma, benign chondroblastoma, chondromyxoid fibroma. These are all cartilage based benign tumours which may occur in any long bone, or in the pelvic bones. *Chondromas* are particularly common in the phalanges or metacarpals and are often disclosed for the first time by pathological fracture (Fig 35.55). These tumours usually develop during the first two decades of life, and the commonest sites are the short bones of the hands or feet. At first there is painless expansion near the end of the bone, sometimes extending throughout the shaft. The well-defined cystic area is demarcated from normal bone

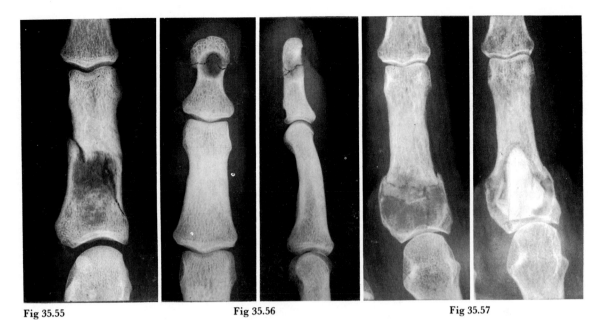

Fig 35.55   Fig 35.56   Fig 35.57

Figs 35.55 to 35.57 Tumours and cysts of the phalanges. Figure 35.55 shows a chondroma with crack fracture; Figure 35.56 is an implantation dermoid with fracture; and 35.57 shows another chondroma treated by curetting and grafting.

and surrounded by an intact but thin cortex. Crack fractures may be sustained from trivial injury, and indeed this is one of the most frequent causes of pathological fracture because chondromas of the phalanges are common tumours and about 40 per cent of them are complicated by fracture.

Treatment of fracture through a chondroma of a phalanx. The finger should be immobilised for two or three weeks by means of a finger splint or light plaster slab applied to the flexor surface of the slightly flexed digit. Some weeks later, when joint movement has been restored, the tumour should be excised and grafted through a lateral approach (Figs 35.56 and 35.57). Fractures through chondromas of the phalanges always unite, and the tumours respond well to surgical treatment. They are not radiosensitive.

Massive chondromas of long bones and bones of the pelvis. Large chondromas sometimes develop in the metaphyseal region of long bones, or in the pelvis or other bones of the trunk. Multiple chondromas in dyschondroplasia and diaphyseal aclasia have already been discussed. Solitary tumours, no less massive, may arise even when there is no developmental disease, and they often continue to increase in size long after cessation of epiphyseal growth. When they occur in the long bones they are often responsible for pathological fractures. In the pelvis they may grow to

gigantic proportions and can compress the bladder or cause ureteric or intestinal obstruction. These massive tumours are all potentially malignant although it is often difficult histologically to distinguish between relatively benign lesions and frankly malignant chondrosarcomas that will eventually metastasise. The distinction must often be made on clinical grounds and any cartilage tumour in an adult which continues to grow, or becomes painful, should be regarded as a probable chondrosarcoma. Treatment is essentially surgical. No cartilage tumour, either benign or malignant, is radio-sensitive, and their growth cannot be controlled by X-ray treatment. Massive chondromas should therefore be treated by local excision with replacement graft or prosthesis, or if that is impossible by amputation of the limb. Large cartilage tumours of the pelvis can only be treated by hindquarter amputation.

Benign chondroblastoma and chondromyxoid fibroma are basically cartilage tumours which are usually sited in or near to an epiphysis. On occasions they can produce a large osteolytic defect in the end of a long bone, but it is extremely rare for them to present with a pathological fracture.

Haemangioma of bone. Haemangioma usually occurs in the vertebrae or skull of young adults. There may be honeycombed rarefaction of one vertebra with collapse and wedging of the body which must be distinguished from the crushing of a simple compression fracture. Haemangioma also arise in the short bones of the hand and foot with characteristic soap-bubble appearance (Figs 35.58 to 35.61). As a rule the bone is destroyed so completely that it bends rather than fractures. The tumours respond well to irradiation, and surgical excision with bone grafting is seldom indicated. Indeed, because of the extremely vascular nature of this tumour, any attempt at local excision and grafting can be a very hazardous undertaking. If, because of repeated fracture, surgery becomes necessary complete excision with prosthetic replacement of the whole or part of the bone may be indicated.

'Disappearing bone disease'. This rare and unexplained condition is thought to be related to a haemangiomatous change in bone.[60] It can affect any bone and has been commonly associated with pathological fracture and progressive absorption of bone (Figs 35.62 to 35.64). The treatment of this disease is difficult—fractures fail to unite and grafts are absorbed by invasion of haemangiomatous tissue.

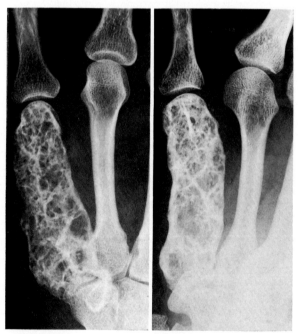

Fig 35.58   **Fig 35.59**

Figs 35.58 and 35.59 Angioma of bone. An angioma of the fifth metacarpal bone was treated by radiotherapy. The symptoms were relieved and the bone reossified. (London Hospital case.)

In the past amputation has been an all too frequent outcome, but successful results have been reported from prosthetic replacement of the diseased bone[61, 62, 63] (Figs 35.64 and 35.65).

MALIGNANT TUMOURS PRESENTING WITH PATHOLOGICAL FRACTURES

Giant cell tumour of bone. There is still disagreement about whether giant-cell tumours should be considered as malignant, and confusion is increased by the variability of aggression that may occur in tumours of apparently similar histological type. On the one hand there seems to be a link between aneurysmal bone cysts (Fig 35.66) with giant cells in their lining wall and solid giant cell tumours with multinucleated cells distributed evenly through a stroma of spindle cells; and on the other hand it is difficult to distinguish between giant cell tumours that are essentially benign and tumours that show gross aggression locally after excision or even, in very rare instances, cause metastases. All these varieties may present with pathological fractures, but there is usually some previous history of local pain. Thus a 'giant cell tumour process' has been postulated with every stage of benignity, aggression and malignity from cystic lesion at one end of the scale to frankly malignant tumours at the other.[64] Giant cell tumours seldom, if ever, occur before the age of 20. It is a tumour more common in women. It always begins in the epiphysis and extends to the area immediately under the articular surface. The late George Perkins[65] described the tumour as 'standing in a corner'—a phrase which aptly sums up the characteristics of extension to a cortex and extension right up to the end of a bone, combined with initial eccentricity. Rare cases have been reported where the tumour has crossed a joint.[66] The bone is expanded, at first asymmetrically, the common sites being the upper end of the tibia, upper end of the fibula, lower end of the femur, and lower end of the radius. There is no subperiosteal new bone formation such as occurs in Brodie's abscess and many osteosarcomas. Radiographs show trabeculation throughout the tumour with thinning and sometimes perforation of the cortex; there is usually a line of condensation separating the tumour from the normal bone of the shaft. At operation the tumour is bright red in colour and often very vascular.

The choice of surgical treatment lies between local excision, complete excision with graft,[67, 68, 69] prosthetic replacement,[70] and amputation. At one end of the scale the fast growing aggressive tumour with a

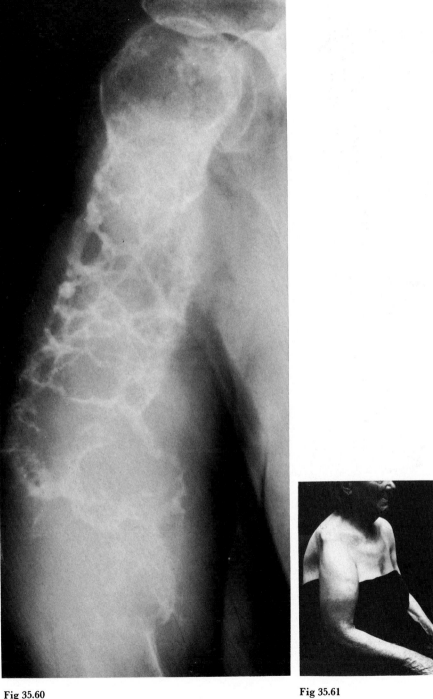

Fig 35.60

Fig 35.61

Figs 35.60 and 35.61 Angioma of bone. Angioma of the shaft of the humerus showing characteristic soap-bubble appearance. There was a pathological fracture, but the old lady lived happily to a ripe age.

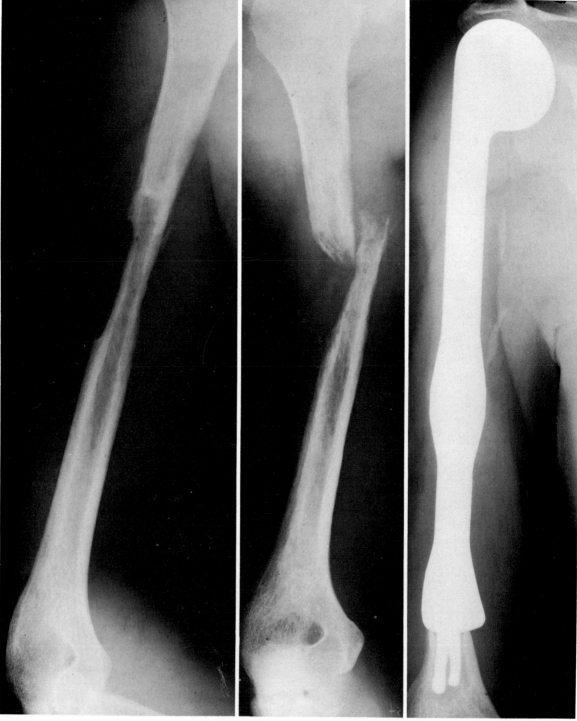

Fig 35.62   **Fig 35.63**   **Fig 35.64**

Figs 35.62 to 35.64 Figure 35.62 is an X-ray of 'disappearing bone disease' (haemangiomatous osteolysis of bone) affecting the humerus. Figure 35.63 shows the pathological fracture which occurred as a result of a minor injury. This case was successfully treated by major prosthetic replacement of the superior three-quarters of the shaft of the bone (Fig 35.64). The late Mr H. Jackson Burrows' case reported by Mr H. Poirier in his article (1968) Massive osteolysis of the humerus treated by resection and prosthetic replacement. *Journal of Bone and Joint Surgery*, 50–B, 158. (Reproduced by kind permission of the author and the editor.)

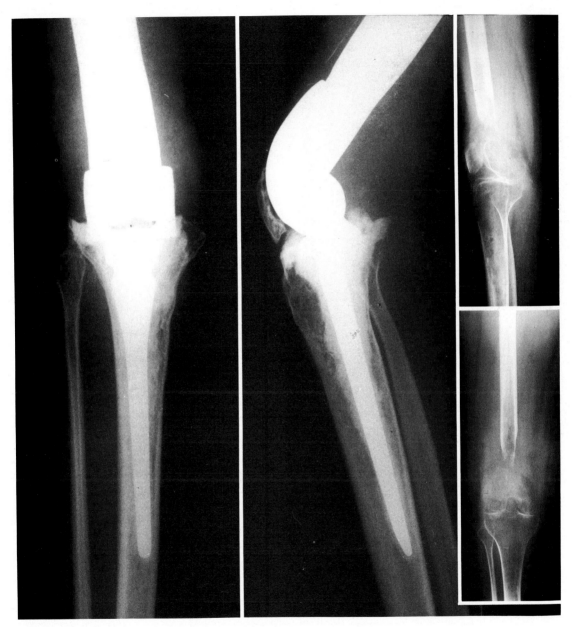

Fig 35.65 X-rays taken four years after prosthetic replacement of the lower third of the femur and knee for non-union of a pathological fracture through an area of 'disappearing bone disease' (see inset).

very cellular stroma and few giant cells must be regarded as potentially malignant and is unsuitable for local excision and curettage. It should be treated by complete excision of the bone or by primary amputation. At the other end of the scale the slow growing tumour with a well-ordered fibrous stroma and many giant cells can often be treated successfully by local curettage and bone graft (Figs 35.67 and 35.68). Good results have also been reported from the use of acrylic cement to fill the defect after curettage.[16] But it must be emphasised that supporters of this method of treatment stress the importance of a meticulous and thorough curettage; and even then they admit to 50 per cent recurrence rate.[71]

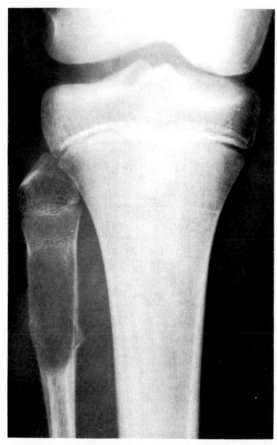

Fig 35.66 Is this a pathological fracture through a giant cell tumour? It was previously reported as so, but it is not! The patient is too young (epiphysis not yet closed) and the lesion has not affected the epiphysis. This is either a simple bone cyst or an aneurysmal bone cyst.

Complete excision of giant cell tumours is certainly the treatment of choice when it can be done without causing functional incapacity. The lower end of the radius can be excised and replaced by a transplant of the upper end of the fibula, or by a graft from the tibia implanted into the carpal bones; the upper end of the tibia can be excised and the knee joint fused; and the lower end of the femur has been replaced by using the anterior half of the upper end of the tibia as a graft.[69] These operations are justified when there is extensive invasion of articular cartilage. In other cases better results may be achieved by more conservative treatment. It must be emphasised, moreover, that even after complete excision of the tumour, islands of osteoclastomatous tissue may remain in the soft tissues and continue to grow, invading the bone that has been transplanted.

A number of cases have been reported of successful long term results from prosthetic replacement of large segments of bone destroyed by slow growing tumours, such as osteoclastoma or chondrosarcoma.[70,72] There is undoubtedly a place for this type of surgery in cases of pathological fracture which would otherwise require ablation or extensive bone reconstruction (Figs 35.69 and 35.70); but it must be remembered that very careful selection of patients is needed and any suggestion that there is extensive tumour involvement of the soft tissues is an absolute contraindication.

Although giant cell tumours can be treated by radiotherapy, there are a number of reported cases of post-irradiation sarcoma of tumours which have been irradiated. In these instances the soft tissue damage by radiation may considerably hamper further surgical treatment. If the diagnosis of giant cell tumour is beyond doubt the treatment should be surgical. Radiation therapy should be reserved for those sites which are inaccessible to surgery, and occasionally for recurrence after surgery.

Osteosarcoma is the most common of the primary malignant tumours of bone, two-thirds of the cases occurring between the ages of 10 and 30 years. The clinical and radiographic features and the incidence of pathological fracture vary according to the bone-producing or bone-destroying qualities of the tumour. In the rare sclerosing type of osteosarcoma (parosteal sarcoma) the tumour may be stony-hard and of slow growth. This variety of tumour never presents with fractures. The more usual radiographic appearance is with periosteal new bone formation, 'sun-ray spicules' of ossification at right angles to the shaft and a 'Codman's reactive triangle' of bone laid down beneath the raised periosteum at the margin of the tumour. The tumours are growing rapidly and usually present with severe, unremitting pain rather than pathological fracture. In the rare osteolytic and telangiectatic osteosarcomas and in Paget's sarcoma the tumour is predominantly destructive and pathological fracture is not uncommon. Although osteogenic sarcoma vary in their response to radiotherapy (they are relatively radio-resistant) the treatment that offers greatest hope of survival is immediate amputation followed by aggressive tumour chemotherapy.

Chondrosarcoma occurs usually between the ages of 30 and 50 in the long bones, pelvis and ribs. The tumours may arise *de novo* or at the site of pre-existing

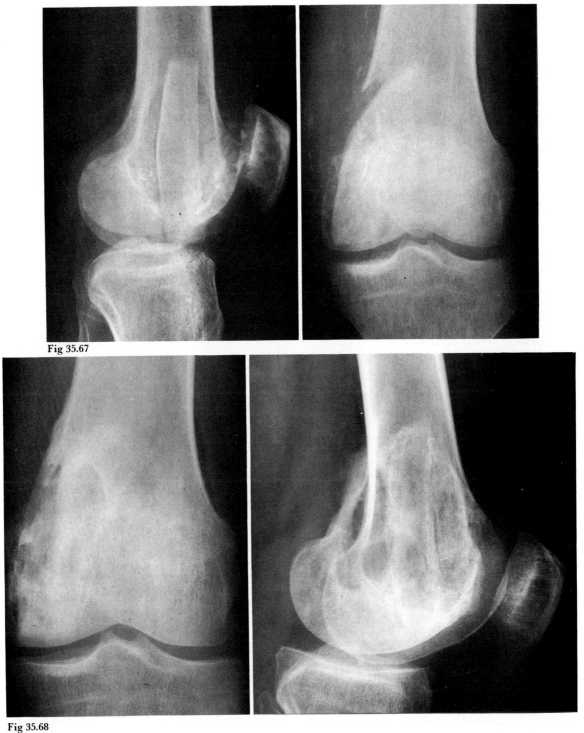

Fig 35.67

Fig 35.68

Figs 35.67 and 35.68 This extensive giant cell tumour had replaced the whole of the medial femoral condyle and caused an infraction into the knee joint. It was successfully treated by thorough curettage of the bone defect and the insertion of cancellous and strut grafts. Strut grafts are important for stabilising a fracture into the articular surface. Figure 35.68 shows the healed lesion four years after grafting.

chondroma, and any cartilage tumour in an adult which is painful and increasing in size should be regarded with suspicion. Growth is usually slow, metastases late, and the prognosis is more favourable than in many other sarcomas of bone. A pathological fracture is sometimes the first major presenting sign, particularly when the tumour occurs in the upper end of the femur, but it is usually preceded by pain of a deep and vague distribution, often mistakenly attributed to a disorder of the low back (Figs 35.71 to 35.73). Chondrosarcoma is not radio-sensitive and should be treated by amputation, or by wide resection using a prosthesis or a large homograft. Curettage with bone grafting is quite useless in the treatment of this tumour and will always result in recurrence (Figs 35.74 and 35.75). Incomplete resection, with or without prosthetic replacement, can lead to disastrous recurrence (Figs 35.76 and 35.77).

Fibrosarcoma of bone is a comparatively rare tumour, occurring usually in adult life. Pain is nearly always the presenting feature and swelling is sometimes minimal. Although there is often a history of trauma shortly before onset of pain, pathological

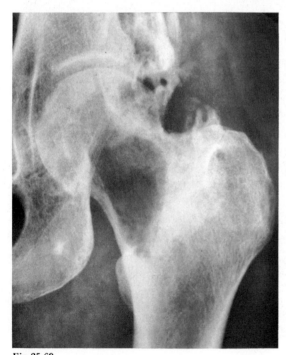

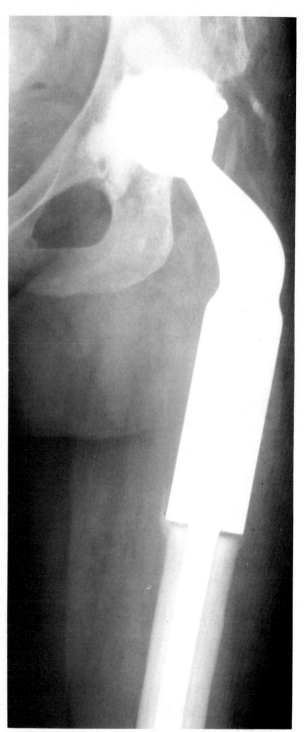

Fig 35.69   Fig 35.70

Figs 35.69 and 35.70 This patient underwent three operations in an attempt to eradicate the giant cell tumour of the upper end of the left femur. A pathological fracture occurred after the third operation. The lesion was successfully removed by prosthetic replacement of the upper third of the femoral shaft and the hip joint. Figure 35.69 shows the prosthesis four years after operation.

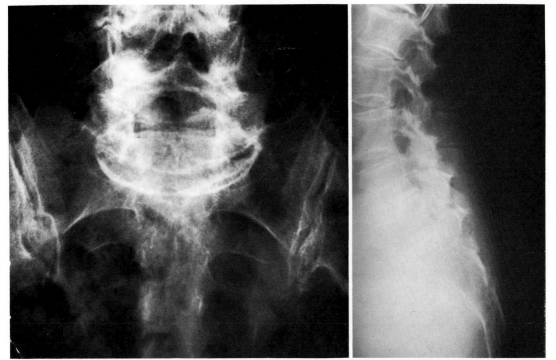

Fig 35.71

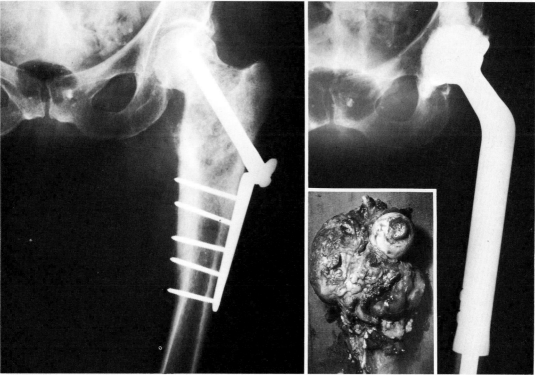

Fig 35.72   **Fig 35.73**

Figs 35.71 to 35.73 Pathological fracture in chondrosarcoma. This patient's complaint of pain around the left hip and thigh had been attributed for many months to a root irritation from degenerative changes in the low back (Fig 35.71). No pelvic X-ray had been taken until the pathological fracture through the neck of the femur revealed the true nature of the disease. The fracture was temporarily fixed with a pin and plate at the time of biopsy (Fig 35.72) and then treated by complete excision of the upper third of the femur and prosthetic replacement (Fig 35.73). The inset shows the very large tumour which was excised at the time of prosthetic replacement.

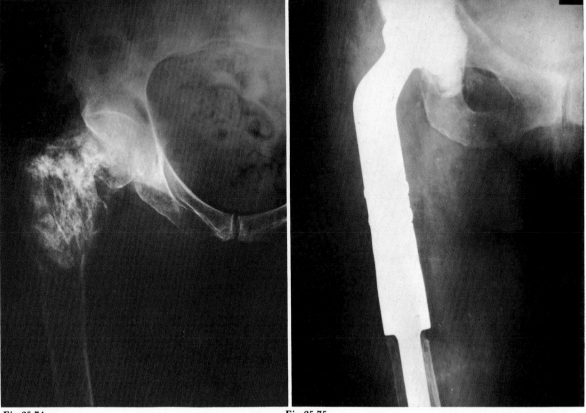

Fig 35.74   **Fig 35.75**

Figs 35.74 and 35.75 Chondrosarcoma—local recurrence and pathological fracture after curettage. Curettage and bone grafting are contraindicated in the treatment of chondrosarcoma. Figure 35.74 shows a pathological fracture of the neck of the femur occurring through tumour proximal to the site of a curettage. This case was successfully treated by excision and prosthetic replacement of the upper half of the femur (Fig 35.75).

fracture is not common and occurs only in fast growing tumours, such as those complicating Paget's disease. The X-ray appearance can be difficult to interpret and varies from one of patchy osteolytic disease to gross osteolysis with the formation of large translucent areas breaking through the cortex. In the early phase the appearance may be confused with infection. The treatment of choice is amputation; the tumour is not radio-sensitive and X-ray therapy should be reserved for palliative treatment only. Chemotherapeutic agents are of questionable value. Local resection and prosthetic replacement has such a high incidence of recurrence that it cannot be offered as a reasonable alternative to amputation.

Malignant fibrous histiocytoma. This malignant connective tissue tumour, which typically occurs in the fifth and sixth decades, may be found in bone or soft tissue. It grows more slowly than a true fibrosarcoma and therefore sometimes presents as a pathological fracture (Figs 35.78 and 35.79). It is characterised by the whorled and 'storiform' (mat like) pattern of its fibroblasts and its bizarre cells with a vacuolated cytoplasm.[73] The degree of malignancy of the tumour is related to the variable neoplastic potential of the tissue histiocyte.[74] If the tumour is in a long bone and is well defined from the soft tissues it can be treated by wide excision of the tumour bearing part of the bone, followed by major prosthetic replacement (Figs 35.80 and 35.81). However, it must be remembered that this tumour tends to spread along fascial planes,[74] and once it has broken into soft tissues it has a high incidence of local recurrence. Therefore prosthetic replacement after pathological fracture is likely to carry a higher risk of recurrence (Fig 35.79).

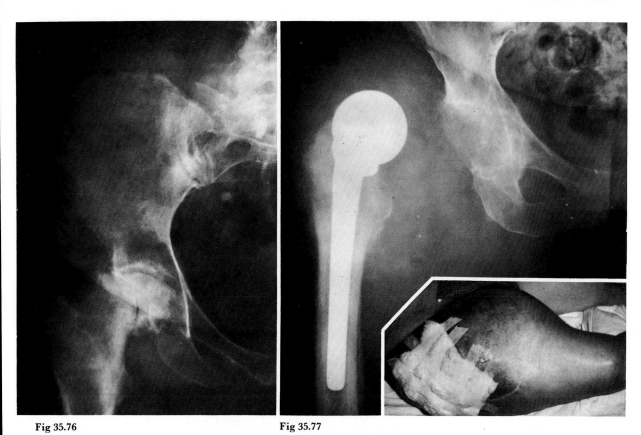

Fig 35.76   Fig 35.77

Figs 35.76 and 35.77 Chondrosarcoma—local recurrence after inadequate excision. This patient sustained a subcapital fracture of the neck of the right femur at the site of a chondrosarcoma (Fig 35.76). The femoral head replacement which was carried out inevitably left much of the tumour still *in situ.* Chondrosarcoma is highly radio-resistant, so that subsequent radiotherapy had no effect on the massive local recurrence (Fig 35.77 and inset). Chondrosarcomas must be treated by very wide excision or by amputation.

Malignant round-cell tumour occurs early in life, usually between the ages of 10 and 20 years, in the shafts of long bones and almost equally commonly in the innominate bone. The name 'Ewing's sarcoma' is often applied to certain types of this tumour. Severe pain and swelling are the usual presenting symptoms and pathological fractures are extremely rare. Although the tumour is very sensitive to radiotherapy and chemotherapy the final outcome is gloomy. There is, however, a suggestion that the prognosis is improved if the primary focus can be removed in addition to giving chemotherapy.[75]

Multiple myelomatosis and secondary neoplasms of bone. When considered together these are by far the most common cause of pathological fracture in the elderly patient; and often the most distressing to treat. With few exceptions the outcome will always be fatal and the remaining period of life may be very short. However, this does not mean that fractures, when they occur, should not be treated. To the contrary, every effort should be made to stabilise fractures as they happen, and prophylactic intramedullary nailing should be undertaken when indicated to reduce their further incidence.

Multiple myelomatosis commonly presents as an acute episode due to pathological fracture of the spine. The tumour arises from cells of the marrow, usually in the second half of life from the ages of 40 to 70 years. The tumours are almost invariably multiple and they show a curious predilection for the bones of the trunk—the spine, ribs, sternum, and then in order of frequency the skull, femora, pelvis and

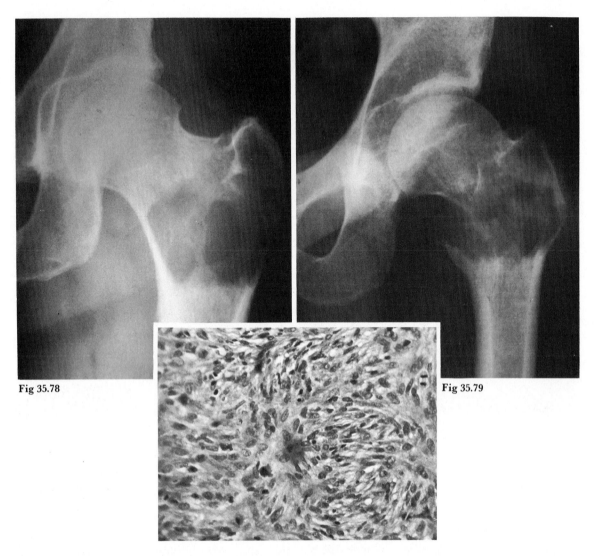

Fig 35.78   Fig 35.79

Figs 35.78 and 35.79 Fig 35.78 shows the X-ray of a 35-year-old patient presenting with a history of pain in the left hip for six months. Biopsy showed the lesion in the femoral neck to be a malignant fibrous histiocytoma. (Inset shows the typical storiform pattern of the fibrous tissue.) Despite crutch walking the patient developed a pathological fracture within a few weeks of biopsy (Fig 35.79). Prosthetic replacement was carried out but the margins of the tumour were difficult to define and there was local recurrence within nine months.

clavicle. Of all malignant tumours of bone it is the one with the highest incidence of pathological fracture. Crush fractures of vertebrae, spontaneous fractures of ribs, or fractures of the shafts of one or both femora may occur in the terminal stages of this disease (Figs 35.82 to 35.85). Pain is the first manifestation and it is usually in the back. In so far as the patients are usually elderly, and pain in the back from senile osteoporosis or intervertebral arthritis is to be expected at this stage, the diagnosis is sometimes

overlooked. A marked rise in the blood sedimentation rate should arouse suspicions that the case is not one of simple osteoporosis. In myelomatosis the sedimentation rate may reach over 100 mm/hr. There may be a considerable increase in the serum-calcium and this carries with it a very bad prognosis. The radiographic evidence of multiple cystic tumours, most of them $\frac{1}{2}$ to 1 inch (1.3 to 2.5 cm) in diameter, occurring not only in the vertebrae but also in the skull and other bones, may make the diagnosis fairly

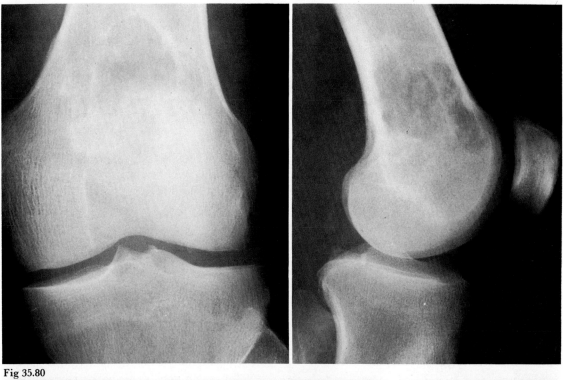

Fig 35.80

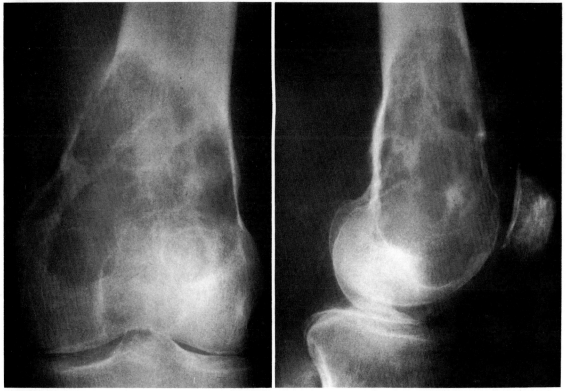

Fig 35.81

Figs 35.80 and 35.81 A 60-year-old man presented with temporary aching in the left knee and X-rays showed a well defined osteolytic lesion within the femoral medulla (Fig 35.80). This was considered a non-osteogenic fibroma of bone. Three years later pain returned and X-rays at that time showed a considerable extension of the femoral lesion (Fig 35.81). Biopsy revealed the typical histological appearance of malignant fibrous histiocytoma. In this case there had been no pathological fracture and the lesion was well contained within bone. It was successfully treated by major prosthetic replacement of the lower third of the femur, using a hinged knee joint.

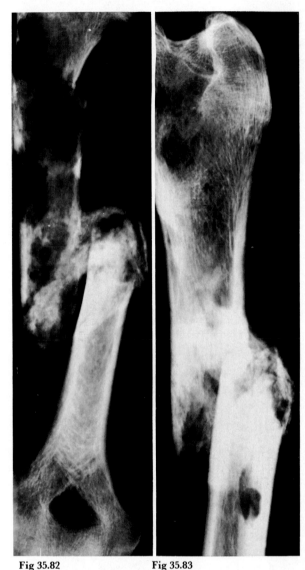

Fig 35.82   Fig 35.83

Figs 35.82 and 35.83 Multiple myelomatosis. Pathological fractures of the shafts of humerus and femur from multiple myelomatosis. There were Bence-Jones proteoses in the urine; the serum-globulin was raised (see Figs 35.84 and 35.85).

clear, but in other cases the tumours are more confluent and there is generalised destruction of all vertebral bodies (Figs 35.86 to 35.88). In these cases confirmation of the diagnosis depends on analysis of the urine for Bence-Jones protein, estimation of serum proteins with the presence of a reversed albumen-globulin ration, and punch biopsy of the marrow

either of the sternum or iliac crest (see Fig 35.88 inset).

Treatment. Multiple myelomatosis is a fatal disease and most patients die within a few months or at the most within a few years. When a myeloma appears to be solitary the expectation of life may be longer, especially if the tumour is irradiated. The tumours are radio-sensitive and after treatment there is usually regression and reossification. If the disease is widespread chemotherapy with one of the cytotoxic group of drugs may be helpful in relieving pain and improving the well-being of the patient.[76, 77, 78]

Multiple fractures of the spine should not be reduced, but a light posterior spinal support may be fitted. In the rare cases where there may be a single deposit with neurological signs decompression and bone graft by the antero-lateral approach is indicated.[79] Fractures of the long bones should be treated by internal fixation whenever practicable, and intramedullary nailing of fractures of the shafts of long bones augmented by acrylic cement fixation has been a major contribution in the terminal management of this condition. It does not preclude the use of radiotherapy later on.

Metastatic tumours of bone. Skeletal metastases can occur in the later stages of any cancer, but particularly the breast, kidney, prostate, thyroid and lung. As a rule generalised bone metastases represent the terminal stages of visceral carcinoma, but sometimes a solitary metastatic tumour is found even before the first symptom or clinical sign of the primary tumour. Indeed, Geschickter and Maseritz found no clinical evidence of a primary growth in one-sixth of the metastatic bone tumours they studied.[80] The differential diagnosis of these solitary metastases presents considerable difficulty because they can resemble primary growths so closely, but the age of incidence is usually much higher than in primary tumours; and the bones most often involved by spread through the blood stream are those with the highest proportion of marrow—the vertebrae, pelvis, upper end of the femur, upper end of the humerus, and the skull and ribs. Intramedullary lesions arising in the middle of long bones should always arouse the suspicion that they are due to a metastasis and as a result the first presenting sign may be a pathological fracture arising from trivial injury, especially in tumours of osteolytic type from primary carcinoma of the breast, kidney and thyroid. *Biopsy of such a lesion may precipitate a fracture,* and it is always wise to protect the limb by a splint or internal fixation

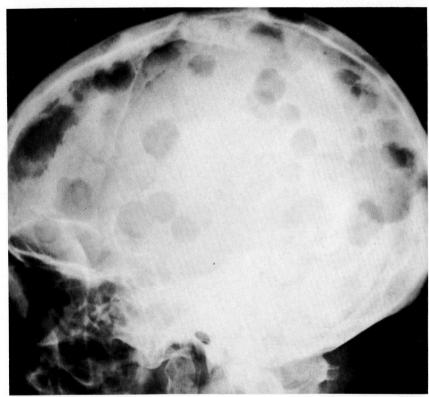

Fig 35.84

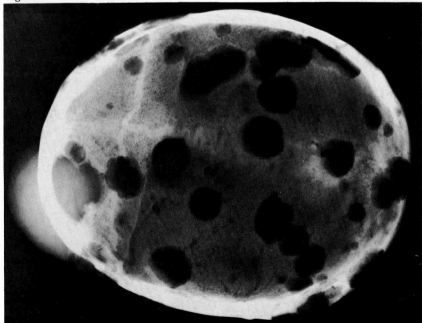

Fig 35.85

Figs 35.84 and 35.85 Multiple myelomatosis. Same case as that shown in Figures 35.82 and 35.83. The patient died. Post-mortem radiographic examination of the skull shows multiple tumours with typical punched-out defects. In the frontal region there is a shadow of the tumour associated with one of the bone defects (Fig 35.85).

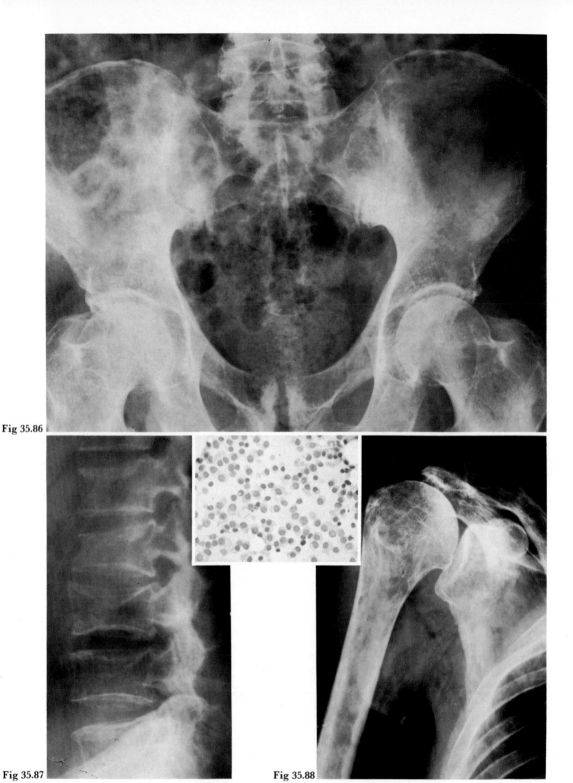

Fig 35.86

Fig 35.87

Fig 35.88

Figs 35.86 to 35.88 Myelomatosis simulating senile osteoporosis. A man aged 78 years sustained compression fractures of the spine simply from lifting weights. Radiographs showed general porosis of the pelvis and spine with cupping of vertebral bodies resembling senile osteoporosis (Figs 35.86 and 35.87). But the plasma globulin was found to be greatly raised (9.9 g per cent, the normal being not more than 2 g per cent). There was depletion of plasma albumen from the normal 4 to 2.1 g per cent. Serum-calcium was raised to 12.6 mg per cent. There was no Bence-Jones proteoses in the urine but radiographs of the humerus and other long bones suggested that in addition to general porosis there were multiple small cysts (Fig 35.88). Sternal marrow puncture showed typical plasma myeloma cells (see inset).

until definitive treatment can be instituted (Figs 35.89 and 35.90).

As a rule the lesions from carcinomatosis are multiple and they are usually osteolytic, but sometimes osteogenic secondaries occur such as in carcinoma of the breast or prostate, which can both be a cause of increased density of a vertebral body, but this in no way prevents pathological fracture (see Figs 35.89 and 35.90). The deposit is first in the medulla and there is then secondary invasion of the cortex, sometimes with diffuse mottling within the area of destruction, but with no periosteal reaction (Figs 35.91 and 35.92). The lesions are less clearly punched out than are the typical deposits of diffuse

myelomatosis. In the spine, there is sometimes destruction of a vertebral body without collapse, indicating that destruction has been accompanied by replacement with tumour tissue, and this serves to differentiate metastatic deposits from tuberculosis and other inflammatory diseases (Fig 35.93). It is sometimes helpful to remember that when a vertebral body collapses as a result of a tumour deposit *both* disc plates collapse, whereas in simple trauma only the upper plate is depressed. When pathological fractures of long bones are sustained they should be immobilised if possible by internal fixation—usually an intramedullary nail with acrylic cement, because this is the best way of relieving pain and it eases the problem of

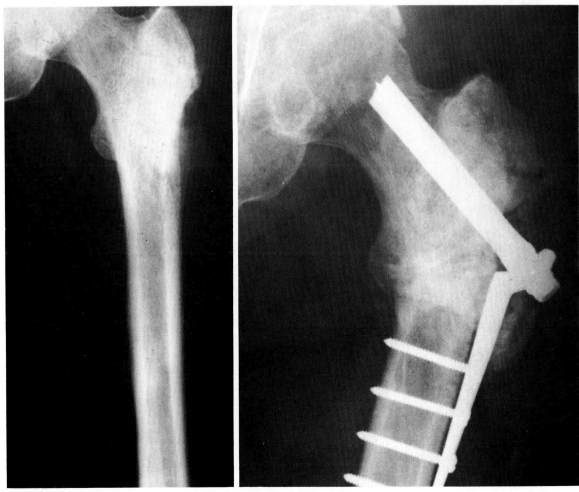

Fig 35.89   **Fig 35.90**

Figs 35.89 and 35.90 An elderly patient presented with a painful sclerotic lesion of the upper end of the left femur (Fig 35.89). Biopsy was carried out and the diagnosis of prostatic carcinoma was made. Five days after biopsy while still in bed he fractured through the tumour. It would have been wise to have applied the internal fixation as a prophylactic measure at the time of biopsy (Fig 35.90).

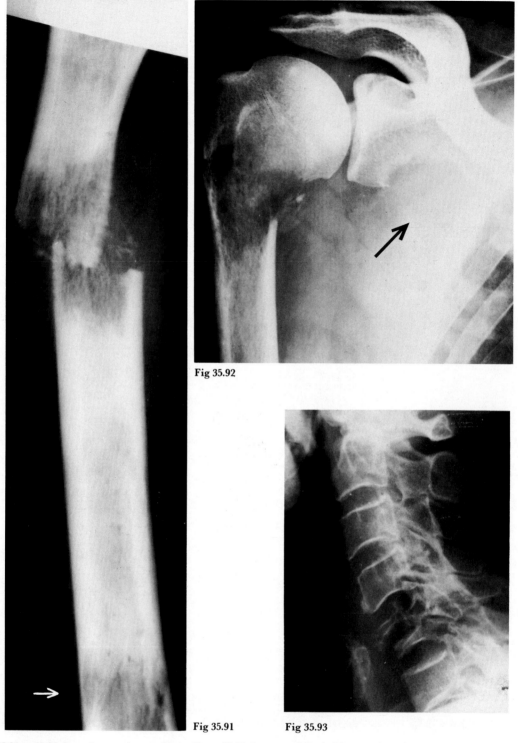

Fig 35.92

Fig 35.91   **Fig 35.93**

Figs 35.91 to 35.93 Secondary carcinoma of bone. Figure 35.91 shows a pathological fracture through a metastasis in the upper shaft of the femur from carcinoma of the breast. There is a second deposit in the lower shaft. The pathological fracture in Figure 35.92 is from a secondary hypernephroma in the humerus associated with another deposit in the scapula. Figure 35.93 shows the typical appearance of secondary carcinoma of the spine; despite extensive bone destruction there is minimal collapse because the bone is replaced by tumour tissue.

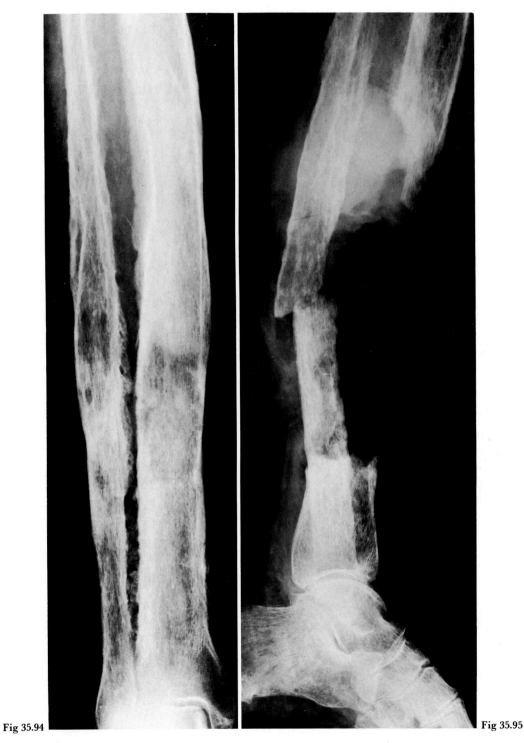

Fig 35.94

Fig 35.95

Figs 35.94 and 35.95 Epithelioma of bone. An epithelioma of the skin occurring at the site of chronic varicose ulceration invaded the tibia and eventually destroyed a very large part of it, the fibula also sustaining fracture (Fig 35.95). (Robert Jones and Agnes Hunt Orthopaedic Hospital case). Pathological fractures of the tibia with similarly extensive destruction is often seen after tropical ulceration with malignant transformation.

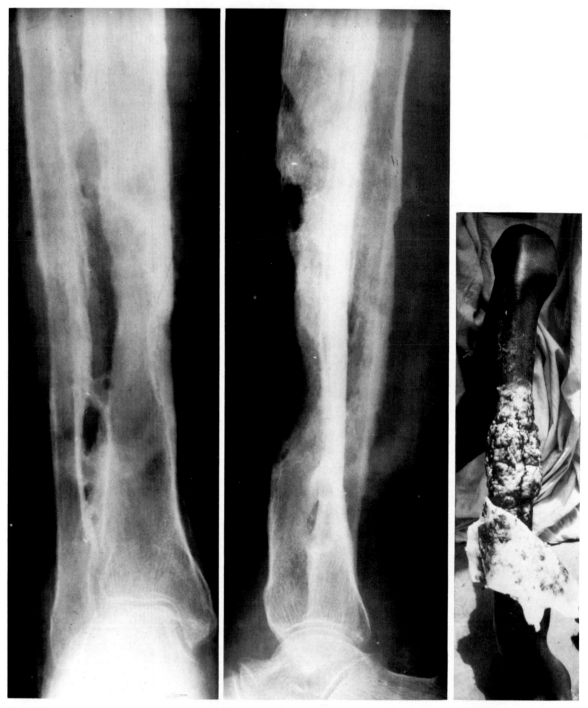

Fig 35.96

Fig 35.97

Figs 35.96 and 35.97 A Nigerian patient had suffered from tropical ulceration of the lower leg for many years. He eventually attended hospital because the ulcer had become very painful due to invasion of the tibia and fibula by epithelioma (Fig 35.96). The very obvious epitheliomatous change in the ulcer is shown in Figure 35.97.

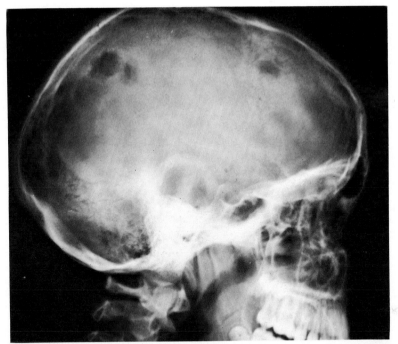

Fig 35.98

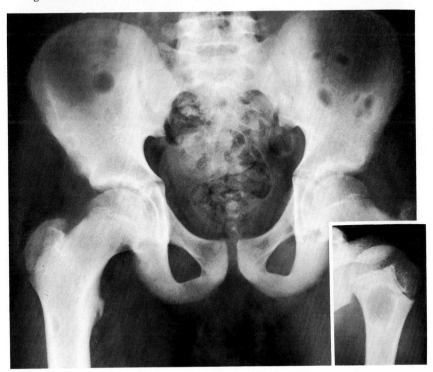

Fig 35.99

Figs 35.98 and 35.99 Histiocytosis X. A boy sustained an injury to the hip joint and radiographs showed small cystic areas in the femora and pelvis. Further radiographs showed similar granulomatous cysts in the neck of the humerus and skull. The diagnosis was confirmed by punch biopsy.

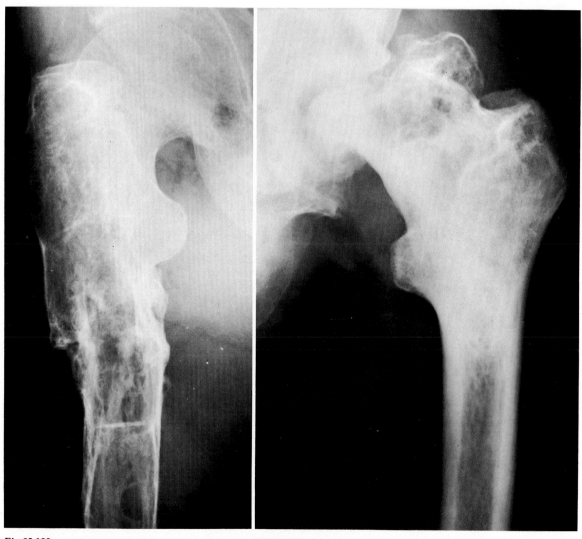

Fig 35.100   **Fig 35.101**

giving radiotherapy. The fractures always unite and good function may be restored. In fractures of the neck of the femur through the site of a metastatic deposit there should be no hesitation in introducing a three-flanged nail, or better still, in carrying out a replacement with a femoral head prosthesis (for techniques see section on General Management of Pathological Fractures).

Most secondary deposits causing pathological fractures in bone can be treated by radiotherapy and many will recalcify after treatment. Tumours such as the prostate, breast and thyroid are hormone dependant and should be given the appropriate therapy. The metastases from renal carcinoma (hyperne-

phroma) are sometimes isolated lesions and there are well documented cases of long term survival after excision of the primary tumour and its secondary deposit.[81] Unfortunately it is also true that bone metastases with pathological fractures have appeared as late as eight years after removal of primary kidney tumour.[82]

Epitheliomatous invasion of bone. Direct invasion of the mandible or maxilla from epithelioma of the lip or tongue is well known, but similar invasion may occur in the shafts of long bones and cause pathological fracture. Examples are illustrated in Figures 35.94 to 35.97. The epithelioma invariably develops at the site of long-standing skin infection and can be the

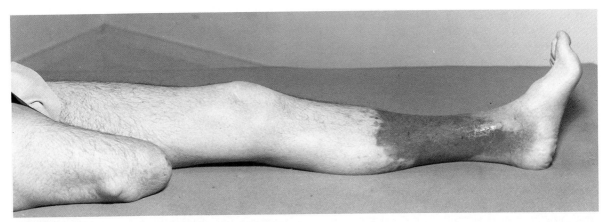

Fig 35.102

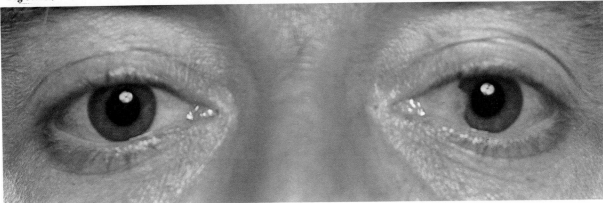

Fig 35.103

Figs 35.100 to 35.103 Lipoid granulomatosis of bone—Gaucher's disease. This Israeli boy sustained so many spontaneous fractures of the shaft of the right femur that the limb was amputated; the condition had been diagnosed as 'chronic osteomyelitis'. There were typical changes of lipoid granulomatosis of Gaucher's type (Fig 35.100) with expansion of the opposite femoral shaft and avascular necrosis of the femoral head (Fig 35.101), pigmentation of the skin (Fig 35.102) and lipoid deposits in the conjunctiva (Fig 35.103).

outcome of chronic varicose ulceration or tropical ulcer. If left untreated the tibia and fibula become involved and may fracture (Fig 35.95). The only treatment is amputation accompanied by excision of affected lymph nodes.

PATHOLOGICAL FRACTURES FROM MARROW CELL DISORDER (GRANULOMA OF BONE)

There is a group of blood and marrow diseases, sometimes known as the granulomatoses of bone, the pathology of which is uncertain, where bone is replaced by infiltration with histiocytes (Histiocytosis X), or by lipoid tissue (Gaucher's disease) in which pathological fractures are common.

Histiocytosis X. (*Eosinophilic granuloma, Hand-Schüller-Christian disease, Letterer-Siwe disease*). These three conditions are almost certainly all manifestations of the same disease in varying degrees,[83] where bone is infiltrated by histiocytes with plump nuclei and a diffuse eosinophil cytoplasm.[84] The maximum age of onset is in the first decade. The mildest form is a solitary lesion, the eosinophilic granuloma of bone, where there is secondary infiltration by eosinophilic leucocytes. This commonly affects the spine and may be responsible for a localised compression of a vertebral body. In the classical Hand-Schüller-Christian disease the histiocytes become swollen with lipid producing a rise in the cholesterol content of the affected tissues and the disease is more widespread. The Christian triad is skull defects, exophthalmus and diabetes insipidus. In Letterer-Siwe disease the histiocytes come to resemble reticulum cells. The deposits are usually small (Figs 35.98 and 35.99), but sometimes in the skull they may coalesce to form larger areas of destruction, giving a 'map-like' picture.[84] Deposits may also be spread widely through the soft tissues affecting lymph nodes, liver and spleen. Deposits from all these three conditions are very radio-sensitive.

Gaucher's disease.[85] (Figs 35.100 to 35.103). This condition, which occurs especially in the Hebraic races, is characterised by the infiltration of the liver, spleen and marrow by large cells filled with kerasin and thought to be derived from the reticulum cells. The deposits are widespread, especially throughout the lower shafts of the femora, which have a characteristic flared and rarefied appearance, usually likened to an Erlmeyer flask.[86] The bone lesions are commonly misdiagnosed as a simple osteomyelitis, but the almost constant finding of enlargement of the liver and spleen should alert the surgeon to the possibility of an underlying Gaucher's disease. Pathological fractures through the weakened bone are very common and should be treated by intramedullary nailing. There may be pigmentation of the skin and lipoid deposits in the conjunctiva. Deposits in the upper end of the femur can result in extreme crushing of the femoral head from avascular necrosis.

PARASITIC DISEASE OF THE BONE CAUSING PATHOLOGICAL FRACTURE

Hydatid disease, though rare in Great Britain and the United States, still occurs not infrequently in the great sheep-raising countries of Australia, South America and South Africa. The taenia *Echinococcus granulosus* inhabits the small intestine of the dog. Many thousands of ova are passed daily in the faeces, thus contaminating food and water and infesting sheep or man—the intermediate hosts in which the larval stage of the worm develops with cyst formation.

Clinical features. Man is usually infested directly from the dog which he pets, caresses or allows to lick his hand. Primary cysts develop in bone in about 1 per cent of cases, first appearing near the epiphyses, usually in the femur or humerus, and less often in the vertebrae, tibia or pelvis. They grow so slowly over a latent period of many years that the diagnosis is seldom established before adult life. The cysts are multilocular, without sclerosis and with minimal bone expansion. Periosteal reaction does not occur unless associated with infection or trauma.[87] A fracture sustained without injury is very often the first clinical manifestation. Non-union is almost inevitable. Within a few months after fracture, as a result of the shedding of parasitic elements from bone into surrounding soft tissues, a large, cystic, painless swelling develops. Because there is little or no inflammatory reaction the clinical picture may resemble a cold abscess, and a number of cases have been misdiagnosed as a tuberculous infection.[88] The diagnosis may be confirmed by the Casoni intradermal test and hydatid complement fixation tests, and if necessary by diagnostic puncture. Microscopic examination of aspirated fluid shows fragments of laminated membrane, small daughter-cysts and sometimes scolices or hooklets.

Treatment of pathological fractures in hydatid disease of bone. The prognosis is very grave because there is usually non-union of the fracture, and extension rapidly occurs in soft tissues, neighbouring joints being involved; there is also a considerable risk of pre-operative or post-operative infection, which may be fatal. Once a fracture has occurred no useful purpose is served by simple incision into the cysts, curettage or the application of formalin; these measures are almost invariably followed by recurrence. In one case of hydatid disease of the innominate bone some measure of success has been claimed from curettage and daily irrigation with 30 per cent hypertonic saline,[89] although in another case report where this method was used to treat a pathological fracture of the femur there was an early recurrence requiring amputation.[90]* Prophylactic excision of the cyst bearing bone, or part of the bone with prosthetic or homograft replacement,[91] may have a place in preventing the disastrous results of pathological fracture. This form of treatment however is contra-indicated after fracture has occurred because of the high incidence of recurrence and infection. Usually, if pathological fracture has taken place amputation above the involved area is the only measure that offers hope and it should be undertaken forthwith (Figs 35.104 and 35.105).

---

*Regression has been reported in liver hydatid disease treated by mebandazole (up to 50 mg/kg/day). (Morris D L 1981 Management of hydatid disease. British Journal of Hospital Medicine 25 : 586). It is possible that this drug may have a place in the management of inoperable disease of the pelvic bones or as an adjunct to local surgery, but at present there is no product licence for its use in the treatment of hydatid disease.

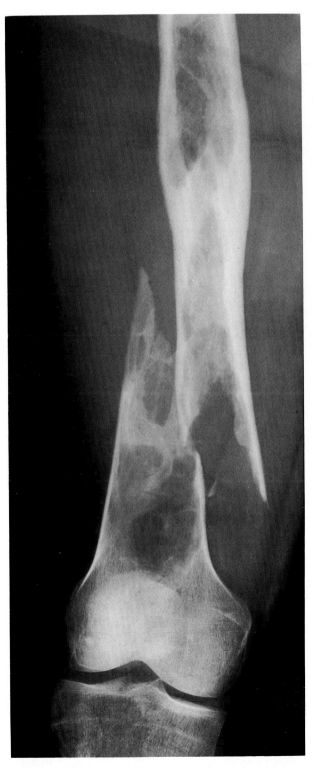

Fig 35.105

Fig 35.104

Figs 35.104 and 35.105 A patient who was known to have hydatid disease of the liver developed a pathological fracture of the right femur (Fig 35.104). She was referred for possible prosthetic replacement of the lower half of the femoral shaft. The decision not to proceed with this was amply justified by examination of the gross specimen after disarticulation of the hip (Fig 35.105). The extensive involvement of the soft tissues, inevitable after pathological fracture, would have certainly resulted in local recurrence with all its attendant complications. Hydatid disease of a long bone with pathological fracture should be treated by amputation.

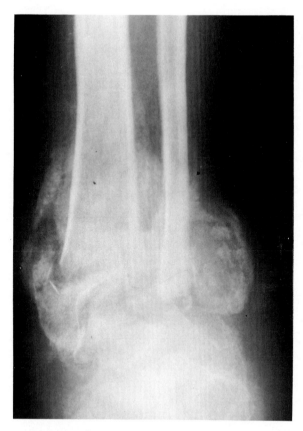

Fig 35.106 Neuropathic fracture. The patient whose ankle X-ray is shown in this Figure sustained a minor injury six weeks before. He walked happily on the limb until swelling became pronounced. He was known to have suffered from tabes for many years and had already been unsuccessfully treated for Charcot's arthropathy of the knee. The explosive nature of the fracture with minimal trauma, and the excessive callus formation, is typical of a neuropathic fracture.

NEUROTROPHIC DYSTROPHIES OF THE BONE CAUSING FRACTURE

Tabes dorsalis and syringomyelia. The degenerative process in the posterior columns of the spinal cord from syphilitic infection, and the peculiar cystic lesion of the cord in syringomyelia, produce bone and joint changes which are indistinguishable. The neurological lesion destroys the sensory nerve tracts in the cord, and both joint sense and sensation of pain in the affected areas are lost. Neuropathic arthropathy is characterised by enlargement of the joint, effusion, laxity of ligaments, dislocation and subluxation, fracture, and deposition of new bone. The characteristic feature of the lesion is that it is painless; gross joint changes may occur without the patient complaining of pain. Fractures may have marked comminution and yet minimal pain (Fig 35.106). In this type of neuropathy bone does not behave as in a normal fracture and bizarre complications may be encountered. When there is neurotrophic disturbance of bone, union—either of a fracture or of an elective arthrodesis—is usually slow, and metallic internal fixation is not well tolerated.

Bone lesions in diabetic neuropathy. That lesions at the ends of the extremities, usually the lower limbs, may occur as a complication of diabetes from vascular changes is well known. It is possibly less well known that diabetes may also cause a neuropathy which produces bone and joint changes similar to those seen in neurosyphilis and syringomyelia. This complication is distinguished from that of vascular degeneration by the fact that the lesions are painless, hairs are present on the skin and the pulses are palpable.[92] Further, diabetic neuropathy does not occur as an acute hazard of diabetes, like acidosis, coma or diabetic gangrene, but as the result of many months or years of uncontrolled or insufficiently controlled diabetes (Figs 35.107 to 35.111). This, indeed, is a most important diagnostic point. The neuropathic bone or joint lesion is often preceded by parasthesia, motor weakness, or other neuritic symptoms. The treatment depends essentially on expert diabetic management. If this can be achieved the prognosis is good, and fractures heal without difficulty. Joint disorders may however be permanent.

IATROGENIC PATHOLOGICAL FRACTURES

There are a number of orthopaedic procedures and treatments which weaken the structure of bone and lead directly to pathological fractures. Post-immobilisation fractures and cortisone induced fractures are good examples of this form of iatrogenic disease, and they have already been discussed under atrophic fractures. There are, however, several examples of local bone weakness brought about by a variety of surgical operations, and these are now discussed briefly.

Fracture through screw holes. Unsupported screw holes are known to act as stress raisers in the bone and expose it to the hazard of pathological fracture[93] (see Figs 16.37 and 16.38). This effect,

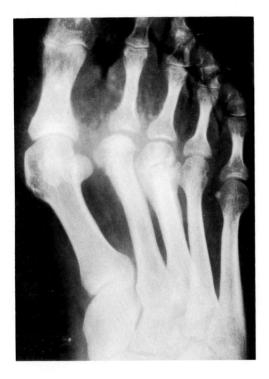

Fig 35.107

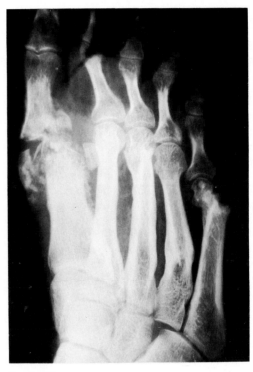

Fig 35.108

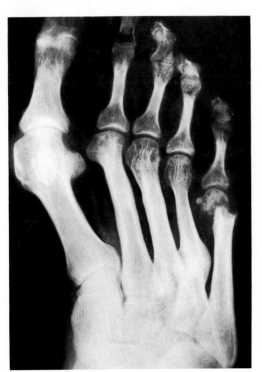

Fig 35.109

Figs 35.107 to 35.109 Neuropathic dystrophy of bone—diabetes and peripheral neuritis. For 21 years this patient was treated for diabetes. Although it was partly controlled by diet and insulin there was vascular disturbance in the feet and peripheral neuritis with impairment of sensation. A fracture of the neck of the second metatarsal bone occurred after 15 years and a fracture of the third metatarsal shortly thereafter (Fig 35.107). These fractures united; but at an unknown date there had also been a fracture of the shaft of the fourth metatarsal. Eight months later there was a fracture of the neck of the fifth metatarsal (Fig 35.108). These fractures united, but were followed by arthropathy of the first metatarso-phalangeal joint (Fig 35.109). (London Hospital case.)

combined with mineral loss induced by the very rigid fixation produced by some of the modern bone plates, demands that patients who have recently had plates removed should avoid strenuous physical exercise until there is radiological evidence of consolidation of the screw holes.

Fracture through biopsy. Generous removal of cortical bone in order to obtain access to an intramedullary lesion may result in a pathological fracture. This is particularly likely to occur in the upper end of the femur (see Figs 35.89 and 35.90) and it is often wise to anticipate the fracture by the insertion of prophylactic internal fixation.

Fracture after removal of infected bone. The necessary removal of sclerotic bone to gain access to sequestrum may so weaken the remaining cortex that fracture occurs with minimal trauma. Weight-bearing bones in particular should be protected by external fixation if a large amount of cortical bone has been removed (Fig 35.112).

Fracture through a donor site for a bone graft (Fig 35.113). This was a common occurrence in the days when cortical bone grafts were popularly used in the treatment of ununited fractures. Most grafts for this purpose are now composed of cancellous bone and are taken from the iliac crest. If a large tibial graft is removed the leg must be protected from weight-bearing stress, or put into a plaster cast for six weeks.

Fracture through areas of cement erosion. The advent of the prosthetic joint into orthopaedics has been responsible for yet another type of iatrogenic fracture—that due to acrylic cement erosion. Loose cement fixation of the intramedullary stem of a joint prosthesis can result in severe endosteal erosion and thinning of cortical bone, which may lead to pathological fracture (Fig 35.114). If such a fracture occurs it should be allowed to unite on conservative treatment and then the loose prosthesis replaced with a long stem variety.

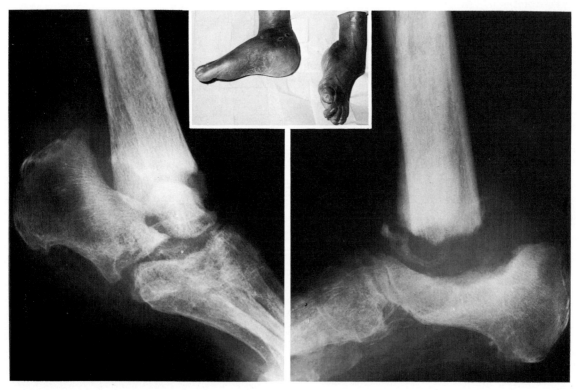

Fig 35.110

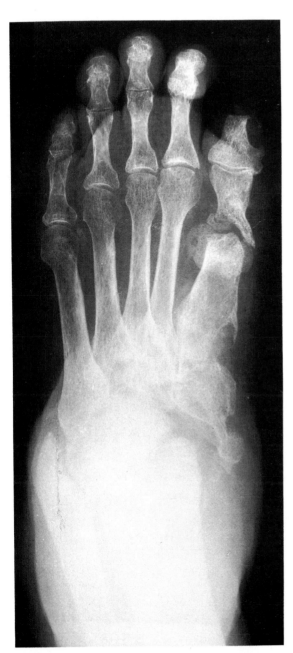

Fig 35.111

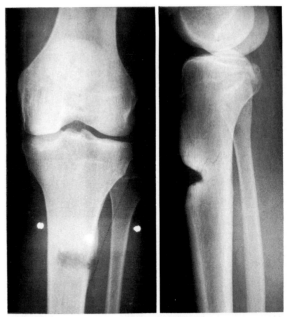

Fig 35.112 This stress crack of the tibial shaft occurred through an area weakened by the removal of the anterior tibial crest. This was excised to gain access to a ring sequestrum which had developed around a badly positioned Steinmann's pin.

Figs 35.110 and 35.111 Diabetic and syphilitic neuropathic dystrophy of bone. This man of 54 had been treated for many years as a diabetic with inadequate dietary and oral therapy. He was also found to have a positive W.R. Neuropathic fractures and arthropathy occurred in both ankles, with secondary infection (Fig 35.110 and inset). Years before he had had a neuropathic joint in the first metatarso-phalangeal joint of the left foot which healed after extensive debridement (Fig 35.111 and compare with Fig 35.109).

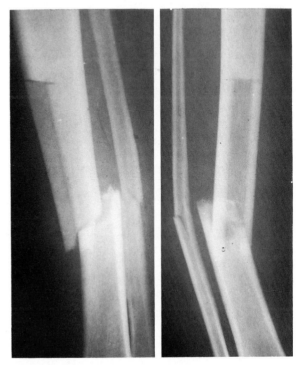

Fig 35.113 Cortical grafts cut from the tibia render the bone vulnerable to pathological fracture. The donor bone should be protected in plaster for six weeks after taking the graft.

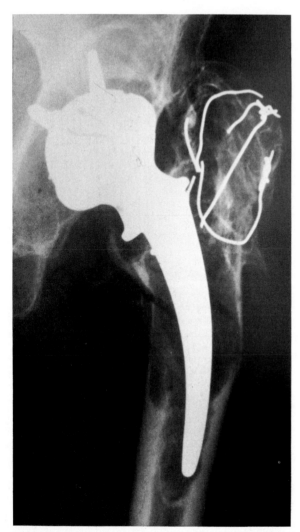

Fig 35.114 The upper femoral component of this patient's total hip replacement became loose along with its cement. There was marked endosteal erosion of bone caused by the movement of the cement and pathological fracture was the result.

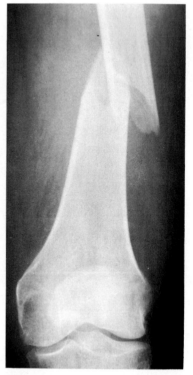

Fig 35.115 In attempting to manipulate this patient's Girdlestone resection of the hip the lower third of the femur was fractured. Forcible manipulation of joints can result in pathological fracture when bones are osteoporotic.

Fractures resulting from joint manipulation. It must always be remembered that a bone which has been exposed to a long period of immobilisation or disuse will have become osteoporotic and may fracture if strained during a forceful joint manipulation. Figure 35.115 shows a fracture of the lower third of the femur which occurred while manipulating a pseudarthrosis after failure to remove an osteotomy plate prior to total hip replacement.

Fractures of prostheses. Although not strictly pathological fractures of bone, fractures of artificial joint implants are in every way fatigue fractures associated with a surgical procedure, and may occur quite unexpectedly and with minimal trauma. The total hip replacement is particularly vulnerable, and as these implants age we must be ready for an increasing incidence of fractures of the stem of the femoral component. There is often a history of a minor fall, or possibly involvement in a road traffic accident, which is followed by vague pain in the hip or thigh for a week or two before a sudden catastrophic

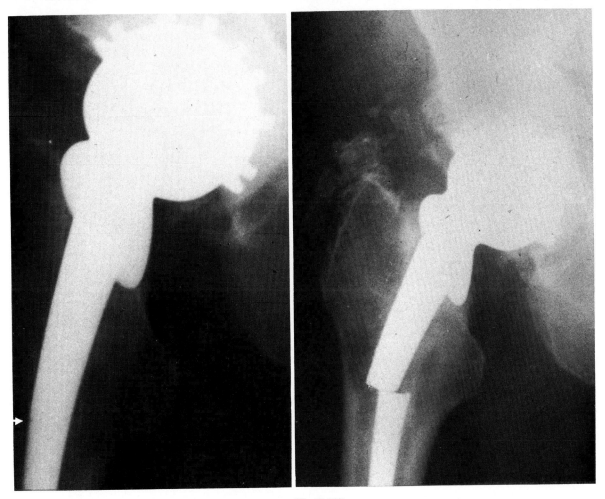

Fig 35.116   **Fig 35.117**

Figs 35.116 and 35.117 A 15½ stone man who had had bilateral McKee arthroplasties of the hips carried out 10 years previously slipped and twisted his right leg. He felt the leg was weak after this and there was vague pain in the upper thigh. X-rays at that time were reported as normal (Fig 35.116). Two weeks later he developed sudden and severe pain in the upper right thigh and he was unable to walk. The X-ray at that time showed an obvious fracture of the metal stem of the femoral component (Fig 35.117). Re-examination of the original X-ray showed a faint linear defect at the site of this fracture, and it is clear that the fatigue fracture of the metal had occurred at that time.

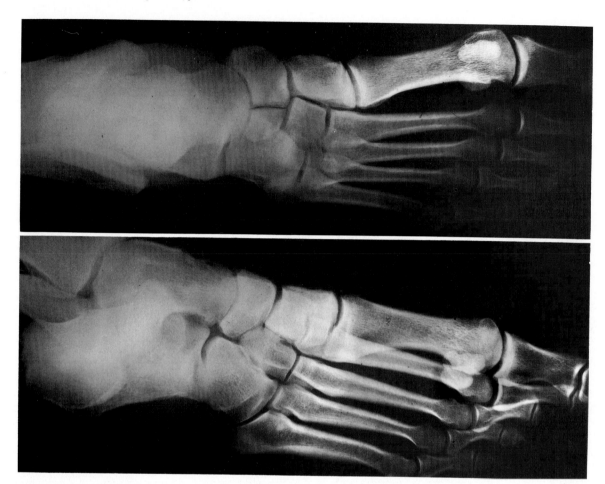

Fig 35.118 Fatigue fractures may present at the most unexpected sites. A woman champion long-distance runner was training strenuously for the Olympics when she developed pain in the right foot. There was no history of injury and the pain was thought at first to be due to ligamentous strain. It was not for some weeks that X-rays eventually showed the real cause—a stress fracture of the tarsal scaphoid. The constantly repeated trauma of landing with the right foot on a hard road surface had been responsible for a stress fracture at the apex of the longitudinal arch. (Two examples of an exactly similar fracture have been reported previously, one occurring in a young athlete, the other in a teenage drummer who used his right foot to strike the bass drum.[94])

break occurs which makes the diagnosis obvious. Often the patient is overweight and expects the artificial hip to stand up to abnormal loading, and in retrospect it may be possible to see the defect of the metal stem in X-rays taken before the break becomes apparent (Figs 35.116 and 35.117).

FATIGUE OR STRESS FRACTURES

A fatigue fracture occurs through apparently normal bone and results from a summation of stresses, any one of which by itself would have been harmless. It may present at the most unexpected sites,[94] but always where maximum repeated stress might be expected (Fig 35.118). There is a precise analogy in the fatigue of metals. A metal rod may be strong enough to resist a stress of certain magnitude, but not strong enough to resist repeated applications of the same stress; the summation causes fatigue fracture of the metal. Detlefsen[95] described a stress fracture of the lower shaft of the fibula in a woman whose work demanded firm pressure of one foot on the vibrating pedal of a machine for eight hours each day. Such fractures may also develop in the lower shaft of the fibula in middle-aged women whose domestic life demands long periods of standing and walking; or in the metatarsal necks of the inexperienced hiker; or in the upper shaft of the fibula in adolescents and young recruits who engage in gymnastics and jump repeatedly from the crouched position.[96] These injuries are commonly missed unless the surgeon is aware of this mechanism (Fig 35.119). In the records of German Army Hospitals for the year 1935–1936[97] there were nearly 600 fractures ascribed to overloading injuries, including metatarsals, 488; tibia, 70; fibula, 12; shaft of femur, 7; neck of femur, 6; os calcis, 4; and pelvis, 3. Fatigue fractures have also been described in the clavicle, first rib and ulna.[98] A recent survey of individuals of both sexes undergoing military training showed only a 1 per cent incidence of fatigue fractures in men but an incidence as high as 10 per cent in women.[99]

March fracture of the metatarsal. A march fracture of the metatarsal may arise from a single stumbling movement; but more generally it is a true fatigue fracture occurring in soldiers during long route marches, or sometimes in holiday-makers unused to long periods of country walking. The fracture is usually in the distal part of the second metatarsal near the neck. Symptoms may develop so gradually that the patient cannot believe that he has

suffered injury, and sometimes it is obvious that the fracture is many weeks old when advice is first sought. It may even be the 'lump' of which the patient complains—a lump consisting of ensheathing callus. Congenital shortening of the first metatarsal is a possible predisposing cause because the first meta-tarso-phalangeal joint lies at a proximal level and may even be in line with the necks of the second and third metatarsals. In this situation the axis of movement between the first and fifth metatarso-phalangeal joints crosses the necks of the second and third metatarsals; and as the patient steps forwards there is an angulatory stress on these bones with the full body weight superimposed (Fig 35.120). Other predisposing architectural weaknesses of the forefoot include hypermobility of the first metatarsal, adduction of the first metatarsal, and transverse flat foot.

The first sign of march fracture is tenderness over the neck of the second metatarsal bone with slight oedema and swelling of the forefoot. The thickening then becomes harder, and after several weeks a lump can be felt at the site of callus formation. In the early stages reliance must be placed on the clinical signs. If a patient complains of pain in this situation after strenuous exercise, and there is localised tenderness and swelling, he has indeed sustained a march fracture of the metatarsal no matter what the radiologist may report. A walking plaster should be applied for a month.

One case has been recorded of amputation of the foot for a march fracture that was mistaken for a sarcoma,[100] but it should be remembered that sarcoma at this site is very rare, whereas stress fracture of the metatarsal is not uncommon. In sarcoma the new bone formation and destruction is very much more extensive (Fig 35.121). A more difficult differential diagnosis is from Panner's disease of the second metatarsal—an allied disorder in which there is periosteal thickening of the shaft of the second and sometimes the third metatarsals. In this condition the blood supply of the distal part of the bone is impaired and there is usually avascular necrosis of the metatarsal head with rigidity of the joint (Fig 35.122).

Fatigue fracture of the calcaneus. This has been previously reported in military recruits.[99] One case is recorded in a 3-year-old spastic child occurring after a period of immobilisation for heel cord lengthening.[101] It should be remembered as a possible cause of pain and stiffness of the foot in a patient suffering from osteoporosis. It has been reported that in athletes the fracture is usually a compression type and always follows the curved line of the posterior

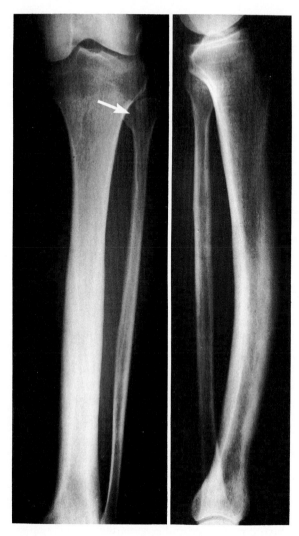

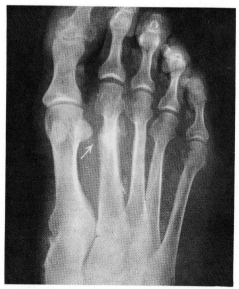

Fig 35.120 March fracture of the second metatarsal with considerable callus formation when first seen—the fracture was several weeks old. Note congenital shortening of the first metatarsal which predisposed to the fracture (see text).

Fig 35.119 Repeated jumping into the fully crouched position can result in a fatigue fracture of the neck of the fibula. Figure 35.119 shows a fracture which occurred in an elderly patient who jumped down from a boat and landed with his knees fully bent. The radiologist's eyes were focused so hard on the Paget's changes in the tibial shaft that he missed the fibula fracture!

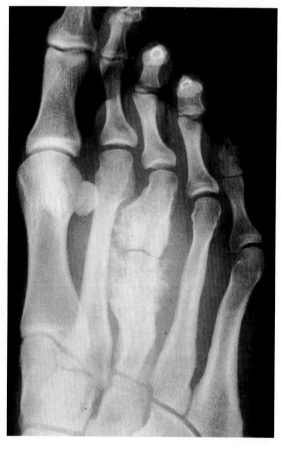

Fig 35.121 A case of parosteal osteosarcoma affecting the shaft of the third metatarsal in which the differential diagnosis of stress fracture was considered. It is true that a pathological fracture has occurred, but the extensive new bone formation combined with destructive bone changes make the diagnosis of tumour beyond doubt.

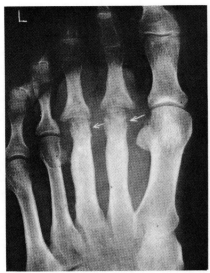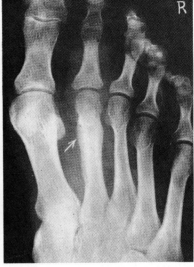

Fig 35.122 Panner's disease of the metatarsals. In the right foot thickening of the second metatarsal shaft simulates an old march fracture, but in the left foot the changes in the second and third metatarsal heads make the diagnosis clear.

surface of the tuberosity but about one inch (2.5 cm) anterior to it.[102]

Fatigue fracture of the lower shaft of the fibula. This fracture occurs in active and hard-pressed women of middle age and also in young athletes. The site of fracture in middle-aged women is usually through cancellous bone just distal to the interosseous ligament, about 1½ inches (3.8 cm) above the tip of the lateral malleolus; in young male track-racers, cross-country runners and marathon racers, the fracture may occur through the more slender cortical bone at a slightly higher level, but the majority are found near to the interosseous liga-ment.[103] In each case the patient complains of discomfort and stiffness of the ankle. There is local tenderness and swelling, but radiographs may show no more than slight condensation of the bone. After a few weeks there is subperiosteal bone formation, and the line of fracture, which is usually directed upwards and medially[102] becomes more evident. It usually suffices to support the ankle with adhesive strapping and to limit weight-bearing activity, but several months may elapse before the pain is entirely relieved, and in the athlete return to training must be carefully graduated.

Fatigue fracture of the upper shaft of the fibula. Fatigue fractures of the upper shaft of the fibula develops in military recruits from repeated jumping. Many of the cases have been reported in German literature. In one report nine artillery men sustained fatigue fracture of the upper shaft of the fibula after practising jumping from the knees-bend position for five minutes several times a day.[104] In another study of 120 military recruits who were made to jump across a gymnasium holding their knees in the fully flexed position 40 per cent (48 recruits) were found to have stress fractures of the upper tibia.[105] It is interesting to note that acute fracture of the upper shaft of the fibula occurs with unexpected frequency in parachute jumpers, who usually land with the knees in flexion. In one series* of 56 bone and joint injuries sustained by parachutists under training there were no less than 11 crack fractures of the upper shaft of the fibula. The relationship between acute fractures from parachute landing and fatigue frac-tures from military training was examined by Jackson Burrows.[96] He pointed out: 'As the metatarsal fracture is the typical march fracture, and the low fibular fracture is perhaps a running fracture, so the high fibular fracture appears to be typically a jump fracture' (see Figure 35.119).

Fatigue fracture of the tibia. There have been many case reports of fatigue fracture of the upper shaft of the tibia, usually an incomplete crack situated about 3 inches (7.6 cm) below the knee joint.[106] The patient complains of pain in the calf or in the upper part of the shin on the medial side. Early radiographs may show an ill-defined area of sclerosis across the

* Studied by Watson-Jones.

shaft of the bone, sometimes with raising of the periosteum from both cortices. The diffuse bone pain, local swelling and increased warmth may lead the unwary to the mistaken diagnosis of osteomyelitis or even sarcoma of bone[102] (Figs 35.123 and 35.124). Later there is a more clearly defined fracture extending incompletely through the bone with a knuckle of subperiosteal callus. The fracture may be bilateral.

The site of lesion may vary with its cause. Ballet dancers have been shown to sustain a fatigue fracture of the anterior border of the mid-third of the bone.[107] Athletes, on the other hand, produce a typical lesion in the postero-medial cortex of the lower third of the tibia ('shin soreness'). Very often an area of periosteal reaction is seen, and if a fracture line does appear it is directed proximally and medially and only involves one cortex[108] (Fig 35.125).

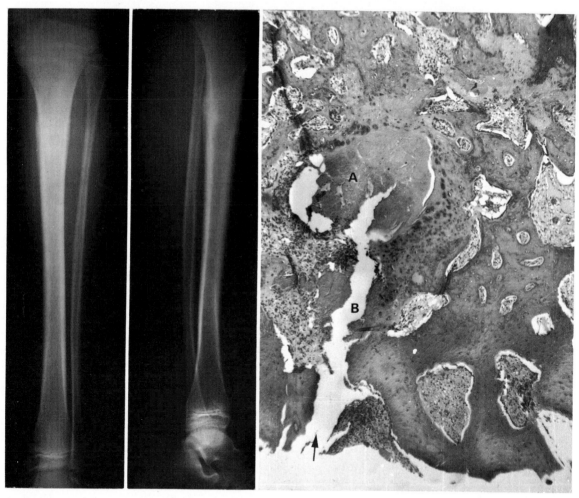

Fig 35.123   **Fig 35.124**

Fig 35.123 and 35.124 Stress fracture of the tibia. A young boy complained of pain and swelling over the shaft of the tibia. X-rays showed an area of bone sclerosis at the main site of tenderness, with overlying periosteal reaction (Fig 35.123). Pain was so severe that infection or bone sarcoma was suspected. Biopsy was performed and showed the bone pattern of fracture callus reaction (Fig 35.124), see separate legend), confirming the diagnosis of stress fracture which should have been made from the characteristic X-ray appearance. At the bottom of the photograph there is a thin band of cortical bone which has been fractured (see arrow). The active resorption of the fractured surfaces indicates that this is not an artefact. The cortex is overlain by fracture callus in which there is a cyst (A) connected to the fracture line by a cleft (B): both cysts and cleft are filled by fibrin which is artefactually disrupted. The callus is composed of immature bone trabeculae, islands of cartilage, and granulation tissue. (H.E. ×45). (The photomicrograph and legend prepared by Dr P. D. Byers, The Institute of Orthopaedics, London.)

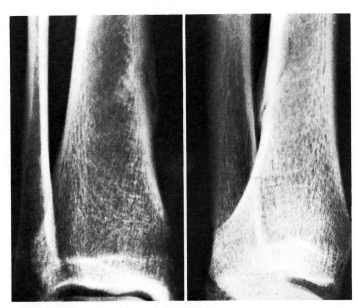

Fig 35.125 Stress fracture of the tibia. 'Shin soreness' in the athlete may eventually show up as an incomplete fracture line, involving only one cortex and directed proximally and medially. The X-ray shown in figure 35.125 was taken four months after the onset of symptoms. Previous films had shown only the minimum of periosteal reaction. (Reproduced by kind permission of the *Journal of Bone and Joint Surgery* and of Mr M. B. Devas from his paper (1958). Stress fractures in the tibia in athletes or 'shin soreness'. *Journal of Bone and Joint Surgery*, 40–B, 227.

Fatigue fracture of the femur. Fatigue fractures of the femoral neck are well recognised in the literature and fairly large series have now been recorded. In a collection of 41 fractures occurring in young men undergoing military training most were undisplaced but in nine there was gross displacement.[109] Fatigue fracture of the femoral shaft is less common, but it is important to recognise the early signs if complete dissolution of the fracture is to be avoided.[110] The fracture has been mainly reported in young military recruits who have previously been white collar workers. The predominant symptom is a poorly localised pain in the knee with stiffness in the morning, the pain gradually building up during the day.

Fatigue fractures of the upper limb. Fatigue fractures have been reported in the clavicle, first rib and forearm bones but with less frequency than in the bones of the weight-bearing lower limbs. The fibula, is not, of course, a weight-bearing bone, and fractures of this bone are probably dependent on the stresses of muscular action. Experiments have shown that powerful contraction of the flexor muscles of the calf produces approximation of the fibula to the tibial shaft.[103] It is probable that excessive muscle action plays an important part in the more rare stress fractures of the upper limb. A fatigue fracture of the

coracoid process has been reported in clay pigeon shooters and attributed to repeated direct and muscular violence to the coraco-brachialis and pectoralis minor attachments;[111] and non-union of a stress fracture of the olecranon epiphysis has been described in an adolescent baseball pitcher.[112] Figures 35.126 and 35.127 show an unusual fatigue fracture of the ulna sustained by a farm-worker aged 20 years who complained of pain after forking and carting manure.[98] There had been no specific injury, but there was local tenderness and swelling over the middle third of the ulna accompanied after 10 weeks by the typical radiographic evidence of a crack fracture with abundant callus which consolidated slowly. There had never been a recognisable injury; but it was the left ulna that developed a fracture, and it was the left forearm that was the fulcrum in the physical activity of supporting the downward thrust of the fork and thereafter resisting the pull of the heavy load.

A case of bilateral stress fracture of the shaft of the radius has been reported in a naval rating who was training with the Fleet Air Arm field gun team. This team takes part in an arduous competition which involves catching and running with a heavy gun barrel carried across the forearms of two men. Bilateral periosteal fractures of the midshaft of the bone occurred in one of the competitors.[113]

Figs 35.126 and 35.127 Fatigue fractures of the ulna which developed without history of injury after forking and carting manure. Ten weeks after the first onset of symptoms (Fig 35.125) there is typically abundant callus which consolidated slowly (Fig 35.127). Reproduced by kind permission of the *Journal of Bone and Joint Surgery* and of Mr Kitchen from his article (1948) Fatigue fracture of the ulna. Journal of Bone and Joint Surgery, 30–B, 622.)

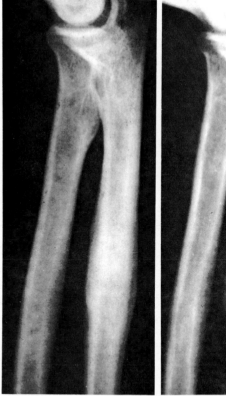

Fig 35.126

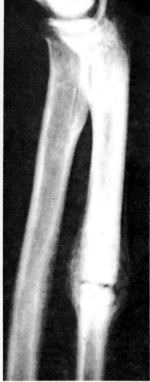

Fig 35.127

REFERENCES

1. Bonarigo B C, Rubin P 1967 Non-union of pathologic fracture after radiation therapy. Radiology 88: 889
2. Blake D D 1970 Radiation treatment of metastatic bone disease. Clinical Orthopaedics and Related Research 73: 89
3. Coran A G, Banks H H, Aliapoulios M A, Wilson R E 1968 The management of pathological fractures in patients with metastatic carcinoma of the breast. Surgery, Gynecology and Obstetrics 127: 1225
4. Devas M B, Dickson J W, Jelliffe A M 1956 Pathological fractures: treatment by internal fixation and irradiation. Lancet 2: 484
5. Zickel R E, Mouradian W H 1976 Intramedullary fixation of pathological fractures and lesions of the subtrochanteric region of the femur. Journal of Bone and Joint Surgery 58–A: 1061
6. Huckstep R L 1975 An intramedullary nail for rigid fixation and compression of fractures of the femur. Journal of Bone and Joint Surgery 57–B: 253
7. Huckstep R L 1976 Early mobilisation of patients with neoplastic bone disease. Journal of Bone and Joint Surgery 58–B: 262
8. Fidler M W, Stollard G 1977 The management of secondary neoplastic deposits in long bones by prophylactic internal fixation. Archivum Chirurgicum Neerlandicum 29(3): 177
9. Beals R K, Lawton G D, Snell W E 1971 Prophylactic internal fixation of the femur in metastatic breast cancer. Cancer 28: 1350
10. Ryan J R, Rowe D E, Salciccioli G G 1976 Prophylactic internal fixation of the femur for neoplastic lesions. Journal of Bone and Joint Surgery 58–B: 1071
11. Sim F H, Daugherly J W, Ivins J C 1974 The adjunctive use of methylmethacrylate in fixation of pathological fractures. Journal of Bone and Joint Surgery 56–A: 40
12. Yablon I G, Paul R G 1976 The augmentative use of methylmethacrylate in the management of pathologic fractures. Surgery, Gynecology and Obstetrics 143: 177
13. Harrington K D, Sim F H, Enis J E, Johnson J O, Dick H M, Gristina A G 1976 Methylmethacrylate as an adjunct in internal fixation of pathological fractures. Experience with 375 cases. Journal of Bone and Joint Surgery 58–A: 1047
14. Murray J A, Bruels M C, Lindberg R D 1974 Irradiation of polymethylmethacrylate in vitro. Gamma radiation effect. Journal of Bone and Joint Surgery 56–A: 311
15. Harrington K D, Johnson J O, Turner R H, Green D L 1972 The use of methylmethacrylate as an adjunct in the internal fixation of malignant neoplastic fractures. Journal of Bone and Joint Surgery 54–A: 1665
16. Wouters H W 1974 Tumeur à cellules géantes de l'éxtremité distale du fémur avec fracture intra-articulaire du genou. Revue de Chirurgie orthopédique et réparatrice de l'Appareil Moteur 60, supp 11: 316
16a. Lane J M, Sculco T P, Zolan S 1980 Treatment of pathological fractures of the hip by endoprosthetic replacement. Journal of Bone and Joint Surgery 62–A: 954
17. Seedorff K S 1949 Osteogenesis imperfecta: a study of clinical features and heredity based on 55 Danish families

comprising 180 affected members. Translated by Elizabeth Aegeson. Universietsforlaget, Arhus

18. Wynne-Davies R 1973 Heritable disorders in orthopaedic practice. Blackwell, Oxford, p 80

19. Murray R C, Jacobson H G 1971 The radiology of skeletal disorders. Churchill Livingstone, Edinburgh, p 36

20. Murray A M, Cruickshank B 1960 Dyschondroplasia. Report of a case. Journal of Bone and Joint Surgery 42–B: 344

21. Siffert R S 1966 The growth plane and its affections. Journal of Bone and Joint Surgery 48–A: 546

22. Stamp T C B, Round J M 1974 Seasonal variations in human plasma levels of 25 hydroxyvitamin D. Nature 247: 563

23. Puschett J B, Moranz J, Kurnick W S 1972 Evidence for a direct action of cholecalciferol and 25 hydroxy-cholecalciferol on the renal transport of phosphate sodium and calcium. Journal of Clinical Investigation 51: 373

24. Puschett J B, Fernandez P C, Boyle I T, Gray R W, Ohmdahl J L, De Luca H F 1972 The acute renal tubular effects of 1.25 dihydroxycholecalciferol. Proceedings of the Society of Experimental Biology and Medicine 41: 379

25. Jackson W P U 1967 Calcium metabolism and bone disease. Arnold, London; p 86

26. Dent C E, Round J M, Stamp T C B 1973 Treatment of sex-linked hypophosphatemic rickets (SLHR). In: Frame B, Parfitt A M, Duncan H (eds) Clinical aspects of metabolic bone disease. International Congress Series, No. 270. Excerpta Medica, Amsterdam, p 427

27. Nassim J R et al 1959 The effects of vitamin D and gluten-free diet in idiopathic steatorrhoea. Quarterly Journal of Medicine NS 28: 141

28. Saville P D et al 1955 The Fanconi syndrome—metabolic studies on treatment. Journal of Bone and Joint Surgery 37–B: 529

29. Chalmers J et al 1967 Osteomalacia—a common disease in elderly women. Journal of Bone and Joint Surgery 49–B: 403

30. British Medical Journal 1968 Osteomalacia in Britain (leading article). British Medical Journal ii: 130

31. Hosking D J 1978 Changes in the serum alkaline phosphatase after femoral fracture. Journal of Bone and Joint Surgery 60–B: 61

32. Fourman P, Royer P 1968 Calcium metabolism and the bone, 2nd edn. Blackwell, Oxford, p 81

33. Albright F, Reifenstein J E C 1948 Parathyroid glands and metabolic bone disease. Williams and Wilkins, Baltimore, p 57

34. Davies D R, Dent C E, Watson L 1968 Tertiary hyperparathyroidism. British Medical Journal iii: 395

35. Copp D E et al 1962 Evidence for calcitonin—a new hormone from the parathyroid that lowers blood calcium. Endocrinology 70: 638

36. Lancet 1978 Ten years treatment of Paget's disease (Leader) Lancet 1: 914

37. Evans G A, Slee G C 1977 Calcitonin for multiple fractures in Paget's disease. British Medical Journal 1: 357

38. Otani 1960 The effects of adreno-cortical hormone on healing of experimental fractures. Journal of Bone and Joint Surgery 42–A: 541

39. Murray R O 1961 Steroids and the skeleton. Radiology 77: 729

40. Griffiths W E G, Swanson S A V, Freeman M A R 1971 Experimental fatigue fracture of the human cadaveric femoral neck. Journal of Bone and Joint Surgery 53–B: 136

41. Todd R C, Freeman M A R, Pirie C J 1972 Isolated trabecular fatigue fractures in the femoral head. Journal of Bone and Joint Surgery 54–B: 723

42. Casuccio C 1962 Concerning osteoporosis (symposium on osteoporosis). Journal of Bone and Joint Surgery 44–B: 453

43. Nassim J R 1968 Personal communication

44. Stone K H 1968 Personal communication

45. Agerholm J C, Goodfellow J W 1965 Simple cysts of the humerus treated by radical excision. Journal of Bone and Joint Surgery 47–B: 714

46. Scaglietti O, Marchetti P G, Bartolozzi P 1979 The effects of methylprednisolone acetate in the treatment of bone cysts. Results of three years' follow-up. Journal of Bone Surgery 61–B: 200

47. Lichtenstein L 1950 Aneurysmal bone cyst: a pathological entity commonly mistaken for giant cell tumor and occasionally for haemangioma and osteogenic sarcoma. Cancer 3: 279

48. Henry A 1969 Monostotic fibrous dysplasia. Journal of Bone and Joint Surgery 51–B: 300

49. Albright F et al 1937 Syndrome characterised by osteitis fibrosa disseminata. New England Journal of Medicine 216: 727

50. Jaffe H L 1958 Tumours and tumorous conditions of the bones and joints. Henry Kimpton, London, p 117

51. Huvos A G, Higinbotham N L, Miller T R 1972 Bone sarcomas arising in fibrous dysplasia. Journal of Bone and Joint Surgery 54–A: 1047

52. Paget Sir James 1877 Osteitis deformans. Medico-chirurgical Transaction 60: 37

53. Collins D H 1966 Pathology of Bone. Butterworth, London, p 230

54. Purves M J 1962 Some effects of administering sodium fluoride to patients with Paget's disease. Lancet ii: 1188

55. De Rose J et al 1974 Response of Paget's disease to porcine and salmon calcitonins. American Journal of Medicine 56: 858

56. Redden J, Hosking D J, Vennart W 1977 Fissure fractures in Paget's disease. Journal of Bone and Joint Surgery 59–A: 251

56a. Dove J 1980 Complete fractures of the femur in Paget's disease of bone. Journal of Bone and Joint Surgery 62–B: 12

57. Jaffe H L 1958 Tumours and tumorous conditions of the bones and joints. Kimpton, London, p 464

58. Price C H G, Goldie W 1969 Paget's sarcoma of bone. Journal of Bone and Joint Surgery 51–B: 205

59. Geschickter C F, Copeland M M 1949 Tumours of bone, 3rd edn. Lippincott, Philadelphia

60. Gorham L W, Stout A P 1955 Massive osteolysis (acute spontaneous absorption of bone, phantom bone, disappearing bone). Its relationship to haemangiomatosis. Journal of Bone and Joint Surgery 37–A: 985

61. Seddon H J, Scales J T 1949 A polythene substitute for the upper two-thirds of the shaft of the femur. Lancet ii: 795

62. Aston J N 1958 A case of massive osteolysis of the femur. Journal of Bone and Joint Surgery 40–B: 514

63. Poirier H 1968 Massive osteolysis of the humerus treated by resection and prosthetic replacement. Journal of Bone and Joint Surgery 50–B: 158

64. Russell D 1949 Malignant osteoclastoma. Journal of Bone and Joint Surgery 31–B: 281

65. Perkins G 1968 Personal communication

66. Windeyer B W, Woodyat P B 1949 Osteoclastoma. Journal of Bone and Joint Surgery 31–B: 532

67. Ottolenghi C E 1966 Massive osteoarticular bone grafts.

Transplant of whole femur. Journal of Bone and Joint Surgery 48–B: 646

68. Wilson P D, Lance E M 1965 Surgical reconstruction of the skeleton following segmental resection for bone tumours. Journal of Bone and Joint Surgery 47–A: 1629

69. Merle D'Aubigne R, Dejouany J F 1958 Diaphyso-epiphyseal resection for bone tumours at the knee with reports of nine cases. Journal of Bone and Joint Surgery 40–B: 385

70. Burrows H J, Wilson J N, Scales J T 1975 Excision of tumours of humerus and femur with restoration by internal prostheses. Journal of Bone and Joint Surgery 57–B: 148

71. Eyre-Brook A L 1964 Symposium on the treatment of giant cell tumours of bone. Journal of Bone and Joint Surgery 46–B: 796

72. Burrows H J 1968 Major prosthetic replacement of bone. Lessons learnt in seventeen years. Journal of Bone and Joint Surgery 50–B: 225

73. Mirra J M, Bullough P G, Marcove R C, Jacobs B, Huvos A G 1974 Malignant fibrous histiocytoma and osteosarcoma in association with bone infarcts. Journal of Bone and Joint Surgery 56–A: 932

74. Spector D B, Miller J, Viloria J 1979 Malignant fibrous histiocytoma. An unusual lesion of interest to the orthopaedic surgeon. Journal of Bone and Joint Surgery 61–B: 190

75. Pritchard D J, Dahlin D C, Dauphine R T, Taylor W F, Beabout J W 1975 Ewing's sarcoma. A clinicopathological and statistical analysis of patients surviving five years or longer. Journal of Bone and Joint Surgery 57–A: 10

76. Speed D E, Galton D A G, Swan A 1964 Melphalan in the treatment of myelomatosis. British Medical Journal i: 1664

77. Council on Drugs 1965 Alkylating agent for multiple myeloma—Melphalan. Journal of the American Medical Association 191: 547

78. Griffiths D Ll 1966 Orthopaedic aspects of myelomatosis. Journal of Bone and Joint Surgery 48–B: 703

79. Valderrama J A F, Bullough P G 1968 Solitary myeloma of the spine. Journal of Bone and Joint Surgery 50–B: 82

80. Geschickter C F, Maseritz I H 1939 Skeletal metastasis in cancer. Journal of Bone and Joint Surgery 21: 314

81. Albrecht P 1905 Beiträge zur Klinik und Pathologischen Anatomie der Malignen Hypernephrome. Archiv fur Klinische Chirurgie, 77: 1073

82. Broster L R 1923 A case of secondary hypernephroma in the femur with spontaneous fracture. British Journal of Surgery 11: 287

83. Schajowicz F, Slullitel J 1973 Eosinophilic granuloma of bone and its relationship to Hand-Schüller-Christian and Letterer-Siwe syndromes. Journal of Bone and Joint Surgery 55–B: 545

84. Cheyne C 1971 Histiocytosis X. Journal of Bone and Joint Surgery 53–B: 366

85. Amstutz H C, Carey E J 1966 Skeletal manifestations and treatment of Gaucher's disease. Journal of Bone and Joint Surgery 48–A: 670

86. Geschickter C F, Copeland M M 1949 Tumours of bone, 3rd edn. Lippincott, Philadelphia, ch 20, p 567

87. Booz M K 1975 Radiological diagnosis of hydatid disease of bone. Journal of Bone and Joint Surgery 57–B: 111

88. Alldred A J, Nisbet N W 1964 Hydatid disease of bone in Australasia. Journal of Bone and Joint Surgery 46–B: 260

89. Parker D, Chapman R 1965 Hydatid disease of the innominate bone. With a report of a case successfully treated by irrigation with supersaturated salt

solution. Journal of Bone and Joint Surgery 47–B: 292

90. Hooper J, McLean I 1977 Hydatid disease of the femur. Report of a case. Journal of Bone and Joint Surgery 59–A: 974

91. Ottolenghi C E 1966 Massive osteoarticular bone grafts. Transplant of the whole femur. Journal of Bone and Joint Surgery 48–B: 646

92. Catterall R C F 1964 Orthopaedic aspects of diabetic gangrene. Journal of Bone and Joint Surgery 46–B: 260

93. Brooks D B, Burnstein A H, Frankel V H 1970 The biomechanics of torsional fractures. The stress concentration of a drill hole. Journal of Bone and Joint Surgery 52–A: 507

94. Towne L C, Blazina M E, Cozen L N 1970 Fatigue fracture of the tarsal navicular. Journal of Bone and Joint Surgery 52–A: 376

95. Detlefsen M 1941 Ermüdungsbruch der Fibula bei ein Industriearbeiterin. Munchener Medizinische Wochenschrift 88: 303

96. Burrows H J 1948 Fatigue fractures of the fibula. Journal of Bone and Joint Surgery 30–B: 266

97. Asal W 1936 Uberlastungsschaden am Knochensystem bei Soldaten. Archiv für Klinische Chirurgie 186: 511

98. Kitchin J D 1948 Fatigue fractures of the ulna. Journal of Bone and Joint Surgery 30–B: 622

99. Protzman R R, Griffis C G 1977 Stress fractures in men and women undergoing military training. Journal of Bone and Joint Surgery 59–A: 825

100. Dodd H 1933 Pied forcé or March foot. British Journal of Surgery 21: 131

101. Stein R E, Stelling F H 1977 Stress fracture of the calcaneus in a child with cerebral palsy. Journal of Bone and Joint Surgery 59–A: 131

102. Devas M 1980 Stress fractures in athletes. Medisport (The Review of Sports Medicine) 2: 227, 262

103. Devas M B, Sweetnam R 1956 Stress fractures of the fibula. Journal of Bone and Joint Surgery 38–B: 818

104. Scherf 1933 Frakturen oder Umbauzonen an der Fibula im Anschluss an besondere sportliche Beanspruchung? Zentralblatt für Chirurgie 60: 2739

105. Symeonides P P 1980 High stress fractures of the fibula Journal of Bone and Joint Surgery 62–B: 192

106. Hartley J B 1942 Fatigue fractures of the tibia. British Journal of Surgery 30: 9

107. Burrows H J 1956 Fatigue infraction of the middle of the tibia in ballet dancers. Journal of Bone and Joint Surgery 38–B: 83

108. Devas M B 1958 Stress fractures in the tibia in athletes or 'shin soreness'. Journal of Bone and Joint Surgery 40–B: 227

109. Blickenstaff L D, Morris J M 1966 Fatigue fracture of the femoral neck. Journal of Bone and Joint Surgery 48–A: 1031

110. Provost R A, Morris J M 1969 Fatigue fracture of the femoral shaft. Journal of Bone and Joint Surgery 51–A: 487

111. Boyer D W 1975 Trapshooter's shoulder: stress fracture of the coracoid process. Journal of Bone and Joint Surgery 57–A: 862

112. Torg J S, Moyer R A 1977 Non-union of a stress fracture through the olecranon epiphyseal plate observed in an adolescent baseball pitcher. Journal of Bone and Joint Surgery 59–A: 264

113. Farquharson-Roberts M A, Fulford P C 1980 Stress fractures of the radius. Journal of Bone and Joint Surgery 62–B: 194

Index
Volumes I and II

Note: Illustrations occurring on a different page from the relevant text are indicated by italics: *f* following an entry indicates footnote.

Ankle
operative approaches (*continued*)
postero-lateral, 356, *358*
postero-medial, 355, *357*
ossification, traumatic, 66, *67*
partial diastasis of inferior tibio-fibular joint, 1107, *1110*
passive dorsiflexion, excessive, 1159, *1164*
peroneal tendons, recurrent dislocation, 1139, *1140*
plantigrade position, manipulation, 1128, *1129*
radiography, different joint positions, 267, *270*
rehabilitation, 92
sprains, diagnosis and treatment, 1117
radiography, 267, *271*
subluxation, radiography, 267, *271*
recurrent, 1120
subtalar joint, torque convertor effect, 1111–1112, *1115*, 1127
weight bearing properties, 1130
Ankylosis, mandibular condyle fracture, 166
Anoxia, in chest injuries, 199
Antacid, prophylactic, following injury, 106
Antibiotics
bacteraemic shock, 110
compound injuries, 131
contraindication in post-traumatic renal failure, 109
detergent solution, 369
endotoxic shock, 110
facial fractures, 182
gunshot wound toilet, 398
local, in open injuries, 410
mandibular fracture, 167
open injuries, 407, 410
preoperative protection, 405
prophylactic, in head injuries, 156
tetanus, 412
shock therapy, 116
Anticoagulants, contraindications, post-operative, following oedema, 233
venous thrombosis, 239
Anticonvulsants, in head injuries, 157
Antiserum, gas-gangrene, 411
tetanus, 412
AO bone plating. *See* Bone, plating, compression
Aorta, rupture, 140, *141*, 199
Arch bar wiring, teeth, 169
Arm
exercise, in above-elbow plaster, 48
injuries, 572–582
sling, cause of gravitational oedema, 54
Arterial injuries. *See also specific part*
arteriography, 224
axillary, 213
closed, 220
management, 227, *228*

Arterial injuries (*continued*)
compression, 220
subfascial syndromes, 223
division or laceration, 219
external distortion, 220
instruments for repair, 226
intimal tears, 220
management, 227, *229*
laceration, management, 227
management, 224
open, 219
patch arterioplasty, 229
spasm, management, 227, *228*
traumatic, 223
surgical treatment, 225
exposure of artery, 227
technique, 226
traumatic false aneurysm, 219
types, 219
Arteries. *See also names of specific arteries*
extradural haematoma, 149
ligation, hazards, 212
Arteriography, arterial injury, 224
Arteriovenous aneurysm, *472*
Arteriovenous fistula, management, 234, *235*
Arthritis
ankle, degenerative, *31*
arthrodesis, 1186, *1191*
hip
cystic signs of, 913, *915*
degenerative, differentiation from traumatic, 913, *914*
traumatic, 903
following hip dislocation, 911
radiocarpal, styloidectomy for, 723
traumatic, following ligament injury, 30
Arthrography. *See also under specific joints*
ligament injury, 40, *41*
semilunar cartilage injuries, 1050
Arthroplasty, elbow dislocations, 634
Arthroscopy, ligament injury, 40
semilunar cartilage injury, 1050
Arthrotomy, open joint injuries, 407
Ascorbic acid, 7, 1214
Asphyxia, traumatic, 197, *198*, 200
Austin Moore, femoral stem prosthesis, 956
operative approach to hip, 337
Avascular necrosis, indication for bone grafting, 449, *454*
Aviator's fracture, 1172
Avulsion injury
accompanying ligament damage, 30, *33*, 34
cause of traumatic ossification, 65
Axonotmesis, 242

Bacteraemic shock, 110
'Bag of bones' treatment, *58*, *59*, 60, *61*, 281, 926

Balance, disturbed, following head injury, 94
Bandaging
acromioclavicular joint, 529
'boxing glove', *50*
eversion stirrup, 1117, *1118*
figure-of-eight, for clavicle, 523
stump, 429
Bankart's operation, 561, *562–563*
Barton fracture, 701, *703*
Baumann's angle, 593, *596*
Bed, fracture 977, *979*
Bed rest, spinal injury, 849, *840*, 841
Bedford support, finger, *744*
Behaviour, in head injury, 93
Bence Jones protein, in multiple myelomatosis, 1254
Bennett's fracture, 760–764
programme of treatment, 764
Bentzon's operation, 725
Betadine antiseptic technique, 369
Biceps tendon, rupture, 520, 522
Bier's regional block, 698
Bile leakage, following liver injury, 202
Bilirubinaemia, post-traumatic, 105
Biological dressings, 11
Biopsy, pathological fractures, *1257*, 1268
Birth injury fractures, 484
frame, *487*
Bjork and Engstrom, tracheostomy technique, 137
Bladder
catheter, visceral injury, 201
control, in spinal injury, 832, 833
involvement in pelvic injury, 867
neurogenic, 804
paralysis, care of patient, 842
late management, 845
rupture, 206
Blisters, fracture, 8, 294
Blood
coagulation mechanism, in shock, 110
examination, in pathological fractures, 1208
secondary, after injury, 128
intravascular circulating volume, 114
platelets, administration, 115
pressure
arterial, monitoring, in shock, 112
factor in acute arterial ischaemia, 213
first examination after injury, 122
visceral injury, 200
products, in fluid replacement, 115
supply, factor in fracture healing, 21, *22*
in callus formation, 17
periosteal, 23
transfusion, early, following injury, 124
Blood gas analysis, 107, 113
Bohler Braun frame, 300, 983